Heart in Fours

Heart in Fours

CARDIOLOGY

for Residents and Practitioners

Third Edition

Pothuri Radha Krishna Murthy
MBBS FCGSP DNB FIAMS

Practitioner
Vijayawada, Andhra Pradesh, India

Foreword

IV Rao

JAYPEE BROTHERS MEDICAL PUBLISHERS (P) LTD

New Delhi • Panama City • London • Philadelphia

Jaypee Brothers Medical Publishers (P) Ltd

Headquarters
Jaypee Brothers Medical Publishers (P) Ltd
4838/24, Ansari Road, Daryaganj
New Delhi 110 002, India
Phone: +91-11-43574357
Fax: +91-11-43574314
Email: jaypee@jaypeebrothers.com

Overseas Offices
J.P. Medical Ltd
83 Victoria Street, London
SW1H 0HW (UK)
Phone: +44-2031708910
Fax: +02-03-0086180
Email: info@jpmedpub.com

Jaypee-Highlights Medical Publishers Inc.
City of Knowledge, Bld. 237, Clayton
Panama City, Panama
Phone: + 507-301-0496
Fax: + 507-301-0499
Email: cservice@jphmedical.com

Jaypee Brothers Medical Publishers Ltd
The Bourse
111 South Independence Mall East
Suite 835, Philadelphia, PA 19106, USA
Phone: + 267-519-9789
Email: joe.rusko@jaypeebrothers.com

Jaypee Brothers Medical Publishers (P) Ltd
17/1-B Babar Road, Block-B, Shaymali
Mohammadpur, Dhaka-1207
Bangladesh
Mobile: +08801912003485
Email: jaypeedhaka@gmail.com

Jaypee Brothers Medical Publishers (P) Ltd
Shorakhute, Kathmandu
Nepal
Phone: +00977-9841528578
Email: jaypee.nepal@gmail.com

Website: www.jaypeebrothers.com
Website: www.jaypeedigital.com

Inquiries for bulk sales may be solicited at: jaypee@jaypeebrothers.com

Heart in Fours: Cardiology for Residents and Practitioners

First Edition: 1995

Second Edition: 2002

Third Edition: **2013**

ISBN 978-93-5090-493-0

Printed at Rajkamal Electric Press, Plot No. 2, Phase-IV, Kundli, Haryana.

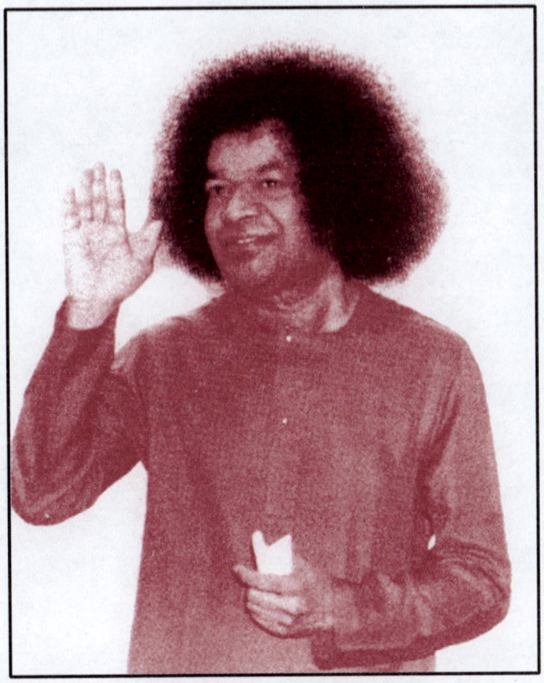

'Heart in Fours'

is humbly and reverentially dedicated to Bhagawan

Sri Sri Sri Satya Sai Baba

Foreword

డా॥ ఎన్.టి.ఆర్. ఆరోగ్య విజ్ఞాన విశ్వవిద్యాలయము, ఆంధ్రప్రదేశ్

Dr. N.T.R. University of Health Sciences, Andhra Pradesh

VIJAYAWADA - 520 008

Dr. I.V. RAO,
M.D. (General Medicine)
VICE - CHANCELLOR

Phone : 0866 - 2451374 (O)
Fax : 0866 - 2450463
E-mail : drivrao@hotmaill.com
Website: http://ntruhs.ap.nic.in

Dr Pothuri Radha Krishna Murthy is a family physician who has been practicing medicine, surgery, obstetrics and gynecology and taking good care of the health needs of the people in Krishna district, Andhra Pradesh, India. He graduated from Guntur Medical College and obtained DNB qualification in family medicine, the first in Andhra Pradesh to gain this distinction and the first few in the country.

He devotes his time in teaching general practitioners for FCGP examination in medicine, surgery, obstetrics and gynecology and preventive medicine. In spite of his busy schedule in family practice, he still takes time to give Guest lectures and orations to teach students, general practitioners and members of IMA in topics related to medicine, cardiology and ECG.

Though he is not a cardiologist himself, he acquired a thorough knowledge of the subject and his interpretation of ECG was appreciated by one and all including the noted cardiologists. His analysis and approach to ECG became a big hit and he is being approached by several student communities for taking regular training classes. In short, he has a passion for cardiology.

He is the author of *'Heart in Fours' Cardiology*, which won many accolades from students, specialists and teachers. Presently, he is bringing out the third edition and I had the opportunity to scan through the chapters of Hypertension and Cardiac Arrhythmias. I am thoroughly impressed by his work particularly, the subject being dealt in "Fours" meaning four salient points for every aspect of the topic concerned.

I greatly appreciated his vision, knowledge and style of presentation and I hope this edition turns out to be the most sought-after book in cardiology by students, practitioners, physicians and cardiologists alike as was the case with his previous work.

I wish him all success in his future endeavors.

IV Rao MD (General Medicine)
Vice Chancellor
NTR University of Health Sciences
Vijayawada, Andhra Pradesh, India

Preface to the Third Edition

By the grace of God and blessings of my well-wishers, I have been able to bring out this third edition, which is a stupendous task. I am extremely happy to bring this third edition of *Heart in Fours: Cardiology for Residents and Practitioners*. It is indeed, heartening to note the overwhelming response given to this by the students, practitioners as well as the consultants.

A picture is worth ten thousand words --- Chinese proverb

Many additional pictures are added in this edition.

The value of experience is not in seeing much but in seeing wisely --- William Osler

Immense popularity and wide acceptability of this book among the students, family physicians and consultants have encouraged me to prepare this third edition.

Readers have appreciated that this is the only of its kind in the medical literature, which can help to remember it easily and to reproduce it easily in 'Fours'. It is easy for the teachers to teach and more easy for the students to remember in 'Fours'.

This book has been updated and a new chapter on 'Pregnancy and Cardiovascular Disease' is an addition.

I did not elaborate the subjects on cardiac catheterization, interventions in cardiology and surgery as they are beyond the scope of this book and they are mostly for the superspecialists.

Pothuri Radha Krishna Murthy

Preface to the First Edition

This book is the outcome of my curious but significant observation of both the theoretical and practical aspects concerning heart as a four-dimensional system. Incidentally, the idea surfaced at the time of preparing myself for Diplomate of National Board (DNB) Final Examination in Family Medicine, in 1983, a couple of decades after leaving the teaching institution as a practicing physician and surgeon. I have discovered this fact after making sufficient headway in the process of writing this book. Now, I am convinced that the idea of number 4, which I have picked up is workable and stable all through my writing. Hence, the title *Heart in Fours*. Surprisingly, in the process, I have found out that all the points (more than 2,000) included herein, have suitably teamed and arranged themselves into four each, and here and there occasionally in multiples of four too! This pattern eventually facilitates a student, a teacher and a physician to recall to his memory, any piece of information without much effort.

My number 'Four' indicates definite parameters in various contexts. In the selection of drugs, drugs may change but the parameters do not. Their number may grow, but the existing parameters do not change. In other places, the number 4 remains as an indomitable classification of symptom complex or complications of heart diseases. This book is written not as a textbook of heart and heart disease. It is aimed at simplicity and practical use rather than theory. I have strained every nerve to make the subject more concise and to the point and to serve as a typical ready reckoner. One can understand the subject with ease and can remember it with greater ease. The causes, diagnosis, treatment, and prevention of various cardiac complaints relevant to the topic are discussed in every chapter and a little overlapping could not be avoided. Diagnostic cardiology has made great strides and its use has become imperative. Care is taken to reach the students and practitioners the knowledge in roentgenology, electrocardiography, echocardiography and cardiac catheterization chapters. Since the chapter on ECG requires pictorial explanation, a good number of diagrams are added. Medicine is an ever-changing subject. The drug schedules given are in accord with the standard accepted at the time of publication. However, changes can be brought after continuous research and clinical experience. Therefore, the readers are advised to check the product information supplied with the drug, so that they can notice the changes that are brought in the dosage and complications, etc. This is of particular importance with newer and infrequently used drugs. The newer drugs need not be better than previous ones. Medical science has undergone revolutionary changes, particularly in the field of cardiac surgery. What was thought impossible is now made possible. An attempt is made to throw open a window on interventional cardiology, surgery in ischemic heart diseases, valvular diseases and congenital heart diseases. However, it is suggested that an appraisal is a must at every stage of management.

Pothuri Radha Krishna Murthy

Acknowledgments

I thank innumerable students, colleagues, general physicians and cardiologists throughout the country who have inspired me with encouragement and suggestions. I should like to place on record in expressing my deep sense of gratitude to the great medical luminaries of national and international repute like *Padmabhushan* Dr MS Valiathan, *Padmas*ri Dr Kakarla Subbarao and Dr R Alagappan and many others for their letters of appreciation.

I thank once again to Dr KP Mishra and Dr S Thanikachalam, renowned cardiologists who wrote foreword to the first and second editions.

I thank Dr IV Rao, Vice-Chancellor of NTR University of Health Sciences, Vijayawada, Andhra Pradesh, who has immediately accepted to write foreword to the third edition.

I thank IMA, Vijayawada branch, where good number of lectures are arranged in various subjects, from which I learned much and also IMA College of General Practitioners and other branches of IMA who arranged my ECG lectures.

I thank the organizers of Sri Satya Sai Temple, Vijayawada, where I have been serving the poor and needy at the free medical camp on every Sunday since two decades where I have the benefit of attending many cardiac patients. Bhagawan Sri Satya Sai Baba gave me the opportunity by appointing me as Chief Medical Officer-in-Charge of postoperative care of patients in Krishna district who underwent heart operations at Sri Satya Sai Institute of Higher Medical Sciences at Puttaparthi and Bengaluru. I have learned much in postoperative follow-up care with satisfaction of free service.

I thank Mr Kotha Durga Prasad, Potti Subramanian, Mr Sanjeev, medical students and Dr P Adinarayana for typing the manuscript.

I thank Dr KV Chalpatirao, Dr P Giriaja, Dr TV Ramanamurthy, Dr Jayakarbabu and Dr P Pullarao, All India Dean IMACGP, for their encouragement.

My thanks are due to Mr Venkataeswar Rao Vakkalagadda (USA), Padmaja Vakkalagadda (USA), and Dr Venkatadura Prasad Pothur (USA), for their computer help of the final proof.

My thanks are due to Dr P Sudharani for proofreading and P Sridhar for computer help.

Finally, I thank my wife Dr P Raja Rajeswary, BAMS, who is the source of motivation to bring out the third edition.

I like to thank Shri Jitendar P Vij (Group Chairman), Mr Ankit Vij (Managing Director) and Mr Tarun Duneja (Director-Publishing) of M/s Jaypee Brothers Medical Publishers (P) Ltd, New Delhi, India, for accepting to bring out the third edition in a beautiful way with color photographs. I thank Mr Suresh of Hyderabad branch, Mr Venugopal of Bangalore branch, Ms Sunita Katla and Mr Rajesh Sharma of Delhi branch, and other staff of Jaypee Brothers for bringing out this stupendous work in time.

Contents

Abbreviations

+	Positive
–	Negative
↓	Decreased or Depressed
	Increased or Elevated
>	More or greater
<	Less or smaller
2D	Echo two-dimensional echocardiography

A

ABG	Arterial blood gases
ACEI	Angiotensin converting enzyme inhibitors
ACS	Acute coronary syndrome
AF	Atrial flutter/fibrillation
AICD	Automatic implantable cardioverter/ defibrillator
AMI	Acute myocardial infarction
AR	Aortic regurgitation
AS	Aortic stenosis
ASD	Atrial septal defect
ASO	Antistreptolysin O
AV	Atrioventricular node

B

BB	Beta blocker
bid	bid in die (Twice in a day)
BMI	Body mass index
BP	Blood pressure
BPH	Benin prostatic hypertrophy
BPM	Beats per minute

C

CABG	Coronary artery bypass graft
CAD	Coronary artery disease
CBC	Complete blood counts
C/I	Contraindications
CCB	Calcium channel blocker
CCF	Congestive cardiac failure
CI	Cardiac index
CK,CPK	Creatine phosphokinase
CO	Cardiac output
COPD	Chronic obstructive pulmonary disease
CPB	Cardiopulmonary bypass
CPKMB	Creatine phosphokinase-MB isoenzyme
CT	Computerized tomography
CVD	Cardiovascular diseases
CVP	Central venous pressure
CVS	Cardiovascular system

D

DBP	Diastolic blood pressure
DCM	Dilated cardiomyopathy

E

e.g.	For example
ECG	Electrocardiography
Echo	Echocardiogram
EDRF	Endothelial derived relaxing factor
EF	Ejection fraction
EMS	Emergency medical services
EPS	Electrophysiological studies
ESR	Erythrocyte sedimentation rate

F

FA	Fatty acids
FBC	Full blood count

G

g	Gram
GFR	Glomerular filtration rate

GIT	Gastrointestinal tract
GP	General practitioner

H

h	Hour
H/O	History of
Hb	Hemoglobin
HF	Heart failure
HOCM	Hypertrophic obstructive cardiomyopathy
HR	Heart rate

I

ICCU	Intensive coronary care unit
IE	Infective endocarditis
IHD	Ischemic heart disease
IM	Intramuscular
IMA graft	Internal mammary artery graft
IMR	Infant mortality rate
ICA	Intensive care unit
IU	International unit
IV	Intravenous
IVI	Intravenous infusion
IWMI	Inferior wall myocardial infarction

J

JVP	Jugular venous pressure

K

kg	Kilogram

L

L	Left
L	Liter
LA	Left atrium
LAFB	Left anterior fascicular block
LAH	Left atrial hypertrophy
LAHB	Left anterior hemiblock
LBB	Left bundle branch
LBBB	Left bundle branch block
LDH	Lactic dehydrogenase
LFT	Liver function test
LPFB	Left posterior fascicular block
LPHB	Left posterior hemiblock
LV	Left ventricle
LVEDP	Left ventricular end-diastolic pressure
LVF	Left ventricular failure
LVH	Left ventricular hypertrophy
LVSWI	Left ventricular stroke work index

M

MAP	Mean arterial pressure
MCCU	Mobile coronary care unit
mg	Milligram
MI	Myocardial infarction
min	Minute(s)
mL	Milliliter
mm Hg	Millimeters of mercury
M-mode Echo	M-mode echocardiography
MMR	Maternal mortality rate
MR	Mitral regurgitation
MS	Mitral stenosis
MVO_2	Myocardial oxygen consumption
mcg/µg	Microgram

N

NSAIDs	Nonsteroidal anti-inflammatory drugs
NSTEMI	Non-ST elevated myocardial infarction
NTG	Nitroglycerin

O

OD	Once a day

P

$PaCO_2$	Partial pressure of CO_2 in arterial blood
PaO_2	Partial pressure of O_2 in arterial blood
PAI	Plasminogen activator inhibitor
PCI	Percutaneous coronary intervention
PCWP	Pulmonary capillary wedge pressure
PDA	Patent ductus arteriosus
PIH	Pregnancy induced hypertension
PMBV	Percutaneous mitral balloon valvuloplasty
PO	Per orem (by mouth)
PS	Pulmonary stenosis
PTCA	Percutaneous transluminal coronary angioplasty
PVBs/PVCs	Premature ventricular beats/premature ventricular contractions
PVR	Pulmonary vascular resistance

R

R	Right
RA	Right atrium
RAAS	Renin angiotensin aldosterone system
RBB	Right bundle branch
RBBB	Right bundle branch block
RBC	Red blood cell
RCM	Restrictive cardiomyopathy
RF	Rheumatic fever
RHD	Rheumatic heart disease
rt-PA	Recombinant tissue plasminogen activator
RUD	Rashkind umbrella device
RV	Right ventricle
RVF	Right ventricular failure
RVH	Right ventricular hypertrophy
RVMI	Right ventricular myocardial infarction

S

S/E	Side effects
SA	Sinoatrial node
SBE	Subacute bacterial endocarditis
SBP	Systolic blood pressure
SC	Subcutaneous
SL	Sublingual
SS	Statum summendum (To be taken immediately)
STEMI	ST elevated myocardial infarction
Stratum	Stratum (Immediately)
Stk	Streptokinase
SV	Stroke volume
SVR	Systemic vascular resistance

T

TC	Total white blood cell count
Tds	Tes die summendum (To be taken thrice a day)
TG	Triglycerides
Tid	Tes in die (To be taken thrice a day)
TPA	Tissue plasminogen activator
TPR	Temperature, pulse and respirations
TS	Tricuspid stenosis
TR	Tricuspid regurgitation

U

U/S	Ultrasound
Uk	Urokinase

V

VSD	Ventricular septal defect

W

WBC	White blood cell
wk	Week(s)

Y

y	Year(s)

Common Hematologic Values

Common hematologic values if outside this range, consult;

Hemoglobin	Men:	13–18 g/dL
	Women:	11.5–16 g/dL
Mean cell volume, MCV		76–96 fL
Platelets		150–400 × 10^9/L
White cells (total)		4–11 × 10^9/L
Neutrophils		40–75%
Lymphocytes		20–45%
Eosinophils		1–6%

Blood gases	κPa	mm Hg
pH	7.35–7.45	
PaO_2	> 10.6	75–100
PaO_2	4.7–6	35–54
Base excess	± 2 mmol/L	

U and E (urea and electrolytes) if outside this range, consult;

Sodium	135–145 mmol/L
Potassium	3.5–5 mmol/L
Creatinine	70–150 µmol/L
Urea	2.5–6.7 mmol/L
Calcium	2.12–2.65 mmol/L
Albumin	35–50 g/L
Proteins	60–81 g/L

LETs (liver function tests)

Bilirubin	3–17 µmol/L
Alanine aminotransferase, ALT	3–35 IU/L
Aspartate transaminase, AST	3–35 IU/L
Alkaline phosphatase	30–300 IU/L (adults)

Cardiac enzymes

Creatine kinase 2	5–195 IU/L
Lactate dehydrogenase, LDH	70–250 IU/L

Lipids and other biochemical values

Cholesterol	4–6 mmol/L desired
Triglycerides	0.5–1.9 mmol/L
Amylase	0–180 somogyi IU/dL
C-reactive protein, CRP	< 10 mg/L
Glucose, fasting	3.5–5.5 mmol/L
Prostate specific antigen, PSA	0–4 mg/mL
T4 (total thyroxin)	70–140 mmol/L
TSH	0.5–5 mU/L

Normal Values

Normal hemodynamics

Right atrial pressure	0–8 mm Hg
Right ventricular	15–30 mm Hg
systolic and diastolic	0–8 mm Hg
Pulmonary artery	15–30/4–12 mm Hg
systolic/diastolic	9–16 mm Hg
mean	
PCWP	2–10 mm Hg
LVEDP	8–12 mm Hg
Cardiac output	5–9 L/min
Cardiac index	2.8–4.2 L/min/m^2
Systemic vascular resistance	770–1500 dyne.s/cm^5
Pulmonary vascular resistance	100–250 dyne.s/cm^5
Left ventricular ejection fraction	55–75%

ATP III classification of LDL, total, and HDL cholesterol

LDL cholesterol, mg/dL (mmol/L)	
< 100 (2.58)	Optimal
100–129 (2.58–3.33)	Near or above optimal
130–159 (3.36–4.11)	Borderline high
160–189 (4.13–4.88)	High
≥ 190 (4.91)	Very high

Total cholesterol, mg/dL (mmol/L)	
< 200 (5.17)	Desirable
200–239 (5.17–6.18)	Borderline
≥ 240 (6.20)	High

HDL cholesterol, mg/dL (mmol/L)	
< 40 (1.03)	Low
≥ 60 (1.55)	High

ATP III criteria for diagnosis of the metabolic syndrome

≥ 3 out of 5 criteria must be satisfied for diagnosis

Variable	**Threshold**
Waist circumference	> 40 inch (men) > 35 inch (women)
Fasting glucose	> 100 mg/dL
Blood pressure	> 130/> 85 mm Hg
HDL cholesterol	< 40 mg/dL in men < 50 mg/dL in women
Triglycerides	> 150 mg/dL

Note

Our knowledge in clinical medicine is constantly changing. As the clinical experience and research are growing, new information is obtained, which may change the treatment and the use of drugs. The drug schedules given are in accordance with the standard accepted at the time of publication. While every step is taken to check drug dosage in this book, it is still possible that errors have been missed. Furthermore, dosage schedules are being continually revised and new side effects identified. Therefore, the readers are advised to check the printed instructions supplied by the drug companies for dosage, complications, etc., before administering any of the drugs recommended in this book. This is of particular importance with newer and rarely used drugs.

Reviews

Padmabhushan Dr MS Valiathan MCh FRCS FRCS FRCP DSc
(Formerly, Director, Chitra Tirunal Institute, Thiruvananthapuram)
Honorary Advisor, Manipal Academy of Higher Education
Madhav Nagar, Manipal, Karnataka, India

I have now had the pleasure of going through many chapters of your *Heart in Fours*. Yours is an amazing, perhaps unique, book on cardiology. Far from preparing a mere aid to examiners, you have compressed all the clinically useful information in cardiology in remarkable series of quartets. I should not have thought such a feet possible.

I have no doubt your book will be of much interest and value to medical students and general physicians. Its mine of information and uniqueness of presentation would have an enduring appeal.

I have placed your book in our Kasturba Medical College Library to bring it to the attention of a large academic community.

Padmasri Kakarla Subbarao MBBS MS FRCR FACR
Director, NIMS, Hyderabad
Former Advisor, Ministry of Health, Medical and Family Welfare, Andhra Pradesh, India

I wish to profusely congratulate you for having brought the concise and informative book on cardiology. Unfortunately in this country, we have specialists and super specialists but their interest in spreading their knowledge to the general practitioner or a student is very little. No doubt, they can address their colleagues and specialists and enrich them with their experience but that is not adequate in the present situation in our country. Please keep it up in other areas also such as "Radiology for General Practitioners".

Dr S Thanikachalam MD DM (Cardiology)
Director, Cardiac Care Center
Professor and Head, Department of Cardiology
Sri Ramachandra Medical College and Research Institute
Chennai, Tamil Nadu, India

Foreword to the second edition:

I had the opportunity to go through the manuscript of *Heart in Fours: Cardiology for Residents and Practitioners* in-depth and enjoyed every chapter for exemplenary way it is written. It is presented in simple fashion avoiding ambiguity. I have no doubt that this creation is useful, not only to medical practioners but also for consultants.

I appreciate the mammoth efforts taken by Dr Pothuri Radha Krishna Murthy in completing this stupendous task of crating this voluminous book.

Dr KP Misra MD FACC FCCP FISE
Consultant Cardiologist, Director Medical Education
Apollo Hospitals, Chennai, Tamil Nadu, India

Foreword to the first edition:

.... In his unusual interest in pursuing academic growth, he came with a novel idea of writing a book on "Cardiology in Fours". This book gives entire subject of cardiology very comprehensively in a simple and unusual format—all items arranged in 4s. Four is a very auspicious number in our country—from Vedas to the paths to salvation—all are actually in 4. Dr Pothuri Radha Krishna Murthy has been inspired by the fact that in cardiology most of the things are all four types or can be expressed in four. This is a delightful way of learning cardiology. He has more than succeeded in presenting the entire subject in this manner. I have gone through the manuscript and enjoyed it thoroughly. I have also presented many times various topics in cardiology emphasizing this role of four. I have no doubts that the readers will find it interesting at the same time comprehensive and simple enough to learn cardiology……….

Dr PC Bhatla BSc MBBS FCGP FRCGP (Australia) FIAMS FAMS
Formerly, National President, IMA
Director, IMACGP, Chairman
Health Care Promotion Trust and National Institute of Primary Health Care
New Delhi, India

I have great pleasure in greeting Dr Pothuri Radha Krishna Murthy as a crusader in initiating and following an innovative approach in presenting cardiology as a condensed capsule. Only through in depth study and understanding could this extensive facts be compiled in such a manner that exhibits extraordinary style of compilation as almost a 'ready reckoner' and useful also for self-assessment.

The presentation is distillate of medical facts, easy-to-grasp and easy-to-remember and apply. There is fluency in description and the comprehensive contents make easy readability by the students of cardiology. The book would meet the needs of the teachers as well who could guide the teacher—learning process as a SYSTEM. I recommend the book to find its place on the desks of all doctors, which in itself will be a tribute to the author for his scholarship.

Professor R Alagappan MD FICP
Director, Professor and Head of Department, Institute of Internal Medicine, Madras Medical College
Senior Civil Surgeon and Physician, Government General Hospital, Chennai, Tamil Nadu, India

I went through the book and found your unique presentation of clustering the points in fours or its multiple very interesting. This approach gives a bird's eye view of the various disciplines in cardiology and at the same time is presented in a simple and easy-to-remember format. I am sure that your book, with its comprehensive text, will serve as a practical guide in the field of cardiology for students and practitioners alike.

Professor CS Bhaskaran MD FRC PATH (LOND) FAMS
Vice Chancellor, University of Health Sciences, Vijayawada, Andhra Pradesh, India

……. I have gone through several of the chapters on different aspects in cardiology and I am much impressed with the presentation. You have chosen the title of the book in most appropriate manner by projecting the day-to-day problems that are encountered by a general practitioner dealing the cardiac ailments. The subject has been dealt extensively and in a simple manner with the presentation of differential points in Fours.

I am confident that this book will serve as a useful practical guide for not only general practitioners but also to other specialists. I once again congratulate you for the excellent work you have done in bringing out this book.

Professor BM Hegde MD FRCP (Lond) FRCP (Edin) FRCP (Glasg) FRCP (Dublin) FACC
Vice Chancellor, Manipal Academy of Higher Education (Deemed University), Manipal, Karnataka, India

Your book is an excellent compilation of present knowledge in the field of heart diseases.

This would be a ready reckoner for students preparing for the examinations and also practicing doctors dealing with cardiovascular problems.

I hope that in the next edition you would give a very strong Indian bias to the text.

I wish your book all success.

Book Review

JIMA (Journal of the Indian Medical Association)—Volume 94, Number 9, September 1996

……….This is a good manual with a practical bedside approach. Particularly the tips on clinical cardiology are going to be helpful for aspiring general practitioners with a cardiological bias as many will desire benefit from indexed approach. I am sure it will gain acceptance from those for whom it is intended….. Mantosh Panja

AP Journal of Practical Paediatrics—Volume 5, Number 2, April to June 1997

....This unique book on cardiology *Heart in Fours* has probably evolved from the fact that it is easier to recall to memory a topic, which is systematically read and registered in our mind. The author has utilized the number "four" in an obsessive style and has approached the relevant topics in clinical cardiology from congenital heart disease to coronary artery disease in a rather simplified manner. Other topics relating to diagnostic and therapeutic cardiology have also been included in similar vein. Though this book is not recommended as regular textbook, it will serve as 'ready reckoner' for the students especially preparing for their practical and viva. The practical aspects of the book is also a good reference for general practitioners.

Review on Second Edition

JIMA (Journal of the Indian Medical Association)—Volume 101, Number 08, August 2003, Page 1999

It is a great pleasure to see that the second edition of *Heart in Fours*: *Cardiology for Students and Practitioners* has been published. It reflects the wide acceptance of the first edition of the book to the readers, for whom the book has been prepared with meticulous efforts and utmost care. The author has expressed his own realization and experience rather than just compiling information from several textbooks.

The book is really an example of the simplest way of presentation of a tough subject in the face of rapid advances in the field. However, there is scope of improving the book in certain places.

....

....

In spite of few limitations, the second edition of the book is excellent and I hope it will be very useful for the practitioners and the students in their day-to-day practice. This book will inspire consultants of cardiology for reproducing their assimilated knowledge in a different way—Mantosh Panja

A Heart Functions in Health and Disease

1. There are only 4 chambers in the heart.

1. Right atrium
2. Left atrium
3. Right ventricle
4. Left ventricle

2. There are only 4 valves in the heart.

1. Mitral
2. Tricuspid
3. Aortic
4. Pulmonary

3. There are only 4 heart sounds.

1. 1st sound
2. 2nd sound
3. 3rd sound
4. 4th sound

4. There are only 4 types of murmurs.

1. Systolic
2. Diastolic
3. To and fro
4. Continuous

5. There are 4 main causes of diseases affecting the heart.

1. Congenital (Balyam—Childhood)
2. Rheumatic (Kaumaram—Adolescent age)
3. Hypertensive (Yavvanam—Middle age)
4. Ischemic (Vardhakyam—Old age)

Like 4 stages of man, Balyam, Kaumaram, Yavvanam and Vardhakym. There can be overlapping. Congenital heart diseases mainly affect the right side of the heart as the strain is more on the right side during intrauterine life. Acquired heart diseases mainly affect the left heart chambers as they are subjected to ten times the pressure compared to the right heart chambers since the left ventricle has to pump the blood into the greater circulation. Majority of chronic valvular diseases upto middle age are of rheumatic origin. Though rheumatic fever affects in childhood, the valvular affection is seen in young age. Hypertension commonly is the disease of middle age, and ischemic heart disease commonly is of old age.

6. There are 4 steps in clinical examination.

1. Inspection
2. Palpation
3. Percussion
4. Auscultation

7. There are 4 main investigations.

1. X-ray
2. ECG
3. Echocardiography
4. Cardiac catheterization

1, 2, 3, are noninvasive, 4 is an invasive procedure.

8. There are 4 groups of drugs to treat heart diseases.

1. Anticongestive (Digoxin and Diuretics)
2. Antihypertensive
3. Antiischemic
4. Antiarrhythmic

9. There are 4 steps in the management of a disease.

1. Etiology
2. Pathology
3. Diagnosis
4. Treatment

10. There are 4 steps in clinical approach of cardiovascular system for correct and complete diagnosis.

1. *First step:* Physiological disturbances.

   Recognize:

   i. Whether there is any overload or strain or hypertrophy?

   ii. Whether there is any heart failure?

   iii. Whether there is any arrhythmia?

   iv. Whether there is any myocardial infarction or ischemic changes?

   Recognise first whether there is any heart failure or not. Whatever may be the cause, the end result of cardiovascular disease may culminate in heart failure. More than 75% of cardiovascular diseases need management of heart failure. So, it is very essential either for the general practitioner or specialist to recognize heart failure in the early stages so as to give the best results.

2. *Second step:* Physical anomalies if any.
   Recognize the anatomical abnormalities:
   i. Endocardium—Affection of the valve
   ii. Myocardium—Enlargement of chambers, Cardiomyopathies
   iii. Pericardium—Pericarditis
   iv. Vascular—Myocardial ischemia or infarction.

   These physical anomalies can be corrected in some cases by surgery. For example mitral stenosis, aortic stenosis, pulmonary stenosis, coarctation of aorta, constrictive pericarditis, coronary artery stenosis, etc.
3. *Third step:* Elicit the etiology; when it could be recognized in the early stage or in its acute (active) stage, something can be done to prevent the causative factor that leads to the heart failure. Most often, the etiological factor has already damaged the heart. Is it
   i. Congenital
   ii. Rheumatic
   iii. Hypertensive
   iv. Arteriosclerotic (Ischemic)
4. *Fourth step:* Elicit the extent of functional disability. The amount of strenuous activity required to elicit the symptoms helps in rehabilitation of the patient. Is he or she
   i. Not aware, no subjective symptoms
   ii. Unable to exert
   iii. Uncomfortable even at rest
   iv. Completely bedridden (impending death)
   (see New York Heart Association (NYHA) functional and objective classification E 52 and 53)

11. Normal Heart.

1. Heart is a mere fist-sized organ weighing around 350 g.
2. It is among the most powerful muscles in the body.
3. Every heart beat pumps blood through 1,50,000 km of vascular bed in the body against the 120 mm Hg pressure.
4. Beats 2,869,776,000 times over an average life span of 75 years.

12. It seems to be marvel. If anything could go wrong?

1. Congenital heart disease—defects since birth.
2. Acquired diseases—rheumatic heart disease where heart valves turn narrow or leak.
3. Coronary artery disease (CAD)/Ischemic heart diseases (IHD)—where heart muscle is deprived of oxygen.
4. Rhythm disorders—where heart rhythm is affected.

CAD/IHD has the highest morbidity and mortality of them.

13. There are 4 important symptoms in the history.

1. Dyspnea/Breathlessness
2. Precordial pain or distress
3. Palpitation
4. Symptoms of general venous congestion, e.g. swelling of feet, cough, digestive disturbance, etc.

One of the symptoms may come earlier than other and may be prominent than other symptom depending on the cause. For example—

Breathlessness is the main symptom wherever there is raise in pulmonary capillary pressure as in left ventricular failure, mitral stenosis, pulmonary hypertension, etc.

Pain is the main symptom of myocardial infarction or in any ischemic heart disease such as angina. (See Chapter E—IHD/CAD, Chapter F—AMI)

Palpitation is the main symptom in arrhythmias such as paroxysmal atrial tachycardia (PAT), premature ventricular beats, etc. (See Chapter D—Cardiac Arrhythmias)

Edema feet or symptoms of systemic venous congestion are prominent in right sided heart failure or in both left and right sided (combined) heart failure besides breathlessness. (See Chapter C—Heart Failure)

Other symptoms like syncope may be seen in diseases where the cardiac output is very less, e.g. aortic stenosis.

DYSPNEA

14. Dyspnea is defined as an abnormally uncomfortable awareness of breathing. It is one of the main symptoms of cardiac and pulmonary disease. Dyspnea is mainly due to the lung becoming stiff as blood accumulates in the pulmonary vasculature behind the failing ventricle. As a result, the work performed and the tension developed by the respiratory muscles increases which leads to the sensation described as breathlessness.

The following terminology is used for describing various types of breathlessness.

Table A-1

1. Dyspnea	Uncomfortable breathing
2. Tachypnea	Rapid breathing
3. Hyperpnea	Increased ventilation due to increased metabolic needs
4. Hyperventilation	Ventilation in excess of metabolic needs
5. Platypnea	Dyspnea related to upright position
6. Trepopnea	Dyspnea related to lateral position
7. Orthopnea	Dyspnea related to supine position
8. Paroxysmal nocturnal dyspnea	Dyspnea related to sleep—wakes up from sleep with shortness of breath

15. There are 4 grades of dyspnea.

Table A-2

Grade	Degree of exertion	PVP (mm Hg)
Grade I	Dyspnea on severe exertion	<12 (normal)
Grade II	Dyspnea on moderate exertion	12–18
Grade III	Dyspnea on mild exertion	19–24
Grade IV	Dyspnea at rest	>25

(PVP = Pulmonary venous pressure)

It is important to ask specially about nocturnal breathlessness which patients often forget to mention this.

It may be a symptom of cardiac failure although more commonly it is a symptom of bronchial asthma.

16. The pattern of breathlessness associated with left ventricular failure can be described under 4 stages.

1. Breathlessness on exertion.
2. Orthopnea: It is due to pulmonary congestion occurring as a result of redistribution of fluid from the periphery to the pulmonary circulation in recumbent position and also in part due to abdominal organs pushing on the diaphragm.
3. Paroxysmal nocturnal dyspnea (PND): It is associated with patient waking from sleep and fighting for breath. It is possibly due to venospasm of capacitance vessels during the REM (rapid eye movement) sleep causing blood to move to the pulmonary circulation from areas of pooling in the veins of the limbs and gut.
4. Acute pulmonary edema occurs when the hydrostatic pressure within the pulmonary capillaries rising to more than 25 mm Hg and is sufficiently greater than oncotic pressure exerted by the plasma proteins to cause marked interstitial edema and the accumulation of free fluid in the alveoli. The mucosal edema and bronchospasm give rise to wheeze.

Wheeze is due to narrowing of the airways due to mucosal edema and bronchospasm commonly seen in bronchial asthma.

The presence of orthopnea and paroxysmal nocturnal dyspnea (PND) strongly suggests pulmonary venous hypertension in contrast to other causes of dyspnea.

Cheyne-Stokes Respiration

It is a disturbance of respiratory rhythm characterized by gradually increasing depth of respiration, till a maximum is attained then followed by gradually diminishing respiratory effort, until a pause of apnea occurs for few seconds to a minute to be followed again by another wave of gradually deepening and then diminishing. It is seen in severely ill patient with very low cardiac output due to heart failure. Neurologist commonly sees in cerebrovascular disease with increased intracranial pressure, narcotic drug poisoning. It is exaggerated when dozing, the hyperpneic phase causes cerebral stimulation to prevent sleep.

It causes insomnia in a patient with heart failure.

Also seen in renal failure, severe pneumonia, alkalosis, after severe vomiting.

Kussmaul's breathing: Deeping singing, rapid breathing at a regular rate should immediately suggest metabolic acidosis commonly seen in diabetic ketoacidosis or uremia.

17. Dyspnea in supine position is due to following mechanism:

1. Increased venous return
2. Increased end-diastolic volume of ventricles
3. Increased wall tension
4. Increased myocardial oxygen requirement

18. Cardiac causes of dyspnea are:

1. *Heart failure of any cause:* Start as dyspnea on exertion (DOE) followed by classic orthopnea, paroxysmal nocturnal dyspnea, cough and wheeze on exertion or on assuming supine position. Dyspnea precedes the cough
2. *Acute myocardial infarction:* It can present as acute shortness of breath (SOB) associated with chest pain.
3. *Ischemic heart disease:* Angina equivalent can present with shortness of breath instead of pain. Paroxysmal nocturnal dyspnea can occur with nocturnal angina with dyspnea as angina equivalent.
4. *Arrhythmias:* Dyspnea begins suddenly with or without palpitation.

Sudden development of dyspnea while sitting rather than lying or whenever a particular position is assumed, suggests the possibility of a myxoma or ball-valve thrombus. When dyspnea is relieved by squatting in children, the most common cause is 'tetralogy of Fallot'.

19. Noncardiac causes of dyspnea are:

1. Pulmonary disease or dysfunction
   a. Associated with much weight gain/obesity
   b. Bronchial asthma associated with cough and wheeze
   c. Chronic obstructive pulmonary disease (COPD): H/o chronic cough with sputum, smoking—easier to breath on bending forward
   Inspiratory dyspnea suggests obstruction of the upper airways whereas expiratory dyspnea suggests obstruction of the lower airways. Cough precedes the dyspnea.

d. Pneumothorax—dyspnea at rest
e. Pulmonary embolism—sudden onset associated with faintness or syncope, hemoptysis or pleuritic chest pain
f. Pulmonary edema
g. Post nasal discharge when attendant with severe cough
h. Sleep apnea with arousal

2. Severe anemia
3. Compression of pulmonary artery or bronchi, e.g. lung tumor
4. Anxiety neurosis or unknown cause: H/o 'nervous breakdown'

Dyspnea associated with numbness, tingling, dizziness, pain at apex, cold perspiration or palpitations. This is suggestive of Da Costa's syndrome or neurocirculatory asthenia. It becomes worse when the patient is upset and is helped by sedatives/tranquilizers.

Dyspnea that occurs only at rest and is absent on exertion is almost always functional.

Dyspnea in patients with panic attacks is usually accompanied by hyperventilation.

20. Whenever there is h/o paroxysmal nocturnal dyspnea (PND), the severity of left ventricular failure/left atrial pressure can be assessed by asking the following 4 questions.

1. When did it first begin?
2. How frequent it is? (number of times per night, week, month or year)
3. Lowest and shortest time between attacks?
4. How it is relieved?

Dyspnea may begin within a minute of lying flat. It may appear whether the patient lies on the back, left side or right side. Sometimes, it appears when the patient slips of pillows accidentally. Usually, it takes about 2 to 4 hours for tissue fluid to fill the intravascular space enough to rise the left atrial pressure to a high level. If fluid accumulates rapidly the patient will be awaken within 2 to 4 hours and may have a recurrence in the same night. If fluid accumulates slowly, the patient may awake after 4 to 6 hours. It takes at least 10 to 30 minutes for fluid to be redistributed into the extravascular space.

The patient must dangle, get out of bed or take a rapid-acting nitrate. It is improved by digitalis or diuretics.

When there is cough—cough precedes the dyspnea in asthma, chronic obstructive pulmonary disease, bronchitis – with frothy or pink sputum.

21. The paroxysmal nocturnal dyspnea may manifest by the following mechanisms:

1. Absorption of edema fluid with increase in right ventricular output overfilling the lungs
2. Diminished sympathetic drive of sleep decreasing left ventricular contractility
3. Sleep induced dreams with the attendant increase in emotional activity with increased catecholamine release
4. Nocturnal arrhythmias

Chest Pain

(*See Chapter E Table E-2 and Chapter F-15 to 18)

Chest pain can originate not only in heart but also in other intrathoracic organs, tissues of the thoracic wall and neck, and from subdiaphragmatic organs.

It is the main symptom in ischemic heart disease/coronary artery disease.

Several terms are used by the patient to describe the chest pain such as discomfort, squeezing, tightness, gripping, compression, burning, gases, acidity, uneasiness, inconvenient feeling, etc.

22. There are 4 steps in evaluation of chest pain.

1. First differentiate the cardiac from noncardiac causes. If the patient voluntarily points with one finger, it suggests non-anginal chest pain. If the patient shows with fist or sweeps across the chest, it is suggestive of angina.
2. If it is cardiac, is it due to
   a. Ischemic heart disease/coronary artery disease
   b. Hypertrophic cardiomyopathy
   c. Aortic stenosis
   d. Aortic dissection
   e. Mitral valve prolapse
   f. Pericarditis
3. If it is due to coronary artery disease, is it
   a. Stable angina
   b. Unstable angina
   c. Printzmetal angina
   d. Variant angina
   e. Acute myocardial infarction
4. If it is noncardiac, is it due to
   a. Pulmonary: Pneumothorax, pulmonary embolism, pluritis.
   b. Esophageal: Reflex esophagitis, acute esophageal tear.
   c. Chest wall: Osteoarthritis, osteochondritis, costochondritis
   d. Gastritis
   e. Pancreatitis
   f. Cholecystitis
   g. Herpes zoster
   h. Functional—anxiety/depression

23. Table of differentiation between cardiac and noncardiac chest pain.

Table A-3

Feature	Favoring ischemic origin (cardiac)	Against ischemic origin (noncardiac)
1. Site	Diffuse, substernal across mid-thorax anteriorly In left arm, shoulders In the left forearm, fingers In the neck, lower jaw, teeth Patient shows with fist or sweeps across the chest	Localized left inframamary area, left hemithorax Patient points with one finger
2. Nature	Chest discomfort, tightness, squeezing, crushing, choking, burning, heaviness, heavy feeling, pressing. Sudden onset with acute myocardial infarction, gradual onset with angina "I think I am going to die" particularly if the patient says with a clichéd fist placed over the sternum (LeVeen sign positive)	Dull ache 'Knife-like' sharp Stabbing Shooting
3. Intensity	Mild to moderate with gradual fluctuation	Rapidly fluctuating
4. Duration	Minutes to hours	less than 5 sec, split of a second
5. Radiation	Left arm, left shoulder, medial side of the left forearm, little finger, lower jaw	No typical radiation
6. Precipitating or provoking factors	Exercise, excitement, Any stress Cold weather or changing weather After heavy meal Sexual activity	Pain after completion of exercise Specific body movement Deep respiration, worse on inspiration with restriction of movement. The patient may "catch his breath", it implies the inflammation of the pleura and localizes the lesion
7. Relieved by	Rest, Nitroglycerin	Lengthy rest and most other measures–antacids for gastritis, analgesics for chest wall pain
8. Accompanying symptoms	a. Related to loss of contracting myocardium and conducting tissue Dyspnea, palpitation, syncope b. Symptoms of autonomic excess Sympathetic excess–Tachycardia, sweating Parasympathetic excess–Bradycardia, vomiting	Hyperventilation

SYNCOPE

Syncope is a common medical problem that accounts for approximately 6% of medical admissions and 3% of causality room visits. Syncope is defined as a sudden transient loss of consciousness associated with decrease in cerebral blood flow and loss of postural tone. Recovery is spontaneous, without neurological deficits and without requiring electrical or chemical cardioversion.

Cerebral blood flow usually decreases with aging, making the elderly at higher risk for syncope.

Differentiating true syncope from other "nonsyncopal" conditions that cause loss of consciousness is important because the mechanism of syncope ranges from nearly normal (physiological) to abnormal and life-threatening.

24. The patient describes syncope or faintness in several ways in his own terms as dizziness, loss of balance, light-headedness, blurred vision, sinking feeling, floating, unsteadiness, swaying, giddiness and vertigo. It results most commonly from reduced perfusion of the brain.

Cardiac causes of syncope can be described under 4 groups.

1. *Acute myocardial infarction:* Massive AMI or myocardial infarction associated with arrhythmias. It is usually preceded by chest pain, dyspnea or palpitation. The patient is immediately taken to hospital with 'heart attack' diagnosis after. Cardiac syncope is associated with increased mortality and may lead to sudden death.
2. *Obstruction of flow through the heart:* Fixed aortic stenosis, pulmonary arterial hypertension, hypertrophic obstructive cardiomyopathy, Takayasu's arteritis mitral stenosis, etc. Aortic stenosis and mitral stenosis are most common.

   Atrial myxoma or ball-valve thrombus is suggested by embolic phenomena or dyspnea with change of posture.

3. *Arrhythmias:*
   Bradyarrhythmias: Stokes-Adams syndrome, sick sinus syndrome or III degree block, drugs like β-blockers, calcium blockers pacemaker malfunction.
   Tachyarrhythmias: Torse de pointes, ventricular tachycardia, ventricular fibrillation, arrhythmias with prolongation of QT interval –most common and potentially dangerous. VT accounts for 11% of all causes of syncope.
4. Cyanotic congenital heart diseases in children (see appropriate chapters for cardiovascular syncope for details).

25. Noncardiac causes of syncope.

1. CNS Causes: Vasovagal syncope, epilepsy, cerebrovascular accident (strokes), autonomic disturbances, vertebrobasilar insufficiency, subclavian steel syndrome, carotid insufficiency, carotid sinus hypersensitivity, vaso vagal causes, 'Drop attacks', etc.
2. Respiratory causes: Acute pulmonary embolism, cough syncope with strenuous cough.
3. Metabolic: Hypoglycemia, hyperventilation.
4. Situation syncope:
   Urinating (micturition syncope)
   Defecating (defecation syncope)
   Swallowing (deglutination syncope)
   Coughing (cough syncope)
   Post-exercise syncope
   Postprandial syncope
5. Postural syncope: Prolonged standing at attention.
6. Dehydration/volume depletion causing a decrease in blood volume.
7. Drug induced syncope: Blood pressure medications include nitrates, ACEI, BB, CCB, quinidine, procainamide, amiodarone, diuretics, vincristine, insulin, cocaine, and dioxin, etc. leading to low blood pressure. Alpha-blockers, prazosin are potent causes of orthostatic hypotension.
8. Autonomic failure: Some patients with Parkinson's disease, diabetic neuropathy.
9. Trauma to abdomen: Ruptured spleen, etc.
10. Excessive bleeding: Menorrhagia, piles.
11. Carotid sinus syndrome
12. Miscellaneous:
    Psychogenic causes: Hysterical, depression.
    Anticoagulants, glossopharyngeal neuralgia.

26. Clinical features suggesting specific causes of syncope.

Table A-4

Symptoms	*Diagnostic consideration*
1. During or immediately after micturition, cough, swallow, or defecation	Situation syncope
2. After sudden unexpected pain, unpleasant sight, sound or smell	Vasovagal syncope
3. With neuralgia–trigeminal or glossopharyngeal	Bradycardia or vasodepressor
4. Upon standing	Orthostatic hypotension
5. Taking hypotensive medicines	Drug induced syncope
6. Symptoms within one hour after meals	Postprandial hypotension
7. Prolonged standing at attention, well trained athlete after exertion	Vasovagal
8. Changing position (from sitting to lying, bending, turning over in bed)	Atrial myxoma, thrombus
9. With head rotation, pressure on carotid sinus	Carotid sinus syncope
10. Associated with vertigo, dysarthria, diplopia	Transient ischemic attack-stroke
11. With arm exercise	Subclavian artery syndrome
12. Exertion causing syncope	Aortic stenosis, pulmonary hypertension, hypertrophic obstructive cardiomyopathy, coronary artery disease

27. Medical management for some noncardiac syncope.

Table A-5

Causes	*Treatment*
1. Situation syncope	Stool softeners, urinate while sitting down
2. Vasodepressor syncope	B-blocker, disopyramide, fluoxetine, dual-chamber pacing, theophylline, and scopolamine
3. Dysautonomic syncope	Elastic support hose, water exercise, increased salt intake, fludrocortisone, ephedrine, midodrine, erythropoietin, and methylphenidate
4. Carotid sinus syncope	Avoidance of tight collars, surgical removal of carotid sinus tumor, pacemaker in patients with predominantly cardioinhibitory syncope

(see cardiac syncope treatment in appropriate chapters)

28. Vasovagal syncope (Neurocardiogenic syncope).

It is the most common form of syncope in young people.

Vagus nerve transmits efferent signals from the aortic arch baroreceptors regulating arterial pressure.

Increase in arterial blood flow stimulates the vagus nerve, inhibiting sympathetic drive and lowering the blood pressure.

When a person stands in an upright position, blood pools in the lower limbs and activates autonomic cycle. The resulting increase in sympathetic nervous activity causes vasoconstriction, increases heart rate, and maintains the blood pressure.

In vasovagal syncope, vasodilation and bradycardia occur rather than the appropriate physiological responses of vasoconstriction and tachycardia.

Vasovagal syncope may be triggered in some situations:

1. Situational syncope: For example, urination, defecation, coughing, sneezing, swallowing, etc.
2. Causes that induce fainting: For example, standing in attention, fasting.
3. Causes of fear: Having an injection, visiting the dentist.
4. Excess alcohol.

The triggering event stimulates adrenergic tone, followed by vagal over activation and then sympathetic withdrawal.

29. Carotid sinus hypersensitivity (CSH).

The fainting may be induced by looking up, turning the head, or just wearing a tight collar. Mechanical deformation of the carotid sinus (located at the bifurcation of the common carotid artery) leads to an exaggerated response with bradycardia or vasodilatation resulting in syncope.

One way of testing is by manually massaging the carotid sinus while taking an ECG but this should only be done by an experienced physician in controlled conditions. In the cardiac inhibitory CSH, asystole lasting more than three seconds may occur. In vasodepressor CSH, the systolic blood pressure may fall more than 50 mm Hg without a decrease in the heart rate.

Patients are advised:

1. Not to massage their neck.
2. Not to wear shirts with tight collars.
3. Not to wash the front of the neck vigorously.
4. People with recurrent attacks may benefit from a pacemaker.

Carotid massage should be avoided in patients with history of stroke or transient ischemic attack within three months. These patients may have carotid bruit heard over the vessels. Carotid Doppler is advised.

30. Orthostatic syncope (Postural hypotension)

It is common in elderly people. Normally when a patient stands the systolic blood pressure drops only 5 to 10 mm Hg, and diastolic pressure rises slightly. Orthostatic hypotension is due to abnormal blood pressure regulation triggered by different things. In orthostasis, the fall in systolic blood pressure exceeds more than 20 mm Hg, frequently the diastolic blood pressure drops by more than 10 mm Hg. This finding demands search for a potential cause.

The gravitation stress of rising quickly to a standing position causes blood to pool in the legs and trunk. This in turn leads to a decrease in venous return and cardiac output and a fall in blood pressure. In healthy persons, autonomic reflexes are activated and rapidly normalize the blood pressure by increasing the heart rate. When the response is impaired, however, cerebral perfusion may be reduced and leads to syncope.

The most common causes are:

1. Volume depletion: Hypovolemia, often induced by excessive use of diuretics
2. Diabetes
3. Infection—Diarrhea with dehydration
4. Alcohol and varicose veins.

31. Investigations.

ECG—To identify arrhythmias, ischemic heart disease.

Echocardiogram—All valvular lesions, congenital lesions, tumors, etc.

Holter's monitor—For arrhythmias.

Special investigations for syncope

1. Tilt-table testing.
2. Loop recorder—effectively couple arrhythmias syncope.
3. SAECG (signal averaged electrocardiography).
4. EP: Electrophysiological studies, e.g. WPW syndrome.

Comprehensive evaluation should include funduscopic examination, carotid bruit, assessment of carotid upstroke, subtle neurological deficits, cardiac murmur, peripheral pulses, dermatological changes for collagen diseases, etc.

Palpitation

(See Chapter D-Cardiac Arrhythmias)

Palpitation is defined as an unpleasant awareness of the forceful or rapid beating of the heart.

32. Palpitation is brought about by the following 4 conditions.

1. Changes in cardiac rhythm or rate, including all forms of tachycardia, ectopic beats, compensatory pause.

2. Increased stroke volume due to valvular regurgitation, e.g. aortic regurgitation, mitral regurgitation, tricuspid regurgitation, left to right shunt.
3. Hyperkinetic state of high cardiac output state such as anemia, fever, thyrotoxicosis, AV fistulae.
4. Sudden onset of bradycardia—Complete heart block, tachy-brady arrhythmia (SSS), sinus block.

33. Following points should be asked in the history of patients with palpitation which may suggest the diagnosis.

Table A-6

Does the palpitation occur	Suggested condition
1. As isolated 'jumps' or 'skips'	Extra systoles, multiple ectopics
2. With sudden onset and end?	Paroxysmal atria tachycardia may start suddenly but often end gradually because sinus tachycardia follows them
3. Independent of exercise or excitement, while the patient is resting, sitting quietly	Atrial flutter, atrial fibrillation, thyrotoxicosis, anemia, pyrexia, hypoglycemia, anxiety neurosis
4. Attacks developing rapidly without any relation to exertion or excitement	Hemorrhage, hypoglycemia, pheochromocytoma
5. Always with exercise	Sinus tachycardia
6. Comes on standing	Postural hypotension, vasodilators, nifidipine, hypertension
7. Any precipitating factors	Tea, coffee, alcohol, tobacco, cocaine
8. Drugs	Digitalis – dose—(digitoxicity) Diuretic without potassium sparing agents Tachycardia producing drugs such as hydralazine or anticholinergic ulcer drugs Antiarrhythmic drugs—Proarrhythmic—Prolonged QT interval Sympathomimetics/parasympatholytics–adrenaline, ephedrine, atropine Monoamine oxidase inhibitors—tricyclic antidepressants –prolonged QT interval Miscellaneous–aminophylline, thyroid extract
9. In middle-aged women with flushing and sweating	Menopausal syndrome
10. With normal or rapid rate and rhythm	Anxiety state
11. With faintness or syncope, weakness or fatigue. Has the patient been told of slow pulse rate	III degree block, sick sinus syndrome
12. In conjunction with angina or syncope	Myocardial ischemia or myocardial infarction. Syncope in association with palpitation is considered a danger signal as it may indicate large area of myocardial infarction
13. With dyspnea with mild exertion	Heart failure, atrial fibrillation, anemia, thyrotoxicosis
14. With valvular disease	Mitral stenosis with atrial fibrillation (digoxin is the choice), mitral valve prolapse, with throbbing in the neck in aortic regurgitation
15. With thyroid disease	Atrial fibrillation with rapid ventricular response (β-blockers are the choice)
16. With depression	Tricyclic antidepressants, prolonged QT interval, ventricular arrhythmias
17. Any pulsations in the neck come and go	A giant 'a' wave of pulmonary hypertension or tricuspid stenosis disappears with atrial fibrillation. Cannon 'a' waves occur whenever there is AV dissociation or retrograde P waves
18. Any maneuvers by either patient or physician, change or stop it by induced gagging or breath holding or vomiting or by carotid massage	Supraventricular arrhythmias—sinus tachycardia, paroxysmal atrial tachycardia, atrial flutter
19. Has the patient been told of abnormal ECG	WPW syndrome—Reentrant supraventricular tachycardia, AF with wide QRS/rapid rates digoxin contraindicated
20. With prosthetic heart valve or pacemaker?	

34. Palpitation in systemic hypertension can occur with the following 4 causes:

1. Use of vasodilators
2. Hypokalemia by potassium loosing diuretics, primary aldosteronism
3. Pheochromocytoma
4. Associated coronary artery disease

35. Palpitation in congenital heart disease: This may be a both sign or a symptom. Increased precordial motion is observed by the parent.

1. Left to right shunt—VSD, PDA—occur in infancy or childhood, later in life with ASD (uncommon with tetralogy of Fallot or with similar etiology)
2. Palpitation as a dominant symptom with cyanosis in Ebstein anomaly, prone to atrial arrhythmias due to large right atrium

3. Cyanotic heart diseases with increased pulmonary blood flow: Transposition of great vessels (TGA) and total anomalous pulmonary venous connection (TAPVC)
4. After Mustered operation (redirecting the venous blood in TGA) due to atrial arrhythmia.

"All those palpitations are not arrhythmias and many arrhythmias do not palpitate."

Edema

36. Peripheral edema is a symptom as well as a sign. Press the skin over the bony area for 10 sec with at least three fingers spread slightly apart and feel for valleys between hills after release. If the 'pitting' is present for more than 1 minute, it is considered as 'slow edema' and is most possible of congestive edema (always need not be). If the 'pitting' disappears in less than 40 sec—it is considered as 'fast edema'. The cause is mostly low albumin level.

Cardiac causes of peripheral edema should be distinguished from other causes:

1. *Cardiac causes*: First appears in the feet
   a. Heart failure: Edema may be decreased by low-salt diet, diuretics whatever the cause may be. Helped by digitalis or after load reduction.
   b. High left atrial pressure: Symptoms of low cardiac output, fatigue, dyspnea or cold extremities
   c. Pericarditis or tamponade: Edema is preceded by dyspnea by days, weeks or months.
2. *Renal causes:* Facial and hand edema, worse on awakening. First starts in the face (puffiness of face). History of renal disease.
3. *Cirrhosis:* First starts in the abdomen. H/o hepatitis, alcoholism or jaundice: Anorexia, fatigue, weakness or ascites; H/o bleeding varices. If polycythemia vera is present, consider hepatic vein thrombosis as a cause of ascites (Budd-Chiari syndrome)
4. *Hormonal causes:*
   a. Myxedema: Weight gain, watery or puffy eyes, voice changes, dry skin, absent sweating, cold intolerance, constipation, sleepiness, menorrhagia, diminished hearing, etc.
   b. Premenstrual: Associated with fullness of breast, headache, and mood changes
   b. On estrogen contraceptive pill
   c. Aldosteronism: Hypertension, weakness, tetany, parasthesias or high licorice intake.
5. *Lymphatic obstruction:* Abdominal swelling or mass such as ovarian cancer, prostatic carcinoma, foot fungus.
   Filarial leg is very common in India, especially in endemic areas. Usually it is unilateral but it can be bilateral (pitting edema in the beginning, later non-pitting)
6. *Stasis or obstructive edema:* With weight gain, obesity or pregnancy. H/o varicose veins or phlebitis in unilateral edema. Superior vena cava obstruction—swollen face.
7. *Drug-induced:* Antihypertensives such as clonidine, hydralazine or rauwolfia derivatives.
   Calcium blockers—especially nifedipine
   Nonsteroidal anti-inflammatory drugs such as ibuprofen, phenylbutazone or indomethacin
8. Intermittent idiopathic edema of women; H/o menstrual disorders, emotionally labile, unrelated to menses.

37. Localization of edema is helpful in finding the etiology. Cardiac edema starts in the legs, as it progresses, it ascends to involve the thighs, genitalia and abdominal wall. Any visible edema of both lower extremities is preceded by weight gain of at least 7–10 lbs. Cardiac edema is generally bilaterally symmetrical.

There are 4 points to rule out cardiac disease quickly as a cause of peripheral edema.

1. A normal jugular venous pulse is incompatible with a cardiac cause unless diuretics have been given. Diuretics may lower the jugular venous pressure before the edema subsides.
2. Edema in face and hands only rule out a cardiac cause.
3. Presacral edema is present in patients confined largely to bed for long periods. History of edema on prolonged standing is observed in patients with chronic venous insufficiency.
4. Mild peripheral edema is a common complaint in normal persons, especially in women during premenstrual period or when they wear tight garments. It is seen in any obese person due to obstructed lymphatic drainage. Idiopathic cyclic edema is associated with menstruation. Intermittent edema occurs in angioneurotic edema with emotional stress and with certain foods.

38. A history of puffiness of the face in early morning is characteristic of:

1. Nephrotic syndrome, acute glomerulonephritis
2. Angioneurotic edema
3. Hypoproteinemia
4. Myxedema

History of ascites preceding edema suggests cirrhosis of liver whereas history of ascites following edema suggest cardiac or renal origin.

39. There are 4 important questions to be asked about the past history.

1. History of rheumatic fever–sore throat, fleeting arthritis, growing pains.
2. History of chorea
3. History of scarlet fever
4. History of diphtheria

(In a child ask for sore throat and growing pains, i.e. nocturnal pains in the legs, cyanotic spells).

SOME CARDIAC CLUES FROM PHYSICAL APPEARANCE

General Appearance

The general built, appearance of the patient, skin color, presence of pallor or cyanosis, as well as the presence of shortness of breath, orthopnea, Cheyne-Stokes breathing and distension of the neck veins should be noted.

40. If the patient is with chest pain

1. Sitting quietly—is suggestive of angina pectoris
2. Moving about, trying to find a more comfortable position—suggests acute myocardial infarction
3. Most comfortable sitting upright—suggest heart failure
4. Leaning forward—suggests pericarditis

41. If the patient appears with

1. Marked weight loss, malnutrition, cachexia – suggests severe heart failure
2. Cold sweaty palms and frequent sighing respirations—suggestive of typical neurocirculatory asthenia
3. Marked obesity, somnolescence and cyanosis and peripheral edema suggests the Pickwickian syndrome (obesity hypoventilation syndrome)
4. Marked abdominally localized obesity is associated with adult onset diabetes and coronary artery disease.

42. The distinctive general appearance of Marfan's syndrome is quiet glaring by

1. Long extremities with an arm span that exceeds the height
2. Longer lower segment (pubis to foot) than upper segment (head to pubis)
3. Arachnodactyly (spider fingers)
4. Narrow and/or sharp feature face with tremulous iris (iridodonesis) in which iris is not supported by the lens because of dislocation or weakness of suspensory ligament. The cardiac lesions associated with are aneurysm of aorta or pulmonary artery or myxomatous degeneration of the aorta or mitral valve with consequent regurgitation.

Head and Face

43. The facial appearance that aids in the diagnosis of cardiovascular disorders are

1. Myxedema: It is characterized by dull expressionless face, periorbital puffiness, loss of outer third of eyebrows, scanty dry hair, coarse dry skin and enlarged tongue. These patients may have cardiomyopathies due to increased interstitial fluid and mucoid infiltration. They may also have pericardial effusion.
2. An ear lobe crease occurs more frequently with coronary artery disease. There is an oblique crease in the ear lobe. Ninety percent of patients over the age of 50 years with significant triple vessel disease have a deep crease. An unilateral ear crease in one study was found to be associated with an intermediate degree of coronary obstruction. However, in Japanese, it is associated more with obesity than with coronary artery disease. Almost 50% of patients with diabetic retinopathy have a diagonal ear lobe crease.
3. Bobbing of the head with each heart beat (de Musset's sign) is characteristic of severe aortic regurgitation.
4. Facial edema may be seen in patients with tricuspid valve disease or constrictive pericarditis.
   Muscular dystrophies may also affect facial appearance.

44. There are 4 cardiac conditions that may be associated with exophthalmos.

1. Thyrotoxic heart disease which can cause high output failure.
2. Advanced congestive heart failure in which there is high venous pressure and weight loss. The stare is probably due to lid retraction caused by increased sympathetic tone accompanying the low cardiac output and exaggerated by the slight proptosis.
3. Sever tricuspid regurgitation can cause systolic pulsations of the eyeballs (pulsatile exophthalmos) as well as earlobes.
4. Carotid-cavernous sinus fistula can cause pulsatile exophthalmos in which case a murmur can be heard over the eye ball.

45. There are 4 cardiac conditions associated with blue sclera.

1. Osteogenesis imperfecta which may be associated with aortic regurgitation, aortic dilatation and dissection
2. Marfan's syndrome which is associated with great vessel aneurysms and mitral or aortic regurgitation
3. Ehlers-Danlos syndrome with its hyperelastic fragile skin, hyperextensible joints and kyphoscoliosis is associated with atrial septal defect, tetralogy of Fallot or regurgitant valves.
4. May be associated with mitral valve prolapse.

46. Cardiac lesions are suspected when the following features are striking in the eyes

1. *Epicanthus:* Down's syndrome (Trisomy 21)—is associated with endocardial cushion defect
2. *Hyperteleorism:* Widely set eyes. It is associated with pulmonary stenosis with atrial septal defect, supravalvular aortic stenosis, Noonan's syndrome, multiple lentigines syndrome, Hurler's syndrome or gargoylism with mitral regurgitation
3. *Argyll- Robertson pupil:* Characterized by retention of accommodation and loss of light reflex. It is associated with leutic aortic aneurysm, leutic aortic regurgitation with coronary osteal stenosis.
4. *Corneal arcus:* Circumferential light gray or yellowish ring around the rim of the iris. It is associated with hypercholesterolemia or coronary artery disease.

A thick band begins inferiorly and is inside the limbus, allowing a thin rim of iris pigment to be seen between the arcus and sclera.

The usual 'arcus senilis' begins superiorly and extends to the rim or limbus of the iris. As the name indicates, it is a sign of old age and is not necessarily associated with hyperlipidemia or coronary artery disease.

An arcus may be absent or diminished on one side if there is reduced flow to that side due to carotid occlusion or previous inflammation.

(Examination of fundi are discussed in Chapter B—Hypertension)

Skin and Mucous Membranes

47. Cyanosis aids to distinguish cardiac conditions. The cyanosis can be described under 4 types.

(See Chapter L-Congenital Heart Diseases-Cyanotic heart disease from L- 22–24, 244–248)

1. *Central cyanosis:* It is due to intracardiac or intrapulmonary right-to-left shunt. The blue or purple discoloration involves the entire body, including well-perfused sites such as conjunctiva and the mucous membrane of the oral cavity (see the tongue). If the nails are cyanotic and the hands are warm, cyanosis is central, e.g. tetralogy of Fallot. Clubbing usually accompanies central cyanosis.
2. *Peripheral cyanosis:* It is due to reduction of peripheral blood flow such as occurs in peripheral circulatory failure and peripheral vascular disease. It is seen in cool, exposed areas such as the nail beds, nose, cheeks, earlobes and outer surface of the lips.
3. *Differential cyanosis:* When the hands are pink and the feet are blue, pulmonary arterial hypertension is present with a right to left shunt through patent ductus arteriosus (See Chapter L Congenital Heart Diseases -123)
4. *Reversed differential cyanosis:* When the cyanosis and clubbing of the fingers are greater than those of toes—suggests complete transposition of great vessels, with either a preductal coarctation or complete interruption of the aortic arch. Slightly less cyanosis of the left arm compared to the right arm favors coarctation rather than complete aortic interruption.

48. The 4 causes of cyanotic cheeks are:

1. 'Malar flush' in mitral stenosis. It can be seen in any condition with low cardiac output.
2. Chronic heart failure with loss of weight—cardiac cachexia.
3. High pulmonary vascular resistance
4. High venous pressure

49. Cardiac conditions that are associated with discoloration of the skin are:

1. Cyanosis (already mentioned)
2. *Jaundice:* It is seen in patients with congestive hepatomegaly, cardiac cirrhosis, pulmonary infarction.
3. Bronze pigmentation of the skin and loss of pubic and axillary hair occur in hemochromatosis which may cause cardiomyopathy due to iron deposits in the heart.
4. Lentigines are small brown macular lesions on the neck and trunk that begin at about the age of six and do not increase in number with sunlight that occur in patients with pulmonary stenosis and hypertrophic obstructive cardiomyopathy.

Hereditary telangiectases are multiple capillary hemangiomas that occur in the skin, lips, nasal mucosa and upper respiratory and gastrointestinal tract and appears like spider nevi. They occur in liver disease but when they occur in lung, they are associated with pulmonary arteriovenous fistulas and cause central cyanosis.

50. Skin temperature aids to differentiate the following 4 cardiac conditions.

1. Warmer than normal skin suggests high output circulation as seen in thyrotoxicosis, severe anemia, beer drinker's acute beriberi.
   Cold hands or feet
2. Moist hands and feet with chest pain, palpitation and fatigue are seen in neurocirculatory asthenia. (Da Costa's syndrome)
3. If only the feet are cold with history of intermittent claudication—suggest peripheral arteriolar obstruction with poor collateral circulation.

4. If cold extremities are of recent onset—a low output cardiac state is suggested. The cold hands of low output state can become warm when palmar erythema develop secondary to cardiac cirrhosis.

51. Xanthomas are cholesterol-filled nodules found either subcutaneously or over tendons in patients with hyperlipoproteinemia. Premature atherosclerosis frequently develops in these patients.

There are 4 types of xanthomas.

1. Xanthoma tendinosa (tendon xanthomas) are nodular swellings of the tendons especially of the extensor tendons of hands, elbows, and Achilles tendon, plantar tendons of soles of feet and patellar tendons. Usually, xanthomas in these sites indicate Type I hyperlipoproteinemia.
2. Xanthoma striatum palmarae—produces yellowish, orange or pink discoloration of the palmar and digital creases; seen most commonly in patients with Type III hyperlipoproteinemia.
3. Tuberoeruptive xanthomas—present subcutaneously or on the extensor surfaces of the extremities
4. Eruptive xanthomas are tiny yellowish nodules 1 to 2 mm in diameter on an erythematous base, which may occur anywhere on the body and are associated with hyperchylomicronemia. They are seen in patients with Type I and V hyperlipoproteinemia.

52. There are 4 skin signs that occurs secondary to small emboli of infective endocarditis (See Chapter J-19)

1. Clubbing and splinter hemorrhages in the nails
2. Janeway lesions
3. Osler's nodes
4. Livido reticualris

Most splinter hemorrhages are not embolic, they move with the nail as grows. They are seen in the nail substance and usually extend to the nail edge.

Splinter hemorrhages of infective endocarditis are sublingual and usually do not extend to the distal nail edge.

Janeway lesions are painless or slightly tender, circular or oval, pink to tan macules about 5 mm in diameter on the palms and soles that do not blanch with pressure.

Osler's nodes are small, painful, tender, reddish-brown raised areas of 3–15 mm diameter occasionally with a whitish center due to infected microemboli and occurring frequently on the finger pads, palms or soles.

Livido reticularis-like mottling of palmar or plantar aspects of the digits may occur in acute bacterial endocarditis. This term indicates a marbling reticulation or fishnet type of mottling of the lower trunk, buttocks and extremities which is exaggerated by cold or emotional upsets. It can also occur in 20% of patients with lupus, periarteritis nodosa or cryoglobulinemia. If it occurs recently in a person over 50 years age, it suggests cholesterol embolization from an abdominal aortic aneurysm.

Extremities

A good number of congenital and acquired heart diseases are associated with characteristic changes in the extremities.

(See Chapter L-Congenital heart diseases 14, 15, 16 for characteristic changes in extremities)

Clubbing

53. The soft tissues of the terminal phalanges of the fingers or toes become hypertrophied and the nails finally curve excessively, giving a drumstick appearance.

Clubbing of the digits is characteristic of central cyanosis, e.g. cyanotic congenital heart disease or pulmonary disease with hypoxia.

1. Clubbing in cyanotic congenital heart diseases: It occurs in right to left shunt, e.g. tetralogy of Fallot, transposition of great vessels.
2. Clubbing with differential cyanosis occurs in complete transposition of great vessels with either preductal coarctation or complete interruption of the aortic arch. Slightly less cyanosis of the left arm compared to right arm suggests coarctation than complete aortic interruption.

   Clubbing and cyanosis more in toes than fingers suggests patent ductus arteriosus with reversal of shunt.
3. Unilateral clubbing of fingers is rare but can occur when an aortic aeurysm interferes with the arterial supply of one arm.
4. Clubbing with splinter hemorrhages occur in the nails in infective endocarditis. Clubbing without cyanosis suggests infective endocarditis of few weeks duration.

Clubbing is seen in conditions other than cardiac diseases and is common with pulmonary disease with hypoxia, e.g. suppurative lung lesions, anoxic cor pulmonale, COPD, pulmonary tuberculosis, carcinoma lung, etc.

Severe clubbing with bony changes occur in hypertrophic pulmonary osteoarthropathy. The changes involve the terminal digits and in rare instances even wrists, ankles, elbows and knees. Clubbing occurs rarely in ulcerative colitis or may even be familial.

Chest

54. See for respirations – Note their

1. Rate/frequency
2. Regularity—regular or irregular
3. Depth

4. Relative effort required during inspiration and expiration

Compare the respiratory rate and pulse rate. It should be 1:4 in normals.

Tachypnea, and tachycardia—see for the cause. Always try to find out the cause when there is change in ratio of respiratory and pulse rate, like 1:3, 1:2.

This gives an idea for respiratory or metabolic acidosis or alkalosis besides respiratory causes itself.

See for characteristic breathing such as Cheyne-Stokes respiration, Kussmaul's respiration, etc.

55. Shape of the chest.

Some cardiac abnormalities are suggested by the chest deformities.

1. Barrel-shaped chest with low diaphragm suggests severe obstructive airway disease, e.g. cor pulmonale, emphysema, chronic bronchitis
2. Pectus excavatum (funnel chest)—Marfan's syndrome—sternum is displaced posteriorly. It rarely compresses the heart to elevate the systemic and pulmonary venous pressure and signs of heart disease are more apparent than real.
3. Pectus carinatum or Pigeon chest—Marfan's syndrome
4. Bulging of left anterior chest—Atrial septal defect with hyperkinetic pulmonary hypertension. Right ventricle never enlarges to the right, i.e. right border of the heart on chest roentgenogram is never due to right ventricle, no matter how big it becomes and right ventricle never bulges the right anterior chest.
5. Bulging of right of the upper sternum can be caused by an aortic aneurysm, superior vena caval obstruction producing venous collateral pattern.
6. Kyphoscoliosis of any etiology can cause cor pulmonale.
7. Shield chest is a broad chest with an increased angle between the manubrium and body of the sternum as well as widely separated nipples. In a female with webbing of the neck, wide carrying angle, and short stature suggests—Turner's syndrome which is associated with coarctation of aorta. In male, it is called Noonan's, or Ullrich's syndrome associated with pulmonary stenosis.
8. Straight back syndrome: Compression of the heart due to loss of the normal dorsal curvature of the spine. This may cause pulmonary ejection murmur but is usually mistaken for pulmonary stenosis or atrial septal defect. Scoliosis as well as pectus excavatum are commonly seen with straight back syndrome.

56. Pectus excavatum is a condition in which the sternum is displaced posteriorly. It is observed in 4 conditions

1. Marfan's syndrome
2. Homocystinuria
3. Ehlers-Danlos syndrome, Hunter-Hurler syndrome
4. Mitral valve prolapse (small fraction)

57. There are 4 steps in examination of cardiovascular system that is to be carefully evaluated.

1. Arterial pulses
2. Jugular venous pulse
3. Precordial palpation
4. Cardiac auscultation

58. There are 4 order of sequences to be followed in the examination.

1. Arterial pulses
2. BP
3. Venous pulses
4. Finally examination of the precordium

ARTERIAL PULSE

59. The arterial pulse represents the pressure pulse transmitted along the arterial system as each bolus of blood is ejected by the left ventricle into the proximal aorta. There are 4 points to be noted while reading the pulse.

1. Rate and rhythm
2. Character
3. Volume
4. Condition of the vessel wall—Normally the radial pulse is soft on palpation. In patients with widespread atherosclerosis, it is often firm and less easily compressed.

60. 4 is the normal ratio of the pulse rate to respiratory rate.

Pulse rate 72 : Respiratory rate 18 = 4:1

61. There are 4 points to assess while applying pressure on radial pulse wave (or carotid pulse) concentrating on separate phases.

1. Sharpness of upstroke
2. Systolic peak
3. Diastolic slope

(1–3 referred as trisection)

4. Thickness of the vessel wall

62. A normal arterial pulse consists of 4 parts (See Fig. A-1: N)

1. *P-Percussion wave:* It is caused by the upstroke. It comes out with the first sound and the peak is reached well before the second sound. It is due to left ventricular ejection.

2. *T- Tidal wave:* It is a smaller wave due to aortic recoil of a reflected wave from the periphery
3. *N- Dicrotic notch:* It indicates end of diastole
4. *D- Dicrotic wave:* It follows dicrotic notch

These waves are better recorded in carotids. The dicrotic notch and wave are not clearly seen as it goes to periphery.

63. There are 4 types of pulse in aortic disease.

1. A slow rising pulse (Pulsus tardus) in aortic stenosis (AS) (Fig. A1-A). It is due to left ventricular systole being prolonged as a result of the mechanical outflow obstruction.
2. A bounding pulse—Water-hammer, collapsing or corrigan pulse in aortic regurgitation (AR) (Fig. A1-B) (High volume pulse falling away quickly). It is due to ejection of large volume of blood into the aorta in early systole and the regurgitation of part of it back into the heart in late systole and diastole.
3. Pulsus bisferiens (double peak) in combined aortic stenosis and regurgitation (Fig. A1-C). This is characterised by two peaks in systole and a mid-systolic dip. Should not be confused with dicrotic pulse in which the second peak is in diastole immediately after the second heart sound.
4. Diminished, delayed or absent femoral arterial pulsations in coarctation of aorta. Femoral arterial pulsations may feel normal in patient with coarctation of aorta associated with severe aortic regurgitation. However, pulsations proximal to the coarctation, radial, brachial or carotid show even greater amplitude. Thus simultaneous palpation of radial (brachial or carotid) and femoral arteries reveal the greater amplitude in the radial pulse. In solitary severe aortic regurgitation without coarctation, the femoral pulsations are greater in amplitude.

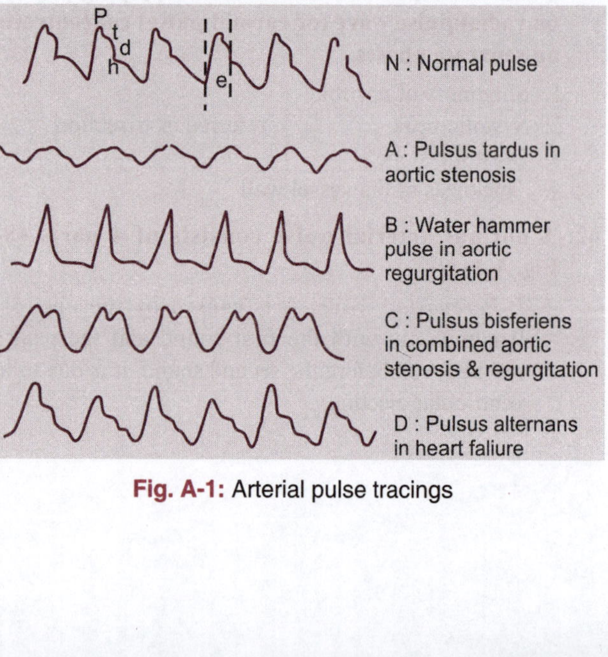

Fig. A-1: Arterial pulse tracings

Diminution of amplitude of radial pulse on one side usually on right side is seen in aneurysm of arch of aorta.

64. There are 4 characteristic pulses other than in the aortic disease.

1. 'Pulsus paradoxus'—Pulse weakening in inspiration in pericardial effusion, constrictive pericarditis and in cardiac tamponade. This is an exaggeration of normal variation of systolic blood pressure during the respiratory cycle and is not in any way paradoxical.
2. 'Pulsus alternans'—when heart muscle is severely damaged. This is characterized by alternate strong and weak beats.
3. 'Pulsus bigeminus'—A normal sinus beat is followed by a ventricular extra systole accompanied by a compensatory pause. The beats may occur in pairs followed by a compensatory pause. Digitalis often causes coupling.
4. 'Irregularly Irregular' pulse with pulse deficit in atrial fibrillation.

65. There are 4 common conditions where bounding pulse (water-hammer or collapsing pulse) is felt.

This is due to an increased stroke volume, a wide pulse pressure and decreased peripheral vascular resistance.

1. Aortic regurgitation (AR)
2. Patent ductus arteriosus (PDA)
3. Large arteriovenous fistulae

} due to abnormally rapid run-off of blood from the high pressure systemic arterial system to the relatively low pressure pulmonary artery in PDA and low pressure venous system in A-V fistulae.

4. Minor degrees in conditions such as anxiety, fever, anemia, pregnancy, thyrotoxicosis and marked bradycardia.

66. There are 4 common causes of pulsus parvus a small weak pulse. This is found in conditions in which the stroke volume is decreased.

1. Diminished left ventricular stroke volume due to myocardial infarction or any myocardial disease, cardiac failure.
2. Diminished left ventricular stroke volume due to restricted filling, e.g. constrictive pericarditis, mitral stenosis.
3. Narrow pulse pressure, e.g. Aortic stenosis.
4. Increased peripheral vascular resistance, e.g. peripheral circulatory failure, shock or hypovolemia of any cause.

67. There are 4 common causes of 'Pulsus paradoxus'.

1. Pericardial disease—Cardiac tamponade, constrictive pericarditis, pericardial effusion.

2. Airways obstruction—Asthma, chronic obstructive airways disease (COAD), severe emphysema, severe upper respiratory obstruction.
3. Hypovolemic shock.
4. Cardiac failure.

68. There are 4 common causes of 'pulsus alternans' (Fig. A1-D).

1. Any cause of ventricular dysfunction, heart failure
2. Severe aortic stenosis
3. Severe aortic regurgitation with left ventricular failure especially after aortic valve replacement
4. Dilated cardiomyopathy or myocarditis

69. There are 4 main causes of irregular pulse.

1. Atrial ectopic beats
2. Ventricular ectopic beats
3. Atrial fibrillation
4. Heart beat varying from beat to beat, e.g. atrial flutter with variable block or Wenkebach phenomenon.

70. There are 4 points to differentiate the irregular pulse clinically at the bed side (assuming that you do not have ECG).

1. *Pulse:* If the pulse is basically regular with intermittent irregularities, the rhythm is likely to be sinus rhythm with extrasystoles. The extrasystoles may be of atrial, junctional or ventricular. If the pulse is grossly irregular (irregularly irregular with pulse deficit), the rhythm is likely to be atrial fibrillation.
2. *Exercise:* Gentle exercise like attempting to touch their toes a few times. In a healthy person with sinus rhythm the tachycardia produced by exercise leaves insufficient time between beats for ectopic beats to develop. Therefore, the ectopics disappear and pulse becomes regular. On the other hand in atrial fibrillation, the tachycardia produced by exercise becomes more irregular as heart speed up.
   Limitations: Remember, in the presence of diseased myocardium, e.g. cardiomyopathy, despite the underlying sinus rhythm exercise may increase ectopic activity resulting in more irregular pulse.
3. *Carotid sinus massage:* Though it is named as carotid massage, it is a massage over the vagus nerve. Pressure over the vagus nerve slows the heart rate temporarily. Pressure should be applied vertically over vagus on one side first for few second and then on the other side (do not apply vagus pressure on both sides at a time). Pulse rate is slowed down in sinus tachycardia, atrial flutter. The rate should be down by 8–12 beats in sinus tachycardia. The rate is decreased in atrial flutter in arithmetic proportion from 2:1 to 3:1, from 3:1 to 4:1, whereas no change is seen with atrial fibrillation or ventricular ectopics (All or none phenomenon in paroxysmal atrial tachycardia - either becomes normal or no response).
4. Other methods to increase vagal tone such as Valsalva maneuver or pressure over the eye balls. These methods help to differentiate supraventricular tachycardias.

71. There are 4 causes of rapid regular pulse.

1. Paroxysmal supraventricular tachycardias (PSVT)—may be atrial, nodal or related to accessory pathway.
2. Atrial tachycardia with fixed block
3. Atrial flutter with 2:1 block in which alternate beats are conducted to the ventricles.
4. Ventricular tachycardia.

72. Causes of sinus tachycardia:

1. Hyperdynamic circulation
2. Congestive cardiac failure
3. Drugs (adrenaline, atropine, and nitrites, etc.)
4. Hypovolemic shock (acute hemorrhage, etc.) constrictive pericarditis.

73. There are 4 causes of rapid irregular pulse.

1. Atrial fibrillation
2. Atrial flutter with varying block
3. Atrial tachycardia with varying block
4. Multiple ventricular ectopics

74. The causes of slow pulse (< 60/min):

1. Sinus bradycardia
2. Heart block, 2:1, 3:1
3. Complete heart block
4. When the weak beat is impalpable as in pulsus alternans or bigeminal rhythm with premature beat impalpable.
5. Atrial flutter or fibrillation with high degree AV block.
6. Sinus arrest with idonodal rhythm.
7. Antihypertensive drugs like β-blockers.
8. Inotropic drug, e.g. digoxin.

Always see the heart rate in your outpatient department (OPD) clinic when a patient is on drugs like β-blocker or digoxin and adjust the dose. This should be followed routinely.

75. Causes of sinus bradycardia:

1. Congenital
2. Physical training (athletics)
3. Convalesce from fever
4. Jaundice
5. Myxedema
6. Hypothermia
7. Raised intracranial pressure
8. Drugs (digitalis and β-blockers).

9. Rapid rise in blood pressure
10. Transiently increased vagal tone (vomiting)
11. Glaucoma
12. Relative bradycardia, e.g. enteric fever.

76. There are 4 causes of high volume pulse.

Table A-7

1. Hyperkinetic circulation	Anemia, thyrotoxicosis	Stroke volume ↑
2. Conditions of aortic run off:	Low diastolic pressure, e.g. aortic regurgitation	Stroke volume ↑
3. Nondistensible arteriosclerotic arterial system	Hypertension in old age	Systemic resistance ↑
4. Anxiety state		Stroke volume ↑

The amplitude of the excursion of pulse indicates the volume of pulse and generally correlates with the stroke volume. In old age and in systemic hypertension, the pulse volume is high due to nondistensible atherosclerotic arterial system. In these conditions, the pulse volume does not truly reflect the stroke volume.

77. There are 4 routine observations to be made while feeling the pulse of the following.

1. *Radial pulse*: For rate, rhythm, volume, character and thickness of the vessel wall.
2. *Carotid pulse:* For any thrill (palpable murmur)
3. *Femoral pulse:* Feeble and delayed compared with radial pulse in coarctation of aorta.
4. *Brachial pulse:* Feel before auscultation while checking for blood pressure.

78. There are 4 places to palpate arterial pulse in the lower limbs (on both sides).

1. Femoral
2. Popliteal
3. Posterior tibial
4. Dorsalis pedis

BLOOD PRESSURE

79. There are 4 ranges of blood pressure that are normal.

1. Neonates—80/50 mm Hg
2. Children—100/60 mm Hg
3. Adults—120/80 mm Hg
4. High normal when diastole is 85–90 mm Hg.

Average systolic pressure in healthy adults is 100–140 mm Hg.

Average diastolic pressure in healthy adults is 60–90 mm Hg.

In children it approximates to the lower figure and in elderly it may reach or exceed the higher level.

The difference between systolic and diastolic pressure is called pulse pressure. It is 30–60 mm Hg. Average pulse pressure is 40 (120–80).

80. Patient is advised the following 4 instructions before recording the BP especially in cardiovascular patients.

1. No drugs like sympathomimetics, even nasal decongestant drops, which may contain ephedrine, etc. should be administered.
2. No tea or coffee at least one hour before should be taken.
3. No smoking at least 15 min. before recording the BP.
4. 5 min. rest or relaxation before recording the BP.

81. 4 types of instruments are available at present to record the blood pressure routinely.

1. *Mercury sphygmomanometer:* This is the most commonly used instrument. By far the most accurate and sensitive instrument with very few chances of getting an erroneous reading. From the practical point of view, the sphygmomanometer has not been replaced by any other gadget.
2. *Aneroid sphygmomanometer:* It is small and handy. It is based on lever mechanism. This instrument needs to be checked every six months as the lever and the stops get displaced due to physical jolts.
3. *Electronic blood pressure instrument:* It does not require a stethoscope. It is utilized for self measurement of blood pressure.
4. Electronic instrument for ambulatory blood pressure monitoring (ABPM). It monitors the blood pressure during 24 hours.

82. There are 4 technical points to be observed while recording the blood pressure.

1. Measurement should be made with a mercury sphygmomanometer, a recently calibrated aneroid manometer or a calibrated electronic device.
2. The appropriate cuff size should be used to ensure an accurate measurement. The bladder should nearly (at least 80%) or completely encircle the arm.
   Spurious high blood pressure readings can be recorded in obese individuals. Largest size cuff should be used in obese individuals which may show a normal BP. In the same way small sized blood pressure cuffs should be used for infants and children.
3. Both systolic blood pressure (SBP) and diastolic blood pressure (DBP) should be recorded. The disappearance of sound (Phase V) should be used for the diastolic reading.
4. Two or more readings separated by 2 minutes should be averaged.

Several blood pressure readings should be taken on each patient examined. It is not uncommon to see a drop of 10–15 mm in systolic blood pressure and 5–10 mm Hg in diastolic blood pressure over a period of 5–10 minutes. Take the blood pressure in both arms. If there is difference, go back to the first one to make sure that it was not an insignificant fast drop.

Hypertension should not be diagnosed on the basis of a single measurement. Initial elevated readings should be confirmed on at least 2 subsequent visits during one to several weeks unless SBP is 210 mm Hg or greater and/ or DBP is 120 mm Hg or greater.

Management of hypertension depends on well-documented data base. This consists of numerous and accurate measures of blood pressure. Even single readings may have predictive value for stroke or premature death if the reading is very high but the multiple readings are more reliable.

83. There are 4 methods of recording the blood pressure.

1. *Palpatory method for systolic pressure:* Palpate the radial artery pulse. Inflate the sphygmomanometer cuff slowly 30 mm Hg or above the level at which radial pulse is no longer felt. Slowly release the pressure concentrating on return of the pulse. Note the reading where the pulse returns. This reading is the systolic pressure in millimeters of mercury.
2. *Auscultatory method:* For systolic pressure and diastolic pressure.

   Systolic Pressure: Raise the pressure 30 mm or above the systolic pressure as noted by the palpatory method, i.e. cuff is inflated 30 mm or above where the Korotkoff sounds disappear. Place the diaphragm of the stethoscope over the brachial artery immediately below the armlet and auscultate the brachial artery while slowly releasing the cuff about 5 mm pressure at a time until the first sound is heard which is taken as the systolic pressure.

   Diastolic pressure: Continue to lower the pressure slowly, the sounds become louder and then quiet suddenly become muffled (phase 4 of Korotkoff sounds) and then inaudible (phase 5 of Korotkoff sounds). This reading is taken as the diastolic pressure. Systolic pressure reading taken by auditory method is usually slightly higher 5–10 mm Hg than taken by palpatory method. The auditory method is recommended for general use.

   Silent Gap: Occasionally sounds disappear below 200 mm Hg for some time and then reappear and then again disappear, e.g. sounds may first appear when the mercury falls to 210 (systolic pressure) and disappear from 180–160—Silent gap. Again reappear and finally disappear at 120—diastolic pressure.

   The importance is that the armlet pressure should be raised well above at the beginning of an estimated blood pressure.

   Silent gap is found in some hypertensive patients.
3. *Doppler method:* After the ultrasonic transducer is placed over the artery, the cuff pressure is deflated slowly as in auscultatory method. An appreciable signal is audible over the artery when the cuff pressure is lower than the intravascular pressure. The sound signal disappears when the cuff pressure drops below the diastolic blood pressure. It gives accurate systolic pressure but not the diastolic blood pressure.
4. *Oscillometric method:* This method helps in measuring systolic pressure, diastolic pressure, mean arterial pressure and heart rate digitally. Recording can be automatically repeated. Mean arterial pressure is automatically repeated. Mean arterial pressure is more accurate with this method.

84. Auscultatory gap or silent gap: some facts one should start taking blood pressure by feeling the radial pulse and inflating the cuff until the radial pulse disappears to get the correct systolic blood pressure because the auscultatory gap is eliminated if Korotkoff sounds are elicited properly. It takes extra time to feel for a radial pulse and to note its disappearance in patients with low volume pulse.

1. The auscultatory gap has been said to occur only when there is venous distension in the arm, i.e. the Korotkoff sounds may be faint when the tissue pressure is high distal to the cuff.
2. The evidence is that it can be elicited in old patients with coronary artery disease by using a tourniquet above the cuff to decrease the flow to the arm.
3. It can be eliminated by exercising the hand by repeated clenching and extending the fingers for about 10 seconds before taking the blood pressure, by inflating the cuff rapidly or by elevating the arm during cuff inflation.
4. An anacrotic pulse contour is necessary as seen in aortic stenosis or in elderly subjects with sclerotic aorta or hypertension.

85. Phase 4 of Korotkoff sounds is taken as diastolic pressure in children.

86. The 4th intercostal space is the ideal space to keep the arm at that level while recording the BP, i.e. arm should be at the same level of the heart. Keep the sphygmomanometer at the same level.

87. There are 4 sources of error in measuring the BP

1. The patient
2. The instrument
3. The observer
4. Training

Source of Error: 1. The patient: A frightened patient shows higher BP readings. False high readings are caused by fear, pain, a full bladder and a chilly consulting room. Tachycardia is an useful indicator of fear and a pulse rate is always recorded at the same time of BP False low readings are caused by tightly rolled sleeves/clothing above the cuff. So, clothing should be removed from the patient's arm.

Source of Error: 2. The instrument: Mercury sphygmomanometers are simple and reliable. Common errors are mostly due to inadequate cuffs and leaking valves. The cuff is an inelastic cloth that encircles the arm and encloses the inflatable rubber bladder. Partial encirclement of cuff causes a false high reading whose error is more or less proportional to the area uncovered. A false high readings of about 20 mm Hg above the true value leads to misdiagnosis and mistreatment in consequence. Bladder lengths vary from 22–36 cms, there being different lengths for obese arm and thigh. Cuffs of smaller size must be used for infants and children.

A full range of well-designed cuffs are available. Cuff width is not important above a minimum width of 11 cm. It is secured round the arm by wrapping its tapering end into the cuff, by velcro surfaces or by hooks. Velcro surfaces must be effective and when they loose their grip the cuff should be discarded. The center of the bladder must be placed directly over the artery to be compressed.

The rubber parts must be in good condition and free of leaks. The tubing must be at least 76 cm long and connections must be air tight and easily disconnected.

The control valve is a common source of error. The filter may become blocked with dirt which demands excessive squeeze on the pump. The control valve must allow the passage of air without much squeeze on the bulb. When closed after raising the mercury, it should hold the mercury column at a constant level for half a minute and when released it must allow controlled fall in the mercury. If it does not hold the mercury column, there is a leak. This can be anywhere in the bag or its connections.

It is usually due to the rubber washer against which the control valve engages being spoiled and needing replacement. Another common site of leak is at the junction of valve nozzle and rubber tube. The leakage effect produces a rapid and uncontrollable descent of the mercury column during reading leading to false readings. Rubber bulb itself sometimes causes leak due to a hole or a crack, or the valve in the bulb may be slipped from its position and is not effective while squeezing- which must be replaced.

The hole or passage connecting the bottom of the tube with the mercury reservoir must open, should show zero level of mercury before the cuff is connected. If it is below this, the mercury needs to be added to the reservoir. The glass tube should be properly cleaned at least once in six months or year. When dust gets accumulated on the inner surface of glass tube, it is difficult to find the exact column of mercury and is guessed at.

The pin hole at the top of the glass tube connecting the mercury column with the atmosphere must also be open. If it is blocked, false high readings are produced because the mercury will not fall freely as pressure is reduced in the cuff.

It is not surprising, if a spot check is made of the BP instruments in use, above 25–30% in regular use may found fault, some of which have not been checked or cleaned from the day they were bought.

Aneroid sphygmomanometers have levers which can stick and are affected by jolts, altitude and atmospheric pressure. They loose their sensitivity frequently. They usually have a small dial which make accurate reading difficult. They are convenient to carry for home visits when exact measurements are seldom important.

Number of electronic BP instruments started coming in the market. Several of them proved to be unreliable. They may show fairly compatible systolic readings but not diastolic readings. In general, electronic instruments still perform poorly compared to mercury manometers.

Source of Error: 3. *The observer:* The correct readings depend on the doctor-patient interaction, motivation and training. Recording by professors gives false high readings than nurses. The higher the hierarchy of the doctor, more the patient frightens giving false high readings, "white coat hypertension'. The soothing and pleasant looks of nurses do not give rise to false high readings. The medical students and nurses readings show close relation. Motivation and patient interaction plays a role in reading the BP the home readings give normals similar to reading by nurses. Sometimes, it is better to delegate the BP recording to nurse or other staff who are trained well. Many a times, the systolic pressures correctly recorded. Systolic pressure is more easily understood and read particularly by nurses and patients, because it is the first regular sound that is heard as the mercury column descends. The diastolic pressure readings varies because it is ambiguous softening, muffling or disappearance. The point at which the sounds become soften—cease to be tapping in quality—is taken as diastolic reading (Korotkoff's phase 4). Disappearance of sound (Korotkoff's phase 5) is 5 to 10 mm Hg lower than the muffling. Framingham study used fourth phase recording whereas Veteran administration study used the fifth phase. Fifth phase is easy to follow by nurses or patients. Phase 5 is an on an average about 2 mm Hg higher than intra-arterial measurement of diastolic pressure, and phase 4 is about 8 mm Hg higher by various studies. In some individuals, phase 5 does not exist, the sounds are audible down to zero. In most of these cases the cause is tightly rolled sleeves above the cuff, but in a few, the sound persists even with bare arm. In such cases use the phase 4 and make a note of the fact in the record. Systolic pressure over 40 years of age has greater predictive value than diastolic pressure, which may show subsequent effect on cardiovascular disease. Converse occurs in youth with hypertension. Use either the left or the right arm on all patients but not both indiscriminately.

Source of Error: 4. Training: Most doctors and nurses measure the BP badly because they have never been properly trained. The teaching of BP reading is given with five or ten minutes of cursory instructions by some seniors who had learned in the same fashion. The student in his view mainly learns that accurate readings are neither feasible nor important. So variation in measurements occurs. A study rate of fall of 2 mm Hg per second is essential, i.e. about a beat per division on glass scale. If the column falls fast with an average interval of 0.8 seconds between beats, it is easy to drop 5 mm Hg before the next signal or even more in bradycardia. It is a tendency to read toward the zeros rather than fives or toward fives instead of other intermediate points. Digit preference can be eliminated by proper training. Firm pressure over the diaphragm may give false low readings and when it is slipped under the cuff, may itself partially occlude the brachial artery and gives false reading. Proper training of medical students and nurses are essential to maintain the correct reading instead of average readings.

Commonest error is surprisingly, not measuring the blood pressure at all!

All patients who visit the clinic or hospital should have their blood pressure checked irrespective of their symptoms.

By measuring the blood pressure, you made a most important cardiovascular diagnosis, i.e. systemic hypertension

By not, measuring the blood pressure, the commonest cardiovascular disease in adults, i.e. systemic hypertension is missed.

88. Common causes of false high readings are:

1. Fear, pain and apprehension
2. A full bladder
3. Cuffs that don't fit or are badly applied to the arm
4. Blocked pin-hole at the top of the glass tube.

89. Common causes of false low readings are:

1. Tightly rolled clothing above the cuffs
2. Dropping the mercury column too fast
3. Pressing hard with the stethoscope over the artery
4. Leakage effect produces rapid and uncontrollable fall of mercury leading to false low readings.

90. There are 4 situations where pressure differences between right and left arm are present.

Table A-8

1. Normal variation	Right arm pressure is usually higher by ≤ 10 mm Hg
2. Arterial occlusion	Atherosclerosis Takayasu's arteritis Subclavian steal syndrome Cardiogenic embolism Arterial catheterization
3. Diseases of aorta	Coarctation: Left subclavian arising from coarct segment aberrant right subclavian artery distal to coarct segment Dissecting aneurysm of aorta: Involvement of right innominate or left subclavian arteries Supravalvular aortic stenosis: Jet of aortic ejection directed to right innominate artery
4. Thoracic outlet syndrome	Arterial compression

If the reading is higher in one arm, that arm should be used for future measurements. Blood pressure is usually lower in the left arm in subclavian steal syndrome caused by reversal of flow down a vertebral artery distal to an obstructed subclavian artery. Blood pressure may be either higher or lower in paretic arm of a stroke patient.

91. The arterial pressure is maintained within physiological limits in all positions in a normal person. When a person changes from supine to standing position, a slight fall, not exceeding 5 mm Hg in systolic blood pressure occurs and the diastolic blood pressure remains constant or may slightly rise. These changes come to normal levels within 3–5 min in a normal person.

The circulatory changes with standing position includes:

1. Diminished venous return
2. Fall in stroke volume
3. Fall in cardiac output
4. Lesser distension of carotid stretch receptors

5. Less reflex inhibition from carotid baroreceptor on the vasomotor center on the brain stem
6. Sinus tachycardia
7. Fall of systolic blood pressure less than 5 mm Hg
5. Constant or rise of diastolic blood pressure less than 5 mm Hg.

92. Postural hypotension results when the compensatory mechanism is inefficient in standing posture.

The patients have symptoms of

1. Extreme weakness
2. Light headedness
3. Dizziness or syncope
4. Blurring or transient loss of vision

Postural hypotension is defined as a fall of 20 mm Hg of systolic BP or 10 mm Hg of diastolic BP or more in standing posture. If the patient is symptomatic even a lesser fall of blood pressure should be considered as significant.

The most common causes of postural hypotension are drug induced (especially antihypertensives) and hypovolemia, elderly and in diabetes.

Postural hypotension is an early sign of hypovolemia due to any cause.

The blood pressure should be taken immediately upon standing and after standing at least 2 minutes to check for spontaneous or drug induced postural changes, particularly in the elderly and in diabetics.

In most of the patient the systolic pressure falls and diastolic pressure rises a few mm of Hg on changing from supine to standing position.

Significant postural fall of 20 mm of Hg or more is common in 10% of people over 65 years age and in more in those with elevated supine systolic blood pressure. Blood pressure should be checked after 5 minutes supine, then immediate 2 minutes after standing particularly in patients above 65 years age, diabetes, on antihypertensive therapy.

For routine blood pressure checkup, the patient should sit quietly for 5 minutes with the arm supported on the table at the level of the heart and the back resting against the chair.

93. Effect of respiration on blood pressure–some facts.

1. Systolic blood pressure decreases in inspiration because the lung capacity increases with inspiration and the volume of pulmonary vascular bed increases, less blood goes from the lungs to the left heart. It causes decrease in systolic blood pressure.
2. Intrathoracic pressure decreases with inspiration. Since the aorta is an intrathoracic organ, its pressure also will drop. So, the systolic blood pressure decreases with inspiration.
3. Systolic BP falls
   a. with normal inspiration—2 to 6 mm Hg
   b. with deep inspiration—up to 10 mm Hg
   c. with very deep inspiration—up to 15 mm Hg
4. A fall of BP between 8 and 10 mm with normal inspiration is considered to be pathological.

The term 'Paradoxus' is used by Kussmaul in late 1800s when he found a drop of blood pressure on auscultation in constrictive pericarditis. It is only an exaggeration of normal physiological effect. He described it as 'Pulsus Paradoxus' because he did not find any change in the apex beat despite the loss of radial pulse with inspiration. Kussmaul also thought it was paradoxical that although the peripheral pulse seems at first to be irregular, it directly comes and goes regularly.

94. There are 4 other uses of sphygmomanometer.

1. *Sphygometric paradoxus:* 'Pulsus paradoxus' is best elicited by this method. It is an exaggeration of normal fall in SBP during inspiration. Any fall of SBP > 8 mm Hg during inspiration is considered a positive sign.
2. *Blood pressure alternans:* When the weak beat is too weak to be palpable, auscultatory method is appreciable. Reducing the venous return by head tilting or nitroglycerine usually exaggerate pulsus alternans and assist in its detection. Palpable alternans over the peripheral pulse is detectable only when the aortic pressure alternate by more than 20 mm Hg. It is easier to appreciate sphygmomanometer than by palpation of the peripheral arterial pulse. The Korotkoff sounds are heard in alternate intensity with alternate beats.
3. *As a venous tourniquet:* Rotating tourniquets are applied to the extremities. This method is helpful in treating acute pulmonary edema by reducing the venous return. The cuffs are tied around both thighs and one of the arm and is inflated to just below the level of diastolic pressure or 80 mm Hg. The cuffs are kept inflated for about 15 minutes a time and rotated through the other extremity.
4. *In thrombocytopenia (Hess sign):* This is to assess the capillary fragility. The cuff is tied around the arm and inflated to a pressure between systolic and diastolic pressure for 5 minutes. More than 20 petechiae appear in an area of 2.5 sq cm. on the inner aspect of the arm is considered as abnormal.

JUGULAR VENOUS PULSE

Arterial pulse reflects the left ventricular function but it cannot give filling pattern of left ventricle. Right ventricular performance cannot be assessed externally by the pulmonary arterial pulse but the filling pattern of right atrium and right ventricle is readily available through the jugular venous pulse. The dynamics of left side of the heart is obtained by arterial pulse, while the right side of the heart is obtained by jugular venous pulse. (for the right side of the heart—see on the right side of the neck). JVP mainly yields information about central venous pressure and type of wave pattern.

95. There are 4 observations to be followed while getting information from jugular venous pulse (JVP).

1. Internal jugular vein rather than external jugular vein is usually used in assessment of JVP. Free communication between the superior vena cava (SVC) and the external jugular vein is often interrupted by valves and fascial planes. So, the internal jugular vein is preferred. External jugular vein may be used if there is a free rise and fall and visible pulsation within it.
2. The jugular venous pulse is more readily observed on the right side than on the left side of the neck because the right innominate and jugular vein extend in an almost straightline cephalad to the superior vena cava, thus favoring the direct transmission of hemodynamic changes in the right atrium. The left innominate vein is not in a straightline and may be kinked or compressed by many structures such as dilated aorta or by aortic aneurysm.
3. Sternal angle is taken as the reference point while measuring the JVP because it is easily seen and is at a fixed height of about 5 cm, above the right atrium regardless of whether the patient is upright or flat. The pressure is measured vertically. Normally, it is about 3 cm above the sternal angle that is up to 8 cm above the right atrium. Observe an abnormal elevation of JVP.
   Vertical height of column is higher than that of the manubrium in the presence of increased hydrostatic pressure in venous congestion. In severe cases, it may be distended throughout its length with the patient upright.
   By convention clinical examination of the heart and JVP is conducted with the patient lying at an angle of 45°. A lower position may be better if the pressure in the jugular vein is low, whilst a higher position may be best in patients in whom the pressure is greatly increased.
4. Another method of eliciting venous congestion is to apply light pressure over the right hypochondrium. In the presence of venous congestion, pressure on the engorged liver produces a rise in the level of the venous column in the neck called hepatojugular reflex.
   Normally the JVP falls during inspiration as more blood is drawn into the thorax. JVP often rises paradoxically with inspiration known as 'Venous Paradoxus' or 'Kussmaul's Sign'. In cardiac tamponade or chronic constrictive pericarditis venous paradoxus occurs due to impaired venous return to the heart.
   The phrase 'distended neck veins', which is widely used as a sign of high venous pressure is a poor way of expression.
   This expression suggests that the observer is probably used looking mainly at the external jugulars, because the internal jugular are rarely visibly distended. A high rise in JVP may be associated with invisible (non-distended) external jugulars.

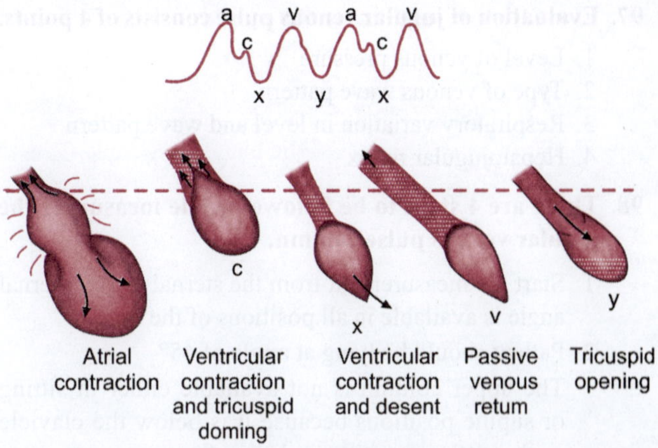

Fig. A-2: Jugular venous pulse

96. There are 4 features to be noted in jugular venous pulse (JVP).

1. 'A' wave: It results from venous distension and is due to atrial contraction, and atrial pressure is raised causing a small volume of blood to pass backwards into the veins—it is presystolic and dominant wave in the JVP
2. 'X' descent: It is due to fall in venous pressure as a result of atrial relaxation during atrial diastole and downward movement of the tricuspid valve during ventricular systole. Atrial pressure is decreased.
3. 'V' wave: or 'venous stasis' is due to the filling of right atrium and great veins whilst the tricuspid is still closed below. Atrial pressure is raised (Remember V-illing wave, i.e. right atrial filling wave).
4. 'Y' decent or "diastolic collapse"—a final depression in the curve, AV valves open allowing sudden flow of blood from the auricle to the ventricle resulting in lowering of right atrial pressure.

'C' wave—so-called carotid pulse—is an inconstant wave. It is not appreciated at the bed side easily and is related to the transmitted carotid pulse when recorded in the neck, and due to tricuspid valve closure when recorded in the right atrium.

'C' and 'V' together known as ventricular complex.

X and Y are troughs of JVP.

97. Evaluation of jugular venous pulse consists of 4 points.

1. Level of venous pressure
2. Type of venous wave pattern
3. Respiratory variation in level and wave pattern
4. Hepatojugular reflex

98. There are 4 steps to be followed while measuring the jugular venous pulse column.

1. Start the measurement from the sternal angle. Sternal angle is available in all positions of the body
2. Patient should be lying at angle of 45°
   The upper column is not available either in sitting or supine positions because it is below the clavicle in the sitting position and therefore cannot be seen and whereas in supine position, the whole column moves beyond the angle of the jaw where it cannot be reached. To bring out the column from below the clavicle in the sitting position, the patient is positioned at approximately 45° angle on the bed.
3. The pulsations of the internal jugular vein are transmitted to the skin of the neck. The top level of the neck pulsations are taken as the jugular venous pressure. Thus, the jugular vein is used as a "pulsation manometer".
   Two imaginary horizontal lines are drawn, one from the sternal angle and the other from the upper level of venous column and the vertical measurement is noted. If the venous column is seen above the clavicle in sitting or standing position, direct vertical measurement is made.
   One of the difficulties in deciding the top level of pulsations is that they tend to diminish toward the upper level. At 45°, the upper limit is 4.5 cm (easy way to remember is 4.5 cm at 45°)
4. Jugular venous pulse is expressed as the number of centimeters above the sternal angle. The right atrial pressure is obtained by adding 5 cm to it. Normal JVP does not exceed 4 cm above the sternal angle (i.e. not more than 9 cm of right atrial pressure). 1.3 cm column of water or blood is equal to 1 cm, Hg. Normal right atrial mean pressure does not exceed 7 mm of Hg or 9 cm of JVP by blood.

99. Normally, right atrial pressure rises to 4 (4 to 6) during contraction while left atrial pressure rises to 8 (7 to 8) during contraction.

100. The upper limit of normal jugular venous pulse is 4 cm. Above the sternal angle which corresponds to a central venous pressure of approximately 9 cm H_2O, since the right atrium is approximately 5 cm below the sternal angle.

101. Examination of the jugular vein wave pattern

1. Normal JVP consists of **4** waves to study clinically
   Two positive waves or ascents – A and V waves
   Two negative waves or descents – X and Y descents
2. 'A' wave in JVP occurs before the first sound but in actual bed side practice, A wave occurs along with first sound. This is due to time delay in between atrial systole and transmission of the wave into the neck and also the intrinsic delays with left and right events.
   The descent that follows the A wave is X descent.
3. V wave occurs along with second sound. The Y descent follows V wave.
   The V wave is not always visible in the normal JVP even though it is usually seen on a jugular pulse tracing. It is because the right atrium is very complaint or distensible chamber, i.e. the right atrium is too distensible to allow its pressure to rise very much when the tricuspid valve is closed.
   In practice, either the ascents or descents are impressive. One can follow either ascent or descent depending on the visibility
4. The 'atrioventricle' or diastasis period is the period of relatively slow filling of the atrium representing between the bottom of Y descent and beginning of the A wave. The wave built up during the diastasis is the H wave. The H wave height wave also reflects the stiffness of the right atrium.
   Position the patient in such a way that the wave pattern is clearly visible.
   Sitting position can be used in case of raised JVP 45° inclination is needed to bring about the venous column and wave pattern in the absence of raised JVP.

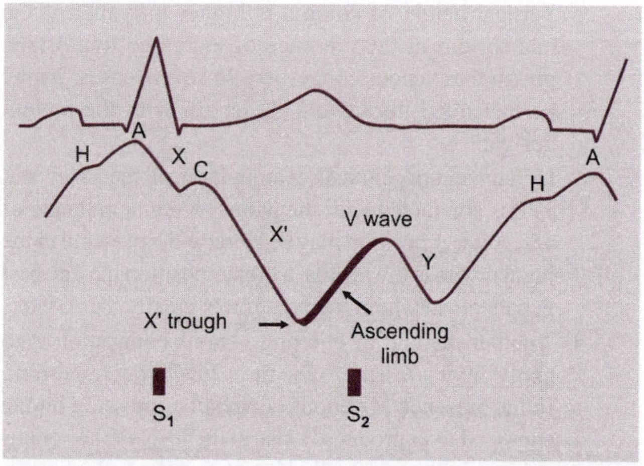

Fig. A-3: Normal jugular venous wave and its relation to ECG wave and normal sounds A = A wave; X = X descent; C = C wave; V wave; Y = Y descent H-H wave represent the 'atrioventricle' or diastase period, between the bottom of the Y descent and beginning of the A wave

102. Following information is obtained from the jugular venous pulse

Table A-9

Information obtained from JVP	Clues in JVP
1. Level of right atrial pressure Right ventricular filling pressure Central venous pressure JVP may reveal the contour and pressures in right atrium and right ventricle without the need for catheterization	Level of jugular venous pulse
2. Pattern of right ventricular filling and right atrial emptying a. Rapid filling, e.g. RVF, TR, CP b. Slow filling, e.g. TS c. Little or no filling, e.g. Tamponade	Y descent Rapid Y descent Slow Y descent Obliterated Y descent
3. Resistance to presystolic right atrium emptying e.g. TS. Noncomplaint right ventricle	Prominent 'a' wave
4. Sequence of atrioventricular contraction, e.g. AV dissociation, complete heart block, junctional rhythm	Analysis of rhythm
5. Obstruction to superior vena cava	Raised JVP with absent pulsations
6. Hyperkinetic circulatory state, e.g. anemia, thyrotoxicosis	Venous hum
7. Central venous pressure in normal breathing in horizontal position	Veins in the neck collapse
8. Edema caused by obstruction of veins in the lower extremities	Not raised, abdominal jugular reflex absent

103. In the beginning one should differentiate venous pulsations from arterial pulse.

Table A-10: Differentiation of venous pulsations from arterial pulsations in the neck

Feature	Venous pulsations	Arterial pulsations
1. Site	Laterally; located, superficial and widespread	More medial, deeper, localized
2. Number of pulsations	Multiple—Two peaks (ascents) and two troughs (descents) per cardiac cycle in sinus rhythm	Single upstroke
3. Level	Has definitive upper level	No definitive upper level
4. Change with position and respiration	Alters with change in posture. Find out by making the patient to sit up higher or lay him lower—alters with angle of the patient. Alters with respiration—falls during inspiration because the blood is drawn into the heart	No alteration
5. Visibility and palpability	Better seen than palpation. More sinuous, and less sharp easy to obliterate	Better palpable than visible. Sharp, thrusting in character. Difficult to obliterate
6. Ascents and descents	The descents are equally impressive or more impressive	The ascent or upstroke is impressive; the descent or down stroke is not impressive
7. Associated feature	Pulmonary arterial hypertension, pulmonary stenosis, tricuspid regurgitation, tricuspid stenosis, right ventricular hypertrophy, right ventricular failure	Hyperkinetic states, aortic regurgitation
8. Compression of the root of the neck	Usually abolishes except in the presence of extreme venous hypertension	Does not affect

104. There are 4 conditions where JVP raises.

1. Usually in right heart failure Reduced compliance of right ventricle, pericardial disease, tricuspid stenosis, ASD with mitral valve disease.
2. Physiologically—when there is increased blood volume such as pregnancy, hypervolemia due to intravenous fluid overload.
3. Pathologically when there is increase in blood volume such as nephritis, Cirrhosis liver.
4. Occasionally due to mechanical obstructions such as superior vena cava obstruction or constrictive pericarditis. Superior vena cava (SVC) syndrome is usually due to carcinoma of the bronchus.

105. All conditions producing elevated JVP give rise to pulsations in the neck veins except superior vena cava obstruction.

There are 4 causes of pulseless elevation in JVP.

1. When external jugulars are used
2. Superior vena caval obstruction—commonest cause with little or no pulsations
3. Cardiac tamponade
4. Constrictive pericarditis

106. There are 4 conditions where 'A' wave is prominent with regular cardiac rhythm (Atrial pressure may be elevated even up to 20 mm Hg).

1. A giant 'A' wave is seen in obstruction to the outflow from the atrium as in tricuspid stenosis or right atrial myxoma.

2. Right ventricular hypertrophy or Right heart failure—A poorly compliant (stiffness or noncomplaint) right ventricle as seen in pulmonary hypertension or pulmonary stenosis.
   A giant 'A' wave can produce a presystolic sound if auscultated over the jugulars.
3. Bulging of hypertrophied interventricular septum into the right ventricle as a result of left ventricular hypertrophy interfering with right ventricular filling. As a consequence right atrium contracts against increased resistance due for instance aortic stenosis, hypertrophic obstructive cardiomyopathy.
   A giant 'A' wave in the presence of an aortic ejection murmur suggest hypertrophic subaortic stenosis. Right ventricular outflow obstruction due to an excessively thick septum is suggested.
4. Tricuspid regurgitation: In this, the blood regurgitates into the right atrium and great veins during ventricular systole. For historical reasons this wave is known as 'v' wave although occurs during 'c' wave.

107. There are 4 conditions where A wave helps in differentiating cardiac arrhythmias. (large A waves also occur in arrhythmias where right atrium contracts while the tricuspid valve is closed by right ventricular systole—such as 'Cannon' 'a' waves.). Cannon 'a' waves occur whenever there is AV dissociation or retrograde P waves.

1. Regular 'Cannon' 'a' wave in junctional rhythm, when the atrium and ventricle are activated simultaneously and the right atrium contracts on a closed tricuspid valve.
2. Irregular 'Cannon' 'a' waves in AV dissociation with ventricular tachycardia or independent 'a' waves in complete heart block, multiple extrasystoles.
3. Increased delay between the 'a' wave and the carotid arterial pulse is seen in 1st-degree AV block (If the arterial pulse is abnormally slow—see for 'Cannon' 'a' waves in the neck).
   Progressive delay between the 'a' wave and the carotid pulse with missed beat is called Wenckebach phenomenon seen in second-degree mobitz type-I block. Wenckebach described this before the advent of ECG by observing jugular and carotid pulse in the neck.
4. 'a' wave is absent in
   a. atrial fibrillation. (Irregularly irregular carotid pulse with pulse deficit). There are only two waves, the c wave and the v wave, as there is no coordinated contraction of the atrium to produce an 'a' wave.
   b. Post DC conversion of atrial fibrillation
   c. Sinoventricular conduction in hyperkalemia

108. There are 4 conditions where X' descent is smaller or even absent.

1. A poor RA or RV contraction: Heart failure, atrial flutter or fibrillation or right atrial standstill
2. Tricuspid regurgitation (TR). The X' descent is encroached on in proportion to the degree of regurgitation
3. Congenital absence of pericardium or loss of pericardium when the surgeon fails to close the pericardium after open heart surgery
4. Build up of the V wave earlier than usual: seen with loss of capacitance of the RA, e.g. right atrial myxoma, or loss of compliance due to hypertrophy, e.g. tricuspid stenosis, stiffened by sutures in the right atrium after open heart surgery.
   X' descent is prominent in pericarditis, cardiac tamponade.

109. V wave represents the filling pattern of right atrium and depends on the venous return through the vena cava. Therefore, the V wave is exaggerated in conditions where there is increased filling of right atrium due to any cause and where the venous pressures are high.

Causes of prominent V wave or relatively deep Y descent are:

1. Tricuspid regurgitation (TR): If one calls regurgitant wave a V wave due to increased filling by more than one source. Right atrium is filled by regurgitant blood. With increasing severity of TR, the X descent becomes more and more shallow and the Y descent increases deep. The systolic right ventricular pressure may be transmitted to the peripheral veins and a palpable venous pulse simulating collapsing pulse of brachials may be felt. In such cases, V wave may measure as high as 60 mm Hg and is difficult to obliterate in the neck.
2. Atrial septal defect –increased filling of right atrium by more than one source
3. Congestive cardiac failure or severe pulmonary hypertension where there is high venous pressure
4. Loss of compliance of right atrium as in pericarditis. A calcified pericardium may constrict only the atria without constricting the ventrticles giving rise to prominent V wave. A severe pectus excavatum may also restrict atrial filling.
5. Loss of capacitance of right atrium as in right atrial myxoma
6. A pluro pericaridial defect
7. A severe mitral regurgitation possibly by displacing atrial septum with the right atrium during ventricular systole.

8. After open heart surgery in which sutures are placed in the right atrium.

If the X descent is smaller than Y descent after surgery, it indicates that the myocardium has probably been damaged during surgery or was depressed before surgery or the pericardium is not closed during surgery.

V waves are diminished in hypovolemia, venodilators (nitrates).

All conditions that cause prominent 'v' waves give rise to rapid Y' descent

Slow Y' descent occurs in tricuspid stenosis, precordial tamponade, tension pneumothroax.

110. Venous hum: Bruit over the neck veins is called venous hum. It occurs whenever there is increased velocity of flow (hyperkinetic states) or diminished viscosity of blood (anemia).

1. It is normally heard in children and pregnancy
2. Hyperkinetic states—Anemia, thyrotoxicosis, beriberi
2. Intracranial arterio-venous fistule
3. Compression of the jugular veins by fascia or bony structures in the neck

No hum is heard in supine position, with the veins distended, there occurs little or no turbulence. Examination of the patient is done in the sitting position with the bell lightly applied at the base of the neck, in between the two heads of sternomastoid. Venous hum is heard as a continuous murmur. It disappears by applying pressure above the stethoscope.

111. Kussmaul's sign:

Normally jugular venous pulse falls during inspiration as more blood is drawn into the thorax. Venous return to the right side of the heart increases. But it is accommodated by the pulmonary vascular impedance. This causes the fall in pulmonary artery, right ventricle and right atrium pressures in spite of increase in venous return. Expiration causes the lungs to squeeze their air and pulmonary circulation is compressed by the thoracic cage increasing the pulmonary impedance and pressures. This results in venous column to rise in expiration and fall in inspiration. When there is increased venous return during inspiration, it cannot be translated as more pulmonary filling, inspiratory filling of the neck veins occurs. This is called Kussmaul's sign. This occurs in

1. Constrictive pericarditis
2. Restrictive cardiomyopathy
3. Tricuspid stenosis
4. Severe right ventricular failure

The JVP is better seen in expiration than inspiration. This sign suggests right ventricular infarction in a patient with acute inferior myocardial infarction and with no signs of left ventricular failure because it will be present in majority of such patients.

112. Some bedside diagnostic clues of jugular venous pulse.

1. Examine the jugular venous pulse in the patient with 45° angle.
2. JVP cannot be measured in supine position
3. When the JVP is not seen above the clavicle in sitting or standing position, the jugular venous pressure is not elevated
4. The first heart sound coincides with A wave and the second heart sound with V wave. The X descent follows the first sound and the Y descent follows the second sound.
5. Elevated jugular venous pressure with no history of dyspnea, orthopnea, paroxysmal nocturnal dyspnea generally means right heart failure
6. Prominent A wave, slow Y descent, no right ventricular impulse, no palpable pulmonary second sound means tricuspid stenosis
7. Elevated jugular venous pressure, rapid Y descent, diastolic outward movement of the whole precordium coinciding with Y descent and pericardial knock means constrictive pericarditis
8. Venous hum is a valuable sign of hyperkinetic circulatory disease in adults.

113. There are 4 areas to be examined carefully over the precordium.

1. Mitral area
2. Aortic area
3. Pulmonary area
4. Tricuspid area

114. There are 4 points to be noted during inspection.

1. Shape of the precordium
2. Pulsations in the precordium
3. Bulging and pulsations outside the precordium
4. Distended veins on the chest wall or in the neck.

CARDIAC IMPULSE

Apex beat or apical impulse is formed by the region of the left ventricle adjacent to the interventricular septum. All the walls of the left ventricle move inwards reducing the ventricular size during systole except the region of the apex which rotates and moves outward lifting the chest wall over it. This normal apical impulse comes out along with the first sound and stays as an outward movement as long as the ventricle contracts ejecting blood into aorta. At the end of ejection (systole), the apex retracts from the chest wall.

The right ventricular events underlying the parasternal area are not palpable unless the right ventricle is enlarged or the chest wall is very thin.

In very large right ventricle, the apex beat may be due to movement of the right ventricle. Therefore, the apex beat really means the most lateral palpable ventricular movement or most lateral cardiac impulse.

The left lateral decubitus position, however, the actual apex beat may be palpated, provided the left ventricle rather than the right ventricle dominates the area.

115. Apex beat is displaced in 4 conditions.

1. Congenital—Dextrocardia—it is seen on the right side
2. Deformities of the chest—usually scoliosis
3. Due to diseases of the surrounding viscera 'Pushing' occurs in plural effusion, pneumothorax; 'Puling' occurs in pulmonary fibrosis, collapse of the lung.
4. Diseases of the heart.

LVH - AR, MR, Double mitral, AS, - Apex is displaced downwards and outwards.

Apex is displaced laterally and downwards into 6th or 7th intercostal space in left ventricular hypertrophy (LVH). Lateral displacement is generally due to more dilatation of the left ventricle than to hypertrophy. Thus in aortic stenosis the apex beat may remain in the mid-clavicular line despite considerable hypertrophy. As the apex moves laterally it is often described as being in the anterior axillary line, the mid-axillary line or even the posterior axillary line.

Left ventricular hypertrophy without dilatation is called concentric hypertrophy. The apex is not displaced significantly in concentric hypertrophy of pressure loaded states like aortic stenosis and impulse may remain at 5th place. Dilatation of the left ventricle is needed to displace the apex downwards and outwards as in moderate to severe volume loaded states.

RVH - Apex is displaced outwards

116. Palpability of the apex beat or most lateral ventricular impulse:

1. Apex beat or apex impulse is palpable in about 1 out of 5 in normal subjects over the age of 40 years.
   It is palpable in children and adolescents in the sitting position in about 50% of persons.
2. It is palpable in about 4 out of 5 older adults and in almost all children or young adults in lateral decubitus position
3. It is palpable in the sitting position than in the supine position because the heart falls away from the anterior chest wall. Cardiac impulse is best felt in the sitting position with the feet up on the bed because the lateral impulse often moves slightly more to the left and against the chest wall in this position. Sitting position with the legs up is probably due to upward push by the compressed abdominal contents and diaphragm. In standing position the apex does not shift to the left.
4. The finger tips or the area just proximal to them are best for feeling faint localized movements.

In patients with a large ventricle, the apex beat may be due to movement of right ventricle. Therefore, the apex beat really means the most lateral palpable ventricular movement or most lateral cardiac impulse.

117. There are 4 important causes of impalpable apex beat.

1. Obesity or thick muscular chest wall
2. When apex lies behind the rib
3. Obstruction to transmission of impulse - Emphysema (barrel-shaped chest), plural or pericardial effusion
4. Feeble heart, e.g. coronary artery disease with decreased apical motion.

Obese, muscular, emphysematous and old persons may have weak or undetectable cardiac pulsations in the absence of cardiac abnormality, and chest deformities.

118. One should see the entire chest for cardiovascular pulsations but particularly in 4 regions.

1. Mitral area—for cardiac apex—for enlargement of left ventricle
2. Left parasternal region—for enlargement of right ventricle—right ventricle produces parasternal heave. Definite 'lift' is felt when hand is placed firmly lateral to the lower left parasternal border in right ventricualr Hypertrophy (RVH). Occasionally, a heaving sternum may result from the great enlargement of the left atrium or left ventricle associated with severe mitral regurgitation.
   RVH—displaces apex beat laterally.
   The lifts or heaves are best felt with the proximal part of the palm (thenar & hypothenar areas).
3. Second left intercostal space—for enlargement of pulmonary artery—pulmonary artery pulsations are seen and felt in the left 2nd intercostal space when enlarged as in pulmonary hypertension, increased pulmonary blood flow or poststenotic pulmonary artery dilatation. Pulmonary artery pulsations may be normal in children and thin persons.
4. Second right intercostal space—for enlargement of aorta—Aortic pulsations are palpated when it is enlarged in aneurysmal dilatation of the ascending aorta or right sided aortic arch.

119. The term point of maximum impulse (PMI) as synonym for apex beat has the disadvantages. PMI may be due to other abnormalities. There are 4 conditions where prominent impulse is seen on the left border of the heart—from above downwards

1. Aortic aneurysm
2. Pulmonary artery dilatation
3. Ventricular aneurysm
4. Apex beat from left ventricle

120. There are 4 places where pulsations should be seen outside the precordium.

1. Suprasternal notch
2. On the neck
3. On the thorax
4. In the epigastric area

121. There are 4 positions where the pulsations of the affected aorta are noted. Pulsations in the thorax are rare, but seen in diseases of the aorta.

1. Seen mainly on the right of the sternum above the level of the 4th rib when ascending aorta is affected
2. Seen under the manubrium sternum, less distinctly when arch of aorta is affected
3. Seen on the left side of sternum when descending aorta is affected
4. Seen in superficial arteries over the chest wall due to collateral circulation in coarctation of aorta. May be best seen over the back when the patient bends forwards to touch his toes.

122. There are 4 important causes of pulsations in the epigastrium besides excitement or nervousness in a thin person.

1. Right ventricular hypertrophy
2. Distensible pulsations of liver in tricuspid incompetence
3. Transmitted pulsation from a tumor (like carcinoma stomach)
4. Expansile pulsation of aneurysm of abdominal aorta.

123. There are 4 points to be noted in any cardiac impulse on precordial palpation.

1. Location
2. Timing (systole or diastole)
3. Duration
3. Contour

124. There are 4 points to note in the normal apex beat on palpation.

1. *Position:* Normal apex beat is located at or medial to the left midclavicular line in the 4th or 5th intercostal space.
2. *Force or amplitude:* Normally tapping
3. *Timing:* Early systolic in duration.
4. *Direction:* Outward thrust localised to a point not more than 2 to 3 cm in diameter.

The apical impulse is usually in the 5th intercostal space inside or at midclavicular line. It may be in the 4th intercostal space in children.

125. The force or amplitude of the apex is described in 4 types.

Left ventricle produces apex beat.

1. Tapping apex is seen in normal persons with loud first sound. It occurs in mitral stenosis, atrial septal defect, etc.
   Tapping apex is due to the velocity of closure of the mitral valve being sufficiently fast to cause a palpable tapping at the apex. It is a sign of mitral stenosis which should therefore be suspected in any patient with tapping apex.
2. Forceful apex beat is present in volume overloaded states where there is increase in preload and decrease in afterload e.g. aortic regurgitation, mitral regurgitation, left to right shunts such as VSD, PDA and in hyperkinetic states like thyrotoxicosis, anemia, pregnancy and may be due to nervousness, excitement.
3. Forceful and sustained 'thrust or heave' is felt in left ventricular hypertrophy due to systolic overload as in aortic stenosis, hypertension. Normally the apex beat moves out for the first third of systole only, and thereafter retracts. As the heart hypertrophies the outward movement is prolonged giving rise to a sustained or heaving apex. The impulse stays for more than half of systole to near to second sound.
   Forceful but less sustained impulse is felt in diastolic overload as in aortic and mitral regurgitation.
4. Systolic retraction: As already mentioned, the apex is formed by the interventricular septum adjacent to the left ventricle; therefore, the movement of interventricular septum naturally influence the apex beat. The normal interventricular septum behaves as a part of left ventricle. In conditions with right ventricular volume overload as in atrial septal defect, tricuspid regurgitation, pulmonary regurgitation, the interventricular septum behaves as a part of right ventricle and their anterior motion of interventricular septum is called paradoxic septal motion in the echo. When the interventricular septum moves along with right ventricle anteriorly, the apex retracts in systole and moves out in diastole.
   Left ventricular enlargement is unlikely in the presence of apical retraction. Apical retraction is the palpable equivalent of paradoxic septal motion in the echo.
   If the region of apex is involved in ischemic heart disease/coronary artery disease, a larger and longer impulse may occur simulating a pressure overload due to dyskinesia. If the impulse appear along with chest pain but disappear after the subsidence of pain, it is diagnostic of ischemia as the cause of chest pain. This is more diagnostic value than Tredmill test or coronary

angiogram. Coronary angiogram reveals anatomical obstruction but fails to predict whether the patients chest pain is related to the lesion at hand.

126. There are 4 conditions where palpation of right ventricular outflow, i.e. infundibulum of right ventricle and main pulmonary artery help to differentiate.

1. Normal pulmonary artery may be palpable in thin chest persons
2. A palpable pulmonary artery and pulmonary component of second heart sound generally mean pulmonary arterial hypertension
3. A palpable pulmonary artery with no palpable pulmonary component of second sound may mean large flow into pulmonary artery without rise in pulmonary pressure as in left to right shunt, e.g. ASD
4. Systolic thrill in the pulmonary artery with no palpable pulmonary artery or pulmonary second sound associated with a sustained parasternal heave means pulmonary stenosis.

127. Apical impulse helps to differentiate the 4 types of cardiomyopathies one from the other.

(Ref: K 21)

1. In dilated cardiomyopathy (DCM)—Apex beat is not often felt because of feeble heart
2. In restrictive cardiomyopathy (RCM)—Apex is usually palpable -(it helps to differentiate from constrictive pericarditis)
3. In hypertrophic cardiomyopathy (HCM)—Double or triple apex is felt.
4. In obstructive cardiomyopathy (OCM)—Apical impulse is not often felt. It may be obliterated by thrombus or fibrous tissue.

128. A double apex or an apex beat consisting of two components is an unusual sign. There are 4 conditions where double apex may be seen.

1. Mitral stenosis (MS)
2. Aortic stenosis (AS)
3. Hypertrophic obstructive cardiomyopathy (HOCM)
4. Left ventricular aneurysm.

In 1, 2, 3 a palpable atrial impulse occurs late in diastole and preceding the main outward movement of the apex. This type of apex is due to unusually powerful atrial contraction in response to the resistance offered to the flow. In 4, the apex is due to bulging during late systole, when the apex would normally be retracting in left ventricular aneurysm.

129. 4 miscellaneous pulsations over the precordium

1. Ventricular aneurysm: Surprisingly, it occupies larger area than normal area of left ventricular apical movement. It is difficult to distinguish from the impulse of dilated and hypertrophied left ventricle. Sometimes, aneurysm is felt as a sustained systolic bulge separately from left ventricular impulse. The aneurysmal pulsations are described as paradoxical pulsation.
2. Aortic aneurysm: Pulsations are felt in the right or left sternoclavicular joint area.
   It is occasionally suspected if it depresses the left bronchus with each pulsation. Depression of left bronchus will in turn pull down trachea. Stand behind the seated patient, and study upward pressure is applied on the cricoid cartilage with the tip of one forefinger, you will readily detect the downward pull on the trachea with each expansion. This is called tracheal tug.
3. A dilated right aortic arch also can give rise to right sternoclavicular pulsation. This occurs in congenital cyanotic heart disease.
4. Coarctation of aorta produces pulsations on the chest wall. Pulsations are better visible by making the patient to bend forward and let his arms dangle to stretch the skin of the back.

130. Shaking of the entire precordium with each heart beat may occur with—

1. Severe valvular regurgitation
2. Large left to right shunts especially patent ductus arteriosus
3. Complete AV block
4. Hypertrophic obstructive cardiomyopathy

Various hyperkinetic states in patients with thin chest wall may be seen.

131. There are 4 abnormal loud sounds which are often palpable and felt like a shock.

1. Loud first sound in mitral stenosis is often palpable.
2. Aortic second sound is often palpable in systemic hypertension.
3. Pulmonary second sound is often palpable in pulmonary hypertension.
4. Third sound or atrial sound (4th sound) is sometimes easier to feel than to hear.

132. Thrills are low frequency vibrations associated with heart murmur. Thrill is a palpable murmur.

Thrills are best felt with the distal palm.

There are 4 places where thrill is commonly felt.

1. *Mitral area:* Systolic thrill in mitral regurgitation radiates toward axilla. Diastolic thrill in mitral stenosis.
2. *Aortic area:* Systolic thrill in aortic stenosis radiates to the right side of the neck.
3. *Pulmonary area:* Systolic thrill in pulmonary stenosis radiates to the left side of the neck.
4. 3rd or 4th intercostal space near the left sternal border in ventricular septal defect.

133. The 4th left intercostal space is the place to purcuss that extends from the left lung towards the heart for the left border which is 1/2″ medial to the midclavicular line.

134. The 4th rib level is ideal to percuss for the right border which is just at right lateral sternal line.

135. There are 4 principles to be kept in mind to obtain maximum information by auscultation.

1. Examination should be in a quiet room free from noises.
2. Concentrate on the phase of cardiac cycle to hear even a faint sound or murmur.
3. Accurate timing of the sound or murmur is ascertained by noting other events in the cardiac cycle like carotid pulse, JVP or apex beat.
4. Significance of cardiac sound or murmur is determined by observing the alteration of its timing or intensity with
   - i. respiration
   - ii. posture
   - iii. handgrip exercise
   - iv. vasodilators like amyl nitrite.

136. There are 4 pitfalls to be kept in mind while hearing the sounds that depend on:

1. *Production of sounds:* This is constant in that particular patient whether low or high pitch, etc. fault may be in the production of the sounds.
2. *Transformation of sound:* Sounds may not be transformed due to pathology in the myocardium, pericardium or chest wall (obesity).
3. *Transformation from the chest wall to the ear:* Fault may be in the stethoscope.
4. *Transformation from the ear to the brain:* That is, brain may not appreciate the correctness of sounds.

Regarding the stethoscope and choice of chest piece:

Use all chest pieces on the same patient. The diaphragm chest piece is good for analysis of heart sounds, systolic clicks, ejection sounds and most systolic murmurs and is best for detecting a faint, early blowing aortic diastolic murmur. The bell is best as a rule to detect a low frequency diastolic murmur and faint gallop sounds. The diaphragm can be used to detect low frequency sounds, although it is not as good as the bell type chest piece. The diaphragm should touch the chest wall lightly to pick up the low frequencies and the low frequency sounds of a gallop or diastolic murmur some times surprisingly can be detected, but this procedure is used when the bell piece is not available.

137. There are 4 steps in cardiac cycle in continuous rotation. Clear idea of cardiac cycle is essential. Auricles and ventricles are both relaxed after the completion of a beat. Then

1. Auricles contract—to force the blood into the ventricles through the AV valves.
2. Then the ventricles contract in turn to expel the blood into great vessels through the semilunar valves.
3. While the auricles begin to relax to refill with blood, i.e. auricular diastole commences during ventricular systole.
4. Finally, the ventricles relax. Thus, the cycle is completed, i.e.

   Auricular systole

   Ventricular systole

   Auricular diastole commencing during ventricular systole.

   Ventricular diastole continuing through auricular systole.

HEART SOUNDS

Heart sounds are relatively brief, discrete auditory vibrations of varying intensity (loudness), frequency (pitch) and quality (timbre). The first sound identifies the onset of ventricular systole and the second sound identifies the onset of diastole. These two heart sounds constitute a framework in which other heart sounds and murmurs can be included.

138. There are 4 causes of heart sounds. They are caused by vibrations of structures.

1. *Valvular:* Mainly by the closure of cusps of the valves. Mitral and tricuspid valve closure in first sound. Aortic and pulmonary valve closure in second sound.
2. *Myocardial:* Vibrations of walls of the cardiac chambers.
3. *Vascular:* Vibrations of walls of the great vessels.
4. *Cardiohemic system:* Vibrations of the column of blood.

139. The 4 heart sounds are produced by:

1. *1st sound:* Produced by AV valves closure

   Mitral and tricuspid valves closure + contraction of the ventricular muscle. So, the beginning of the ventricular systole is noted by the first sound and occurrences of the apex beat.

2. *2nd sound:* Produced by semilunar valve closure Aortic and pulmonary valves closure. Tension in great vessel walls.
3. *3rd sound:* Produced by rapid ventricular filling. Arises from vibrations in the atrioventricular valve structures and in the ventricular muscle.
4. *4th sound:* Produced by forceful atrial contraction. Carotid pulse or the apex beat should be used to time the events in cardiac cycle but not radial pulse which occurs sometime later.
   Clinically, systole begins with the first sound and apex beat, i.e. closure of the AV valves, and ends immediately before the second sound, i.e. closure of the semilunar valves.

3rd and 4th are diastolic sounds.

140. There are 4 structural factors of the AV valve that play their role in producing the 1st sound of the heart.

1. Papillary muscles
2. Chordae tendinae
3. Valve leaflets
4. Valve ring

141. At the 4th left costal cartilage behind its inner edge and adjoining part of the sternum the mitral valve lies.

142. At the 4th cartilage or interspace tricuspid valve lies.

Upper end at 4th cartilage or interspace and its lower end near the lower border of 5th right sternocostal junction. (Pulmonary valve lies horizontally at upper border of 3rd left costal cartilage. Aortic valve lies near left half of the sternum near the lower border of the 3rd costal cartilage).

143. Listen the valve closure in 4 areas.

The valves lie so close to each other that the sounds from all of them would reach the chest piece of stethoscope and it is difficult to distinguish them. So,

1. Listen the mitral valve—at cardiac apex, i.e. mitral area at left 5th intercostal space (ICS) in the midclavicular line where left ventricle is near the surface.
2. Listen the tricuspid valve, i.e. tricuspid area where the right ventricle is just beneath the chest wall, left sternal edge.
3. Listen the aortic valve—over the aorta at 2nd right costal cartilage, i.e. aortic area—2nd right intercostal space (ICS) at the parasternal end.
4. Listen the pulmonary valve—over the pulmonary artery at 2nd left intercostal space, i.e. pulmonary area at the left parasternal end.

The sounds of the respective valves are heard mostly in these areas. Therefore, they are called as Mitral, tricuspid, aortic and pulmonary areas. It is therefore best to concentrate on the first heart sound at the apex and left sternal edge and to ignore the second sound in these areas. Concentrate on the second heart sound in both second intercostal spaces and to ignore the first heart sound in areas. Third and fourth heart sounds should be listened for over the ventricles that is between the apex and left sternal edge.

144. The 4 areas are to be auscultated in a systematic way. First begin with

1. Mitral area—note the timings at which the sounds are heard in the cardiac cycle by feeling apex beat or carotid pulse. Then
2. Tricuspid area followed by
3. Aortic area and finally
4. Pulmonary area.

Auscultation may be done in MA, AA, PA, TA when mitral systolic murmur is associated with an aortic murmur.

145. There are 4 types of deviations from normal heart sounds in disease.

1. Sounds may have different intensity, absolute or relative to that in health.
2. Sounds may be split.
3. There may be triple rhythm.
4. May have adventitious sounds.

146. High frequency or high pitched sounds or murmurs are described in 4 terms.

1. Soft
2. Blowing
3. Musical
4. Cooing

147. Low frequency or low pitch sounds and murmurs are described in 4 terms.

1. Rough
2. Rumbling
3. Dull
4. Thud

148. There are 4 conditions where sounds are heard in diminished intensity or scarcely audible.

1. Normally in thick chest wall patients.
2. In severe degree of emphysema
3. Sounds are distant or inaudible in pericardial effusion or chronic constrictive pericarditis.
4. In diseases where the myocardium is involved, e.g. acute myocardial infarction, cardiomyopathies.

Conversely, the sounds may be normal in serious heart disease. Thus, the alteration in intensity is considered in relation to all other features.

149. There are 4 points to describe with the sounds.

1. Is there splitting
2. Is there opening snap
3. Is there ejection sound (from semilunar valves)
4. Is there nonejection systolic clicks

First Heart Sound

150. The 4 conditions that influence the intensity or loudness of S_1.

1. Position of mitral leaflet at the beginning of systole
2. Rate of rise of LV pressure
3. The presence or absence of disease of mitral valve
4. The amount of tissue, air or fluid between the heart and stethoscope.

Loudness of heart sounds depend more upon the velocity of closure of the valves than upon the strength of ventricular contraction.

151. Main abnormalities of the first heart sound relate to its intensity or loudness rather than the timing.

There are 4 conditions where the intensity or loudness of first heart sound is increased.

1. When the cardiac output is high and pulse is fast: Tachycardia of any cause, e.g. anxiety, anemia or hyperthyroidism, and in all hyperkinetic states. The diastole is shortened.
2. When AV flow is increased—because of high cardiac output, e.g. LVH. A high velocity closure of the valve causes loud sound affected by the full force of left ventricular contraction
3. When AV flow is prolonged because of mitral stenosis, high pressure is generated in the left atrium in order to push blood through the narrowed valve. The valve is held open for longer than normal into the early part of ventricular systole. A high velocity of closure of the valve, causing a loud sound, is then affected by the full force of left ventricular contraction.
4. When atrial contraction precedes ventricular contractions by a short PR interval.

The aortic ejection click is often mistaken for loud S_1. When the S_1 is louder at the base than apex, an ejection click is likely.

With a normal heart rate, normal PR interval, if the S_1 is loud, one should consider mitral stenosis.

152. The 4 conditions where intensity or loudness of first sound is quiet or diminished in which the velocity of closure of the valve is low.

1. Rigid or calcified AV valve
   (loud in mobile AV valves, e.g. mitral stenosis (MS), diminished when they become rigid
2. Imperfect closure due to reduced valve substance, e.g. mitral regurgitation (MR).
   Chordae tendinae have become shortened and so prevent proper closure of the valve.
3. When the rate of rise of ventricular pressure is low, e.g. myocardial infarction (MI)
4. Long PR interval.

153. There are 4 causes of loud S_1 in mitral stenosis.

1. Open mitral valve at end diastole
2. Delayed closure of mitral valve
3. Mitral valve closure at higher pressure of left ventricle
4. Thickened but mobile mitral valve

154. There are 4 causes of normal or diminished S_1 in mitral stenosis.

1. Heavily calcified mitral valve with or without subvalvular fusion
2. Associated mitral regurgitation
3. Associated severe aortic regurgitation
4. Marked left ventricular events due to severe right ventricular hypertrophy

155. There are 4 causes of reduced loudness of S_1 in mitral regurgitation.

1. Loss of isovolumic systole
2. Fibrosis and shortening of leaflets
3. Failure of leaflets to close
4. Myocardial dysfunction as in secondary mitral regurgitation

156. If the S_1 is loud, either mitral regurgitation is unlikely or one of the following conditions likely

1. Loud ejection click of aortic stenosis mistaken for S_1.
2. Severe tricuspid regurgitation of silent mitral stenosis mistaken for mitral regurgitation
3. Associated mitral stenosis
4. Mitral regurgitation of mitral valve prolapse

When aortic stenosis is mistaken for mitral regurgitation, the accompanying ejection click will be mistaken for S_1.

In mitral valve prolapse, when prolapse occurs early, the click stimulates loud S_1. In some children with rheumatic mitral regurgitation S_1 is loud with well-preserved anterior leaflet. This is of importance because these valves can be repaired and valve replacement can be avoided. S_1 is diminished out of proportion to the severity of mitral regurgitation in papillary muscle dysfunction of coronary artery disease and functional mitral regurgitation of cardiomyopathy.

157. The following 4 causes may be attributed for abnormal splitting of the first sound due to mechanical or electrical factors.

1. Mitral stenosis } Mechanical
2. Left atrial myxoma } Mechanical
3. Arrhythmias } Electrical
   a. BBB
   b. PVB
   c. Tachycardia
   d. Idioventricular rhythm
4. Ventricular pacing

The split of the first sound does not have the same significance as that of second sound and is heard in 40% of normal.

Second Heart Sound

158. Out of all the heart sounds and murmurs, the most important is the assessment of second sound

There are 4 points to know about the normal second heart sound S_2.

1. They are mainly caused by the closure of semilunar valves of aortic and pulmonary valves - A_2 and P_2 components. Normally P_2 follows A_2.
2. They have high pitched harmonics and both the components can be heard separately in the pulmonary area by using the diaphragm.
3. Aortic valve closure is audible in all areas whereas pulmonary valve closure (P_2) is audible only in pulmonary area.
4. Normally second heart sound heard in the pulmonary area is louder than in aortic area in the young whereas second heart sound heard in the aortic area is louder in the old age.

159. Normal second sound has two components—the aortic closure sound (A_2) and pulmonic closure sound (P_2)

During quiet breathing both the components are superimposed on each other during expiration. Thus only a single sound is heard.

During inspiration, aortic component comes slightly early whereas the pulmonary component is delayed, resulting in splitting of the second sound in which aortic second precedes pulmonary second sound.

A loud second sound is due to abnormally high pressure causing the valve to shut with greater force than normal velocity. As a consequence A_2 is often loud in systemic hypertension and P_2 is louder in pulmonary hypertension.

A soft S_2 occurs in situations in which stiffness of the valves interferes with their closure. As a consequence A_2 is often soft in aortic stenosis and P_2 is soft in pulmonary stenosis.

The aortic component is louder than the pulmonary component except in infants below the age of 6 to 12 months.

Intensity of the second sound is accentuated or diminished

Aortic second sound is accentuated in

1. Systemic hypertension of any cause
2. Aortic regurgitation

   Diminished or absent in
3. Fibrosis or calcification of aortic valve when it becomes immobile
4. Aortic valve atresia or aortic valve is absent, A_2 is absent.

160. The aortic second sound A_2, can come late or early. The following are situations where A_2 is delayed or comes early

Delayed in conditions when ventricular ejection is prolonged in

1. Aortic valvular or subvalvular stenosis LVH
2. In large left to right shunt as in PDA
2. Aortic regurgitation
3. Left bundle branch block
4. systemic hypertension

A_2 comes early in

5. Mitral regurgitation
6. Ventricular septal defect
7. Constrictive pericarditis

161. Abnormalities of the pulmonic component P_2 of the second sound P_2 may be accentuated or diminished in intensity or delayed in timing in the following conditions. Although it may occur early in tricuspid regurgitation, it is not recognized as such on the bed side since tricuspid regurgitation as an isolated lesion (without pulmonary arterial hypertension) is rare.

1. P_2 is accentuated in pulmonary arterial hypertension of any cause
2. Diminished in intensity in pulmonary stenosis
3. Absent in pulmonary valve atresia where the pulmonary valve is absent
4. Delayed in pulmonary stenosis, ASD, RBBB and pulmonary arterial hypertension, RVH

162. The 4 situations when split of the pulmonary second sound (P_2) occurs as pressure of blood in the pulmonary circulation rises.

1. Normally, in young people
2. Mitral stenosis
3. Primary pulmonary hypertension
4. Emphysema, fibrosis or collapse of lungs progressing to cor pulmonale.

P_2 split is an important sign to differentiate the hypertrophy of ventricles. It should be remembered that second sound has aortic and pulmonary components (A_2 and P_2). When there is hypertrophy of one ventricle, there is an asynchronous closure of the semilunar valves. The closure of the semilunar valves of the hypertrophied ventricles lags behind and causes the splitting of the second sound. It changes with respiration also. Blood is drawn into the thorax during inspiration followed by a relative increase in right atrial pressure and right ventricular stroke volume. The right ventricular systole measured from the first sound to P_2 is increased and so P_2 is slightly delayed.

On the left side, the left ventricular stroke volume falls during inspiration because of the increased negative pressure in the thorax. It increases the capacity of the left atrium and pulmonary veins reducing the left atrial pressure and left ventricular stroke volume. Thus, the left ventricular systole is shortened and A_2 comes earlier. Thus, the A_2 comes earlier and P_2 later and so the splitting widens during inspiration.

Reverse mechanism occurs during expiration.

So, in right ventricular hypertrophy the splitting widens with inspiration and closes with expiration. In left ventricular hypertrophy, the splitting widens with expiration and closes with inspiration.

If the RVH is recognized, the diseases causing resistance in the lesser pulmonary circulation like mitral stenosis, pulmonary hypertension, emphysema, fibrosis, collapse of the lung can be thought of and others are excluded. If the LVH is recognized, the diseases causing resistance in the greater circulation like systemic hypertension either essential, renal or endocrinal, or aortic valvular disease AS or AR), aneurysm of the aorta near the aortic valve can be thought of and others are excluded (see Fig. A.9).

163. Normal second sound is single (or closely split less than 0.03 sec) in expiration and split in inspiration with louder A_2 preceding the P_2. Wide splitting of the second sound is defined as splitting during expiration due to early A_2 or late P_2, i.e. A_2-P_2 interval is 0.03 sec or more during expiration.

The following 4 conditions where in P_2 split may show difference.

P_2 split is due to delay in closure of one of the semilunar valves. It may result from delayed conduction or mechanical factors.

1. Loud narrow P_2 split in pulmonary hypertension.
2. During inspiration, if the A_2-P_2 interval increases further, it is called wide variable splitting. Wide and variable splitting of second sound is seen in pulmonary stenosis, mitral regurgitation and ventricular septal defect. In pulmonary stenosis, it is due to delay in P_2 whereas in mitral regurgitation and ventricular septal defect, it is due to an early A_2
3. Wide splitting of second sound occurs in RBBB and total anomalous pulmonary venous connection due to delay in P_2

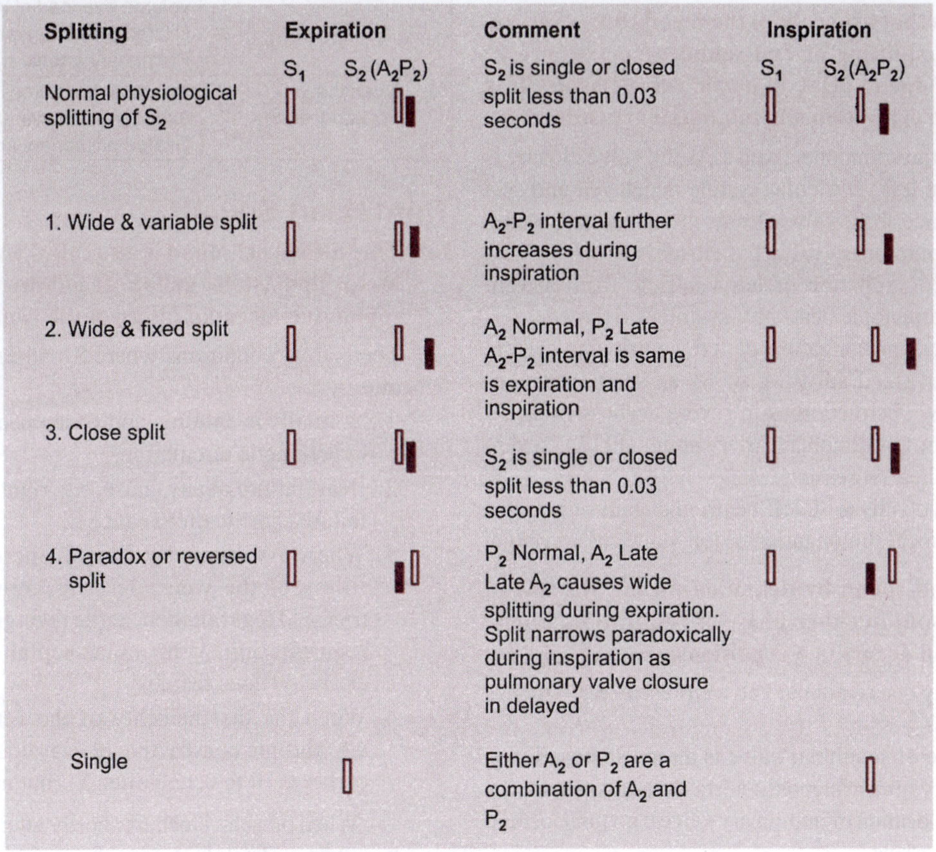

Fig. A-4: Splitting of the second heart sound

4. If the A_2-P_2 interval is same in expiration and inspiration it is called widely split and fixed second sound. Wide and fixed P_2 split is seen in ASD.

Pulmonary valve closure is delayed by an increased R V stroke volume due to L to R shunt in ASD. There is splitting of second sound throughout respiratory cycle. As a consequence of both pulmonary hypertension and increased blood flow in ASD, P_2 may be both loud with wide fixed split.

A single second sound means that it is either A_2 or P_2 or a combination of both A_2 and P_2. The decision whether A_2 or P_2 or a combination of both A_2 and P_2 depends on analysis of total clinical picture. For example, generally, in Tetralogy of Fallot, only a single second sound is heard and it is A_2 since P_2 is so soft that it is not audible. In ventricular septal defect with pulmonary arterial hypertension and right to left shunt in Eisenmenger's complex, again a single second sound is heard and represents a combination of A_2 and P_2. In these situations, one cannot differentiate TOF and Eisenmenger's complex. However, history and roentgenogram can easily separate them. Thus, the interpretation of the single second sound is not dependent on auscultation alone.

164. The 4 causes that bring about the reversed P_2 split are, paradoxical splitting of 2nd sound occurs where P_2 precedes A_2 due to delay in aortic valve closure. It is maximum in expiration and minimum in inspiration).

1. LBBB is the commonest cause. Aortic valve closure is delayed in left ventricular systole is delayed and as a consequence aortic valve closure is delayed and occurs after the pulmonary valve has closed.
2. In delayed excitation of left ventricle from a right ventricular ectopic beat—LV systole is delayed.
3. Mechanical prolongation of left ventricular systole causes reversed splitting of S_2 as seen in severe aortic flow obstruction as in severe aortic stenosis, a large aorta-to-pulmonary artery shunt (PDA), severe ischemic heart disease.
4. Cardiomyopathy with left ventricular failure because of mechanical prolongation of left ventricular systole.

165. Single second sound by definition means absence of an audible split in either phase of respiration. Single second sound occurs in 4 conditions.

1. When only one semilunar valve is present, e.g. Truncus Arteriosus
2. When one of semilunar valve is atretic/stenosed, e.g. pulmonary atresia/stenosis, aortic atresia/stenosis.
3. Posterior location of pulmonary valve e.g. transposition of great vessels
4. Extreme loudness of one of the sounds, e.g. single loud P_2 in extreme pulmonary arterial hypertension.

166. There are 4 conditions where aortic second sound is accentuated.

Table A-11

Condition	Mechanism
1. Systemic hypertension	Elevated pressure beyond the valve Dilated ascending aorta
2. Aneurysm of aorta	Dilatation of vessel
3. Aortic regurgitation	Aortic root disease Free mobility of the leaflets Increased flow across the valve Dilated ascending aorta
4. Congenital bicuspid aortic valve	Thickened but mobile aortic valve

167. There are 4 conditions where pulmonic second sound is accentuated.

Table A-12

Condition	Mechanism
1. Normally in infants and children, and in thin chest wall	Higher pulmonary arterial pressures Stethoscope is nearer to the pulmonary artery
2. Pulmonary arterial hypertension	Higher closing pressure of valve Dilated pulmonary artery
3. Left to right shunts	Increased flow across the valve due to volume overload of right ventricle. Dilated pulmonary artery. Pulmonary arterial hypertension.
4. Hyperkinetic circulatory states	Increase flow across the valve with exaggerated valve excursion. Dilated pulmonary artery.

Third Heart Sound

168. The third heart sound is also called a ventricular gallop are protodiastolic gallop. It follows the second heart sound during rapid filling of the ventricle.

There are 4 conditions where S_3 is heard (0.14 to 0.16 s after A_2).

1. Normally in children and young people where there is hyperkinetic circulation.
2. Heart failure of any cause, e.g. right or left ventricular failure shortly after acute MI.
3. Where AV diastolic flow is increased with rapid filling of the ventricles, e.g. mitral regurgitation, tricuspid regurgitation, aortic regurgitation, pulmonary regurgitation, ventricular septal defect, systemic arterio-venous fistulas.
4. When the distensibility of the ventricle is altered, e.g. chronic constrictive pericarditis - early and sharp earlier 0.10 to 0.12 s after A_2 (but not tamponade).

When present, it occurs shortly after the second sound. It occurs in diastole during the period of rapid filling of the ventricles and may be thought of as creaking of a stiff diseased ventricle (usually left) as it fills.

Left sided S_3 is best heard in mitral area with the bell in left lateral position during expiration. Right sided S_3 is best heard at left sternal border or just below the xiphoid during inspiration.

Third heart sound usually does not occur in AV valve stenosis.

S_3 disappears with the treatment of heart failure.

It is uncommon in conditions in which the left ventricle is hypertrophied but not dilated, e.g. aortic stenosis.

169. The range of interval between second and third heart sound at ordinary heart rate is 0.12 to 0.16 sec.

170. An early third heart sound with normal heart rate of 70–90 /min, is considered to be a feature of constrictive pericarditis. Besides constrictive pericarditis, any condition that cause high venous or atrial pressures and quick reversal of pressures in early diastole may give rise to early third heart sound.

Early third heart sound occurs in the following 4 conditions.

Table A-13

Condition	Mechanism of early S_3
1. Constrictive pericarditis	Small ventricular cavity with high filling pressures as in constriction
2. Severe mitral regurgitation with large V wave	Very rapid reversal of pressures during early diastole
3. Severe tricuspid regurgitation with large V wave.	Very rapid reversal of pressures during early diastole
4. Any severe ventricular failure	High venous or atrial pressures

171. Third heart sound is almost always heard in congestive heart failure. An absent of third sound in the presence of congestive heart failure may suggest the following possibilities.

1. Pericardial tamponade
2. Mitral stenosis
3. Tricuspid stenosis
4. Acute myocardial infarction with left ventricular failure in some patients.

Diagnosis of heart failure should be rechecked.

172. Third heart sound is correlated with the presence of heart failure. The ventricular end-diastolic pressure is usually above 25 mm Hg on the left side. The right sided third heart sound correlates with a rapid 'Y' descent in the JVP.

Correlation of third heart sound with heart failure.

Table A-14

1. Symptoms	Dyspnea, Orthopnea, PND
2. Structural	Dilated ventricle
3. Functional	Systolic dysfunction - (EF < 40%)
4. Hemodynamic	LVEDP > 25 mm Hg

173. There are 4 differentiating features of left ventricular third heart sound and right ventricular third heart sound.

Table A-15

Features	LVS_3	RVS_3
1. Site	Mitral area - Apex	Left lateral border
2. Position	Left lateral decubitus	Supine Passive leg rising
3. Respiration	Better heard during expiration	Inspiration
4. Associated features	Left sided causes for S_3	JVP Rapid Y descent

174. Third heart sound in valvular heart disease help to differentiate 4 distinctive features.

The presence of third heart sound in patients with valvular heart disease is often regarded as a sign of congestive heart failure, but it may also depend on the type of valvular disease. Folland and participants in the Veterans Affairs Cooperative study on valvular disease assessed the prevalence of third heart sound and cardiac function.

1. The prevalence of third heart sound was higher in patients with mitral regurgitation (46%) than in those with mitral stenosis (8%). The prevalence of S_3 is increased with the severity of MR.
2. The presence of S_3 is higher in aortic regurgitation (28%) than in those with aortic stenosis (11%).
3. LVEF was significantly lower when a third heart sound was present in patients with AS (0.38 versus 0.56) in those without third heart sound or mixed aortic valve disease (0.4 versus 0.55). In patients with AS third heart sounds are uncommon but usually indicate the presence of systolic dysfunction and elevated filling pressure. However, EF was only slightly lower in patients with MR and third heart sound (0.5 versus 0.57). In patients with MR third heart sound is common but do not necessarily reflect LV systolic dysfunction or increased filling pressure.
4. Pulmonary artery wedge pressure was higher when a third heart sound was detected in patients with AS (18.6 mm Hg versus 12.1 mm Hg) than in those without S_3. There was no association between the PA wedge pressure and third heart sounds inpatients with MR.

Fourth Heart Sound

175. Fourth heart sound is also called atrial or presystolic gallop.

There are 4 points to know about 4th heart sound.

1. It is caused by auricular systole.
2. It occurs before the 1st heart sound, i.e. late diastole/presystolic and is low pitched (low frequency).
3. When it is loud, it often shows a prominent 'a' wave in JVP.
4. A large 'P' (auricular wave) is seen in ECG.

(S_4 is not heard in health by ordinary auscultation.)

S_4 should be differentiated from a split first sound and an ejection sound. This could be easily done by following Inching' technique.

By auscultating at the left lower sternal border or apex, S_4 is eliminated by pressure on the stethoscope. Pressure eliminates S_4 but does not eliminate the ejection sound or splitting of the S_1. S_4 is usually not heard over the aortic area whereas the ejection sound is heard. The normal split of S_1 is heard in mitral and tricuspid areas—which is caused by mitral and tricuspid components and they sound alike and only one component of the S_1 is generally heard over the aortic area.

Third and fourth sounds from the right ventricle become louder during inspiration as more blood is drawn into the right side of the heart.

176. There are 4 requirements for 4th heart sound.

1. Healthy atrium
2. Sinus rhythm
3. Nonstenotic AV valves
4. Noncomplaint nondilated ventricle as in
   a. Ischemia/infarction
   b. Concentric hypertrophy
   c. Restrictive myopathy
   d. Acute volume load

177. There are 4 conditions where 4th heart sound occurs.

1. All conditions of concentric left ventricular hypertrophy.
   a. Systemic hypertension (moderate/severe)
   b. Aortic stenosis (moderate/severe)
   c. Hypertrophic obstructive cardiomyopathy
   d. Restrictive cardiomyopathy
2. All conditions of concentric right ventricular hypertrophy.
   a. Pulmonary stenosis (moderate/severe)
   b. Pulmonary arterial hypertension (moderate/severe)
   c. Restrictive cardiomyopathy
3. Coronary artery disease
   Ischemia/infarction
4. Acute regurgitant lesions
   a. Acute aortic regurgitation
   b. Acute mitral regurgitation
   c. Acute tricusspid regurgitation

In contrast to the third heart sound, which may mean heart failure, 4th heart sound does not mean heart failure. It only means a 'hard working ventricle'.

178. 4th heart sound (S_4)

1. Does not occur in health (Vs/S_3)
2. Not always a sign of heart failure (Vs/S_3)
3. Always indicate that the heart is abnormal (Vs/S_3)
4. Never occurs in atrial fibrillation.

S_4 presystolic gallop—is most frequently found in patients with coronary heart disease. It should be searched carefully as it is an expected sign in patients with coronary heart disease and in patients with history of myocardial infarction. S_4 is a consistent finding in patients with hypertension for many years without cardiac decompensation.

Additional Sounds–Opening Snap, Ejection Clicks, Nonejection Clicks

179. There are 4 points to know about opening snap.

(Since the opening of normal mitral and tricuspid valve is silent, the presence of opening snap is always abnormal. It is a brief high pitched early diastolic sound).

1. Heard only with AV valve stenosis. Most commonly with mitral stenosis.
   The tricuspid stenosis patients also have severe mitral valve disease. The tricuspid opening snap is often overshadowed by mitral opening snap.
2. It indicates mobile AV valve.
3. Mitral opening snap in mitral stenosis is heard maximum at the lower left sternal border and radiates to the base of the heart, often mistaken with P_2. Careful auscultation at the upper left sternal border will identify both components of second sound followed by OS.
   Opening snap of tricuspid stenosis occurs later in diastole than mitral opening snap.
4. Closeness to 2nd sound indicates severity of stenosis. (OS may also occur when there is increased flow across the AV valve with left to right intracardiac shunts and in AV valve regurgitation).

180. The normal opening of the semilunar valves is noiseless. But when the aortic or pulmonary valve opening is associated with noise, ejection clicks occur.

The 4 features of ejection sounds - systolic ejection sounds (clicks)

1. Are caused by semilunar valves. Valve is usually abnormal. It may be trivial as in bicuspid valve without stenosis.
2. Coincides with the opening of the valve in early systole—Occur in early systole closely following S_1.
3. Are sharp, high pitched, heard better during expiration.
4. Aortic ejection sound is heard best at the apex and 2nd right intercostal space (RICS). Pulmonary ejection sound is best heard at upper left sternal border.

181. The 4 conditions where ejection sounds occur in:

Valvular

1. Aortic stenosis like opening snap of aortic valve
2. Pulmonary stenosis like opening snap of pulmonic valve.

Vascular

3. Dilatation of aorta in systemic hypertension.
4. Dilatation of pulmonary artery in pulmonary hypertension.

182. There are 4 points to note about nonejection systolic clicks.

1. They are due to prolapse of posterior leaflet of mitral valve resulting from functional unequal length of chordae tendinae
2. They occur with or without late systolic murmur. Often denote mitral regurgitation.
3. They are best heard along the left sternal border and apex.
4. They may be single or multiple.

They occur in systole later than systolic ejection sound. Often, midsystolic click is mistaken as 2nd sound and the actual 2nd sound is called as OS or S_3.

183. Effect of maneuvers cause alteration in first sound, nonejection click interval. This is caused by change in ventricular size.

Table A-16

Decrease in ventricular size occur in	*Increase in ventricular size occur in*
1. Standing, squatting	Supine
2. Valsalva phase II	Valsalva phase II
3. Inspiration	Expiration
4. Drugs like nitroglycerin, amylnitrate	Phenylephrine

184. Whenever an extra sound is heard in systole, the possibilities are varied. The loud first sound and split first sound may be mistaken for ejection click. First sound is best heard at the apex and split first sound is heard only at the tricuspid area.

Whenever there is clicky sound in systole, approach to the patient should be in the following way.

Table A-17

1. Changes significantly with posture	Nonejection click (MVP) Look for murmur of mitral regurgitation
2. No change with posture	Ejection click either aortic or pulmonary
3. Best heard in aortic area but also widely audible at left sternal border and apex	Aortic ejection click
4. If aortic-A_2 normal or accentuated, second sound normally split	Aortic vascular click
5. If aortic-A_2 diminished S_2 reversibly split	Aortic valvular ejection click
6. Best heard in pulmonary area, not widely audible	Pulmonary vascular or valvular click
7. Loud P_2, palpable pulmonary artery	Pulmonary vascular click
8. Wide split S_2, diminished P_2, impalpable pulmonary artery with systolic thrill at pulmonary area	Pulmonary valvular click, mild to moderate or severe

185. There are 4 sounds which can cause confusion around first heart sound.

1. Split S_1
2. S_1- ejection click.
3. S_1- nonejection click.
4. S_4- S_1

Right sided ejection clicks are not confused with other sounds as they are localized to the pulmonary area.

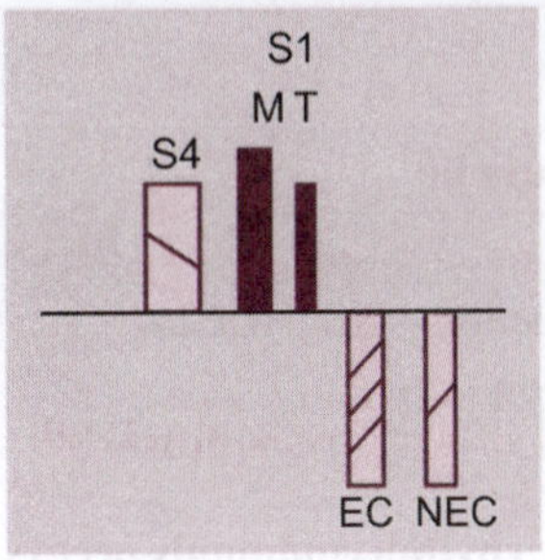

Fig. A-5: Confusion around first heart sound M: mitral component of S_1; T: tricuspid component of S_1; EC: ejection click; NEC: nonejection click

186. There 4 sounds which can cause confusion around second sound.

1. S_2 split
2. S_2 - OS
3. S_2 - S_3
4. Nonejection click - S_2 (rare)

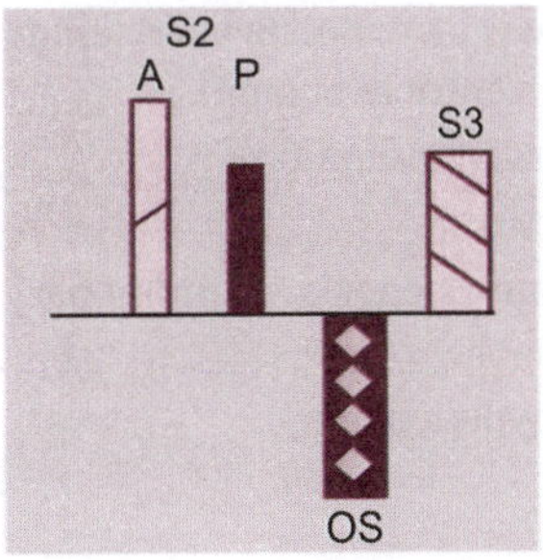

Fig. A-6: Confusion around second heart sound A: aortic component of S_2; P: pulmonary component of S_2; OS: opening snap

187. Differentiation of sounds around first heart sound.

Table A-18

Feature	*Split S_1*	*S_1-EC*	*S_1-NEC*	*S_4-S_1*
1. Sight and audibility	Tricuspid area localized	Base widely audible	Apex widely audible	Apex localized
2. Character	Low frequency	High frequency sharp, clicky	High frequency sharp, clicky	Low frequency often palpable
3. Relation to physiological act	Best audible during inspiration	No change in aortic click	NEC loud and earlier with standing	Isometric hand grip increases S_4
4. Associated features	– Normal – RBBB – ASD – Ebstein's anomaly	– Aortic stenosis – Bicuspid aortic valve	– Mitral valve prolapse	– Coronary artery disease – Cardiomyopathy – LVH with hypertension

188. Differentiation of sounds around second heart sound.

Table A-19

Feature	*S_2 split*	*S_2-OS*	*S_2-S_3*	*NEC-S_2(rare)*
1. Sight and audibility	Pulmonary area localized	Medial to apex widely audible	Apex localized	Apex variable
2. Character	High pitch may be palpable	High pitch not palpable	Low pitch palpable	High pitch not palpable
3. Relation to physiological act	Inspiration	No change	Expiration	Posture
4. Associated features	– Normal – RBBB – ASD – Ebstein's anomaly	– Mitral stenosis	– Normal – Heart failure mitral regurgitation	– Mitral valve prolapse

189. Reversed splitting of S_2 occurs in

1. LBBB
2. Aortic outflow tract obstruction—AS, HOCM
3. Severe systolic hypertension
4. Right ventricular ectopic

190. The 4 conditions where triple rhythm commonly occurs when S_3 or S_4 are prominent. They give a cadence of sounds known as triple rhythm. Triple rhythm often occurs in 4 conditions.

Triple rhythm from S_3 occurs in

1. Heart failure of any cause. It is an important sign of heart failure. Atrial pressure is increased in heart failure and the early filling of the ventricle is rapid.
2. Shortly after acute myocardial infarction.

Triple rhythm from S_4 occurs in

3. Right heart from pulmonary stenosis or pulmonary hypertension.
4. Left heart from systemic hypertension.

Both ventricular S_3 and atrial S_4 diastolic gallops may be present in a patient. This is common in heart failure patients associated with coronary heart disease, hypertension, and dilated cardiomyopathy. When S_3 and S_4 occur in close proximity, a short low frequency diastolic rumbling murmur may be heard. However, when diastole is shortened with increased heart rate (above 100 per min) in patients with S_3 and S_4 gallops, these two gallops occur exactly at the same time, S_3 overlying on S_4 producing a single loud sound in diastole, often louder than S_1 or S_2. This is called Summation gallop which is rare. The gallop occurring in close proximity should not be called as summation gallop.

A faint gallop of S_3 or S_4 can easily be missed in a patient who has an emphysematous chest. Anteroposterior diameter is increased in condition such as chronic obstructive pulmonary disease COPD. The S_3 or S_4 gallop is missed if examined over the usual areas of precordium, lower left sternal border and apex. This can be easily detected by listening over the xiphoid area or epigastric area.

HEART MURMURS

191. Murmurs in contrast to sounds are prolonged sound vibrations. Murmurs are due to disturbance in blood flow which manifests as turbulence. Turbulence is known as an irregular state of motion in which velocity and pressures show a random variation in relation to space. The site of maximum intensity correspond to the site of turbulence. For example,

1. Root of the aorta in aortic stenosis
2. Root of pulmonary artery in pulmonary stenosis
3. Left atrium in mitral regurgitation
4. Cavity of left ventricle in aortic regurgitation

192. The following causes due to which murmurs or abnormal sounds are heard along with or replacing normal sounds. They are due to

1. Narrowing of the valves, e.g. MS, AS
2. Incompetence of the valve, e.g. MR, AR
3. Abnormal apertures, e.g. ASD, VSD
4. Abnormally high blood flow through a normal valve, e.g. anemia, thyrotoxicosis—flow murmer.

A thrill is a palpable vibration. A loud murmur may produce a palpable vibration or thrill.

193. The age of the patient helps to differentiate the cause of murmur in 4 types.

1. Murmurs in neonates and children of congenital valvular disease are from right side origin. The strain is more on the right side during the intrauterine life.
2. Murmurs of the postnatal origin (acquired) are often of the left side origin than from the right side.
   The left side chambers are subjected to ten times the pressure compared to the right side chambers. Therefore, most of the acquired heart diseases affect the left side of the heart.
3. Murmurs in the aortic area in adults are common from valvular disease.
4. Murmurs in the pulmonary area in adults are rare from valvular disease.

194. Description of murmur with following features is important.

1. Sight/location of best audibility of murmur
2. Timing and configuration of murmur
3. Intensity of the murmur—Grading
4. Length of murmur
5. Character of murmur
6. Selective radiation or propagation of the murmur
7. Relation to a physiological act or maneuver
8. Accompanying features

195. There are 4 timings of murmur to determine.

Timing of the murmur is noted with reference to heart sounds and in turn compare the time of occurrence of apex beat.

1. Systolic murmur: Occurs in between the first and second sound, i.e. in systolic phase. It can be early, mid or late or holo systolic, e.g. MR, AS. They may be functional also.
2. Diastolic murmurs: Occurs in between the second sound and first sound, i.e. in diastolic phase. Diastolic murmurs are always significant. They may be early, mid, late or holo diastolic, e.g. MS, AR.
3. To and fro murmur. There is systolic murmur as well as diastolic murmur - but second sound (S_2) is heard in between them, e.g. AS + AR.
   AS gives systolic murmur which precedes S_2, AR gives diastolic murmur which follows S_2 and S_2 is heard in between.
4. Continuous murmurs (or machinery murmur). There is systolic and diastolic component. Murmur starts somewhere in systole and ends somewhere in diastole passing through second sound. It passes through S_2 and so it is masked, e.g. patent ductus arteriosus.

196. Systolic murmurs starts with or after first sound and ends before or at second sound.

The 4 types of systolic murmurs are described depending on their time of occurrence.

1. Early systolic—starts with first sound; doesn't reach second sound

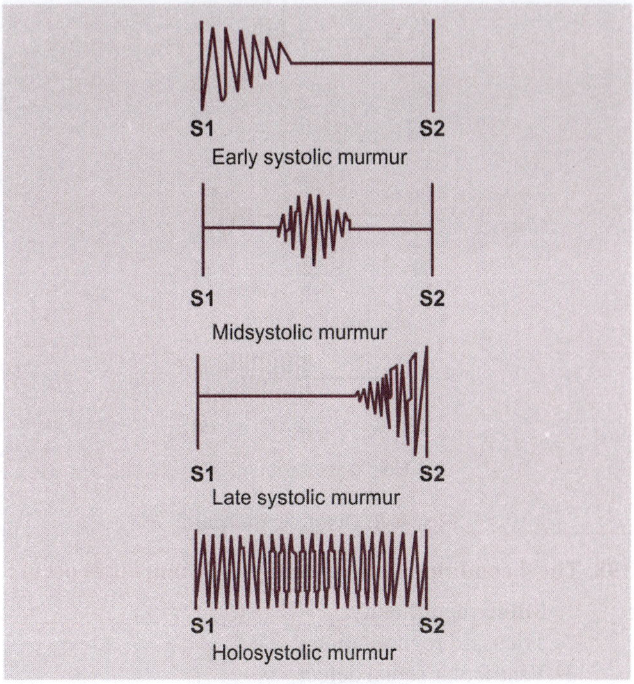

Fig. A-7: Systolic murmurs

2. Mid systolic–starts sometime after first sound and reaches peak by mid systole or later and ends before second sound of that side (A_2 or P_2)
3. Late systolic—starts after first sound; ends with second sound of that side (A_2 or P_2)
4. Holosystolic (Holo = entire)–starts with first sound occupying all of systole up to the second sound on that side (A_2 or P_2).

197. Diastolic murmurs starts with or after second sound, ends at or before first sound.

The 4 types of diastolic murmurs are described according to their time of occurrence.

1. Early diastolic—starts with second sound (A_2 or P_2); duration in diastole is variable
2. Mid diastolic—starts after second sound; ends before first sound
3. Late diastolic—starts late after second sound and extends to the first sound of that side (mitral and tricuspid)
4. Holodiastolic—early diastolic murmurs occupying whole of diastole from second sound to first sound.

Diastolic murmurs for all practical purpose are organic.

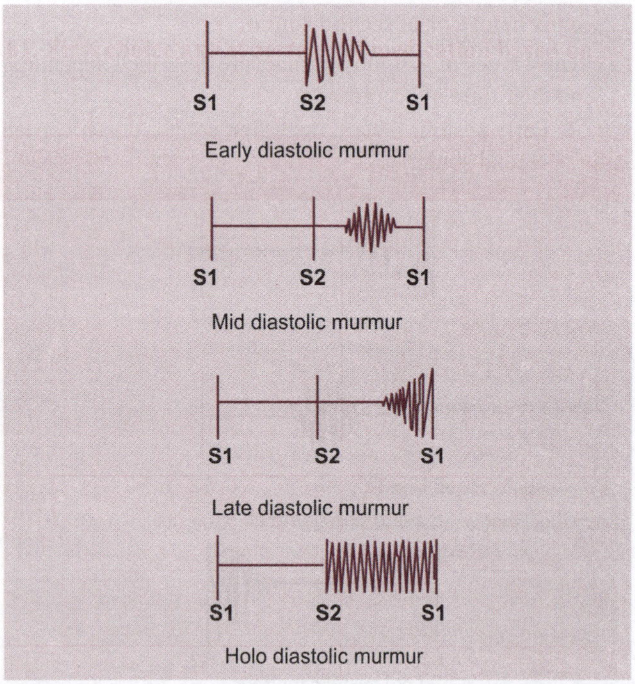

Fig. A-8: Diastolic murmurs

198. The 4 conditions where holosystolic murmurs occur:

1. Mitral regurgitation
2. Tricuspid regurgitation
3. Ventricular septal defect
4. Patent ductus arteriosus with pulmonary hypertension.

It begins with first sound and occupies whole of systole and ends with second sound–left sided murmur ends with aortic component and right sided murmur ends with pulmonary component of the second sound.

199. The intensity or loudness of the murmur may be described in 4 grades as follows; (Usually systolic murmurs are described in 6 grades)

Grade I—Faint—heard only with special effort

Grade II—Heard easily without effort

Grade III—Loud—associated with palpable thrill.

Grade IV—Heard with the stethoscope removed from contact with the chest wall.

Systolic murmurs are classified on a loudness scale of 1–6. Diastolic murmurs are classified on a loudness scale of 1–4.

Remember, the stenotic murmurs are usually tend to be rough and rumbling while the regurgitation murmurs are soft and blowing.

The loudness of a murmur does not determine its importance. A very loud murmur may be less significant than a faint murmur which is significant. High pitch indicates large pressure difference across small orifice, e.g. AI.

Low pitch indicates small pressure difference across large orifice, e.g. MS.

Systolic murmurs are graded based on their intensity and the presence or absence of a thrill. Systolic murmurs often occur even in the absence of organic heart disease. Therefore, it is important to differentiate organic murmurs from functional. Murmurs above Grade III are usually organic. Presence of a thrill is always organic.

A palpable vibration of the pulmonic sound in the pulmonary area and first sound at the apex are often mistaken for a thrill. A clue is that in the presence of a thrill, the accompanying murmur is always loud. If the murmur is faint, an associated thrill is unlikely.

200. The 4 configurations of a murmur are described as follows:

1. Crescendo intensity is low in the beginning and slowly rises
2. Decrescendo intensity is high in the beginning and slowly falls (diamond shaped)
3. Crescendo decrescendo intensity rises first and slowly falls.
4. Plateau—No rise or fall.

201. Character of the murmur generally gives a clue to the diagnosis of the lesion. In general, the murmurs with a high pressure difference between two chambers are of

high frequency or pitch, and those with a low pressure difference are of low frequency. For example,

Table A-20: Character of the murmur

Feature	Mechanism
High pressure difference between two sites	*High frequency (high pitch)*
1. Mitral regurgitation (LV 120 to LA 12 mm Hg)	Soft
2. Aortic regurgitation (Aorta 80 to LV 12 mm Hg)	Blowing
Low pressure difference between two sites	*Low frequency (low pitch)*
3. Mitral stenosis (LA 20 to LV 5 mm Hg)	Rough
4. Tricuspid stenosis (RA 15 to RV 5 mm Hg)	Rumbling

202. There 4 conditions where high pressure difference between two sites give rise to mixed frequency. For example:

1. Aortic stenosis (LV 200 to Aorta 120 mm Hg) - Rough
2. Pulmonary stenosis (RV 120 to PA 25 mm Hg) - Harsh
3. Ventricular septal defect (LV 120 to RV 25 mm Hg)
4. Aortic regurgitation, pulmonary regurgitation (rare)

In general, all regurgitant murmurs (MR, AR, TR, PR) are of high frequency and all stenotic murmurs are rough as a rule. The murmur of AV valve stenosis (MS, TS) are of low frequency, but murmurs of semilunar valves stenosis are mixed in frequency.

A pansystolic murmur means a pansystolic pressure difference between two chambers. This pressure difference exists with left ventricle and left atrium as in mitral regurgitation, right ventricle and right atrium as in tricuspid regurgitation, and between two ventricles as in ventricular septal defect. Pansystolic murmurs present only in these conditions because no where else in the heart a pansystolic pressure difference exists. The murmur of mitral regurgitation, tricuspid regurgitation are dealt in Chapter I and ventricular septal defect in Chapter L.

203. Observe the 4 variations of murmur.

1. With respiration: Intensity of all the murmurs of right side origin increases with inspiration because the blood flow to the right side of the heart increases during inspiration, e.g. TS, TR, PS, PR, ASD. Intensity of all the murmurs of left side origin increases with expiration, eg, MS, MR, AS, AR, Watch the abdominal movements for respiration keenly while changing with respiration. The murmur is of constant intensity when the heart lesion is severe and the stroke volume does not vary with respiration.
2. With posture (see next point)
3. With hand grip exercise: It increases the systemic arterial pressure and heart rate. Often accentuates the murmurs of MS, MR, AR. Diminishes those of AS, subaortic stenosis.
4. With Valsalva maneuver.

204. There are 4 effects of posture on heart sounds and murmurs.

1. Left lateral recumbent position: Mitral systolic and diastolic sounds are accentuated. Left atrium is in posterior position and it goes more posteriorly in left lateral decubitus position and the mitral murmurs are well heard. Turn the patient to left lateral decubitus position, wait for 6 or 7 beats and hear the murmur.
2. Supine posture: Functional systolic murmurs are accentuated. They may disappear on standing, e.g. anemia. The blood flow to the heart in lying position is more and there is increase of blood volume (preload) which causes functional murmur.
3. Sitting posture with forward bending: Aortic and pulmonary murmurs, clicks, pericardial rub are accentuated.
4. Upright position: Venous hum is heard only when upright. Functional murmurs disappear. 1/3rd of the circulating blood goes to lower limbs on standing and so the circulating blood volume to the heart decreases and the functional murmurs disappear.

Standing decreases heart size, so accentuates the murmur of hypertrophic cardiomyopathy, occasional murmur of mitral valve prolapse.

(Squatting increases venous return and increases systemic arterial resistance–it accentuates murmurs except those due to hypertrophic cardiomyopathy and mitral valve prolapse which often decreases)

205. There are 4 causes of midsystolic ejection murmur in aortic area.

1. Aortic stenosis, noted by decreased pulse pressure and thrill.
   (Patient bending forward in expiration)
2. Increased rate of flow
3. Systemic hypertension
4. Valve thickening or sclerosis without stenosis.

206. There are 4 causes of midsystolic ejection murmur in pulmonary area.

1. Functional in young people
2. Pulmonary stenosis
3. Pulmonary hypertension
4. Increased rate of flow, e.g. ASD, TAPVD (Total anomalous pathway venous drainage), hyperdynamic circulation.

207. There are 4 causes of loud systolic murmur with a thrill.

1. at apex—mitral regurgitation
   (Pansystolic extends from 1st to 2nd sound, radiates to the axilla, heard well with the bell)
2. at 4th left intercostal space—VSD.
3. at pulmonary area—pulmonary stenosis
4. at aortic area—aortic stenosis

208. The 4 valvular murmurs should be differentiated from functional murmurs as seen in

1. Atrial myxoma
2. Hypertrophic obstructive cardiomyopathy (HOCM)
3. Ruptured papillary muscle or chordae tendinae
4. Aneurysm of sinus of Valsalva

209. The 4 areas where functional murmurs (Haemic murmurs in anemia) occur over the precordium (and vessels also) as follows:

1. Usually heard in the 2nd left intercostal space over or just lateral to pulmonary artery
2. Frequently heard in mitral area
3. Much less frequently in tricuspid area
4. Uncommon in aortic area.

They are systolic, become less distinct or inaudible when the patient stands. Many systolic murmurs are functional and of no clinical significance but have to be sorted from those that represent serious underlying pathology.

210. There are 4 conditions where functional systolic murmurs are common in the pulmonary area. They are due to increased flow in the pulmonary artery.

1. Anemia
2. Hyperthyroidism
3. ASD
4. Chest deformity

A systolic 'flow' murmur is due to high flow through a normal valve. It is heard in early systole and has a similar quality of aortic stenosis. In severe cases of high output failure may also be seen.

The term 'innocent murmur' is currently accepted. The innocent murmurs are better heard in young people who have thin chests rather than obese or muscular. The innocent systolic murmur is early to mid systole and generally grade 1 to 3 on a scale of 6.

211. The 4 distinguishing points of functional systolic murmur from systolic murmur of mitral regurgitation in mitral area are:

1. They are localized to mitral area and do not have the direction of selective propagation of mitral regurgitation murmur.
2. They are never loud and they never fill the systole as they are usually confined to early to mid systole.
3. They are not accompanied by a thrill.
4. They become less distinct or inaudible when the patient assumes standing position or disappear if the breathing is held in inspiration.

212. There are 4 causes of diastolic murmur.

1. Stenosis: Mitral and tricuspid stenosis.
   Mitral stenosis: Lightly apply the bell at the apex. Better heard in left lateral decubitus position; accentuated in expiration. Presystolic accentuation occurs in pure stenosis but is absent once atrial fibrillation occurs.
   Tricuspid stenosis: becomes louder in inspiration.
   (Murmurs on left side origin accentuate in expiration and murmurs on right side origin accentuate in inspiration).
2. Regurgitation
   Aortic regurgitation: Often missing, listen with diaphragm for soft whispered R' murmur with patient leaning forward in expiration.
   Austin-Flint murmur (functional mitral stenosis) may occur in aortic regurgitation.
   Pulmonary regurgitation: Usually due to pulmonary hypertension.
   Graham-Steel murmur (pulmonary regurgitation) may occur in mitral stenosis due to back pressure resulting into pulmonary hypertension.
3. Thickening: Mitral or tricuspid thickening, e.g. Carry-coombs murmur in active rheumatic carditis.
4. Increased AV flow rates—
   Mitral in VSD and PDA
   Tricuspid in ASD and TAPVD
   Diastolic murmur is organic for all practical purpose.

213. In 1900, Gibson described the diagnostic continuous murmur of patent ductus arteriosus and the murmur is appropriately named after him. Continuous murmur overlap (or pass through) the second heart sound and spill over to diastole with no respect to the boundaries of cardiac cycle. It need not change in character of its murmur from systole to diastole.

There are 4 situations where 'Continuous' or 'machinery' murmur is heard.

1. Patent ductus arteriosus (PDA)
   Common, heard in 2nd LICS or under clavicle.
   Rare
2. Aorto-pulmonary septal defect (2nd or 3rd LICS)
   Over the lungs (rare)
3. Pulmonary AV fistula
   Bronchial artery anastamosis in pulmonary atresia.
   Over the large veins

4. Venous hum.
   (Artificial ductus in Blalock or Waterston shunt)

The continuous murmur differs from a 'to and fro murmur' by the above features. The murmur of ventricular septal defect + aortic regurgitation, aortic stenosis + regurgitation, mitral stenosis + mitral regurgitation belong to the category of 'to and fro murmur' where S_2 is heard.

214. The 4 sounds or murmurs that are heard over the peripheral vessels

1. Aortic systolic murmur conducted into the carotids.
2. Aortic regurgitation pistol - shot sounds heard over the femorals.
3. Continuous murmur of humping quality was heard over the aneurysm and arteriovenous aneurysm.
4. In children, continuous 'venous hum' may occasionally be heard in the neck and conducted down into the upper chest diminished by slight change in posture.
   (Murmur is heard over the thyroid gland in thyrotoxicosis)

215. The simple technique called 'INCHING' is the best to follow for more accurate timing of the heart sounds and murmurs. The clinician uses the fact that the second sound is the louder of the two over the aortic area. This fact of loud second sound in aortic area is taken as a reference point as the examiner 'Inches' the stethoscope from the aortic area down to the apex.

There are 4 points to be followed by keeping the second sound in mind, as the stethoscope is inched downwards from the aortic area.

1. An extra sound that occurs in systole before the second sound is a systolic click.
2. If the sound occurs after the S_2, then it is a diastolic sound either S_3 or S_4 - diastolic gallop.
3. If a murmur occurs before the S_2, then it is a systolic murmur.
4. If a murmur occurs after the S_2, then it is a diastolic murmur.

This technique gives an accurate timing.

A ventricular diastolic gallop S_3 is usually absent at the base. As the 'Inching' downwards from aortic area to the apex occurs the S_3 appears after the S_2 and is easily identified.

On the other hand when there is S_4, which is a presystolic atrial gallop, the Inching' is done from below upwards, from the apex and lower border of the sternal border upwards to the base. The first heart sound is taken as a reference point because the extrasound is occurring in presystole before the first sound. S_4 disappears as the stethoscope is 'Inched' up. This way S_4 is easily identified as the sound being presystolic than early diastolic.

Mammary Souffle

216. The 4 features of mammary souffle—

1. It is an arterial murmur due to large flow of blood into the breast during later pregnancy and early postpartum period in lactacting women.
2. It is usually begins in the second or third trimester, or it may not begin until the first postpartum week. It usually lasts from several weeks to two months of postpartum.
3. It is usually heard along the left sternal border and is rarely more than 3/6 grade.
   It may disappear when the patient sits up.
4. It is usually late systolic and the murmur often passes through second sound into early diastole. Therefore, it must be distinguished from other causes of continuous murmur.

Valvular diseases

(See Chapter I-Valvular Heart Diseases for Details)

217. There are 4 common causes of valvular disease.

1. Congenital—usually affects on right side
2. Rheumatic—usually affects on left side
3. Syphilitic
4. Infective endocarditis. (Bacterial or Mycotic)
   (There are several other causes which are not frequent, e.g. Litman-Sach's endocarditis (SLE), carcinoid, ankylosing spondylitis, Marfan's, atheroma, dissecting aneurysm, trauma, etc.)

218. There are 4 congenital valvular lesions that are responsible for

1. Most cases of pulmonary valve disease
2. Some cases of aortic valve disease
3. Occasionally tricuspid valve
4. Rarely mitral valve.

219. The 4 valves that are being effected by rheumatic endocarditis in order of frequency.

1. Most frequently the mitral valve
2. Next the aortic valve
3. Infrequently tricuspid valve
4. Very rarely pulmonary valve.

220. The 4 age groups that help to know the etiology of valvular disease.

1. *Children:* Pulmonary valve stenosis is always congenital.
   Aortic stenosis may be of congenital origin, it may be a late development of accelerated aging process in congenital bicuspid valve disease.

2. *Young age:* Valvular involvement is mostly of rheumatic origin: Mitral valve is the commonest multiple valvular involvement always favors rheumatic origin. Aortic stenosis may arise from fusion of aortic valve cusps from rheumatic damage. Aortic regurgitation with stenosis always suggestive of rheumatic origin.
Arteriosclerosis mainly involves aortic valve—resulting in both stenosis and regurgitation. When it occurs in younger, it is always better to investigate for collagen diseases like periarteritis nodosa, disseminated lupus erythematosus, or thromboangitis obliterans in addition to syphilitic aortitis occluding the mouths of coronaries.
3. *Middle age:* Syphilis affects the aortic valve resulting in aortic regurgitation. Associated organic aortic stenosis denies syphilitic etiology. Syphilis never affects mitral or tricuspid.
4. *Old age:* Arteriosclerosis mainly involves aortic valve resulting in both stenosis and regurgitation. Mitral valve also may be affected. See for other evidence of arteriosclerotic changes in peripheral vessels. Hypertension and arteriosclerosis are mainly responsible for ischemic heart disease).

221. There are 4 types of valvular regurgitations as follows:

A diseased valve may be narrowed (stenosis) or may fail to close adequately (regurgitation) permitting regurgitation of blood. Regurgitation may be present without structural damage to the cusps as in

1. Mitral regurgitation from dilatation of mitral valve ring in left ventricular failure.
2. Tricuspid regurgitation—from dilatation of tricuspid valve ring in right ventricular failure.
3. Pulmonary regurgitation from dilatation of pulmonary valve ring in pulmonary hypertension.
4. Aortic regurgitation from dilatation of aortic valve ring in aortic aneurysm.

Mitral Stenosis
(See Chapter I - Valvular Heart Diseases)

222. The 4 Inspection and palpation findings in mitral stenosis are:

1. Soft pulse
2. Tapping apex
3. BP normal or slightly low
4. Presystolic thrill may be present (See for the signs of RVH also).

223. The 4 cardinal auscultatory features of mitral stenosis are:

1. Loud first heart sound.
2. Opening snap—Occurs relatively late in mild stenosis, early in severe mitral stenosis
If the mitral valve is rigid and calcified, there will be no accentuation of first sound and opening snap will be absent.
3. Mid-diastolic murmur, which is crescendo in nature, well localized, not conducted and best heard in the left lateral recumbent position with the bell.
4. Presystolic murmur due to increase in blood flow across the narrowed mitral valve during atrial contraction.
Murmurs can be absent when atrial fibrillation develops.

224. The 4 characteristic features of 'Opening snap' are:

Opening snap is heard only with AV valve stenosis.

1. Opening snap is a loud sound heard just after the second sound caused by abrupt checking of the valve opening (like the crack of a sail struck by a strong wind)
2. Closeness to second sound indicates severity of stenosis; 0.10 sec after second sound in mild to moderate stenosis; 0.06 sec after second sound in severe stenosis.
3. It indicates mobile AV valves, if the valve is rigid or calcified, there is no opening snap or accentuation of first sound.
4. It is maximal medial to apex, louder in expiration, thereby differentiating from P_2 split.

225. The following 4 characteristic features of mitral diastolic murmur in mitral stenosis are to be remembered.

1. It is best heard at the apex or medial to it, sharply localized without any direction of relative propagation.
2. Presystolic murmur (PSM) in mild cases, full length mid-diastolic murmur (MDM) due to increased flow through narrowed valve during atrial contraction. Murmur will be absent when atrial fibrillation develops.
3. Harsh, low pitched and rumbling because the blood is flowing through a narrowed orifice.
4. Crescendo in character intensity is low (in the beginning and slowly rises) best heard with the bell while the patient lies on left lateral recumbent position and is accentuated in expiration.
(sometimes associated with a thrill.)

226. There are 4 X-ray findings in mitral stenosis.

1. Straightening of the left border
2. Prominent pulmonary conus
3. Right ventricle and right atrial enlargement
4. Sickle shaped esophagus shadow in barium swallow of RAO chest X-ray caused by enlarged left atrium.

227. The 4 findings of ECG in mitral stenosis shows.

1. Atrial hypertrophy notched 'M' 'Mitrale' -P more than 2.5 mm wide in left atrial enlargement. When severe pulmonary hypertension etc. complicates, tall and more peaked P 'Pulmonale' more than 2.5 mm height in right atrial enlargement, more than 2.5 mm height and wide indicated biatrial enlargement.
2. Right axis deviation
3. Right ventricular hypertrophy
4. Fibrillary waves when atrial fibrillation develops.

Baseline shows coarser undulation in atrial fibrillation of mitral stenosis origin than the coronary artery disease origin.

When left ventricular hypertrophy is present it suggests that additional lesion is present such as mitral regurgitation, aortic valvular disease or hypertension.

228. The following 4 findings are seen in echocardiogram which is the most specific noninvasive method for diagnosing mitral stenosis.

1. M-mode echo shows: Anterior and posterior leaflet do not show wide separation in early diastole, i.e. less than 15 mm and they maintain fixed relation throughout diastole.
2. Reduction in EF slope This slope is related to the severity of obstruction. It reflects failure of anterior leaflet of the mitral valve to float back to mid position in mid diastole.
3. Multilayered echos or thickening of echo pattern in calcified and thickened mitral valve—which restrict the movement.
4. Two-dimensional echocardiogram determines the area of mitral orifice.

The left atrium is usually enlarged.

229. The following 4 clinical features indicate the severity of the mitral stenosis.

1. When dyspnea becomes worse
2. When left atrium is enlarged
3. When diastolic murmur is longer
4. When 'Opening snap' is closer to second sound.

230. The 4 steps for the management of mitral stenosis are:

1. Digoxin and diuretics (For failure and atrial fibrillation)
2. Anticoagulants to prevent emboli
3. Antibiotics to prevent infective endocarditis
4. Balloon valvuloplasty/surgery (valvotomy or valve replacement depending on the condition).

231. There are 4 common complications of mitral stenosis.

1. Pulmonary hypertension
2. Congestive cardiac failure
3. Atrial fibrillation
4. Embolism.

Mitral Regurgitation (See Chapter I- Valvular Heart Diseases)

232. The 4 signs of mitral regurgitation.

1. Collapsing pulse
2. Apex beat displaced laterally and heaving
3. Systolic thrill may be present
4. Muffled mitral first sound because mitral valve could not close due to incompetency. Presence of third heart sound indicates severe mitral regurgitation. A blowing pan systolic murmur best heard in the mitral area, conducted toward the axilla and angle of left scapula.

233. The 4 characters of systolic murmur in mitral regurgitation are:

1. It is heard in full systole—'Pan systolic' because the blood is leaking through the mitral valve as ventricle contracts. So, it starts with first sound and continues throughout systole.
2. It is best heard at the mitral area, radiates toward the axilla and angle of left scapula.
3. It is blowing, best heard in left lateral recumbent position.
4. It increases in intensity with expiration.

234. The 4 different names of systolic click-murmur syndrome

1. Prolapsing mitral; valve leaflet syndrome
2. Barlow's syndrome
3. Floppy valve syndrome
4. Billowing mitral leaflet syndrome.

235. The 4 findings of systolic clickmurmur

1. Mid or late systolic click which occurs 0.14 sec - or more after first sound. Clicks may be multiple.
2. High pitched late systolic crescendo-decrescendo murmur best heard at the apex in left lateral recumbent position, occasionally 'whooping or honking'.
3. Click and murmur occur earlier in standing, valsalva maneuver or inhalation of amylnitrite all of which reduces left ventricular volume.
4. Click and murmur may be delayed or disappeared by squatting isometric exercises which increase left ventricular enddiastolic volume.

236. The 4 usually associated features of late systolic murmur in the mitral area systolic click murmur syndrome indicates mitral regurgitation).

1. Prolapse of floppy valvular cusps -
   Posterior leaflet of mitral valve prolapses during systole to give a late systolic 'Click' and murmur. It may be

an incidental finding (in 5% of people) or associated with Marfan's syndrome.
2. Diseases of chordae tendinae
3. Papillary muscle dysfunction
4. Ruptured papillary muscle following myocardial infarction.

AORTIC STENOSIS

(See Chapter I- Valvular Heart Diseases)

237. There are 4 causes of obstruction to the left ventricular outflow.

1. Aortic stenosis
2. Hypertrophic obstructive cardiomyopathy (HOCM)
3. Discrete congenital subvalvular aortic stenosis.caused by membranous diaphragm or fibrous ridge below the aortic valve.
4. Supravalvular aortic stenosis caused by narrowing of ascending aorta or fibrous diaphragm above the aortic valve.

238. The 4 etiological factors of aortic stenosis are:

1. Congenital
2. Rheumatic—almost always associated with involvement of mitral valve. Often accompanies aortic regurgitation.
3. Accelerated aging process in a congenital bicuspid valve—it is a late development—found in 0.5% of routine postmortems in elderly.
4. Idiopathic calcific aortic stenosis in old age due to degenerative process—a 'wear-and-tear' phenomenon.

239. About 1/4 of all patients with chronic valvular disease suffer from aortic stenosis.

240. There are 4 symptoms in aortic stenosis.

1. Breathlessness—exertional dyspnea—caused by increased pulmonary capillary pressure which in turn is caused by increased left atrial and left ventricular end diastolic pressures.
2. Chest pain anginal pain caused by compression of coronary vessels.
3. Syncope—caused by low cardiac output.
4. Dizziness and sudden death is common when associated with severe aortic stenosis.

Obstruction of any one of the heart valves can cause syncope and dizziness. Aortic stenosis is the most common cause since it is more close to the brain—the closer the valve to the brain, the more likely it can cause syncope.

Eighty percent of patients with symptomatic aortic stenosis are male.

Valve must be replaced, if aortic valve disease gives symptoms.

241. The 4 Inspection and Palpation findings of Aortic stenosis are

1. Slow sustained small pulse (anacrotic)
2. Apex is heaving and sustained throughout systole and is displaced downwards and outwards, characteristic of left ventricular hypertrophy.
3. Low systolic and high diastolic blood pressure with low pulse pressure.
   (A systolic pressure of more than 200 mm Hg. practically excludes aortic stenosis)
4. A systolic thrill over the aortic area or in the neck above the clavicle.

242. The 4 auscultatory findings in aortic stenosis are:

1. Aortic ejection click (like 'opening snap' of mitral stenosis) due to opening of aortic valve in aortic stenosis. It is therefore heard just after the first sound at the beginning of ejection murmur. No click is heard if the valve is fibrosed or calcified.
2. Absent or feeble aortic second sound: A_2 is feeble because of delayed and soft closure of aortic valve. Left ventricle takes longer time to expel its blood through narrowed aortic valve. Pulmonary valve closure may precede, which causes reversed splitting of the second sound. Second sound widens on expiration, narrows on inspiration 'paradoxical splitting' of second sound. The paradoxical (or reversed) splitting of the second sound may be present with severe degree of obstruction and it is much more common in hypertrophic obstructive cardiomyopathy.
3. A high pitched rough mid systolic ejection murmur best heard over the aortic area and may be heard at the apex, increase on expiration.
   All murmurs due to ejection of blood through abnormal semilunar valves (e.g. in aortic stenosis or pulmonary stenosis) or abnormally high blood flow through normal semilunar valves, e.g. in systemic hypertension or pulmonary hypertension) are called ejection systolic murmurs.
   Both aortic and pulmonary ejection murmur have the same pattern.
4. Systolic murmur radiates with the blood stream to the carotid as in so-called 'Carotid shudder'.

The murmur is at least grade III/IV with significant obstruction.

Occasionally, when the murmur is transmitted downward and to the apex, it is confused with the murmur of mitral regurgitation. However, it can be differentiated as the mitral regurgitation systolic murmur is holosystolic, whereas, aortic stenosis murmur is diamond-shaped and of ejection type.

AORTIC REGURGITATION
(See Chapter I- Valvular Heart Diseases)

243. ¾ of all patients with pure aortic regurgitation are males. Females predominate among patients with aortic regurgitation associated with mitral valve disease).

244. The 4 common causes of aortic regurgitation are:
1. Congenital from abnormal bicuspid valve
2. Rheumatic
3. Tertiary syphilis
4. Infective endocarditis.

Rheumatic etiology is less common in isolated aortic regurgitation. Coexistence of significant aortic stenosis with aortic regurgitation usually excludes all rarer forms of aortic regurgitation because it occurs almost in rheumatic or congenital basis.

245. The 4 less common or rare causes of aortic regurgitation are:
1. Atheroma
2. Cystic medial necrosis of ascending aorta with or without manifestations of Marfan's syndrome
3. Ankylosing rheumatoid spondylitis
4. Severe hypertension.

246. Search for the 4 causes predisposing to aortic regurgitation
1. Syphilis
2. Essential hypertension
3. Marfan's syndrome
4. Ankylosing rheumatoid spondylitis

247. The 4 findings on inspection and palpation are:
1. See for the following signs in peripheral vessels.
   a. Corrigan's pulse a rapidly rising 'water-hammer pulse' which collapses suddenly in diastole 'Collapsing pulse'.
   A quick rise or flip' of the radial pulse may even better be felt by rising the arms over the head. This simple maneuver makes this type of pulse more evident in aortic regurgitation.
   b. Corrigan's neck sign—pulsatile neck vessels—caused by abrupt distension and collapse of larger arteries.
   c. de Musset's sign—sobbing or nodding motion of the head with each systole.
   d. Quncke's pulse capillary pulsation in nail beds on applying pressure to nail tips.
   e. Pistol shot sounds can be heard over the femoral artery or to and fro murmur (Duroziez's murmur or sign) due to retrograde flow of blood audible by lightly pressing with stethoscope.
2. High systolic and low diastolic BP with wide pulse pressure.
   How important this wide pulse pressure is surprising. For example in some patients an aortic systolic murmur followed by aortic diastolic murmur was heard—the characterstic of 'to and fro' murmur. The systolic murmur in some cases was accompanied by aortic systolic thrill. Because of these findings aortic stenosis was diagnosed in addition to aortic regurgitation. However, subsequently at operation or autopsy, stenosis was not present but only regurgitation. In such conditions where there is a loud systolic murmur even with a palpable thrill, if a wide pulse pressure exists—the SBP of 170 to 180 or above and DBP of 40 to 30 or down to 0, the patient has only regurgitation—no stenosis.
3. Heaving apex beat in 6th or 7th left intercostal space in the anterior axillary line is suggestive of left ventricular hypertrophy.
4. A diastolic thrill may be palpable.
   (Thrill is not common.)

248. The 4 auscultatory findings in aortic regurgitation are:
1. An early diastolic murmur, high pitched, soft, blowing, whisphered decresendo diastolic murmur heard in the aortic area or 3rd left intercostal space which is conducted down and to the left toward mitral area. The murmur is short in mild regurgitation, becomes louder and longer as the severity increases and is usually holodiastolic in free aortic regurgitation.
2. Listen carefully with diaphragm, best heard in patient sitting up, leaning forward in expiration—often it is missed. Murmur is intensified by isometric exercise such as handgrip, reduced by inhalation of amyl nitrite.
   When it is best heard along the right sternal border, it is suggestive that regurgitation is caused by aneurysm of aortic root.
3. An associated ejection systolic murmur can be present. When aortic regurgitation is large, the left ventricle has to pump double the normal volume of blood during systole, which gives rise to aortic systolic ejection murmur; So, presence of ejection systolic thrill or murmur in aortic regurgitation need not necessarily indicates associated aortic stenosis.
4. Austin-Flint murmur (functional mitral stenosis) may occur in aortic incompetence. It is a soft low pitched, rumbling presystolic or mid diastolic murmur caused by the displacement of anterior leaflet of mitral valve by the aortic regurgitant flow.

Therefore, three murmurs were heard in severe aortic regurgitation, 'to and fro' murmur of early diastolic murmur, an ejection systolic murmur and Austin-Flint murmur occurring in mid diastole with some components of presystole.

"Cooing" or musical diastolic murmur is caused by vibration of everted aortic cusp in the regurgitant stream.

249. A quickrise in pulse, water-hammer or Corrigan pulse is a consistent finding of aortic regurgitation—a diagnostic possibility either to accept or refuse. When we auscultate for diastolic murmur with the patient sitting, leaning forward with breath holding in expiration at the left 3rd sternal border, a systolic murmur is heard instead of diastolic murmur — then suspect hypertrophic cardiomyopathy. Ask the patient to stand, the murmur becomes louder, then listen in squatting position, the murmur decreases in intensity. This standing and squatting maneuver is repeated several times because the characteristic change may occur after three or four times. So to differentiate from hypertrophy the 4 steps are:

1. A quick rise in pulse, water-hammer, Corrigan pulse is felt.
2. Look for aortic regurgitation which is conspicuous by its absence of diastolic murmur.
3. Systolic murmur is heard instead of diastolic murmur in hypertrophic cardiomyopathy.
4. Listen in squatting position—repeat standing and squatting for several time—the murmur becomes louder in standing diminishes in intensity in squatting in hypertrophic cardiomyopathy.

These patients have symptoms of coronary artery disease. These patients may not have symptoms of syncope or dizziness. Sudden death in young athelets under 30 years age is due to ventricular fibrillation—hypertrophic cardiomyopathy is most likely cause. Squatting maneuvar helps to identify this condition early.

Tricuspid Stenosis
(See Chapter I- Valvular Heart Diseases)

250. The 4 inspection and palpation signs of tricuspid stenosis are:

1. Small pulse
2. Giant 'a' wave in the JVP with presystolic hepatic pulsations.
3. Quiet heart without parasternal lift or pulsations.
4. BP within normal limits.

251. The 4 auscultatory findings of tricuspid stenosis are:

1. Presystolic or mid-diastolic murmur of the same characteristics as in mitral stenosis but
2. Located in tricuspid area with no selective propagation
3. Accentuated during inspiration
4. Usually associated with other valvular involvement most commonly rheumatic mitral stenosis or with combination of mitral stenosis and aortic stenosis.

TRICUSPID REGURGITATION
(See Chapter I - Valvular Heart Diseases)

252. The 4 etiological factors of tricuspid regurgitation is

1. Ebstein's anomaly: It is the downward displacement of tricuspid valve ring and leaflet into the right ventricle.
2. Usually functional—Secondary to marked dilatation of right ventricle and tricuspid valve ring. Complicate right ventricular failure of any cause.
   a. Congestive cardiac failure of any cause—rheumatic or congenital heart disease.
   b. Ischemic heart disease—Inferior wall infarction of right ventricle.
   Infarction of right ventricle papillary muscle.
   c. Cardiomyopathy, e.g. endomyocardial fibrosis.
   d. Pulmonary hypertension, chronic cor pulmonale.
3. Infective endocarditis
4. Carcinoid heart disease.

253. Signs of tricuspid regurgitation: They are usually functional wherever there is dilatation of the heart.

The 4 findings on inspection and palpation are:

1. Venous throbbing in the neck.
2. Pulsating jugular veins in the neck.
   A large 'V' wave in the JVP which may move the ear lobes with the patient reclining at 45°. The diagnosis is often made from the neck veins. The characteristic changes in the venous pulse disappear or diminish when the heart failure is controlled.
3. Pulsatile liver—systolic hepatic pulsations present
4. Hyperdynamic right ventricular thrust, i.e. right ventricular heave is present.

254. The 4 auscultatory findings in tricuspid regurgitation are (mechanism is similar to mitral regurgitation)

1. Pan systolic murmur
2. Best heard in the tricuspid area
3. With or without a thrill
4. Murmur is accentuated during inspiration which draws more blood into right side during inspiration. Murmur is reduced during expiration or Valsalva maneuver.

Pulmonary Stenosis

Signs of pulmonary stenosis: usually congenital and so present from birth.

255. The 4 findings on inspection and palpation are:

1. Small pulse
2. Slapping apex beat
3. Right ventricular heave at the left sternal border
4. Systolic thrill in the pulmonary area.

256. The 4 auscultatory findings in pulmonary stenosis are:

1. Rough ejection systolic murmur best heard in the pulmonary area
2. Increased during inspiration
3. Conducted towards the middle of the clavicle
4. Absent or feeble second sound.
(Pulmonary regurgitation is very rare. Occasionally present in mitral stenosis or pulmonary hypertension.)

HEART FAILURE
(See Chapter C - Heart Failure for Details)

257. Heart failure can be described in 4 types.

1. Right heart failure
2. Left heart failure
3. Conbined heart failure

} Central circulatory failure

4. Peripheral circulatory failure

More than 75% of the management of heart diseases consists in treating the heart failure. Most of the heart diseases first cause either right or left sided heart failure. Therefore, it is imperative to know which type of heart failure is present.

Following anatomical principles are born in mind for clear understanding of heart failure.

Though anatomically, the heart has evolved to be one organ, physiologically it consists of two pumps. The right heart pumps blood into the lungs through the lesser circulation and the left heart to all other tissues through the systemic circulation.

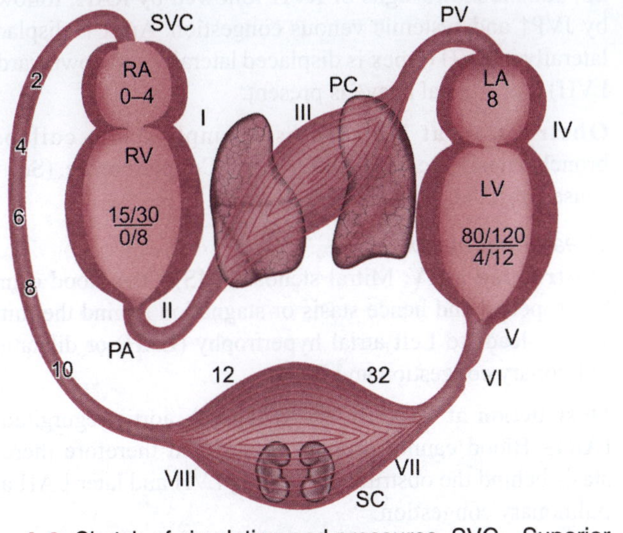

Fig. A-9: Sketch of circulation and pressures. SVC—Superior vena cava: RA—Right atrium; RV—Right ventricle; PA—Pulmonary artery; PC—Pulmonary circulation; PV—Pulmonary vein; LA—Left atrium; LV—Left ventricle; SC—Systemic circulation

The study of the Figure A-9 of the heart will illustrate the point clearly. In diseases, these pressures are disturbed and dilatation or hypertrophy of one chamber or other is caused. The right heart encounters the resistance offered by the lesser circulation as shown in the diagram at the levels I, II and III, while the left heart encounters the resistance offered by the greater circulation as shown in the diagram at the levels IV, V, VI, VII and VIII.

258. Obstruction at various levels of circulation causes the following:

Lesser Circulation

1. At I: Tricuspid stenosis leads to right atrial hypertrophy, dilatation and ischemic lung fields.
2. At II: Pulmonary stenosis leads to right ventricular hypertrophy, and ischemic lung fields.
3. At III: Fibrosis, emphysema, collapse, bronchiectasis etc. lead to right ventricular hypertrophy and cor pulmonale.

Greater Circulation

4. At IV: Mitral stenosis leads to left atrial hypertrophy, dilatations, pulmonary congestion and right ventricular hypertrophy.
5. At V: Aortic stenosis, aortic regurgitation lead to left ventricular hypertrophy and later pulmonary congestion.
6. At VI: Coarctation of aorta leads to left ventricular hypertrophy and later pulmonary congestion.
7. At VII: Essential hypertension leads to left ventricular hypertrophy and later pulmonary congestion.
8. At VIII: Acute nephritis, chronic nephritis, polycystic kidney, pyelonephritis, etc. lead to renal hypertension resulting in left ventricular hypertrophy and later pulmonary congestion.

When the right heart or left heart fails, it fails to propel the blood forwards and therefore there will be stasis or stagnation of the blood immediately behind it.

259. The 4 signs of left ventricular failure.

1. Breathlessness as the main symptom.
Pulmonary crepitation
Pulmonary edema
Plural effusion
} Depending on congestion of pulmonary circulation
2. Gallop rhythm
3. Pulsus Alternans
4. Cheyne Stokes respiration
} Depending on failing left ventricle

260. The 4 signs of right ventricular failure.

1. Engorged neck veins (JVP) and of the upper limb and those of the superior vena caval territory.

2. Enlarged and tender liver
3. Edema feet or other dependent parts of inferior vena caval territory

} Depending on systemic venous congestion

4. Right ventricular gallop rhythm—depending on a failing ventricle.

Combination of both signs may be present in combined failure.

261. Peripheral circulatory failure is caused when there is disparity between the circulating blood volume content and the volume capacity of blood vessels.

1. Severe hemorrhage of whatever origin
2. Severe diarrhea or vomiting leading to dehydration.

} Depending on the diminution of volume content

3. Shock
4. Collapse

} Depending on the increase of volume capacity following paralyzed capillaries.

262. The 4 main signs of peripheral circulatory failure are:

1. Apathy or symptoms of restlessness
2. Pale, cold, clammy skin
3. Rapid and thready pulse
4. Low BP

Pericardial Disease (See Chapter N for Details)

263. The 4 signs of pericardial disease are:

1. Pulsus paradoxus—Rotch's and Ewart's sign
2. Increased cardiac dullness—left border is far away from, the apex beat.
3. Distant heart sounds
4. Pericardial rub—This is heard when there is dry pericarditis and disappears when there is effusion.

It is a to and fro rub frequently associated with pain appearing and disappearing easily gives quadruple rhythm, which gives the impression of the cadence of a running train.

SUMMARY

CLINICAL APPROACH TO THE DIAGNOSIS OF HEART DISEASE

(This is mainly for the family physician (FP)/general practitioner (GP) who have no access to the latest equipments—especially those working in rural primary health center (PHC) or tribal areas and those independent FP/GPs of under developed countries. This is followed during our student days in 1950s and 1960s when there were no facilities for advanced equipments like echocardiogram, etc.)

264. This can be conveniently described in 4 steps.

I. First Step

Follow Point A-10

i. Is there any physiological disturbance?
ii. Whether there is any overload or strain or hypertrophy.

How to recognize whether there is any overload or strain or dilatation or hypertrophy of any chamber?

Follow Figure A-9

Careful study of the diagram gives average pressures of each chamber and blood vessels. In diseases, these pressures are disturbed and dilatation or hypertrophy of chamber one or other is caused.

The right side of the heart encounters the resistance offered by the lesser circulation as shown in the figure—At the level I, II, and III.

While left side of the heart encounter the resistance offered by the greater circulation as shown in the figure—At the levels IV, V, VI, VII and VIII.

Obstruction at various levels of circulation causes the following:

Lesser circulation:

Obstruction at I—Tricuspid stenosis (TS): Leads to right atrial hypertrophy (RAH), dilatation and ischemic lung fields, JVP↑.

Obstruction at II—Pulmonary stenosis (PS): Leads to right ventricular hypertrophy and ischemic lung fields (Pulmonary oligemia). The right ventricle cannot propel the blood forward and therefore there will be stasis or stagnation of blood behind. So, patient shows signs of RVH followed by RAH, followed by JVP↑ and systemic venous congestion. Apex is displaced laterally in RVH (Apex is displaced laterally and downward in LVH). Parasternal heave is present.

Obstruction at III: Fibrosis, emphysema, collapse, bronchiectasis, etc. leads to RVH and Cor pulmonale. (See for causes of RVH, S/S of RVH).

Greater circulation

Obstruction at IV: Mitral stenosis (MS)—the blood cannot be propelled and hence stasis or stagnation behind the mitral valve—leads to Left atrial hypertrophy (LAH) or dilatation, pulmonary congestion and RVH.

Obstruction at V: Aortic stenosis (AS), aortic regurgitation (AR)—Blood cannot propel forward and therefore there is stasis behind the obstruction causing LVH and later LAH and pulmonary congestion.

Obstruction at VI: Coarctation of aorta—leads to LVH

Obstruction at VII: Essential hypertension due to increased peripheral vascular resistance → leads to LVH → later pulmonary congestion.

Obstruction at VIII: Acute nephritis, chronic nephritis, polycystic kidney, pyelonephritis, etc. leads to renal hypertension (secondary hypertension) resulting in LVH → and later pulmonary congestion.

See for the apex—LVH

See for the causes of LVH

LVH is followed by → LAH → followed later by pulmonary congestion.

Auscultation of P_2: which has aortic and pulmonary component.

P_2 abnormalities – P_2 split, P_2 loudness gives an idea whether there is LVH or RVH is present (A 162 & 163). P_2 split is an important sign to differentiate the hypertrophy of ventricles. When there is hypertrophy of one ventricle, there is an asynchronous closure of the semilunar valves. The closure of the semilunar valves of hypertrophied ventricle lags behind and causes the splitting of the second sound. The splitting widens during inspiration and shortens with expiration in RVH. In LVH splitting widens with expiration and closes with inspiration.

If the RVH is recognized, the diseases causing resistance to the lesser circulation like mitral stenosis, pulmonary hypertension, emphysema, fibrosis, collapse of the lung, etc. can be thought of and others are excluded. If the LVH is recognized the diseases causing resistance to the grater circulation like hypertension either essential or renal, or endocrinal or aortic valve disease (AS), etc. are thought of and others are excluded.

Once RVH or LVH is recognized, search for the causes that gives rise to P_2 split in relation to other characters—it gives an idea that which chamber is enlarged.

When the right heart or left heart fails, it fails to propel the blood forward and therefore there will be stasis or stagnation of the blood behind it.

After recognizing LVH or RVH, see whether there is any heart failure (HF) or not.

Whatever the etiology is, the ultimate result of cardio-vascular disease (CVD) is heart failure. More than 75% of the management of heart disease consists in treating the heart failure. Therefore, it is important either for the specialist or the FP/GP that he should recognize the heart failure in the early stages so that he can give the best results.

Most of the heart diseases cause either right side or left side heart failure. Therefore, it is necessary to know which type of heart failure is present. For clear understanding of heart failure, it is better that the following important anatomical principles are born in mind.

Though, anatomically the heart has evolved to the one organ, physiologically it consists of two separate pumps. The right heart pumps blood into the lungs through lesser circulation and left heart to all other parts through the systemic circulation (See Figure A-9).

Following are the signs of each type of failure.

1. Signs of left ventricular failure (LVF)—See A-259
2. Sings of right ventricular failure (RVF)—See A-260
3. Sings of combined heart failure (CHF)
4. Peripheral circulatory failure—See A-261

II. Second Step

1. How to recognize the physical defects which lead to the heart failure?

As already mentioned, the physical defects can be from

- i. Endocardium—Valvular
- ii. Myocardium
- iii. Pericardium
- iv. Vascular

Is it valvular?

Signs of mitral stenosis (MS) (See A-222–223, 224)

- i. Soft pulse
- ii. Tapping apex
- iii. BP normal or slightly low
- iv. Presystolic thrill
- v. S_1 loud
- vi. Opening snap
- vii. Mid–diastolic murmur
- viii. Presystolic murmur

Murmurs can be absent when atrial fibrillation (AF) develops.

2. Signs of mitral regurgitation (See A-232–234, 235)

- i. Collapsing pulse (Corrigan/Water hammer pulse)
- ii. Apex beat tends to be heaving
- iii. A blowing, pansystolic murmur, best heard in the mitral area conducted toward the axilla and behind
- iv. Systolic thrill may be present
- v. Muffled mitral S_1—because the mitral valve could not close due to mitral incompetence
- vi. S_3 occasionally heard

3. Signs of aortic stenosis (See A-239–241)

- i. Slow sustained small pulse (anacrotic)
- ii. Heaving apex—displaced downwards and outwards – forceful and sustained throughout systole.
- iii. A systolic thrill over the aortic area or in the neck above the clavicle.
- iv. A rough mid systolic ejection murmur best heard over the aortic area conducted along the carotid arteries and may be heard as well at the apex.
- v. Absent or feeble aortic second sound—aortic valve cannot close, no spring door action because the aortic pressure is greater than left ventricular pressure.

vi. LVH sings (in X-ray and ECG)
vii. Low systolic and high diastolic BP with low pulse pressure.
viii. Aortic ejection click, $P_2\uparrow\uparrow$, paradoxical P_2 split.

4. **Signs of aortic regurgitation: (See A-246, 247).**
 i. Collapsing or water hammer pulse (Corrigan pulse)
 ii. Pulsatile neck vessels (Corrigan neck signs)
 iii. Heaving apex located in the 6th or 7th LICS usually in the anterior axillary line (Heaving but not sustained)
 iv. An early diastolic murmur, soft and blowing in quality best heard in the aortic area or 3rd LICS which is conducted down and to the left toward the mitral area.
 v. Pistol shot sounds or Duroziez's murmur heard over the femorals.
 vi. Signs of LVH (X-ray and ECG)
 vii. High systolic and low diastolic BP with wide pulse pressure.

5. **Signs of tricuspid stenosis (TS) (See A-250, 254).**
 i. Small pulse
 ii. Giant 'a' wave in the jugular pulse with presystolic hepatic pulsation.
 iii. Quiet heart without a parasternal lift or pulsations.
 iv. Presystolic or mid diastolic murmur of the same characteristics as that of mitral stenosis but located in the tricuspid area, and is accentuated during inspiration.
 v. X-ray with enlarged right atrium and oligemic lung fields.
 vi. BP within normal limits.
 vii. Usually associated with other valvular involvement

6. **Signs of tricuspid incompetence (See A-253, 254).**
 i. Venous throbbing in the neck
 ii. Pulsatile jugular veins in the neck
 iii. Pulsatile liver
 iv. Hyperdynamic right ventricular thrust
 v. A pan systolic murmur with or without a thrill localized over the tricuspid area and which increases during inspiration.
 vi. Usually functional whenever there is dilatation of the heart.

7. **Signs of pulmonary stenosis (PS) (See A-255, 256).**

 This is usually congenital in origin and so present from birth.
 i. Small pulse
 ii. Slapping apex beat
 iii. Wide left parasternal pulsations.
 iv. Right ventricular lift
 v. Systolic thrill in the pulmonary area
 vi. Rough ejection systolic murmur best heard in the pulmonary area increased during inspiration and may be conducted toward the middle of left clavicle.
 vii. Absent or feeble pulmonary second sound.
 viii. Oligemic lung fields with RVH (in X-ray and ECG)

8. **Signs of pulmonary regurgitation.**
 i. Very rare
 ii. Occasionally present in mitral stenosis or with pulmonary hypertension.
 iii. Early diastolic murmur indistinguishable from that of aortic regurgitation well localized without conduction and without circulatory changes as in aortic regurgitation.

III. Step of Approach is to know the Etiological Factor

Known from birth—Congenital
Young—Rheumatic
Middle age—Hypertension, syphilis
Old age—Ischemic

Congenital heart disease as already mentioned involve the right side of the heart.

The 4 common congenital heart disease seen in practice are:

1. Atrial septal defect (ASD)—which is recognized by RVH, with wide P_2 fixed split.
2. Ventricular septal defect (VSD)—is recognized by loud pan systolic murmur in the left 3rd and 4th ICS, associated with a thrill and shows no preponderance of one ventricle over the other.
3. Patent ductus arteriosus (PDA)—is know by continuous machinery murmur in the left 2nd ICS, associated with a thrill and with signs of left ventricular hypertrophy (LVH).
4. Fallot's tetralogy—is the commonest cyanotic heart disease and is recognized by its cyanosis. Clubbing and signs of pulmonary stenosis.

Pulmonary stenosis: with or without other defects is almost always congenital.

Majority of chronic disease of the heart up to middle age is due to rheumatic heart disease. Next common cause is ischemic heart disease presenting either from hypertension or from atherosclerosis. In advance countries where the ravages of acute rheumatic fever could be controlled, the hypertension and ischemic heart diseases are top in the list as an etiological factor. In India rheumatic heart disease is still prevalent as we could not fully control during the acute rheumatic fever stage.

Presently, in India IHD/CAD cases are increasing in number along with increasing number of hypertension and diabetic patients.

In the young age, rheumatic fever makes us an extensive damage of the layers of the heart in acute stage resulting in myocardial failure and death. A few cases may going for pericardial effusion.

Pericardial effusion of this rheumatic etiology is rarely troublesome as spontaneous recovery is the rule with or without treatment. On the other hand, damage to the endocardium during the acute stage is the one that is responsible for the frequently occurring valvular disease. Almost all cases of pure mitral stenosis or combination of mitral stenosis with other valvular diseases are due to rheumatic fever.

In the middle age, aortic incompetence due to syphilis is not frequently seen as before. Association of aortic stenosis denies the luetic etiology. Mitral and tricuspid valves are never affected by syphilis.

In old age, atherosclerosis mainly involves the aortic valve resulting in both stenosis and regurgitation. Mitral valve may also be affected. In this cases, there is some evidence of arteriosclerotic changes in the peripheral vessels. Hypertension and arteriosclerosis are mainly responsible for ischemic heart disease (IHD). When it occurs in the younger age group, it is always better to bear in mind the collagen diseases like periarteritis nodosa, disseminated lupus erythematosis or thromboangiitis obliterans in addition to syphilitic aortitis occluding the mouths of coronaries.

Anemia, beriberi, thyrotoxicosis, alcohol, etc. lead to generalized involvement of the myocardium and results in hyperdynamic circulatory failure. Smoking is another common important cause of IHD/CAD.

They are easily recognizable and reversible with proper treatment.

IV. Step: To Elicit the Extent of Functional Disability

(NYHA —functional disability – E 50, 51)
This helps in rehabilitation of the patient, to decrease the cardiac neurosis, apprehension, etc. and make the patient to do his normal routine work. Breathing exercises, physical exercises like walking, etc. is advised to IHD/CAD, post MI, post CABG, to bring to as near as normal activity.

265. Steps to a healthy heart

Table A-21

Do's	*Don'ts*
1. Reduce salt intake	Avoid smoking
2. Exercise regularly	Avoid alcohol
3. Take enough rest	Avoid fatty foods
4. Eat high fiber diet, green leafy vegetables and fresh fruits	Avoid hurry, worry and curry (curry means diet)

(The aim of this summary is to give only few salient points which help in the diagnosis of heart diseases and details are given in respective chapters).

B Hypertension

Since its description by William Harvey in 1628, blood pressure and other hypertensive studies have been progressed tremendously to the present knowledge.

The most common circulatory disorder is hypertension. This is a common disease especially when one gets older. It is estimated that more than 60 million people in USA have hypertension and one billion worldwide have hypertension. This is a common disease in the old age. As the population ages, the prevalence of hypertension increases. It presents the biggest single problem in continuing primary health care. It is much widely published in the United States as 'the silent killer' a title which greatly adds discomfort in the minds of some patients. There are many books written as a whole or some aspects of it but may be very few written by a primary care physician, general practitioner, family medicine specialist for his colleagues. Since this is essentially a malady for family doctors—it is time to work to prevent the complications mainly of target organs—heart, brain, kidneys and eyes. What is expected in this chapter is mainly the account how to manage the condition besides dealing with the intellectual and technical aspect.

1. Prevalence and risk of hypertension.

1. Hypertension prevalence is 60 million people in US
2. Blood pressure relation to risk in cardiovascular diseases (CVD) is continuous, consistent and independent of other risk factors.
3. Each increment of 20/10 mm Hg doubles the risk of CVD, across the entire blood pressure range starting from 115/75 mm Hg.
4. Prehypertension signals the need for education to reduce blood pressure in order to prevent hypertension.

2. An attempted definition of hypertension is given since the factors to give precise definition make it difficult.

1. Probable best definition of hypertension is that it is a sustained blood pressure above the average for the person's age. Blood pressure is the lateral pressure exerted on the vessel wall by the blood contained within.

   Many textbooks state that in practical terms the hypertension is a sustained blood pressure of systolic BP (SBP) 140 mm Hg or greater and/or diastolic BP (DBP) 90 mm Hg or greater.

   The WHO definition of high blood pressure is as under:

   - A systolic pressure equal to or above 160 mm Hg and a diastolic pressure equal to or greater than 95 mm Hg is hypertension.
   - A normal blood pressure is a systolic blood pressure equal to or less than 140 mm Hg and a diastolic pressure equal to or less than 90 mm Hg. Blood pressure in between are labeled as borderline hypertension. However, this is an over simplification for the following reasons.
2. The average blood pressure of apparently healthy persons increases with age, indicating that it is fallacious to choose any one blood pressure reading as normal or abnormal for all ages.
3. At any particular age in a society, there is a scatter of blood pressure among apparently healthy persons. The pressure is high in non-white population of the same age. It varies not only with age but with race, sex also.

4. There is no cut-off level beneath which the complications of hypertension do not occur. The risk of cardiovascular complications such as heart failure, myocardial infarction, stroke increases as the blood pressure increases.

However, at any age a high blood pressure carries a greater risk of adverse events than a low blood pressure.
Treating systolic blood pressure (SBP) and diastolic blood pressure (DBP) to targets that are <140/90 mm Hg is associated with decrease in cardiovascular disease complications. *In patients with diabetes mellitus and renal disease the BP goal is 130/80 mm Hg.*

3. There are 4 factors that determine the blood pressure.

The two main physiological factors:
1. Multiple of cardiac output
2. Peripheral vascular resistance.
   And
3. Neuronal autonomic reflexes—both sympathetic and parasympathetic.
4. Chemical: Renin-angiotensin-aldosterone system.
   Each of these parameters are in turn dependent upon other factors.

4. Main factors that determine the systolic and diastolic pressure are systolic pressure.

1. The volume of blood ejected during systole and the response to it.
2. The compliance or elasticity of the walls of the arterial tree. If systolic pressure is low the stroke volume is small or alternatively if the arterial walls are very dispensable. By contrast systolic pressure will be high if the stroke volume is large or the walls of the vessels are rigid.
   Diastolic pressure is determined mainly by:
3. Diameter of the lumen.
4. Elasticity of the arterial walls—gripping and exerting pressure upon the blood whilst the aortic valve is closed and the heart is not pumping. Diastolic pressure determines flow of blood during diastole as well as systole. It is also responsible for filling of the coronary arteries during diastole.

5. Cardiac output depends on 4 factors (see Chapter C-Heart Failure, Point No. 10).

1. Length of the muscle fiber at the end of diastolic phase (EDV)—i.e. length of the cardiac muscle just at the onset of contraction—preload.
2. Inotropic state of the muscle, i.e. ability of the cardiac muscle to develop tension and force, i.e.—myocardial contractile state.
3. The resistance against which the heart has to work—afterload, i.e. peripheral vascular resistance—afterload.
4. Heart rate.

Cardiac output is the multiple of stroke volume and pulse rate. Stroke volume depends upon the preload, intrinsic contractility of the heart muscle and afterload.
It has been postulated that in very early hypertension, the rise in blood pressure is caused by raised cardiac output which is related to sympathetic over activity. The subsequent rise in peripheral vascular resistant developed as a compensatory manner to prevent the rise in pressure being transmitted to the capillary bed.

6. Peripheral vascular resistance depends on 4 factors.

1. Diameter of the lumen.
2. Thickness of the vessel wall (ratio of lumen to wall thickness). Elasticity of the arterial walls, gripping and exerting pressure upon the blood whilst the aortic valve is closed and the heart is not pumping.
3. Effects of vasoconstrictors like noradrenaline, angiotensin II.
4. Effects of vasodilators like acetylcholine, kinins and prostaglandins.

They act on vascular smooth muscle.
In the great majority of patients with an established hypertension an increase of peripheral vascular resistance is the main hemodynamic abnormality. On the other hand, in some patients cardiac output is normal or slightly reduced, although in a few cases it is increased initially.
Peripheral vascular resistance is determined not by large arteries or the capillaries but by small arterioles, the walls of which contain smooth muscle cells. Rise in intracellular calcium concentration is related to the contraction of smooth muscle cells, which may explain the vasodilator effect of calcium channel blockers. This may explain the action of calcium channel blockers in peripheral vascular resistance.
In very early hypertension, the elevation of the blood pressure is caused by a raised cardiac output, which is related to sympathetic over activity. Subsequently, peripheral vascular resistance rises in a compensatory manner to prevent the raised pressure being transmitted to the capillary bed where it would substantially affect cell homeostasis. Prolonged smooth muscle constriction is thought to induce structural changes with thickening of the arteriolar vessel walls possibly mediated by angiotensin, leading to an irreversible rise in peripheral resistance. ACEI helps in preventing the structural changes and they play a role in hypertensive treatment where there is peripheral vascular resistance is high.

7. There are 4 neural and chemical factors that influence the BP:

1. Altered function of CNS.
2. Altered function of sympathetic nervous system.
3. Altered renin-angiotensin-aldosterone system.
4. Deficiency of renal vasodilator substances.

8. Autonomic nervous system maintains its role on BP by influencing the 4 factors that determine cardiac output by the activation of adrenergic receptors on:

1. Venules and veins—determine the return of blood—(EDV—Preload)
2. Myocardium—determines the degree of contractile state (inotropic state).
3. Smooth muscle of the arteriolar walls—determines the degree of peripheral vascular resistance (afterload).
4. SA node—determines the heart rate.

Hypertension is probably related to an interaction between the autonomic nervous system and renin-angiotensin system together with other factors including sodium, circulating volume and some recently described hormones.

9. The autonomic reflexes that regulate arterial pressure arises in stretch receptors (baroreceptors) from 4 sites.

1. Carotid sinus.
2. Aortic arch.
3. Heart chambers.
4. Lungs.

10. The abnormal action of the sympathetic system (brain-stem sympathetic centers) affect the BP in 4 ways.

1. *By its action on the heart:* The heart rate and its contractility increases resulting in increased cardiac output and rise of BP.
2. *By its action on veins:* It causes venoconstriction which thereby increases the venous return resulting in increased cardiac output and rise in BP.
3. *By its action on arterioles:* It causes vasoconstriction which increases the peripheral vascular resistance resulting in rise of BP.
4. *By its action on kidneys:* It increases renin secretion thereby activating renin-angiotensin-aldosterone mechanism. Angiotensin II increases peripheral vascular resistance resulting in rise of BP aldosterone increases sodium reabsorption, venous return, cardiac output—resulting in rise of BP.

11. Angiotensin II rises BP in 4 ways.

1. By direct vasoconstrictor action on systemic arterioles.
2. Acts indirectly through hypothalamic adrenergic activity.
3. By stimulating adrenal cortex to synthesize aldosterone which acts on renal tubules to cause sodium and water retention.
4. By converting into angiotensin III which is a more active stimulator of aldosterone release.

12. Summary of regulation of blood pressure.

BP = Cardiac output × Peripheral vascular resistance.

Cardiac Output

1. Blood volume
   i. Sodium
   ii. Mineralocorticoids
   iii. Atriopeptin
2. Cardiac factors
   i. Contractility
   ii. Heart rate

Peripheral Vascular Resistance

3. Humoral factors

Constrictors	*Dilators*
– Angiotensin II	– Prostaglandins-PGI, PGE, PGD
– Catecholamines	– Bradykinins
– Thromboxane	
– Leukotrienes	– Nitric oxide (NO)
– Endotheline	– Endothelium-derived relaxing factor (EDRF)
– Ouabain	

4. Neural factors

Constrictors	*Dilators*
α-adrenergic	β-adrenergic

Local factors like autoregulation, ionic (pH, hypoxia) also have a role.

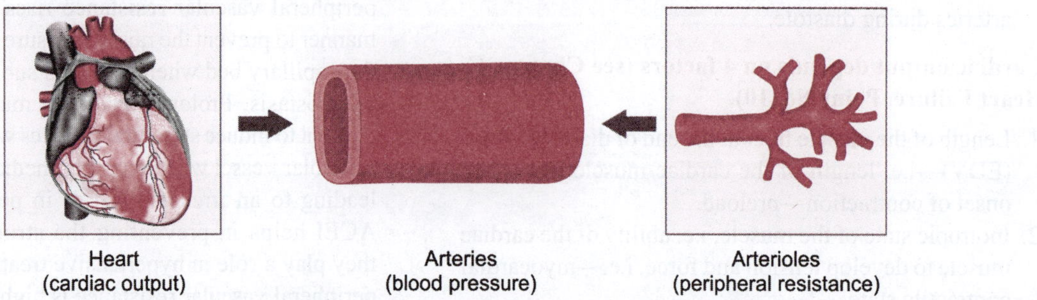

Fig. B-1: The heart, arteries, and arterioles in hypertension

13. Regulation of blood pressure

Table B-1

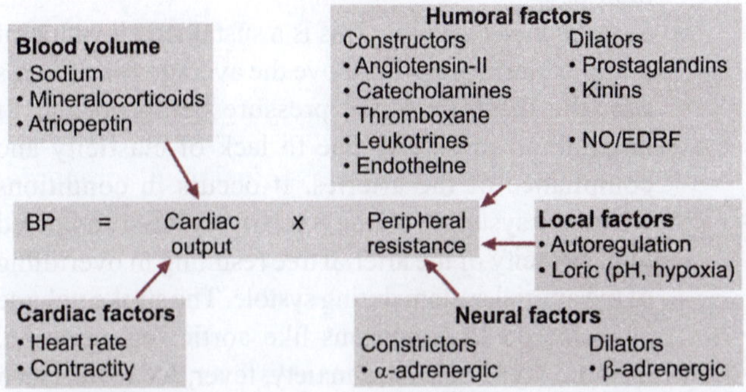

14. Atrial natriuretic peptide.

1. Also known as atrial natriuretic factor.
2. Secreted by cardiac atria in response to volume distension.
3. It is a natural hypovolemic agent.
4. Acts on renal vasculature to cause powerful vasodilation and diuresis.

15. Changes in blood vessels in hypertension.

1. Increase in muscle elastic tissue of arterial wall.

↓

2. Replacement by fibrous tissue.

↓

3. At bends and bifurcations—tendency to fibrin/platelets to be deposited.

↓

4. Risk of thrombosis is increased; small arteries become hard and inflexible large arteries loose elasticity and dilate.

16. Role of angiotensin II in maintaining blood pressure during fall of BP (shock).

Table B-2

Site of action of angiotensin II	Effect
1. Vascular smooth muscle	Constriction; increase in peripheral vascular resistance
2. Renal efferent arteriole	Constriction; maintenance of glomerular filtration rate
3. Proximal renal tubule	Increased sodium reabsorption
4. Adrenal cortex	Increased aldosterone secretion
5. Central adrenergic activation	Increased release of norepinephrine
6. Ganglion facilitation	Increased release of norepinephrine
7. Presynaptic receptors	Increased release of norepinephrine; decreased re-uptake
8. Baroreflexes	Withdrawal of vagal tone

17. 'Renin Profile' (High renin, low renin, normal renin) in essential hypertension does not hold good for diagnosis, prognosis because of the following 4 reasons:

(Useful in secondary hypertension)

1. 'Renin status' may change with age and also with stimulus used to rise plasma renin activity.
2. Patient with low renin hypertension may respond well to β-blockers also.
3. All patients with high renin hypertension may not show substantial reduction in BP for β-blockers.
4. In 'Conn's syndrome' (Primary aldosteronism) PRA level is very low and only small increase in plasma volume. The elevation of BP mostly depends on vasoconstriction. It shows that hypertension seldom depend only on vasoconstriction or volume—both mechanisms combinedly act irrespective of renin status.

18. Hypertension cannot simply be divided by renin or blood volume content into the following 4 types:

1. High renin.
2. Low renin.
3. Increased blood volume.
4. Decreased blood volume.

19. Salt retention helps in raising the BP in 4 ways:

1. By retaining water along with sodium.
2. By retaining sodium in arteries of hypertension.
3. By associating with high level of ionized calcium in the arterial smooth muscle.
4. By increasing peripheral vascular resistance.

20. The following 4 conditions may cause reduced sodium excretion at normal BP due to abnormal renal function:

1. Primary tubular defect.
2. Mild increase in the activity of mineralocorticoids.
3. Decreased activity of renal kallikrein-kinin-prostaglandins.
4. Increase in local vasoconstrictor activity reducing the renal blood flow secondary to sodium excretion (by angiotensin II or sympathetic system).

21. Serotonin causes aggregation of platelets which in turn causes release of free serotonin at the periphery which could initiate the viscous cycle by:

1. Increasing platelet aggregation.
2. Serotonin release.
3. Vasoconstriction and vascular damage.
4. Hypertension.

(Serotonin blockers in hypertension are under trial)

22. Following terms are used for different forms of hypertension:

1. [1*]*Essential (Idiopathic or primary hypertension):* This is the term applied to hypertension for which the etiology is currently not known. It may not be of one cause and may have several etiologies which result in increased peripheral vascular resistance. Over 80–85% of hypertensives fall into this group.
2. *Secondary hypertension:* This hypertension is due to specific identifiable cause. About 10–15% of hypertensives fall into this group. More and more hypertensives fall into this category as knowledge in understanding of hypertension increases and availability of latest investigations. It is more likely in persons aged under 30–40 years. Its importance lies in the fact that it can be completely curable in some cases where the causes are reversible. So, the possibility of secondary hypertension is thought of in every hypertensive patient and investigated accordingly.
3. *Malignant hypertension:* It is defined as severe hypertension accompanied by papilledema with retinal hemorrhages and exudates. Usually the BP is more than 200/140 mm Hg. The importance of malignant hypertension lies in fact that without treatment it carries a very poor prognosis with one year mortality of 95% usually from cardiac and/or renal failure.
4. *Accelerated hypertension:* It is the term used for significant recent increase over previous hypertensive levels associated with evidence of vascular damage on fundus examination but without papilledema.
5. *Labile hypertension:* It is the term used to describe hypertension associated with more variation in blood pressure readings than usually found. Some believe that it is not a separate entity by itself but merely represent an excessive changes of blood pressure that occurs in normotensives or hypertensives throughout the day with exercise, emotion, etc.
   (So, labile hypertension is labeled for patients who sometimes but not always have arterial pressures within hypertensive range. These patients are often considered to have borderline hypertension).
   Labile blood pressure is the term used to describe blood pressure that is normal at times and abnormally high at other times. Some believe that labile BP is a risk factor for the later development of sustained hypertension.
6. *Sustained hypertension:* It is the term used to describe when the diastolic pressure always exceeds the normal levels. Sustained hypertension can become accelerated or enter into a malignant phase.
   Individuals are said to be normotensives if the arterial pressures are equal or less than the normal levels for their age.
7. *Systolic hypertension:* This is a sustained elevation of systolic blood pressure above the average for person's age, the diastolic blood pressure being normal. It is common in elderly due to lack of elasticity and compliance of the arteries. It occurs in conditions where the systolic volume is relatively large compared with capacity of the arterial tree resulting in overfilling of the arterial system during systole. The stroke volume is increased in conditions like aortic regurgitation, anemia, thyrotoxicosis, anxiety, fever, AV fistula such as PDA, hyperkinetic circulation such as beriberi, Paget's disease of bone.
8. *Renal hypertension:* This is the term used to describe hypertension associated with kidney disease. Kidney is both a culprit as well as a victim in hypertension. It plays a greater role in the causation of hypertension. Both renal parenchymal as well as renovascular disease can cause hypertension.

23. The causes of essential hypertension (primary or idiopathic) is unknown. It is a multifactorial disease. So several causes are suggested. The etiological factors suggested are:

1. Genetic disposition.
2. Salt intake.
3. Overactivity of sympathetic nervous system.
4. Baroreceptor insensibility.
5. Kidney and control of fluid volume.
6. The renin-angiotensin system.
7. Endothelial dysfunction.
8. Atrial natriuretic hormone.
9. Hypercoagulability.
10. Insulin sensitivity.
11. Intrauterine influence.
12. Snoring.

1. Genetic disposition: This is suggested by the familial tendency. Hypertension runs in families. It is observed that patients with essential hypertension and their relatives but not patients with secondary hypertension, have a defect of sodium efflux from their cells resulting in abnormal high levels of intracellular sodium. It is possible that it may result in an increase of intracellular calcium that in its turn may increase the contractility of arteriolar smooth muscle which results in increase of peripheral vascular resistance and hypertension. Although, there is a clear familial component in hypertension, a genetic basis is definable in less than one in every 100 patients. Interestingly, these are some of the rare causes of hypertension where single drugs

[1*] It is obvious the term 'essential' used in this context is false since it is not essential that one should have hypertension. But this cannot be replaced since it is followed from many years.

are most effective often lowering the blood pressure by 30–40% compared with the average of 10% for drugs in essential hypertension. For example, alpha-blocker phenoxybenzamine in pheochromocytoma and spironolactone in Conn's syndrome or the genetic syndrome of apparent mineralocorticoid excess. All the genetic causes of hypertension so far identified are due to increased sodium retention. So, salt restriction in high-risk families during growth could forestall development of complications or even hypertension itself.

Transmission of high blood pressure does not follow the classic Mendelian rules of inheritance attributable to a single gene locus (except few rare forms given in Table B-2).

Hypertension appears to be a polygenic and multifactorial disorder in which the interaction of several genes with each other and with the environment is important. The candidates prone for the genetic transmission suggested in those that affect the various components of the rennin-angiotensin-aldosterone system, the kalli-krinine -kinin system, and the sympathetic nervous system.

The angiotensin gene may be related to hypertension. The angiotensin-converting enzyme gene may be related to left ventricular hypertrophy or hypertensive nephropathy.

Adducin gene may be related to salt sensitive hypertension. Experimental model of genetic hypertension have shown the inherited tendency primarily resides in the kidneys. For example, that a transplanted kidney from a hypertensive donor to a 'normotensive' families shows raise in blood pressure and need antihypertensive drugs in the recipient. Conversely, a kidney form a normotensive donor does not raise the blood pressure in the recipient.

2. *Salt intake:* There is strong relation between the salt intake of a population and the prevalence within it of hypertension and its complications. Although strict restriction of salt to about 10 mmoles per day result in significant lowering of blood pressure, moderate restriction of salt that is acceptable to the patients has not shown improvement on hypertension. The blood pressure of individuals have not shown any relation to the intake or excretion of salt. So, it is possible that yet an unidentifiable subgroup of hypertensives are sensitive to salt intake.

   Abnormalities of sodium handling:
   i. Decrease in natriuresis.
   ii. Excess retention of sodium in smooth muscle.
   iii. Operation of sodium: Calcium exchange leading to increased cytosolic calcium and vasoconstriction.
   iv. Membrane defect in sodium transport, hence intracellular retention.

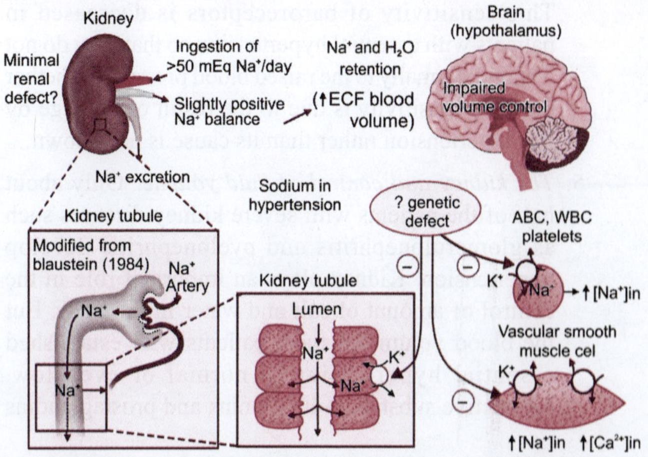

Fig. B-2: Hypothesis for salt-sensitivity hypertension

Salt sensitive hypertension: Wide relation between salt intake and main blood pressure levels due to abnormal salt handling by kidney.

Hypothetically, in the presence of minimal degrees of a genetically determined renal defect, small amounts of sodium are retained so that extracellular fluid (ECF) volume is increased with release of the proposed natriuretic hormone from the hypothalamus. This hormone inhibits sodium-potassium exchange in vascular smooth muscle. Cell sodium in the myocyte increases to increase calcium via the sodium—calcium exchange to enhance vascular tone.

Sodium transport across vascular smooth muscle cell walls is also thought to influence blood pressure via its interrelation with calcium transport. Ouabain may be a naturally occurring steroid-like substance which is thought to interfere with cell sodium and calcium transport, giving rise to vasoconstriction.

3. *Overactivity of sympathetic nervous system:* Chronic overstimulation of sympathetic nervous system by stress increases the circulating catecholamines which in turn leads to chronic vasoconstriction, an increase of peripheral vascular resistance and increase in cardiac output resulting in hypertension.

   Neurogenic theory:
   – Enhanced adrenergic activity
   – Increased cardiac activity.

4. *Baroreceptor insensitivity:* Normally, baroreceptors respond to a rise of blood pressure which stimulates pressure sensitive stretch receptors in the carotid sinus and aortic arch. They respond by discharging impulses that inhibit the sympathetic outflow from the brain to the peripheral arterioles which in turn, results in vasodilatation, decrease in peripheral vascular resistance and lowering of blood pressure.

This sensitivity of baroreceptors is decreased in patients with essential hypertension so that they do not respond normally to the raised blood pressure. Whether this less sensitivity is due to the result of damage by the hypertension rather than its cause is not known.

5. *The kidney and control of fluid volume:* Only about half of the patients with severe kidney diseases such as glomerulonephritis and pyelonephritis develop hypertension. Kidney plays an important role in the control of amount of salt and water in the body. But the blood volume of most patients with established essential hypertension is normal or even low. Vasoactive substances like kinins and prostaglandins acting locally within the kidney may have some effect on the blood pressure.
   There can be abnormal salt handling by the kidney.
6. *The renin-angiotensin system:* Whenever the perfusion pressure in the renal artery falls, the enzyme renin is released from the juxtaglomerular apparatus. Renin acts on the plasma protein, angiotensinogen to produce angiotensin I which in turn, is acted upon by converting enzyme to produce angiotensin II. Together with thromboxane, angiotensin II is one of the most known powerful vasoconstrictor. They also stimulate the release of aldosterone from the adrenal cortex.

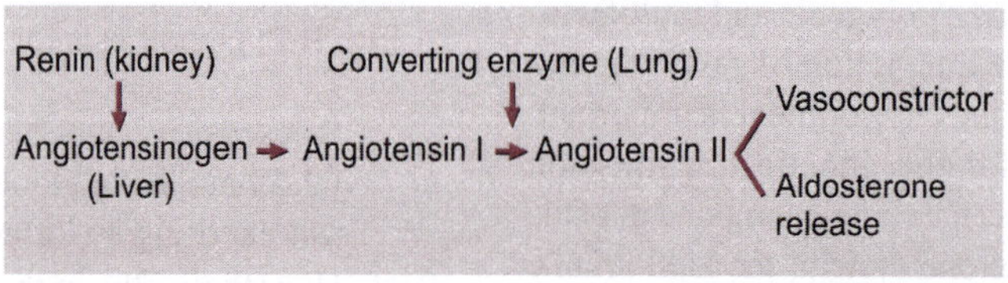

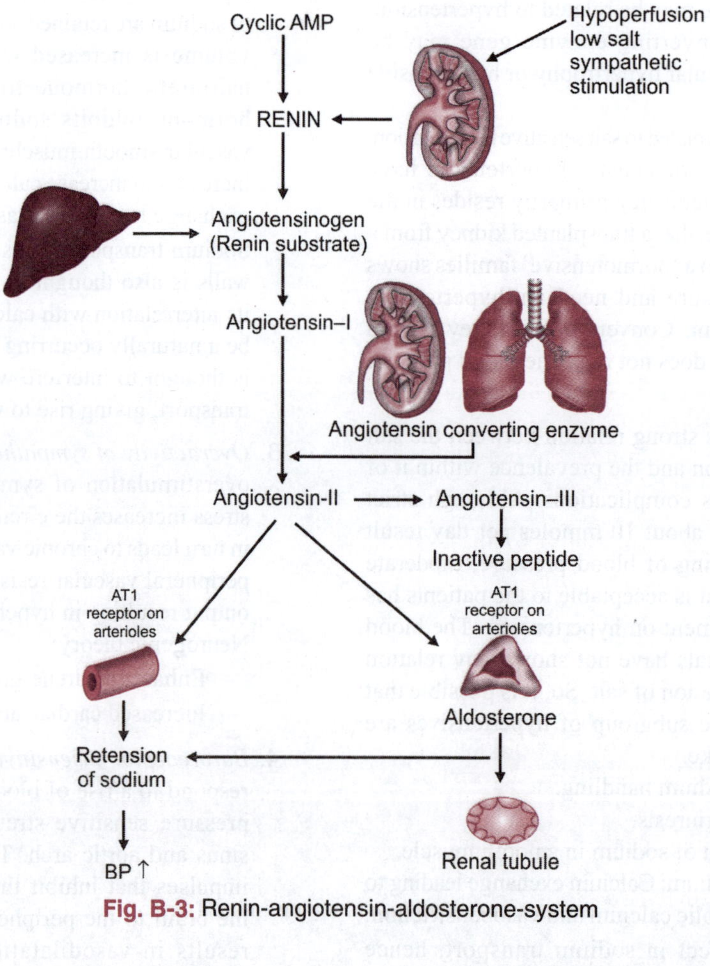

Fig. B-3: Renin-angiotensin-aldosterone-system

The role of renin in essential hypertension is doubtful because plasma renin levels are high in only about 10%, intermediate in about 60% and low in about 30% of patients.

On the other hand, diuretics have a paradoxical effect causing blood pressure to fall and plasma renin levels to rise. Renin is also released in response to stimulation from the sympathetic nervous system.

Renin-angiotensin-aldosterone system (RAAS) has a definitive role in the secondary hypertension and is associated with conditions such as renal artery stenosis and coarctation of aorta in which the kidney is undeperfusid to release renin.

The circulatory renin-angiotensin system is not directly responsible for the essential hypertension. In particular, many hypertensive patients have low level of renin and ACE II (especially in elderly and black people) and ACEI are not particularly effective.

However, there is increasing evidence of important noncirculating "local" renin-angiotensin autoerine or paracrine systems which also control blood pressure. Local renin systems have been reported in the kidney, the heart, and the arterial tree. They may have important roles in regulating regional blood flow.

Now, the existence of local RAAS in the blood vessels, heart, kidney, brain and elsewhere is known where it may mediate local effects (such as tissue remodeling) independent of circulating renin or angiotensinogen levels. Actions of angiotensin II are mediated mostly by AII subtype (AT1) receptor and less certainly by subtype AT2 receptor. AT1 receptors are responsible for vascular smooth muscle contraction and hypertrophy, cardiac contractility, stimulating SNS and CNS inhibition of endothelial function and thus mediate renal tubular sodium reabsorption. The role of AT2 receptors in healthy adults and even in those with cardiac and vascular damage is still uncertain.

7. *Endothelial dysfunction:* Most powerful vasoactive mediators, nitric oxide and endothelin have been identified recently, and both occur within endothelial cells. Nitric oxide is the principal physiological vasodilator while endothelin is the most potent vasoconstrictor. Superoxide easily breaks down nitric oxide, so balance between oxygen and nitric oxide is likely to be one of the control mechanisms of vascular tone. Free radicals in the body cause various types of damage including lipid peroxidation and subsequent endothelial cell injury and damage to proteins and nucleic acids. Cells and tissues are usually protected from the effects of lipid peroxidation by several naturally occurring antioxidents. A balance between peroxide generating and peroxide removing may control cyclooxygenase activity and the rate of generation of prostaglandins. Prostacyclin is an extremely potent vasodilator and antiaggregatory agent synthesized in the vascular endothelium. Its actions are usually balanced by those of thromboxane, a potent locally acting vasoconstrictor and proaggregatory agent. Peroxides inhibit prostacyclin synthesis and not influence thromboxane synthesis. Inhibition of prostacyclin synthesis causes the formation of foam cells, the accumulation of cholesterol esters, and atherogenesis. The overall effect is a clear diminution of vasodilator effect. Lipid peroxidation in cell membrane increases their permeability to calcium, so intracellular free calcium also is raised. which also increases vascular resistance.

8. *Atrial natriuretic hormone*
   i. Also known as atrial natriuretic factor.
   ii. Secreted by cardiac atria in response to volume distension.
   iii. It is a natural hypovolemic agent.
   iv. Acts on renal vasculature to cause powerful vasodilation and diuresis.

It is recently isolated. This is secreted from the right atrium when it is stretched. It causes salt and water loss via the kidneys and it also causes vasodilatation. There are conflicting reports of high levels and normal levels of the hormone in hypertension. Its role in hypertension is not clear.

9. *Hypercoagulability:* Hypertensive patients show a prethrombotic or hypercoagulable state. Besides abnormalities of vessel wall (endothelial dysfunction are damage). They show abnormal blood constituents (abnormal levels of hemostatic factors, platelet activation and fibrinolysis) and blood flow (rheology, viscosity and flow results). These appear to be related to target organ damage, and long-term prognosis and same may be altered by antihypertensive treatment.

10. *Insulin sensitivity*: This has a group of risk factor including hypertension, obesity, glucose intolerance, diabetes, dyslipidemia, etc. It is suggested as single syndrome—metabolic syndrome X or Raven's syndrome with a common pathway to cause hypertension and vascular damage. Some patients who are not obese also may show resistance to insulin. There are many objections to this hypothesis but it explains the CVS risk factors which are synergistic or multiple than additive.

11. *Intrauterine influences:* Neonates who are small at birth are more likely to be hypertensive adults. Babies who are small for the age are also likely to

have metabolic abnormalities that are associated with later development of hypertension, cardiovascular disease, insulin resistance, diabetes, dyslipidemia and abdominal obesity. Intrauterine nutrition, low birth weight, neurovascular anomalies, etc. may be a cause.

12. *Snoring:* Regular snoring is also reported as a risk factor for the development of hypertension presumably because it results in anoxia causing vasoconstriction.

It is probable that a great many interrelated factors contribute to the raised blood pressure in hypertensive patients and their relative roles may differ between individuals. Among the factors that have been widely studied are salt intake, obesity, insulin resistance, the renin-angiotensin system, and the sympathetic nervous system. In the past few years, other factors have been evaluated including genetic, endothelial dysfunction, low birthweight and intrauterine nutrition and neurovascular anomalies.

Research on causation remains wide open.

24. Four examples of genetic causes of hypertension where single drugs are most effective.

Table B-3

Syndrome	Genetic defect	Treatment
1. Glucocorticoid remediable aldosteronism	Chimuric gene between aldosterone synthase and 11 β-hydroxylase, exposing aldosterone synthesis to stimulation by adrenocorticotropic hormone	Dexamethasone
2. Ladle's (Pseudohyper-aldosteronism)	Activating mutations in epithelial sodium channel distal tubes or collecting ducts to conserve sodium and excrete potassium despite the virtual absence of aldosterone	Amiloride
3. Conn's (Primary aldosteronism) Apparent mineralo-corticoid excess	Inactivating mutations in 11 β-hydroxysteroid dehydrogenase, exposing mineralocorticoid receptor to cortisol	Spironolactone
4. Pheochromocytoma: Chromaffin tumor from adrenal medulla	Stores and secretes catecholamines	α-blocker -phenoxybenza-mine

Ladle's syndrome: BP ↑, plasma renin ↓, aldesterone ↓, potassium ↓—all of which respond to amiloride, an inhibitor of distal renal epithelial sodium channel.

25. Organs affected in angiotensins

The classic pathway of biosynthesis that produces angiotenins in the bloodstream are shown on the left side of the figure.

Angiotensin receptors in the principal organs affected by the action of angiotensin are shown on the right hand side of the figure.

1. Angiotensinogen is synthesized by the liver and released into the blood where it is cleaved to form angiotensin I by renin secreted from juxtaglomerular apparatus in the kidneys.
2. Angiotensin-converting enzyme (ACE) in the lung catalyzes the formation of angiotensin II from angiotensin I, and the same enzyme destroys bradykinin.
3. Further proteolytic cleavage generates angiotensin III
4. Generates angiotensin IV.
   (Remember, angiotensins are four: I, II, III, IV).

Two renal actions are shown—the stimulation of proximal tubular function and the vasoconstriction of efferent arterioles.

Left dashed arrow is the inhibition by angiotensin II of the release of renin by the kidneys.

All the receptors shown are of the AT1 subtype except certain receptors in the brain.

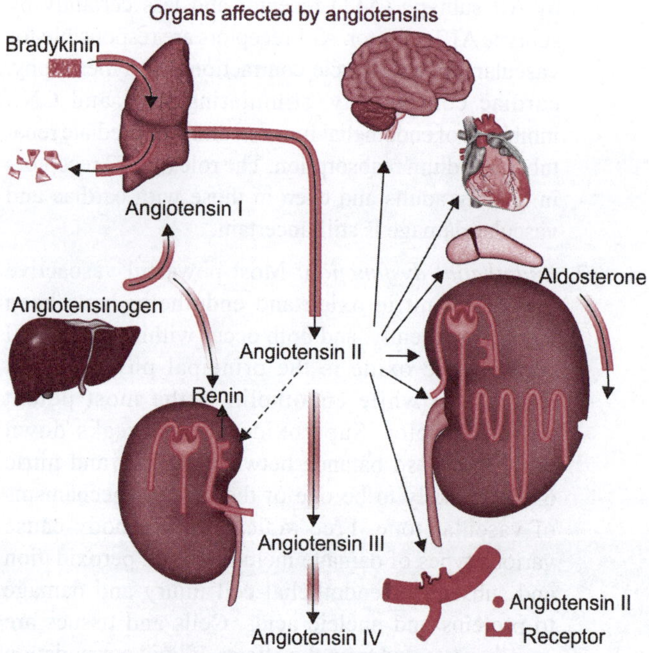

Fig. B-4: Formation of angiotensins and organs affected by their actions

26. Angiotensin II stimulates a variety of physiologic responses that support arterial blood pressure and renal function. Angiotensins contribute to the pathogenesis of:

1. Hypertension.
2. Arterial disease.
3. Cardiac hypertrophy, heart failure.
4. Diabetic renal disease.

27. Actions of angiotensin II tissue affected action.

Table B-4

1. CVS	
a. Heart	Increases contractility and ventricular hypertrophy
b. Arteries	Stimulates contractions and growth
2. CNS	
a. Brain	Stimulates thirst and the release of vasopressin
b. Sympathetic nervous system	Increases central sympathetic outflow Increases adrenal release of epinephrine Facilitates peripheral sympathetic transmission
3. Kidney	Inhibits release of renin Increases tubular reabsorption of sodium Stimulates vasoconstriction Releases prostaglandin Affects embryogenesis
4. Adrenal zona glomerulosa	Stimulates secretion of aldosterone

28. Abnormal sodium handling causes 4 manifestations:

1. Decreased natriuresis.
2. Excess retention of sodium in smooth muscle.
3. Operation of sodium calcium exchange leading to increased cytosolic calcium and vasoconstriction.
4. Membrane defect in sodium transport, hence intracellular retention.

29. Atrial natriuretic hormone.

1. Also known as atrial natriuretic peptide or atrial natriuretic factor.
2. Secreted by cardiac atria in response to volume distension.
3. It is a natural hypovolemic agent.
4. Acts on renal vasculature to cause powerful vasodilatation and diuresis.

30. Natural history of untreated early essential hypertension has the following 4 steps in its development.

1. Hereditary: Environment (including salt intake, obesity, occupation, family size, crowding, interpersonal relationship, etc.)

↓

2. Prehypertension

↓

3. Increased cardiac output

↓

4. Early hypertension

31. Early untreated essential hypertension leads to complicated hypertension in 4 stages (shortens the life span by 10–20 years).

1. Increased peripheral vascular resistance

↓

2. Established hypertension

↓

3. Accelerated arteriosclerosis

↓

4. Complicated hypertension

Table B-5

CVS	*Renal*	*Cerebral*	*Eye*
Angina of effort LVF, LVH Myocardial infarction Aortic aneurysm/ aortic dissection Embolization Occlusion of branches Peripheral vascular disease	Arteriosclerosis Insufficiency Microalbuminuria Proteinuria Microscopic Macroscopic Hematuria Renal failure	Stroke due to thrombosis Embolization Hemorrhage Encephalopathy Transient ischemic attack (TIA), lacunar infarcts, cognitive impairment Dementia	Retinopathy Malignant phase (1–5%) Papilledema Clinically blurring of vision

32. Untreated hypertension damages mainly 4 end organs.

Table B-6

1. Heart 60–70%	a. Left ventricular hypertrophy, left ventricular strain b. Ischemic changes in ECG, IHD c. Myocardial infarction, sudden death d. Congestive cardiac failure LVH →LVF→Stasis of blood in the lungs →RVH→RVF Aortic aneurysm, aortic dissection. Embolization and occlusion of branches.
2. Brain 32%	Cerebrovascular accidents thrombosis, hemorrhage, embolization, hypertensive encephalopathy Subarachnoid hemorrhage Multiple microaneurysm → Multiple infarcts → Progressive disability
3. Kidneys	Arteriosclerosis, insufficiency resulting in proteinuria, hematuria, azotemia further HT→Progressive loss of kidney function and renal failure
4. Eye	Retinopathy Hemorrhages and exudates Retinal detachment, papilledema Blindness

In malignant or accelerated hypertension—diastolic BP > 130 mm Hg with progressive organ damage—LVF, convulsions, proteinuria, retinopathy, etc. are seen.

Control of blood pressure of a hypertensive patient reduces the likelihood of heart failure by 55% transient ischemic attack, stroke by 35–40%, renal failure but it has little or no effect on the incidence of myocardial infarction which is a common occurring in good number of patients. However, it is observed that the incidence of myocardial infarction is reduced in the subgroups namely the elderly and also non-smoking males treated with β-blockers, by 22–25%.

33. Cardiovascular mortality risk doubles with each 20 mm Hg SBP or 10 mm Hg DBP increment.

1. Normal range 155/75 mm Hg
2. 135/85 mm Hg—2 times
3. 155/95 mm Hg—4 times
4. 175/105 mm Hg—8 times

34. Following are the main histological effects of hypertension upon the 4 organs—1. Arteries, 2. Heart, 3. Brain, 4. Kidneys.

1. Medium sized arteries such as radial artery show
   - Thickening of the media and intima
   - Accelerated atherosclerosis.

   Both these changes lead to narrowing of the lumen of the vessel and increase in peripheral vascular resistance. Small arteries and arterioles: In addition, these show accelerated atherosclerosis.

   There is tendency of fibrin/platelets to be deposited at bends and bifurcation's which in turn increases the risk of thrombosis/embolism.

A. Deposition of hyaline-plasma proteins and lipids being forced into the vessel wall. B. Reduplication of elastic lamina of the vessel wall.	Changes seen in essential hypertension
C. Fibroid necrosis: Deposition similar to hyaline often in association with an inflammatory infiltrate. D. Onion skinning reduplication of smooth muscle of the arterial wall.	Changes seen in malignant hypertension

2. *The heart:* Hypertension is often associated with hypertrophy of the muscle cells of the heart. As a consequence of it, the heart 'outgrows' its blood supply or the walls of the coronary arteries become narrowed, leading to relative ischemia of muscle fibers resulting in degenerative changes and patchy fibrosis.
3. *The brain:* There are microaneurysms of upto about 1 mm diameter in the small arteries of the brain known as 'Charcot Bouchard' aneurysms of hypertensive patients but not normotensives. These were described about 100 years ago by Charcot and Bouchard. Rupture of these aneurysms is probably a major cause of cerebral hemorrhage.
4. *The kidney:* Besides the changes described in small arteries and arterioles, the kidney in hypertension is associated with sclerosis of glomeruli, tubular atrophy and fibrosis of the interstitium.

35. There are 4 major non-modifiable risk factors:

1. Age
2. Sex
3. Race
4. Family history

36. There are 4 major modifiable risk factors:

1. Smoking
2. Diabetes
3. Dyslipidemia
4. Obesity

37. There are 4 factors which contribute to the hypertension in women who take oral contraceptive pills:

(The estrogen component stimulates hepatic synthesis of renin substrate angiotensinogen which in turn, produces angiotensin II)

1. Presence of mild renal disease with increased vascular sensitivity to angiotensin II.
2. Family history of hypertension.
3. Over 35 years age.
4. Obesity.

38. Obesity causes hypertension by

1. Increase in blood volume.
2. Increase in cardiac output.
3. Increase in intra-abdominal fat and pressure→ impaired renal function.
4. Insulin resistance

Obesity is defined as weighing 120% or more of one's acceptable or standard weight. Overweight is defined as weighing 110–119% of one's acceptable weight. Contribution of obesity makes the difference of incidence of death from cardiovascular diseases. It is now recognized that abdominal obesity giving the person an 'apple' shape is indicated by an increase in the ratio of abdominal/hip girth is an independent risk factor. Whereas obesity around the buttocks and thighs giving the person a 'pear' shape is not a risk factor. The obesity needs perfusion of excess body mass which otherwise increases demand on the heart. 50 mL of blood flows in the vessels for every 1 lb of extra weight. *Longer the waistline, shorter the lifeline.* Higher death rate in obese may be a direct or indirect consequence of hypertension. Weight reduction appears to be an effective first line therapy for about 50% of patients with mild to moderate hypertension.

For each 9.3 calories excess energy entering the body, 1 gram of fat is stored.

When greater quantities of energy (in the form of fat) enter the body than expected the body weight increases. It is often said that obesity result from too high a ratio of food intake to daily exercise (expenditure).

Body mass index (BMI) is a good measure of obesity this is calculated as weight in kilograms divided by square of height in meters, for example, BMI of a person who is

90 kg weight and 1.66 meter height is

$$90/(1.66)2 = 90/2.75 = 32.7$$

Normal and abnormal ranges of BMI are:

• Normal	21–27 (Adult male) 18–25 (Adult female)
• Overweight	27–29.9 (Adult male) 25–27.9 (Adult female)
• Obese	30–40
• Severe (morbid)	Above 40
• Obese	

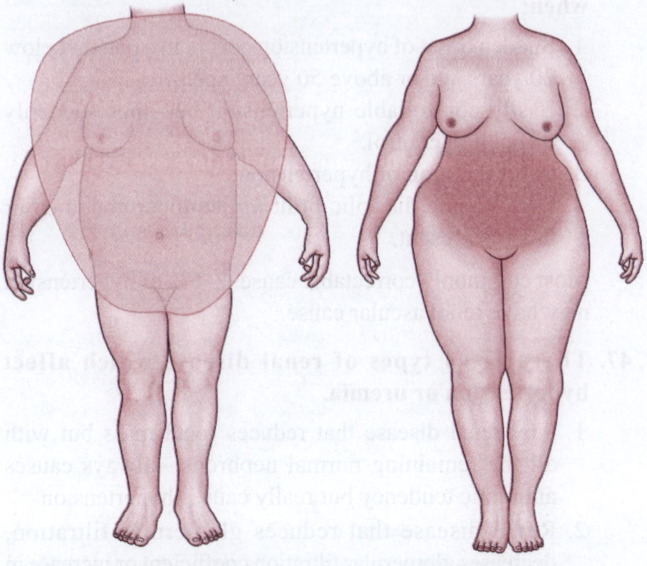

Fig. B-5: Body shapes in obesity

39. Complications of obesity

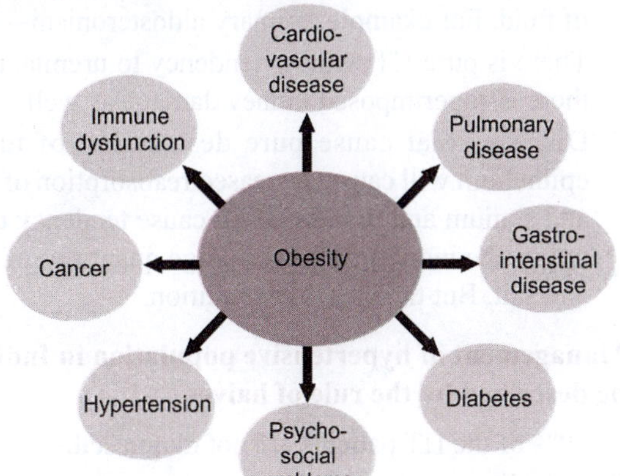

Fig. B-6: Complications of obesity

40. There are 4 CVS changes that are closely associated with obesity.

1. Hypertension.
2. Left ventricular hypertrophy and heart failure.
3. Ischemic heart disease.
4. Cardiomyopathies.

41. The causes of secondary hypertension (10–15%) can be classified into 4 groups.

1. *Renal causes*
   a. Congenital: Renovascular stenosis, polycystic kidney.
   b. Infective: Chronic pyelonephritis, acute and chronic glomerulonephritis.
   c. Vascular: Arteriolar nephrosclerosis, renal artery stensosis, diabetic nephropathy.
   d. Neoplastic: Renin producing tumors.
   e. Obstructive uropathy: Renal stones.
   f. Analgesic nephropathy.
2. *Endocrinal*
   a. Adrenocortical hyperfunction,
   e.g. Cushing's syndrome
   Primary hyperaldosteronism
   (Conn's syndrome).
   b. Pheochromocytoma.
   c. Hyperthyroidism or hypothyroidism.
   d. Acromegaly.
3. *Neurogenic*
   – Psychogenic-depression.
   – Bulbar poliomyelitis.
   – Increased intracranial pressure (Acute).
   – Brain tumor, encephalitis, respiratory acidosis.
   – Polyneuritis (acute porphyria, lead poisoning).
   – Sympathomimetic amines, monoamine oxidase inhibitors (MAOI).
4. *Miscellaneous*
   • ***Iatrogenic***
   – Sympathomimetic amines
   – Oral contraceptives
   – Steroid therapy
   – Carbenoxolone
   – Tyrosine containing food
   – Excessive IV fluids
   – MAO inhibitors
   – Anorectic agents: should be used with caution because many can raise BP and some may increase the risk of valvular heart disease and pulmonary hypertension

- *Toxic*
  - Lead and cadmium poisoning
  - Toxemia pregnancy
  - Raised intracranial pressure
  - Coarctation of Aorta
  - Polycythemia vera
  - Hypercalcemia
  - Polyarteritis nodosa
  - Acute intermittent porphyria
  - Familial dysautonomia
  - Sleep apnea.

Steroid therapy, primary aldosteronism, oral contraceptives, carbenoxolone cause hypertension due to salt and water retention.

Secondary hypertension is suspected in patients < 20 years age, h/o renal disease, urinary tract infections, drug h/o and in clinical signs like abdominal bruit, endocrinal features, etc.

42. The proportion of secondary hypertension attributable to specific known causes varies according to:

1. The mode of ascertainment.
2. Selection of cases.
3. Intensity of investigation.
4. Credibility of investigators.

The more we know about hypertension, the more we find the specific causes. Hospital records are notoriously biased by the selection of primarily or secondarily referred cases that suits the special interests of the head of departments concerned.

43. Kidney is both a culprit as well as a victim in hypertension. Hypertension can cause:

1. Acute renal disease.
2. Acute renal failure.
3. Chronic renal disease—polycystic disease, chronic interstitial nephritis.
4. Chronic renal failure.

44. There are 4 probable ways of action in renal parenchymal disease that cause hypertension.

1. The damaged kidneys may produce an unidentified vasopressor substance other than renin.
2. It may fail to produce vasodilator substance like prostaglandin or bradykinin.
3. It may fail to inactivate circulating vasopressor substances.
4. Ineffective disposal of sodium resulting in sodium retention which may be responsible for hypertension.

45. There are 4 points to differentiate between hypertension caused by renal parenchymal disease and renovascular disease.

1. Peripheral plasma renin activity is less in renal parenchymal disease than in renovascular hypertension.
2. Cardiac output is normal in renal parenchymal disease (unless uremia or anemia is present).
3. Blood volume is high in renal parenchymal disease and low in renovascular hypertension.
4. Circulatory response to tilting and Valsalva maneuver are exaggerated in renovascular hypertension.

Uric acid levels are correlated indirectly with renal blood flow and directly with renovascular disease. Unexplained uremia in essential hypertension is likely to reflect early renovascular involvement. If uric acid is high, see for renovascular involvement.

46. Renovascular hypertension is suspected in patients when:

1. Sudden onset of hypertension occurs in a patient below 20 years age or above 50 years age.
2. Easily controllable hypertension becomes suddenly difficult to control.
3. Short duration of hypertension.
4. Systolic and diastolic bruit in the upper abdomen or flank is present.

Most commonly correctable cause. 2–6% of hypertension may have renovascular cause.

47. There are 4 types of renal disease which affect hypertension or uremia.

1. Any renal disease that reduces renal mass but with all the remaining normal nephrons—always causes anuremic tendency but really causes hypertension.
2. Renal disease that reduces glomerular filtration, decreases glomerular filtration coefficient or increase in peripheral vascular resistance will cause hypertension but no uremic tendency when all glomeruli are affected equally.
3. Any factor that causes excessive tubular reabsorption of fluid. For example, primary aldosteronism—HT. There is pure HT with no tendency to uremia, unless there is superimposed kidney damage as well.
4. Diseases that cause pure destruction of tubular epithelium will cause decreased reabsorption of water and sodium and therefore will cause tendency to HT, unless the individual ingests large quantities of water and salt. But this is a rare condition.

48. Management of hypertensive population in India can be described by the rule of halves.

1. 50% of the HT patients are not diagnosed.
2. 50% diagnosed but do not have treatment.
3. 50% under treatment are inadequately treated and their hypertension is not under control.

4. 50% of the remaining hypertensives under adequate treatment are well-controlled.

For the essential cause of failure or discontinue of treatment is that in the early stages, the patient feels perfectly well, resents the nuisance of a regime which often makes him unwell. Avoidance of unnecessary restrictions, choice of least unpleasent pills and understanding by the patient of what the issue is for him are essential components of successful compliance.

49. There are 4 groups of hypertensive population in India as shown by the survey done in some centers in Bombay and Chandigarh.

1. 50% unknown or latent.
2. 25% identified but untreated
3. 12.5% inadequately treated.
4. 12.5% adequately treated.

Prevalence of hypertension is very high in India, 111/1000 above the age of 30 years. But in any given time only 10% of hypertensive patients are on treatment with antihypertensive medication. The prevalence of coronary artery disease and hypertension is fast catching up with western trends.

According to one survey:

1. 34% not aware.
2. 12% aware but not taking treatment.
3. 32% receiving treatment but poorly controlled.
4. 22% under control.

50. When the life expectancy of a person with high blood pressure left untreated is compared with a person similar in age, sex, race and exposed to the same environment but with a normal pressure, it is seen that the person with untreated high blood pressure lives shorter.

The following 4 are examples of life expectancy.

A 35-year-old male:

1. With a BP of 130/90 mm Hg dies 4 years earlier.
2. With a BP of 140/90 mm Hg dies 9 years earlier.
3. With a BP of 150/100 mm Hg dies 17 years earlier.
4. With a BP of more than 160/110 mm Hg dies more than 20 years earlier.

As compared with a person of same age, exposed to a similar environment. This is why hypertension is regarded as a 'Silent Killer'.

51. The hypertension patients may present in any of the following 4 ways:

1. As an asymptomatic—found during routine examination (for recruitment, LIC, etc). The person may not be aware of it for years. It is detected on a routine physical examination. Hypertension seldom causes symptoms until organ damage has occurred, which may be irreversible.
2. May present with unrelated disease or indirectly related disorder (MI) who has hypertension on examination.
3. May present with symptoms of hypertension.
4. May present with hypertensive emergency.

52. Hypertension is classified into 4 groups as per the fifth report of Joint National Committee (JNC) (USA) on detection, evaluation and treatment of high blood pressure for adults aged 18 years and older.

53. JNC 7 report as published in JAMA May 21, 2003 on

1. Prevention
2. Detection
3. Evaluation
4. Treatment of high blood pressure.

54. Classification and management of blood pressure for adults—by JNC 7 report.

Table B-7

BP classification	SBP	DBP	Lifestyle modification	Initial drug treatment	
				Without compelling indication	With compelling indication
Normal	< 120	< 80	Encourage	No antihypertensive drug indicated	Drugs for the compelling indications
Prehypertension	120–139	80–89	Yes		
Stage I hypertension	140–159	90–99	Yes	Thiazide-type diuretics for most, may consider ACEI, ARB, BB, CCB, or combinations	Drugs for the compelling indications, other antihypertensive drugs (Diuretics, ACEI, ARB, BB, CCB) as needed
State II hypertension	≥ 160	> 100	Yes	Two-drug combination for most (Usually thiazide-type diuretic and ACEI, ARB, or BB or CCB	

ACEI, angiotensin-converting enzyme inhibitor; ARB, angiotensin receptor blockers; BB, β-blocker; CCB, calcium channel blocker

55. Note the following 4 points while categorizing the BP.

1. Hypertension grading is based on an average of two or more readings taken at each of two or more visits during the next 1 to 2 months after the initial reading except when the initial blood pressure corresponds to stage 4.
2. When SBP and DBP fall into different categories, the higher category should be selected to classify; the individual's blood pressure status.
   For example, 160/92 should be classified as stage 2 and 180/120 should be classified as stage 4.
3. Isolated systolic hypertension is defined as a SBP of 140 mm Hg or more and DBP of less than 90 mm Hg.
4. The physician should specify the presence or absence of risk factors and target organ disease. For example, a patient with BP 144/94 mm Hg with diabetes and left ventricular hypertrophy should be classified as having stage I hypertension with diabetes risk factor and target organ disease of left ventricular hypertrophy.

56. Hypertension is graded according to the diastolic pressure as:

1. Mild hypertension when diastole is 90–104 mm Hg.
2. Moderate hypertension when diastole is 105–114 mm Hg.
3. Severe hypertension when diastole is above 115 mm Hg.
4. Systolic hypertension so-called casual hypertension is found on routine examination is a feature of non-compliant arteries of old age. Diastolic pressure of 80 mm Hg or less with elevated systolic pressure of 160 mm Hg or above is also important in assessing cardiovascular morbidity.

Abnormal blood pressure should be considered in relation to the age of the patient. A BP of 140/90 mm Hg would indicate severe hypertension in a child whereas it is considered as high normal in an adult.

57. The blood pressure is recorded in:

1. Supine position.
2. Upright position.
3. Both upper and lower extremities.
4. Left lateral position in pregnant woman.
   High BP is a sign.

How does this help?

A rise in diastolic pressure when the patient changes from supine to the standing position is most compatible with essential hypertension.

A fall of BP in the absence of antihypertensive medication suggests other forms of secondary hypertension.

The shift of the body position from lying to standing is usually associated with cardiovascular adjustment which tries to compensate for the effects of gravity on the circulatory system by the action of capacitance vessels (veins). The compensatory mechanism is inefficient in some who show orthostatic intolerance to standing exhibited by:

i. Increase in heart rate.
ii. Fall in systolic BP.
iii. Decreased pulse pressure.
iv. Few subjective symptoms of cerebral ischemia.

Orthostatic hypotension and tachycardia may be suggestive of reduced blood volume while resting tachycardia may be a clue to the severe heart failure.

Seated pressures cannot be used to assess progress because good control of DBP < 90 mm Hg, usually represents syncope levels of hypertension in the standing position or after exercise. The best target pressure to use is the standing pressure. It is a great help to exercise the patient and measure one standing pressure, using a step-test or a stairway. Results from this help in evaluating the control of BP.

Patients with aortic incompetence may show higher systolic pressure in the legs than in the arms, while patients with coarctation of aorta may show lower systolic pressure in legs and some elevation of blood pressure in the arms.

Blood pressure in pregnancy should be measured with the woman seated or lying on her left side. This is because profound hypotension can occur in late pregnancy if a woman lies supine because of the mechanical obstruction of the inferior vena cava by the gravid uterus. It is probably advisable to take the BP after taking the history and before other clinical examination.

Roll-over-test in pregnant women: Record the BP in left lateral position. After 5 min, record the BP in supine position. If diastole goes up by 20 mm, she goes into toxemia. It starts after 24 weeks of pregnancy. If positive, 90% go into toxemia pregnancy.

Do not take the BP on the hemiplegic side due to autonomic imbalance.

58. The standing blood pressure should be measured in

1. All patients on antihypertensive therapy on follow-up.
2. All patients on vasodialator therapy for heart failure.
3. All patients with syncope or near syncope.
4. Hypovolemia due to any cause.

59. BP should be checked about 4 times in patients with arrhythmias like atrial fibrillation, ventricular ectopics, etc. for correct reading.

60. The reporting system of blood pressure should also be defined. There are 4 points to specify while reporting blood pressure:

1. Lying or sitting or standing.
2. Left arm or right arm.
3. Morning or evening.
4. During activity or after adequate physical or mental rest and with or without medication.

Diurnal variation of blood pressure occurs in both normotensive and hypertensive people being lowest in the early part of the night and highest in the hour or so before waking in the morning. It rarely shows with reading taken by the sphygmomanometer but it can be revealed by continuous intra-arterial pressure recording. The diurnal variation is exaggerated in hypertensives. Changes in blood pressure do occur throughout the day in response to activity or emotion.

61. A new concept in the management of hypertension has been the recent introduction of ambulatory blood pressure monitoring (ABPM) which gives an assessment of:

1. The average BP during 24 hours.
2. The number of abnormal BP readings in 24 hours.
3. BP at work.
4. BP response to stress and changes in circadian pattern of BP.

62. The indications of ABPM at present are:

1. Recording circadian fluctuations of BP and association with target organ damage, white coat hypertension, episodic hypertension.
2. Evaluation of BP changes in unstable angina, pulmonary congestion, myocardial infarction, episodic rise of BP associated with pheochromocytoma.
3. Evaluation of drug resistance to see if ABPM shows good control.
4. Evaluation of hypotensive episodes with antihypertensive drugs.

Exact role of ABPM in the treatment of hypertension remains to be defined.

63. Ambulatory BP monitoring (ABPM)—according to JNC 7 report:

1. ABPM is warranted for evaluation of "white coat" hypertension in absence of target organ damage.
2. ABPM values are usually lower than clinical readings.
3. Awake individuals with hypertension have an average BP of > 135/85 mm Hg and during sleep > 125/75 mm Hg.
4. BP drops by 10 to 20% during the night, if not, signals possible increases risk for cardiovascular events.

64. Hypertensives may give the pulse a hard atherosclerotic quality and cause hypertensive retinopathy. It is the first visible sign of arteriolar damage and therefore provides the principle means to assess the urgency of treatment in individual case. The changes in the vascular tree of the body can be directly visualized within the eye using an ophthalmoscope. The retinal vessels are the only vessels of the body which can be visualized directly, more or less in their naked form. This provides a clue to the changes simultaneously occurring in other organs of the body.

The retinal 'arteries' are really arterioles, their walls are thin and transparent with a mean diameter of just over 1 mm. The retinal veins are 10–40% larger than arterioles and cross behind them. The caliber of veins and arterioles uniformly diminish as they branch out from the disk to the periphery; and this is shown by a uniform central light reflex along their length.

Normal fundus shows the column of blood they contain. At the arteriovenous crossings, the contents of veins is seen clearly through the transparent arteriolar walls without any 'nipping' effect.

The following 4 changes occur in hypertensive retinopathy:

1. *Variation in caliber of retinal arterioles:* This is the earliest and most constant sign of retinopathy. These variations are permanent. They are not caused by spasm, but by thickening of the intima which narrows the column of blood. Fibrosis and elastosis of the media cause more opacity.
2. *Arteriovenous 'nipping':* It is not a true 'nipping' which would produce thicker vein on the proximal side of the crossing. It is an effect of the increased thickness and opacity of the retinal arteriolar wall, through which the venous blood at the crossing is no longer easily visible. This sign is seen at a more advanced stage of arteriolar thickening.
3. *Changes in the arteriolar light reflex:* Develop as arteriolar thickening advances. It is seen first as a 'copper' or 'silver' wire appearance in which blood column becomes less and less visible and the arteriolar wall more and more opaque.
4. *Narrowing of the retinal arterioles:* Though it is unreliable, this is estimated in practice always as relative to the much more variable caliber of the veins. Arteriolar narrowing eventually produces a pale fundus.

These changes are well seen and interpreted without difficulty with a dilated pupil. It is difficult to follow several arterioles from each of the optic disks through undilated pupil, particularly by those who seldom see a grossly abnormal fundus.

65. Fundoscopic changes in hypertension are classified into 4 grades by Keith-Wagener-Barker (from Mayo Clinic 1939).

1. Grade I - Spasm and narrowing of the lumen, increased light reflex (silver wiring).
2. Grade II - Tortuosity and arteriovenous (AV) nipping.
3. Grade III - Hemorrhages and soft or cotton wool exudates.
4. Grade IV - Papilledema, hard exudates fanning out from the macula, usually developing after papilledema.

(Grades III and IV: Malignant hypertension)

The grading has been proved to have direct relation with the prognosis. For practical purposes Grade I and II are usually clubbed together as one and Grade III and IV which are obvious are also clubbed as one hypertensive retinopathy of Grade I and II are associated with mild to moderate hypertension, Grade III and IV with malignant hypertension. This grading has been proved to have direct relation with the prognosis. The antihypertensive measures especially in malignant hypertension can spare the heart, brain, kidneys and the other organs.

66. The optic fundi are one of the important targets for hypertensive damage. Transient or permanent loss of vision in one or both eyes is one outcome of uncontrolled hypertension.

Sudden loss of vision is usually from any of the following 4 causes

1. Vitreous hemorrhage.
2. Central retinal artery occlusion (CRAC).
3. Central retinal vein occlusion (CRVO) (Hemorrhage retinopathy) and branch vein occlusion.
4. Retinal detachment.

Each is a fairly common presentation of hypertension in an unscreened population.

67. Hypertensives are graded into 4 stages by hemodynamic alterations of CVS.

Stage I – Normal-sized heart with no evidence of cardiac involvement by chest X-ray or ECG.

Stage II – Early LVH as detected by ECG left atrial abnormality (S4).

Stage III – Clinically evident LVH by X-ray or ECG.

Stage IV – Left ventricular failure (LVF).

68. There are 4 points in evaluating the hypertensive patients during history taking, clinical examination and laboratory tests.

1. Find the correctable cause of secondary HT.
2. Establish the baseline before starting treatment.
3. Assess the factors which may influence the type of treatment or adversely modified by the therapy.
4. Identify the other risk factors responsible for the development of arteriosclerotic cardiovascular disease.

69. Symptoms of hypertension.

Uncomplicated hypertension may be asymptomatic and the person may not be aware of it for years. Common nonspecific symptoms which a person suffering from hypertension may have:

1. Headache: Headache is no more common in hypertensive than normotensive.
2. Epistaxis.
3. Tinnitus or dizziness.
4. Visual disturbance or syncope.

70. The symptoms that may occur with malignant hypertension are:

1. Headache—mostly morning occipital headache.
2. Blurred vision due to retinopathy.
3. Chest pain of ischemic heart disease.
4. Shortness of breath due to stiffness or failure of left ventricle.
5. Claudication due to peripheral vascular disease.
6. Symptoms of uremia of renal failure.
7. Congestive cardiac failure.
8. Stroke.

71. The 4 symptoms that may occur with hypertensive encephalopathy are:

1. Drowsiness.
2. Confusion.
3. Dysphagia.
4. Minor strokes or fits.

Hypertensive encephalopathy may occur with or without the retinal changes of malignant hypertension. The diastolic blood pressure is usually greater than 120 mm Hg but occasionally may be as low as 110 mm Hg. It is associated with focal swelling of the brain most probably due to leakage of plasma from damaged arterioles and capillaries. It is an emergency where rapid lowering of the blood pressure is indicated.

72. Secondary hypertension is suspected when there is following clinical features:

1. Onset at < 20 or > 50 years age.
2. Extreme hypertension, particularly if refractory to standard treatment.
3. Accelerated or malignant hypertension.
4. Recent elevation of serum creatinine that is unexplained or reversibly induced by an ACEI.
5. Unprovoked hyperkalemia—muscle cramps, weakness.
6. Abdominal bruit.
7. Labile paroxysms of hypertension with headache.
8. Weight loss, tachycardia, sweating, tremor.
9. Abdominal or flank mass.
10. Delayed or absent femoral pulses with lower blood pressure in lower extremities.
11. Truncal obesity with purple striae.
12. Joint pains/swelling/facial or peripheral edema.

73. A person with secondary hypertension may complain of symptoms of his underlying disease for example.

Table B-8

1. Abdominal pain, dysuria, frequency, nocturia	May signify renal disease
2. Joint pains/swelling facial or peripheral edema	Connective tissue disorder/or forms of nephritis
3. Weight loss, failure to gain weight, sweating, flushing, fever, palpitation	Pheochromocytoma
4. Polyuria, polydipsia, muscle cramps, weakness, constipation	Hypokalemia in patients with primary aldosteronism

74. The 4 points that help in the personal history are:

Table B-9

1. H/o diet containing tyrosine	Tobacco chewing, snuff powder, smoking, *pan-parag*
2. H/o injection of drugs	Drug induced hypertension—some cough syrups containing ephedrine, nasal drops containing ephedrine/ pseudoephedrine, anoretic agents
3. Occupational h/o	Lead and cadmium poisoning
4. H/o abdominal trauma, hematuria	Renovascular hypertension
5. H/o claudication	Peripheral vascular disease
6. H/o loss of close relative, financial loss, etc.	Depression
7. Previous H/o chest pain	IHD, MI
8. Previous H/o transient ischemic attack, stroke	CNS complications

75. The 4 points that help in the family history are:

Table B-10

1. Toxemia pregnancy/ Eclampsia	Important in essential hypertension
2. Renal disease	Inherited renal disease
3. Tumors	Endocrinal disease
4. Strokes or sudden death	Hypertensive heart disease, IHD, MI

76. Physical examination.

General appearance: It may give a clue to some causes of secondary hypertension.

Table B-11

1. Pallor, puffiness of face or pedal edema	Renal disease
2. Pallor, sweating at rest, swelling, loss of weight	Pheochromocytoma
3. Inappropriate muscle development of upper limbs	Coarctation of Aorta
4. Round face, hirsutism, buffalo hump, truncal obesity, striae	Cushing's syndrome
5. Webbing of neck, low hairline, wide spaced nipples, wide carrying angle	Turner's syndrome
6. Coarse, oily skin, large tongue, prominent supraorbital ridge, increased teeth space, increase in shoe size, thick spade fingers	Acromegaly
7. Exophthalmos, thyroid swelling or nodule	Thyrotoxicosis
8. Expressionless face, dry skin and hair, non-pitting edema of eyelids, hands, feet	Myxedema

77. Signs for causes of secondary hypertension should be looked for—for example,

Table B-12

1. Abdominal bruit, particularly those that lateralized to the renal areas or have a diastolic component	Renal artery stenosis
2. Abdominal or flank masses	Polycystic kidney
3. Delayed or absent femoral arterial pluses and decreased blood pressure in the lower extremities	Coarctation of aorta
4. A pulsatile expansile mass	Abdominal aortic aneurism

78. Some clues from the laboratory tests.

1. *Unprovoked hypokalemia:* Primary aldosteronism.
2. *Hypercalcemia:* Hyperparathyroidism .
3. *Rised creatinine or abnormal urine analysis:* Renal parenchymal disease.
4. *T3, T4, TSH:* TSH raised in hypothyroidism, TSH decreased thyrotoxicosis.

79. The main features of the physical examination in hypertension are to assess the organ damage. In most of the cases, there are no specific signs. The 4 commoner signs of CVS when present are:

1. Apex: Apical impulse is sustained and non-displaced in early stage. Apex is laterally displaced in late stages due to left ventricular hypertrophy/dilation.
2. S1 is normal in intensity and character.
   S2 is louder at the right upper border because of accentuated aortic component (A2). It can have a reverse or paradoxical split either due to increased after load or to associated left bundle branch block (LBBB).
3. S4 is frequently palpated and audible indicating the stiffened hypertrophied and noncompliant left ventricle due to chronic pressure overload. S3 is present when there is heart failure
4. Murmurs: Aortic systolic flow murmur may be present. An early mid systolic murmur of aortic sclerosis is commonly present.

An early decrescendo diastolic murmur of aortic insufficiency may be heard along the mid left parasternal area especially in the presence of an acutely elevated blood pressure, frequently disappearing once the blood pressure is better controlled.

A pansystolic murmur of mitral insufficiency may be present in patient with dilated mitral annulus and advance heart failure S4 is a typical constant finding in a patient with mild to severe hypertension. He or she may have S4 even for 10–15 years without any cardiac failure. If heart failure develops S3 occurs for the first time. A tambour second sound is heard particularly with high BP which is previously thought as a sign of leutic aortitis. It is now known that it is most common in hypertension. Aortic systolic murmur is another sign.

The auscultatory finding of S4 gives a clue as to when to start antihypertensive treatment in a patient with a mild hypertension. Some may start treatment when the BP is 150/90, others when the BP is 158/102, 160/100, 160/110 and so on and so forth. The decision varies from one physician to another. A clue to start treatment is that if a patient has an atrial presystolic S4 sound alone and if the BP is constantly around 140/90 or above, medical therapy is indicated, if the patient is not overweight.

The presence of S4 indicates that the heart has already been sufficiently affected and the treatment should be started immediately. It further justifies, if a tambour S2 and an aortic systolic murmur are present even if the BP is constantly 140/90. These clinical auscultatory findings helps in deciding the medical therapy.

80. Never treat a hypertensive patient without examining the vessels at the 4 places.

1. Carotid pulse—to rule out occlusion or stenosis. Bruit over great vessels—for coarctation or arteritis.
2. Femoral pulse—absent or delayed femoral pulses, low leg pressure relative to arm BP—coarctation of aorta.
3. Auscultation over the abdominal aorta—occlusion or stenosis. Bruit for renal artery stenosis.
4. Auscultation over both flanks for renal arteries.

Otherwise, you may miss a curable surgical condition if the above examination is not done.

81. The features that contribute to the high morbidity and mortality of hypertension are:

1. Black race.
2. Younger age.
3. Male sex. Women tolerate and suffer less morbidity and mortality than men.
4. Height of the BP: The risk is related to both the systolic and diastolic BP. Risk is high with DBP > 115 mm Hg.
5. State of the arteries. For example, Grade III and IV hypertensive retinopathy carry 95% of mortality in one year without treatment.
6. Smoking.
7. Obesity.
8. Hypercholesterolemia.
9. Diabetes mellitus.
   Hypertension increases the risk of ischemic heart disease. The main effect of each of the 6, 7, 8 and 9 add to the risk. The risk is very high if there is combined effect in a patient of hypertension who is obese, smoker with elevated plasma lipids and glucose intolerance.
10. Alcohol: Regular consumption of smaller quantities of alcohol three times a day raise the blood pressure by about 5–9 mm Hg. This effect can be rapidly reversed within a week or so by simply stopping alcohol. Limit the alcohol consumption to no more than 2 drinks (30 mL of ethanol, for example 24 oz of bear, 10 oz of wine or 3 oz of whisky) per day in most men and to no more than one drink per day in women and lighter weight person. Pressor effect of large amounts of alcohol result from increase in cardiac output and heart rate.

11. Evidence of left ventricular hypertrophy.
12. Evidence of renal impairment.

Proper treatment with drugs can improve heart and kidney function.

82. Investigations: The investigations should be planned separately for each patient after getting clues from the clinical features. Certain basic investigations may provide a pointer toward the underlying condition for which more advanced studies may then be done in certain cases. More sophisticated tests are done in complications of hypertension. Main aim is to provide baseline data for future events.

The investigations can be taken up in 4 phases.

Phase-I. Broad screening

In the first phase, the baseline data are designed to determine if there is underlying cardiac or renal disease and to determine physiological sequel of blood pressure and future events.

1. Hemogram for associated anemia, infections, etc.
2. Urine analysis: To rule out renal parenchymal disease. The presence of proteinuria, hematuria, cells and casts indicate renal damage. See for glucose and bacteriuria. Urine for albumin and sugar, microscopic examination is a must in every case.
3. Biochemical: Urine culture in girls and selected boys. Urinary infections are common in children. Cystitis, pyelonephritis, etc. may be a cause of hypertension in children.
4. Chest X-ray: The heart is often normal in the early stages but enlarges after. The aorta may dilate and become elongated and tortuous as a result of increased pressure within it. Unfolding of aorta and calcification is commonly seen in old people with hypertension. Rib notching of coarctation of aorta may be seen perhaps once in a lifetime.
5. ECG: It helps as a baseline for evaluation of future chest pain or left ventricular failure. This may be normal and give more or less constant pattern over a five-year span and detection of significant changes is mulch easier where there is a previous record.

   Presence of pathological Q waves may reveal a previous silent infarct. Mortality from reinfarction and sudden death may be prevented by taking sufficient precautions.

   This may be normal or show left ventricular hypertrophy with or without strain pattern, left axis deviation. In Framingham study, definite left ventricular hypertrophy with ST and T wave changes was associated with a ninefold in five-year mortality in men and tenfold increase in women. This increased risk is independent of risk from hypertension alone. The voltage changes reflect muscular hypertrophy alone, whereas the ST and T wave changes reflect ischemic (coronary) artery disease.
6. Ultrasound abdomen: To check for kidney size and assess the type of renal disorder if any is present.
7. Echocardiography: To check for left ventricular function and any evidence of ischemic damage to the muscle by checking regional wall motion. For establishing baseline left ventricular mass for possible target organ damage and prognosis of drug therapy is justified.
8. IVP for evaluation of renal hypertension. It gives information of anatomy and function. It may show a small kidney and delay the excretion of contrast on the affected side.
9. Serum creatinine and urea—for renal status and any effect of the hypertension upon it.
10. Plasma potassium concentration: Hypokalemia in a patient not taking diuretics is a pointer toward excess mineralocorticoid secretion, for instance primary or secondary hyperaldosteronism.
11. Serum sodium: High in hyperaldosteronism.
12. Blood sugar fasting and postprandial: Rule out diabetes. To assess for any additional cardiac and renal risks associated with hypertension.
13. Serum cholesterol and lipid profile: At least crude lipid profile is done to assess and predict additional risks over and above that due to hypertension alone. Reliable results for total cholesterol and HDL can be obtained from non-fasting casual samples which can predict the outcome. VLDL results are reliable only after 18 hours fasting.
14. Plasma uric acid: In pregnant hypertension to rule out chronic hypertension. Increased levels are found in eclampsia. Hyperuricemia probably reflects decrease in renal blood flow presumably a reflection of nephrosclerosis.

Phase-II. Specific screening and non-invasive diagnostic procedure. Appropriate selective procedure may be done following data obtained from Phase-I. In patients with secondary hypertension, the underlying cause can be identified. Usually, the patients are aged under 40 years.

Secondary hypertension:

1. T3, T4, TSH—to rule out any thyroid dysfunction.
2. Plasma renin and serum aldosterone for evaluation of renal hypertension.
3. Plasma catecholamines and their metabolites with/without clonidine suppression—for pheochromocytoma. Vanillylmandelic acid (VMA) 24 hours urine for
   — VMA and catecholamines

– 17 keto and 17 hydroxysteroids

– Aldosterone excretion.

Catecholamines are elevated in pheochromocytoma. Aldosterone is raised in adenoma or bilateral hyperplasia of the adrenal cortex.

4. Voiding cystourethrogram—if IVP shows findings suggestive of cystoureteric reflux.
5. Computed tomography of kidneys and adrenals
6. Isotope renography complicated hypertension.
7. EEG and CAT scan for cerebral complications.
8. Color Doppler study of carotid arteries.

Young hypertensives under 30 years need thorough search for secondary causes including routine urography and estimation of 24 hours VMA. Routine urography above the age of 30 years may not be useful in the absence of renal disease.

Measurement of renin and plasma renin activity (PRA) are of no proven clinical value except for research purpose.

Phase-III. Invasive

In patients with hypertension in whom a likely organic cause is not diagnosed in Phase-I and II and in patients with severe hypertension and its complications.

1. Aortography—coarctation of aorta.
2. Coronary angiography.
3. Cerebral angiography.
4. Renal angiography.
5. Adrenal angiography.
6. A venography for renal vein renin levels: A comparison of renin produced by each kidney is measured by catheterizing the renal veins. This is often used in proven renal artery stenosis to assess the likely outcome of surgery. A ratio of 1.5:1 is indicative of possible success. There can be success with smaller ratio also. While others with higher ratio do not, because the other kidney has been damaged by the hypertension.
7. Caval catecholamines.
8. Digital subtraction arteriography.

Aortography is justified only if medical control of hypertension has been tried and failed.

Phase-IV

1. Renal biopsy
2. Split renal function studies.

Isotope renography: For renal blood flow and the excretory function of the kidney. It may show delayed excretion of isotope from the kidney. However, as both IVP and isotope renography are normal in about 20% patients of renal artery stenosis, this is usually done in patients in whom the renal artery stenosis is suspected before proceeding to renal arteriography.

83. Brief guide to work-up for secondary causes of hypertension.

Table B-13: Investigative procedure

Diagnosis	*Initial tests*	*Additional tests*
1. Chronic renal disease	Urinalysis, serum creatinine scanning of kidney	Isotopic renogram, renal biopsy
2. Renovascular disease	Plasma renin level before and 1 hour after enalapril	Aortogram
3. Coarctation	BP in legs, X-ray chest	Aortogram
4. Primary aldosteronism (Conn's disease)	Levels of plasma potassium, and sodium, plasma renin and aldosterone (ratio)	Urinary potassium, plasma or urinary aldosterone after saline load, CT of adrenal
5. Cushing's syndrome (Adrenocortical hyperfunction)	AM plasma cortisol level after 1 mg of dexamethasone at bedtime	Urinary cortisol level after variable doses of dexamethasone CT of adrenal
6. Pheochromocytoma	Spot urine test for metanephrine	Levels of urinary catechols, plasma catechols, basal and after 0.3 mg of clonidine, adrenal CT and scientiscans
7. Hyper-or hypothyroidism	T3,T4, TSH	Radioactive scanning of thyroid
8. Acromegaly, brain tumor	X-ray skull	CT of brain

84. Main aim of the treatment of hypertension is to reduce the likelihood of complications. This is achieved by 4 principles.

1. *Assessment of the patient and the need for treatment:* The most important assessment in any hypertensive patient is to collect more readings of casual pressure. To start on a lifelong drug treatment and medical dependence, because of one or two slip shot measurements using a standard sphygmomanometer cuff applied below a tightly rolled sleeve on the fat arm of an apprehensive patient, is clinically, scientifically and humanly indefensible. To interfere with moderately deviant pressures in the diastolic range of 90–100 mm Hg in middle-aged people whose pressures are unrelated to their symptoms or to 'treat' the transient ataxias of old age by inappropriate use of antihypertensive drugs is questionable. On the other hand, we come across younger people without symptoms walk about with untreated diastolic pressures of 120, 130 or even 160. 170 mm Hg, who needs immediate investigation before the start of treatment.

2. *Treatment of modifiable risk factors*
   For example, stop smoking and alcohol
   Reduction in weight
   Treatment of DM and hypercholesterolemia
   Smoking is an avoidable risk factor for hypertension and as well as coronary artery disease. Action on smoking should generally precede any antihypertensive treatment. Full history of smoking should be obtained like number of cigarettes a day, how long, pattern of smoking at home, at work, and at social gatherings, etc. This should be followed by a ***'smoking examination'***—measurement of peak flow rate with a flowmeter, or FEV1, if you have a spirometer. The readings should be compared from a nomogram giving normal values for sex, age, and height. Flow rate readings always improve after stopping smoking. In patients with advanced chronic obstructive pulmonary disease (COPD) with flow rate below 300 liters a minute, substantial improvement is unlikely, but it prevents further deterioration. Peak flow rate also helps in assessment of airway obstruction with β-blockade. If the doctor is a smoker, a nurse or other health worker who is a non-smoker should advise the patient to stop smoking . The smoking doctor, advising the patient to stop smoking is as effective as an alcoholic running a clinic for his fellow sufferers. An alternative for the doctor is to stop smoking first. Just changing from cigarettes to pipe or cigars probably does not reduce the risk.
3. *Identification and rectification of the causes of secondary hypertension where possible:* The first requirement of good management was to exclude secondary hypertension. The commonly met 4 causes of secondary hypertension should always be sought and excluded.
   The first is iatrogenic—oral contraception in women.
   The second is depression—depression is a common symptom with many hypertensives and with all antihypertensive drugs. Cause and effect is very difficult to prove and here is little reliable evidence for basic clinical decisions. It is useful to start treatment for depression before antihypertensive drugs are started. If the patient is seen with complaint of depression who is on antihypertensive drugs should be investigated empirically by gradually withdrawing it.
   The third is renal artery stenosis—Auscultate over both flanks for renal arteries. Bruit is heard in renal artery stenosis.
   The fourth is coarctation of aorta. The diagnosis is easy if it is remembered that femoral pulses are always reduced and delayed in relation to the radial pulse.
4. *Reduction of the blood pressure.*

85. The management of hypertension in the population over the last 10–15 years has resulted in marked reduction in the incidence of following 4 conditions:

1. Left ventricular failure.
2. Renal failure.
3. Cerebrovascular strokes (almost halved).
4. Coronary heart disease (not much reduced as others).

86. Chances of success in fighting against hypertension varies from:

1. Country to country (more in Japanese, less in Eskimos).
2. Urban to rural (more in urban population).
3. Literate to illiterate (more in literates).
4. Social customs, etc.

The hypertension in urban population is high in comparison to the rural population in India.

The differences in rural and urban population in India and other places, clearly due to lifestyle and dietary factors. Hypertension is rarely found in rural or "tribal" areas of Africa, but it is very common in African cities and in Black people in Britain and the United States.

87. The proportion of hypertensives likely to be receiving adequate treatment is best expressed by the 'rule of 4s' which implies that for every:

1. First, adequately treated hypertensive
2. Second, who is inadequately treated
3. Third, who is known to have hypertension but not receiving any treatment
4. Fourth, who is not even known to have hypertension.

88. There are 4 principles in the management of hypertension.

1. General Measures: Non-drug treatment
2. Antihypertensive drugs
3. Treatment of complications
4. Treatment of underlying cause if detected.

89. Non-drug treatment (Lifestyle modification) consists of 4 observations.

It is beneficial in mild hypertension between 90–104 mm Hg diastolic and in those whose therapy has been stopped. It is also beneficial in moderate and severe HT along with drugs.

1. *Rest:* Physical, mental and psychological relaxation to avoid stress. Practice relaxation techniques—like Savasana, transcendental meditation)
2. *Diet:* (DASH—dietary approaches to stop hypertension)
   Restrict salt to 4–5 g/day (Less than 1 g/day reduces BP but difficult to practice)
   Restrict calories; restrict cholesterol and saturated fats to reduce weight.

Weight reduction: 1 kg loss of body weight = 1.6/1.3 mm Hg fall in BP. Weight loss also reduces sensitivity to sodium thereby improving further response to non-drug therapy.
Potassium supplementation (by fruits).
Vegetarian diet—it causes low glomerular filtration rate (GFR) whereas non-vegetarian diet increases GFR. GFR is more in hypertension. Non-vegetarian diet still increases GFR and causes more damage to the kidneys. Vegetarians have low BP than non-vegetarians.
$Na^+ \downarrow K^+ \downarrow Ca^{++} \downarrow$ in the diet.
Pure fish oil can be taken—commercial fish oil contains additional vitamin D. Take pure fish oil without vitamin D. Fish oil is the precursor of vasodilator. It acts through essential fatty acids—arachidonic acid chain system by blocking.
Caution on diet should be advised, particularly for those with high total cholesterol or low HDL.
A prudent diet, low in animal fats, using polyunsaturates where fats are unavoidable with a relative increase in vegetable and cereal content, within a reduction in total calories should be advised.
The fiber content of diet may have an important affect on plasma lipids.

3. *Avoid:* Stress, smoking, alcohol, excessive tea or coffee, drugs like corticosteroids, MAO inhibitors, oral contraceptive pills in females, etc.
4. *Exercise:* Advise dynamic (isotonic) exercises like walking, jogging, skipping, running, cycling, swimming, etc. Avoid static (isometric) or strenuous exercises like weightlifting, bull-worker, etc. since they increase peripheral vascular resistance.

90. Exercise: Exercise is continued till the target heart rate (HR) is reached.

Maximum HR = 220 – Age
Target HR = 75% of maximum heart rate unless there are limitation due to other caused like coronary artery disease (CAD) hypertension.
At any given time, blood glucose in circulation is not enough to meet with the ongoing glucose demands. Lot of glucose is taken up by the skeletal muscle during exercise. Hence, the liver starts a process of gluconeogenesis wherein glycogen stores are converted into glucose.
In continuous exercise: From ammonic acids to glucose.
High sympathetic activity: Mobilizes from free fatty acids from adipose tissue which also helps to generate ATPs – the energy units

Sympathetic activity ↑ ______→ releases epinephrine
glucagon
↓ inhibits
Insulin output from islets.

This along with gluconeogenesis—helps in maintaining the glucose hemostasis.
This explains the rarity of hypoglycemia during exercise in non-diabetics.
Increase uptake by skeletal muscle: Increases the sensitivity to insulin. This can lost for more than 12–24 hours. Regular exercise also increases insulin receptors and requirements of exogenous insulin.
This effect can last for more that 12–24 hours.
Blood lipids: Reduces cholesterol, triglycerides increases HDL. The effect of triglycerides is more pronounced.
Each session: 5–10 min. Warming up and cooling down gradually increased from mild, simple activation.

In diabetes – 5 km walk in 45 min, or
8 km cycling in 15 min.
500 spot running steps (left and right continue as in 11 min. Undertaken with lower intensity and longer time.

Each session should be 20 to 25 min, at 5 to 6 times a week or minimum 3 times a week.

About 1/3rd of energy used each day by a normal person goes into muscular activity and in the laborers as much as 2/3rd, and occasionally 3/4th is used in this way.

91. Regular aerobic exercise have the following 4 favorable cardiovascular effects.

1. Improves endothelial function.
2. Improves peripheral vasodilatation.
3. Reduces plasma catecholamines.
4. Reduces resting heart rate and improves heart rate variability.

92. Our ancient medicine ayurveda, stresses the following 4 principles for the well-being of an individual

1. *Aachaar:* (Conduct and character)
2. *Vichaar:* (Thought process)
3. *Vyavahaar:* (Person to person dealings)
4. *Ahaar and nidra:* (Food and sleep habits)

These principles hold good even today not only to the causes of essential hypertension but for other diseases too.

93. The 4 relaxation techniques that are commonly followed are:

1. Transcendental meditation.
2. Yoga (Savasana).
3. Biofeedback.
4. Psychotherapy.

Stress is an essential challenge in life for progress. There should be no immediate reaction to mental stress. By sitting calm, analyzing and taking appropriate action, one can convert bad stress (distress) into good stress (eustress).

Studies have shown that a person who works even 16 to 18 hours a day with social and mental satisfaction will be without mental fatigue and lower BP recordings than an individual who works 6–8 hours per day for purely selfish purposes. Transcendental meditation does not mean meditation for 20 minutes in the morning. It means that the meditator is always happy, enjoys his work, is more alert and more productive. Meditative mood is maintained while walking, talking or working. This avoids fears, prejudices, unwanted stress, self-destructive habits such as smoking or alcohol. Mild to moderate hypertension becomes normal in people who practice transcendental meditation.

94. Restriction of salt: A reduction in sodium by 5–6 g sodium chloride results in a fall of BP of 5.4/6.5 mm Hg. Rigid salt restriction is not recommended. Moderate reduction of 2 g per day is achieved by the following:

1. Avoid processed foods, substitute with natural foods.
2. Do not add extrasodium during cooking or at the table.
3. Substitute salt with mixed sodium and potassium preparations.
4. Avoid fast foods, antacids with high sodium content.

Elimination of salt shaker at table (Na = 1.6–2.8 g).
Elimination of salt in cooking and at table (Na = 1.2–1.8 g).
Institution of A and B + low sodium diet (Na = 0.2–1.0 g).

95. The stress can be subdivided into 4 types.

1. Stress by dynamic exercise.
2. Stress by static exercise.
3. Cold stress.
4. Mental stress.

In dynamic exercise and mental stress, the surge involves largely the systolic BP and it can be easily controlled by β-blockers. In static exercise and cold stress surge involves mainly the diastolic pressure and it can be easily controlled by α-blockers.

96. The use of antihypertensive drugs should be lifelong or it should be maintained until pressure falls in the aged failing heart. It is difficult to predict with certainty, the response of any individual to long- term antihypertensive medication. Each patient is different, because each person has a unique metabolic inheritance, experience and environmental adaptive nature. In few patients whose pressures remain controlled after stopping drugs will usually found to have begun treatment on poorly thought indications. The aim of treatment is to reduce the pretreatment pressure to a target pressure, verified at regular intervals with side-effects tolerable to the patient.

Following 4 values must be known within reasonable limits:
1. Initial pressure.
2. Target pressure.
3. Follow-up compliance.
4. Side-effects tolerable to the patient.

Better to take at least 3 or 4 readings before starting treatment. If this record is not maintained, the extent of reduction in pressure is uncertain. Follow-up pressures should be frequently measured but not once in 6 months or a year. If there is very high pressure, rapid fall for the first three months followed more slowly for next 6 months is maintained.

If the initial pressure is only 10 mm Hg moreover the target pressure, apparent successful treatment can be guaranteed for at least the first year of treatment with any antihypertensive drug or even sometimes with a placebo. This type of 'treatment' is now happening on a mass scale with borderline hypertension in diastolic range of 90–100 mm Hg.

97. There are 4 overall guidelines to start drug therapy:

1. Patients with diastolic blood pressure above 100 mm Hg if associated with an end organ damage should be started on drugs immediately.
2. Patients with diastolic blood pressure below 100 mm Hg who are otherwise at low-risk should be encouraged to loose weight if obese, reduce sodium intake, exercise regularly and relax.
3. Patients with diastolic blood pressure in low 90s should be observed for 6 months and if the level goes above 100 mm Hg, the drug therapy should be started.
4. Patient should be maintained in low 80s of diastolic pressure after starting the drug therapy, provided there are no side-effects.

98. Antihypertensive drugs can be classified into 4 groups:

I. ***Diuretics:* Drugs that alter sodium and water balance**
   a. *Thiazides and related agents:* Hydrochlorothiazide, chlorothiazide, chlorothalidone.
      Thiazides have a greater hypertensive effect than the loop diuretics. They act in two phases. They reduce the plasma volume in first phase and peripheral vascular resistance in long-term second phase due to changes in electrolyte and intracellular fluid resulting in reduced contractility of the smooth muscle cells of the arterial wall.
   b. *Loop diuretics:* Furosemide, ethacrynic acid, bumetanide, etc.
   c. *Potassium-sparing diuretics:* Spironolactone, triamterene, amiloride, etc.
   d. *Other diuretics:* Indapamide, xipamide, metolozone.

II. ***Adrenergic inhibiting drugs***

a. *Centrally acting agents:* Methyldopa, clonidine, guanabenz, guanfacine.

b. *β-adrenergic antagonists (β-blockers):* Selective and non-selective, propranolol, atenolol, metoprolol

c. *α-adrenergic antagonists:* Prazocin, terazocin, phenoxybenzamine, phentolamine.

d. *α and β-blockers:* Labetalol—it is particularly useful in patients with renal failure. It is largely metabolized and excreted by the liver.

e. *Adrenergic-neuron blocking agents:* Guanethidine, teserpine, etc.

f. *Ganglion-blocking agents:* Trimethaphen.

III. ***Vasodilators***

a. *Arterial:* Calcium channel blockers (Nifedipine, amlodipine, felodipine, nicardipine, verapamil, diltiazem, hydralazine, prazosin, minoxidil, diazoxide, etc.

b. *Arterial and venous:* Sodium nitroprusside, nitroglycerin.

Prazosin is a vasodilator as well as α-blocker

IV. ***Selective enzyme inhibitors***: Captopril, enalapril, lisinopril, ramipril, perindopril, etc.

These drugs inhibit the conversion of angiotensin I to angiotensin II and also suppress the secretion of aldosterone and inhibit the synthesis of kinins.

For example, captopril acts on converting enzyme, saralasin acts on angiotensin II.

Losartan potassium is an angiotensin II receptor blocker ARBs: Losarten, candisarten, irbesarten, telemesarten, olmasarten, etc.

99. Other way of classification into 4 groups:

1. ***Volume depleting drugs***
   - Benzothiadiazine and related compounds
     Thiazides, metolazone, xipamide, indapamide
   - Loop diuretics
     Furosemide, ethacrynic acid, bumetanide
   - Potassium sparing agents
     Spiranolactone, triamterene, amiloride.
2. ***Renin-lowering antivasoconstrictors*** (adrenergic or sympathetic blocking drugs).
   - *β-blockers:* propranolol, atenolol, metoprolol
   - *Alpha-receptors:* phenoxybenzamine, phentolamine
   - *Alpha and β-blocker:* Labetalol
   - *Central:* Alpha-methyldopa, clonidine
   - *Peripheral:* Reserpine, guanethidine, debrisoquine,
   - *Autonomic ganglion blockers:* Mecamylamine, pentolinium, trimethaphan.
3. ***Renin-independent direct vasodilators.***
   - *Hydralazine:* These drugs act by directly relaxing vascular smooth muscle.
     - Diazoxide
     - Sodium nitroprusside
   - *Prazocin:* This drug competitively inhibits post-synaptic alpha-1 adrenoreceptors.
     - Minoxidil
     - Natrilix, guanethedine.
4. ***Miscellaneous***
   - Calcium channel blockers—nifedipine
   - Selective angiotensin-converting enzyme inhibitors—enalapril, captopril
   - Angiotensin II receptor antagonist—losartan potassium
   - Angiotensin II—Sarlasin
   - Renin-independent adrenergic blockers: Guanethidine, bethnidine pargyline, debrisoquine.

100. Drugs used in the treatment of hypertension dosage and route of administration, selected side effects and comments

Table B-14

Drug	*Dosage*	*Route*	*Selected side effects and comments*
Diuretics thiazide diuretics			
1. Hydrochlorothiazide (Esodry)	12.5–50 mg/od or bd	Oral	$K^+\downarrow$, $Na^+\downarrow$ Magnesium ↓
2. Chlorothiazide (Deursil)	12.5–50 mg/od	Oral	Uric acid ↑ $Ca^{++}\uparrow$
3. Chlorthalidone	12.5–50 mg/od	Oral	Short-term; cholesterol↑
4. Bendrofluazide	2.5–5 mg/24 h po	Oral	glucose↑
Loop diuretics			Short duration of action
5. Furosemide	40–80 mg/2–3 times a day	Oral/IM/IV	
6. Ethacrinic acid	25–50 mg/od/bd	Oral	
7. Bumetanide	1–2 mg/od	Oral	
8. Torsemide	5–100 mg/od	Oral	

Contd...

Contd...

Drug	*Dosage*	*Route*	*Selected side effects and comments*
Potassium sparing diuretics 9. Spiranolactone 10. Triamterene 11. Amiloride	25–100 mg/2–4 times a day 50–100 mg/1–2 times a day 5–20 mg/od	Oral Oral Oral	Hyperkalemia (Gynecomastia)
Other diuretics 12. Xipamide 13. Indapamide 14. Metolozone	20 mg/od 2.5 mg/od 2.5–5 mg/od	Oral Oral Oral	Lipid neutral
Adrenergic inhibiting drugs *Centrally acting agents* 15. Methyldopa 16. Clonidine 17. Guanabenz	250–1000 mg/tid qid 5–10 mg/kg IVI (IV, 250–1000 mg/4–6 hours) 0.2–1.2 mg/bd or qid 4–16 mg/bd	Oral/IV Oral Oral	Sedation,dry mouth, bradycardia, withdrawal hypertension (Hepatic and autoimmune disorders) Postural hypotension
Adrenergic neuron blocking agents 18. Guanethidine 19. Reserpine 20. Prazocin terazocin 21. Phentolamine 22. Phenoxybenzamine	10–300 mg/daily 0.1–0.5 mg/daily 0.07 mg/kg, (maximun 2.5 mg) mg/daily 1–5 mg/bd or tid 2.5 mg/od 1–5 mg 10–50 mg/od/bd	Oral Oral IM/IV Oral Oral /IV Oral	Nasal congestion, sedation, depression, activation of peptic ulcer
Alpha-blockers 23. Prazosin 24. Terazosin 25. Doxazosin	1–20 mg/day 1–20 mg/day 1–16 mg/day	Oral Oral Oral	
β-blockers 26. Propranolol 27. Atenolol 28. Metoprolol 29. Timolol 30. Nadolol 31. Esmolol	10–120 mg/2–4 times a day 50–100 mg/od/bd 25–125 mg/bd 20–60 mg/od/bd 40–320 mg/od 200–500 mg/kg/min for 4 min then 50–300 mg/kg/min	Oral/IV Oral Oral Oral Oral Oral	Bronchospasm, Bradycardia, heart failure masking of insulin-induced hypoglycemia; Impaired peripheral circulation Insomnia, fatigue Decreased exercise tolerance Hypertriglyceridemia (except agents with intrinsic sympathomimetic activity)
Alpha-and β-blockers 32. Labetalol 33. Carvedilol	100–600 mg/bd 3.125–12.5 od/bd	Oral/IV Oral	Postural hypotension Bronchospasm
Ganglion blocking agents 34. Trimethaphan	1–10 mg/min	IV	
Direct vasodilators arterial 35. Hydralazine 36. Minoxidil 37. Diazoxide	50–75 mg/qid/6h 0.1 to 0.2 mg/kg. Repeat 6th hrly (tolerance may develop)	Oral IM/IV	Headache, fluid retention, tachycardia (Lupus syndrome) (Hirsutism)
Arterial and Venous dilators 38. Sodium Nitroprusside	0.5 to 8 mg/kg/min IVI	IVI	
Calcium channel blockers nondihydropyridines 39. Diltiazem 40. Verapamil	30–60 mg/bd/td 40–240 8th hourly 0.15 mg/kg as bolus IV and 0.005 mg/kg/min as IVI	Oral Oral IV	Conduction defects, worsening of systolic dysfunction, gingival hyperplasia Nausea, headache Constipation

Contd...

Contd...

Drug	*Dosage*	*Route*	*Selected side effects and comments*
Dihydropyridines 41. Amlodipine 42. Nifedipine	 2.5–10 mg/od 10–20 mg/od/bd	 Oral Oral	Ankle edema, flushing, headache, gingival hyperplasia
Angiotensin-converting enzyme inhibitors (ACEI) 43. Captopril 44. Enalapril 45. Ramipril 46. Lisinopril 47. Benazepril 48. Quinapril 49. Trandolapril 50. Fosinopril 51. Perindopril	 12.5–75 mg/bd/tds 5–40 mg/od/bd 1.25–5 mg/od/bd 5–40 mg/od 5–40 mg/od 5–80 mg/od/bd 1–4 mg/od 10–40 mg/od 1–16 mg/od	 Oral Oral Oral Oral Oral Oral Oral Oral Oral	Common: cough Rare: angiedema, hyperkalemia, rash, loss of taste. Leukopenia
Angiotensin II Receptor blockers 52. Losartan Potassium 53. Valsartan 54. Irbesartan 55. Olmesartan 56. Telmisartan	 25–100 mg/od 80–320 mg/od 150–300 mg/od 20 mg/od 20 mg/od	 Oral Oral Oral Oral Oral	Angioedema (very rare) Hyperkalemia

For doses and side effects—the physicians are requested to see the package literature for additional information. All side effects are not included.

101. First choice antihypertensive medication based on patient characteristics.

Table B-15

Drug class	*Specially beneficial for*	*Increased risk in patients with*	*Contraindications and side effects*
1. ACE inhibitors For example, Captopril Enalapril Lisinopril Ramipril Benazepril	Younger age Associated HF Diabetes Nephropathy Unilateral Renovascular disease Provides renal protection Safe in peripheral vascular disease. Improves quality of life regression of LVH	Bilateral renal artery stenosis	Pregnancy Allergy to Sulfahydryl group, Cough Rash Loss of taste Leukopenia Proteinuria
2. β-blockers For example, Propranolol Atenolol Metaprolol Pindolol Esmolol	Young, high renin levels, recurrence of coronary artery disease. Anxiety co-existing angina migraine, glaucoma, arrhythmias	Bronchial asthma, Peripheral vascular disease, diabetes, hyperlipidemia, allergy, depression	Asthma Heart block Glucose Intolerance
3. Calcium channel blockers: Nifedipine Nicardipine diltiazem Amlodipine Felodipine Verapamil, nimodipine	Older Salt sensitive No CNS side effects Coronary Vasodilatation, LVH Unstable angina	Heart failure Bradycardia or AV conduction delay	Conduction defects Systolic dysfunction Gingival hyperplasia

Contd...

Contd...

Drug class	*Specially beneficial for*	*Increased risk in patients with*	*Contraindications and side effects*
4. Diuretics For example, Thiazide Furosemide Spiranolactone Indapamide	Elder, obese Salt sensitive Low renin Enhance effectiveness of all other agents	DM, gout, digitalis toxicity hyperlipidemia, Cardiac arrhythmias	Pre-existing volume contraction S/E electrolyte disturbance Metabolic disturbance
5. Centrally acting agents for example, Methyldopa Clonidine	Adjuvant in Refractory Hypertension	Orthostatic Hypotension	C/I Liver disease Depression S/E sedation Dry mouth Withdrawal syndrome Autoimmune syndrome
6. Alpha-blocker Prazocin Terazosin Doxazocin	No decrease in cardiac output No alteration in blood lipids No sedation	Orthostatic hypotension Elderly, severe coronary artery disease	First dose hypotension lassitude, syncope sedation, fluid retention
7. Alpha + β-blocker Labetalol Carvedilol	Pregnancy	Orthostatic hypotension Elderly, severe coronary artery disease	First dose hypotension Lassitude, syncope sedation Fluid retention
8. Direct vasodilators For example, Hydralazine Minoxidil Diazoxide Sodium nitroprusside	Severe malignant hypertension Hypertensive emergencies	Severe coronary artery disease DM	Fluid retention Tachycardia Angina Lupus like symptoms

102. Selection of initial antihypertensive drug in special circumstances.

Table B-16

Coexisting condition or entity	*Preferred drugs*	*Relatively or absolutely Contraindicated/care required*	*Remarks*
1. Older age > 75 years	Diuretics, BBs, ACE inhibitors	CCB, guanethidine methyldopa	
2. Bronchial asthma /COPD	Calcium blockers, clonidine, prazocin	β-blockers, labetalol, reserpine	
3. Acute MI	BB, CCB, ACEI, NTG, Diuretics	Diazoxide, hydralazine,	BBs are cardioprotective and antiarrhythmic. CCB are antiarrhythmic and reduces afterload and LV mass NTG increases coronary blood flow. Diuretic reduces preload
4. Ischemic or coronary artery disease	β-blockers, calcium blockers	Direct vasodilators (Hydralazine, minoxidil)	
5. LV dysfunction/congestive heart –failure	Diuretics, ACE inhibitors, NTG, alpha-and β-blockers with care	β-blockers, calcium blockers	

Contd...

Contd...

Coexisting condition or entity	*Preferred drugs*	*Relatively or absolutely Contraindicated/care required*	*Remarks*
6. Post-MI	β-blockers, ACEI , NTG	Diazoxide, hydralazine, nifedipine	
7. Aortic stenosis/Hypertrophic obstructive cardiomyopathy (HOCM)	β-blockers, ACEI	Calcium blockers, alpha-blockers	
8. Aortic dissection	Nitroprusside, β-blockers	Diazoxide, hydralazine, NTG	Diazoxide, hydralazine, NTG causes tachycardia and hence are avoided
9. Cardiac arrhythmias (PAT, AF)	β-blockers, verapamil, clonidine, ACEI	Pindolol, acebutol, vasodilators	Adenosine in PAT is better
10. Pulmonary hypertension	ACEI, calcium blockers, alpha-blockers, vasodilators	β-blockers	
11. Insulin dependent diabetes type-I	ACEI, calcium blockers, central alpha agonists, alpha blockers	Diuretics, β-blockers	
12. Diabetics mellitus Type-II	ACEI, CCB, low dose diuretic	β-blockers	
13. HTN, DM, DCM, HF, CRF	Direct vasodilators prazosin, hydralazine along with insulin dezocine, carvedilol.	ACEI if serum creatinine > 3 mg	
14. DM + Dyslipidemia	ACEI, CCBs	Diuretics, β-blockers	ACEI and CCBs are lipid neutral
15. DM, resistant HTN	ARBs + CCB + HCTZ along with insulin		
16. Renal insufficiency/failure	Loop diuretics, ACEI , β-blockers, hydralazine	CCB, nitroprusside	
17. Diabetic nephropathy	ACEI/ARBB, cardioselective alpha-blockers, Diuretics, (2nd line–CCB)	ACEI/RBBB when serum creatinine > 3 mg; renal artery stenosis	
18. Diabetic nephropathy, dilated cardiomyopathy (DCM)	Prazosin/hydralazine – Direct vasodilators, ACEI, ARBB, alpha-and β-blockers. (Labetalol, cardivas, diuretilcs nitroglycerine)	ACEI when serum Creatine > 3 mg	
19. Diabetes, chronic renal failure (CRF), DCM, with heart failure	Prazosin, alpha-and β-blockers, nitroglycerin, diuretics		Hydralazine may cause tachycardia
20. Diabetes, CRF, DCM with hyperkalemia	Prazosin, alpha-and β-blockers, nitroglycerin, diuretics with loop–diuretics, hydrochlorothiazide.	Potassium sparing diuretics are not given	
21. Renal artery stenosis	Diuretics, calcium blockers	ACEI, ARBs	
22. Hyperlipidemia	Alpha-blockers, calcium blockers, ACEI	Diuretics, β-blockers, (except pindolol, acebutolol)	ACEI, CCBs are lipid neutral
23. Hyperuricemia	ACEI calcium blockers, alpha-blockers	Diuretics, β-blockers Central acting agents	
24. Chronic liver disease	Clonidine, diuretics, direct vasodilators, ACEI, calcium blockers	β-blockers (hepatic - metabolism) methyldopa	
25. Migraine headache	β-blockers, (nonselective without ISA) clonidine, ACEI	Vasodilators	
26. Cerebrovascular disease	ACEI, calcium blockers, diuretics	β-blockers, methyldopa, reserpine, guanethedine	

Contd...

Contd...

Coexisting condition or entity	*Preferred drugs*	*Relatively or absolutely Contraindicated/care required*	*Remarks*
27. Hypertensive encephalopathy	Nitroprusside, furosemide, β-blockers	Alpha-methyldopa	Methyldopa and reserpine cause sedation and hence are avoided
28. Subarachnoid hemorrhage	Nitroprusside, β-blockers	Diazoxide, hydralazine	BP should be reduced only 25% in first 24 hours especially if DBP is above 130 mm Hg
29. Spinal card syndrome	β-blockers, nitroprusside, phentolamine.		
30. Pregnancy	Methyldopa, hydralazine, labetalol, CCB	ACEI	
31. Toxemia of pregnancy	Methyldopa, hydralazine, labetalol CCB, diuretics	ACEI	
32. Eclampsia	Hydralazine, methyldopa, magnesium sulfate, diuretics	Reserpine, guanethidine, diazoxide, ACEI, β-blockers	
33. Pheochromocytoma A. Preoperative B. Intraoperative i. For hypertension ii. For arrhythmias iii. For hypotension C. Postoperative	 Alpha-blockers, prazosin 1 to 2 mg 6th hourly or nitroprusside followed by β-blockers Phentolamine or nitroprusside β-blockers IV fluids Nifedipine, nitroprusside, diazoxide, NTG ointment		The antihypertensive treatment should not be abruptly stopped
34. Hyperthyroidism	Nonselective β-blocker		
35. Glaucoma	β-blockers, clonidine, diuretics		
36. Sinusitis/rhinitis	Clonidine methyldopa, ACEI, CCB	β-blockers, reserpine	
37. Peripheral vascular disease	ACEI calcium blockers, alpha-blockers, β-blocker, vasodilators	β-blockers	
38. Depression/psychogenic	ACEI, CCB, β-blockers, alpha-blockers, vasodilators	Methyldopa, reserpine	
39. Acid peptic disease	Clonidine, β-blockers, calcium blockers clonidine	Reserpine, guanethidine	
40. Menopausal symptoms	Clonidine	Vasodilators	
41. Impotence	ACEI, calcium blockers, alpha-blockers	β-blockers, diuretics methyldopa, reserpine	
42. Benign prostatic hypertrophy (BPH)	Alpha-blockers		
43. Alcoholic withdrawal tremor	β-blockers	β-blockers	
44. Catecholamine excess (recreational drugs induced	β-blockers		

ACEI: Angiotensin-converting enzyme inhibitor, ARBs: Angiotensin receptor blockers, BB: β-blocker, CCBs: Calcium channel blockers, DCM: Dilated cardiomyopathy, HCTZ: Hydrochlorothiazide

103. There are 4 important points to be noted about the action of antihypertensive drugs:

1. Action on peripheral vascular resistance.
2. Action on plasma volume.
3. Action on plasma renin activity.
4. Action on cardiac output.

104. An ideal hypertensive drug should possess 4 characteristic features:

1. It should restore the cardiovascular functions to normal.
2. It should confirm to compliance so that it is given once or twice a day.
3. It should have limited contraindications so that it can be used in the presence of frequently associated diseases with hypertension. For example, diabetes mellitus, arthritis, etc.
4. It should be efficient as monotherapy without second drug and with less side effects.

105. The following 4 general rules should be observed while giving drugs:

1. BP should be lowered gradually reduce the SBP < 150 mm Hg and DBP < 90 mm Hg, through the day, in all postures, and in all states of normal activity.
2. Treatment should be individualized according to the severity of hypertension, hemodynamic disturbances and other associated diseases. Reduce or at least not to increase the risks of the major outcomes of hypertension.
3. The treatment should be continued indefinitely in most patients. Treatment should be as simple as possible, single tablet a day if possible. The treatment should not be hanged unless there is absolute need.
4. One should be familiar with thorough knowledge of limited number of drugs and use them correctly. The newer drugs need not necessarily be a better one. Competent treatment can be given by becoming familiar with and sticking to one or two drugs from each group of medication.

106. The following 4 rules should be followed in the treatment of hypertension with drugs:

1. Drugs should be given in a stepwise pattern starting with a single drug except in severe hypertension.
2. Combination of drugs is preferable to high dose monotherapy because one can use lower doses of the individual drugs with lesser side effects.
3. Drugs which do not interfere with mood and mind are preferable since they interfere least with daily activities.
4. Never stop treatment abruptly or withdraw one drug suddenly.

It is a good rule, both to start and to stop all drugs slowly. If they are stopped suddenly all antihypertensive drugs except diuretics and reserpine produce dangerous side effects in some patients. To stop any antihypertensive drug suddenly is an invitation to trouble. Sudden withdrawal may be dangerous with β-blockers and methyldopa, and very dangerous with clonidine.

107. There are 4 steps in the management of high blood pressure:

The original 'stepped care' program for managing essential hypertension put forward in 1978 by WHO and subsequently extended by the United States Joint National Committee has undergone a number of important changes during the last two decades.

Diuretic induced affects on plasma potassium glucose tolerance, and lipids that occur both with diuretic and β-blockers may argue whether these drugs should still be used as first-line therapies in hypertension. However, JNC 7 report published in JAMA May 21, 2003 recommended that thiazide diuretics should be used in drug treatment for most patients with uncomplicated hypertension, either alone or combined with drugs from other classes.

1. **STEP I:** One should start β-blockers (if no contraindication) or diuretic or other sympathetic blocking drugs alone.
   For example, start with propranolol if there are no contraindications like asthma, heart failure, Raynaud's phenomenon or insulin dependent diabetes mellitus. 10–40 mg po/day, one should slowly increase the dose upto 160 mg/qid or if any contraindication—begin with cardioselective β-blocker. For example, atenolol 50–100 mg/po/od.
   Thiazides are an alternative.
   Cheap and long-acting thiazides are more useful with potassium supplement, for example, bendrofluazide 5 mg/po/od, if necessary add potassium sparing diuretic—triamterene, spiranolactone.
   Rapidly acting diuretics are less useful unless it is associated with cardiac or renal failure.
   Diuretics alone are useful in old people where the renin is low.
   Check serum potassium.
   Avoid diuretics in diabetes.
   The efficacy and overall safety of both either a β-blocker or thiazide diuretic is about the same. Therefore which is to be choosed is somewhat arbitrary but may be helped by considering the following.
   A β-blocker is preferable in sexually active males particularly in non-smokers. Since it is less likely to cause impotence and has cardioprotective effect. Because of their role in angina, β-blocker

is preferable in patients with both angina and hypertension.

If you start with thiazide, no titration is needed and the full antihypertensive effect is seen in few days. If you start with a β-blocker, titration must be continued for at least 3 to 4 weeks, either to the point of bradycardia (heart rate < 60) or of stable control of pressure, except with atenolol.

Other sympatholytic agents, e.g. methyldopa 125–250 mg/bd to qid rise upto 3 g/day.

If no response.

2. **STEP II:** Combine diuretics + β-blocker or other sympatholytic agents.

   Most hypotensive drugs take upto 3 weeks to have their full effect.

   If the blood pressure remains very high before or after that time, the β-blocker or thiazide diuretic chosen is not working, then add the other that is a β-blocker to a thiazide or vice versa.

   Diuretics increases renin secretion secondary to volume depletion.

   β-blockers blunt the renin secretion and the action of β-blockers is increased in the presence of renin when combined with diuretic. If no response.

3. **STEP III:** Add vasodilators

   Hydralazine or calcium channel blockers or prazocin propranolol or atenolol with hydralazine 25 mg/12 hours 50 mg/8 hours po.

   Hydralazine reduces peripheral vascular resistance (afterload), causes reflux tachycardia which is prevented by a β-blocker.

   Diuretic is further added.

   If no response

4. **STEP IV:** Enzyme inhibitors.

   Act on renin-angiotensin-aldosterone mechanism

   Captopril inhibits angiotensin-converting enzyme (ACE) 25–150 mg/8 h. With furosemide 40 mg—1 g/24 h po give potassium supplements since captopril reduces aldosterone secretion as well.

   Enalapril 2.5 mg, 5 mg or 17.5 mg.

   Or add additional adrenergic inhibiting drugs to step III or alpha-and β-blocker, e.g. Labetalol may be tried.

Selection of Drug is Individualized

One need not follow the step method.

108. Selection of the first drug in the stepped care treatment is based on.

1. Patient's history and physical findings.
2. Demographic criteria—age, sex, race, body habits.
3. Laboratory findings.
4. Coexisting disease—coronary artery disease, previous myocardial infarction, diabetes mellitus, gout.

In combination therapy β-blockers and nifedipine is a sound combination. Powerful afterload reduction by nifedipine offsets the bradycardia and negative ionotropic effect of β-blocker. A combination of ACE inhibitors and calcium channel blockers are increasingly being used as they attack both renin-angiotensin and the increased peripheral vascular resistance. β-blocker and ACE inhibitor do not add to the effectiveness of any single agent.

109. Diuretics: All presently used diuretics impede the reabsorption of sodium in the renal tubule. They differ mainly in the extent to which they increase or decrease renal tubular loss of potassium, and the speed, duration and intensity of their diuretic effect. All diuretics lower the arterial pressure, even the old mercurial diuretics that had to be given parentally.

Thiazide diuretics are most frequently used and extensively investigated for many years. Thiazide diuretics form the corner stone in many of the therapeutic programs designed to reduce hypertension.

Mode of action of thiazides and related agents.

1. They act primarily on the distal tubule and cortical portion of the collecting tubules to prevent active reabsorption of sodium and chloride ions. Reduce arterial pressure primarily by sodium diuresis resulting in volume depletion. In long-term use, they reduce peripheral vascular resistance.
2. They cause as much a 8% of the glomerular filtrate to pass into urine under favorable conditions.

   Thiazides are excreted unchanged in urine. Thiazide diuretics are ineffective in patients with less than 20% renal function. (Furosemide is a safe alternative)
3. They are effective in 3 or 4 days
4. They have a flat dose response curve.

The daily recommended doses have been progressively reducing. Today, as small as 6.25 mg to 12.5 mg are recommended as most of the hypertensive effects are obtained with the small doses without hypokalemia and other side effects.

It is noted that blacks and elderly respond well to diuretics than younger and nonblocks.

110. Following are the uses of diuretics:

1. Hypertension.
2. Congestive heart failure, acute myocardial infarction, coronary heart disease.
3. Cirrhosis of liver.
4. Renal insufficiency, chronic renal failure, nephrotic syndrome.

5. Pulmonary edema.
6. Cerebral edema.
7. Glucoma.
8. Certain epilepsies like petitmal.

Carbonic anhydrase inhibitors, e.g. acetazolamide is useful.

Diuretics are very useful in heart failure or accelerated hypertension.

111. There are 4 advantages of diuretics in hypertension.

1. If properly used, they are still be the appropriate initial choice for many patients and second choice for even more.
2. Thiazide diuretics are cheap and can be given once daily. No need of frequent dose titration.
   Thiazide diuretics are the only antihypertensive drugs that can be used optimally in a fixed dose. All others with possible exception of atenolol show variability in effective dose.
3. Thiazide diuretics are exception to the rule that antihypertensive drugs produce dangerous side affects if stopped suddenly. Interestingly, they do not affect normal blood pressure. Thiazides are less potent antihypertensive agents than furosemide.
4. Diuretics can be combined among their subgroups and with other groups of drugs used in hypertension. They enhance the effectiveness of all the antihypetensive drugs.

112. Some diuretic combinations available among their subgroups.

1. Hydrochlorothiazide 5 mg + Amiloride 5 mg—1 tab. od.
2. Furosemide 40 mg + Amiloride 5 mg—1 to 2 tab daily
3. Furosemide 40 mg + Triamterene 50 mg—1 tab od.
4. Furosemide 20 mg + Spironolactone 5 mg—1 to 4 tab daily for 7 to 10 days, later adjust the dose according to response.
5. Furosemide 20 mg/40 mg + Hydrochlorothiazide 5 mg + Amiloride 5 mg/or spironolactone 5 mg.
6. Furosemide 40 mg + controlled release of potassium chloride 600 mg 1 tab od.
7. Triamterene 50 mg + Benzathiazide 25 mg—1 to 2 tab daily.
8. Spironolactone 25 mg + Hydrochlorothiazide 25 mg —3 to 4 tab daily.

113. Some diuretic combinations available with other groups of drugs for the treatment of hypertension.

β-blocker + diuretic are very good combinations

1. Propranolol 40 mg + Hydrochlorothiazide 20 mg
2. Propranolol 40 mg + Hydroflumethiazide 25 mg
3. Propranolol 40 mg + Xipamide 10 mg
4. Atenolol 50 mg/100 mg + Chlorthiazide 25 mg
5. Atenolol 50 mg/100 mg + Hydrochlorothiazide 25 mg + Amiloride 2.5 mg

Others

6. Enalapril 5/10 mg + Hydrochlorothiazide 25 mg
7. Lisinopril 5 mg/10 mg + Hydrochlorothiazide 12.5 mg
8. Clonidine HCl 100 mg + Chlorthalidone 15 mg

Diuretics when combined with other antihypertensive drugs greatly increase their effectiveness, reduces necessary dosage and thereby increases tolerability. Potassium supplements are not needed in patient without advanced heart damage and combined preparations with potassium should not be used. Potassium sparing diuretics are rarely helpful. Serious side effects are common in over 30 to 40 years of continuous treatment.

If they are not sought, they will not be found.

114. Following are some of the disadvantages with thiazide diuretics:

1. Like with many drugs include anorexia, nausea, vomiting, headache and dizziness.
2. Hypokalemia due to renal potassium loss. Some of the unabsorbed sodium is subsequently absorbed in the distal tubule where it is exchanged for potassium and hydrogen ions which pass out in the urine subsequently resulting in hypokalemia. Plasma potassium should never be allowed to fall below 3.0 mEq/L. Estimation of potassium is safe in a patient on thiazide diuretic. Routine estimation of potassium is neither necessary nor possible in many uncomplicated hypertension provided that treating physician remembers that hypokalemia is the cause of tiredness and muscle fatigue which the patient complains. Plasma potassium is measured when this common complaint arises. It is essential to separate serum or plasma from RBC before sending to the laboratory, otherwise potassium levels may be grossly elevated. T-wave changes in ECG represent advanced and dangerous stage of hypokalemia and therefore cannot be used as a screening test. 10% of reduction of body potassium is to be expected over 3 years without potassium supplements.
   The potassium losses caused by diuretics may be maintained by using low doses, reducing sodium intake, and increasing potassium intake or adding potassium supplements. Hypokalemia is much important in hypertensive patients with heart complaints. Patients with severe heart complaint seem to have a reduced total body potassium even without diuretics, perhaps mainly from muscle wasting and indifferent diet.

Hypertensives with heart disease have been found to have 30% fall in total body potassium compared with only 10% in those without heart complications. In all these patients, potassium is required to maintain above 3.5 mEq/L.

Digitalis toxicity is greatly increased by hypokalemia. Most of the patients do not need potassium supplements. Those who need them usually require much larger doses. Potassium supplements are given whenever necessary. Dietary potassium can be effectively increased by coconut water, fruits, canned or frozen orange juice.

It is necessary to drink 500 mL of this to provide 24 mmol of potassium, involving a considerable caloric load. But in sick patients, this may be more acceptable than even more tablets.

Potassium sparing diuretics: Amiloride, triamterene, spironolactone.

The risk of potassium shift, upward or downward is sudden in cardiac arrhythmias or arrest. Renal failure leads to potassium retention, and in these patients, potassium sparing diuretics can be dangerous. Patients with heart complications that create a risk of hypokalemia are also at high-risk of renal failure. Use of potassium supplements with potassium sparing diuretics is very dangerous.

None of the potassium sparing diuretics when used alone are potent diuretics or effective antihypertensive agents. They are usually used in combination with thiazide or loop diuretics to limit hypokalemia or hyperuricemia. To avoid anticipated hypokalemia in patients on digitalis, or to restore diuretic response in those who have become refractory. Otherwise, they are rarely a sensible first choice except perhaps in the elderly.

3. Thiazides can precipitate uremia and therefore should be used in elderly patients after estimation of baseline creatinine.
4. They may cause hyperuricemia due to uric acid retention and may precipitate clinical gout in patients with latent hyperuricemia. Probenecid should be used to increase renal excretion of uric acid. Allopurinol should be avoided as it can cause serious toxicity.
5. They may precipitate hepatic coma in patients with impending liver failure, and should not be used in alcoholics without liver function tests.
6. Thiazides can cause carbohydrate intolerance. Hypoglycemia appears in the long-term use of diuretics and disappears when diuretics are stopped. Thiazides and less commonly loop diuretics may precipitate or worsen diabetes mellitus.
7. Hyperlipidemia: Thiazides may cause hyperlipidemia on long-term use. Unlike other diuretics, indapamide does not seem to cause any negative changes in lipid profile. Indapamide may be better than hydrochlorothiazide in inducing regression of left ventricular hypertrophy.
8. Electrolyte imbalance: Besides hypokalemia caused by thiazide or loop diuretics, hyperkalemia and metabolic acidosis may be caused by potassium sparing diuretics. Hyponatremia may occasionally result from increased excretion of sodium.

   Hypomagnesemia may be caused by thiazide or loop diuretics although predominantly by the later. Rarely occurs with thiazide dose below 100 mg/day. Symptoms range from mild muscular weakness to tetany, convulsions, and finally coma. Resistant ventricular arrhythmias may also occur. Hypomagnesemia can be controlled by small doses of diuretics and potassium, sparing diuretics. Oral magnesium oxide 200–400 mg/day can be used as replacement when required.

   There is a dose response for all metabolic effects—namely hypokalemia, hyperuricemia, hyperglycemia, and hyperlipidemia but not for hypertensive effect. So, lower doses of diuretics are recommended.

115. Drug induced hypokalemia by diuretics is common in:

1. Hypertension.
2. Heart disease.
3. Nephritis.
4. Cirrhosis liver and others.

The thiazide drugs actually cause sodium diuresis primarily but secondarily affects potassium loss.

116. In hypertension on diuretics—hypokalemia is known by:

1. Polyuria.
2. Muscle cramps/muscle weakness.
3. Premature heart beats.
4. Fatigue.

117. Natural causes of hypokalemia (Metabolic diseases).

1. Diabetes.
2. Renal.
3. Cushing's syndrome.
4. Hyperaldosteronism (Hypersecretion of aldosterone).

Diuretics block or limit the sodium reabsorption.

In the tubules 99% of sodium and chloride are reabsorbed and returned to the body fluids. One percent of sodium and chloride is finally eliminated in the urine.

118. Potassium sparing diuretics.

Aldosterone regulates potassium balance, helps in increased sodium and water reabsorption.

Table B-17

Spironolactone	*Triamterene*
1. Aldosterone antagonist. No action in adrenalectomy patients	Independent of hormone whether aldosterone present or not
2. Works on distal tubule, gradual onset	On distal tubule
3. S/E gynecomastia	
4. Impotence, hirsutism, reversible on withdrawal of the drug, drowsiness, lethargy, maculopapular eruptions	Vomiting, dry mouth, photosensitivity, anaphylaxis, uric acid rise, weakness

- Potassium loss: Diet and drug supplementation
- Mild: Bananas (16 bananas); 14 glasses of orange juice
- High potassium diet—not effective way
- Limiting sodium helps in potassium loss
- Potassium supplements—potassium chloride.

119. Potential serious significant affects occur when thiazide diuretics interact with:

1. *Adrenal steroids:* Potassium loss with thiazides is increased by steroids and its risks are increased by digitalis.
2. They potentiates the action of muscle relaxants used in anesthesia
3. *Anticoagulants:* They impair response to anticoagulants, so that they can precipitate bleeding when withdrawn.
4. *Lithium compounds:* They reduce lithium clearance by 24%. So, they must be used with caution, if at all used in patients with manic depressive psychoses.

β-BLOCKERS

120. β-blockers control the hypertension in 4 ways.

1. By its central action—suppressing the control of sympathetic outflow.
2. On CVS—by reducing heart rate and cardiac output
3. On kidneys—by decreasing the renin secretion.
4. At the periphery—it lowers the norepinephrine release at postganglionic sympathetic nerve endings.

β-blockers started in 1966 with propronolol and many are available now.

121. β-blockers are suitable for:

1. Young patients.
2. Anxious patients.
3. Patients with concomitant angina, post MI.
4. Non-smokers.

122. β-blockers are the drugs of choice in hypertension in patients.

1. Below 50 years age.
2. Systolic HT or hyperkinetic circulation. (Tachycardia with wide pulse pressure).
3. Labile hypertension.
4. Hypertension associated with other conditions where β-blockers are indicated, e.g. HT with exertional angina
   Old MI
   AF with fast ventricular rate
   Ventricular arrhythmias responding to β-blockers.
5. Hypertrophic obstructive cardiomyopathy (HOCM).
6. Cynotic spells of Fallot's tetralogy.
7. Thyrotoxicosis.
8. Pheochromocytoma.
9. Digitalis induced arrhythmia.
10. For reduction of rate of spontaneous depolarization of SA node and junctional pacemakers.
11. Slowing of the conduction within the atria and AV node—can abolish PSVT in AV node reentrant pathway.
12. Prevention of recurrent VF in congenital QT syndrome.
13. Prevention of sudden cot death in children with family h/o.
14. Useful in prophylaxis of sudden CVS death following acute MI, should be used cautiously in patients with latent or overt failure because of negative inotropic effect.
15. Migraine.
16. Schizophrenia.

123. Long-term use of β-blockers show cardioprotective and vasculoprotective effects such as:

1. Reduction of tachycardia.
2. Reduction of arrhythmias.
3. Reduction of infarct size in MI.
4. Reduction of recurrence of MI.

124. Cardioprotective doses of β-blockers:

Table B-18

	Before addition of diuretics (mg)	*Maximum dose with diuretics (mg)*
Atenolol	50	100
Metoprolol	150–200	300
Propranolol	160–240	240
Acebutolol	400	600

125. Classification of β-blockers based on cardioselectivity and ISA.

Table B-19

Cardioselective	
1. Without ISA (PAA)	Atenolol, metoprolol, bisoprolol, esmolol, carbonolol, betaxolol, berantolol
2. With ISA (PAA)	Acebutolol
Non-cardioselective	
3. Without ISA (PAA)	Nadolol, propranolol, timolol, sotalol
4. With ISA	Pindolol, oxyprenolol, penbutolol

ISA = Intrinsic sympathomimetic activity
PAA = Partial agonistic activity
(The term PAA is preferable to ISA)

Propranolol is not suitable for the emergency treatment of hypertension. It should not be given intravenously in hypertension.

126. There are 4 absolute contraindication to β-blockers:

1. Severe bronchial asthma.
2. Heart block greater than first degree, heart failure.
3. Peripheral vascular disease.
4. Unstable insulin dependent diabetes.

Better to have a baseline peak flow rate record in all patients before starting β-blockers, as latent asthmatics are commonly revealed for the first time by treatment. Mild asthmatics should have their flow rate monitored frequently.

Irreversible airways obstruction: An impaired peak flow rate or FEV1 that does not improve after inhalation of isoprenaline—is not an absolute contraindication for β-blockers.

So, it is important to know the nature of wheezing if the history is not clear. Many patients with hypertension and/or angina, who also have chronic obstructive pulmonary disease may benefit from cardioselective β-blocker such as atenolol. However, dosage must be titrated with extra caution. Many patients are so exhausted by their respiratory disability that they simply cannot cope with the diminished effort tolerance that commonly accompanies β-blockers. Better drugs are now available to control hypertension in asthmatics (see Calcium blockers) avoid β-blockers in chronic bronchitis, emphysema, chronic obstructive pulmonary disease.

β-blockers block the adrenergic β-receptors in the AV node which results in increase of: PR interval (first degree block); therefore, they can increase AV block to any degree.

First degree block is not a contraindication.

Peripheral vascular disease Raynaud's phenomenon due to reduction of cardiac output and blockade of vasodilator B2 sympathetic receptors in the walls of arterioles, claudication may be made worse. Gloves and bed socks are very effective for cold hands and feet.

β-blockers can be dangerous in brittle diabetics because it suppresses the normal warning symptoms of hypoglycemia. Glycogenolysis is under control of alpha-receptors in the liver and of β-receptors in the skeletal muscle. There are sufficient glycogen stores in stable diabetics. But in childhood diabetes or in diabetic ketoacidosis β-blockers can precipitate hypoglycemia. Hypoglycemia can occur both in diabetes and non-diabetics. It is less likely and less severe with β-1 selective blocker. Hypoglycemia may not be recognized because the usual tachycardia but not sweating is suppressed. Whenever a patient on a β-blocker presents in coma, hypoglycemia should be considered.

β-blockers rise scrum triglycerides, and lower HDL cholesterol but less with cardioselective agents. These changes are due to reduced lipoprotein lipase activity. Chromium supplements 200 mg tds corrects them.

127. Following are some of the side effects of β-blockers

1. Bronchospasm.
2. Bradycardia, heart failure.
3. Cold hands and feet.
4. Depression and psychosis.
5. Impaired response to hypoglycemia in insulin dependent diabetes.
6. Hyperlipidemia.
7. Fatigue, reduction of libido and impotence (1 to 5%).
8. Vivid dreams.

128. β-blockers are the excellent antihypertensive drugs because of the following reasons:

1. If there are no contraindications, β-blockers produce no major side effects on the cardiovascular, hepatic, renal or hematological systems.
2. Once a day dosage allows for good compliance.
3. They can be used alone as first-line therapy in more than 60% of hypertensive patients, under the age of 65 and used successfully in the majority of patients in combination with a diuretic or with a dihydropyridine calcium antagonist.
4. Useful in patients with increased adrenergic activity namely:
   a. Younger age group.
   b. Hyperdynamic β-adrenergic circulatory state, hyperkinetic heart syndrome.
   c. Alcohol withdrawal hypertension.
   d. Patients with labile or elevated blood pressure and palpitation.

5. β-blockers are particularly indicated for patients with proven or suspected ischemic heart disease, left ventricular hypertrophy, aneurysms, supraventricular or ventricular arrhythmias.
   They significantly reduce sudden cardiac death from whatever cause. Hence, β-blockers are useful in primary prevention of coronary artery disease and stroke.
6. They do not cause significant postural hypotension unlike most other antihypertensive drugs.
7. Patients with hypertension and hypercholesterolemia are at high-risk for manifestations of ischemic heart disease and should be treated with a β-blocking drug like acebutolol or pindolol and an appropriate cholesterol lowering drug.
8. It is not necessary to discontinue β-blocking drugs prior to general anesthesia but should be informed to anesthetist.

129. β-blockers have the following 4 maternal disadvantages in pregnancy with hypertension which can also occur with hypertension itself.

1. Decrease in placental circulation.
2. Retard intrauterine growth.
3. Depress neonatal respiration.
4. Sets in hypoglycemia.

130. Some practical points to remember in clinical use of β-blockers.

1. The hypertensive patient is not only worried about his blood pressure but is afraid of stroke, heart attack, or death. β-blockers are the only cardiac agents that have been proven to decrease the incidence of stroke or sudden cardiac death. Despite their differences in cardioselectivity and intrinsic sympathomimetic activity (ISA) all β-blockers seem to be effective as antihypertensive agents.
2. Patients with post Q wave myocardial infarction with hypertension having ejection fraction of 40% or above and especially those with electrical and mechanical complications are a challenging subset in whom β-blockers without ISA, e.g. atenolol, metoprolol, have been clearly shown to reduce long-term mortality and the incidence of nonfatal myocardial infarction.
3. Abnormal lipid metabolism is not seen in those with ISA, e.g. pindolol, acebutolol. These can be used in patients of hypertension with hyperlipidemia.
4. Atenolol and nadolol are among the least lipid soluble β-blockers which escape hepatic inactivation and are excreted through the kidneys virtually unchanged remaining active in plasma for a longer time thus allowing once a day administration.
5. Sotalol, a long acting agent has the unique property of acting as an antiarrhythmic agent due to its Class III antiarrhythmic action like amiodarone, but its adverse effect on lipid metabolism is the limiting factor.
6. In diabetics due to masking of hypoglycemic symptoms propranolol is not advised. Agents, like metoprolol are better suited in this respect.
7. In so-called 'labile hypertensive' patients undergoing surgery, short-acting β-blockers like esmolol have proved very effective.
8. β-blockers should not be stopped abruptly. They should be tapered gradually otherwise rebound hypertension may precipitate a crisis especially in those with coronary artery disease.

131. Alpha and β-receptor blockers.

Labetalol is a nonselective β-1 and β-2 receptor blocker. It is highly selective for α-1 receptor like prazosin. Carvedilol is a non-selective β-blocker with a lesser degree of alpha-blocking effect that is responsible for vasodilating effect. Carvedilol may contribute some of its beneficial effects in heart failure.

The 4 beneficial effects are:

1. Sympathetic inhibition.
2. Vasodilatory.
3. Antioxidant.
4. Antiproliferative.

132. Some follow the routine first line of drugs in order of preference as follows:

1. Diuretic.
2. β-blocker.
3. Calcium channel blocker.
4. Angiotensin-converting enzyme (ACE) inhibitors.

133. Some follow the alternative firstline of drugs in order of preference as follows:

1. **A**—Angiotensin-converting enzyme inhibitors ACEI/ (ARBs).
2. **B**—β-blockers.
3. **C**—Calcium channel blockers (CCB).
4. **D**—Diuretics.

CALCIUM CHANNEL BLOCKERS

134. Calcium channel blockers (CCB): These are very effective antihypertensive agents which are also being increasingly used because of many attractive features. For example, nifedipine, amlodipine, verapamil, diltiazem, cinnarizine, lidoflazine.

With the discovery of calcium channels regulating the entry and exit of calcium from cells to extracellular fluid and vice versa, number of drugs which block these channels have been described. In addition to voltage dependent channels, receptor activated and stretch activated channels have recently been described.

The CCB drugs act by inhibiting the influx of calcium ions through the slow calcium channels into myocardial muscle and vascular smooth muscle cells, thus decreasing the availability of intracellular calcium. This results in reduced activity of the enzyme ATPase within the cells.

The result of their action is:

1. Relaxation of arterial smooth muscle in the periphery resulting in reduction of afterload.
2. Reduces contractility of the heart muscle cells resulting in reduction of cardiac work and output.
3. Reduces oxygen consumption by the heart.
4. Relaxation of coronary vascular smooth muscle of those coronaries which are not irreversibly stenosed.

One of the disadvantages of early CCBs such as nifedipine is their relative lack of selectivity as powerful vasodilator. Unnecessary side effects of excessive vasodilatation with peripheral edema, headache and even reflex tachycardia occur.

135. The calcium channel blockers are classified into 4 major groups depending on their chemistry and type of channel blockade.

1. *Dihydropyridine*: Nifedipine, nicardipine, amlodipine, felodipine, nisoldipine, nitrendipine, nimodipine. They reduce the BP by vasodilatation. They are potent vasodilators and also have some mild diuretic effect. They cause headache and flushing which tend to improve with continued use. Ankle edema is thought to result from direct effect of these drugs on capillary permeability and is not responsive to diuretics. They have little or no effect on AV node.
2. *Benzothiazapine diltiazem:* It has some effect on both cardiac conduction and vascular smooth muscle.
3. *Phenylalkylamines*: Verapamil, emopramil, verapamil slows AV node conduction and reduces myocardial contractility.
4. *Indolizinsulfones:* Fantofarone.

Verapamil and diltiazem are contraindicated in patients with heart block and should be used with care in patients taking digoxin or β-blockers because of the additive effects on cardiac conduction and contraction. Mibefradil's derived from verapamil is a vasodilator with negative chronotropic activity which does not impair cardiac contractile force. Long-term treatment with CCBs may be associated with higher risk of cardiovascular morbidity and mortality.

136. Nifedipine is commonly used in hypertension. It has the following 4 advantages in hypertension:

1. It produces prompt predictable and dependable fall in both SBP and DBP proportional to the pretreatment level but with little or no effect on normotensives.
2. Suitable for long-term management as well as emergency treatment. It can be administered orally for long-term treatment and sublingually for the treatment of hypertensive crisis.
3. Raises cardiac output, increases renal blood flow and sodium excretion.
4. Combination with β-blockers exhibits still greater fall in BP and amelioration of side effects.

Nifedipine and diltiazem are used as antihypertensives while verapamil is mostly used in hypertensive patients concomitantly suffering from cardiac arrhythmias.

137. In contrast to other drugs nifedipine does not produce:

1. CNS disturbances.
2. Sexual dysfunction.
3. Worsening of COPD.
4. Hypokalemia, hyperglycemia and hypercholesterolemia.

138. Nifedipine can safely be given to patients having contraindications to β-blockers such as:

1. Bronchial asthma and other COPD.
2. Congestive cardiac failure, AV block.
3. Peripheral vascular insufficiency.
4. Diabetes mellitus.

It causes some degree of relaxation of bronchial smooth muscle and uterus.

139. Calcium channel blocker, verapamil reduces the oxygen demand of the myocardium by reducing contractility, excitability and conductivity. This drug is therefore employed for cardiac conditions such as:

1. Angina pectoris.
2. Prinzmetal angina (drug of choice).
3. Cardiac arrhythmias (paroxysmal atrial tachycardia).
4. Hypertrophic cardiomyopathy.

Diltiazem effects both cardiac muscle and peripheral vessels.

140. The advantages of calcium channel blockers and ACE inhibitors over diuretics and β-blockers are:

1. Less impotence—(many hypertensives are made sexless by treatment).
2. Better exercise tolerance—they improve the blood flow to the heart, brain and kidneys.
3. No postural hypotension.
4. Can be used in diabetes mellitus where thiazide diuretics are contraindicated. Can be used in chronic obstructive pulmonary disease (COPD), peripheral arterial disease, asthma where β-blockers are contraindicated.

ANGIOTENSIN-CONVERTING ENZYME INHIBITORS

141. Angiotensin-converting enzyme (ACE) inhibitors: These are the most rapidly growing family of antihypertensive drugs and are widely used for all degrees and forms of hypertension.

They act in 4 ways to reduce the hypertension:

1. By inhibiting the angiotensin-converting enzyme thereby preventing the conversion of angiotensinogen I to angiotensin II which is a powerful vasoconstrictor, which leads to vasodilatation.
2. By inhibiting the aldosterone secretion, reduces plasma and urinary aldosterone levels, resulting in reduction of sodium retention, thus lowering the BP. Natriureteric effect as a consequence of inhibition of aldosterone secretion.
3. By preventing the degradation of bradykinin, which is a vasodilator, increases its blood and fluid levels, thus contributing lowering effect of BP. Bradykinin has been shown to have beneficial effects associated with the release of nitric oxide and prostacyclin which make contribute to the positive hemodynamic effects. Bradykinins may also be responsible for some of the adverse effects such as dry cough, hypertension and angioedema.
4. By interfering with central sympathetic system. ACEI reduces the activity of the sympathetic nervous system as angiotensin II, promotes the release of noradrenalin and inhibits the reuptake. In addition, they also improve β-receptor density (causing their up regulation) variation in heart rate, baroreceptor function, and autonomic function (including vagal tone).
5. Decreases the release of norepinephrine from terminal neurons.
6. It is an inhibitor of tissue and vascular renin-angiotensin system.
7. It has antiproliferative action of myocyte and arterial smooth muscle level.
8. Decreases formation of endothelin from endothelium.

142. The 4 commonly used ACE inhibitors are:

1. Captopril 12.5–75 mg/bd or tds.
2. Enalapril 5–40 mg/od or bd.
3. Lisinopril 5–40 mg/od.
4. Ramipril 1.25–5 mg/od.

Besides these, there are many other ACEI like perindopril, benazapril, fosinopril, quinapril, trandolapril, accupril, cerenapril, cilazapril, deapril, zofenopril, spirparil, etc.

143. Angiotensin-converting enzyme (ACE) inhibitors are indicated in the following 4 conditions:

1. In moderate to severe hypertension refractory to traditional drug therapy (reduces the dose of other drugs particularly vasodilators).
   It may even replace IV sodium nitroprusside in the treatment of severe rapidly accelerating hypertension.
   In diagnosing renin dependent hypertension, may be useful in diagnosing primary aldosteronism.
   In diagnosing hypertension that follows percutaneous transluminal angioplasty.
2. In congestive heart failure (it does not substitute digitalis or diuretics).
   In dilated (Congestive) cardiomyopathy.
   They are the ideal choice in patients with left ventricular dysfunction of all grades.
   It has beneficial effect on preload and afterload.
3. In acute myocardial infarction (not on the first day)
4. In post thrombolysis
   Post PTCA
   Postoperative AR, MR, VSD, PDA.
   In post-MI patients, they help in LV remodeling, prevent LV dilatation and cardiac failure
   Thus, in post-MI hypertension, they become the ideal choice.
5. In peripheral vascular disease and HT: Captopril—unlike β-blocked there is no impairment of calf blood flow and no reduction of walking distance in patients with intermittent claudication.
6. In hypertension with diabetes: In view of its neutral effects on carbohydrate metabolism, consistent decrease in microalbuminuria, ACEI are considered as the therapy of choice in diabetes and in diabetic nephropathy in the early stages to prevent microalbuminuria.
7. In hypertension with hyperuricemia: ACEI have a uricosuric effect, they could be a first choice for patients with gout and hypertension or for hypertensive hyperuricemic patients.
8. Hypertension with renal parenchymal disease: Though, it is said to be renoprotective, caution is needed. Safe in chronic renal failure in early stages, high renin or low renin and on low salt diet. Occasionally, deterioration of renal function takes place.
   Before starting, see for any bilateral renal artery stenosis.
   Beware of serum creatinine. Do not use or cautious if serum creatinine is > 3 mg.

(It can be used in hypertension with chronic pulmonary disease provided there is no cough. ACEI may improve pulmonary function by decreasing hypoxic vasoconstriction. However, the high incidence of cough, occurring is a major drawback.)

144. There are 4 precautions to be observed while initiating therapy with ACE inhibitors.

1. Vasodilators should be stopped 48 hours before.
2. Potassium sparing diuretics should be stopped the day before.
3. Nitrates should be stopped the night before.
4. Dose of other diuretics should be reduced 24 hours before. Patient may require half the previous dose.

Testing: It is difficult to predict whether ACEI monotherapy could be effective or not in a given patient. Therefore, an acute test may predict the long-term response. A practical method is to initiate test dose with captopril 6.25 mg and wait for 30 min. If no excessive response or sensitivity to ACEI is observed, then 25 mg of captopril can be given. If the BP comes down within another hour then the patient is potentially responsive to ACEI. It is always essential to initiate therapy with a low dose, because in case, the patient has high renin state, there could be a precipitous fall in BP. It must be stressed at this juncture that the full effect of the drugs may not be seen for 7 to 10 days. To achieve maximum benefit, advise the patient to have low sodium diet. Addition of a low dose diuretic may further potentiate the antihypertensive effect, more than it would, by increasing the dose of ACEI.

145. The angiotensin converting enzyme inhibitors are specially useful in the following:

Four groups of hypertension .

1. Renal parenchymal hypertension.
2. Accelerated or malignant hypertension.
3. Hypertension with heart failure.
4. Hypertension complicated by coexisting conditions such as diabetes mellitus, gout, asthma, peripheral vascular diseases and mental depression.

It was in 1985, that the possibility of using ACEI as the first-line of therapy was proposed.

146. Contraindications for using ACE inhibitors.

1. In bilateral renal artery stenosis.
2. In patients with one kidney or kidney transplant.
3. In significant subaortic stenosis or other obstructive valvular disease.
4. In hypertrophic and restrictive cardiomyopathy and constrictive pericarditis.
5. Severe carotid artery stenosis.
6. Severe renal failure (serum creatinine > 3 mg/dL) Caution is needed when ACE inhibitors are used in patients with renal failure since worsening of renal failure or hyperkalemia may occur.
7. In leukopenia or neutropenia.
8. In pregnancy and lactation.

Pre-existing dry cough is a relative contraindication.

147. There are 4 major adverse effects of ACE inhibitors.

1. *Cough:* A dry ticklish irritating non-productive cough occurs in upto 20% patients and is clearly dose related. The accumulation of bradykinin appears to be responsible for cough. The cough responds to treatment with NSAIDs like aspirin, indomethacin. The new angiotensin II receptor blocker, losartan does not cause cough or angiedema. The onset of cough may be delayed upto 24 months. Inhaled sodium cromoglycate is beneficial in some patients.
2. *Hypotension:* Dizziness may occur in volume depleted patients. So, caution is to be taken while using these agents along with diuretics. To avoid fall of BP, treatment should be started with low doses (for example, first dose—1/2 tablet of lowest strength to be given at bed time) and increased gradually over a few weeks.
3. Angioedema is rare although more common in patients of Afro-Caribbean origin than in other ethnic groups.
4. *Renal failure:* May be precipitated or worsened.

148. Advantages of ACEI over other antihypertensives.

1. Better quality of life.
2. Fewer side effects.
3. No reflex tachycardia.
4. No alteration of carbohydrate, uric acid or cholesterol metabolism.

149. Angiotensin II receptor antagonists: Recently introduced losartan potassium and several similar drugs being developed are not peptides and are orally active.

Some aspects of therapeutic applications are:

1. Like ACEI, angiotensin-receptor antagonists lower arterial blood pressure without inducing tachycardia, probably because they simultaneously reset baroreflexes.
2. Angiotensin II receptor- antagonists do not cause cough in patients who have side effect with ACE inhibitor supporting the hypothesis that the cough is mediated by bradykinins. This can be used in patients who have favorable response to ACE inhibitors but also have a cough.
3. Similarly, this can be used in patients in whom angioedema develops during treatment with ACEI.
4. Until the role of angiotensins in the fetal development is clarified, angiotensin receptor antagonists should not be given to pregnant women or to those who may become pregnant.

150. Saralasin (IV), is another enzyme inhibitor useful in the following 4 conditions:

1. To differentiate renin dependent HT from other HT. Bolus dose of 10 mg will significantly lowers the BP in renin dependent hypertension.

2. To predict reversibility of hypertension in renovascular hypertension before subjecting to surgery.
3. To know the antihypertensive effect of renin lowering drugs.
4. In the management of hypertensive crisis.

151. Alpha-blockers: They are likely to be used much more frequently in the future because of the better advantages they offer. Currently, their use is limited.

The advantages are:

1. They lower the blood pressure by reducing peripheral vascular resistance and at the same time maintaining cardiac output.
2. They have a positive influence on coronary risk factors—blood lipids, blood glucose, smoking, insulin resistance and regression of left ventricular hypertrophy. Selective alpha-blockers are known to antagonise the adverse cardiovascular effects of nicotine.
3. They are also antithrombotic by reducing platelet aggregation and increasing fibrinolytic activity.
4. They also reduce the formation of the precursors of atherosclerosis fatty streaks.

Prazosin and doxazosin are available alpha-blockers. A good alpha-blocker should not produce postural hypotension with the first dose.

Prazosin acts as alpha-blocker and as well as arterial vasodilator. Initially low dose 0.5–1.0 mg is given at night to prevent first dose hypotension followed by 2.5 mg bd or tds up to 20 mg/day β-blockers and diuretics have an additive effect when combined with prazosin. Alpha-receptors are found in the prostate. Thus, alpha-blockers improve clinical symptoms in patients with benign prostatic hypertrophy. Terazosin 1–20 mg od, Doxazosin 1–16 mg od (Trimazosin, Indoramin, Urapidil, Ketanserin are others).

152. Combination antihypertensive therapy

Rational for combination:

1. CCBs have a natriuretic effect which make contribute to rendering BP maintenance angiotension II dependent.
2. Edema caused by CCBs is less when combined with RAAS blockers (Renin angiotensin aldosterone system).
3. Single pill combination of amlodipine and valsartan in the management of hypertension.
4. These antihypertensive agents in combination are associated with greater clinical benefit with either agent alone.

ACEI/ARB with a diuretic reduces sodium retention and vasoconstriction mediated by angiotension and reduces volume hence enhancing the efficacy of both antihypertensive components, e.g. irbesartan with hydrochlorothiazide (HCTZ).

Aliskerin—direct renin inhibitor—blood pressure reduction with aliskerin/valsartan combination are significantly greater than with the monotherapy.

Antihypertensive therapy can be tailored to each individual patient, taking into account underlying disease such as dyslipidemia, diabetes and cardiac or renal insufficiency. The starting dose should be less than the full recommended dose to avoid sudden and marked fall of BP. The dose has to be increased to get the control of BP with minimum side effects. Increasing dose of single drug may cause adverse effects. So, a combination of drugs in small doses can effectively control the hypertension with minimal side effects such as cough with ACEI, fatigue from β-blockers, and pedal edema with dihydropyridine calcium antagonists.

There are four good commonly used combinations of antihypertensive drugs.

Table B-20

1. β-blocker	+ Thiazide diuretic
2. β-blocker	+ Calcium channel blocker
3. ACE inhibitor	+ Diuretic
4. ACE inhibitor	+ Calcium channel blocker

β-blocker and thiazide diuretic combination results in additive antihypetensive effect that permits the effective use of very low dose of thiazide diuretic. The mechanism of action is complimentary to each other. Increased sympathetic outflow and renin angiotensin axis activation induced by diuretic being blunted by β-blockers. Hence, this combination was recommended as first line of treatment by Joint National Committee on the detection, evaluation and treatment of high blood pressure unless contraindicated or unacceptable. However this combination has negative effect in dyslipidemic, gouty and diabetic patients.

β-blockers decrease the heart rate and cardiac output and therefore reduce peripheral perfusion, whereas calcium blockers may marginally increase heart rate and improve peripheral perfusion. Headaches caused by vasodilatation can be attenuated by β-blockers because they reduce the rate and force of cardiac contraction, the prevention of myocardial infarction and sudden death is a difficult proposition. These combinations may be of some help in prevention, since β-blockers are extensively studied for their effect in reducing coronary mortality and sudden cardiac death.

The thiazide diuretics are particularly useful in obese hypertensive patients with concomitant mild heart failure and patients with low renin hypertension. The loop diuretics are useful in hypertension with impaired renal function and in patients with severe hypertension. Diuretic induced sodium depletion stimulates renin secretion and angiotensin II production leading to attenuation of blood pressure reduction. Therefore, in patients with inadequate hypotensive response to diuretic therapy, addition of ACE inhibitor is useful. ACE inhibitors inhibit the counter regulatory activation of renin-angiotensin-aldosterone (RAA) system. This means that the effects of diuretics and ACE inhibitors can be assumed to be at least additive and may even be synergistic, thereby allowing low doses of both drugs to be used. In contrast to thiazide diuretics ACEI are devoid of adverse metabolic side effects such as hypokalemia, hyperglycemia and hypercholesterolemia. A further benefit of the combination is that ACEI reverse the left ventricular hypertrophy. Since the antihypertensive efficacy of an ACEI diuretic combination is greater than individual components, it is possible to use low dose of thiazide diuretic. The combination should result in less side effects on blood glucose, serum cholesterol and serum potassium. Efficacy of ACEI and thiazide diuretics, involving captopril, enalapril, ramipril or lisinopril with hydrochlorothiazide have been widely studied and are found to be greatly useful.

The calcium channel blockers are of particular use in elderly, diabetic, asthmatic or hyperlipidemia patients but are also appropriate when patients require treatment for both angina and hypertension CCB cause vasodilatation, induces reflex activation of sympathetic nervous and RAA system leading to an attenuation of their hypotensive effects. Therefore, in patients who have insufficient response to CCB , an addition of ACEI, which inhibits the activation of these systems may be synergistic. This combination can be termed as 'tandem blockers' because they block the undesired counter regulatory effects in kidney and vessels in complimentary manner, hence a stronger antihypertensive effect is seen. Combination of enalapril 5 mg and felodipine 5 mg in elderly population produced higher normalization than a 10 mg of either monotherapy. Reduction in albuminuria in hypertensive non-insulin dependent diabetic patients with nephropathy has been reported during treatment with a combination of captopril and nicardipine.

153. There are 4 less commonly used combinations.

Table B-21

1. β-blocker	+ Alpha-blocker (Labetalol)
2. β-blocker	+ Vasodilator (Propranolol 40 mg + Dihydralazine sulph 25 mg)
3. Adrenergic neuron blocking agent	+ Vasodilator (Serpasil 0.1 mg + Dihydralazine sulph 10 mg)
4. Adrenergic neurone blocking agent	+ Vasodilator + Thiazide diuretic (Serpasil + Dihydralazine sulph + Hydrochlorothiazide 10 mg)

The usage of these drugs became less as the better drug combinations are available now.

154. There are 4 bad combinations of antihypertensive drugs

Table B-22

1. β-blocker	+ Verapamil → Dangerous (They should not be combined)
2. β-blocker	+ ACE inhibitor
3. Calcium blocker	+ Thiazide diuretic
4. ACEI	+ Potassium sparing diuretic + Potassium supplements

Benefits of ACEI and BB are controversial. Combination requires further studies. ACEI and CCB combination is attractive because both do not exert any metabolic or central effects but are only few studies.

155. Some useful combinations of drugs for treatment of hypertension.

β-blocker + Diuretic:

1. Atenolol 50 mg + Hydrochlorothiazide 25 mg + Amiloride 2.5 mg 1 cap per day
2. Propranolol 40 mg + Hydrochlorothiazide 25 mg 1 to 2 tab per day
3. Metaprolol 100 mg + Hydrochlorothiazide 12.5 mg 1 to 2 tab per day.
4. Atenolol 50 mg + Chlorthalidone 1 to 2 tab per day.
5. Atenolol 100 mg + Chlorthalidone 25 mg 1 to 2 tab per day.

β-blocker + Calcium channel blocker:

6. Atenolol 50 mg + Nifedipine 20 mg 1 to 2 cap or tab per day.
7. Atenolol 50 mg + Amlodipine 5 mg 1 tab per day.

ACEI + Diuretic:

8. Enalapril 10 mg + Hydrochlorothiazide 25 mg 1 to 2 tab per day.
9. Clonidine 100 mg + Chlorthalidone 15 mg 1 to 2 per day.
10. Reserpine + Dihydralazine 1 to 2 tab per day.
11. Reserpine + Dihydralazine + Hydrochlorothiazide 1 to 2 tab per day.
12. Enalapril + Amlodipine 1 tab per day.

156. After a long time usage of drugs, some of the non-diuretic antihypertensive agents may lose their efficacy by renal sodium retention in the following way:

1. Non-diuretic antihypertensive drug, e.g. vasodilators

↓

2. Increased renin secretion

↓

3. Increased aldosterone secretion

↓

4. Increased sodium retention → Increase in fluid volume → raise in BP.

157. There are 4 important IV preparations which act immediately in hypertensive crisis.

(Malignant or accelerated hypertension)

1. *Diazoxide:* 300 mg in 20 mL ampoule by rapid IV infusion.
2. *Sodium nitroprusside:* Initially as (5 mg in 540 cc 5% dextrose) 0.5–1.5 μg/kg/min. Dose adjusted to the requirement of an individual.
3. *Trimethaphan:* 1–10 mg IV/min ganglion blocking agent.
4. *Phentolamine:* 1–5 mg IV acts on alpha receptors—useful in suspected or proved pheochromocytoma. (oral preparations are not available for the above 4 drugs.

Reserpine, methyldopa, hydralazine: Oral, IM or IV preparations are available—but their onset of action is slow.

158. Additional consideration in antihypertensive drug choices.

Potential favorable effects.

1. Thiazide type diuretics are useful in slowing demineralization in osteoporosis.
2. β-blockers are useful in the treatment of atrial tachyarrhythmias / fibrillation, migraine, thyrotoxicosis (short-term) essential tremor or perioperative hypertension.
3. CCBs are useful in Raynaud's syndrome and certain arrhythmias.
4. Alpha-blockers are useful in prostatism.

159. Additional considerations in antihypertensive drug choices.

1. Thiazide diuretics should be used cautiously in gout or in h/o significant hyponatremia.
2. ACEIs should not be used in individuals with h/o of angioedema.
3. Aldosterone antagonists and potassium sparing diuretics can cause hyperkalemia.
4. ACEIs and ARBs are contraindicated in pregnant women or those likely to become pregnant.

160. The following drugs should be avoided in certain conditions with hypertension:

1. Avoid β-blockers in peripheral vascular disorders. Avoid ACE inhibitors in bronchospastic conditions.
2. Avoid centrally acting drugs like clonidine, reserpine, etc. in cerebrovascular disease (symptomatic). Avoid hypotension.
3. Avoid calcium channel blockers in elderly patients aged above 75 years.
4. Avoid ACE inhibitors in bilateral renal artery stenosis or solitary kidney, pregnancy.

161. Hypertensive patients may present with various profiles. Following are some examples:

1. Hypertensive with dyslipidemia.
2. Obese hypertensives.
3. Smokers.
4. Diabetic or prediabetic hypertensives.
5. Hypertensive with angina.
6. Postinfarct hypertensives.
7. Hypertension in elderly.
8. Pregnant hypertensives.

ESSENTIAL HYPERTENSION

It accounts for about 90% of hypertensives in adults.

162. There are 4 points to be noted in the selection of drugs for the treatment of essential hypertension.

1. Follow the method of non-drug treatment.
   Restriction of salt is very essential because the essential hypertension is thought to be due to defective excretion of salt by the kidneys.
2. Hemodynamic assessment is to be done by exercise. For example, in a patient with BP 140/90 mm Hg. If the systolic BP goes up from 140 to 190 or above and diastolic BP comes down from 90 to 80 or below after the exercise—it means, the peripheral vascular resistance is normal and the hypertension is due to volume overload.
   Thus, this patient requires salt restriction and diuretic to eliminate sodium and water—i.e. to reduce volume overload.
   Long-acting diuretic like hydrochlorothiazide or chlorthalidone for long-term therapy are given.
   Use of long-acting diuretics for long-term use of 5 to 10 years may rise triglyceride levels, which increases atherosclerosis. Therefore, give the long acting diuretics in small doses. Do not exceed 25 mg of hydrochlorothiazide or chlorthalidone.
   (Loop diuretic like Furosemide should not be given as the action lasts for 6 hours only).
3. If the systolic BP goes up from 140 and above and the diastolic BP stays normal after exercise. It indicates the cardiac output is increased whereas the peripheral resistance is neither decreased nor increased.

These patients need a drug which dilates the peripheral vessels—peripheral vasodilators.

Calcium blockers block the entry of calcium into the cell for contraction of the vessel wall—so, the vessels get dilated. For example, nifedipine, amlodipine diltiazem. Long-acting nifedipine has 18 hours action. Single dose of long-acting nifedipine may be enough. Hypertensive emergencies are common between 3–5 AM because the long-acting drugs like nifedipine has action for 18 hours. So, the patient needs bd dose. It may have side effects like headache, reactive tachycardia due to intense vasodilatation. amlodipine 5 mg od can be given this can be counteracted by combining with β-blocker. So, next question arises what type of β-blocker-

Propranolol, non-selective β-blocker acts on all the tissues of the body. Therefore, better choose a cardioselective β-blocker, for example, atenolol or metaprolol

Metaprolol has only 8 hours action, so needs repeated dose.

Atenolol is long acting.

Nifedipine 5 to 10 mg and Atenolol 50 to 100 mg can be combined.

4. If the systolic BP and the diastolic BP go on rising—stop the exercise immediately—otherwise, he may go into syncope, tachyarrhythmia, etc.

   It indicates that both volume overload and peripheral vascular resistance are increased.

   These patients need direct vasodilators. For example, prazocin, enzyme inhibitors, e.g. captopril, enalapril, Lisinopril.

   Captopril 25 mg bd

   Enalapril 5 to 10 mg od

   Diuretics are not given with ACE inhibitors.

   Enalapril can prevent diabetic nephropathy.

163. Following 4 low dose combination therapy shows advantage for systemic hypertension:

Low dose of

1. Diuretic + β-blocker
2. ACE + CCB
3. ACE + Diuretic
4. CCB + β-blocker

Subtherapeutic doses of two agents providing additive therapeutic effects cause least side effects. They gradually reduce the BP. They avoid rapid BP lowering which may lead to tissue hypoperfusion. So, non-specific side effects like fatigue, light headedness, dizziness are not felt.

HYPERTENSION AND DIABETES

The prevalence of hypertension among diabetics is twice as compared to non-diabetics. Hypertension and diabetes are both associated with hyperlipidemia. This means that many patients will have three cardiovascular risk factors, even if they do not smoke. Increased adrenergic activity, disturbed lipid profile can cause insulin resistance. The effects of antihypertensive drugs on glucose and lipid metabolism are to be considered in treating hypertension with diabetic patients. Alpha-blockers are safe and may even have beneficial effect on plasma lipids. Calcium channel blockers and ACE inhibitors are lipid neutral and also safe when used carefully. ACE inhibitors can cause significant reduction in urinary albumin excretion and slows the deterioration of renal function and can be used in diabetes with nephropathy. This effect seems to be independent of blood pressure control. Thiazide diuretics may disturb the lipid profile and worsen insulin resistance and are to be avoided. β-blockers are to be used with caution because of lack of awareness of hypoglycemic symptoms.

All patients should follow the non-pharmacological measures before the drug treatment (See B-89).

All patients should have complete workup including detailed clinical examination documenting the CVS status, peripheral circulation, fundus examination and assessment of body mass index. Basic investigations should include glycemic status, lipid profile, renal profile, serum electrolytes, urinary protein estimation.

In Type 1 diabetes, hypertension develops many years later. On the other hand, Type 2 diabetics may have hypertension before the development of the diabetes or may develop during the course of the disease till the development of nephropathy. The non-renal causes of hypertension may be contributed by advancing age, obesity, ethnicity and insulin resistance.

The presence of hypertension in diabetes increases the incidence of nephropathy, coronary artery disease, stroke, peripheral vascular disease, retinopathy and lower limb amputations. In fact, diabetes account for more than 40% of patients undergoing dialysis or renal transplantation.

164. Always see for any secondary hypertension in diabetes mellitus; following 4 points are to be looked for:

1. Endocrinal diseases that cause both hypertension and diabetes, for example, acromegaly, Cushing's syndromes, Conn's syndrome, pheochromocytoma.
2. Drugs that cause both hypertension and diabetes: For example, oral contraceptives (combined preparation, glucocorticoids).

3. Antihypertensive drugs causing diabetes: Potassium loosing diuretics, (especially chlorthalidone, diazoxide).
4. Hypertension secondary to diabetes complications: Nephropathy, renal scarring following recurrent urinary tract infection, isolated systolic hypertension due to atheroscleroses.

165. The best way to choose the initial drug for diabetic hypertension is to see for the comorbid condition and then select the one favorably affect that condition and avoid those drugs that make the condition worse. For example:

1. If the patient has IHD/CAD, the initial drug can be a cardio selective β-blocker or ACEI.
2. If the patient has cardiac failure—diuretics, ACEI and β-blocker. Avoid CCBs.
3. If the patient has frequent hypoglycemia or has hyperlipidemia—go for ACEI and CCBs; Avoid β-blockers and diuretics.
4. If the patient has impotence—go for ACEI and CCBs avoid β-blocker, methyldopa.

If the first drug works only partially additional drugs can ba added on a step-wise manner. At present the ACEI have an edge over the other drugs in view of its favorable effects on the accompanying comorbid conditions and emerging has the first line of drug in diabetes with hypertension. A low dose diuretic like thiazide will often prove to be the second drug in many situations. CCBs like amlodipine is another drug to be added to others.

Type 2 diabetes are relatively resistant to antihypertensive drugs in view of the associated obesity, hyperinsulinemia and many may require three drugs for tight BP control.

166. ACEI have the most beneficial affect in diabetes.

1. They appear to enhance the insulin sensitivity and improve glycemic control.
2. Reduce the total cholesterol and triglycerides.
3. Reduces lipoprotein.
4. Reduces microalbuminuria and proteinuria and retard the progression of diabetic nephropathy in both normotensive and hypertensive diabetic patients.

167. Antihypertensive drugs and diabetes in general without other complications.

Table B-23

1. Alpha-blockers	Beneficial effects on plasma lipids
2. β-blockers	Safe if used carefully. Cardioselective are better
3. ACEI	Safe if used carefully
4. CCB	Generally safe

168. There are 4 types of hypertension in diabetic patients.

1. Surgically curable—its prevalence is similar to non-diabetic population.
2. Diabetics mellitus without nephropathy
   - Essential hypertension
   - Systolic hypertension with varying degrees of diastolic pressure.
3. Diabetes mellitus with nephropathy—renal ('Diabetic') hypertension.
4. Diabetes mellitus with neuropathy.

Hypertension is a common comorbidity in diabetes. In Type I DM, hypertension is often a result of nephropathy whereas in Type II diabetes it often occurs as a part of metabolic syndrome. A target BP of 130/80 mm Hg is recommended.

169. Drugs in the treatment of hypertension in diabetic patients without nephropathy just as in the case of non-diabetic patients.

1. *β-blockers:* Give selective β-blocker if there are no contraindication for example, metaprolol 100 mg/day in two divided doses up to 400 mg/day or atenolol 50–100 mg/day. Theoretically, β-blockers can conceal the clinical manifestations hypoglycemia but in real practice, it is not a problem.
   The major disadvantages of β-blockers in diabetes with hypertension are:
   i. Their adverse effects on exercise tolerance and weight control.
   ii. Adverse effects on metabolic parameters.
   iii. Interference with protective mechanisms for avoiding or recovering from hypoglycemia.
   iv. Their propensity to cause vasoconstriction.
   Isolated systolic hypertension is said to be present when SBP > 140 mm Hg with normal DBP. The basic cause for this is loss of arterial elasticity associated with atherosclerotic process and diabetes is well known to produce premature and extensive atherosclerosis.
2. *Alpha-blockers:* Prazosin, terazosin, doxazocin are effective in controlling hypertension in diabetic patients. Their added advantage is their ability to reduce insulin resistance. However, orthostatic hypotension may be a problem in autonomic neuropathy. More long-term studies on their efficacy are required before they become the drug of choice for diabetic hypertensions
3. ACEIs/ARBs and CCBs can be started as the first-line of drug which are also showing favorable response.
4. *Vasodilators:* Add vasodilatorse depending on other comorbid conditions. Hydralazin 50 mg/day up to 300 mg/day in divided doses or Prazocin 1 mg/day up to 15 mg/day in divided doses.
   Diuretics can be combined in small doses.

Presently, the preferred first-line drugs are ACEI/ARBs as modulation of renin-angiotensin system exerts vascular protective effects beyond blood pressure control by limiting target organ damage. The diuretics, BBs, CCBs may also be used in combination therapy. Most diabetics need 2 to 3 drugs for optimal BP control. ACEI/and ARBs retard deterioration renal function and rate of progression to end-stage renal disease (caution of using ACEI/ARBs if serum creatining > 3 mg%).

First-line therapy should be based on ACEI/ARBs cardio selective BB and diuretics that have been convincingly shown to reduce morbidity and mortality in patients with diabetic nephropathy. CCBs agents can be added as second line therapy.

When the hypertension develops in the absences of nephropathy, genetic and acquired factors may be responsible. Total body sodium is elevated with normal or low activity of RAAS, in some of these cases. The hypertensives may have higher than normal levels of serums insulin, which may lead to increased renal sodium and water reabsorption. Insulin resistant states have decreased vasodilatory response in skeletal muscle and also reduced synthesis of vasodilatory prostaglandins. Insulin resistance state associated with Type 2 diabetes also causes increased secretion of endothelins which are vasopressors.

170. There are 4 steps in the treatment of hypertension in diabetic patients with nephropathy.

The pathogenesis of hypertension in diabetes associated with nephropathy is thought to be volume dependent. In diabetes, there is low renin levels associated with lower serum aldosterone. The nephropathy causes extracellular fluid retention and increase in total body sodium levels, thus reducing the activity of RAAS.

Step I: Thiazide or loop diuretics—adequate diuresis with diuretics should be the sheet anchor in the treatment. Caution: Fall in glomerular filtration secondary to volume depletion might result in further deterioration of renal function. Hence, maintain a trace edema.

Use of potassium sparing diuretics have the risk of precipitating hyperkalemia.

Thiazide diuretics cause natriuresis and vasodilatation and are useful in hypertension. In systolic hypertension in elderly study, the absolute risk reduction, was twice as great as in diabetic subjects compared to nondiabetics. Thiazide diuretics may not be effective in those with GFR less than 60 mL/min/1.73 sq/m. Thiazide diuretics are also not liked friendly and may not be the first agent to be considered in diabetic hypertension. Loop diuretics like furosemide are useful in those with GFR less than 60 mL/min and in combination with other drugs.

If there is no response :

Step II: Vasodilators: Prazocin which does not influence the cardiac output is preferred.

It appears very clear that the interruption of the renin-angiotensin system is warranted in patients with diabetic nephropathy. The use of either ACEI or ARBs are useful in either form of diabetic nephropathy. ACEI or ARBS in Type I or II diabetes protect against progression of chronic renal failure.

Caution: Coexisting cardiac disease is invariably present with diabetic nephropathy. Drugs like hydralazine are avoided because they have a tendency to increase cardiac output and precipitate coronary insufficiency. Hydralazine decreases the afterload without effect on preload and increases the cardiac output whereas prazocin does not influence the cardiac output.

If there is no adequate response:

Step III: Add methyldopa or clonidine.

Clonidine is probably the safest antiadrenergic drug in diabetes with nephropathy.

If there is no response—with progressive renal failure as indicated by serum creatinine of 5 mg.

Step IV: Dialysis and/or kidney transplantation.

171. Step care regimen in hypertension in diabetic mellitus with nephropathy differs from essential hypertension as follows:

Table B-24

Step care regimen in essential hypertension	*Steps in Diabetic hypertension with nephropathy*
1. Diuretic or β-blocker	1. Diuretics-thiazide or loop diuretics
2. Diuretic + β-blocker	2. Alpha-blocker
3. Vasodilator hydralazine	3. Vasodilator—Prazocin (of) Hydralazine
4. Adrenolytics—Methyldopa	4. Adrenolytics—Clonidine (or) Methyldopa

172. There are 4 mechanisms for low plasma renin activity (PRA) in diabetes mellitus with nephropathy.

1. Low synthesis of inactive prorenin.
2. Low catecholamine concentration.
3. Hyalinization of afferent arteriole.
4. Hypervolemia caused as in
   - Progressive nephropathy with water retention
   - Uncontrolled diabetes mellitus, hyperglycemia leading to hypervolemia.

173. Treatment of hypertension in diabetes mellitus with neuropathy consists of (involvement of peripheral and autonomic nerves in a state of supine hypertension with orthostatic hypotension):

1. Correction of hypoaldosteronism by mineralocorticoid replacement—alpha flurohydrocortisone 0.05 to 0.3 mg/day.
2. Single dose of prazocin or hydralazine at bed time to decrease the supine nocturnal hypertension.
3. Elastic stockings to facilitate venous return by potentiating the muscular pump to improve cardiac output.
4. Occasionally, ephedrine 25 mg po 4 times a day to elevate the upright BP.

Paradoxically, it is the orthostatic hypotension which requires therapy rather than the supine hypertension.

174. There are 4 causes of orthostatic hypotension.

1. Blunting of baroreceptor reflexes.
2. Low levels of circulating catecholamines and renin.
3. Hypoalbuminemia due to urinary protein loss and contracted plasma volume.
4. Defective cardiac function.

175. Side effects of antihypertensive drugs need a short discussion especially in diabetes mellitus. Commonly used thiazide diuretics may cause the 4 following side effects.

1. Hypokalemia—diminishes the insulin release and worsen the diabetic state.
2. Hyperuricemia—rarely causes gout but it is certainly toxic to the pancreas due to its structural similarity to alloxan.
3. Hypercholesterolemia.
4. Hypertriglyceridemia.

The above 3 and 4 conditions add some more risk in the already existing cardiac disease in diabetes.

Use of spiranolactone and triamterene in hypoaldosteronism may lead to serious hyperkalemia.

176. Following are the 4 side effects of some antihypertensive drugs used in hypertension associated with diabetes mellitus.

1. β-blockers
   - Mask the hypoglycemic adrenergic symptoms.
   - May precipitate latent cardiac failure.
2. Sympathetic inhibitors like methyldopa, guanethidine may precipitate or accentuate postural hypotension and impotence.
3. Vasodilators like hydralizine may precipitate coronary insufficiency. Severe orthostatic hypotension with the first dose of prazocin must be watched for.
4. Calcium channel blockers like nifedipine can interfere with insulin secretion.

Even though the treatment is individualized, clonidine has been found to be a safe and good drug in hypertension with diabetes mellitus.

INSULIN RESISTANACE HYPERTENSION

A close association between hypertension and insulin resistance (IR) has been reported in a number of studies over the pasts three decades. Many obese as well as non-obese hypertension patients have IR indicated by higher than normal plasma insulin level, both fasting and postglucose load even if they are not overt diabetic.

Decrease in insulin sensitivity among non-obese hypertensives by euglycemic insulin-clamp technique is a gold standard test for insulin sensitivity.

177. Components of insulin resistance syndrome (IRS).

Initial description

1. Resistance to insulin mediated glucose uptake.
2. Hyperinsulinemia.
3. Impaired glucose tolerance (IGT).
4. Hypertension.
5. Increased LDL cholesterol.
6. Decreased HDL cholesterol.
7. Hypertriglyceridemia subsequent additions.
8. Visceral adiposity.
9. Small dense LDL.
10. Increased plasminogen activator inhibitor-1 (PAI-1).
11. Microalbunemia.
12. Increased proinsulin.

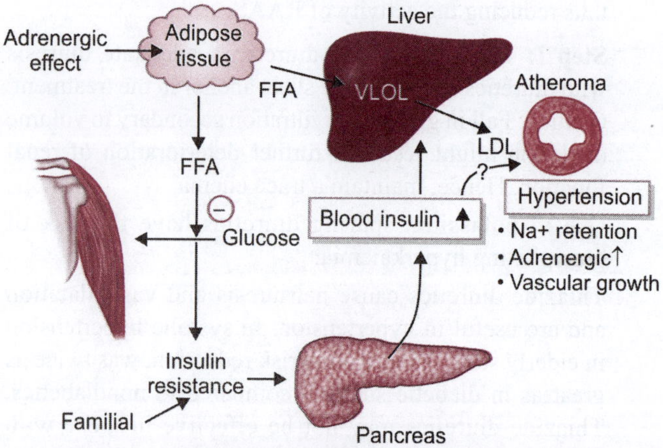

Fig. B-7: Insulin resistance

Proposed sequence of events leading to insulin resistance. Based on inhibition of uptake of glucose by circulating free fatty acids VLDL

178. There are 4 mechanisms by which hyperinsulinemia increases BP.

1. Enhancement of renal sodium and water absorption.
2. Stimulation of sympathetic system which in turn stimulates the renin-angiotensin system. (There is a dose related increase in plasma norepinephrine following insulin infusion).
3. Vascular smooth muscle hypertrophy secondary to mitogenic action of insulin.
4. Modifying ion transport across the cell membrane.

Decreases Na^+-K^+ ATPase activity, increases Na^+-H^+ pump activity and cytosolic Ca^+ level in insulin sensitive vascular and renal tissues.

Insulin stimulated vasodilatation which is mediated through nitric oxide (NO), is impaired in presence of IRS. Still the potential role of insulin in modifying blood pressure is not completely understood. Strong evidence is the patients with insulinoma and polycystic ovary syndrome, who do not have increased incidence of hypertension and there is no change in blood pressure after removal of the tumor.

179. Hyperinsulinemia and hypertension.

1. Hyperinsulinemia causes hypertension. Higher the insulin level, greater the risk of hypertension.
2. Insulin resistance plays an important role in the pathogenesis of hypertension.
3. Insulin resistance starts at an early age and it manifest as full bloom insulin resistance syndrome in later life.
4. Fact: Not all insulin resistants are hyprtensives, and nor all (non-obese) hyprtensives are insulin resistant. However, the two go together more than by chance and there are known mechanisms for their interaction.

180. Therapeutic aspects

While treating, clinician should identify the individuals with other manifestations of IRS. Control of hypertension by drugs does not ameliorate IRS nor any currently available antihypertensive drug result in deterioration of insulin sensitivity.

Better avoid thiazide diuretics and β-blockers which enhance hyperinsulinism during drug therapy of hypertensives with IRS especially diabetics.

Drugs with some beneficial effect are:

1. ACEI
2. Biguanides (Metaformin)
3. Alpha-blockers
4. Amlodipine

HYPERTENSION IN THE OLD AGE

Management of hypertension in the old age (more than 75 years).

Dementia and cognitive impairment occur more commonly in people with hypertension in old age. Effective antihypertensive therapy reduces progression of cognitive impairments.

The pathological features which characterize aging are atherosclerosis and gradual loss of cell mass compared to senile osteoporosis but manifests more importantly is presenile dementia or diffuse cerebral atrophy, first described by Alois Alzheimer in 1906 and named after him, Alzheimer's disease. In some old age patients with hypertension, disabling dementia precede death and they showed independent life impossible.

It occurs in more than 2/3rd of individuals after the age of 65 years this is also the population with the lowest rates of BP control.

There can be multi-infarction brain failure as a late outcome of hypertension as distinct from stroke. Multi-infarction dementia may be preventable in some at least by control of pressure, but we have no evidence for or against this. The principle objective of medical care in the old age is to maintain independence and the quality of life. "Add life to years and not years to life." Longevity is secondary importance. The aim must be to keep the old well from sickness. In view of this, myocardial infarction or aortic rupture diminishes in importance as age advances, because they are as a rule less distressing modes of death compared to stroke or brain failure. Stroke or brain failure cause physical mental and social impairment and they showed independent life impossible.

Stroke occurs much more commonly in the presence of heart failure, so there became two main outcomes, we feel to prevent. Our main aim should be the control of hypertension in middle age and then maintain that control in old age, though with less therapeutic aggressiveness.

Pseudohypertension due to increased arterial rigidity should be suspected in patients with high BP without evidence of end organ damage.

Although primary hypertension is for the most common in elderly. It is important to rule out the secondary hypertension especially in patient who have late-onset of hypertension after the age of 65 years or resistant hypertension despite being on multiple drugs. Atherosclerotic renovascular hypertension, primary aldosteronism may occur frequently in old age especially in patients who have late-onset of hypertension.

CCBs especially immediate release of nifedipine has precipitated ischemic events and in large doses may increase coronary mortality in patients who had MI. Therefore, immediate-release nifedipine should be used with caution, if at all used.

Alpha-blockers may be useful in patients with prostatism with urinary symptoms, but otherwise have no added advantage.

Prazosin is usually not recommended in old age because of high incidence of orthostatic hypotension.

181. Hypertension in older persons.

1. More than two-thirds of people over 65 years have hypertension.
2. This population has the lowest rates of BP control.
3. Treatment including those with isolated systolic hypertension should follow same principles outlined for general care of hypertension.
4. Lower initial doses may be indicated to avoid symptoms—standard doses and multiple drugs will be needed to reach BP targets.

182. Functionally, the following 4 cardiovascular changes are seen in old age with hypertension:

1. Decrease in cardiac output due to fall in stroke volume and slower contractility.
2. Increased risk of cardiovascular complications and other target organs. Narrowing of range of optimal heart rate—any significant bradycardia or tachycardia will impair cardiac output.
3. Increase in peripheral vascular resistance due to atherosclerosis
4. Decreased sensitivity to baroreceptors.
   Failure of vasoconstrictor reflexes to the changes in posture leads to postural hypotension.
   Always check the BP in supine, sitting, and standing positions in elderly patients.

The drugs producing postural hypotension are serious. Symptomatology of the elderly cardiac patient may vary from that of the adult. Left heart failure may suddenly manifest itself as pulmonary edema when provoked by emotional upheaval, sudden unaccustomed exertion, or excessive salt intake. Anorexia, weight loss and emaciation may be pointers to heart failure in the elderly.

183. The following renal changes are seen in the old age with hypertension:

1. Renal blood flow and glomerular filtration are progressively decreased in the old age and they are aggravated in hypertension and predisposes to renal damage and vice versa.
2. Renal concentration power is decreased. Renal conservation of sodium is decreased due to salt restriction. This may increase the possibility of dehydration.
   Hence, use the diuretics with caution preferably in very small doses.
3. Renal tubular function diminishes resulting in defective transport of salt, glucose and acid loads.
4. Decreased activity of juxtaglomerular apparatus results in lowered secretion of renin leading to alteration in renin-angiotensin-aldosterone response.
   - Fall in renin.
   - Fall in aldosterone.
   - Renal blood flow falls by 50%.

184. There is increased risk of complications old age.

1. Stroke.
2. Acute myocardial infarction (AMI).
3. Heart failure.
4. Renal failure.

185. Drug treatment of hypertension in elderly consists of:

1. Thiazide diuretics
   a. Well-tolerated in old age.
   b. Effective in low dosage.
   c. Once a day dose.
   d. Evidence of reduction in CVS mortality and stroke. Decrease in cholesterol level in long-term use.
      - Hydrochlorothiazide 25 mg od (or less 1/2 tab od)
      - Chlorthalidone 100 mg od (or less 1/2 tab od)
      - Indapamide hemihydrate 2.5 mg od (or less 1/2 tab od)
2. β-blockers
   They do not adversely affect the autoregulation of cerebral blood flow.
   Propranolol 10 mg to start with and slowly increased. or cardioselective β-blockers-atenolol 50 mg od.
3. Methyldopa 125 to 250 mg od or bd.
4. ACEI for example, Enalapril 5 to 10 mg od or bd.

The difference in advantages of various drugs are appreciated by reduction in cardiovascular morbidity and mortality, reduction in fatal and non-fatal strokes. Definite advantage is found in the reduction of strokes by 40%, but reduction in coronary heart disease is only 10–15%.

186. The following 4 points may be noted while treating hypertension in the elderly:

1. Benefit in mild hypertension is uncertain.
   Drugs are useful in moderate or severe hypertension.
   Non-drug treatment is given in mild hypertension.
2. Begin with low doses and gradually increase and watch for the side effects.
3. Take extra caution in cerebrovascular and peripheral vascular diseases—since fall in BP may reduce tissue perfusion.
4. Avoid calcium channel blockers.
   Dilatation of stiff atherosclerotic vessels may precipitate transient ischemic attacks.

Elderly hypertensive patients benefit from the treatment upto the age of 84 years even in isolated systolic hypertension. Most physicians tend to be cautious while treating the patients aged over 70–75 years for fear of side effects.

SYSTOLIC HYPERTENSION

Earlier much importance was not given to isolated systolic blood pressure. Nowadays many studies conducted have shown that in patients with isolated systolic hypertension, there is an increase in morbidity and mortality especially from cerebrovascular accidents.

Isolated systolic hypertension can be observed in elderly people due to increased stiffness of the vasculature. It is observed in thyrotoxicosis, atrioventricular fistula (AV fistula), aortic regurgitation, beriberi, Paget's disease and patent ductus arteriosus (due to increase in cardiac output secondary to hyperdynamic circulation).

187. Know the following 4 points in the management of systolic hypertension.

1. It is common in the old age—BP 200/90 mm Hg. Pulse pressure is wide. Aorta and the peripheral arteries become increasingly rigid due to loss of elasticity and calcium deposition in the media in the old age. About 60% of diabetics may show systolic hypertension—diastolic pressure is relatively low.
2. Calcium blockers are totally avoided in systolic hypertension in the old age. Atherosclerosis is already existing. Dilatation of stiff vessels can precipitate transient ischemic attacks.
3. Indapamide 2.5 mg od is to be given as it is a thiazide analogue with diuretic and vasodilator properties but should not be given in severe renal or hepatic insufficiency.
   If there is no response.
4. Cardioselective β-blocker like atenolol 50 mg od is to be given.
   β-blockers do not adversely affect autoregulation of cerebral blood flow.

188. Treatment of chronic Hypotension consists of:

It is worth mentioning here as it is not infrequently seen in the practice specially in women.

1. Usage of elastic stockings is to be advised.
   Toes up exercise to pump the blood up from feet to potentiate the muscular pump and improve cardiac output.
2. More salt in the diet.
3. Injection nandrolone phenylpropionate 25 mg.
   Desoxy corticosterone phenylproprionate 10 mg.
   1 mL IM once in 2 or 3 weeks is to be given to correct hypoaldosteronism by mineralocorticoids.
4. Ephedrine 25 mg po 3 to 4 times a day is to be given.

POSTURAL HYPOTENSION

A decrease in standing SBP > 10 mm Hg when associated with dizziness or fainting is more frequent in older patients with systolic hypertension, diabetes, and those taking diuretics, vasodilators (for example, nitrates, alpha-blockers and sildenafil like drugs and some psychotropic drugs).

Caution is needed to use small doses initially or to avoid volume depletion and excessively rapid dose of titration of antihypertensive drugs.

Orthostatic hypotension: It is defined as a drop of 30 mm Hg in SBP or drop of 20 mm Hg in mean BP (diastolic plus 1/3rd of the pulse pressure) when going from supine to standing position.

Patients usually complain of light headedness, fatigue, unsteadiness, headache, neck tightness or cognitive slowing especially in the elderly. In severe cases, syncope can occur. Asymptomatic orthostatic hypotension does not require intervention but those blood pressure is less than 80/50 mm Hg are usually symptomatic and require treatment.

189. Management

1. As a first step—unnecessary medication should be stopped.
2. Should drink eight or more glasses of water (fluid each day and liberally add salt up to 150–250 mEq to the diet.
3. Pharmacological treatment is to use the drugs to increase the intravascular volume with mineralocorticoid or to increase the vascular resistance through stimulation of alpha-receptors. The mineralocorticoid Fludrocortisone (Florinef) is given at a dose of 0.1 mg od or bd and can be increased to as high as 0.3 to 0.6 mg per day. Supine hypertension and dependant edema are common and not unexpected. Care must be taken to avoid congestive heart failure.
4. Midodrine (Proamatine) is a peripherally acting alpha-1 agonist that produces vasoconstriction of both arterioles and venous capacitance vessels. The initials dose is 2.5 mg bid or tid. The maintenance dose is 30 mg/day in divided doses, with usual maximum dose of 40 mg/day. It is well-absorbed orally and generally well-tolerated. As a selective alpha adrenergic agonist, it is relatively free of β-adrenergic side effects and pulse rate usually does not increase. Patients with supine hypertension on midodrine (> 150/90) should be treated by elevating the head of the bed to a 30° incline. Side effects of midodrine include scalp pruritus, and tingling, pilomotor reactions, GIT complications, headache and dizziness. Because, it does not cross the blood-brain barrier, it is less likely to produce CNS side effects than ephedrine.

Refractory cases may respond to combination therapy with fludrocortisone.

Rarely, ergotamine tartrate (Cafergot) is given to the patient of orthostatic hypotension.

RENAL HYPERTENSION

Renal parenchymal disease is the most common cause of secondary hypertension especially among children and elderly.

190. Kidney and hypertension: The kidney is important in most forms of hypertension.

1. A defect in renal function is almost certain in the pathogenesis of primary hypertension.
2. Renal damage often develops in the course of primary hypertension. Hypertension is a major cause of end – stage renal disease (ESRD) mostly in elderly.
3. Chronic renal disease is the most common cause of secondary hypertension. Present in 2–5% of all secondary hypertensives. It may be said that 50% of all second hypertension are of renal cause.
4. Hypertension in common in all forms of acquired and congenital forms of renal parenchymal disease.

So, control of hypertension is important in preventing progressive renal damage. Thus, it is obvious that some degree of renal damage occurs in hypertension and that hypertension responsible for large portion of renal failure. The kidney is both the victim and the culprit. Clinically, there is often a vicious cycle. There is now strong evidence that the vicious circle can be broken by early and effective antihypertensive treatment particularly diabetic nephropathy and various diseases that cause chronic disease as well.

191. This is usually seen in 4 states.

1. Acute, transient and reversible.
2. Reversible chronic state.
3. Irreversible chronic state.
4. Surgically reversible chronic renal hypertension.

192. Kidney plays a major role in controlling the BP. Maintenance of BP by renal-body fluid system involves the following 4 steps.

1. An increase in arterial pressure causes kidneys to excrete more fluid.
2. Increased fluid loss reduces both extracellular fluid volume and the blood volume.
3. Decrease in blood volume causes decrease in venous return and therefore decreases cardiac output.
4. Reduced cardiac output reduces the arterial pressure back to normal.

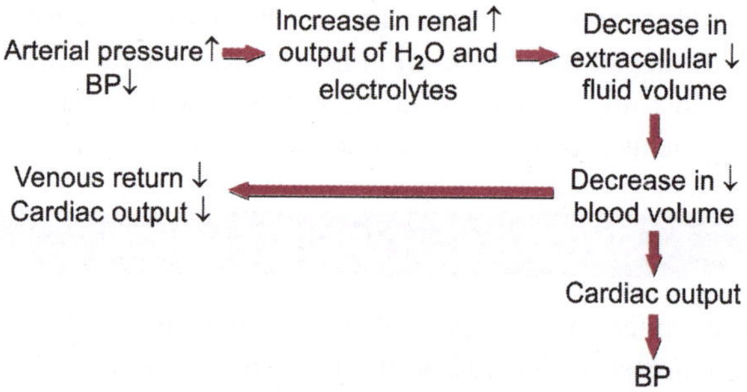

193. Increase in extracellular fluid volume causes the raise in BP in the following way:

1. 2% chronic increase in extracellular fluid volume leads to chronic increase in blood volume.
   ↓
2. Which in turn leads to increase in circulating filling pressure by 5%.
   ↓
3. Which in turn leads to increase in venous return and cardiac output by 5%.
   ↓
4. Which in turn leads to increase in total peripheral vascular resistance by 25–50% leading to raise in BP.

Therefore, chronic increase of few 100 cc of extracellular fluid (ECF) can lead to serious hypertensive effect.

Diuretics reduce the extracellular fluid by about 500 cc per day and reduce the BP.

194. Defect in handling of sodium and water by the kidneys has been suggested as the basis for increase in blood volume (Autoregulation theory).

1. Renal retention of water.
   ↓
2. Increase in extracellular fluid and blood volume.
   ↓
3. Increase in cardiac output.
   ↓
4. Increase in peripheral vascular resistance leading to raise in BP.

Each 1 g of sodium would lead to retention of 200 cc of fluid. Therefore, the restriction of salt in the non-drug treatment of hypertension is emphasized. Sodium retention is the most important factor in the development and maintenance of hypertension in renal disease.

195. The following points are noted:

1. Is there any role of kidney in essential hypertension? Yes

   Aging and hypertension: As the population is aging—The BP is going up. At 60 years age, the kidney has the half the renal function of 25 years age.

2. Can hypertension could be transplanted? Yes
If the kidney donor's both parents are hypertensive, the kidney recipients have more chances of hypertension even though the donor does not have hypertension at the time of donation.
3. Is there any genetic role in renal hypertension? Yes
All genetic causes mostly due to increased sodium retention. Primary increasing in tubular reabsorption sodium was described in animal models.
4. Can decrease in renal blood flow (RBF) cause sustained hypertension? Yes (Gold blott HTN)
Renal artery stenosis is a known cause of curable hypertension.

196. Affects of hypertension on kidney can cause.

1. Acute renal disease.
2. Acute renal failure.
3. Chronic renal disease.
4. Chronic renal failure.

197. Intrarenal hypertension is detrimental to the kidney.

Initially, kidney is causing hypertension, then becoming victim—a viscious cycle develops. Glomerular hypertension plays a major role. Kidney is both a culprit as well as a victim in hypertension.

There are 4 important features in glomerular nephritis.

1. Hypertension is usually associated with varying degrees of renal insufficiency in the form of raised blood urea, serum creatinine and decreased creatinine clearance.
(Azotemia means raised nitrogenous substances in the blood. Blood urea, serum creatinine are raised due to decrease in GFR).
2. Urine shows albumin, RBC (granular) casts, etc.
Microalbuminuria: This is of importance because these indicate impaired function of renal parenchyma, suggesting primary or secondary (in diabetics) renal disease in very early stage. So, quantitative measurement of minute quantities of albumin in the urine is important.
Normal albumin excretion is 30–300 mg/day or 20 to 200 mg/min.
3. Glomerular function is more impaired than tubular renal function.
4. Renal biopsy is needed for the final diagnosis.
In patients with chronic pyelonephritis or polycystic renal disease who are salt wasters do not develop hypertension. The removal of salt and water by diuretics or dialysis is effective in controlling arterial pressure in the majority of patients with renal parenchymal disease.

198. Renovascular hypertension is suspected in:

1. When there is sudden onset of hypertension below 20 years of age or above 50 years age.
2. Easily controllable hypertension becomes suddenly difficult to control.
3. Short duration of severe hypertension.
4. Systolic-diastolic bruit in the upper abdomen or flank.

199. Papilledema in hypertension occurs in:

1. Malignant or accelerated hypertension.
2. Acute glomerulonephritis
3. Eclampsia
4. Hypertensive encephalopathy

(2–4: Transient)

200. When renovascular hypertension is suspected, the following are checked for confirmation:

Renovascular hypertension is important since it is a curable hypertension.

History taking is important.

1. Systole diastolic bruit over the abdomen—it is the important clinical finding in renovascular hypertension.
2. Basal BP is taken.
Captopril (ACE inhibitor) 25 mg tab po is given.
BP is taken again after 1/2 to 1 hour.
If the BP falls to 20 mm Hg systole and diastole suspect renovascular hypertension.
The test can be done by estimating serum creatinine before and 24 hours after giving captopril.
Serum creatinine determines the renal blood flow. If serum creatinine falls after 24 hours suspect bilateral kidney disease or unilateral renal artery thrombosis.
3. Uric acid level unexplained hyperuricemia in essential hypertension is likely to reflect early renovascular involvement. Uric acid levels are correlated indirectly with renovascular disease.
4. Renal angiography.

201. Treatment of renal hypertension consists of:

General measures are as for the essential hypertension. The drugs given should not reduce RBF. Combination is preferable as and when required.

Mild cases:

1. Thiazides or hydrochlorothiazide 25 mg to 50 mg for one week.
In diabetes mellitus, gout—Furosemide is given.
If renal impairment present—Furosemide is given.
If there is no response:
2. Hydralazine is added.
If there is no response to hydralazine, add methyldopa in place of hydralazine.

If there is no response:

Change to β-blockers.

3. In severe cases:

   Diuretic + hydralazine + β-blocker/ Methyldopa.

   The ACE inhibitors and standard triple therapy regimens (Diuretic + Vasodilator + β-blocker) may reduce blood pressure to a similar extent.

4. In resistant cases—add diazoxide, a non-diuretic thiazide.

   Diuretic + Propranolol + Diazoxide.

   Diazoxide 100 to 200 mg qid for 10 to 12 days therapy helps to bring down the BP.

ACEI are more protective in chronic renal disease especially when there is proteinuria.

Increased peripheral vascular resistance may result from activation of RAS secondary to regional ischemia. The hypertension associated with vascular disease such as vasculitis or scleroderma results from ischemia induced activation of RAS. It mimics the clinical findings of acute glomerular nephritis except that the volume expansion and edema that is characteristic of later are absent.

202. ACE inhibitors are now widely used in hypertension with renal disease.

Following points are to be noted while using the ACEI in renal disease.

1. They reduce microproteinuria and macroproteinuria and preserve the renal function.
2. They are useful in hypertension with renal failure associated with other complications such as cardiac failure or diabetes.
3. In patients receiving diuretic therapy, they should be used with caution, because they cause great fall in blood pressure if the patient become dehydrated by diuretic therapy. It should be more guarded when used with potassium sparing diuretics.

   It is dangerous to add potassium supplements to a patient who is already receiving ACEI along with potassium sparing diuretics because of hyperkalemia.
4. ACEI are contraindicated in renal artery stenosis or solitary kidney (after kidney transplantation because they may precipitate renal failure).

203. Guidelines for selecting the antihypertensive drug in hypertension with renal disease.

The drugs that are excreted by the kidney, particularly ACEI and β-blockers are to be given in small doses initially. Calcium blockers are effective and relatively safe. Loop diuretics, e.g. furosemide may be useful especially if there is sodium or water retention. They may have to be given in high doses in edema.

Table B-25

1. ACE inhibitors	Small doses initially, care when used along with diuretic therapy
2. β-blockers	Small doses initially
3. Calcium blockers	Relatively safe in patients with renal failure
4. Loop diuretics	Useful in sodium and water retention

204. There are 4 causes of failure of diuretic therapy:

1. Inadequate dose.
2. Marked reduction in sodium.
3. Very low albumin.
4. Individual susceptibility to diuretics.

205. There are immediate complications during diuretic therapy due to electrolyte disturbance.

1. Hypokalemia
   - Not only by diuretic effect it can also be due to secondary hyperaldosteronism.
   - It may cause even encephalopathy.
   - Diuretics are discontinued.
   - Treat by potassium supplements or add potassium sparing diuretics or aldosterone antagonists.
2. Hyponatremia
   - Diuretic is discontinued.
   - Mannitol, water diuretic or prednisolone is given.
3. Hypochloremic alkalosis.
4. Azotemia.

206. The treatment strategy in hypertensive renal disease consists of the following 4 measures:

1. Restriction of dietary protein intake to less than 0.6 g/kg/day.
   - Avoid potential renal toxicity.
   - Avoid volume depletion, IV contrast agents, aminoglycosides and NSAIDs.
2. Maintenance of BP: Less than 140/90 mm Hg if possible with an ACE inhibitor.

   ACE inhibitors protect the kidneys in patients with diabetes mellitus with or without concomitant hypertension by reducing glomerular capillary pressure and glomerular permeability to protein molecules.
3. Control of blood glucose concentration (less than 7.8 mmol/L).
4. Prevention of hypercholesterolemia—maintain LDL cholesterol less than 3.4 mmol/L).

207. The following 4 guidelines are to be noted for the treatment of end stage renal hypertension.

1. Diet (see diet under non-drug treatment).
2. Dialysis – Peritoneal dialysis

   – Hemodialysis.
3. Drugs – β-blockers, vasodilators.
4. Nephrectomy or kidney transplantation.

HYPERTENSIVE HEART FAILURE

(See Chapter C-Heart Failure)

208. The pathophysiology of hypertensive heart disease is a complex interplay of the following 4 factors:

1. Hemodynamic.
2. Structural.
3. Neuroendocrine.
4. Cellular and molecular.

209. Uncontrolled and prolonged hypertension can lead to the following changes in the heart:

1. Left ventricular hypertrophy (LVH).
2. Coronary artery disease (ischemia or infarction).
3. Conducting disturbances especially atrial fibrillation, Others—ventricular ectopics, ventricular tachycardia.
4. Congestive heart failure.

LVH is defined as an increase in the mass of left ventricle (LV). Concentric LVH is an increase in LV thickness and LV mass with increased LV diastolic pressure and volume, commonly observed in hypertension. While development of LVH has a protective role in response to increased wall stress to maintain adequate cardiac output, later it leads to the development of diastolic dysfunction and ultimately systolic dysfunction.

Left atrial abnormality: Structural and functional changes of left atrium are very common in patients with hypertension. The increased afterload imposed on the left atrium by the elevated LV diastolic pressure secondary to rise in BP leads to increased left atrial size and thickness.

BP ↑ → LVEDP ↑ → ↑ Afterload on LA

↓

↑ LA size and thickness gives rise to structural and functional changes of LA

Increased left atrial size in hypertension in the absence of valvular heart disease or systolic dysfunction usually implies chronicity of hypertension and may correlate with the severity of LV diastolic dysfunction. These LA structural changes predisposes to atrial fibrillation in hypertension. AF in the presence of LV diastolic dysfunction may precipitate overt heart failure.

210. Although valvular disease does not cause hypertensive heart disease, chronic severe hypertension can cause.

1. Aortic root dilatation: Leading to aortic insufficiency.
2. Accelerate the process of aortic scleroses.
3. Dilatation of the annulus causes mitral regurgitation.
4. Tricuspid regurgitation.

211. Left ventricular hypertrophy is related to the increase in cardiovascular mortality.

1. LVH

↓

2. LV diastolic dysfunction → HF.

↓

3. LV failure → Stasis of blood in lungs.

↓

4. RV failure ← Hypertrophy of right ventricle.

Prevalence of LVH by ECG is 2.9% for men and 1.5% for women.

Prevalence of LVH by echocardiography is 15–20%.

Thirty-three of patients without LVH have evidence of asymptomatic LV diastolic dysfunction.

LVH is an independent risk factor that increases the risk of subsequent cardiovascular disease (CVD). Regression of LV H occurs with aggressive BP management including weight loss, sodium restriction and treatment with all classes of antihypertensive drugs except the direct vasodilators hydralazine and minoxidil.

212. Heart failure is a common complication of hypertension. Congestive heart failure is frequently under recognized partly because at the time the heart failure develops, the dysfunctioning of left ventricle is enable to generate the high BP, thus obscuring the etiology of the heart failure. The prevalence of asymptomatic diastolic dysfunction in the patients with hypertension and without LVH may be as high as 33%.

Hypertension causes heart failure in 4 different clinical pathways:

1. Acute left ventricular failure with pulmonary edema.
2. Chronic heart failure in the presence of hypertension.
3. End-stage failure in controlled hypertension.
4. Chronic heart failure in the absence of recognized hypertension.

1. *Acute left ventricular failure with pulmonary edema:* This occurs because the left ventricular output fails against massive peripheral vascular resistance of a narrowed and damaged arteriolar tree. It may be precipitated by increased venous return by simply lying flat while going to sleep in a patient with intercurrent illness or myocardial infarction. If the ischemic or hypertrophied left ventricle pumps only 2 mL less than the right ventricle pumps into the pulmonary artery at each beat, within 2 or 3 minutes extra half liter of blood must accommodate in the lungs resulting in pulmonary edema. Characteristic:
   i. Paroxysmal nocturnal dyspnea.
   ii. Crackles over both bases of lungs.

iii. Pink frothy sputum.
iv. Triple rhythm are present.

Effective treatment with injection morphine, furosemide and others gives satisfactory results. It is dangerous if it is precipitated by myocardial infarction which may not be obvious. The satisfactory result of these cases is deceptive. This should be prevented by good control of hypertension when heart failure is anticipated.

2. *Chronic heart failure in the presence of hypertension:* This develops more gradually with increasing dyspnea, raised jugular venous pressure, crepitations at the lung bases, edema and hepatomegaly. The high BP indicates the reversible cause and needs treatment. Atrial fibrillation is commonly seen and may cause fall in blood pressure, and makes difficulties in measurement of pressure. Atrial fibrillation (paroxysmal, chronic recurrent, or chronic persistent) frequently is observed in patients with hypertension. Hypertension is the most common cause of atrial fibrillation in western hemisphere. In a recent study, nearly 50% of patients with atrial fibrillation had hypertension. Left atrial structural abnormalities, associated with coronary artery disease and left ventricular hypertrophy have been suggested as possible contributing factors. Atrial fibrillation not only can cause decompensation of systolic and more importantly diastolic dysfunction due to loss of atrial click, but it also increases the risk of thromboembolic complications, most notably stroke. Premature ventricular contractions, ventricular arrhythmias, and the risk of sudden cardiac death are observed more commonly in patients with LVH. The etiology of arrhythmias is thought to be due to concomitant CAD and myocardial fibrosis. The presence of left ventricular hypertrophy (LVH) in hypertension is evidence of end organ damage. LVH is an independent risk factor for cardiovascular mortality which is 3 to 4 times higher in those patients with LVH than in those without LVH. Hypertensive patients may develop heart failure as a result of severe hypertension alone or of coronary heart disease. β-blockers and verapamil are contraindicated in hypertension with heart failure and caution should be used with diltiazem. ACE inhibitors with diuretics could bring hypertension under control. ACE inhibitors like captopril, enalapril, lisinopril or ramipril have been proved to prolong life expectancy in heart failure. A similar but less benefit is also seen by using combination of nitrates and hydralazine. However, this combination is not commonly used unless ACE inhibitors are contraindicated or cause side affects.

3. *End-stage heart failure in controlled hypertension:* Elderly patients who have had 20–30 or more years of effective control of severe hypertension ultimately fail if they escape from myocardial infarction or some other intercurrent illness. The problem of stopping treatment at the very old age is different.

4. *Chronic heart failure in the absence of recognized hypertension:* Low output failure due to excessive afterload may reduce pressure in the long run, resulting in failure of tissue perfusion throughout the body. Hypertension is not perceived as a cause if the previous pressure is not known. The diminished tissue perfusion of heart failure increases the risks of most of the recognized complications, particularly stroke, myocardial infarction and fatal pulmonary embolism. Antihypertensives have no place at this stage. It is a commonly seen in elderly women.

HYPERTENSION AND ISCHEMIC HEART DISEASE

213. Angina and myocardial infarction are common in hypertensive patients. Effective control of hypertension improves anginal symptoms regardless of drugs used for angina. However, the antihypertensive drugs of choice are those with antianginal properties.

1. β-blockers.
2. Dihydropyridine CCB—nifedipine.
3. Benzothiazpine—diltiazem is useful in non-Q wave infarction.
4. ACEI useful in MI particularly if there is compromised LV function.

Combination therapy of β-blockers with aspirin has shown definite reduction in reinfarction rates. β-blockers and nifedipine can be combined in angina. Nifedipine should be avoided in post-MI as one study has suggested that nifedipine may increase the risk of reinfarction.

Hypertensive patients on thiazide diuretics admitted with MI should have their serum potassium checked because they may have hypokalemia which may precipitate arrhythmia and sudden death.

In AMI patients admitted with shock, have their BP fallen and hypertension could be masked unless the history is known. Hypertension becomes apparent only after subsequent visits during treatment.

214. Effect of different antihypertensive agents on coronary risk factors.

Table B-26

	Diuretic	β-blockers	CCB	ACEI
BP	+	+	+	+
1. Total/HDL cholesterol	–	–		
2. Left ventricular hypertrophy	+	+	+	+
3. Glucose intolerance	–	–		+
4. Hyperinsulinemia	–	–		+

+ = Positive effect; – = Negative effect

HYPERTENSION AND DYSLIPIDEMIA

215. This combination which is present in about 50% of hypertensives greatly increases CVS risk factors when associated with raised total cholesterol and low HDL levels. The risk is still greater in diabetes patients. Treatment of hyperlipidemia should be with strict diet control, failing diet control , lipid lowering drugs are to be used. The following 4 points should be noted while using drugs in hypertension with hyperlipidemia.

1. Strict diet control failing which lipid lowering drugs.
2. Alpha-blockers have beneficial effects on lipids.
3. ACEI and CCB are lipid neutral.
4. Thiazides and β-blockers have adverse affects on lipids.

HYPERTENSION AND PERIPHERAL VASCULAR DISEASE

216. Peripheral arterial disease (PAD).

1. PAD is equivalent in risk to IHD.
2. Most of the drugs can be used in most PAD patient except β-blockers.
3. Other risk factors should be managed aggressively.
4. Aspirin should be used.

217. There is a strong association between peripheral vascular disease and hypertension. Control of BP is important. The following 4 points are to be noted while treating the patient:

1. β-blockers worsen the symptoms of claudication, therefore should be avoided.
2. There is likelihood of an undiagnosed atheromatous renal artery stenosis.
3. ACEI are to be used only after careful monitoring after excluding renal artery stenosis.
4. Calcium channel blockers are probably the drug of choice because they are relatively safe in this condition and infarct they may improve the symptoms of claudication.

HYPERTENSIVE CRISIS

Hypertensive crisis is defined as severe elevation in BP (SBP > 200 mm Hg, DBP > 120 mm Hg). More than 60 million persons are estimated to have systemic HTN in the united states of whom many are inadequately treated. Approximately 1% of these patients progress to crisis. Patients with secondary causes of hypertension are also at higher risk of hypertensive crisis. Unless it is promptly treated these patients may go into cardiovascular, renal or cerebral organ damage and death. Effective treatment improves the prognosis.

Hypertensive crisis includes hypertensive emergency and urgency. According to JNC, severe hypertension is defined as SBP > 180 mm Hg and DBP >120 mm Hg (Normal 120/80).

Hypertension emergency is defined as severe hypertension with evidence of acute end organ damage and is manifested in a variety of syndromes. Severe hypertension in the presence of chronic organ damage without associated symptoms doesn't constitute an emergency. Hypertension urgency is generally defined as severe hypertension without significant acute end-organ damage.

Pseudoemergencies are acute raise in BP to a physiological trigger (For example, pain, anxiety, postictal state) in response to sympathetic outflow.

218. Some common hypertensive emergencies:

1. Hypertensive encephalopathy.
2. Intracranial hemorrhage includes stroke, subarachnoid hemorrhage, head injury.
3. Eclampsia
4. Acute left ventricular failure with pulmonary edema.
5. Hypertension and myocardial ischemia and infarction. Exception includes LV dysfunction in which low BP may represent an emergency.
6. Immediate postoperative CABG, kidney transplantation.
7. Accelerated malignant hypertension with papilledema (Bilateral retinal hemorrhages and exudates in accelerated hypertension or papilledema in malignant hypertension).

Less common causes:

8. Aortic dissection.

9. Pheochromocytoma crisis.
10. Food or drug interaction with monoamine oxidase inhibitors.
11. Rebound hypertension after sudden drug withdrawal (clonidine).
12. Idiosyncratic reactions, e.g. atropine
In hypertensive emergencies, complications occur over hours to days and hypertensive urgencies over days to weeks.

219. There are 4 hypertensive urgencies.

It includes emergencies without end organ damage.
1. Accelerated or malignant hypertension.
2. Hypertension associated with coronary artery disease.
3. Toxemia of pregnancy.
4. Acute onset of hypertension in children with acute glomerulonephritis.

220. There are 4 rare hypertensive emergencies.

1. Acute aortic dissection.
2. Pheochromocytoma crisis.
3. Monoamine-oxidase inhibitor tyramine interaction.
4. Postoperative hypertension especially after kidney transplantation.

Any form of hypertension can cause hypertensive crisis. The main factor that determines is the level of blood pressure rather than the cause of hypertension.

Sometimes absolute level of blood pressure does not show the seriousness but the associated complications may make even moderate hypertension dangerous as in acute left ventricular failure, acute aortic dissection.

221. Hypertensive emergency vs Urgency

Table B-27

	Hypertensive emergency	*Hypertensive Urgency*
1. End orgon damage	Present	Absent
2. Fundal changes	Grade 3–4	Grade 1–2
3. Medication	IV infusion for first 24 hours	Oral or IV
4. BP reduction	In hours	In hours or days

222. Catecholamine excess giving hypertensive urgency state can occur in:

1. Pheochromocytoma.
2. Clonidine withdrawal.
3. Food or drug interaction with MAO inhibitor.
4. Cocaine ingestion.

223. Factors that aggravate hypertensive crisis are:

1. Discontinuation—withdrawal syndrome. Change over to other systems of medicine.
2. Drugs—steroids, sympathomimetics, amphetamines, LSD, oral contraceptives, diet pills, tricyclic antidepressants, MAO inhibitors, Ergot alkaloids, alcohol abuse.
3. Head injury.
4. Autonomic hyperactivity in Guillain-Barré syndrome, and other spinal card syndromes.

224. Parental drugs for hypertensive crisis.

Table B-28

Drugs	*Route and dose*	*Onset and duration*	*Remarks*
1. Sodium nitroprusside	IV infusion 0.25–8 μg/kg/min	Immediate 1–2 min	Thiocyanate toxicity in high dose infusion prolonged > 48 hours particularly in renal insufficiency Caution with high intracranial pressure or azotemia
2. Diazoxide	IV bolus 50–150 mg every 5 mt or as infusion 7.5–30 mg/min	1–5 min 4–12 hr	Good in cerebrovascular accidents. Should not be used in angina, myocardial infarction, dissecting aneurysm. Now obsolete
3. Nitroglycerin	IV infusion 5–10 μg/min with increments of 5 μg/min until some response Maximum of 10–20 μg/min can be used	2–5 min 3–5 min	Useful in acute myocardial infarction
4. Trimethaphan	IV infusion pump 0.5–5 mg/min	1–5 min 10 min	Drug of choice in aortic dissection
5. Phentolamine	IV 1–5 mg	1–2 min 3–10 min	Useful in pheochromocytoma

Contd...

Contd...

Drugs	Route and dose	Onset and duration	Remarks
6. Hydralazine	IM/IV 10–20 mg every 6 hr	10–20 min 3–8 hrs	Useful in eclampsia
7. Methyldopa	IV 250–1000 mg every 4–6 hr		Tolerance may develop
8. Esmolol	200–500 mg/kg/min for 4 min, then 50–300 mg/min/IVI	1–2 min	Aortic dissection, Postoperative
9. Labetalol	IVI 2 mg/min or 20–80 mg/IV bolus every 10 min	5–10 min	Most hypertensive emergencies except acute heart failure
10. Nicardipine	5–15 mg/hr IV	5–10 min	Most hypertensive emergencies caution with acute heart failure
11. Enalapril	1.25–5 mg IV 6th hrly	15 min	Acute left ventricular failure
12. Fenoldopam			

Sodium nitroprusside: It is the drug of choice in most hypertensive emergencies. It is a potent direct vascular smooth muscle relaxant. It decreases afterload and preload by means of dilating arterioles and increasing venous capacitance.

Thiocyanates levels raise in patients with renal insufficiency and cyanides accumulate in patients with hepatic diseases. Side effects includes muscle spasm, tinnitus and seizures. Thiocyanates toxicity is extremely rare.

Sodium nitroprusside 50 mg is dissolved in a liter of 5% dextrose to give a concentration of 5 μg/mL IV infusion is started delivering 0.5–0.8 μg/kg/min or 0.01–0.16 mL of the solution/kg/minute in IV drip.

Sodium nitroprusside is the drug of choice for the treatment of majority of hypertensive emergencies as it allows controlled reduction of BP but requires continuous intra-arterial monitoring and clinical surveillance. It is dangerous to use without proper facilities for monitoring.

Effective alternatives in less sophisticated settings would be IV bolus administration of diazoxide or labetalol. Diazoxide is not available in India.

However, sodium nitroprusside, diazoxide, trimethaphan, phentolamine are used in institutions where continuous intra-arterial monitoring is possible.

Labetalol, hydralazine, methyldopa IV bolus can be used in family practice or in PHC set-up.

Labetalol is useful in most hypertensive crisis. It is a alpha-blocker and non-selective β-blocker with partial β-2-agonist activity. When given IVI, the relative β-to-alpha-blocking effect of labetalol is 7:1. The main disadvantage is its relatively long duration of action.

Contraindications in acutely decompensated heart failure, cardiogenic shock, bradycardia, heart block (more than first degree) and reactive airway diseases.

Nitroglycerin (see Chapter–F for details): It is the drug of choice in myocardial ischemia, acute MI and congestive heart failure. It is primarily a venodilators and has modest effects on afterload at high doses. The reduction in preload and afterload decreases myocardial oxygen demand. Nitroglycerin also dilates the epicardial coronary arteries, inhibits vasospasm and favorably redistribute blood flow to the endocardium. Nitroglycerin directly increases cerebral blood flow (CBF) raises intracranial pressure (ICP) and is not used in situation initially characterized by high ICP.

Hydralazine (see HTN in pregnancy for details): This is a useful drug in pre-eclampsia and eclampsia. It is a direct vasodilator with no effect on venus capacitance. It crosses the uteroplacental barrier but has minimal affects on the fetus. It decreases systemic vascular resistance (SVR), induces compensatory tachycardia and increases intracranial pressure. It can aggravate angina and is contra-indicated in patients with ongoing coronary ischemia, aortic dissection, or increase ICP.

Nicardipine: It is a dihydropyridine calcium channel blocker. It inhibits vascular smooth muscle contraction but has little or no activity on the heart's AV node or SA node. It is useful in postoperative hypertensive crisis and some neurological conditions. It doesn't raise intracranial pressure and directly reduces cerebral ischemia. It is contraindications in AMI, heart block and renal failure.

Enalapril: It is a short acting IV ACEI. It lowers the BP abruptly. It is not widely used in hypertensive emergencies, as it can precipitate hypertension particularly in volume depleted patients. Enalapril 10 mg bolus followed by 7.5 mg IVI is useful.

Fenoldopam: It is a selective peripheral dopamine-I receptor agonist. It is an arterial vasodilator. It is beneficial in renal insufficiency. It is contraindications in glaucoma. It is a potent systemic vasodilator and is used primarily by anesthetists to control BP intraoperatively.

Methyldopa and *Reserpine* are not recommended for parental use in treating acute crisis as they produce somnolence and drowsiness which interfere with the clinical evaluation of the patients level of consciousness.

225. Drugs in hypertensive emergencies

Table B-29: Drugs useful in various types of hypertensive emergencies

No. Situation	*Drugs useful*	*Drugs Contraindicated*	*Remarks*
1. Acute Myocardial Infarcation	1. BBs 2. CCBs 3. ACEIs 4. NTG 5. Nitroprusside (NP)	Diazoxide (DZ) Hydrallazine (HZ)	BBs are cardioprotective and anti-arrhythmic CCBs are also antiarrhythmic and reduce afterload ACEIs reduce afterload and LV mass NTG increases coronary blood flow
2. Post CABG HT	1. NP 2. NTG	DZ HZ	
3. Cardiac failure	1. ACE Is 2. NTG 3. NP 4. BBs?	BBs?	
4. Aortic dissection	1. NP 2. BBs	DZ HZ NTG	DZ, HZ and NTG cause tachycardia and hence are avoided
5. Hypertensive encephalopathy	1. NP 2. Furosemide 3. BBs	Alpha-methyldopa (MD)	MD and reserpine cause sedation and are hence to be avoided
6. Subarachnoid hemorrhage	1. NP 2. BBs	DZ HZ	BP should be reduced only by 25% in first 24 hr, especially if DBP is above 130 mm Hg
7. Spinal cord syndrome	1. BBs 2. NP 3. Phentolamine		
8. Renal failure	1. BBs 2. HZ 3. Dialysis	NP CCBs	
9. Eclampsia	1. HZ 2. MD 3. Magnesium sulfate	DZ Diuretics Trimethophane	
10. Pheochromocytoma A. Preoperative B. Intraoperative a. For HT b. For arrhythmias c. For hypotension	Alpha-blockers-prazocin 1–2 mg 6 hourly or NP followed by BBs Phentolamine or NP BBs IV fluids 1. Nefidipine SL 2. NP 3. DZ 4. NTG ointment 1. Phentolamine or NP BBs IV Fluids		The antihypertensive treatment should not be abruptly stopped
11. Postoperative	1. Nefidipine SL	DZ	
12. Catecholamine excess (Recreational drugs induced HT	1. BB 2. NP		

BBS: β-blockers; CCBs: Calcium channel blockers; ACEI: Angiotensin-converting enzyme inhibitors; NTG: Nitroglycerin; NP-Nitroprusside; DZ: Diazoxide; HZ: Hydrallazine; MD: Alphamethyldopa

226. IV sodium nitroprusside and IV diazoxide differ in their action in 4 ways in hypertension crisis.

Table B-30

Sodium nitroprusside IV	*Diazoxide IV*
1. Site of action	
Dilates both arterioles and venues	Direct relaxant action on arterioles only
2. Mode of action	
Decreases peripheral vascular resistance with reduction in venous return and cardiac output	Decrease in peripheral vascular resistance is accompanied by reflex tachycardia, increased left ventricular contractility and cardiac output
3. Indications	
In hypertension crisis, associated with left ventricular failure, acute coronary or cerebrovascular insufficiency and pheochromocytoma.	In hypertensive crisis associated with renal or cerebrovascular disease. Used with caution in coronary heart disease. Should not be used in dissecting aneurysm
4.Mode of administration	
Needs continuous IV drip, 50 mg in 500 mL of dextrose (20 mg/min). Action is short lived 1–5 min, needs continuous monitoring of BP	IV bolus 300 mg (5 mg/kg) rapidly/IV infusion Action starts within 1–2 min and lasts for 3–12 hr Can be given intermittently bd or tds

227. Drugs for oral therapy in hypertensive crisis

Table B-31

Drug	*Dose and onset of action*	*Hemodynamics*					*Remarks*
		SVR	*CO*	*GFR*	*CBF*	*HR*	
1. Nifedipine po/sl	10–20 mg 15 min	↓	↑	↑→	↑	↑	Good response short duration S/E, BP ↓ syncope, headache, edema
2. Captopril Po	6.25–12.5 mg	↓	↑→	↑	→	↑→	Unpredictable response, BP ↓ in high renin group
3. Prazosin po/sl	1–2 mg 5–15 min	↓	↑→	↑		↑→	S/E , BP ↓, syncope especially in low renin group. Variable efficacy
4. Clonidine po	1.1–0.2 mg 30 min	↓	↑→	→	↓→	↓	Unpredictable slow onset of action, sedation, dryness of mouth, bradycardia
5. Labetalol po	100–200 mg/po 30–120 min						Well-tolerated
6. Hydralazine po	10–50 mg 20–40 min						Safe in pregnancy
7. Nimodopine po 8th hrly	10–20 mg 15–20 min						Avoid sublingual use as the fall in BP is very rapid
8. Atenolol po/day	50–100 mg 32–60 min						May be an alternative

SVR: Systemic vascular resistance; CO: Cardiac output; GFR: Glomerular filtration rate; CBF: Cerebral blood flow; HR: Heart rate

These drugs are useful in managing hypertension urgencies, when the patient is in less immediate danger, the oral therapy is preferred.

These drugs can be used conveniently in situations in which parental drugs have been used in the past.

The choice of oral versus parental drugs depend on the urgency/emergency of the situation and general condition of the patient. Nifedipine liquid, obtained by biting or swallowing a 10 mg capsule in repeated doses is an easy, safe and rapid way of lowering the blood pressure.

The hypotensive effect is seen in 10 minutes on diastolic blood pressure and 20 minutes on systolic pressure. In cases where the hypotensive urgency is needed due to omission of treatment, a safer course would be to simply restart the old medications and monitor their response closely.

Captopril in doses of 2.5 mg given sublingually usually lowers pressure in about 20–30 minutes.

Maximum effects of captopril, however occurs only 4 hours after administration. Although, oral therapy of captopril is promising, it is difficult in an emergency situation to exclude renal artery stenosis, which could result in a precipitous fall in BP or even serious prolonged renal failure. IV captopril results in smooth BP reduction and the dose required is small with a plasma level of only 15 mg/mL.

Importance of Autoregulation

Understanding of the concept of autoregulation is vital for better management of hypertensive crisis. Blood flow to the most of vital organ like brain, heart, kidney is autoregulated, i.e. blood flow to the organ remain unchanged between a range of mean arterial pressure (MAP) by vasoconstriction at higher MAP and vasodilatation at lower MAP. This autoregulation is last during hypertensive crisis. Hence, perfusion of vital organs will solely depend upon the BP and excessive lowering shall result in hypoperfusion. This concept is well-illustrated in cerebral blood flow which is autoregulated in MAP range of 60–120 mm Hg, in normotensive persons and in the MAP range of 120–160 mm Hg in chronic hypertension. In both normotensive and hypertensive the lower limit of cerebral autoregulation is approximately 25% below the resting MAP. With MAP below the lower limit autoregulation CBF will decrease causing ischemia, with MAP above the upper limit of autoregulation pressure, forced vasodilatation will cause cerebral edema.

BP reduction of hypertensive crisis in acute stroke syndrome, extracranial artery obstruction, history of TIA and elderly are at particular risk of cerebral ischemia. On the other hand, in patients of hypertensive encephalopathy a 25% reduction in MAP is effected over 2–3 hours and patients with acute cerebral infarction or intracranial bleeding, the reduction in MAP should be still slower (over 6–12 hrs) and goal should be to keep DBP 100 mm Hg. MAP should not be lowered below 120 mm Hg, in first 48 hrs. A normal BP shall be achieved gradually over 1–2 weeks especially in intracranial pathologies. Diuretics should be used only during volume overload states.

MAP – ↓ – (CBF) Cerebral blood flow ↓ – Ischemia
MAP – ↑ – → Forced vasodilatation – → Edema.

Principles of Treatment

Aim is to keep a balance between prevention of progressive end organ damage and the risk of significant regional and global hypoperfusion. So, MAP should be reduced by 20–25% over a period of minutes to hours depending on the nature of crisis.

For patients of hypertensive urgency, MAP has to be lowered over 12–24 hours. In patients of LVF, aortic dissection, AMI or unstable angina, the BP should be reduced within 15–30 minuts. The heart can usually tolerate rapid reduction in BP better than brain, even in the presence of coronary atherosclerosis as myocardial oxygen demand is greatly reduced by lowering the BP.

228. The following precautions are to be taken to prevent complications of treatment of hypertensive crisis.

1. Do not introduce oral drugs prematurely.
2. Monitor standing blood pressure in a patient who has been receiving potent antihypertensive agents in supine position.
3. Do not produce acute hypotension and ischemia of the brain causing worsening of the neurological status by overtreating with multiple potent antihypertensive drugs or by lowering the blood pressure rapidly over a period of minutes.

   This complication is avoided by gently reducing the BP over a period of an hour or so and tailoring the drug slowly depending on the patient's condition. In malignant hypertension, the blood pressure should be reduced over a period of few days.

   Drugs with a short duration of action are advantageous.
4. Do not produce complications by nature of therapy.

   Avoid diazoxide in ischemic heart disease.

Avoid centrally acting drugs like clonidine in cerebrovascular accidents or hypertensive encephalopathy because of their sedative effects.

HYPERTENSION IN CHILDREN

Hypertension in infancy and childhood is rare though it is not a recognized concept that roots of essential hypertension starts in childhood. Until a decade back, the hypertension in children were due to secondary hypertension and primary or essential hypertension was thought to be very rare. Because of frequent routine BP readings in children, mild essential hypertension is increasingly diagnosed and is stated to be the most common cause of hypertension in children.

229. Newborn is said to be hypertensive when:

a. Full term
   1. SBP > 90 mm Hg
   2. DBP > 60 mm Hg

b. Preterm
   3. SBP > 80 mm Hg
   4. DBP > 50 mm Hg.

230. Average blood pressure measurement in children by auscultatory method.

Table B-31

Age	Systolic in mm Hg	Diastolic in mm Hg
1. 1–3 months	75 ± 5	50 ± 5
2. 4–12 months	84 ± 5	65 ± 5
3. 1–8 years	95 ± 5	65 ± 5
4. 9–14 years	105 ± 5	65 ± 5

231. Hypertension by age group.

Table B-32

Age group	Blood pressure
1. 1 week–1 month	112/74 mm Hg
2. 3–5 years	116/76 mm Hg
3. 6–9 years	122/78 mm Hg
4. 10–15 years	126–136/82–86 mm Hg

Heavier and /or taller children have higher BP than smaller children of same age (Lauer et al 1984). The correlation of higher BP range associated with height and weight has been important particularly in children of high normal BP. (Borderline or 90–95th percentile. These values being considered normal if the child is taller or obese)

232. Proper cuff size should be used. Narrow cuff gives false high readings.

Appropriate cuff sizes for different age groups are:

1. Infants—2.5 cm
2. 1 month–1 year—5 cm
3. 1–8 years—9 cm
4. Older children—12.5 cm

233. There are 4 methods of measurement of blood pressure in children:

1. Auscultatory method as in adults.
   Blood pressure measurement in infants.
2. *Flush method:* Cuff is applied as usual. Part of the limb distal to the cuff is compressed by elastic crepe bandage. The cuff is inflated. As the pulse is occluded, the pressure bandage is removed and cuff deflated. Return of flush in the limb indicates mean pressure.
3. *Oscillometry:* An oscillometer is applied to record oscillations of brachial artery which increases rapidly at systolic pressure and decreases suddenly at diastolic pressure.
4. *Doppler method:* An electronic transducer is used instead of oscillometer. When systolic pressure is reached, movements of the arterial wall cause a Doppler effect (change in frequency of reflected wave). This is transformer into sounds. Recordings are similar to auscultatory method.

234. Causes of secondary hypertension in children can be described in 4 groups according to age:

Table B-33

1. Newborn—infancy	Renal artery thrombosis Renal artery stenosis Congenital renal malformation Coarctation of aorta Bronchopulmonary dysplasia
2. Infancy—6 years	Renal parenchymal diseases Acute glomerulonephritis Acute pyelonephritis Polycystic disease Renal artery stenosis Coarotation of aorta
3. 6–10 years	Renal artery stenosis Renal parenchymal disease Aorta-arteritis Essential hypertension
4. Adolescence	Essential hypertension Renal parenchymal disease

235. Medical management of hypertension in children.

Drug therapy of hypertension has always been a challenging task. The causes are variable, consisting of renal disorders (75%) and renovascular disorders (12%) accounting nearly 80–90% of cases.

Following steps are to be observed when managing hypertension in children.

1. Appropriate tests are done to find out the primary cause responsible so that specific treatment can be given immediately.
2. After arrival at a specific diagnosis, the basic consideration will be whether the hypertension is 'curable' or not 'curable'.
3. Rise factors are considered before starting drug therapy Family history, obesity, dietary habits, lack of exercise, stress factors, and smoking, etc.
4. Non-drug measures like weight reduction, exercise, dietary changes are given a good trial for nearly 3 to 6 months.
5. The therapeutic options are chosen on the individual merits of a particular case. Appropriate drugs should be selected and given in cautious manner, starting in small doses from minimum therapeutic dose to maximum tolerated dose to avoid side effects.
6. Treatment of complications.
7. Treatment of hypertensive crisis.

8 Consider if there is any surgical conditions of secondary hypertension. Surgical correction though superior to medical treatment has considerable morbidity and mortality. The introduction of percutaneous transluminal renal angioplasty (PTRA) by Gruntzig, et al in 1978, balloon angioplasty techniques have revolutionized the treatment of secondary hypertension. Percutaneous transluminal angioplasty (PTA) has been used for correction of hemodynamically significant renal artery stenosis, aorto-arteritis and coarctation of aorta.

236. Management of hypertensive encephalopathy in children.

1. If child convulsing: Give IV anticonvulsants.
2. For BP: IV labetalol infusion at 1 mg/kg/hr. If adequate response, infusion may be stopped.
   If no response over 30 minutes:
3. Rate may be increased
   1 mg/kg/hr. Maximum of 3 mg/hr
   Hypertensive response up to 6 hours.
   or
4. IV sodium nitroprusside starting dose 0.5 µg/kg/min maximum being 8.0 mg/kg/min

237. Parentral drug therapy of hypertensive crisis in children.

Table B-34

	Drug of choice	Alternate	Avoid
1. Encephalopathy	NP, LB, DZ	HZ	MD
2. Acute heart failure	NP, HZ	DZ	LB
3. Acute renal failure	LB, HZ, DZ	–	NP
4. Subarachnoid hemorrhage	NP, LB	–	DZ, HZ

NP: Nitroprusside; HZ: Hydralazine; LB: Labetalol; MD: Methyldopa; DZ: Diazoxide

238. JNC algorithm for treatment of hypertension.

1. Lifestyle modification

Not at goal BP (< 140/90 mm Hg)
(< 130/80 mm Hg, for those with diabetes or chronic disease)

2. Initial drug of choice

Without compelling indication

Stage I hypertension
(SBP 140–159 or DBP 90–99 mm Hg)
May consider ACEI, ARB, BB, CCB or combination

Stage II hypertension
(SBP > 160 or DBP ≥ 100 mm Hg)
2 drug combination for most usually thiazide type diuretic and ACEI or ARB or BB, CCB

3. With compelling indications

Drugs for the compelling indications.
Other antihypertensive drugs (diuretic ACEI, ARB, BB, CCB) as needed.

4. Not at goal blood pressure

Optimize dosages or additional drugs until goal at BP is achieved
Consider consultation with hypertension specialist

Hypertension associated with toxicemia of pregnancy is obviously omitted in this categories and separately dealt in the Chapter V on pregnancy and cardiovascular disease.

SURGICAL MANAGEMENT OF HYPERTENSION

More than 80% of patients have primary or essential hypertension. A small number of patients suffer from secondary or correctable hypertension. These patients require detailed investigations to pin point the cause of hypertension.

Pathophysiology

Goldblatt (1934) established that reduction in renal blood flow (RBF) in experimental animals could cause reversible hypertension. It is now known that stenosis of renal artery may be responsible in some cases. The patient may develop renovascular hypertension whenever there is reduction in the blood flow to the kidney. It is characterized by elevation of SBP and DBP.

239. Some commonly encountered conditions which are amenable to surgical treatment are:

1. Renovascular hypertension.
2. Unilateral renal parenchymal disease.
3. Obstructive urinary lesions.
4. Pheochromocytoma.
5. Cushing's syndrome.
6. Primary aldosteronism.
7. Coarctation of aorta.
8. PDA (systolic only).

240. Secondary hypertension is suspected when:

1. Hypertension in a child or an young adult.
2. Rapid onset of hypertension in a patient over 50 years of age.
3. Symptomatic, moderate hypertension of short duration not responding adequately to medical treatment.
4. Easily correctable hypertension suddenly becomes difficult to control.
5. Hypertension developing after acute flank pain.
6. Bruit over the renal angle or epigastrium.
7. Angiosplastic changes in the fundus.
8. Clinical presentation suggest the possibility of a disease like.

Pheochromocytoma

Cushing's disease or Crohn's syndrome.

If the hypertension has been present for some duration the removal of the cause does not always lead to complete reversal of hypertension. Mild hypertension requiring some treatment does persist in some cases.

241. Etiology of renal artery occlusive disease:

1. Atherosclerosis—80%.
2. Fibrodysplasia—15–18%.
3. Aneurysm, embolus, dissections.
4. Trauma.

242. Specific investigations.

(Routine investigations such as urine, FBC, BUN, creatinine, electrolytes, etc. are to be done).

1. *Ultrasound examination:* It can pick up suprarenal tumors—pheochromocytoma. It may not pick up if the tumor is less than 1 cm size.
2. *CAT scan:* It can pick up normally located as well as ectopic tumors fairly accurately. CAT scan is now being replacing angiogram.
3. *Intravenous pyelogram (IVP):* This is one of the early investigations done when a surgical condition is suspected. This is not a specific investigation. Following findings indicate the involved side.
   - Delayed visualization of the involved kidney
   - Reduction in the size of one kidney
   - Notching of the ureter.
4. *Renin assay:* It tells the involved side and severity of the lesion. Serum renin assay tells the presence of renovascular hypertension but does not tell the side involved. Selective renal vein sampling gives more specific information. Renin volume 1.5 times higher on one side is generally considered specific of the involvement of the side.
5. *Epinephrine and norepinephrine estimations in blood and urine:* These are fairly accurate and indicate the existence of adrenal tumor. A higher nor-epinephrine level indicates the possibility of an ectopically located tumor.
6. *Estimation of urinary vanyl mandelic acid (VMA):* Epinephrine and norepinephrine are metabolized to vanyl mandelic acid (VMA) which is excreted through the urine. This is also a diagnostic test of high accuracy. A 24 hour urine specimen is collected for VMA estimation. High levels are found particularly after an episode of hypertension.
7. Estimation of plasma cortisol levels (elevated in Cushing's syndrome).
8. Urinary ketosteroid estimation.
9. Serum aldosterone (elevated in primary aldosteronism).
10. Digital subtraction angiography (DSA).
    This is relatively a newer technique. It is replacing the conventional arteriography. The accuracy is of 95% or more.
11. Arteriography
    Renal arteriography: It is a specific investigation and gives the anatomical diagnosis. Generally fibromuscular dysplasia involves the distal two-thirds of the artery. Right side is more frequently involved than the left side. Arteriosclerotic lesions involve the proximal one-third of the artery more often seen as localized areas of the narrowing of the artery.
    Aortography in coarctation of aorta.
12. *Renal biopsy:* It helps in preoperative assessment of the outcome of revascularization surgery.
    Stimulation and suppression tests have now largely been abandoned.
    Homard test and Stamey test have been devised for differential renal function.

243. The hypertension is adequately controlled by medical treatment before doing surgery. The patient is prone to have higher morbidity and mortality if the hypertension is not adequately controlled before surgery.

The surgical procedure depends on the specific lesion. The following surgical procedure are employed in renovascular hypertension:

1. Resection and anastamosis of a segment of the renal artery or endarterectomy.
2. Bypass grafting: Bypass is done between the aorta and the segment of the renal artery beyond the strictured segment. Long saphenous vein graft or prosthesis can be used for bypass grafting.
3. Percutaneous transluminal angioplasty (PTA): It is known as balloon angioplasty. The first PTA was done by Gruntzig in 1978. It carries less risk as compared to open surgery. With increasing technique and experience, the PTA is likely to replace surgery in renovascular hypertension when the cause is non-

ostial atherosclerosis or fibromuscular dysplasia with the diseased segment limited to the main artery or its immediate branches.
4. Nephrectomy.

244. Surgical treatment of pheochromocytoma.

The following precautions are to be taken:
1. Preoperative adequate control of hypertension .
2. Phenoxybenzamine along with β-blockers is used to control the hypertension.
3. Continuous monitoring of the heart and blood pressure is necessary during surgery because handling of the tumor releases catecholamines in the blood which can suddenly rise the blood pressure.
4. There can be sudden fall of blood pressure after the removal of the tumor which needs to be sustained by IV fluids and/or blood or drugs.

245. Some points about surgery for pheochromocytoma.

1. A 'Buckle-handle' incision is used in the epigastrium for adequate exposure. This allows access to palpate the opposite side for any missed lesion. It may be bilateral in small percentage of cases.
2. Always search should be made for any ectopic tumor after finding the tumor at the expected site.
3. Very gentle handling of the tumor is essential while removing the tumor and all the assistants should be refrained from feeling the tumor to satisfy their curiosity until the tumor is safely out of the body.
4. Surgery is curative and results are very encouraging.

Cushing Syndrome

Occurs most commonly in females in 3rd and 4th decade and due to excessive plasma cortisol secreted by the adrenal gland. Hypertension is a constant feature. The patient has a buffalo hump, moon face, abdominal striae, hirsutism, central obesity. In children, Cushing syndrome is usually due to malignant lesion of the adrenal gland. Occasionally, it may present in adult female with amenorrhea.

246. Surgical treatment consists of:

1. Removal of the adrenal gland.
2. Partial or subtotal adrenelectomy if the cause is hyperplasia.
3. Total or subtotal adrenalectomy if there is adrenal tumor.
4. Total adrenalectomy for carcinoma.

There is prompt regression of typical clinical look after surgery. However, hypertension may not regress to normal immediately and the menstrual cycle in a female may take a few months to restore normal.

Primary Aldosteronism or Conn's Syndrome

This is caused by adrenal adenoma which releases excessive aldosterone producing variety of symptoms like muscular weakness, polydipsia, polyuria, transient episodes of paralysis and hypertension. The disease is more common in females and is seen in the 4th or 5th decade. Serum aldosterone levels are elevated. There is low serum potassium level, and some elevation of serum sodium and mild degree of alkalosis. In addition, serum renin levels are low.

Surgical treatment consists of subtotal adrenalectomy for an adenoma and total adrenalectomy for carcinoma.

Coarctation of aorta (See Coarctation of Aorta)

Aortogram

Surgically correctable hypertension can be detected if the clinician has a high suspicion index. Family physician or the first clinician plays the vital role by suspecting the surgically correctable hypertension. A successful outcome is most likely in a large proportion of cases with a surgical cause of hypertension. Surgical hypertension shortens the life span but if diagnosed early and adequately corrected, the patient can have more or less a normal life span.

REFRACTORY HYPERTENSION

247. Hypertension can be considered refractory if blood pressure cannot be brought down to 150/100 mm Hg by a rational triple drug combination including a diuretic, prescribing maximal doses. If the pretreatment blood pressure was above 180–200/150–120 mm Hg, a minimal regimen of drugs for at least 4 weeks though not 6 weeks should be tried before labeling hypertension as refractory as follows.

1. *Oral diuretics:* Equivalent to 50 mg of hydrochlorothiazide, chlorthalidone, furosemide, bumetanide, ethacrinic acid or amiloride, etc.
2. *Adrenergic inhibiting drugs (sympathetic inhibitors):* β-blockers equivalent to propronolol 320 mg, atenolol 100 mg, metoprolol 50 to 100 mg methyldopa 2 g, etc.
3. *Vasodilators:* Hydralazine 300 mg.
   Calcium blockers: Diltiazem 120 mg tds, nifedipine 20 mg 6th hourly, nitrendipine 20 mg, felodipine 10 mg, amlodipine 10 mg.
4. *ACE inhibitors:* Captopril 100 mg tds, enalapril 40 mg, lisinopril 40 mg ramipril.

248. Following are the reasons for hypertension to be refractory:

Blood pressure remaining above goal in spite of concurrent use of 3 antihypertensive agents of different classes.

Ideally one of the three agents should be a diuretic and all agents should be prescribed at optimal dose amounts.

1. Poor compliance by the patient.
   a. Inconvenient dosage, e.g. tid or 6th hourly.
   b. Financial constraints: Many patients in India are unable to buy the drugs regularly.
   c. Adverse affects of drugs by which the patient feels reluctant to take the drugs.
   d. Drop out of patients from treatment and suppression.
2. Related to drugs.
   a. Inappropriate drug selection or drug combination
   b. Interactions with drugs.

NSAIDs nullifies antihypertensive effects by salt retention.
Hormone replacement therapy (HRT) at menopause nullifies antihypertensive effects.
Nasal decongestants/'cold' medicines.
Liquor ingestion (tobacco chewing).
Cocaine, erythropoietin, etc.

Stimulants	*Analgesics*
Methylphenidate	NSAIDs, aspirin, cox-2 inhibitor
Dexmethylphenidate	Sympathomimetic agents
Dextroamphetamine	Decongestants
Amphetamine, methamphetamine	Diet pills
Modanafil	Cocaine

Substance that can interfere with BP control.
- Alcohol
- Oral contraceptives
- Cyclosporin
- Erythropoietin
- Natural liquorice
- Herbal.

3. Volume overload
   a. Increased sodium intake
   b. Renal failure
   c. Diuretic requirement.
4. Weight gain.
5. Alcohol intake > 2 ounces per day.
6. Renovascular hypertension and other causes of secondary hypertension.
7. White coat hypertension: Only when doctor measures BP.
8. Pseudohypertension: Faults in measurement.

249. The drugs that are used may loose their efficiency. The manner by which non diuretic antihypertensive agents may loose their effectiveness by renal sodium retention.

Non-diuretic antihypertensive agent
↓
↓ Blood pressure ↑ Blood pressure
↓ ↑
1. Renal sodium retention → Increased fluid volume
↑
2. Aldosterone
↑
3. Renin secretion
↑
4. Vasodilator

250. Management of refractory hypertension

Fortunately, these cases are rare. What is to be done for the persistent severe hypertension of 200/120 mm Hg despite a thorough trial of treatment with all the usual drugs including triple drug combination. Always review the case:

1. Check whether the patient is taking drugs regularly. This is a common fault on the patient for hypertension to be refractory. When once the doctor tells the patient that his blood pressure has come to normal, the patient discontinue treatment by himself. He comes again after weeks or months only when he develops symptoms and feels uneasy saying that his hypertension has recurred. It is not recurrent hypertension but it is the failure on the part of the patient to continue treatment after significant and sustained reduction of blood pressure. Lack of suppression and maintenance therapy are responsible for most treatment failure.
2. Check whether the patient is using potentially incompatible drugs. These are mainly with asthmatics—who needs change from β-blockers.
   Depressive illness: Depression is a common symptom in all hypertensives and with all antihypertensive drugs. Cause and effect is very difficult to prove, and there is little reliable evidence on which to base clinical decision. All centrally acting antihypertensive drugs particularly those which delete or obstruct catecholamines and serotonin mainly methyldopa, reserpine, and clonidine are liable to cause depression. Some sort of symptoms are described—as depression with reserpine, tiredness with methyldopa, and weakness with propronolol. Depression is a common and an important symptom which should be actively sought in all hypertensive patients under treatment throughout follow-up.
   Women on oral contraceptive pill: The advent of contraceptive pill has not been an unmixed blessing. There is rise in venereal diseases and promiscuity. Sodium retention causing rise in blood pressure and the risk of

thromboembolic episodes are the two serious side effects. The introduction of low estrogen pill has reduced these side effects. The patient with hypertension should stop the oral pill. She needs barrier methods or sterilization for contraception. An effective male contraceptive pill is not yet emerged and the trials are still underway. Some patients may be using cough syrup regularly or using nasal decongestant drops which contain ephedrine. Some may be using tobacco in a different form as snuff powder regularly. Some patients may be using cortisone's regularly for some of the complaints.

3. Check whether the patient is suffering from intractable background of stress. Mechanisms here are complex and doubtful. Many probably overlap and the patient may not take drugs regularly. Good liaison with open and friendly relationship can sort out many problems.
4. Check whether the patient is intolerant to most drugs. It is particularly important to change the drugs and drug combinations in these patients. Change one drug at a time. Allow sufficient time for assessment before changing or adding. Select successive drugs from different pharmacological groups rather than variant brands of the same group.
5. Check whether the patient is resistant to the drugs normally used. These are the hard core and most difficult to treat. It is surprising that the refractory patients are unknown to pharmaceutical manufacturers.
6. Check whether the patient has controlled other risk factors—mainly smoking, obesity salt restriction, stoppage of smoking, reduction in obesity can be of definite help to control the hypertension.
7. Check whether the associated disease are given proper treatment—like diabetes mellitus, chronic renal failure, etc.
8. Finally review again—Check whether the patient is suffering from any secondary hypertension—who has a treatable cause.

Drug treatment in hypertension outcome studies: Over the past 35 years studies the drug treatment of hypertension demonstrated that reduction of blood pressure is associated with reduction of cardiovascular morbidity and mortality.

The second Australian National Blood Pressure Study

It is based on to study the newer drugs compared to the older drugs. The subject of study are the patients aged 65–84 years. The study is to determine whether there is any difference in total cardiovascular events, (fatal and non-fatal) over a 5-years treatment period between antihypertensive treatment with an ACE inhibitor based regimen and treatment with a diuretic-based regimen.

To study—cost/benefit analysis, quality of life analysis, impact of left ventricular hypertrophy, genetic involvement (association of ACE gene and the angiotensinogen gene to cardiovascular outcome), ambulatory blood pressure monitoring, etc.

GP/Family Medicine Specialist Involvement

This study is being undertaken in general practice because this is where the majority of hypertensive patients are seen and managed. Indeed, because of the number of patients required to give statistically significant results, it is the only place for research of this nature can take place.

(For Pregnancy and Hypertension—see Chapter on CVD in Pregnancy)

C Heart Failure

Heart failure is defined as inability of the heart to maintain sufficient output necessary for adequate oxygenation of tissues at rest or during stress. Every cardiac patient has a potential for developing heart failure.

Heart failure is not a diagnosis. It is a manifestation of an underlying anatomical or pathological cause affecting the heart.

1. This complex clinical syndrome is characterized by 4 components:

1. Impaired myocardial performance
2. Progressive activation of neuroendocrine system leading to
3. Circulatory insufficiency and
4. Congestion.

The major pathophysiologic process in the progression of heart failure appears to be cardiac remodeling often referred as progressive chamber enlargement resulting in obligatory reduction of ejection fraction.

2. Epidemiology of heart failure:

1. About 4.7 millions (NHANES III data) of heart failure patients are in United States and once HF develops, 6 year mortality approaches 80% in men and 65% in women.

   With continued raise in population, improved survival of patients with acute myocardial infarction and reduced mortality from other diseases (stroke), the incidence of heart failure continue to increase. The lifetime risk of developing heart failure is about 20%.
2. The death rate attributed to HF in USA rose by 64% from 1970 to 1990 while death rate from coronary artery disease dropped by 40% during the same period. As the population ages, the incidence of HF and its mortality rate will continue to increase.
3. Heart failure mortality is about twice as high for African Americans as Whites for all age groups.
4. People age 65 and older represent the fastest growing segment of the population and the rise of HF increases with age. The condition affects 1% of people age 50 years but about 5% of people age 75 years.

3. Heart failure can be clinically classified into 4 groups.

Table C-1

I. High output failure	*v/s*	*Low output failure*
The heart maintains normal or above normal output but this is not sufficient for adequate oxygenation of tissues		i. Intrinsic muscle disease, e.g. acute myocardial infarction, ischemic heart disease, restricted cardiomyopathy ii. Excessive after load, e.g. aortic stenosis, hypertension iii. Restriction of filling, e.g. constrictive pericarditis hypovolemia iv. Decreased heart rate, e.g. heart block
A. Due to decrease in systemic resistance i. Anemia—myocardial anoxia ii. Pregnancy iii. Thyrotoxicosis		

Contd...

Contd...

iv. Fever—impairs myocardial metabolism. Generalized systemic vasodilatation due to stimulatory effect on metabolism v. Beriberi—profound vasodilatation—impaired myocardial metabolism vi. Atrial or ventricular septal defect vii. AV fistula—blood is shunted directly from arteries to the veins. Occasionally in Paget's disease		
B. Due to increase in systemic filling pressure i. Too rapid and too much transfusion of IV fluids ii. Excess secretion of steroids—especially aldosterone resulting in salt and water retention in renal failure. Symptoms of right ventricular failure predominate at first later followed by left ventricular failure		
II. Acute failure	*v/s*	*Chronic failure*
Large myocardial infarction, High degree A–V block with a very slow ventricular rate (< 35/min) or Tachyarrhythmia with a very rapid ventricular rate (> 180/min) Pericardial tamponade pulmonary embolus with large pulmonary infarction can cause acute valvular catastrophe		Multiple valvular disease, slow progressive dilated cardiomyopathy (DCM). Slow progressive edema occurs with normal BP
i. Acute pulmonary edema ii. Cardiogenic shock iii. Acute decompensation of chronic left HF hypotension with or without peripheral edema. Symptoms are due to inadequate organ perfusion and/or acute congestion of venous bed behind the ventricles iv. Acute valvular catastrophy, malignant hypertension, hypertensive crisis, acute myocarditis. Cardiac tamponade, toxins (alcohol, nonsteroidal anti-inflammatory agents), infection, sodium and dietary indiscretion, medications, non-compliance result in acute failure. It can be clinically grouped into v. Acute decompensation usually refers to episodes of acute or subacute worsening of clinical features due to a wide range of precipitants, the most common causes are dietary indiscretion (especially over usage of salt), medical noncompliance, and arrhythmias (commonly atrial fibrillation)		
III. Right heart failure	*v/s*	*Left heart failure*
This is caused by elevated venous pressure and decreased cardiac output independent of abnormal LV contractility		Clinical features of pulmonary edema dominates. Dyspnea, orthopnea, wheeze, cough, hemoptysis occur as a result of pulmonary congestion, e.g. aortic stenosis due to mechanical overload, myocardial infarction blood accumulates in the lungs in heart failure
JVP is raised, congestive hepatomegaly, systemic venous congestion, edema occur, e.g. pulmonary stenosis pulmonary hypertension, pulmonary embolism tricuspid regurgitation blood accumulates in the great veins in right heart failure Lung causes: Emphysema, asthma, COPD, fibrosis, collapse of lung, pulmonary infarction		
IV. Backward failure	*v/s*	*Forward failure*
e.g. Pulmonary hypertension ↓ Right ventricular end-diastolic pressure (RVEDP) ↑ ↓		e.g. AMI, AS, systemic hypertension of long duration ↓

Contd...

Contd...

Pressure and volume in right atrium and venous system behind the ventricle ↑ ↓ Retention of sodium and water ↓ Systemic venous and capillary pressures ↑ ↓ Transudation of fluid into interstitial spaces ↓ Edema ↓ Angiotensin—Aldosterone mechanism ↓ Fluid retention occurs because the failing ventricle is unable to pump all the blood presented to it, i.e. blood is dammed back behind the failing ventricle ↓ The concept of backward failure was propounded by James Hope in 1832	Cardiac output ↓ ↓ Inadequate discharge of blood into the arterial system ↓ Diminished renal perfusion ↓ Proximal tubular sodium reabsorption ↓ Distal tubular reabsorption ↓ Sodium and water retention by renin ↓ Edema Low cardiac output causes poor perfusion of kidneys that increases retention of sodium and fluid ↓ The concept of forward failure was propounded by Meckenzie in 1913

Heart failure can also be described as unilateral versus bilateral cardiac failure, systolic versus diastolic failure.

Systolic heart failure: This occurs when the heart's ability to contract decreases. The heart cannot pump with enough force to push a sufficient amount of blood into the circulation. Blood coming into the heart from the lungs may back up and cause fluid to leak into the lungs resulting in pulmonary congestion.

Systolic heart failure and diastolic heart failure is somewhat arbitrary and can vary with different imaging modalities. Systolic heart failure is measured by ejection fraction (EF). However, there may not be exact correlation between the symptoms and the degree of cardiac dysfunction, e.g. a patient with markedly reduced EF may have minimal symptoms and can respond favorably to medical treatment.

Diastolic heart failure: This occurs when the heart has a problem of relaxing. The heart cannot properly fill with blood because the muscle has become stiff, loosing its ability to relax. This leads to fluid accumulation, especially in the feet, ankles and legs. Some may have lung congestion.

Congestive heart failure (CHF) is a term that is usually used to mean both left and right heart failure. It is used to describe all patients with heart failure. In reality, congestion (build up of fluid) is just one feature of the condition and does not occur in all patients.

The term congestive heart failure is over used to describe heart failure, as all the patients with heart failure do not have signs and symptoms of congestion. The major pathophysiologic process of heart failure appears to be cardiac remodelling often referred to as progressive chamber enlargement and obligatory reduction of ejection fraction.

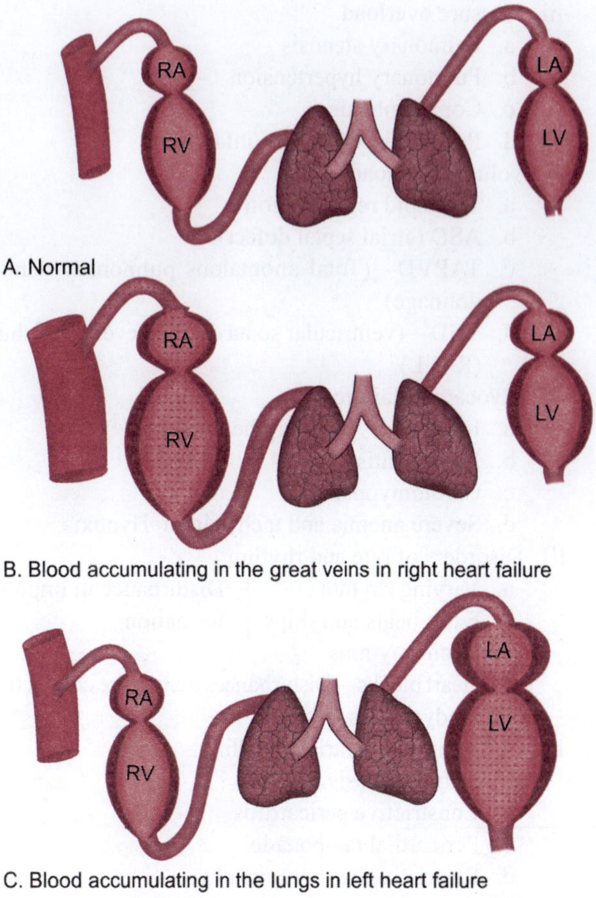

Fig. C-1: Fluid retention in cardiac failure

4. Causes of the heart failure can be classified under 4 headings:

I. Mechanical overload
LVF
i. Pressure over load
   a. Hypertension
   b. Aortic stenosis
   c. Coarctation
   d. Hypertrophic obstructive cardiomyopathy (HOCM)
ii. Volume overload
   a. Aortic regurgitation
   b. Mitral regurgitation
   c. VSD or PDA
   d. AV fistula or anemia
   e. Excess transfusion
   f. Sodium retention drugs (Phenylbutazone, carbonoxalone, corticosteroids)
   g. Primary aldosteronism
   h. Secondary aldosteronism
RVF
iii. Pressure overload
   a. Pulmonary stenosis
   b. Pulmonary hypertension
   c. Cor pulmonale
   d. Pulmonary embolism/infarction
iv. Volume overload
   a. Tricuspid regurgitation
   b. ASD (atrial septal defect)
   c. TAPVD—(Total anomalous pulmonary venous drainage)
   d. VSD—(ventricular septa defect) reversal of shunt (R→ L)

II. Myocardial failure:
   a. Infarction—coronary heart disease
   b. Myocarditis
   c. Cardiomyopathy
   d. Severe anemia and tachycardia–Hypoxia

III. Disorders of rate and rhythm
   a. Varying rhythm } Disturbance in impulse formation
   b. Extra beats and skips } Disturbance in impulse formation
   c. Rapid rhythms
   d. Heart blocks—Disturbances of impulse conduction, bradycardias.

IV. Restriction of ventricular filling:
   a. Mitral stenosis
   b. Constrictive pericarditis
   c. Pericardial tamponade
   d. Restrictive cardiomyopathy

In the pediatric population the leading causes of heart failure are significantly different from those in adults. Therefore, therapeutic guidelines in the pediatric group are directed more to specific causes of heart failure. (See Chapter L—Congenital Heart Diseases 220 to 243.) The guidelines for adult's heart failure are associated with ventricular dysfunction with major focus on systolic dysfunction.

5. Causes of heart failure WHO criteria, 1996.

I. Dilated cardiomyopathy (idiopathic), hypertrophic cardiomyopathy, restrictive cardiomyopathy, arrhythmogenic right ventricular cardiomyopathy, unclassified cardiomyopathies, fibroelastosis, systolic dysfunction without dilatation, mitochondrial cardiomyopathy.

II. Specific cardiomyopathies, ischemic valvular obstruction or insufficiency, hypertensive inflammatory (lymphocytic, eosinophilic, giant cell myocarditis) infections (Chagas disease, HIV, enterovirus, CMV, bacterial or fungal infection).

III. Metabolic endocrine (thyroid diseases, adrenal insufficiency, pheochromocytoma, acromegaly, diabetes mellitus) familial storage disease (hemochromatoses, glycogen storage disease, Hurler's syndrome, Fabry's -Anderson disease), electrolyte deficiency syndrome (hypokalemia, hypomagnesemia), nutritional disorders (kwashiorkor, anemia, beriberi selenium), amyloid familial mediterranean fever.

IV. General systemic diseases, connective tissue disorders (SLE, polyarteritis nodosa, rheumatoid arthritis, scleroderma, dermatomyositis, polymyositis, sarcoidosis), muscular dystrophies (Duchenne's, Becker's myotonic), neuromuscular (Friedreich's ataxia, Noonan's disease), toxins (alcohol catecholamine, cocaine, anthracyclines and other chemotherapeutics, irradiation), peripartum cardiomyopathy.

6. Heart failure is classified into 4 stages by the American College of Cardiology and American Heart Association:

1. *Stage A:* Patients at high risk for developing heart failure with no structural heart disease.
2. *Stage B:* Patients with structural heart disease who have not yet developed symptoms of heart failure.
3. *Stage C:* Patients with past or current symptoms of heart failure associated with underlying structural heart disease.
4. *Stage D:* Patients with end-stage heart failure who require specialized advanced treatment.

Heart failure staging can go only in one direction, that is, once symptoms occur, patients will be considered at "stage C" even if their symptoms may resolve.

7. New York Heart Association functional classification:

Class I: Patients have cardiac disease but without resulting limitations of physical activity. Ordinary physical activity does not cause undue fatigue, palpitations, dyspnea or anginal pain.

Class II: Patients have cardiac disease resulting in slight limitation of physical activity. They are comfortable at rest. Ordinary physical activity results in fatigue, palpitation, dyspnea, or anginal pain.

Class III: Patients have cardiac disease resulting in marked limitation of physical activity. They are comfortable at rest. Less than ordinary physical activity causes fatigue, palpitations, dyspnea, or anginal pain.

Class IV: Patients have cardiac disease resulting in an inability to carry on physical activity without discomfort. Symptoms of cardiac insufficiency or of the anginal syndrome may be present even at rest. If any physical activity is undertaken, discomfort is increased.

Some patients may have cardiac dysfunction (e.g. low EF) without any symptoms who are referred to having asymptomatic heart failure or asymptomatic LV dysfunction. Some other may have preserved LV systolic function but, demonstrate typical signs of heart failure, which is called heart failure with preserved LV function.

The New York Heart Association (NYHA) functional classification, looks some what vague, but remains the most commonly used standard to describe severity of signs and symptoms.

KILLIP Classification of heart failure in acute myocardial infarction into 4 groups (see Chapter F-171).

8. Risk factors

1. Hypertension
2. Diabetes
3. Coronary artery disease
4. Smoking
5. Hyperlipidemia or
6. Obesity
7. Alcohol
8. Advanced age.

Hypertension and diabetes are particularly important among prominent risk factors.

Uncontrolled hypertension increases the risk of heart failure by 200 percent compared with those who do not have it.

i. Diabetics have about two to eight fold greater risk of heart failure then those without diabetics.
ii. Women with diabetics have a greater risk of heart failure then men with diabetes.
iii. Part of the risk also comes from the associated risk factors, such as hypertension, obesity, dyslipidemia. However, the disease process in diabetes also damages the heart muscle.
iv. Genetic abnormalities contribute to the risk for certain types of heart disease, which in turn may give rise to heart failure. However, in most instances, specific genetic link to heart failure has not been indentified.

9. Heart failure usually develops slowly except in conditions like acute heart failure in acute myocardial infarction. Because the heart failure usually develops slowly, the symptoms may not appear until the condition has progressed over years. The heart masks the underline problem by making adjustments that delay—but do not prevent—the eventual loss of pumping capacity.

The heart adjusts or compensates in 4 ways to cope with and hide the affects of heart failure.

1. Enlargement (dilatation), which allows more blood into the heart.
2. Thickening of muscle fibers (hypertrophy) to strengthen the heart muscle, which allows the heart to contract more forcible and pump more blood.
3. More frequent contractions, which increases circulation.
4. Increasing contractile state

   By making this compensatory adjustment the heart can temporarily make up for loses in pumping ability, some times for years. However, compensation has its limits. Eventually, the heart cannot offset the lost ability to pump the blood, and the signs of heart failure develops.

10. There are 4 compensatory mechanisms that follow after the heart failure.

1. *Frank-Starling mechanism:* Elevation of end-diastolic pressure and volume results in increased contractile force through Frank-Starling mechanism.
2. *Increased sympathetic/Adrenaline stimulation:* It tends to increase the contractile state.
3. *Myocardial hypertrophy/dilatation:* May provide more contractile elements.
4. *Redistribution of blood:* The renin angiotensin system increases its activity in response to decrease in cardiac output.

11. However, each of the above 4 compensatory mechanisms has a price when they become excess.

1. Excessive raise in ventricular end-diastolic pressure and volume cause pulmonary or peripheral edema.
2. Excessive sympathetic tone causes undesirable tachycardia.
3. Excessive hypertrophy or dilatation causes increased oxygen consumption.
4. Excessive sympathetic tone and renin-angiotensin systems, increase the peripheral vascular resistance.

Increased myocardial oxygen consumption tends to occur with all the 4 compensatory mechanisms. If the cardiac disease progresses, the contractility diminishes continuously and the compensatory mechanisms become insufficient to maintain cardiac output. The pivotal abnormality in congestive cardiac failure is myocardial dysfunction, which is characterized by decrease in myocardial contractility. The pump function of the heart becomes insufficient to meet the body requirements. Congestive cardiac failure is thus a systemic manifestation of the poor pump function.

12. **Compensatory mechanism for inadequate cardiac output is by arteriolar and venous constriction mediated through catecholamines. Arteriolar constriction maintains blood pressure increasing the systemic vascular resistance, which increases the work of the heart. Venoconstriction results in decreased venous capacitance and increased venous return, thereby increasing the filling pressure of the ventricles to increase the cardiac output.**

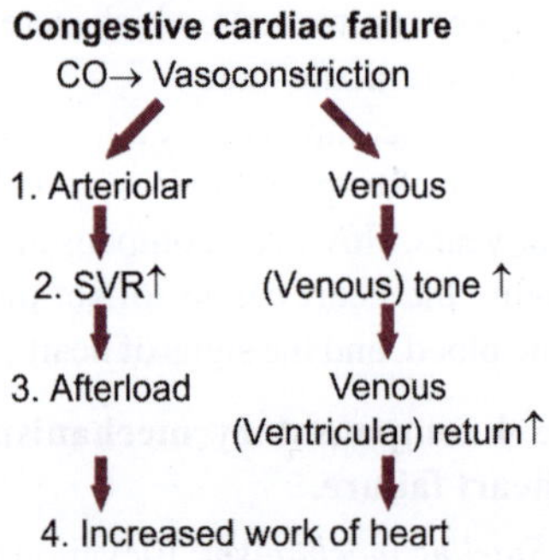

Fig. C-2

13. **There are 4 types of circulatory reflexes which respond immediately to compensate acute cardiac failure:**
    1. Mainly sympathetic reflexes become strongly stimulated increasing the circulatory catecholamines (the parasympathetic become reciprocally inhibited at the same time.).
    2. Baroreceptor reflexes are activated by diminished arterial pressure.
    3. Chemoreceptor reflexes of the CNS are activated by chemical response.
    4. Reflexes originating from the damaged heart itself are also activated.

    Sympathetic and renin angiotensin system activation occurs to improve the cardiac output and maintain perfusion of vital organs, which is essential for survival. Unfortunately, the compensatory mechanisms over react resulting in an inappropriate increase in systemic vascular impedance, which further increases the work on ventricles. This result in further impairment of cardiac contractility, establishing a vicious cycle.

14. **There are 4 subtypes of myocardial receptors:**
    1. β-I adrenergic receptors—which mediate positive inotropic response are reduced in congestive cardiac failure. The decrease in number is proportional to the degree of myocardial dysfunction. The decrease is probably related to the increased catecholamines in congestive cardiac failure.
    2. β-II receptors—remain normal. This suggests that β-II receptors may be still useful in increasing the myocardial contractility and are not affected in congestive cardiac failure.
    3. Postsynaptic alpha-I receptors are also capable of increasing myocardial contractility.
    4. H-2 receptors are not affected in congestive cardiac failure. They are potentially available for enhancing the myocardial contractility.

15. **There are 4 important neurohormonal derangements in chronic heart failure:**
    1. Activation of sympathetic nervous system.
    2. Activation of renin angiotensin system.
    3. Increase in endothelin.
    4. Increase in vasopressin.

    In addition to the activation of vasoconstrictor hormonal system, the activity of the several hormonal systems with vasodilator activity is also altered in patients with chronic heart failure.

    These hormonal systems exert hemodynamic effects that can alter cardiac function, prolonged activation may also exert direct deleterious effects on cardiac muscle cells. This has led to the development of therapeutic interventions designed to block the effects of endogenous vasoconstrictor systems as well as enhance the affects of vasodilator systems. The clinical utility of many of these interventions (e.g. ACEI, β-blockers) in selected patients is well established. Whereas the efficiency of others, e.g. vasopressin antagonists and endothelin antagonists are still under trial.

16. **4 changes occur during adrenergic stimulation of the myocardium such as exercise:**
    1. Increase in cardiac output (CO).
    2. Increase in aortic flow velocity.
    3. Increase in stroke volume.
    4. Increase in ventricular pressure.
       (Note—relatively little change occurs in ventricular EDV).

17. **There are 4 adrenergic effects on the myocardium:**
    1. Tachycardia—(chronotropic effect)
    2. Reduction in cardiac dimensions.
    3. Increased velocity of ejection.
    4. Increased force of contraction (inotropic effect).

18. **Cardiac output depends on 4 factors:**
    1. *Preload:* Length of the muscle fiber at the end of diastolic phase (EDV)—Preload, i.e. length of the cardiac muscle at the onset of contraction.

2. *Contractility:* Inotropic state of the muscle. It is the ability of cardiac muscle to generate tension and force, i.e. myocardial contractile state.
3. *After load:* The resistance against which the heart has to work to maintain circulation, i.e. after load, i.e. peripheral vascular resistance, elasticity of the blood vessels.
4. *Heart rate:* The frequency of ejection.

Cardiac output is defined as the output of blood delivered to the systemic circulation per unit of time. It is generally expressed in liters per minute. Cardiac output is the product of stroke volume × heart rate.

Cardiac index is the cardiac output related to the body size. It is expressed in liters/minute/square meter of body surface area.

1, 2, 3 represent the stroke volume, and may be calculated by subtracting the volume of the heart at the end of systole (end systolic volume) from the volume of the heart when it is full of blood at the end of diastole (end diastolic volume).

(*Note:* Diuretics act at No 1—EDV reduced. Digoxin acts at No 2—Inotropic state. Vasodilators act at No 3—After load reduction occurs. No 4—Heart rate is automatically corrected by controlling the others.)

(β-blockers reduce heart rate.)

19. 4 to 8 liters is the normal cardiac output in a healthy adult at rest.

20. Cardiac reserve is 4 times the normal cardiac output.

The maximum percentage that the cardiac output can increase above normal is called cardiac reserve. This can be easily estimated by exercise test or treadmill test. Cardiac output ranges from 4 to 8 liters per minute at rest to 20 liters per minute with vigorous exercise.

Normal heart can increase its cardiac output 4 times the normal under stress in young persons.

Cardiac output may rise to 4 to 8 times during exercise in a trained athlete (16 to 30 liters).

21. The cardiac output may fall as low as 1/4th in cardiac failure, i.e. 1 to 2 liters per minute.

22. Cardiac output is approximately distributed to the 4 main organs as follows.

Table C-2

To the brain	1/5th of cardiac output (1000 mL/min)
To the heart	5% of cardiac output (225 mL/min)
To the kidneys	1/4th cardiac output (1300 mL/min)
To the liver	1500 mL/min

Remember the kidneys receive 1/4th of cardiac output

23. Ejection fraction is the fraction of end-diastolic volume that leaves the ventricle during systole as stroke volume. A typical ejection fraction is 0.60.

Ejection fraction is calculated as the difference between left ventricular end-diastolic volume and end systolic volume divided by end-diastolic volume × 100.

There are 4 simple steps to calculate the ejection fraction, e.g.

1. *LVEDV:* 140 mL
2. *LVESV:* 50 mL
3. *Stroke volume:* 140–50 = 90 mL
4. *Ejection fraction:* 90/140 × 100, i.e. 64%.

Normal ejection fraction is 60–70% in a healthy adult. In severe cardiac failure, it may be as low as 10-20%.

24. Ejection fraction

Table C-3

1. Normal range	55–80%
2. Mild LV dysfunction	40–50%
3. Moderate LV dysfunction	30–40%
4. Severe LV dysfunction	< 30%

25. Left ventricular end diastolic pressure is less than 12 mm Hg in a healthy person and is equal to:

1. Left atrial mean pressure is < 12 because when the mitral valve opens the left ventricle and left atrium behaves like a common chamber.
2. Pulmonary venous pressure is < 12 because the pulmonary veins are in continuity with left atrium.
3. Pulmonary wedge pressure is < 12 because it is same as pulmonary venous pressure.
4. Pulmonary arterial diastolic pressure is < 12 because it is equivalent to pulmonary capillary wedge pressure.

Thus, in practice, the measurement of Pulmonary artery pressure reflects the pulmonary wedge pressure, pulmonary venous pressure, left atrial pressure and left ventricular diastolic pressure.

Similarly the right ventricular diastolic pressure is eqivalent to mean right atrial pressure and jugular venous pressure (< 7–8 mm Hg)

Peak right ventricular systolic pressure is equivalent to mean pulmonary arterial systolic pressure.

26. Preload is defined as the force, stretching the muscle fibers of the heart when it is resting and full of blood at the end of diastole.

There are 4 factors which determine the preload:

1. Functioning venous return.
2. Compliance of the ventricles.
3. End-diastolic volume.
4. End-diastolic pressure within certain limits.

The relationship between the force of contraction and the resting length of the muscle fibers is known as Frank-Starling mechanism. Increase in preload increases the force of myocardial contractility.

27. There are 4 common causes where the left ventricular end-diastolic volume (LVEDV—Preload) may be elevated.

1. Myocardial failure.
2. When there is LV high load, e.g. aortic regurgitation (AR), mitral regurgitation(MR).
   In AR, MR there is an increase in the column of blood filling the heart, that is an increase in preload and end-diastolic pressure. The increased filling pressure causes stretching of the walls of the heart and dilates over a period of time in the same way as a balloon dilates when it is blown up.
3. When the ventricle is hypertrophied and relatively non-compliant, e.g. restrictive cardiomyopathy.
4. When there is restriction of ventricular filling, e.g. constrictive pericarditis, cardiac tamponade secondary to pericardial effusion.

28. Inotropic effect or myocardial contractility is the inherent capacity of the myocardium to contract and it is independent of the loading conditions. Inotropic effect strengthens systole and lengthens diastole. This inherent contractility is reduced in diseases of the cardiac muscle.

Inotropic state of the myocardium can be influenced by 4 factors:

1. Sympathetic activity.
2. Certain chemicals like caffeine, theophylline, digitalis, isoprenaline, alupent, calcium, etc. increase force velocity relationship.
3. Certain chemicals depress the inotropic state, e.g. general anesthesia, quinidine, procainamide, β-blockers—all antiarrhythmic drugs.
4. Permanent damage, such as myocardial infarction.

Though it is not possible to assess the myocardial contractility clinically, it is now possible to assess by echocardiogram. It is useful to find out the status of the myocardium which determines the long-term prognosis following surgical correction of cardiac anomalies.

29. After load is defined as the force against which the heart has to contract during systole to eject the stroke volume.

There are 4 factors which determine the ventricular after-load:

1. Force of contraction at a given level of diastolic muscle length is inversely related to the after load, i.e. greater the after load less effective is the myocardial contractility. After load for a dilated heart is greater than for a heart of normal size.
2. Tension in the myocardial fiber.
3. Intracavity pressure.
4. Ventricular radius.
   (*Note:* Laplace's law - 2, 3 and 4).

For example, at the same given level of aortic pressure, the enlarged LV has a greater after load than a normal sized heart.

Frank-Starling law: The contractile activity of myocardium depends on length of the muscle fiber at rest, i.e. at the diastolic phase of the cardiac cycle (EVD) and the inotropic state of the heart (ability of the muscle to contract) within the physiological limits.

In a simple way it states that if the heart muscle is stretched before it contracts, it will contract with more energy. This is equivalent to a bow-and-arrow effect, i.e. the more taut the bow, the farther the arrow will go.

Beyond limits, this is not true.

In principle, it is a measure of all the forces against the ejection of the stroke volume. In practice these forces are

- blood pressure or peripheral vascular resistance,
- viscosity or stickiness of the blood,
- resistance in the walls of the heart itself.

30. Frank-Starling relationship: It is useful in understanding the basis of treatment of left ventricular failure. The relationship between the left ventricular filling pressure and cardiac index (CI) in normal and failing heart depends on it. Based on this relationship the patients can be divided into 4 subsets.

1. *Subset I:* Patients with normal hemodynamics with normal CI at normal filling pressure.
2. *Subset II:* Patients with normal CI but have excessive filling pressure which manifests as pulmonary congestion. These patients should be treated with diuretics and/or vasodilators.
3. *Subset III:* Patients with low CI due to hypovolemia. These patients usually respond to volume replacement.
4. *Subset IV:* Patients with pulmonary congestion and low CI. These are the sickest patients. These patients require treatment with inotropes and vasodilators.

The intra-aortic balloon pump (IABP) counter pulsations may be required in these patients who are unresponsive to this therapy. Thus, the primary goals of therapy with CCF are a) to reduce pulmonary congestion by lowering the pulmonary capillary wedge pressure (PCWP) and b) to improve CI by improving the contractile function of the myocardium.

31. The following 4 measurements help to determine the accurate left ventricular performance:

1. Left ventricular end-diastolic pressure (LVEDP)
2. Cardiac output
3. Total body oxygen consumption at rest
4. Total body oxygen consumption during exercise

Normal end-diastolic pressure of the left ventricle is less than 12 mm Hg. In left sided heart failure due to increased weight of the blood column filling the heart, it is greater than 12 mm Hg.

32. There are 4 mechanisms in the retention of fluid in chronic heart failure:

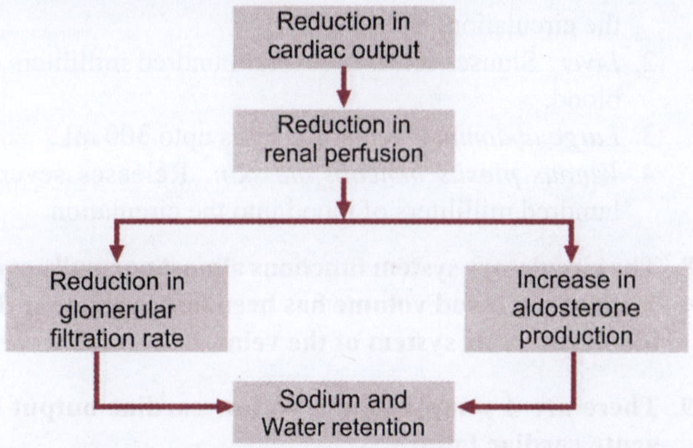

Fig. C-3: Effect of reduction in cardiac output on: (1) Glomerular filtration rate (2) aldosterone production leading to sodium and water retention

1. Reduction in cardiac output reduces renal perfusion, which consequently results in reduction in renal perfusion pressure and sympathetic constriction of the afferent arterioles, it causes reduction in glomerular filtration, leading to retention of sodium and water.
2. A secondary effect is activation of renin angiotensin system. The activated renin-angiotensin-aldosterone axis results in antidiuresis.
3. Aldosterone augment sodium and therefore water retention. The inadequate cardiac output results in other systemic effects besides activating the sympathetic and renin angiotensin system. It increases sympathetic tone of arterioles.
4. The hypervolemia from antidiuresis is also a compensatory mechanism since it increases the circulating volume thereby increasing the cardiac output.

33. There are 4 events by which fluid retention causes further myocardial damage producing a vicious cycle:

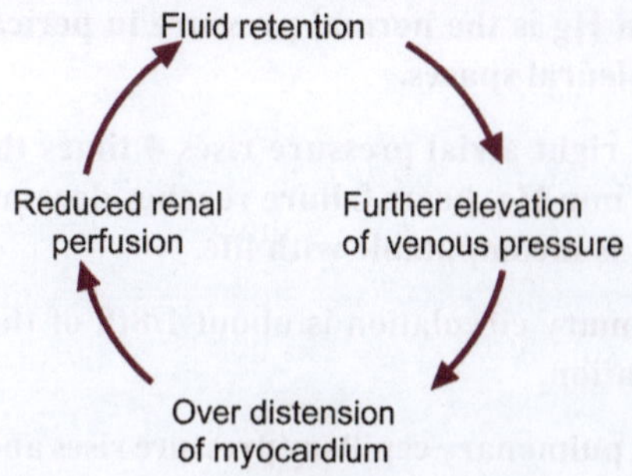

Fig. C-4

Author Query: Kindly provide legend

34. Peripheral edema is the result of imbalance between the following 4 factors:

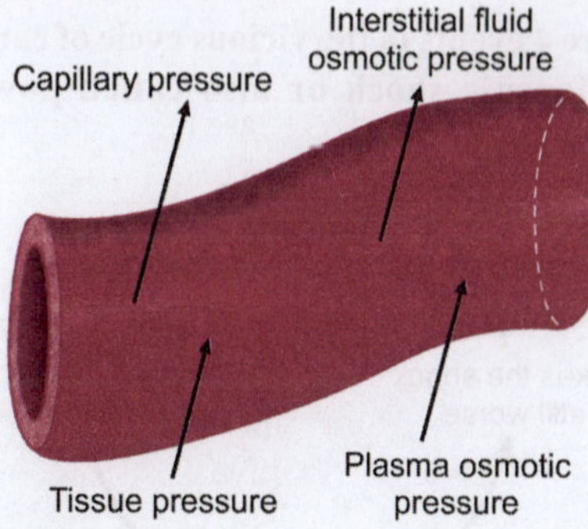

Fig. C-5: Balance between mechanisms tending to force fluid out of vascular bed and those retaining fluid in vessels

1. Plasma osmotic pressure 2. Interstitial tissue pressure	Mechanisms for retaining fluid in the capillary bed
3. Interstitial fluid osmotic pressure 4. Capillary pressure.	Mechanisms favoring the exudation of plasma fluid into the tissues.

(See chapter A-36, 37 for edema)

35. 0 to 4 mm Hg is the normal right atrial pressure.

The normal right atrial pressure is 0 mm Hg, which is equal to the atmospheric pressure around the body. The right atrial pressure is frequently called as central venous pressure (CVP).

36. –4 to –5 mm Hg is the lower limit of right atrial pressure—when the flow of the blood from the peripheral vessels to the heart is greatly reduced as in severe hemorrhage.

37. 4 to 8 mm Hg is the pressure in the peripheral veins—usually greater than the right atrial pressure because they are offered some resistance.

38. Peripheral venous pressure is not elevated until the heart is weakened to rise right atrial pressure to as high as 4 to 6 mm Hg.

39. –4 mm Hg is the normal pressure in pericardial and intrapleural spaces.

40. When right atrial pressure rises 4 times the normal, i.e. 16 mm Hg, heart failure reaches decompensation, which is incompatable with life.

41. Pulmonary circulation is about 1/8th of the systemic circulation.

42. When pulmonary capillary pressure rises above 28 mm Hg, i.e. above the colloid osmotic pressure of plasma—pulmonary edema results.

43. 24 to 32 mm Hg is the normal colloid osmotic pressure of plasma when the lungs remain dry.

44. There are 4 events in the vicious cycle of cardiac shock or cardiogenic shock or also called power failure syndrome.

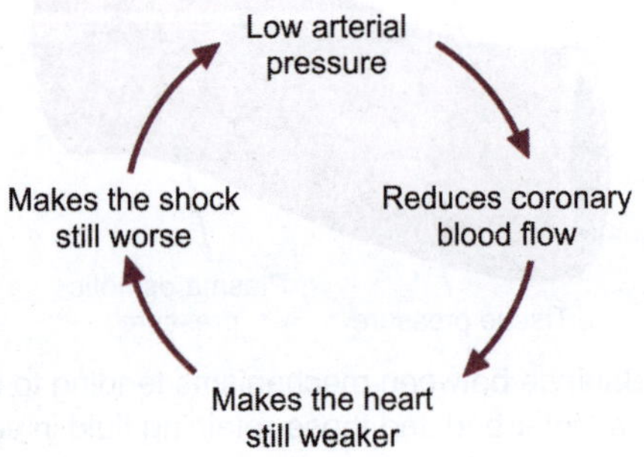

Fig. C-6:

In myocardial infarction already coronary atherosclerosis is there—deterioration sets in when systolic pressure falls as low as 80–90 mm Hg. Whereas in normal heart, it must reach below 45 mm Hg. So, it is extremely important to prevent short periods of hypotension in acute MI.

45. The 4 causes of decreased myocardial contractility in chronic heart failure:

1. Excessive stretch causes damage to the muscle fibers and sometimes give rise to growth of excessive fibrous tissue in the ventricular walls.
2. Diminished number of capillaries in relation to excessive myocardial mass.
3. Diminished stores of norepinephrine vesicles in the sympathetic nerve endings—decreases the sympathetic drive of the myocardium, which is especially necessary in times of stress.
4. Defective excitation—contraction coupling caused by diminished ATP energized pump for calcium absorption into sarcoplasmic reticulum.

46. Redistribution of blood in acute cardiac failure is brought in such a manner that more important organs like brain and heart receive normal or near normal supply—and less important organs have reduced blood supply causing symptoms.

The 4 organs affected and the consequences are as follows:

1. Reduction of cutaneous blood flow—Causes pale, cold, clammy skin, peripheral cyanosis and even low grade fever.
2. Reduction of muscle blood flow—Causes fatigue.
3. Reduction of Gastrointestinal tract blood supply—Causes anorexia, indigestion, etc.
4. Reduction of kidney blood supply—Causes sodium and water retention.

47. There are 4 specific "blood reservoirs" of the systemic veins:

1. *Spleen:* Releases as much as 1500 mL of blood into the circulation.
2. *Liver:* Sinuses releases several hundred milliliters of blood.
3. *Large abdominal veins:* Releases upto 300 mL.
4. *Venous plexus beneath the skin:* Releases several hundred milliliters of blood into the circulation.

48. The circulatory system functions almost normally even 1/4th of the blood volume has been lost because of the blood reservoir system of the veins.

49. There are 4 symptoms due to low cardiac output in acute cardiac failure:

1. Generalized weakness.
2. Fainting.
3. Symptoms of increased sympathetic activity, such as feeble and thready pulse, cold and clammy skin, sweating, so on and so forth.
4. Congestion: Pulmonary congestion alone can occur in left sided heart failure. Systemic congestion alone can occur in pure right sided chronic heart failure.

50. There are 4 types of circulatory failure.

1. Right heart failure
2. Left heart failure
3. Combined heart failure

(1–3: Central circulatory failure)

4. Peripheral circulatory failure (See Chapter A-257)

51. Clinical features of cardiac failure depends on the following 4 factors:

1. *Right atrial hypertension*

   JVP is raised.

   Systemic congestion: Congestion of systemic veins may lead to swelling of the legs and even the trunk.

   Tricuspid regurgitation—characteristic systolic wave which often moves the ears—when patient reclines at

45°, epigastric pain, pain in the right hypochondrium due to stretching of the liver capsule as a result of congestion of the liver. Palpable, tender sometimes pulsatile liver.

Jaundice in late cases due to hepatic congestion, hepatocellular hypoxia associated with central lobular atrophy.

In long standing cases, centrilobular necrosis—give rise to 'nutmeg liver' may progress to cardiac cirrhosis.

Splenomegaly results from chronic venous congestion or portal hypertension secondary to cirrhosis, but splenomegaly with hypertension should rise the suspicion endocarditis.

Ascites and plural effusion may be a future of chronic heart failure. In the presence of plural effusion, search for pulmonary embolism with infarction.

2. *Left atrial hypertension*

Dyspnea, orthopnea, paroxysmal nocturnal dyspnea, pulmonary congestion, pulmonary edema.

Atrial fibrillation may develop in mitral stenosis. Atrial fibrillation is the commonest arrhythmia associated with cardiac failure.

Persistent coughing is another common symptom, especially coughing that regularly produces mucus or pink blood stained sputum. Some patients develop wheezing.

X-ray evidence of LAH.

3. *Restriction of cardiac output:* Reduced exercise tolerance.

Fatigue or easy tiring is another common symptom, is probably due to oxygen debt resulting from the blood supply to the muscles and other tissues being insufficient for their need due to low cardiac output. Without proper "fuel" the body cannot performer as much work, which translates into fatigue.

Syncope—e.g. Aortic stenosis, pulmonary arterial hypertension, complete heart-block.

Coldness, pallor, peripheral cyanosis—due to compensatory peripheral vasoconstriction.

Impairment of renal function—Oliguria, proteinuria , increased specific gravity, prerenal azotemia.

Impairment of hepatic function—Loss of appetite and change of bowel habit in part due to congestion and poor perfusion of the gastrointestinal tract.

Weight loss due to cardiac cachexia is seen in advanced cases.

Cheyne-Stokes respiration

Venous thrombosis, pulmonary embolism

Cerebral symptoms, such as confusion, headache, insomnia, anxiety, impairment of memory.

4. *Precipitating factors:* should be looked for particularly in refractory heart failure.

i. Systemic hypertension.
Discontinuation of medicines
Rapid elevation of Hypertension.

ii. Anemia

iii. Thyrotoxicosis
Heart failure actually may be one of the first clinical manifestation of hyperthyroidism in a patient with underlying thyroid disease.

iv. Pregnancy
Heart failure frequently recognized for the first time in pregnancy with valvular disease—in which cardiac compensation may return following delivery.

v. Myocardial infarction: In patients with compensated myocardial infarction—a fresh infarct can cause heart failure.

vi. Arrhythmias: There are 4 precipitating factors that cause heart failure in arrhythmias:
a. No proper ventricular filling due to lack of time in tachyarrhythmias.
b. The AV dissociation results in loss of atrial booster pump mechanism.
c. Loss of normal synchronocity of ventricular contraction in any AV conduction defect.
Marked reduction in cardiac output in bradycardia associated with AV block

vii. Rheumatic and other forms of myocarditis: Further effect in patients with pre-existing heart disease.

viii Infective endocarditis—e.g. diphtheria.

ix. Pulmonary infection—Patients with pulmonary vascular congestion are more prone but any infection may precipitate heart failure.
Fever, tachycardia, hypoxemia, increased metabolic demands may further overload the myocardium of chronic heart failure patient.

x. Pulmonary embolism: From thrombi in the veins of lower limbs.
→ results in increased pulmonary arterial pressure
→ results in right heart failure (RHF).
In the presence of pulmonary vascular congestion —such emboli may cause infarction of the lung.

xi. Diet and drugs—Beriberi
Excess sodium intake, administration of salt retaining drugs.
Administration of cardiac depressant drugs.
Discontinuation of medicines for heart failure.

xii. Physical, environmental and emotional excesses.
Over exertion.
Excessive heat or humidity.
Emotional crisis.

52. Framingham criteria for the diagnosis of congestive heart failure consists of:

Major Criteria

1. Dyspnea—paroxysmal nocturnal dyspnea or orthopnea
2. Raised JVP—Increase in venous pressure > 16 cm of water
3. Rales
4. Cardiomegaly
5. Acute pulmonary edema
6. S3 gallop
7. Circulation time >25 sec
8. Hepatojugular reflex.

Minor Criteria

1. Edema—ankle edema
2. Night cough
3. Dyspnea
4. Hepatomegaly
5. Pleural effusion
6. Decreased vital capacity to one third of maximum
7. Tachycardia >120/min
8. Weight loss of > 4.5 kg in 5 days in response to treatment.

53. The patterns of breathlessness associated with left ventricular failure may be described in 4 stages. (See Chapter A-14-21)

Breathlessness is defined as an abnormal and uncomfortable awareness of breathing. This is seen when the demand on the lungs is greater than their capacity to respond or when the tension developed by the respiratory muscles is excessive in relation to their movement.

1. Breathlessness on exertion
2. Orthopnea
3. Paroxysmal nocturnal dyspnea
4. Acute pulmonary edema.

54. Pulmonary edema produces complex effects, which include:

1. Interference with gas exchange.
2. Alteration in the ventilation—perfusion ratio with 'shunting' of unoxygenated blood through the lungs.
3. Decrease in the lung compliance (stiff lung).
4. Increasing the work of breathing.

55. Other common symptoms of heart failure include:

1. Fatigue and low exercise tolerance are common complaints in patients with heart failure.
2. Dizziness may occur due to impaired perfusion but more commonly iatrogenic, related to the use of heart failure medicines.
3. Palpitation and syncope may occur when there is associated arrhythmia, which needs prompt evaluation.
4. Anorexia and abdominal pain are due to congestion of liver in the heart failure especially with right heart failure.

Commonly seen but seldom considered symptoms are cough, insomnia and depressed mood.

56. There are 4 clinical signs by which heart failure can be diagnosed:

1. *Raised jugular pressure:* Hepatojugular reflux present.
2. *Pulsus alternans:* Palpating the radial pulse may reveal that it alternate in amplitude with each beat—strong beat, weak beat, strong beat, weak beat. Every other beat is weaker than the preceding one and is more stronger after a premature beat. This cannot be detected if very firm pressure is applied over the artery; instead, a very light pressure is needed to reveal.
   When the pulsus alternans is identified, then alternation of the second sound will be heard on auscultation in most patients if we listen carefully.
   If a murmur is present, it too will alternate in intensity.
3. *A ventricular diastolic gallop S3 should be heard:* A faint third heart sound is present occurring in early to mid-diastole—the timing of the ventricular gallop (S3). Patient is turned to the left lateral position and the point of maximum impulse of the left ventricle is located (Apex). The bell of the stethoscope is lightly placed over this area. The ventricular gallop is now louder and clearly heard when the patient turns from supine to left lateral position. The gallop may also show alternation with every other beat. Pressure on the stethoscope can eliminate this gallop. It signifies increased LVEDP in patients with decrease in LV function.
4. *Pulmonary edema:* Signs of retention of sodium and water—edema, pleural effusion, ascites.
   Pulmonary edema due to accumulation fluid in the pulmonary interstitium and alveoli from high left atrial pressures are commonly referred to as acute cardiogenic pulmonary edema (ACPE).
   Plural effusion gives rise to dullness at the lung bases. Sometimes, edema, ascites and hepatomegaly may occur even with pulsatile liver palpable during late stage of congestion.
   These clinical signs establish the diagnosis of cardiac decompensation in the outpatient or at bedside without much expensive tests.
   More of these findings are prominent and are easier to find, the greater the degree of heart failure is the rule. Therefore, pulsus alternans can be treated as one of the most subtle signs of heart failure and once it is found, search for the ventricular gallop (S3), alternation of sounds and murmurs. Clinical features of HF varies markedly among the patients. 50% of patients with LV systolic dysfunction may be asymptomatic.

57. Vital signs are often important:

1. Pulse—tachycardia.
2. Temperature—Cold and clammy skin.
3. Respiration—tachypnea.
4. BP—narrow pulse pressure is often a sign of poor prognosis or advanced disease, BP monitoring and its management is also very important in the treatment of heart failure.

Body weight is often useful in compensatory state.

58. Clinical features of heart failure varies markedly among the patients. About 50% of patients with LV systolic dysfunction may be asymptomatic. So well compensated systolic heart failure may not reveal any abnormalities. A high index of suspicion based on symptoms must be needed. The physical signs in heart failure varies depending on the compensation, chronicity (acute versus chronic) and chamber involvement (right heart failure versus left heart failure).

Fluid or volume overload is the hallmark sign for heart failure essentially in the setting of acute decompensation and right heart failure.

The typical physical signs of volume overload in heart failure includes:

1. Pulmonary edema due to accumulation of fluid into pulmonary interstitium and alveoli from high left atrial pressure commonly referred to as acute cardiogenic pulmonary edema (ACPE), this gives rise to pulmonary rales.
2. Plural effusion—this gives rise to dullness at the lung bases.
3. JVP rise—Elicited at 45° inclination although when JVP is elevated it may be apparent only when the patient sitting up right.
4. Edema, ascites, hepatomegaly, may occur, even with a pulsatile liver palpable during congestion.

59. Often neglected is the subtle sign of peripheral perfusion which is noted by:

1. Color
2. Warm or cool extremities
3. Capillary refill
4. Anemia.

This is important in assessing adequacy of perfusion in patients with advanced heart failure.

60. Valsalva maneuver is useful in the diagnosis of heart failure.

Performance of this maneuver—forced expiration against a closed glottis causes the following 4 changes:

1. Raise in intrathoracic pressure.
2. Raise in venous pressure.
3. Decrease in venous return to the heart.
4. Decrease in heart size—Fall in stroke volume and pulse pressure.

61. Valsalva maneuver test has been standardized. The patient is requested to blow against an aneroid manometer and maintain a pressure of 40 mm Hg for 30 second. Atrial pressure tracings taken normally show 4 distinct phases.

1. An immediate raise in arterial pressure. It represents the transmission of increased intrathoracic pressure into the periphery.
2. Continuation of the strain accompanying reduction of venous return results in reduction in systolic, diastolic and pulse pressures followed by a reflex increase in heart rate.
3. Release of the strain causes sudden drop of arterial pressure equivalent to the fall in intrathoracic pressure.
4. Combination of sudden rush of blood that had been dammed in the venous bed into the heart and reflex vasoconstriction and tachycardia causes overshoot of arterial pressure to above control levels with wide pulse pressure.

Phase 1 and 3 are normal in heart failure. The impedance of venous return during phase 2 does not affect the stroke volume.

Therefore, the baroreceptor reflex is not activated and there is no overshoot on release of the strain. This gives a 'square wave' appearance of the tracing.

62. Investigations:

I. Routine bold tests: TC, DC, ESR, Hb, TRBC, PCV, MCV, MCH, MCHC,

Routine urine for albumin, sugar, and microscope tests, etc. for associated diseases.

Hematocrit (PCV, MCV, MCH, MCHC), helps in the diagnosis of anemia.

Anemia should be corrected by iron, folic acid, B_{12}, by PO or parenteral or by blood transfusion (whole blood or packed cells).

Anemia is prevalent in heart failure patients up to 15–25% and contribute to the development of high output heart failure. Hemodilution from fluid retention may also cause anemia and should be treated with diuretics.

TC, DC, ESR helps in suspected associated acute or chronic infections which should be cleared. Direct peripheral blood smear gives a broad idea of type of anemia. Platelets, malaria parasites may be seen.

II. Routine urine for albumin, sugar gives an idea of associated renal pathology, and diabetes, which should be further worked out.

Microscopic urine should be examined to see for pus cells, RBC, casts, etc.

The edema can be due to congestive heart failure or hypoalbuminurea.

Do not come to a conclusion by normal serum creatine. Serum creatine starts raising after 50% of the kidney is damaged. So check the urine for albumin by boiling test for early diagnosis of kidney pathology.

III. Routine biochemical tests: Blood sugar for diabetes

Lipid profile for dyslipidemia because the coronary artery disease may be the predominant cause of heart failure.

Blood urea, serum creatine for renal pathology.

Serum bilirubin for liver pathology.

Special test for thyroid: T3, T4, TSH, they are needed in patients with new onset heart failure.

Electrolytes: To see abnormalities, which are common in heart failure particularly potassium—hyperkalemia.

Acidosis: Metabolic acidosis is common in heart failure.

A patient with breathlessness without any rales in the lungs—suspect metabolic acidosis.

Hypokalemia, hypomagnesia and metabolic alkalosis are common with diuretics.

Hyperkalemia is more dangerous in heart failure. It can occur from drugs inhibiting the RAAS or common and should be monitored owing to their arrhythmogenic property. Adding potassium sparing diuretics, and oral potassium will increase the chances of hyperkalemia.

Hyponatremia typically signifies fluid retention. Electrolytes monitoring is important before initiation of aldosterone receptor antagonists.

LFT: Elevation of transaminase levels, or altered coagulation indices can occur when right sided heart failure is predominant due to hepatic congestion.

IV. Biomarkers: Natriuretic peptide, such as B—type natriuretic peptide (BNP) or aminoterminal pro- B-type natriuretic peptide (pro-BNP) are two important methods developed in heart failure to diagnosis and treatment.

63. There are 4 known natriuretic peptides.

1. ANP—Atrial natriuretic peptide (from atrium)
2. BNP—Betanatriuretic peptide (from ventricles)
3. CNP—From endothelium
4. DNP

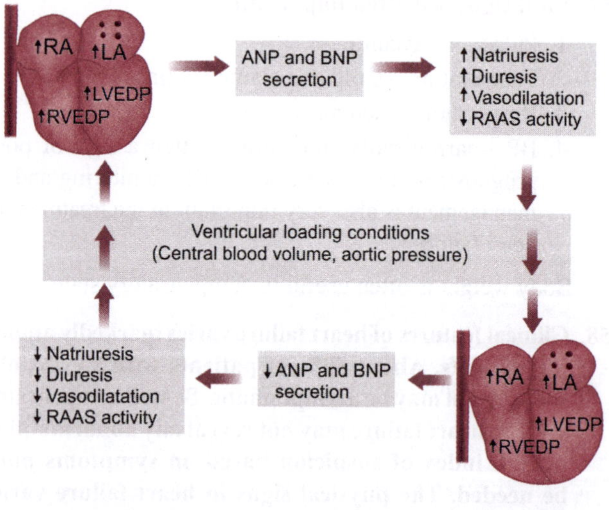

Fig. C-7: Cardiac secretion of natriuretic peptides which serves to maintain intervascular volume homeostasis

LA, Left atrium; LVEDP, Left ventricular end-diastolic pressure; RA: Right atrium; RAAS, renin-angiotenisn-aldosterone system; RVEDP, right ventricular end-diastolic pressure.

64. BNP—(first thought BNP is from the brain) and pro-BNP or proteins produced by the ventricles are now available for clinical use. BNP is released from the cardiac ventricles especially from left ventricle, during pressure or volume overload. It has the following physiological action.

1. It dilates arteries and veins.
2. It acts as a beneficial neurohormonal modulator by decreasing the levels of vasoconstrictors.
3. It decreases the sodium retaining neurohormones.
4. Along with atrial natriuretic peptide (ANP) it maintains, hemostasis by promoting diuresis and natriuresis.

65. The BNP assay has become the most important blood test in cardiology.

Table C-4

BNP levels pg/mL	Clinical condition
< 100	Normal
< 500	Goal at hospital discharge
≥ 700	Decompensated congestive HF
≈ 3000	During nesiritide infusion

Normal pro-BNP level—< 125 pg/mL

There is wide variation of BNP depending on patient's age, (secreted more as we age), gender (more in women), medical therapy, body mass index, renal function, perioperative status, and other comorbid disease (like thyroid).

Recent guidelines have been established with their use in the clinical setting.

BNP differs from troponin, which rises when there is ischemia or necrosis.

66. BNP is useful in heart failure in 4 ways:

1. Screening for HF.
2. Diagnosing HF.
3. Monitoring HF therapy.
4. Evaluating prognosis of HF.

1. *Screening for HF:* Though the BNP or pro-BNP levels are elevated in cardiac dysfunction, the sensitivity is relatively low in asymptomatic patients and it is highly dependent on the cutoff levels chosen. Strategies to screen BNP for HF in asymptomatic patients in several setting (e.g. Patients with stage A and B HF, such as post MI) are still in development.
2. *Diagnosing HF:* It is especially useful to distinguish dyspnea due to HF from dyspnea due to other causes (or from breathing not perfectly (BNP). Normal levels are < 100 pg/mL. The test has a negative predictive level of at least 96%. So, HF can be confidently ruled out for patients with dyspnea. However, BNP levels in acute cardiogenic pulmonary edema may not rise until a few hours later.
   BNP levels can be used to determine severity of HF. When symptoms are either vague or excessive, patients in renal failure or on dialysis or waiting for dialysis may have elevated levels whether HF present or not. As a rule, the BNP assay is not useful in renal failure patients. Patients with right-sided HF (due to pulmonary hypertension, chronic cor pulmonale, or pulmonary emboli) also have elevated BNP levels (usually 300–400 pg/mL)
3. *Monitoring HF therapy:* BNP levels are complimentary to clinical assessment and should not replace at bed side or hemodynamic assessment. A single BNP or pro-BNP value should not be used. The BNP levels should be tested at intervals while assessing the response to therapy.
   In general, diuretics and drugs inhibiting the renin-angiotensin-aldosterone system (RAAS) lower the BNP and response to β-blockers may vary.
4. *Determining the prognosis of HF:* BNP and pro-BNP levels correlate closely with morbidity and mortality of HF, perhaps better than many standard prognostic tools. A high BNP or pro-BNP levels indicate high risk.

67. Synthetic BNP (Nesiritide): A recombinant form of BNP is an intravenous agent approved in 2001 to treat decompensated HF.

Nesiritide's primary physiological effect is vasodilatation, both in the arteries and veins. It acts,

1. By binding to specialized receptors on the surface of smooth muscle and endothelial cells.
   ↓
2. When the receptors are activated, the concentration of cyclic GMP increases resulting in vasodilation.
3. It promotes diuresis, by its hemodynamic effect on both in the vasculature and in the kidneys.
4. Though, it has no inotropic properties it increases cardiac output via reflex vasodilation.

Since it has no direct electrophysiologic properties, it will not precipitate ventricular tachycardia or other arrhythmias. It lowers pulmonary capillary wedge pressure more effectively than IV nitroglycerine and improves dyspnea faster than standard therapy.

68. Nesiritide is indicated in:

1. Decompensated HF.
2. Fluid overload.
3. Dyspnea at rest or minimal activities.
4. Evidence of elevated filling pressures (e.g. Bulging neck veins).

Nesiritide is not given to everyone. It should be regarded as "up-front" care for decompensated HF, not as a last resort for cachectic, terminally ill patients who are ready for hospice.

69. Contraindications of nesiritide are:

1. Low cardiac output state (e.g. "Overdiuresed", "cold and dry").
2. Hypotension (< 90 mm Hg/SBP).
3. Cardiogenic shock.
4. Low filling pressures.

In addition, nesiritide is contraindicated in other conditions in which vasodilating agents do not help, e.g. AS, obstructive cardiomyopathy, restrictive cardiomyopathy, pericardial constriction and cardiac tamponade. Clinical judgement is important in selecting the patients.

70. Nesiritide has a rapid onset of action seen within 15 minutes. It has longer half life (15–20 min) than other intravenous agents. Affect lasts for 2–4 hours after stopping.

Inactivation occurs in the vasculature, when the drug binds to a clearance receptor or neutralized by endopeptidase, unlike other drugs, which requires liver metabolism or renal clearance.

BP should be monitored during nesiritide infusion.

Table C-5

Time from start	Frequency of measurement
1st hour	Every 15 min
2nd hour	Every 30 min
3rd and 4th hour	Every 1 hour
5th hour on	Every 4 hours

It can be given for an average of 29 hours to recovery. It does not require pulmonary artery catheters. Cardiac monitoring is enough. Always check electrolytes to avoid hypokalemia, hyponatremia, or azotemia because of vigorous diuresis. It is not associated with tachyphylaxis. Nesiritide is expensive (about 375$ per day) but worth it. Additional cost is small compared to savings of avoiding on extended hospital stay and time spent on ICU.

71. BNP—adjusting with other medications:

Baseline therapy may be augmented:

1. An ACE inhibitor should be started, or if the patient is already on one, it should be increased to target level.
2. If the maximum is already on, one should add something else, such as a nitrate, hydralazine, or spironolactone.
3. Diuretics should be used with care with BNP infusion. Usually given for first two days then cut back on day three to avoid prerenal azotemia.
4. β-blockers therapy should be left unchanged β-blockers should only be started when a person is euvolemic. They should be neither started nor discontinued when a patient has fluid overload and is decompensated.

72. There are 4 main abnormalities that are likely to be seen on plain chest X-ray in cardiac failure: (Refer Chapter P-Roentgenology; Fig. P-10)

1. *Stag's horns sign:* Prominence of the upper lobe veins often likened to stag's horns. This is due to increased pulmonary venous pressure in left ventricular failure causing a relative diversion of blood from the lower to the upper zones in the erect posture. Prominence of the upper lobe veins is a characteristic radiological feature of pulmonary congestion.
2. *Bat's wing sign:* Enlargement of the hila and a ground glass appearance of perihilar region often likened to a bat's wing. It is due to frank pulmonary edema or rarely uremic lung.
3. *Kerley B lines or Septal lines:* Most commonly seen in the lower lobes near the costophrenic angles. They are fine dense lines thought to be due to edema in the lymphatics. When horizontal, these are known as Kerley B lines. Pulmonary lymphatics seen radiologically as transverse linear opacities at the lung bases as Kerley B lines.
4. Plural effusion seen, as obliteration of costophrenic angles in mild effusion.

   Cardiomegaly: Transverse diameter of the heart is increased.

   The ventricle, which is enlarged may not be accurately appreciated on plain chest X-ray. As a rule, heart size is never normal in chronic congestive heart failure.

   Calcification of valves, such as aortic valve may be seen occasionally in a lateral view.

73. Normal sized heart in X-ray in heart failure is seen in:

1. Mitral stenosis.
2. Cor pulmonale.
3. Acute mitral regurgitation.
4. Acute aortic regurgitation.
5. Acute myocardial infarction.
6. Constrictive pericarditis.
7. Diastolic heart failure.
8. Intracardiac masses (myxoma).

74. There are 4 ECG changes that are likely to be seen in heart failure. ECG may be normal despite severe acute left ventricular failure. It is abnormal in chronic heart failure.

1. Left ventricular hypertrophy. S in V1 + R in V5 = > 35 mm.
2. Left ventricular strain or pressure overload pattern suggested by ST depression that looks like a tick drawn backwards in the lateral leads V4–V6, LI and a VL. These changes may be seen in ischemia or digitalis effect. Symmetrical T inversion in V5, V6 is suggestive of left ventricular strain.
3. Height of R wave may be varying in alternate beats showing the evidence of pulsus alternans.
4. Arrhythmias: Most commonly atrial fibrillation.
5. There may be evidence of pastmyocardial infarction. (QS waves).
6. Pericardial affusion: voltage < 5 mV in frontal leads and <10 mV in pericardial leads.
7. Cardiac amyloidosis (low voltage and pseudoinfarction pattern in anterior leads).
8. Heart blocks: There may be evidence of left bundle branch block, indicated by wide QRS complexes in left pericardial leads (i.e. iatrogenic or infiltrative diseases in particular LBBB morphology with QRS >130 m).

   Recent understanding of the role of impairment of cardiac synchrony in the evolution of heart failure has led to the management of QRS duration and morphology. This helps to determine the potential benefits of cardiac resynchronization therapy particularly in LBBB with QRS > 130 m.

   Congestive heart failure cannot be diagnosed by ECG.

75. Echocardiography is particularly useful in heart failure for which no cause has been found out. This is helpful to obtain the following 4 points of information:

1. *Valves of the heart:* Whether moving normally, thickened or stenosed or incompetent. An unsuspected, yet correctable valvular lesion may be found. Because of low cardiac output and low flow past the valve it may not produce an audible murmur.
2. *Size of the chamber and movements of their walls:* Ventricular function can be assessed by size of the chambers and movement of their walls. Reduced movement of the walls may suggest low cardiac output. Ejection fraction determines the degree of cardiac decompensation. Ejection fraction is low in advanced heart failure. Ejection fraction becomes higher as the patient starts improving and it becomes normal when the cardiac decompensation is eliminated.
3. *An unsuspected cardiac aneurysm:* It is seen as an abnormal outward movement of the ventricular wall during systole.
4. Obstructive cardiomyopathy suggested by thickening of the ventricular septum.

76. Following tests are indicated in special cases:

1. Right heart catheterization gives information of cardiac index filling pressures, pulmonary atrial pressure, pulmonary capillary wedge pressure, systemic vascular resistance, pulmonary vascular resistance, etc. useful in patients isolated right heart failure of unknown cause.
2. Left heart catheterization: Useful in patients with history of coronary artery disease, elevation of coronary artery anatomy to identify the cause of decompensation and guide the treatment. To identify whether the decompensation is caused by ischemia and to determine whether the revascularization (percutaneous angioplasty or stent or bypass) is indicated.
3. Endomyocardial biopsy: Indicated only when primary myocardial disease is suspected and when other causes of decompensation have been ruled out. It may be helpful in prognostic information in cases like cardiac amyloidosis.
4. Left ventricular scintigraphy.

77. Left ventricular scintigraphy:

This gives information about the circulation of blood as it flows through the chambers of the heart. It differs from thallium scintigraphy, which give information about the circulation of the myocardium.

Procedure: The 4 steps are:

1. Isotope technetium-99 labeled red blood cells are injected intravenously.
2. Images are recorded as the isotope labelled RBC pass through the chambers of the heart.
3. Difference in size and density of images are assessed in systole and diastole.
4. Ejection fraction and cardiac output are measured.

   It is also useful to assess the prognosis following myocardial infarction. Mortality in the first year after myocardial infarction is greatly increased in those with ejection fraction less than 40%.

   Cardiac aneurysm can also be diagnosed by the presence of bulging of the left ventricle during systole.

78. There are 4 broad principles in the management of heart failure.

1. Improving the coronary blood flow by "bypass surgery".
2. Improving myocardial function by correcting precipitating or aggravating causes like
   i. Metabolic defects (acidosis, alkalosis, anoxia and electrolyte imbalance).
   ii. Thyrotoxicosis, hypertension, myxedema.
   iii. Anemia, beriberi.
   iv. Arrhythmia, etc. (see precipitating factors).
3. Correcting or removal of the underlying cause like structural abnormalities, such as acquired valvular defects, congenital malformations, etc.
4. Control of congestive cardiac failure itself.

The treatment consists in relieving the patient from congestive cardiac failure as well as identifying and correcting the cause, which resulted in CCF.

79. The following 4 risk factors should be controlled in congestive heart failure:

1. Restriction of salt.
2. Stoppage of smoking.
3. Avoidance of alcohol.
4. Reduction of obesity (diet and exercise).
5. Treatment of hypertension.
6. Treatment of hyperlipidemia.
7. Treatment of diabetes mellitus.
8. Treatment of coronary artery disease—ischemic heart disease.

80. There are 4 principles in the treatment of congestive cardiac failure itself:

1. Reduction of cardiac workload, e.g. rest, reduction in weight by 'Diet and Habits'.
2. Improving pump performance by increasing myocardial contractility by positive inotropic action, i.e. digitalis.
3. Reduction of preload (EDV) by controlling excessive fluid and water retention, e.g. diuretics.
4. Reduction of after load, e.g. vasodilators.

81. Remember 4 D's in the treatment of heart failure.

1. Diet and habits—to reduce cardiac workload.
2. Digitalis—to increase cardiac contracitlity by positive inotropic action.
3. Diuretics—to reduce preload.
4. Dilators—both venous and arteriolar dilators.
   - Venous dilators—to reduce preload.
   - Arteriolar dilators—to reduce after load.

82. There are 4 principles to reduce or remove the cardiac workload:

1. Physical and emotional rest.
2. Treatment of obesity—restriction of fats and caloric intake, monitored by regular weighing.
3. Vasodilator therapy.
4. Assisted circulation.

83. Restriction of physical activity is advised depending on the severity of heart failure by the following 4 ways:

1. Absenting from sports and heavy labor.
2. Absenting from full-time work or equivalent activity and allowing rest periods during the day time.
3. Confine to house.
4. Confine to bed, chair.

Use bedside commode, avoid staining at stool, use stockings to reduce risk of deep vein thrombosis.

84. There are 4 guidelines to follow to achieve physical and emotional rest:

1. A good patient-doctor relationship and use of drugs like diazepam 2.5 mg twice daily. Fluzepam 15–30 mg may go a long way in providing mental rest.
2. Reduced physical activity plays a critical role in the treatment of heart failure throughout the entire course. The intensity of reduction in physical activity depends on the severity of heart failure.
3. Deep breathing exercises, leg exercises and elastic stockings are advisable to prevent the hazards of thrombephlebitis, pulmonary embolism. Carefully supervised exercise programs are useful in improving symptomatic state and exercise tolerance of patients with stable and compensated chronic heart failure.
4. Patients with left ventricular ejection fraction of less than 20% are at high risk for systemic or pulmonary embolism when they are bedridden for long time. Long-term anticoagulants may be considered in such patients if there is no contraindication. The use of anticoagulants in low doses of heparin 5000 units subcutaneously twice daily or coumadin should be considered with heart failure with or without previous history of thromboemobolic disease.

85. There are 4 methods to improve pump performance:

1. Digitalis.
2. Sympathomimetic amines, e.g. dopamine, dobutamine.
3. Other positive inotropic agents (newer cardiotonic agents), e.g. amrinone.
4. Pacemaker.

86. There are 4 methods to control sodium and water retention:

1. Restriction of salt in the diet.
2. Restriction of water intake.
3. Diuretics.
4. Mechanical removal of extracellular fluid.

87. There are 4 guidelines to follow in restriction of salt and water in heart failure patients:

Restriction of sodium intake remains one of the cornerstones of treatment of congestive heart failure. Sodium restriction becomes a critical strategy for the treatment of heart failure as the disorder progresses.

1. Modest restriction of sodium intake is recommended in most patients with heart failure with good response to diuretic regime to prevent retention of fluid. There is no need of elimination of salt in the cooking unless fluid retention occurs despite diuretics. Sodium intake is restricted by eliminating salt shaker from the table so that dialy intake of sodium will be restricted to 1.6 to 2.8 g per day.
2. Reduction of salt intake to 1.2 to 1.5 g per day can be achieved to simply eliminating salt from cooking and from the table.
3. Reduction of salt intake to 0.2 to 1.0 g per day by low sodium diet is advised in Class IV congestive heart failure patients.
4. In advanced cases of congestive heart failure, the concentration of antidiuretic hormone may be increased and the ability to excrete free water load may be impaired. Water intake should be restricted under these circumstances so that sodium concentration does not fall below 130 mEq/L. In other cases, water intake may be left free to the patient's desire.

88. There are 4 methods of mechanical removal of extracellular fluid:

1. Thoracentesis.
2. Paracentesis.
3. Dialysis—hemodialysis or peritoneal dialysis.
4. Phlebotomy.

Patients with advanced congestive cardiac failure who have become resistant to diuretic therapy may recollect the fluid following thracocentesis/paracentesis. Removal by peritoneal or hemodialysis with ultrafiltration may be done successfully in patients resistant to diuretic therapy.

DIGITALIS

89. The 4 fundamental observations of inotropic action of cardiac glycosides are:

1. Digitalis exerts a positive inotorpic action on cardiac muscle but not on skeletal muscle.
2. They increase the force velocity of contraction of the normal as well as the failing heart.
3. The positive inotropic action is dependent on contraction frequency declining on either side by an optimum value.
4. The rate of onset and magnitude of inotropic action are dependent on the available concentrations of ions including potassium, sodium, calcium and magnesium. Cardiac glycosides by some mechanism increase the availability of calcium to the contractile element at the time excitation-contraction coupling.

Digitalis inhibits the enzyme Na^+/K^+ activated ATPase and thus inhibits the transport of sodium and potassium ions across the cell membrane. This results in a net potassium exit from the myocardium and an increase in the calcium released to the contractile element at the time of excitation-contraction coupling.

90. Digitalis (Foxglove) is first described in Fuch's herbarium in 1543. An account of Foxglove was published in 1785 by William Withering—Physician in Birmingham.

Digitalis still holds good in the treatment of heart failure though it has 4 disadvantages:

1. Dubious bioavailability.
2. High toxicity—complicated dosage regime.
3. Narrow therapeutic index—the margin between therapeutic dose and toxic dose is very narrow.
4. Host of interactions.

91. Digitalis acts at the following 4 sites:

1. *SA node:* In patients with heart failure with sinus rhythm, it slows the SA node mainly by its action on the vagus. It has direct effect on the SA node at higher concentrations. Its effect on the SA node in healthy person is negligible—stimulates vagus.
2. *AV node:* It slows the conduction through AV node and increases the refractory period mainly by it's effect on the vagus. This action is useful in blocking the numerous impulses passing down from the atria in atrial fibrillation.
   It has direct effect on AV node in higher concentrations as on the SA node—depresses AV node
3. *Purkinje conducting tissue:* It has direct effect. It slows-the conduction which may result in prolongation of P-R interval and lengthening of refractory period.
4. *Cardiac muscle cells:* It has direct effect. It increases conduction rate and shortens the refractory period in atria and ventricles. It has the opposite action to those on AV node and Purkinje system.

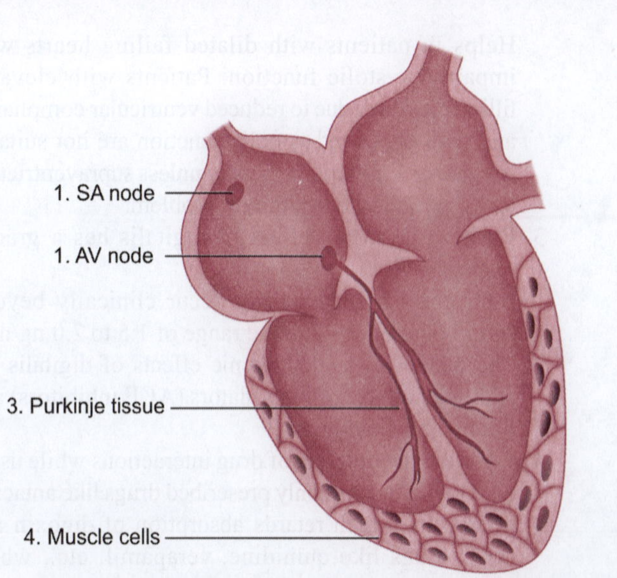

Fig. C-8: Digitalis action at various sites upon the failing heart

Digitalis has positive inotropic action by inhibiting the enzyme Na^+-K^+ ATPase in the walls of the cardiac muscle fibers. Normally this enzyme pumps sodium out of the cells whereas digitalis pumps the sodium into the cells through a separate sodium/calcium exchange mechanism. The sodium that enters the cell is then exchanged for extracellular calcium. As a result intracellular calcium is increased resulting in increased contractility of the cardiac muscle fibers.

92. Digitalis has 4 major effects on the heart:

1. It increases contractility and irritability acting on myocardium. It exerts inotropic action by increasing intracellular calcium availability.
2. Changes the electrical properties of AV conduction, thereby lowering the heart rate.
3. Potentiates vagal influence on the heart (chronotropic action—rate is reduced—partly by action on SA node.)
4. Important effect on cardiac muscle is to shift its force-velocity upwards.
   In short, it strengthens systole and lengthens diastole.

93. Digitalis is the most potent drug used in congestive heart failure because of its 4 advantages:

1. It improves depressed cardiac contraction.
2. It increases cardiac output.
3. It promotes diuresis.
4. It reduces filling pressure of the failing heart.

94. There are 4 guidelines to follow while using the digitalis in congestive heart failure:

1. Its use is undisputed in patients with congestive heart failure complicated by supraventricular arrhythmias.
2. It shows sustained improvement in cardiac function in congestive heart failure patients with sinus rhythm.

Helps in patients with dilated failing hearts with impaired systolic function. Patients with elevated filling pressures due to reduced ventricular compliance and with preserved systolic function are not suitable candidates for digitalis therapy unless supraventricular tachycardia is a concomitant problem.

3. Positive inotropic effect of digitalis has a graded response.
   Inotropic benefit may not occur clinically beyond serum digoxin level in the range of 1.5 to 2.0 ng/mL. The beneficial hemodynamic effects of digitalis are additive to those of vasodilators (ACE inhibitors) and β-adrenergic agonists.
4. Consider the problem of drug interactions while using digoxin with commonly prescribed drugs like antacids, neomycin, which retards absorption of digoxin and other drugs like quinidine, verapamil, etc., which increases serum digoxin levels.

95. Digitalis is particularly useful in the following 4 varities where the heart failure is associated with:

1. Increased ventricular end-diastolic pressure, such as hypertension, valvular or congenital heart disease.
2. Tachyarrhythmias, such as atrial flutter or fibrillation in slowing the rapid ventricular rate by its action of AV node. It is the drug of choice in controlling the ventricles to fill in between beats thereby increasing the cardiac efficiency. It is useful in certain supraventricular arrhythmias.
3. Impaired ventricular contractility secondary to chronic ischemic heart disease. It is ineffective when there is extensive ventricular damage from ischemic heart disease.
4. Depressed myocardial function by drug therapy with β-blockers or quinidine.

Relatively little beneficial effect in most forms of cardiomyopathy, myocarditis, beriberi with heart failure and mitral stenosis.

Thyrotoxicosis with sinus rhythm is usually adequately controlled by diuretics alone or diuretics plus vasodilators. Most patients of cardiac failure with sinus rhythm do not need maintenance with digitalis. (Digitalis is not useful in acute heart failure).

96. Patients with elevated filling pressures due to reduced ventricular compliance but with preserved systolic function at rest are not usually appropriate candidates for digitalis therapy unless supraventricular tachycardia is an associated problem. The effects of digitalis are not much beneficial in the following 4 conditions:

1. Digitalis is not of much benefit in isolated mitral stenosis with normal sinus rhythm unless right ventricular failure has supervened.
2. Digitalis has little benefit in patients with precordial tamponade or constrictive pericarditis except when there is invasion of the myocardium in the later.
3. Digitalis is of little use and may even be harmful in hypertropic obstructive cardiomyopathy because it can increase left ventricular outflow obstruction by augmenting the contractility of the hypertropic outflow tract segment.
4. Digitalis may not be beneficial in patients with left ventricular hypertrophy and well-preserved left ventricular ejection fraction in the presence of symptoms relating to filling pressures. Digitalis may be beneficial in later stages of hypertropic obstructive cardiomyopathy in which ventricular dilatation and congestive problems dominate over obstructive hemodynamics. Digitalis may improve symptoms of angina when it is associated with cardiomegaly and congestive heart failure. Patients with dilated failing hearts, impaired systolic function often manifesting S3 gallop show much benefit with digitalis.

97. There are 4 types of supraventricular arrhythmias where digitalis is of potential use:

1. *Atrial fibrillation:* It is one of the most common conditions. It is used to slow the ventricular rate and this gives time for the ventricles to fill between the beats and thereby increase the efficiency of ventricles in atrial fibrillation. All patients of cardiac failure with atrial fibrillation should be digitalized. Atrial fibrillation with rapid ventricular rate will respond to digitalis and may be converted to normal sinus rhythm. Atrial fibrillation of recent origin shows good response.
   Addition of β-blockers or verapamil may be useful in cases where ventricular rate is difficult to control without emergence of toxic symptoms. For example, untreated thyrotoxicosis when congestive heart failure is absent or minimal.
2. *Atrial flutter:* Usually with 2:1 AV block can be managed with digitalis in doses sufficient to produce a degree of AV block that results in ventricular rate of 70–100 min. Digitalis by its direct action on atrial muscle tends to convert into atrial fibrillation, which occasionally results in sinus rhythm if the drug is stopped.
3. *Paroxysmal supraventricular tachycardia—whether of atrial or atrioventricular junction origin:* This arrhythmia usually responds to digitalis when simple methods like carotid sinus pressure alone have failed. Combination of carotid sinus pressure and digitalis will often work better. It probably acts by vagal effect. Adenosine and verapamil 5–10 mg intravenously are the drug of choice. Other drugs used include quinidine, disopyramide, flecainide and amiodarone.

4. *Wolff-Parkinson-White syndrome:* Tachyarrhythmias associated with this form of conduction may be terminated or prevented by digitalis. Other antiarrhythmic drugs may be more effective.

98. The 4 differences between the two most commonly used preparations of digitalis are:

Table C-6

	Digoxin	*Digitoxin*
1. Usual daily maintenance dose	0.125 mg to 0.25 mg/ od to tds	0.1 to 0.2 mg
2. Excretion	85% renal	85% hepatic
3. Half-life	1.6 days	5 days
4. Protein binding	20%	90%

Digoxin is more commonly prescribed drug than digitoxin. Digitoxin is mainly administered in renal impairment. In uremia, the half life of digoxin is about 4 1/2 days whereas of digitoxin is about 7 days.

99. Following is the dosage schedule of most commonly prescribed digoxin. The 4 methods followed are:

1. 0.25 mg to 0.5 mg per day is the usual maintenance dose with normal renal function and with reasonable absorption of the drug. Digitalization can be obtained over a period of one week without loading dose with normal renal function. The digoxin is usually given for five days a week in order to prevent the toxic affects.
2. Oral digitalization of digoxin: Loading dose of 1–2 mg in divided doses depending on the speed of necessity of the clinical condition.
   1 mg immediately followed by 0.25 mg 6–8 hourly for 3–4 doses
   0.5 mg 6–8 hourly for 3–4 doses.
   0.25 mg 6–8 hourly for 3–4 doses.
3. Urgent digitalization by intravenous route.
   0.5 to 0.75 mg IV for 40 kg body weight (100 lb) as loading dose or can be given over half to one hour in 200 mL of 5% dextrose. Intractable life-threatening acute left ventricular failure is the main indication.
4. Dosage in children—Digoxin elixir is administered in children as follows:
   35 to 60 µg/kg for infants up to 1 year.
   30 to 40 µg/kg for 2 to 5 years.
   20 to 35 µg/kg for 5 to 10 years.
   10 to 15 µg/kg for children over 10 years.
   Digoxin is safe at 0.125 mg dose od is needed to treat patient with normal renal function. Serum digoxin levels have no correlation with clinical response. Therefore, monitoring is unnecessary unless toxicity is suspected or in the setting of worsening of renal failure, usually levels of less than 1 nmol/L are desirable. Withdrawal of digoxin have often shown worsening of clinical status.

100. The digitalis dose requirement is adjusted by 4 factors:

1. State of renal function (because 85% is excreted unchanged).
   Dialysis or exchange transfusion does not remove digoxin from the tissues.
2. State of GIT which affect the absorption (about 60% of the oral drug is absorbed in the gut).
3. State of liver function (because it is metabolized in the liver).
4. Conditions, which potentiates digitalis action, e.g. hypokalemia, hypoxia, hypomagnesemia and hypothyroidism.

Note: For a person of 70 kg weight—1.5 to 2.5 mg is required for full digitalization 0.25 to 0.5 mg is the usual maintenance dose, IV dose is 2/3rd of the total dose recommended. Digitalis maintenance dose should be reduced in elderly people when renal impairment is present and when used with drugs, which increases digoxin concentration as with amiodarone, verapamil.

101. Following factors influence the patients sensitivity to digitalis:

1. Advanced age : Partly due to decreased renal clearance of the drug.
2. Severity of underlying cardiac disease:
   – Advanced ventricular disease
   – Sick-sinus syndrome
   – AV node disease
3. Renal impairment: Especially with digoxin.
4. Electrolyte and acid-base imbalance: Most commonly caused by diuretic therapy.
5. Thyroid state:
   – Hypothyroidism—The half-life of the drug is prolonged
   – Hypothyroidism with cardiac failure
   – Cardiac failure with sinus rhythm
   – Cardiac failure with atrial fibrillation.
6. Respirotary disease: Mainly due to hypoxia, e.g. cor pulmonale.
7. Autonomic nervous system tone.
8. Concomitant drug administration, anesthetics, catecholamines and sympathomimetic amines, antiarrhythmic drugs.

Carotid sinus massage can give bed-side clue to impending digitalis toxicity. The common disorders that occur in response to carotid stimulation before they occur spontaneously are rhythm disorders such as second degree AV block, accelerated AV junctional rhythm, premature ventricular beats or bigeminy.

102. Digitalis side effects can be described under the following 4 groups:

Digitalis may cause almost any type of arrhythmia. Ventricular and junctional arrhythmias are more common than supraventricular arrhythmias.

1. *Four types of ventricular arrhythmias:* The following are the common ventricular arrhythmias in an ascending order of frequency and seriousness.
   i. Ventricular extra systoles (premature ventricular beats).
   ii. Pulsus bigeminus/Trigeminus.
   iii. Ventricular tachycardia.
   iv. Ventricular fibrillation.

   These are due to drug action on ventricular muscle cells causing increase in excitability by increasing the speed of conduction and reducing the refractory period. Hypokalemia partly potentiates this effect by the drug competing with potassium for binding sites on the enzyme Na^{+}-K^{+} ATPase. More amount of drug is bound to the enzyme and so potentiates the drug side effects.
2. *Four types of supraventricular arrhythmias:*
   i. Sinus arrhythmias.
   ii. Atrial extrasystole, (atrial premature contractions).
   iii. Paroxysmal supraventricular tachycardia with variable block.
   iv. Atrial flutter/fibrillation often with a very slow ventricular rate due to increased refractory period of the AV node.
3. *Four types of bradyarrhythmias:*
   i. Sinus bradycardia
   ii. Sinus block
   iii. Sinus arrest
   iv. Heart block of any degree including third degree heart block.

   These are due to slowing of the SA node and conduction along the bundle of His and increasing refractory period of AV node.
4. *Four types of noncardiac side effects:*
   i. Gastrointestinal distrubances :
      a. Anorexia/nausea and vomiting due to stimulation of vomiting center. This may give rise to cardiac cachexia in chronic digitalis intoxication.
      b. Diarrhea.
   ii. Visual disturbances including blurring of vision, or yellow vision known as cinchonism.
   iii. Nervous system changes including fatigue and restlessness.
   iv. Gynecomastia.

It is important to check for side effects frequently in every patient receiving digitalis. The therapeutic and toxic dose of digitalis are very narrow. One tablet of digitalis a day may be life saving whereas two tablets may be life-threatening. In most of the patients, the toxicity can be controlled by omitting the next one or two doses. It is a common practice to prescribe digitalis for 5 days a week. Better control of therapy and avoidance of toxicity is possible with serum digoxin assays.

103. There are 4 drugs that are useful in tachyarrhythmias resulting from digitalis intoxication after withdrawal of the drug:

1. *Phenytoin:* Useful in AV block, hyperkalemia, and in ectopic arrhythmias, such as PVBs. It has little adverse effect on the sinoatrial rate, atrial conduction, atrioventricular conduction of bundle of His conduction. 100 mg IV administered slowly every 5 minutes until control of arrhythmia occurs, followed by maintenance dose of 400 to 600 mg/day if the arrhythmia is controlled.
2. *Lidocaine:* Useful in ventricular tachyarrhythmias in the absence of preceding AV block. 100 mg IV bolus doses every 3 to 5 minutes followed by continuous infusion of 15 to 50 mg/kg weight per minute as required to control the arrhythmia.
3. *Potassium:* Useful in hypokalemia with ectopic tachyarrhythmias. Should be given in AV block.
4. *β-Blockers:* Useful in digitalis-toxic arrhythmias. They decrease the automaticity, shortens the refractory period of atrial muscle, ventricular muscle and purkinjee fibers and slow the conduction velocity. They should not be given in the presence of severe heart failure or AV block. β-blockers of short duration of action, such as esmolol may be preferable as an initial step.

   Quinidine and procainamide are not useful.

   Cardiac glycoside-binding resins, hemoperfusion, cardiac glycoside antibodies are on clinical trials.

   Direct current counter shock is not useful and may induce more serious arrhythmias. It should be tried when all other methods have failed in the presence of life-threatening arrhythmias. The risk is low when lower energy levels are used.

   Cardiac pacemaker may be required in digitalis induced AV block.

104. There are 4 commonly used antiarrhythmic drugs that cause elevation of serum digitalis levels:

1. Verapamil
2. Amiodarone—which competes with digitalis for protein binding
3. Nifedipine
4. Quinidine.

105. There are 4 common serum electrolyte disturbances.

1. Hypokalemia or Hyperkalemia
2. Hypomagnesemia
3. Hypercalcemia
4. Hyponatremia.

These are commonly caused by diuretic therapy.

The side effects are more in the setting of hypokalemia.

106. Hypomagnesemia caused by digitalis toxicity can induce:

1. Premature ventricular beats and ventricular tachycardia
2. Prolongation of PR and QT intervals
3. T-wave flattening
4. Atrial fibrillation and supraventricular tachycardia
5. Torsades de pointes
6. Coronary artery spasm
7. Ventricular fibrillation/sudden death in IHD
8. More extensive myocardial infarction.

107. Digitalis—some practical aspects:

1. Ensure a maintenance dose of 125—375 µg (0.125–0.375 mg) daily (5/7 days). Concentration should be monitored especially in cases of uncertainty about therapeutic levels have been achieved (range 6 h after dose 1.2–1.9 ng/mL).
2. Maintenance dose should be reduced in elderly people when renal impairment is present and when used with drugs that increase digoxin concentrations (amiodarone, verapamil).
3. Monitor potassium to avoid hypokalemia and renal function (S creatinine).
4. Digoxin toxicity.

Serious toxicity should be treated by correcting potassium concentration and with drugs, such as β-blockers and glycoside binding agents (cholestyramine) and in severe cases specific digoxin antibodies (digibind).

INOTROPIC DRUGS

The number of inotropics available has increased from the time, when we only had adrenaline, noradrenalin, and isoprenaline. The inotropic drugs can be divided into two main groups based on whether or not their actions depend upon increase, in intracellular cyclic adenosine monophosphate (cAMP)

108. There are 4 cAMP dependent groups of inotropic drugs.

1. Catecholamines
2. Cyclic nucleotide phosphodiesterase inhibitors (PDI)
3. Thyroid hormone
4. Glucagon

The cAMP independent agents include digoxin, calcium salts and α adrenergic agonists.

Sympathomimetic Amines

109. The effects of adrenergic nervous system are mediated by both α and β-adrenoceptors. These have been subdivided into 4 groups:

1. α-*1 receptors:* They cause peripheral vasoconstriction and increased myocardial contractility.
2. α-*2 receptors.*
3. β-*1 receptors:* They predominate in the myocardium and cause increased contractility, and heart rate (HR).
4. β-*2 receptors:* They predominate in the skeletal muscles and bronchi and cause muscle vasodilatation and bronchodilatation.

110. There are 4 sympathomimetic amines in use which act largely on β-adrenargic receptors to improve the pump performance:

1. Epinephrine and norepinephrine.
2. Isoprenaline.
3. Dopamine—immediate precursor of norepinephrine.
4. Dobutamine—synthetic catecholamine.

111. Epinephrine; It stimulates the β-1 receptors. There are 4 feature of epinephrine:

1. It improves myocardial contractility: It increases the force of systolic contraction, thereby shortening the systole.
2. It improves conduction through the AV node and therefore reduces the degree of AV block, if present.
3. It minimises the cardiac distension.
4. It optimizes coronary perfusion.

By its stimulation of β-1 receptors, it increases the heart rate (HR). These actions markedly increase the cardiac work and myocardial oxygen consumption (MVO_2).

Epinephrine in a dose of 0.02 to 0.08 mg/kg/min is predominantly, a β-agonist and it is only with higher dosage that peripheral constriction occurs.

112. Epinephrine is useful for the treatment of:

1. Acute heart failure.
2. Peripheral vascular collapse or anaphylaxis: It can be used as a bolus 2 to 10 mg for treating sudden episodes of hemodynamic compromise leading to hypotension.
3. Depressed ionotropic function at the end of cardio-pulmonary bypass (CPB). It is considered a drug of choice at the end of CPB. In higher doses, peripheral vascular effects predominate and arrhythmias may develop. Vasodilators can be used concomitantly during such times.
4. Coronary artery bypass grafting (CABG): It is safely used where internal mammary artery (IMA) has been used in CABG. It increases the flow in IMA proportional to the increase in systolic blood pressure and the patency of IMA graft is maintained.

It is useful after CPB in cardiac surgical patients in the dose of 0.04 mg/kg/min. Epinephrine improves cardiac index (CI) in all patients with increase in mean arterial pressure (MAP), heart rate (HR) and left ventricular stroke work index (LVSWI) without change in systemic vascular resistance (SVC). In addition, no arrhythmias occurred with its use.

113. Norepinephrine: It is a naturally occurring catecholamine. It has 4 features:

1. It has a predominantly alpha stimulating effect (vs epinephrine-β-1 stimulator)
2. It increases systemic vascular resistance (SVR) by arteriolar constriction.
3. It is indicated primarily to maintain BP when there is marked decrease in SVR (peripheral vascular failure).
4. It is frequently used during normothermic by-pass to maintain satisfactory mean arterial pressure (MAP).

It can be used as bolus of 2 to 5 mg followed by infusion, if necessary. Once the MAP has risen to satisfactory level, it can be discontinued and some other inotrope, such as dopamine can be substituted.

114. There are 4 features of isoprenaline.

1. It is a synthetic catecholamine.
2. It has a β-adrenergic receptor activity. It stimulates both β-1 and β-2 receptors leading to profound cardiac stimulation that is accompanied by significant dilatation of vascular smooth muscle.
3. It increases myocardial contractility and HR. The CO, however, may not be increased due to impairment in cardiac filling resulting from tachycardia and peripheral vasodilatation. It increases myocardial oxygen consumption (MVO_2). Due to these effects, it is not considered as a suitable choice in the presence of coronary artery disease.
4. It has pulmonary vasodilator property.

115. Isoprenaline is useful in the following conditions:

1. It is very effective in the management of acute bradyarrhythmias or AV block. It can be administered as a bolus of 5 to 10 mg followed by an infusion (0.02 to 0.04 mg/kg/min), if necessary.
2. It is useful as a potent chromotropic agent in the presence of profound β-blockade that may be seen in some patients of CAD.
3. It is useful in the management of increased pulmonary vascular resistance (PVR) due to any cause thus helping to control right ventricular failure.
4. It is useful in mitral valve disease with pulmonary hypertension. It is useful in some patients undergoing mitral valve surgery.
5. Cardiogenic shock.
6. Endotoxic shock.
7. Acute Stokes-Adams attack.
8. Evaluation of congenital heart defects.

116. Dobutamine has the following 4 features:

1. It is a synthetic catecholamine
2. It is a powerful β-1 stimulator
3. It, therefore improves
   i. Ventricular contractility
   ii. Stroke volume (SV)
   iii. Cardiac output (CO)
   iv. Systemic pressure.
4. It is also a β-2 receptor stimulator causing peripheral vasodilatation.

It has wide acceptance in clinical practice due to these effects of improved myocardial contractility and a degree of peripheral vasodilatation.

It has no effect on the dopaminergic receptors in the kidney, so it does not produce specific renal vasodilatation. However, renal blood flow is improved by increasing CO.

117. Dobutamine is useful in the treatment of following 4 conditions:

1. Low cardiac output states associated with chronic congestive failure (CCF), refractory failure.
2. Cardiogenic shock in severe acute MI (see chapter F 194, 195).
3. Cardiac surgery—cardiogenic shock during surgery/ spasm of internal mammary artery.
4. Excessive β-blockade.

It has favorable effects on coronary blood flow and myocardial oxygen consumption (MVO_2). It also decreases wall stress by reducing diastolic and systolic ventricular volumes while increasing mean arterial pressure (MAP) and maintaining HR relatively unchanged.

Due to these beneficial hemodynamic effects, its use during and immediately following cardiac surgery is common. It has been compared with epinephrine in patients following CABG. It was found that both drugs (epinephrine 0.01d to 0.03 mg/kf/min and dobutamine (2.5 to 5 mg/kg/ min) significantly improve hemodynamics. However, dobutamine increases HR, significantly more than epinephrine. It can be administered in the dosage of 2.5 to 5 mg/kg/min that can be increased up to 15 mg/kg/min.

Previous trials evaluating intermittent dobutamine IV infusion in patients with chronic heart failure was stopped prematurely because of excess mortality in the group taking dobutamine.

118. The 4 features of dopamine are:

1. It is the naturally occurring catecholamine. It is an intermediate compound in the synthesis of epinephrine and norepinephrine.
2. It produces ionotropic effect by stimulating β-1 receptors.
3. It also stimulates α-1 receptors by releasing endogenous norepinephrine to produce considerable vasoconstriction.

4. It has an unique action of stimulating dopaminergic receptors in the renal, mesenteric and coronary arterial beds. This results in smooth muscle relaxation and vasodilatation.

119. Dopamine has the following 4 actions:

1. Systemic vascular resistance (SVR): It causes greater increase in SVR as compared with dopamine. It does not stimulate vascular β-2 receptors and therefore, its unopposed stimulation of α-1 receptors is responsible for overall vasoconstriction. It may, therefore be necessary to combine vasodilator along with dopamine infusion.
2. It also increases pulmonary artery (PA) pressure.
3. It increases PVR.
4. It increases left ventricular filling pressure.

Dopamine is frequently administered in combination with other inotropes for its beneficial effect on renal function at low dose (2 to 4 mg/kg/min). The higher doses should be avoided as they cause increase in HR and vasoconstriction. The maximal dopaminergic receptor stimulation is observed in the dose of 2 to 3 mg/kg/min. In the intermediate dose range of 2 to 6 mg/kg/min, cardiac β-1 receptors are stimulated leading to increase in CO. This further improves the renal blood flow. α adrenergic stimulation begins at the dose of 5 mg/kg/min producing vasoconstriction. In critically sick patients, dopamine is combined with more potent inotropic drugs to improve renal blood flow.

120. Dopexamine: The quest for 'ideal' inotropic agent has resulted in the development of many new agents. A new synthetic catecholamine, dopexamine is one among them. It is strictly related to dopamine and dobutamine. Dopexamine has the following 4 features.

1. It stimulates DA1 receptors.
2. It stimulates DA2 receptors.
3. It stimulates β-2 receptors.
4. It is a mild stimulator of β-1 receptors.

It has no effect on α-receptors. It has also an inhibitory action in the neuronal catecholamine uptake mechanism that is most probably responsible for the positive inotropic action of this drug.

121. Dopexamine is indicated in the following 4 conditions:

1. *Chronic congestive cardiac failure (CCF):* It reduces after load through systemic arterial vasodilatation. The cardiac stimulation is achieved by direct and indirect (i.e. inhibition of catecholamine uptake) positive inotropic mechanism.
2. *Following cardiac surgery:* It is similar to chronic CCF.
3. *Septic shock:* It can safely be used to improve myocardial performance in shock.
4. *When there is need for renal vasodilatation:* It increases renal perfusion by selective renal vasodilatation and mild cardiac stimulation.

Its effect is most pronounced when used as a continuous infusion of 1 to 4 mg/kg/min. However, HR can be substantially raised in higher doses leading to myocardial oxygen consumption (MVO_2). Thus, dopexamine can be used where its systemic and renal vasodilators properties are useful. It is not available in India.

DIURETICS

122. Diuretics can be classified into 4 groups:

1. *Thiazide diuretics:* Act at the cortical portion of distal end of the ascending limb of loop of Henle. They are moderately effective.
   For example, chlorothiazide 0.5 to 1 mg daily. Hydrochlorothiazide 25 to 100 mg daily, chlorthalidone 2.5 to 10 mg daily.
   They act by inhibiting the reabsorption of sodium and chloride ions just proximal to the distal tubule. Some of the unabsorbed sodium is subsequently absorbed in the distal tubule where it is exchanged for potassium and hydrogen ions, which pass out in the urine. As a consequence, thiazide diuretics may cause hypokalemic alkolosis.
2. *Loop diuretics:* They act at the ascending limb of loop of Henle mainly by inhibiting the chloride ions in the ascending loop.
   For example, furosemide 40–160 mg daily, ethacrynic acid 50–100 mg daily, bumetanide 1 to 4 mg daily.

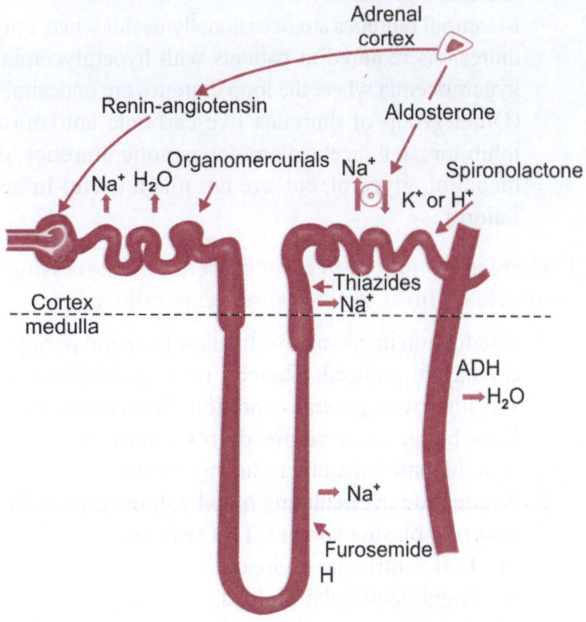

Fig. C-9: Diagram of salt and water exchange in the kidneys. Major sites of action of diuretics

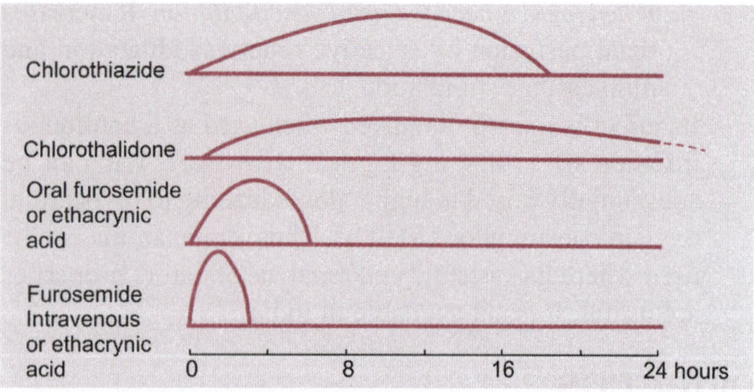

Fig. C-10: Comparison of duration of action of commonly used diuretics

3. *Potassium sparing diuretics or distal tubular diuretics.* For example, spironolactone 25–200 mg daily, triamterene 50–200 mg daily, amiloride 5–20 mg daily.
   i. Spironolactone is a true aldosterone antagonist—acts by antagonizing aldosterone action. It is inactive in adrenalectomized persons.
   ii. Triamterene and amiloride act by directly reducing potassium transport mechanism.

   Potassium sparing diuretics act by inhibiting the reabsorption of sodium from the distal tubule. As a consequence, reduced amounts of potassium and hydrogen are exchanged for sodium.

   In the presence of renal impairment, this can result in metabolic acidosis and hyperkalemia that occasionally may be dangerous.
4. *Organomercurials:* Act on proximal convoluted tubules, e.g. mersalyl.

   Mercurial diuretics are occasionally useful when a rapid diuresis is required in patients with hyperglycemia or hyperuricemia where the loop diuretics are undesirable. (Other group of diuretics like carbonic anhydrase - inhibitors, e.g. acetazolamide; osmotic diuretics, e.g. mannitol, glycerol, etc. are not much useful in heart failure).

123. There are 4 major effects of diuretics in improving the clinical features of congestive heart failure:

1. A reduction in edema: Both pulmonary and peripheral edema are reduced. Thereby relieves breathlessness and improves general condition. Sometimes, patient feels better even before diuresis starts because of venodilatation thereby reducing preload.
2. A reduction in circulating blood volume especially by lowering plasma volume. This reduces:
   i. Left ventricular preload.
   ii. Right ventricular preload.
   iii. Jugular pressure.
   iv. Hepatic congestion.
3. A slight reduction in ventricular size so that ventricle contracts more effectively.
4. A reduction in left ventricular after load to a less but significant extent as a result of peripheral vasodilatation. It improves left ventricular function.

124. There are 4 guidelines in using diuretic therapy:

Diuretics remain the cornerstone of the treatment of congestive cardiac failure.

1. Bed rest combined with moderate salt restriction and a diuretic alone may result in a clinically important degree of fluid loss and decline in ventricular filling pressure. Vasodilators may be ineffective if not administered with a diuretic.
2. Thiazide diuretics may be used in the treatment of mild congestive heart failure but they are ineffective when the GFR is less than 30 mL/min.
3. Furosemide, ethacrinic acid or bumetanide is preferred in moderate to advanced congestive heart failure. Since absorption of loop diuretics by oral route may be reduced in advanced congestive heart failure due to intestinal congestion, intravenous route is preferred initially to achieve control of heart failure.
4. Patients on long-term diuretic therapy should be watched for side effects like hypokalemia, hypomagnesemia, carbohydrate intolerance and hyperuricemia. Combination of loop diuretics like furosemide with potassium sparing diuretics like spiranolactone or amiloride may prevent hypokalemia, hypomegnesemia and should be used.

125. There are 4 points in the selection of diuretics in heart failure:

1. In chronic cardiac edema of mild to moderate degree without hyperglycemia, hyperuricemia or hypokalemia—oral thiazides, e.g. cyclopenthiazide 0.25 to 0.5 mg daily. Potassium supplements are usually necessary. Better guided by serum potassium levels.
2. In severe refractory failure—ethacrinic acid or furosemide either alone or in combination with spironolactone, triamterene or amiloride is useful. Furosemide 40 mg; may require 160 mg or more daily. Intravenous is needed in severe cases.
3. In very severe heart failure rarely combination of thiazide, loop diuretic and potassium sparing diuretics are required, e.g. hydrochlorothaizide 50 mg + furosemide 40 mg + amiloride 5 mg. Do not use potassium supplements and potassium sparing drugs.
4. In heart failure wit h severe secondary aldosteronism spironolactone may be effective.

126. The diuretic like furosemide IV in acute myocardial infarction with heart failure causes fall in left ventricular filling pressure and improvement in orthopnea and dyspnea by 4 ways:

1. By decreasing the plasma volume by massive diuresis.
2. By decreasing cardiac output.
3. By decreasing systemic blood pressure.
4. By improving coronary perfusion.

127. Diuretics may cause the following 4 side effects:

1. *Dehydration:* It may result in hypovolemia and causes postural hypotension.
2. *Electrolyte imbalance:*
   i. Hypokalemia alkalosis may be caused by thiazide or loop diuretics.
   ii. Hyperkalemia and metabolic acidosis may be caused by the potassium sparing diuretics.
   iii. Hyponatremia may occasionally result from increased excretion of sodium.
   iv. Hypomagnesemia may be caused by thiazide or loop diuretics although predominantly by the latter.
3. *Metabolic effects:*
   i. Hyperuricemia—thiazide and loop diuretics commonly cause hyperuricemia and may occasionally precipitate clinical gout.
   ii. Carbohydrate intolerance—thiazides and less commonly loop diuretics may precipitate or worsen diabetes mellitus.
   iii. Lipids—thiazides may cause hyperlipidemia.
4. *Endocrine disorders:* Gynecomastia and impotence in males may be caused by spironolactone by antagonizing androgen activity. Use of thiazides in hypertension has been shown to double the incidence of impotence in middle-aged men.

128. Some points to be noted during diuretic therapy:

1. The lowest possible dose of diuretic should be used to prevent sustained volume overload.
2. A patient of right-sided heart failure often must tolerate some degree of peripheral edema.
3. In some patients of heart failure, a moderate degree of renal insufficiency is tolerated to maintain relative euvolemic (urine albumin may be 1+ or 2+ with normal serum creatinine level).
4. In some relatively asymptomatic patients who have no signs of fluid retention supported by a relatively low level of BNP level may not need any diuretic therapy.

The concept of diuretic therapy is evolving. In such cases, check the dietary sodium indiscretion and medication noncompliance.

A combination of loop diuretic plus potassium sparing diuretic plus thiazide diuretic may be helpful.

Add thiazide diuretics 30 minutes before loop diuretics for synergistic response if necessary.

129. Advantages of potassium sparing diuretics.

1. Aldosterone receptor antagonists, such as spironolactone is used in patients with heart failure. Concept of incomplete blockade of renin-angiotensin-aldosterone system (RAAS) by ACE inhibitors have led to the use of aldosterone antagonists, which showed significant benefits in advanced heart failure. Spironolactone is indicated in advanced heart failure (NYHA III and IV), in LVEF less than 35%, already treated with ACEI/and β-blockers without significant renal dysfunction (creatinine > 2.5 mg/dL) or hyperkalemia > 5 mEq/L.
2. It is given in low doses 25 mg per day if creatinine is < 2.0 mg/dL and potassium < 4.5 mEq/L usually no need of increasing the dose. Potassium supplements should be reduced or stopped.
3. Spironolactone should be monitored in one to two weeks after initiation and monitored at regular intervals. Some patients may need lower dose 12.5 mg per day or 25 mg on alternate day at initiation or during follow up. If creatinine is 2–2.5 mg/dL or potassium is 4.50–5 mEq/L. One trial has demonstrated that Eplerenone 25–50 mg per day has shown significant mortality benefits in post MI heart failure.
4. Watch the side effects of hyperkalemia particularly in concomitant renal insufficiency and diabetes with renal tubular acidosis, which requires dose reduction or discontinuation.

Painful gynecomastia or galactorrhea is common with spironolactone, but rare with eplerenone.

VASODILATORS

130. Use of vasodilators in the management of congestive cardiac failure has been introduced in the last decade. Vasodilators act by reducing the arteriolar and venous vasoconstriction thereby reducing the work of the heart.

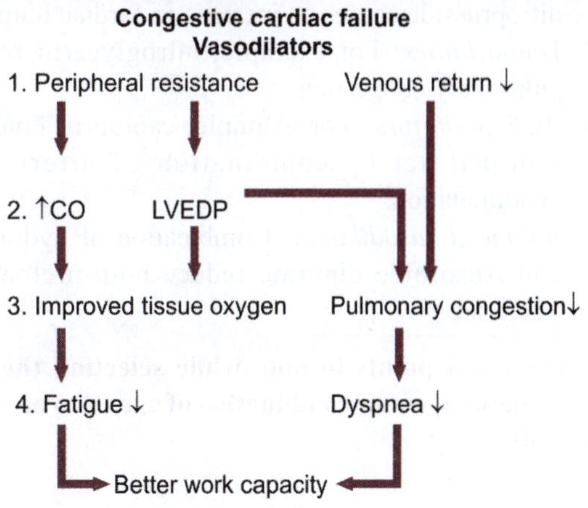

Fig. C-11

131. Vasodilators act in 4 ways to relieve signs and symptoms in acute or chronic intractable heart failure secondary to coronary arterial disease, cardiomyopathy or valvular regurgitation:

1. They reduce the impedance to left ventricular ejection, i.e. after load with only mild reduction in arterial pressure—thereby lowering the cardiac workload.
2. They reduce pulmonary capillary wedge pressure.
3. They reduce elevated left ventricular end-diastolic pressure (LVEDP) which in turn might improve subendocardial perfusion.
4. They increase cardiac output.

The addition of vasodilator drugs to the inotropic therapy of patients with CCF is one of the important advances in the management of heart disease. It has been shown that vasodilators can be used to shift the Starling curve up and to the left, thereby reducing the pulmonary congestion and improving the CO. This improvement in cardiac performance is associated with decrease in MVO_2. In a patient with moderate to severe ventricular dysfunction, SVR is elevated because of increased catecholamine levels. In this situation, addition of vasodilator helps to decrease the outflow resistance, thereby increasing the CO. Simultaneous infusion of volume may be necessary to avoid preload and afterload mismatch as concomitant venodilatation may lead to reduction of intracardiac volume.

132. Vasodilator therapy is particularly useful in the following 4 conditions:

1. In acute cardiac failure due to myocardial infarction.
2. In refractory congestive cardiac failure.
3. In acute pulmonary edema – if it is not precipitated by myocardial infarction is often associated hypertension.
4. In dilated (congestive) cardiomyopathy—(DCM).

133. Vasodilators can be described under 4 groups:

1. *Arterial vasodilators:* For example, sodium nitroprusside causes an increase in cardiac output.
2. *Venodilators:* For example, nitroglycerin reduces pulmonary congestion.
3. *ACE inhibitors:* For example, captopril, enalapril, ramipril act by combination of arterial and venodilatation.
4. *Balanced vasodilators:* Combination of hydralazine and isosorbide dinitrate reduce both preload and afterload.

134. There are 4 points to note while selecting the ideal vasodilator agent or combination of agents to any given patient:

1. Is it acute or chronic heart failure ?
   In acute failure—it should have rapid onset of action and short duration, e.g. IV sodium nitroprusside—but its use requires careful hemodynamic monitoring.
   In chronic congestive heart failure the drug should be orally effective and should last its action at least for 6 hours, e.g. hydralazine, prazocin, captopril.
2. If the primary defect is reduction of cardiac output and/or mitral regurgitation—arterial vasodilator is the drug of choice, e.g. hydralazine (25–100 mg/12 h/po).
3. If pulmonary edema is the main problem—Venodialator is the drug of choice, e.g. nitroglycerin (isosorbide dinitrate 10 mg/8 h/po). Isosorbide and hydralazine combination has shown improvement in the quality of life.
4. If both reduction in cardiac output and pulmonary edema are the principle problems—the drug of choice is that which acts on both arterial and venous side, e.g. prazocin or captopril/enalapril.

Prazocin 5 mg initially then 1 mg/8 h; captopril 25 mg/bd/po, enalapril 5–10 mg/od/po; ACE inhibitors have shown improvement in longevity.

135. Sodium nitroprusside: It acts by direct relaxation of arteriolar and venular smooth muscle, thus decreasing both preload and after load.

The hemodynamic effects of sodium nitroprusside patients with low cardiac output include.

1. Decrease in systemic vascular resistance (SVR).
2. Increase in cardiac output (CO).
3. Decrease in
   i. Pulmonary arterial pressure
   ii. Pulmonary capillary wedge pressure (PCWP)
   iii. Central venous pressure (CVP)
   iv. Pulmonary vascular resistance (PVR)
4. Decrease in mean arterial pressure (MAP) in patients with elevated MAP.

It is administered as an IV infusion in a starting dose of 0.5 mg/kg/min. The dose can be increased further depending upon the hemodynamic response. Reflex tachycardia that is commonly observed in patients with normal CI during nitroprusside infusion for induced hypotension, is rarely a problem in patients receiving nitroprusside for after-load reduction in low cardiac output states. In fact, heart rate may sometimes be decreased due to improvement in SVR and CO.

It can be used during cardiac surgery to control systemic as well as pulmonary hypertension and for the treatment of low output state along with inotropes.

136. Nitroglycerin predominantly affects the venous system with less effects on arteries. It, therefore, decreases preload with little or no effect on after load. In patients with congestive cardiac failure, it causes reduction in:

1. Pulmonary arterial pressure (PAP)
2. Pulmonary capillary wedge pressure (PCWP)
3. Central venous pressure (CVP)
4. Pulmonary vascular resistance (PVR).

The cardiac output may remain unchanged and even decreases, if decrease in preload is significant.

137. It is useful in:

1. Systemic hypertension
2. Pulmonary hypertension
3. Low cardiac output states in combination with ionotrope
4. During CABG: Due to its property on coronary artery dilatation, it may be preferred over sodium nitroprusside. It is not an effective agent for the treatment of systemic hypertension. It is administered as an IV infusion in the dose of 0.5 to 5 mg/kg/min.

138. There are 4 modes of administration of vasodilators in use:

Table C-7

1. Intravenous	Nitroglycerin Sodium nitroprusside Phentolamine	10–20 µg/min IVI 5–15 µg/kg/min IVI 5–15 µg/min IVI
2. Oral	Nitroglycerin Isosorbide dinitrate Hydralazine Phenoxybenzamine Phentolamine Prazocin Captopril Enalapril Nifedipine	5–20 mg q2h po 10–60 mg q4h po 10–100 mg q6h po 10–20 mg q8h po 50 mg q4–6h po 1–5 mg q6h po 6.25–25.0 mg q6–8h po 2.5 mg qid to 15 mg po bid 5–20 mg qid po
3. Sublingual	Nitroglycerin Isosorbide dinitrate	10–40 mg 6 hr sl 5–20 mg 2 hr sl
4. Transdermal	Nitroglycerin	5–60 mg transdermal 1–2 (in ointment) 10–60 cm^2 (patches)

139. There are 4 vasodilators in use which act mainly on arterial site. The arterial dilators reduce the peripheral vascular resistance and helps to increase cardiac output. Therefore, they are particularly useful in relief of symptoms due to low cardiac output such as fatigue.

Table C-8

	Duration of action	Dosage
Phenoxybenzamine	Oral/IV	5–15 mg/kg/min IVI 10–20 mg q8h PO
Phentolamine	Oral	50 mg q4–6h PO
Hydralazine	Oral	10–100 mg q6h PO
Nifedipine	Oral	5–20 mg q PO 10–40 mg 6th h SL

Phenoxybenzamine, phentolamine action is by direct alpha adrenoceptor blockade. Hydralazine acts by direct relaxation of vascular smooth muscle.

Nifedipine acts by calcium channel blockade. Calcium channel blockers usually are not used in heart failure.

140. There are 4 vasodilators in use which act both on arterial and venous sites:

Table C-9

	Route	Duration	Dosage
Sodium nitroprusside	IVI	minutes	5–15 mg/min IVI
Captopril	Oral	hours	6.25–25 mg 6–8 po
Enalapril	Oral	hours	mg to 15 mg bid po
Prazocin	Oral	hours	1–5 mg 6 h po

141. Nitroglycerin is a venodilator. This can be administered by 4 ways:

1. Intravenous
2. Oral (tablets and spray)
3. Sublingual
4. Transdermal.

142. ACE inhibitors (Angiotensin-converting enzyme inhibitors) are indicated in 4 conditions.

1. Hypertension.
2. Cardiac failure even in refractory heart failure.
3. LV dysfunction with compensated cardiac failure.
4. Diabetes mellitus with proteinuria.

Do not give potassium sparing diuretics while giving **ACE Inhibitors (ACEI)**.

143. There are 4 angiotensin-converting enzyme inhibitors (ACEI) that are commonly used in cardiovascular diseases.

Table C-10

1. Captopril	6.25–25 mg 6–8 hr po
2. Enalapril	2.5 to 20 mg bd po
3. Ramipril	1.5–10 mg od/bd po
4. Lisinopril	5–40 mg qid po

144. ACE inhibitors (captopril or enalapril) are effective in patients with mild as well as severe heart failure. The 4 advantages with ACE inhibitors are:

1. They show consistant hemodynamic improvement by increase in cardiac output and ejection fraction.
2. They show improvement in exercise tolerance.
3. They show reduction in cardiac dimensions.
4. They show significant symptomatic improvement by enhancing the sense of well being and prolong the life.

They showed favorable effect on survival in congestive heart failure and may be superior to the combination of hydralazine and isosorbide dinitrate.

145. It is useful in:

1. Asymptomatic LV dysfunction.
   They are effective in asymptomatic LV systolic dysfunction, reduces the development of heart failure.
2. LV dysfunction after AMI: ACEI have shown lower mortality in patients with impaired systolic function after MI irrespective of symptoms.
3. Slows disease progression.
   ACEI influence the natural course of chronic heart failure.
4. In severe heart failure.

146. ACE inhibitors (captopril or enalapril) in cardiac failure help in 4 ways:

(Congestive cardiac failure patients show high plasma renin level, caused by diuretic therapy, increased coronary artery resistance with diminished coronary reserve).

1. LVH is corrected—possibly by reversal of angiotensin mediated stimulation of protein biosynthesis.
   Reduces both end-systolic and end-diastolic ventricular dimensions (seen on echocardiography). Reduces pulmonary wedge pressure, right atrial pressure.
2. Improves coronary blood flow.
3. Lowers angiotensin II, noradrenaline and vasopressin.
   Deficiencies of serum potassium and magnesium are corrected.
4. Ventricular ectopics are diminished.

If forward failure is predominant with low cardiac output, fatigue—ACE inhibitors are useful. Captopril or enalapril cause profound fall in BP due to arteriolar dilatation.

If possible give captopril test dose of 5 mg po and monitor BP

Increase the dose to 25 mg/8 h po 1 hour before food.

Enalapril (5 mg, 10 mg tablets)—initial dose is 2.5 mg od gradually increased to 10–20 mg over a period of 2 to 4 weeks.

Maximum dose is 40 mg od. BP and renal function should be monitored both before and during treatment with enalapril because severe hypotension and rarely consequent renal failure have been reported.

Consider recent diuretic therapy and salt/volume depletion before initiating therapy with ACE inhibitors. Diuretic dose should be reduced before starting ACE inhibitors.

ACE inhibitors are used in conjuction with digitalis and diuretics.

Do not give potassium supplements or potassium sparing diuretic while giving ACE inhibitors. Dangerous hyperkalemia may occur.

Recent randomized placebo controlled study, Randomized Aldactone Evaluation Study (RALES) reported that hyperkalemia is uncommon when low dose spironolactone (< 25 mg daily) is combined with an ACEI. Risk factors for developing hyperkalemia include spironolactone dose more than 50 mg per day, high doses of ACEI, or evidence of renal impairment. Serum potassium and creatinine are measured within 5–7 days when ACEI are combined with potassium sparing diuretics until the levels are stable and then every 1–3 months.

Do not use ACE inhibitors in acute myocardial infarction with low blood pressure. Higher the blood pressure more the advantage. Useful in large myocardial infarction with significant left ventricular dysfunction but not in mild myocardial infarction.

Start after 3 to 16 days after myocardial infarction. Use short acting ACE inhibitors than long-acting.

147. There are 4 precautions to be taken while using ACE inhibitors in congestive heart failure:

1. With potassium supplements
2. With potassium sparing diuretics

} They tend to increase the serum potassium levels

3. Excessive hypotension is the major hazard especially in patients who are already being treated with diuretics and is contraindicated in patients with already marked hypotension.
4. They are contraindicated in intrinsic renal disease with renal failure and bilateral renal artery stenosis. (see chapter B-146)

148. Dangerous hyperkalemia may occur when ACE inhibitors are used in combination with potassium sparing agents or large doses of oral potassium. This combination can:

Precipitate hyperkalemia when used in heart failure. One has to be careful in monitoring serum electrolytes, when such condition exists, ECG shows characteristic tall tented T waves, absent P waves denoting atrial arrest, wide bizarre QRS complexes. Even a pacemaker may not be able to depolarize such a heart in hyperkalemia.

Metabolic correction is an absolute necessity in patients with oliguria, hyperkalemia, acidosis and cardiac abnormalities in ECG.

As an emergency treatment, the following can be instituted for the treatment of hyperkalemia, particularly prior to sending the patient to an advanced center for further management.

Table C-12

	Onset of action	Duration
1. 10% calcium gluconate 10 mL IV slowly followed by a slow infusion of the following	5 min	1–2 hr
2. Glucose and insulin infusion	15–30 min	4 hr
3. 7.5% sodium bicarbonate infusion	15–60 min	4 hr
4. Hypertonic saline	30–60 min	4 hr

The same principle of treatment for hyperkalemia can be modified by giving 10% calcium gluconate, 10 mL IV followed by a slow intravenous infusion of the following:

Table C-13

1. 10% dextrose or 5% dextrose saline	300 mL
2. 7.5% sodium bicarbonate	100 mL
3. 50% glucose	100 mL
4. Regular insulin	20 IU

Calcium ions counteract the neuromuscular effect of potassium on the myocardium. Sodium bicarbonate, hypertonic saline, and glucose with insulin act by transfer of potassium from the extracellular to the intracellular compartment.

Other methods are:

Exchange resin	Rectal	30–90 min
	Oral	2–12 hr
Hemodialysis		1–2 hr

Cation exchange resins like sodium polysterens sulfonate (kayexalate or resonium A, winthrop laboratories) bind potassium. Each gram of resin binds approximately 1 mEq of potassium (approximately 20 mEq of potassium is released from the cells in the body daily). The recommended dose is 15 to 30 g mixed with 20 mL. 50% glucose or 70% sorbitol or along with a laxative orally, the dose being repeated every 8 h. The hypertonic solutions and the laxative help to propel the resins through the gut, since otherwise it tends to get insipissated. Rectally, it is given in a dose of 30 g as a retention enema with a cleansing enema given 2 h later. It should be realised that the patients absorb about 2.5 mEq sodium for each gram of resin taken. Hence, resins in the calcium phase have been tried instead. Hemodialysis is very effective for the removal of potassium from the system. Peritoneal dialysis is less effective.

Hypokalemia rarely requires to be treated, unless severe or unless the patient is receiving digitalis. It is safer to give potassium orally than parentally, When given parentally, concentrations above 60 mEq per liter and rates above 3 mL/min should be avoided.

149. Initial evaluation of heart failure:

1. Note the heart failure staging and NYHA functional class.
2. Note the plasma B-type natriuretic peptide level as an aid to diagnosis, management and prognosis of heart failure.
3. Determine the systolic versus diastolic dysfunction.
4. Determine the cause beyond LV function (other than cardiac cause) by complete metabolic profile, blood counts, thyroid function, ECG and chest X-ray.

150. Nonpharmacological therapies:

1. Fluid restriction—< 2 L/day increase to < 1.5 L/day when serum sodium < 130 mg/dL.
2. Salt restriction—≤ 3 g sodium for mild HF (NYHA I and II) ≤ 2 g sodium diet for advanced HF (NYHA III and IV).
3. Patient education regarding diet, medication, fluid management activity, signs and symptoms of worsening conditions and daily weight monitoring as advised.
4. Cardiac rehabilitation—home health consult recommended.

151. Drug dosing of common medicines in chronic heart failure:

Table C-13

Drug	State (mg)	Target (mg)
I. ACEI/ARBs		
Captopril	6.25 to 12.5 tid	50 tid
Enalapril	2.5 to 5 bid	10 bid
Lisinopril	2.5 to 5 qd	20 qd
Ramipril	1.25–2.5 bid	5 bid
Quinapril	5 bid	20 bid
Fosinopril	2.5 or 5 bid	20 bid
Benazepril	2.5 or 5 bid	20 bid
Moexipril	7.5 qd	30 qd
Trandolapril	1 qd	4 qd
Candesartan	16 qd	32 qd
Valsartan	80 qd	160 qd
Losartan	12.5 to 25 qd	50 qd
Irbesartan	150 qd	300 qd
Telmisartan	40 qd	80 qd

Contd...

Contd...

Drug	*State (mg)*	*Target (mg)*
II. Vasodilators		
Hydralazine	25 qid	50–75 qid
Isosorbide dinitrate	10 to 20 tid	20 to 80 tid
III. Diuretics		
Furosemide	10 qd (IV) 20 qd (po)	As required
Bumetanide	1 qd	As required
Torsemide	10 qd	As required
Ethacrynic acid	50 qd	As required
Hydrochlorothiazide	25 qd	As required
Triamterene	50 qd	As required
Metolazone	2.5 qd	As required
Spironolactone	12.5 to 25 qd	25 qd
Eplerenone	50 qd	100 qd
IV. β-blockers/α–and β blockers		
Metoprolol	25 qd	150 to 200 qd
Bisoprolol	1.25 qd	10 qd
Carvedilol	3.125 bid	6.25 to 25 bid

152. β-adrenergic blockers: Once considered as contraindication to patients with heart failure are now considered first line therapy in heart failure (NYHA II or III) because of consistent decrease in mortality. The exact mechanism is still not well understood though it is said to act on neurohumoral axis.

1. These are particular benefit in patients with post-MI with tachycardia and should be started promptly before or concurrently with ACEI.
2. The general principal is to "start slow and go slow". The initial dose is slowly titrated every 2 to 4 weeks over 3 to 4 months to the target dose provided the patient can tolerate the adverse effects.
3. Only carvedilol, bisoprolol, and metoprolol succinate have been approved for the medical treatment of chronic heart failure. Atenolol and metoprolol are relatively inexpensive but there is no evidence to support this.
4. These drugs are used to prolong the survival and they usually do not improve the symptoms.

153. Side effects of β-blockers are:

1. Light-headedness or dizziness.
2. Significant bradycardia.
3. Advanced heart block is a contraindication unless permanent pacemaker is available.
4. Hypotension, it is managed by lowering the dose of diuretics and ACEI and by adjusting the timing of the drug. β-blockers are given two hours after vasodilator therapy or ACEI are given in the evening and β-blockers in the morning. Carvedilol with its non-selective α-blocking vasodilating effects cause greater BP lowering effect than selective β-blocker such as metoprolol.

154. Guidelines for β-blockers usage:

1. Titrated to target dose as tolerated.
2. Use in NYHA II or III (may be used in NYHA I patients with history of MI or hypertension or NYHA IV patients who are euvolemic, no signs and symptoms of volume overload.
3. Reduce the dose if dizziness or light-headedness, worsening of heart failure (edema, weight gain, dyspnea, or significant bradycardia).
4. Contraindicated in bronchospasm (asthma, bradycardia < 50 beats/min or < 60 beats/min with symptoms, heart block, SSS without permanent pacemaker, overate congestion, or symptomatic hypotension), severe hepatic failure.

Phosphodiesterase Inhibitors

155. The 4 features of phosphodiesterase inhibitors are:

1. They act through inhibition of phosphodiesterase type III (PDE III) that is found predominantly in cardiac muscle →
2. Results in increased levels of cAMP →
3. Leads to an increase in calcium channel entry into the cell.
4. Causes vasodilatation by inhibiting PDE III directly in vascular tissue.

These drugs have a potent positive inotropic effect as well as arterial vasodilatory activity and hence, have also been named as 'inodilators'.

These drugs are classified on the basis of their biochemical properties. They are either bipyridines, e.g. amrinone and milrinone or imidazoles, e.g. enoximone and paroxetine. Among these only amrinone is available in India.

156. Amrinone is a noncatecholamine and nonadrenergic. Therefore, it does not rely upon β-receptor stimulation for its positive inotropic activity. It exerts its inotropic activity by inhibiting PDE III at the cell membrane which results in higher cAMP levels.

Amrinone has the following 4 actions:

1. Increases cardiac index (CI).

2. Decreases pulmonary capillary wedge pressure (PCWP).
3. Decreases systemic vascular resistance (SVR).
4. Decreases pulmonary vascular resistance.

Heart rate and blood pressure generally remains stable.

157. Amrinone is useful in:

1. Heart failure:
   a. Biventricular failure
   b. Right ventricular failure
      i. Acute exacerbation of chronic heart failure
      ii. Refractory heart failure. This is not much useful in long-term treatment of congestive heart failure and may be detrimental.
      iii. Diastolic left ventricular failure due to its property of improving the compliance of the ventricle.
2. Cardiac surgery: In acute heart failure following cardiac surgery. Weaning patients from cardiopulmonary bypass (CPB).
3. In low cardiac output states with IABP.
4. In situations where the heart has a reduction in β receptors, e.g. prolonged sympathetic stimulation in heart failure or when 'stunning' of the myocardium is suspected with down regulation of β receptors. Because of its prolonged half-life, it must be administered as a intravenous loading dose followed by an infusion. A loading dose of 1 to 2 mg/kg followed by a maintenance infusion of 5 to 10 mg/kg/min. It can produce a precipitous fall in BP after the bolus loading dose, especially if the cardiac filling pressures are normal or low.

158. The failure of myocardial function of normal or ischemic areas to return to baseline after periods of hypoxic injury and reperfusion is called the "stunned myocardium" The mechanisms generating stunned myocardium are related to the following 4 changes:

1. Reduced high energy phosphate levels.
2. Intracellular calcium overload.
3. Generation of superoxide radicals.
4. Abnormalities in microvascular flow involving platelets and white blood cells. The contractile performance of stunned myocardium may remain depressed for hours to weeks with gradual recovery of viable myocytes.

Another factor contributing to myocardial dysfunction after CPB is the down regulation of β-adrenergic receptors. Patients undergoing cardiac surgery may also be in chronic congestive failure before operation. Thus, the myocardium may be exposed to high levels of catecholamines before and during CPB. This down regulation of β receptors may lead to myocardial dysfunction following cardiac surgery.

159. Amrinone can be used with the following drug combinations:

1. *Amrinone and dobutamine:* Both have shown to consistently increase cardiac output and decrease pulmonary capillary wedge pressure (PCWP) without significant effects on heart rate. It is useful in severe heart failure.
2. *Amrinone and dopamine:* These increases cardiac output without decrease in PCWP and also produces significant increase in heart rate or BP.
3. *Amrinone and epinephrine:* Used in stable patients just weaned from CPB.
4. *Amrinone with other catecholamines/vasodilators:* Combined administration produces greater improvements in hemodynamic response.

160. Milrinone is a second generation PDE III inhibitor and has similar hemodynamic profile to amrinone. However, positive ionotropic effect is much; more than that of amrinone. Milrinone has the following 4 actions:

1. Improves myocardial relaxation (positive lusitropic effect) and improves coronary perfusion and thereby increases cardiac output. The changes in systemic arterial pressure occur indirectly from an increased cardiac output.
2. Decreases PCWP.
3. Decreases SVR.
4. Decreases pulmonary vascular resistance (PVR). This property can be useful in patients undergoing mitral valve surgery in India who are known to present for surgery at a advanced stage with high PVR.

It can be administered in a loading dose of 50 mg/kg followed by a IV infusion of 0.3 to 0.75 mg/kg/min.

Other Inotropic Drugs

161. Calcium: Calcium salts are used to improve myocardial performance in some situations, such as:

1. Rapid transfusion of large quantities of citrate preserved blood products.
2. Myocardial depression following immediately after termination of CPB associated with residual effects of cardioplegia. This belief is based on the consideration of that infants, young children and adults are often hypocalcemic during and shortly after CPB.
3. Low ionic calcium concentration (calcium levels of < 0.9 mM).
4. Severe hyperkalemia or with calcium channel blockers over dose.

Calcium chloride 5 to 10 mg/kg increases mean arterial pressure (MAP) and blood ionized calcium concentration but has no effect on cardiac index (CI). Thus intravenous calcium salt appear inadequate choice for inotropic drug support. Small doses of calcium chloride (< 5 mg/kg $CaCl_2$) can also be used to increase SVR.

162. Arrhythmias in congestive heart failure can lead to 4 complications:

1. Dilatation or hypertrophy of myocardium.
2. Fibrosis of myocardial fiber.
3. Thrombus formation with embolic complications.
4. Infections.

Antiarrhythmic drugs need not be given unless there are multiple multifocal ectopics or one episode of ventricular tachycardia. Amiodarone is the safe antiarrhythmic drug. It has less negative inotropic effect.

163. Antiarrhythmic treatment in systolic heart failure: sudden cardiac death is unpredictable and accounts nearly one half of deaths among systolic failure patients.

In patients who had acute myocardial infarction, use of conventional antiarrhythmic agents to suppress PVBs leads to increased mortality.

Frequent PVBs are marker of increased mortality.

Amiodarone is helpful in the treatment because:

1. It has low incidence of proarrhythmia.
2. It has favorable hemodynamic effects.
3. It has no harmful effects on systolic heart failure with frequent PVBs.
4. It reduces the incidence of arrhythmic deaths.

164. There are 4 therapeutic goals to improve the quality of life:

1. Relief of symptoms
2. Improving exercise tolerance
3. Lessening the episodes of congestive heart failure
4. Lessening hospitalization for congestive heart failure.

165. Morbidity and mortality in patients with congestive heart failure can be assessed by 4 major criteria:

1. Clinical criteria
2. Hemodynamic
3. Biochemical
4. Electrophysiological.

166. Clinical assessment of prognosis in heart failure consists of 4 factors:

1. Exercise capacity
2. Heart rate at rest
3. Pulse pressure
4. Presence of S3.

The presence of audible third heart sound, low pulse pressure, low systolic pressure with reduced exercise capacity is associated with high mortality.

167. Hemodynamic assessment of prognosis in heart failure consists of:

1. Ejection fraction—both left ventricular and right ventricular ejection fraction
2. Left ventricular stroke work index—left ventricular systolic pressure
3. Left ventricular filling pressure
4. Right atrial pressure
5. Maximal oxygen uptake
6. Mean arterial pressure
7. Cardiac index
8. Systemic vascular resistance.

The above-mentioned factors have been assessed, each one separately by various methods to know whether they indicate prognosis independent of one another. Out of many of them, ejection fraction appears to be the most important factor on survival in patients with long standing advanced heart failure.

Sometimes, ejection fraction is found normal but still show signs of heart failure. These patients have diastolic heart failure. Ejection fraction may be normal in 70–80% of diastolic heart failure. In hypertension, left ventricular hypertrophy, ejection fraction may be normal but show HF. In dilated cardiomyopathy, first show systolic HF, later when muscle cells are replaced by fibrous tissue, goes into diastolic HF. Ejection fraction has shown direct relation with morality whereas systemic vascular resistance and heart rate has inverse relation with mortality. Low stroke work with raised left ventricular filling pressure and increased systemic vascular resistance are indicative of poor prognosis.

168. Biochemical assessment of prognosis in heart failure consists of:

1. Plasma catecholamines
2. Plasma renin
3. Plasma vasopressin
4. Plasma atrial natriuretic peptide—β-natriuretic peptide
5. Serum sodium
6. Serum potassium
7. Total potassium stores
8. Serum magnesium.

1, 2, 3 and 4 have shown strong inverse correlation on survival. High concentration of these reflect the severity of heart failure.

The substances like norepinephrine, angiotensin II are potent vasoconstrictors which increase left ventricular after load and thereby reduce shortening of myocardial fibers. They have direct adverse effect on the myocardium. Increased norepinephrine concentration may cause ventricular arrhythmias, and hypokalemia. Reduction in total body potassium stores can result from the activation of the renin-angiotensin-aldosterone axis and administration of potassium loosing diuretics.

Hyponatremia is directly related with high mortality. Hyponatremic patients appear to show response to angiotensin-converting enzyme inhibitors.

Exercise capacity as reflected by maximal oxygen uptake during programmed exercise test and sympathetic activation as estimated by plasma norepinephrine concentration have contributed important independent information on mortality.

169. Electrophysiological assessment of prognosis in heart failure consists of 4 points:

1. Frequent ventricular asystole.
2. Complex ventricular arrhythmias.
3. Ventricular tachycardia.
4. Atrial flutter/fibrillation.

Death in severe congestive heart failure occurs either by progressive pump failure by sudden unexpected arrhythmias in half of the patients. Arrhythmias like ventricular tachycardias, atrial fibrillation, LV conduction blocks are indicative of poor prognosis. Ventricular arrhythmias have shown independent adverse prognostic effects. Routine treatment with antiarrhythmic drugs for arrhythmias in heart failure do not show independent adverse prognostic effects. Routine treatment with antiarrhythmic drugs for arrhythmias in heart failure do not show much protective evidence in reducing mortality. It is suspected that repletion of potassium and magnesium stores may modify the outcome in these patients.

The administration of ACE inhibitors block the aldosterone induced potassium loss and restores intracellular and extracellular potassium, which may help to reduce the mortality in congestive heart failure. Similar beneficial effects are seen with β-blockers in dilated cardiomyopathy and postmyocardial infarction patients with heart failure in the same manner.

170. There are 4 practical guidelines for the management of congestive heart failure by New York Heart Association (NYHA):

Table C-14

1. Class I (NYHA) patients with mild heart failure	Physical and mental rest Reduce salt and water intake Reduce cardiac work load
2. Class II (NYHA) patients with moderate heart failure	Use above measures of class I and add digitalis and diuretics
3. Class III (NYHA) patients with severe heart failure	Use above measures of class II add vasodilators
4. Class IV (NYHA) patients with intractable heart failure	Use above measures of class III, plus newer inotropic agents like amrinone and mechanical assistance

171. Common clinical predicator of poor survival in systolic heart failure:

1. Old age
2. Functional capacity—high New York Heart Association functional class.
3. Severely reduced LV ejection fraction (LVEF) < 25%, [Left ventricular end-diastolic dimension < 25%], extensive cardiac remodeling (LVED > 65 mm) or reduced cardiac index (CI < 2.5).
4. Concomitant diastolic dysfunction (especially restrictive mitral inflow and dilated left atrium) and increase in pulse pressure.
5. Reduced right ventricular function.
6. Atrial fibrillation, tachycardia, and reduced heart rate variability.
7. Low peak VO_2 with maximal exercise (14 mL/min/kg), low heart rate response to exercise (ventilatory response to hypoxia) and low VE/VO_2.
8. High plasma B-type natriuretic peptide (BNP) and N-terminal pro-BNP levels.
9. Anemia of heart failure.
10. Markers of reduced tissue perfusion:
    a. Low mean arterial pressure.
    b. Renal insufficiency (creatinine clearance < 60 mL/min).
    c. Attenuated response to diuretics and lack of hemodynamic and structural improvement (reverse remodeling) with medical therapy.
    d. Persistent signs of congestion and fluid retention, including hepatic insufficiency.
    e. Serum sodium <135 mg/dL.
11. Cardiac and neurohormonal biomarkers (cardiac troponin, norepinephrine, cytokines, endotheline-1, urotensin II, cardiotropin-1)

Cardiac dyssynchrony (QRS > 130 msec, left bundle-branch block)

172. There are 4 mechanical methods that are used in severe intractable heart failure:

1. Intra-aortic balloon counterpulsation.
2. Implantable cardioverter defibrillator (ICDS).
3. Artificial heart.
4. Transplantation.

Implantable cardioverter-defibrillators are increasingly used now to prevent sudden cardiac death preferably in patients with large MI, systolic HF with EF < 35% with recurrent ventricular tachycardiac (VT).

Many patients with systolic heart failure are suitable to this expensive therapy. Risk and benefits are to be calculated preferably with an electrophysiologist.

173. Cardiac transplantation or artificial heart is considered when the following 4 lines of treatment have failed in heart failure:

1. Failure to respond to treatment with digoxin, diuretics, vasodilatores with strict diet control, physical and emotional rest.
2. Failure of intravenous inotropics—dopamine, dobutamine, amrinone, sodium nitroprusside.
3. Physical removal of fluid by thoracentesis, paracentesis, peritoneal/hemodialysis with ultrafiltration.
4. Failure of interventional procedures like intra-aortic balloon pump, ventricular assisted devices, etc.

ACUTE LEFT VENTRICULAR FAILURE (PULMONARY EDEMA)

174. Acute heart failure can be clinically described into 4 groups

1. Acute cardiogenic pulmonary edema.
2. Cardiogenic shock.
   Acute decompensation of chronic left heart failure.
3. Noncardiac disorders where clinical presentation can be similar in many respects to that of acute heart failure, e.g. noncardiogenic pulmonary edema.
4. Patients with acute heart failure require immediate hospital admission.

175. One should do the clinical assessment quickly to detect the causes of heart failure which are best treated by special therapeutic approaches, e.g.

1. AMI
2. Arrhythmias such as high degree AV block/or VT
3. Pericardial tamponade
4. Pulmonary embolism.

If these have been excluded, further testing to determine the etiology of heart disease is done in more appropriate time.

Clinical presentation of acute heart failure ranges from sudden appearance of dyspnea to frank cardiogenic shock.

176. There are 4 principles in the management of acute left ventricular failure:

1. First check the blood pressure.
   Hypertension—Good prognosis
   Hypotension—Grave prognosis.
2. Start initial treatment.
3. Look for any precipitating factors.
4. Reassess the underlying cause.

177. Initial diagnostic evaluation of acute pulmonary edema:

1. History/Physical examination.
2. 12-lead ECG.
3. Continuous monitoring.
4. Laboratory tests: Blood studies—Complete blood count (CBC), electrolytes, blood urea nitrogen (BUN), creatinine, cardiac enzyme levels, blood sugar, complete urine examination.
5. Chest X-ray.
6. Digital pulse oximetry/arterial blood gases.
7. Transthoracic Doppler 2D-echo.
8. Cardiac catheterization/Coronary angiography for suspected Acute MI to determine cause(s) for refractory acute pulmonary edema.

Transthoracic doppler 2D Echo is indicated in all patients who present with acute cardiogenic pulmonary edema, unless there are obvious precipitating factors and the patients cardiac status evaluated previously. Transesophageal echo may be required to diagnose or more clearly define certain lesions like ruptured chordae tendinae, aortic dissection, etc.

178. There are 4 steps to be followed while initiating treatment in acute left ventricular failure:

1. Oxygen 100% by Mask/Binasal catheter.
2. Decrease cardiac workload.
3. Decrease pulmonary congestion.
4. Improve cardiac performance.

179. Oxygen 100% preferably under positive pressure acts in 4 ways in reducing pulmonary edema.

1. It increases interalveolar pressure.
2. It reduces transudation of fluid from the alveolar capillaries.
3. It impedes venous return to the thorax.
4. It reduces pulmonary capillary pressure.

Intubation with mechanical ventilation is necessary in severe hypoxia that does not respond rapidly to therapy and in those with respiratory acidosis.

180. Cardiac workload is decreased in 4 ways:

1. Bed rest	
2. Propped up position	Injection morphine 3 mg IV repeated
3. Reduce pain	Decreases pain
4. Reduce anxiety by assurance	Decreases anxiety Dilates veins.

181. Morphine acts in 4 ways in reducing acute pulmonary edema:

1. Reduces apprehension.
2. Reduces the release of catecholamines.

3. Reduces vasoconstrictor stimuli to the arterial and venous beds.
4. Results in systemic vasodilatation which allows blood to be sequestrated peripherally.

Do not give morphine if there is significant hypotension or any evidence of respiratory failure. It should be administered with caution to patients with chronic pulmonary insufficiency and those with respiratory or metabolic acidosis in whom suppression of ventilatory drive can cause drastic lowering of systemic pH.

182. There are 4 drugs, which help to decrease pulmonary congestion in acute left ventricular failure:

1. Morphine IV 3 mg to 20 mg IV depending on the severity and route of administration.
   It is a venodilator. Its action is by direct relaxation of vascular smooth muscle. Naloxone should be kept ready for any respiratory depression. Cyclazine is given if there is any vomiting or diamorphine 5 mg IV slowly, unless liver failure or chronic obstructive airway disease is present.
2. Furosemide IV 40–200 mg bolus or ethacrynic acid 40–80 mg.
3. Nitrates—venodilators-nitroglycerin 5–10 mg SL repeated every 5 to 10 minutes 4 times as needed and repeated 4–6th hourly.
   Sublingual nitroglycerin is effective in patients with acute cardiogenic pulmonary edema due to both ischemic and nonischemic causes. If the systolic blood pressure is acceptable (> 95 to 100 mm Hg), nitroglycerin can be administered intravenously as well (starting dose 0.3 to 0.5 μg/kg body weight/min). Choose the route of administration according to the circumstances.
4. Aminophylline IV 5 mg per kg bolus slowly over 20 minutes use only if there is severe bronchospasm. (240 to 480 mg IV slowly).
   If no response
   Mechanical } Phlebotomy
   Tourniquets } rarely indicated

183. Aminophylline acts in 4 ways to reduce the acute pulmonary edema:

1. Diminishes bronchoconstriction.
2. Increases renal blood flow.
3. Increases sodium excretion.
4. Increases myocardial contractility.

184. Mechanical methods:

1. Keep the patient in sitting position with legs dangling along the side of the bed.
2. Phlebotomy-venesection—Removal of 300–350 mL of blood if the patient is plethoric, dyspneic, and markedly cyanozed (alternatively leeching was practiced in olden days).
3. Paracentesis of ascites or hydrothorax.
4. If all methods are failed try mechanical methods. Intubation and mechanical ventilation in patients with severe hypoxia that does not respond rapidly to therapy and in those with respiratory acidosis.

185. The 4 other supplementary methods to be tried if there is no response for the above treatment:

1. Keep the patient in sitting position with legs dangling along the side of the bed which reduces venous return to the heart.
   Apply venous occlusion cuffs on all four limbs. Each cuff should be deflated for every 5 minutes, in every 15 minutes, rotation.
2. Digitalize—if not given before, three-fourth of full dose of digoxin IV is given.
3. If no response—try after load reduction by IV, sodium nitroprusside 20–30 μg/min in patients who have systolic pressure more than 100 mm Hg. Sodium nitroprusside (starting dose of 0.1 μg/kg/min) may be administered for patients not immediately responsive to nitrate therapy and for those whose pulmonary edema is in large part attributable to severe mitral or aortic regurgitation or marked systemic hypertension. The dose is increased as needed to improve the patient's overall clinical and hemodynamic status, using a systemic systolic pressure of 85 to 90 mm Hg as the usual lower limit for dose incremination in patients previously normotensive and as long as adequate perfusion of vital organs is maintained.
4. If all methods are ineffective—try venesection, which may be life saving. Intubation and mechanical ventilation are of value in patients with severe hypoxia that does not respond rapidly to therapy and in those with respiratory acidosis.

186. There are 4 drugs which help to improve the cardiac performance:

1. Digitalis: In atrial tachyarrhythmias like AF/PAT to reduce ventricular rate.
   IV digoxin.

Leeching: In olden days, leeches are applied over liver region, temples, and medial side of the thighs. Parts are scrubbed with ether, soap and water. A drop of milk or blood is applied to the region. The test tube containing leech is inverted over the area. The leech crawls and attached. Consuming capacity of each leech is about 2 drops of blood. 12 leeches about 24 drops. Leeches fall down after drawing the blood. Leeches secretes hirudin (an anticoagulant) and apply it about the site of bite and hence blood continuously looses from the punctures. Bleeding is stopped after about 10–12 oz of blood have been removed.

2. Nonglycoside inotropics—β-adrenergic agonists.
   Dobutamine IV drip
   Dopamine IV drip
3. IV vasodilators.
4. IV sodium nitroprusside—if blood pressure is uncontrolled.

187. Treat the following 4 precipitating factors:

1. Hypertension/hypotension
   Accelerated hypertension: Nifedipine SL 10 mg repeated till BP is stabilized.
   IV nitroprusside if hypertension is uncontrolled.
   Hypotension—bad prognosis. IV dobutamine or IV dopamine drip to maintain blood pressure.
2. Myocardial infarction/ischemia.
3. Infection—give suitable antibiotics.
4. Arrhythmias.

188. Reassessment of the underlying cause. The 4 points to be kept in mind are:

1. Treat the etiology.
2. Look for any surgically correctable lesion.
3. Look for other associated diseases—pulmonary, thyroid, etc.
4. Look, whether the previous treatment was adequate or not:
   Is he/she following the instructions properly (rest, diet)? Has he taken care of the risk factors like smoking?

189. Placement of a pulmonary artery balloon catheter should be considered in the following 4 situations:

1. When the patient's clinical condition is deteriorating, recovery from acute presentation is not proceeding as expected.
2. When high dose nitroglycerin or nitroprusside is required for clinical stabilization.
3. When dopamine or dobutamine are needed to augment systemic blood pressure and peripheral perfusion.
4. When uncertainty exists regarding the diagnosis of acute cardiogenic pulmonary edema.

190. Summary of therapeutic management of pulmonary edema:

1. Oxygen.
2. Nitroglycerin—sublingual or intravenous.
3. IV diuretic (e.g. furosemide) .
4. Morphine sulfate.
5. Administration of cardiovascular support drugs to attain and stabilize clinical hemodynamic status (e.g. IV infusion of nitroprusside, dopamine/dobutamine).
6. Thrombolytic therapy or urgent revascularization (PTCA or CABG) for acute MI.
7. Intubation and mechanical ventilation for severe hypoxia that does not respond rapidly to therapy and for respiratory acidosis.
8. Definitive correction of underlying cause (mitral valve replacement or repair of acute severe mitral regurgitation) when indicated and clinically possible.

CARDIOGENIC SHOCK

(See Chapter F-AMI 186–191)

191. Acute decompensation of chronic congestive heart failure.

There are 4 general principles of management of this group:

1. Clinical evaluation.
2. Hemodynamic stabilization.
3. Diagnostic studies for reversible precipitating factors.
4. Optimization of long-term therapy.

The clinical features of this group of patients generally are secondary to volume overload, elevated ventricular filling pressures and depressed cardiac output.

Mild to moderate symptoms can be treated by intravenous or oral diuretics or both in the long-term therapy of chronic HF unless they are complicated by AMI, or concurrent threatening condition (hypokalemia, moderate to marked azotemia, symptomatic arrhythmia).

Moderate to severe symptoms: Treatment is similar to that of patients presenting with acute HF.

192. Recommendations for intra-aortic balloon counterpulsation in HF:

1. Acute HF conditions such as cardiogenic shock, pulmonary edema not responding to the proper administration of fluid volume or pharmacologic therapy, or both in patients with potentially reversible HF or as a bridge to heart transplantation.
2. Acute HF accompanied by refractory ischemia in preparation for cardiac catheterization/coronary arteriography and definitive intervention .
3. Acute HF in AMI complicated by significant mitral regurgitation (papillary muscle rupture) or rupture of the interventricular septum to obtain hemodynamic stabilization for definitive diagnostic studies or intervention or both. In patients with progressive chronic HF to allow for proper diagnostic procedure and time to consider treatment options and definitive interventions such as cardiac surgery, heart transplantation.
4. Significant aortic insufficiency.
5. Aortic dissection.

6. Patients unresponsive to therapy in whom the cause is known to be uncorrectable or irreversible and who are not candidates for heart transplantation.
7. Patients in the end stage of terminal illness.
8. Bleeding diathesis or severe thrombocytopenia.

193. Recommendations for placement of pulmonary artery balloon catheter in HF:

1. Assessment of the status of intravascular volume, ventricular filling pressures, and overall cardiac functions in patients whose decompensated chronic HF is not responding appropriately to standard therapy—Evaluation of overall cardiac hemodynamic status and exclusion of left heart failure in a patient with decompensated chronic lung disease.
2. As a diagnostic tool to resolve any uncertainty of whether pulmonary edema is cardiogenic or non-cardiogenic in origin. As a diagnostic tool to assess the origin and clinical and hemodynamic significance of a new systolic murmur in acute HF.
3. Cardiogenic shock or near shock that does not respond promptly to the proper administration of fluid volume.
4. Acute pulmonary edema that does not respond to appropriate intervention or is complicated by systemic hypotension or shock/near shock

194. Summary of the management of heart failure:

1. Initial diagnostic testing for patients with acute HF should be limited to those tests necessary to exclude etiologies requiring special therapeutic procedures. Further diagnostic tests are generally deferred until hemodynamic stability and improvement have been attained.
2. Initial laboratory testing generally can be limited to CBC, urinalysis, serum electrolytes, creatinine, cardiac enzymes, blood urea nitrogen, arterial gases and PH, ECG, chest X-ray and transthoracic Doppler two-dimensional echocardiography.
3. Patients with acute heart failure and evidence of AMI/ infarction should be considered for urgent cardiac catheterization, coronary arteriography and definitive interventional procedures. Thrombolytic therapy should be considered if these studies cannot be done expeditiously.
4. Treatment of acute cardiogenic pulmonary edema consists initially of intravenous diuretics, nitrates, oxygen and morphine. Intubation and mechanical ventilation are of value in selected patients.
5. Patients with cardiogenic shock who do not have evidence of volume overload should receive a rapid intravenous infusion initially and the response observed.
6. Patients with cardiogenic shock unresponsive to intravenous fluid administration or who have obvious volume overload should be given intravenous dopamine initially.
7. A pulmonary artery balloon flotation catheter should be inserted in all patients with cardiogenic shock unless there is rapid response to intravenous fluids. Patients with acute cardiogenic pulmonary edema generally do not require a pulmonary artery catheter. However, catheter insertion is indicted in those not responding appreciably to therapy or those in whom it is unclear whether the pulmonary edema is due to cardiac or noncardiac origin.
8. Intra-aortic balloon counterpulsation may be indicated in patients with acute HF not responding adequately to therapy. The device is particularly helpful in attaining hemodynamic improvement and stability while awaiting additional diagnostic or therapeutic interventions.

Chronic and Stabilized Acute Heart Failure in Adults

195. All patients presenting with chronic HF should undergo diagnostic evaluation initially necessary to:

1. Determine the type of cardiac dysfunction—systolic or diastolic dysfunction.
2. Determine the correctable etiologic factors.
3. Determine the prognosis.
4. Determine the mode of treatment.

Two-dimensional echo is of particular benefit in the initial evaluation to specifically assess ventricular mass, chamber size, systolic and diastolic dysfunction and to uncover the correctable etiologic factors best treated by specific therapy (e.g. aortic stenosis, segmental hypokinesia/akinesia suggesting occlusive coronary artery disease). Magnetic resonance imaging (MRI) is promising but is not routinely used because of its cost-effectiveness.

196. The most commonly identified causes of left ventricular systolic dysfuntion in the USA are:

1. Coronary artery disease.
2. Hypertension.
3. Idiopathic dilated cardiomyopathy.
4. Myocarditis.

With large scale detection programs of hypertension and improved modalities, aggressive treatment of hypertension to the general population, ischemic heart disease has become the most common cause of heart failure in adults. Patients whose HF cannot clearly be attributed to hypertension or coronary artery disease should undergo a detailed evaluation for other specific etiologies.

Idiopathic dilated cardiomyopathy (DCM) should only be diagnosed after exclusion of other conditions.

Myocarditis is frequently considered in those with unexplained HF, particularly if the patients are young and the failure is of acute onset. However, myocarditis is an uncommon cause of HF. Biopsy evidence of significant inflammation and myocardial necrosis is required to prove the diagnosis of acute myocarditis.

197. Several noninvasive tests are available now to detect the ischemic or hybernating myocardium that includes:

1. Gold standard positron emission tomography (PET)
2. Thallium scintigraphy
3. Technitium-99 sestamibi
4. Pharmacological means for finding ' ischemia' by using dipyridamole, dobutamine or adenosine (dobutamine echocardiography for assessing myocardial viability).

198. Following investigations are recommended as routine diagnostic studies for adult patients with chronic HF or stabilized acute HF not previously performed.

1. CBC, urine analysis, blood-serum analysis include– glucose, BUN, creatinine, elctrolytes, phosphorous, magnesium, calcium and albumin levels.
2. Chest radiograph.
3. ECG, Treadmill, Holter's monitoring or signal-averaged electrocardiography.
4. T2, T3, TSH hormones in patients with atrial fibrillation and unexplained HF, and in patients with sinus rhythm and unexplained HF.
5. Tansthoracic Doppler two-dimensional echocardiograph.
6. Noninvasive stress testing to detect ischemia in patients without angina but with a high probability of coronary artery disease who would be candidates for revascularization. In all patients with unexplained HF who are potential candidates for revascularization. Noninvasive testing to detect ischemia and assess myocardial viability or coronary arteriography in patients with a previous infarction but with no angina who could be candidates for revascularization.
7. Cardiac catheterization/coronary arteriography in patients with angina or large areas of ischemic or hibernating myocardium, also in patients at risk for coronary artery disease who are to undergo surgical correction of noncoronary cardiac lesions. In all patients with unexplained HF, who are potential candidates for revascularization, less common tests are performed.
8. Endomyocardial biopsy in patients.
   i. With recent onset of rapidly deteriorating cardiac function or other clinical indications of myocarditis.
   ii. Receiving chemotherapy with adriamycin or similar myocardial toxic agents.
   iii. With a systemic disease and possible cardiac involvement (hemochromatosis, sarcoid, amyloid, Loeffler's endocarditis, endomyocardial fibroelastosis).

199. Diastolic function is classically divided into 4 components (4 major components of ventricular diastolic):

1. Active relaxation
2. Early filling
3. Diastasis
4. Atrial systolic filling.

1. Active relaxation is energy dependent and begins just before the closure of aortic valve and ends just after the opening of the mitral valve. Calcium ion influx appears to be related to active relaxation and provides suction effective filling.
2. Early filling—passive rapid filling/on the other hand, begins after the opening of the mitral valve, is pressure-driven and ends with pressure equalization. A later phase of passive filling is most suitable for describing ventricular stiffness since there is no longer a suction effect at this point.
3. Diastasis occurs in the medial of diastole when the AV valve is partially on the pressure gradient between the left atrium and the left ventricle is decreased. Diastasis does not contribute to the flow, and provides important functional reserve in diastole with tachycardia.
4. Atrial systolic filling.

200. Evaluation of diastolic dysfunction.

Majority of patients with HF have reduced left ventricular systolic function and variable degree of diastolic dysfunction. However, a significant subset of about 30% have predominantly diastolic dysfunction with normal or near normal systolic function (normal EF). The management of patients with primarily systolic or diastolic dysfunction is different and it is critical to make the distinction. Diastolic dysfunction impairs ventricular filling by diminishing relaxation (during early diastole) or reducing compliance (early to late diastole) of the ventricles or both. The hemodynamic consequences of diastolic dysfunction include elevation of 4 pressures:

1. Ventricular filling pressure
2. Left atrial pressure
3. Pulmonary venous pressure
4. Pulmonary capillary pressure.

If uncorrected, an eventual increase in pulmonary artery pressure and right heart pressures take place, the elevated filling pressure is frequently sufficient to maintain a normal stroke volume and cardiac output at rest, but they are compromised in situations when the increase in cardiac output is needed, e.g. exercise.

201. Myocardial ischemia, hypertrophy and fibrosis are the usual underlying pathologic processes for ventricular diastolic dysfunction. The common causes of diastolic dysfunction include:

1. Coronary artery disease.
2. Systemic hypertension.
3. Diabetes mellitus.
4. Aortic stenosis.
5. Hypertrophic obstructive cardiomyopathy.
6. Infiltrative cardiomyopathies/obliterative cardiomyopathy/endocardial fibroelastosis.
7. Restrictiave cardiomyopathy (RCM).
8. Constrictive pericarditis.

Passive chamber stiffness is directly related to myocardial mass and myocardial stiffness (due to fibrosis) and inversely related to chamber volume. Constrictive pericarditis and restrictive cardiomyopathy classically give rise to diastolic heart failure due to decreased compliance. In such cases, diuretics help a lot. Pericardiectomy gives dramatic relief of congestive heart failure in patients with constrictive pericarditis.

Impairment of active relaxation of the ventricle is a more important cause of diastolic heart failure than an increase in passive stiffness (diastolic compliance). Heart failure due to impaired relaxation is commonly seen in hypertension, coronary artery disease, aortic stenosis, hypertrophic obstructive cardiomyopathy as well as some other conditions.

202. Clinical manifestations of diastolic dysfunction can range from:

1. No symptoms to dyspnea
2. Pulmonary edema
3. Signs of right heart failure
4. Exercise intolerance.

Diastolic dysfunction usually presents as a chronic condition. Acute diastolic dysfunction producing acute pulmonary edema is not an uncommon manifestation of acute myocardial infarction or uncontrolled hypertension.

203. Diastolic dysfunction should be suspected when a patient presents with symptoms and signs of HF and has normal or near normal ventricular systolic function.

The following investigations help:

1. Two-dimensional echocardiogram to assess systolic function and to detect diastolic dysfunction, later by measuring indexes of the rate of diastolic filling. Constrictive pericarditis, a surgically treatable condition must be excluded in patients whose diastolic dysfunction appears to be secondary to restrictive cardiomyopathy.
2. Radionuclide imaging for IHD/CAD.
3. Endomyocardial biopsy (e.g. myocardial amyloidosis, hemochromatosis).
4. Cardiac catheterization when noninvasive studies are nondiagnostic. Alternatively, one could directly do cardiac catheterizaton/coronary arteriography when there is high suspicion of occlusive coronary artery disease (angina or myocardial infarction).

204. Functional assessment of the patient encompasses many dimensions that include:

1. Physical capacity
2. Emotional status
3. Social function
4. Cognitive capabilities.

Assessment of physical function is most important. Emotional, social and cognitive factors may have a strong effect on the patient's capacity to adhere or respond to a therapeutic regimes. Clinical assessment, especially depression, social support and cognitive capabilities should be performed regularly.

205. Summary of chronic heart failure:

1. Patients presenting with chronic HF and those patients with acute HF in whom the cause was not established during the stabilization period should undergo diagnostic testing to determine the etiology.
2. HF due to diastolic dysfunction must be differentiated from that due to systolic dysfunction. This can be done by 2D Echo, radionucleide imaging or cardiac catheterization.
3. Coronary artery disease must be excluded as the casual factor in patients with HF.
4. Ongoing assessment of functional capacity plays an important role in the management of patients with HF.

206. Therapy of left ventricular dysfunction.

The treatment of chronic HF has changed remarkably in the past one to two decades. Heart failure is no longer considered a simple edematous state that is responsive to intermittent diuretic therapy. Many if not most patients are now nonedematous, but the condition is still disabling and lethal. Many of them showed improvement in the treatment of patients with New York Heart Association functional class I to IV heart failure due to systolic dysfunction.

1. ACE inhibitors for all patients with significantly reduced left ventricular ejection fraction unless contraindicated.

2. Isosorbide dinitrate and hydralazine in patients who cannot take ACEI.
3. Digoxin in patients with HF due to systolic dysfunction not adequately responsive to ACEI and diuretic drugs.
4. Digoxin in patients with atrial fibrillation (AF) and rapid ventricular rates.
5. Diuretics for patients with fluid overload.
6. β-blockers for high-risk patients after an acute myocardial infarction.
7. Anticoagulation in patients with atrial fibrillation, or previous history of pulmonary or systemic embolism.
8. Antiarrhythmic drugs for ventricular arrhythmias.

Oral ACE inhibitors should be given to all patients in functional Class I with significant left ventricular systolic dysfunction (ejection fraction < 35–40%). However, in patients with functional Class I with systolic dysfunction with asymptomatic or minimally symptomatic, use of ACE inhibitors prevents heart failure.

In the studies of left ventricular dysfunction (SOLVD) prevention trial with enalapril, survival and ventricular enlargement (SAVE) with captopril, Gruppo Italiano per lo Studio della Sopravvivenza nellinfarto miocardico (GISSI-III) and International Study of Infarct Survival (ISIS) trials all showed benefit with ACEI. Intravenous enlapril offered no advantage. Contraindications to ACEI include shock, angioneurotic edema, or significant asymptomatic hypotension, i.e. SBP < 70 to 90 mm Hg is not a contraindication to ACEI therapy but clinical judgement must always govern therapeutic decisions. Dosing is very important. It should be started with lower doses and gradually increased. Enalapril should be started at 2.5 mg and titrated to 10 mg twice a day whereas captopril should begun at 6.25 to 12.5 mg tds and gradually titrated to 50 mg tds. Larger doses have shown more effective in reducing mortality. ACEI are given to all patients of functional Class II to IV unless there is contraindication or not tolerated. The dosed should be gradually increased, i.e. enalapril 20 mg; captopril 150 mg; lisinopril 5 to 20 mg; quinapril 5 mg bd, for the treatment of heart failure.

Acute Infarction Ramipril Efficiency (AIRE) study, Ramipril 5 mg twice daily showed reduced mortality.

Once a patients has begun ACEI therapy, the drug should be given for an indefinite period of time, probably for life, if well tolerated.

Although, ACEI are the corner stone of treatment for HF, Isosorbide dinitrate and hydralazine should be considered when ACEI are not tolerated because of symptomatic hypotension, azotemia, hyperkalemia, cough, rash or angioneurotic edema.

Isosorbide dinitrate 5 to 10 mg three times a day and hydralazine 10 mg four times a day should be the initial doses. If tolerated, hydralazine should be increased gradually to 75 mg four times a day and isosorbide dinitrate to 40 mg three times a day. A minimal 10 hour 'nitrate free' period at night should be achieved to prevent nitrate tolerance. Occasionally, isosorbide, diuretic and hydralazine are added to any ACEI when symptoms of dyspnea, or fatigue persists.

Digitalis has been used for more than 200 years to treat HF. Yet controversy still persists regarding their use in patients with HF and normal sinus rhythm. The role of digoxin in patients with HF and atrial fibrillation is accepted and recent studies indicated that it is useful in left ventricular systolic dysfunction and sinus rhythm. It increases left ventricular ejection fraction and exercise tolerance in patients with chronic HF, it may reduce sympathetic activity as a major mechanism of action. Digoxin has not been shown to be efficacious in asymptomatic patients with ventricular systolic dysfunction. Patients receiving long-term digoxin therapy with or without concomitant ACEI therapy may manifest clinical deterioration when digoxin is withdrawn.

Patients with HF and AF should have their ventricular rate controlled. Multiple drugs may be necessary, such as digoxin, diltiazem or a β-blocker. Uncontrolled or recent onset of atrial fibrillation can worsen HF or lead to decompensation. It is usually prudent to convert new-onset AF or AF of uncertain duration to normal sinus rhythm. In some cases amiodarone or occasionally cathter ablation or modification of the AV node may be necessary to prevent uncontrolled rapid ventricular rates.

Initiating diuretic therapy is highly individualized. Thiazide diuretics may be started but reduced renal perfusion may ultimately favor the use of a loop diuretic such as furosemide or bumetanide. Thiazide diuretic drugs are ineffective if the glomerular filtration rate is < 30 to 40 mL/min and actually reduce this rate further.

Patients should be advised to weigh themselves daily and keep record of their weight. An increase of 1 or 2 kg may be an indication to supplement the maintenance diuretic dose. For example, 2.5 mg of metazolone may be added to 2 or 3 days to the loop diuretic drugs, followed by a return to the usual maintenance dose of loop diuretic when the weight stabilizes.

Sodium restriction becomes a critical strategy in the treatment of HF as the disorder progresses. Sodium should be limited to < 2 g per day before starting large doses or multiple diuretic drugs.

When diuretic resistance develops it is advisable to start a combination that act on different nephron segments, e.g. thiazide or metolozone plus a loop diuretic drug, which are often effective. Careful monitoring of BUN, creatinine, electrolytes are necessary when these diuretics are combined. Hypokalemia and contraction alkalosis are frequent accompaniments of vigorous diuretic drug use. Hypokalemia aggravates ventricular arrhythmias which occur in the majority of patients with heart failure. Potassium chloride in doses of 20 to 60 mEq/L dose is frequently required to maintain serum potassium levels of 4.5 to 5.0 mEq/L. Dietary supplementation of potassium is rarely sufficient. Alternatively, potassium sparing agents such as amiloride, triamterene or spiranolactone can be used to maintain serum potassium levels. Dangerous hyperkalemia may occur when ACEI are used in combination with potassium-sparing diuretic drugs or large doses of oral potassium. Serum potassium levels should be carefully monitored (see 124). Hyperkalemia and sodium retention can occur with nonsteroidal anti-inflammatory agents when used in patients with HF. In general, nonsteroidal anti-inflammatory drugs are avoided in patients with HF. Hypomagnesemia (serum magnesium levels < 1.6 m Eq/L) should also be corrected when observed.

Patients with resistant sodium retention with truly refractory HF may require dobutamine IVI (2 to 5 μg/kg/min), dopamine (1 to 3 μg/kg/min) or a constant infusion of furosemide (1 to 5 mg/h); Fluid restriction to 1000 to 2000 mL/d is of value in patients with dilutional hyponitremia.

More recently, β-blockers with additional pharmacological properties have been evaluated extensively. Nebivolol and bucindolol which have both β-blocking activity and vasodilator properties, improved left ventricular performance during long-term therapy.

Carvedilol, which also has combined β-blocker and vasodialtor activity has been shown to improve left ventricular function, symptoms and submaximal exercise tolerance in symptoms of wide ranging activity.

It has been suggested that long-term β-blockers may reduce morbidity and mortality in patients with chronic HF. They have been shown to reduce mortality in high-risk patients after an AMI, including many patients with HF.

The metoprolol in dilated cardiomyopathy (DCM) trial has shown that metoprolol reduces the combined risk of mortality and the need for heart transplantation in patients with idiopathic dilated cardiomyopathy. Initiation of β-blockades may exacerbate HF in some patients. Hence, physicians might consider the use of β-blockers in selected patients with chronic HF.

Anticoagulation with warfarin is frequently used for patients with chronic HF to prevent systemic embolization. The embolic complications are linked to a low ejection fraction and many physicians currently administer anticoagulation to patients with an ejection fraction <20–25%. Many physicians will administer anticoagulation in patients with left ventricular dysfunction and an intracardiac thrombus. Patients with atrial fibrillation should receive anticoagulation to achieve target range of ratio of 2.0 to 3.0. A recent report suggests that optimal range of anticoagulation for patients with a documented embolism should be 2.0 to 3.9.

Ventricular arrhythmias are nearly omnipresent in patients with HF. Asymptomatic ventricular arrhythmias including mild palpitations and nonsustained ventricular tachycardias need not be treated. Antiarrhythmic therapy can worsen ventricular arrhythmias and produce negative inotropic effects in patients with HF. When antiarrhythimic drugs are used in patients with HF, they ordinarily should be initiated in the hospital. Empirical use of type I antiarrhythmic drugs should be avoided for treatment of ventricular arrhythmias with HF. There can be improvement in survival with amiodarone. The empirical use of amidarone for patients with HF needs further study.

Calcium blockers are sometimes used as an antianginal therapy or hypertensive agents in patients with angina or hypertension who have left ventricular dysfunction, but they may worsen HF. The risk of worsening HF is with newer agents like felodipine also. However, in Prospective Randomized Amlodipine Survival Evaluation (PRAISE) trial, the use of amlodipine in HF was not accompanied by any adverse effects on morbidity or mortality, rather, the study reported a favorable effect of amlodipine on the survival of patients with nonischemic DCM. This is evaluated in a following trial.

207. Diastole function depends mainly on 4 important parameters:

1. Heart rate—diastole is disproportionately shortened with faster heart rates.
2. Circulating fluid volume.
3. Anatomic consideration, e.g. LA, MV, pulmonary veins, LV mass, and pericardium.
4. Active myocardial relaxation (i.e. myoenergetics).

208. Diastolic dysfunction therapy.

The treatment of HF due to diastolic dysfunction has both similarities and dissimilarities to the treatment of HF due to systolic dysfunction. The recommendations do not include therapy for HOCM because the pathophysiology of HCOM differs significantly from most other causes of diastolic dysfunction. The goal of drug therapy in diastolic dysfunction is to reduce symptoms by lowering the elevated filling pressures without significantly reducing cardiac output. This can be achieved by the judicious use of diuretics and nitrates. β-blockers may improve diastolic filling by reducing heart rate. Pharmacological treatment of left ventricular dysfunction consists of:

1. Diuretics
2. Nitrates
3. Drugs suppressing AV conduction to control ventricular rate in patients with AF
4. Anticoagulation in patients with AF or previous systemic or pulmonary embolization.

Calcium channel blockers, β-blockers and ACEI may benefit. Agents with positive ionotropic actions are not indicated if systolic function is normal.

REFRACTORY HEART FAILURE

Usually it is not refractory.

Small percentage of congestive cardiac failure patients fail to respond to anticongestive treatment. Be sure that the heart failure is not due to faulty diagnosis or treatment before labelling as refractory or intractable heart failure.

Consider carefully several possibilities before assuming that this state reflects advanced preterminal extreme myocardial impairment.

209. Ask the following 4 questions in order to find out the clue:

1. Are the symptoms due to heart failure?
2. What type of heart failure it is ?
3. What brought on the heart failure ?
4. What is aggravating the failure?

210. Check whether the cardinal signs and symptoms of heart failure are caused by other disorders or not. The 4 points to be kept in mind are:

1. Dyspnea: Sometimes taken as a symptom of heart failure which may be caused by:
   Pulmonary disease—pneumonia, asthma, pulmonary infarction, pleural effusion (noncardiac)
   Obesity
   Acidosis
   Hyperventilation
   Hyperthyroidism
2. Pulmonary rales—may be caused by bronchopulmonary disease.
3. Edema or ascites (noncardiac): may be caused by:
   Renal disease,
   Hepatic obstruction (cirrhosis)
   Hypoproteinemia
   Malignancy
   Vitamin B deficiency especially in chronic alcholics with or without peripheral neuritis.
4. Distended neck veins—may be caused by:
   Hypervolemia,
   Pregnancy
   Superior vena caval obstruction.

   Liver enlargement can be due to hepatic or extrahepatic diseases.
   Tachycardia is nonspecific.
   Heart failure is frequently noticed for the first time in pregnancy with rheumatic valvular disease in whom cardiac compensation may return following delivery.

211. What type of heart failure you are dealing with? it does not mean:

1. Congenital—just because the patient is an infant or child.
2. Rheumatic—just because the patient is young.
3. Hypertensive—just because the patient is middle aged.
4. Coronary Heart disease—just because the patient is old.
   Such assumptions are usually correct, but occasionally they vary.
   Congenital heart disease may be asymptomatic until the age of 45 years or after and hypertension or ischemic heart disease may develop before the age of 35 years.
   Discovery of valvular lesion in older patients with heart failure rather than coronary heart disease may well explain why the digitalis is ineffective.

212. What disorder brought on the heart failure?

It is important to recognize not the cause of heart failure but the precipitating cause of heart failure as well. It is still more important to find out the precipitating disease or disorder which brought on heart failure especially in refractory heart failure. The 4 disorders are:

1. Infections—
   Pulmonary infection—pneumonia
   Rheumatic or other forms of myocarditis
   Infective endocarditis—diphtheria
   Urinary tract infections
   If we fail to identify that the heart failure is brought by pneumonia and assume his lung condition is a consequence of heart failure and allow the pneumonia remain untreated—the heart failure becomes refractory to treatment.
   In patients who are on complete bed rest with low cardiac output and circulatory stasis are more prone for developing thrombi in the lower limbs. Pulmonary embolism from thrombi in the lower extremeties results in raise of pulmonary arterial pressure and right heart failure. Such emboli may cause infarction of the lung in the presence of pulmonary congestion.
   Classical signs of pulmonary infarction may be absent (Pleural pain, changes in chest X-ray, hemoptysis) and the sole clue may be in the form of unexplained fever, leukocytosis, raised ESR, which aggravates the

cardiac problem. Sometimes, transient increase of serum bilirubin or frank jaundice may be present.

Patients with pulmonary vascular congestion are more prone but any infection may precipitate heart failure.

Any infection can affect patients with pre-existing heart disease.

Fever, tachycardia, hypoxemia and any other increased demand may further overload the myocardium of chronic heart failure.

2. Acute myocardial infarction—In patients with chronic but compensated ischemic heart disease—a fresh infarct can bring heart failure.

   Sometimes clinically "silent" myocardial infarction can cause heart failure.

3. Arrhythmias—in congestive cardiac failure.

   The presence of arrhythmias in heart failure may cause difficulty in treating heart failure because:

   a. No proper ventricular filling due to lack of time in ventricular tachyarrhythmias.
   b. Marked reduction of cardiac output in bradyarrhythmias associated with AV block.
   c. AV block dissociation leads to loss of atrial booster pump mechanism.
   d. Loss of normal synchronocity of ventricular contraction in AV conduction defects.

   Recognize them early, find out the cause, treat it properly before the heart failure becomes advanced.

4. Clinically silent—

   Aortic stenosis, mitral stenosis or constrictive pericarditis are amenable to surgical treatment.

   Hypertension, hyperthyroidism, infective endocarditis are amenable to medical treatment.

   Rapid elevation of blood pressure in some patients with hypertension of renal origin or discontinuation of antihypertensive medication may result in cardiac decompensation.

   Precipitation or intensification of heart failure may be one of the first clinical manifestation of hyperthyroidism in patients with underlying heart disease.

   If precipitating cause is properly recognized it can be treated more vigorously and effectively than the underlying cause.

   Prognosis is better in whom the precipitating cause is treated than in whom the underlying heart disease has advanced to the point of chronic heart failure with extreme myocardial impairment.

213. What is aggravating the heart failure?

There are plenty of conditions that aggravate heart failure and many are correctable. The following 4 are easily correctable aggravating causes:

1. Excessive exercise.
2. Excessive intake of salt or fluids.
3. Excessive or inadequate doses of digitalis or diuretics.
4. Electrolyte imbalance.

214. See for the 4 concomitant diseases that are likely to be overlooked:

1. Pulmonary disease—Pneumonia, pulmonary infarction, asthma, emphysema, recurrent pulmonary emboli. Pulmonary infarction is one of the commonest cause of refractory heart failure. If recognized early and treated vigorously with anticoagulants or in suitable cases by venous ligation, the heart may again respond to proper treatment.
2. Advanced renal disease especially with hypertension or bacterial endocarditis.

   During early stages, evidence of congestive heart failure may overshadow the less obvious but often more serious renal disease.

   Presence of nitrogen retention with small output and low specific gravity urine should alert the presence of serious renal impairment. In such cases it is difficult to manage electrolyte disturbance or congestive cardiac failure.
3. Hyperkinetic states such as:

   Anemia
   Fever
   Thiamine deficiency
   Arteriovenous fistula
   Hyperthyroidism.

   Overlooking the hyperkinetic states is serious because they are associated with high output failure. Digitalis is ineffective in these states and it may be contraindicated.
4. An underlying or overlooked cause of heart failure that may be amenable to surgical or medical treatment.

   Congenital—Patent ductus arteriosus or coarctation of aorta.

   Silent rheumatic valvular lesion like aortic stenosis or mitral stenosis, constrictive pericarditis, cardiac tumors.

   Infective endocarditis, hypertension and thyrotoxicosis are amenable to medical treatment.

215. Recognize the following 4 treatable factors which are unrecognized earlier:

1. Thyroid disorders.
2. Chronic arterial hypoxia due to pulmonary disorders complicating congestive heart failure often respond to oxygen therapy.
3. Severe anemia.
4. Thiamine deficiency especially in chronic alcoholics with or without peripheral neuritis and/or edema.

Surgically correctable congenital heart disease, rheumatic valvular disease, constrictive pericarditis, etc. are dealt accordingly.

216. Thyroid disorders:

A. Hyperthyroidism: Severe manifestations of hyperthyroidism include:
1. Heart failure among the elderly and in patients with low ventricular reserve.
2. Atrial fibrillation is a common in 9–22% of patients—suspect especially when it is resistant to digoxin.
3. Angina pectoris, which was previously stable may become unstable.
4. Nonspecific symptoms, such as fatigue, weight loss, and insomnia may predominate.

Masked thyrotoxicosis: It may not show any usual clinical features when it occurs in elderly with congestive cardiac failure. High degree of suspicion reveals the features like unusually soft skin, excess sweating, frequent diarrheas, heat intolerance, sinus tachycardia or atrial fibrillation. Serum PBI (protein-bound iodine) assay should be done. Circulation time helps to differentiate the high output failure from congestive failure.

Treat the thyrotoxicosis—carbimazole 5 mg tab—dose depends on the severity.

Radioactive iodine. Patents with refractory heart failure with normal thyroid gland sometimes improve by radioactive iodine therapy since it lowers the metabolism and hence the heart load.

B. Hypothyroidism is common in patients with heart failure.
1. Severe hypothyroidism, i.e. myxedema may cause decreased cardiac output in heart failure.
2. Bradycardia.
3. Pericardial effusion in severe cases.
4. ECG findings:
   i. Low voltage QRS in all leads.
   ii. Sinus bradycardia.
   iii. Increase PR interval.
   iv. Flat or inverted T waves.

(See Chapter Q-218).

Treatment consists of 50 µg of levothyroxine per day per elderly or 100 µg od for young otherwise healthy patients.

217. There are 4 clues to suspect thyrotoxicosis in refractory heart failure.

1. Atrial fibrillation.
2. Relative increase in circulation time.
3. Increased cardiac output (high output failure).
4. Resistant to the normal treatment of heart failure with digitalis, etc.

218. Severe anemia: High output heart failure occurs from severe anemia. Acute anemia commonly occurs due to rapid blood loss during surgery and major trauma. It is associated with depressed cardiac output caused by hypovolemia. These patients need immediate blood transfusion. However, the symptoms of CHF in chronic anemia are due to the following 4 compensatory mechanisms:

1. Decreased vascular resistance—it is the main compensatory mechanism.
2. Increased 2, 3- diphosphoglycerate (DGP), which shifts the hemoglobin oxygen dissociation curve to the right.
3. Fluid retention.
4. Increased cardiac output caused by resting tachycardia.

Even normal hearts can go into congestive heart failure with chronic anemia of severe proportions (hemoglobin <4 g/dL).

Management depends with severity of anemia. Patients with CHF should be given transfusion (whole blood or packed cells) slowly about 1 or 2 units over 24 hours and undergo diuresis whereas, mild to moderate anemia can be treated with iron, B12, and folic acid depending on the type of anemia.

New parental IV Preparations are also available, which can be given by IV infusion.

219. Thiamin deficiency (beriberi) is rare in western countries but still common in developing and under developed countries. It is common in those who observe fad diets for long periods and in those with alcoholism.

1. Wet beriberi shows the features of high output failure such as marked edema, peripheral vasodilation and pulmonary congestion.
2. Dry beriberi shows glossitis, hyperkeratosis, and peripheral neuropathy.
3. Investigations may show metabolic acidosis caused by lactic acid and depressed ketolase levels in RBC.
4. Treatment—give 100 mg thiamine IV followed by daily po and dietary replacement. Patients show very good improvement.

(See Chapter K-30, 31)

220. Treat the patient strictly and properly in refractory failure. Verify the rest, diet, digitalis and diuretics. The 4 very important steps in treatment are:

1. Strict bed rest—hospitalize the patient. Rest in bed or chair supplemented with a tranquilizer or a sedative. Elevation of the head-end of the bed to lessen the

tendency of pulmonary edema and congestive dyspnea. Short periods of bed rest alone may produce diuresis

2. Strict diet control—check the sodium intake. one liter of milk per day can be taken for few days in severe cases.
   Kempner diet consisting of rice, fruit juice and sugar restricts sodium intake to 200–400 mg/day. Drugs that increase sodium and water retention should not be taken, e.g. coticosteroids, estrogen, phenylbutazone, etc.
3. Digitalis—under digitalization or overdigitalization can contribute for refractory heart failure.
   Underdigitalization is common—patients do not take properly.
   Digitalis excess can cause bradycardia or tachycardia. There is a tendency to increase the dosage in tachycradia which may further increase toxicity and refractory failure.
   In the presence of atrial fibrillation with resting ventricular rate of 90/min. Increase in digitalis dose is needed. Extracardiac factors like hypokalemia, impaired renal or hepatic function needs low digitalis dose. Hypoxia in chronic cor pulmonale potentiates the toxic effects of digitalis and increases refractoriness.
4. Diuretics—A change from oral to IV diuretics may be useful. Most of them are benefited by changing the diuretic regimen alone. Check whether the patient is receiving maximum effective dose. When there is no response, combination is beneficial:
   Chlorothiazide
   Furosemide or ethacrinic acid oral or parentral.
   Potassium sparing diuretic spironolactone 25 mg × 6 hourly or triamterene 100 mg tds can be added to furosemide or ethacrinic acid or amiloride.
   Potassium sparing diuretics are useful in refractory failure with secondary aldosteronism. Triple or quadruple regimen can be used to potentiate the effects because they act by different mechanisms and at different sites in the nephron.
   Patients with resistant sodium retention or truly refractory HF needs IV dobutamine (2 to 5 μg/kg/min), dopamine (1 to 3 μg/kg/min) or a constant infusion of furosemide (1 to 5 mg/h). Fluid restriction to 2000 mL/d is needed in patients with dilutional hyponatremia.

221. Search for the following 4 unsuspected complications:

1. Electrolyte disturbance: Patients on prolonged diuretic therapy and on salt restriction may be suffering from anorexia and electrolyte disturbance. They show lack of response to diuretics and show marked weakness and apathy.
   'Hypochloremic hypokalemic alkalosis' is the common disturbance. Treat with 5 cc of 20% potassium chloride 4 times a day.
   Use of potassium sparing diuretics, spironolactone or triamterene prevent this complication.
   Hyponatremia and hypochloremia.
   In the presence of edema, these values reflect dilutional hyponatremia and not true sodium depletion. This is treated by restriction of water intake to one liter per day and not with addition of sodium chloride.
   When there is no response to water restriction, treat it by peritoneal dialysis.
2. Advanced renal disease—common in those with hypertension or bacterial endocarditis.
   Nitrogen retention with a small output low specific gravity urine should be suspected in the presence of serious renal impairment. It is difficult to manage electrolyte disturbance or congestive heart failure in such cases.
3. Pulmonary infarction: It is one of the commonest causes of refractory heart failure. If it is recognized, treat it vigorously with anticoagulants or by venesection in suitable cases.
4. Extreme myocardial impairments: This should be suspected when all the above causes are satisfied and then the heart failure has become intractable and will remain refractory to any treatment.

222. Treatment of edema in refractory heart failure consists of 4 steps:

1. Diuretics—Most patients require combination of potent diuretics. Thiazide or loop diuretics can be combined with one or more potentiating drugs such as spironolactone, triamterene, aminophylline, acetazolamide, if edema persists.
2. Hemodialysis or peritoneal dialysis.
   - Removes sodium and water while correcting electrolyte imbalance and nitrogen retention.
3. Paracentesis removes fluid from pleural and peritoneal cavities.
4. Ultrafiltration may be considered in late stage of heart failure resistant to conventional treatment.

223. Consider the following 4 groups of drugs in refractory heart failure (after digitalis and diuretics) and use them depending on the severity of the condition.

1. *Vasodilators:* Nitrates, hydralazine, prazocin, minoxidil.
   Nitrates acts on preload.
   Hydralazine acts on after load
   Combination of isosorbide dinitrate and hydralazine acts both on preload and afterload.
   Prazocin acts both on preload and afterload.

Prazocin is particularly useful in valvular regurgitation secondary to congestive cardiac failure.

Exclude stenotic lesions like AS, MS in congestive cardiac failure before starting vasodilators. (Prostacyclin, and prostaglandin PGE are in experimental stage).

2. *ACE inhibitors:* Captopril or enalapril are only arteriolar dilators.

   Consensus trail has shown addition of enalapril reduced mortality rate in class IV type patients of congestive cardiac failure.

3. *Dobutamine and phosphodiesterase inhibitors:* Oral inotropic drugs available after digitalis amrinone, Milrinone are showing promising results.

   Newer inotropic agents also have peripheral vasodilator effect, which are being increasingly used now.

   Dobutamine and phosphodiesterase temporarily improve cardiac output and renal blood flow is sometimes effective in lessening symptoms and relieving refractory salt and water retention. Low dose dobutamine, 2.5 to 5 µg/kg/min is frequently sufficient. Alternatively, IV milrinone (50 µg/kg loading dose, then 0.375 to 0.75 µg/kg/min) may be used. Occasionally, patients may improve symptomatically as a result of long-term low dose dobutamine infusion (2 to 5 µg/kg/min) given through an indwelling central catheter on a long-term outpatient basis. Large doses of dobutamine may produce:

   a. Tachycardia
   b. Ventricular arrhythmias
   c. Hypokalemia
   d. Myocardial ischemia.

   Concerns have been raised about its safety in light of the increase in mortality reported with high dose dobutamine infusions and long-term milrinone therapy.

4. *β-blockers:* Catecholamines can be controlled by the β-blockers. β-blockers can precipitate congestive failure but use of β-lockers in advanced myocardial disease has shown some benefit. Some improvement is shown with metaprolol in DCM, with light increase in ejection fraction also. Metaprolol works in some but does not work in most of the patients. So selection of patient is important when using metaprolol in CHF.

   Small doses of β-blockers may be useful in certain subset of patients with congestive heart failure due to dilated cardiomyopathy (DCM). The benefit is attributed to increase in β receptor density and improvement of diastolic compliance.

   However, they should be used under strict supervision with extreme caution in congestive heart failure. β blockers when given as an addition to a regimen of ACE inhibitor + diuretic showed improvement in HF. They are not given alone. B-blockers are not given in acute HF (calcium blockers nifedipine, diltiazam have no role in congestive cardiac failure). Addition of low dose amrinone to the standard treatment of moderately severe chronic heart failure may show improvement in some patient.

   Use of steroids with immunosuppressive purpose has shown some use. Myocardial biopsy has shown that active myocarditis may persist even up to 2 years after the onset of symptoms. Steroids and immunosuppressive agents control active disease to some extent and thus control congestive cardiac failure.

224. The following 4 changes have occurred recently in the medical management of HF:

1. Diastolic failure—it is not known earlier.
2. Digitalis is the first and last drug in HF—Several new drugs have come in the management of HF
3. β blockers are contraindicated earlier—Now they are given in several cases of HF along with ACEI + diuretics even in refractory HF.
4. Exercise is completely banned—exercises are programmed now.

225. Surgical management of heart failure:

Over the past three decades, the mortality from cardiovascular disease has decreased in industrialized societies while the incidence and prevalence of heart failure has been increasing over the age of 65 years.

The natural course of HF is progressive. Introduction of angiotensin converting enzyme inhibitors showed consistently improved prognosis in the medical management of HF. Some patients are benefited by conventional cardiac surgery like correction of congenital defects, valve repair or replacement, coronary revascularization. Options are increasing with new operative procedures.

1. Cardiac transplantation.
2. Dynamic cardiomyoplasty.
3. Left ventricular volume reduction.
4. Mechanical support—left ventricular assist devices.

1. Heart transplantation (Ref. U Point 50–57) is presently the optimum surgical treatment for many patients. Scarcity of donor organs restricts the allograft transplantation. Recent claims of xenotransplants for transgenic porcine hearts and their potential availability is unlikely to solve the problem by immunosuppressive agents alone.
2. Dynamic cardiomyoplasty (Ref. U point - 49) has attracted because there is no question of rejection and therefore no need for immunosuppressive drugs also. Elective surgery is possible.

However, more than 30% of operative and first year mortality and little objective hemodynamic improvement survivors have not kept up their interest despite improvement in the quality of life.

3. Reduction of left ventricular volume for dilated cardiomyopathy involves surgical resection of a large segment of ventricular muscle. It results in reduction in the radius and increase in wall thickness of the left ventricle. Intraoperative mortality is 15% but with 85% survivors improving from NYHA functional class IV to functional class I and II . The procedure is still on trials and results are awaited.
4. Left ventricular assist devices are now available (The Novocar and HeartMate devices) for long term implantation. They are inherently expensive, but randomized trials comparing with medical management or transplantation my prove them cost effective.

226. The major limitations of left ventricular assist devices are

1. Risk of infection.
2. Thromboembolism.
3. Noise.
4. Batteries to be charged every 8 to12 hours.

The Jarvik 2000 is an axial flow pump about the size of a thumb in contrast to the one liter volume displacement of HeartMate, designed to sit within the apex of the left ventricle and silently deliver non-pulsatile flow rates up to 10 liters per minute. The long-term physiological effects are still under investigation. It is likely to be available for clinical use.

D Cardiac Arrhythmias

Arrhythmias have remained comparatively neglected subject in cardiology. Medical management of arrhythmias are modestly effective. Many a times their impact is short lived and arrhythmias recur or rate control is lost. With the advent of radiofrequency ablation as a cure in some conditions and pacemaker therapy in refractory cases, cardiac arrhythmias have generated new hope of interest and appeal.

1. There are 4 types of cardiac muscle fibers.

1. Atrial muscle fiber 2. Ventricular muscle fibers	Contract in the same manner as skeletal muscle fibers
3. Excitatory fibers 4. Conductive fibers	Specialized fibers for rapid conduction of impulses

2. The 4 electrophysiological properties of cardiac tissue are:

1. Excitability and contractility
   a. "All or None" phenomenon
   b. The force of contraction
2. Automaticity/Rhythmicity.
   The heart has the power of initiating its own impulses without recourse to external agencies. Normally this function is done by the SA node.
   The ability to initiate and maintain the heartbeat over prolonged periods is only present in the specialized tissues–SA node, AV node, bundle of His and its branches.
   The autonomic nervous system regulates the conduction system by both sympathetic and parasympathetic divisions. The sympathetic system innervates the heart as a whole, the parasympathetic innervation is restricted mainly to the supraventricular portion (AV node and above).

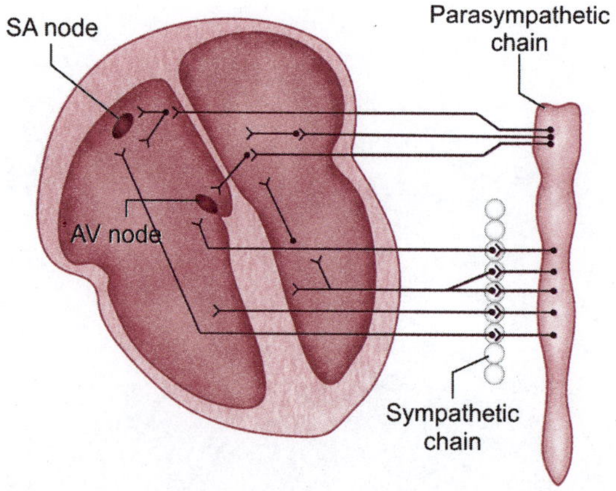

Fig. D-1: Autonomic innervation of the heart

   Automaticity is the ability of a cardiac tissue fiber to generate pacemaker activity spontaneously. It can be both normal and abnormal source of automaticity.
   It should be stressed here that all the cardiac arrhythmias are as a result of increase or decrease in automaticity or conductivity or a combination of both.
3. Conductivity: Speed of conduction in mm/second

Atrial muscle	400
AV node	200
Perking fibers	4000
Ventricular muscle	400

4. Refractoriness: Absolute during contraction 0.2 sec.
   Relative shortly after contraction.
   There is no normal stimulation during the refractory period. Conductivity and refractoriness are characteristics of myocardium even though present to some extent in skeletal muscle.

3. The force of contraction of the heart muscle depends on 4 factors.

1. Initial length of the fiber
2. The duration of diastolic phase
3. The nutrition and oxygen supply of the myocardium
4. Rate: at 72 per minute
   Systolic is 0.25 to 0.3 sec
   Diastolic is 0.55 to 0.5 sec

4. 4 microns is the average diameter of each fiber of the SA node.

(3–5 μ in width and 1 cm length in contrast to the 15–20 μ of surrounding atrial muscle fibers).
SA node is visible to the naked eye.

5. 0.4 meters/sec is the average velocity of conduction of the action potential in both atrial and ventricular muscle (that is 0.3–0.5 sec or about 1/250 of velocity of large nerve fiber, 1/10th velocity of skeletal muscle fiber).

6. 0.04 seconds is the approximate time taken for the impulse to travel from SA node to the AV node through the internodal pathway.

7. 4 meters per second is the conduction velocity of bundle of His.

8. 4 meters per second is the velocity of impulse in Purkinje system.

(1.5–4.0 meters, about six times that of the usual cardiac muscle and 300 times that of the junctional fibers—this allows immediate transmission of cardiac impulse to the ventricular system).

9. 0.4 to 0.5 meters per second is the velocity of transmission of impulse in the ventricular mass by the ventricular muscle fibers themselves.

10. At a normal heart rate of 72/min, the period of contraction is about 0.4 of the entire cardiac cycle.

11. There are 4 stations at which the cardiac impulses are relayed normally.

1. SA node—Rhythmic and self-excitatory—impulse is started
2. AV node—Impulses from the atria are delayed before passing into the ventricles
3. AV bundle or bundle of His conducts from the atria into the ventricles.
4. Purkinje system—Left and right Purkinje fibers conduct the impulse to all parts of the ventricles.

12. The excitatory and conduction fibers are discovered from Purkinje to SA node, i.e. from below upward (microscopic structures are discovered earlier to the structures seen by naked eye).

1. Purkinje system was discovered in - 1845
2. Bundle of His was discovered in - 1893
3. Atrio ventricular node was discovered by Taward - 1906
4. SA node was discovered by Keith and Flack - 1907
   (SA node can be seen by naked eye)
   (Internodal tracts were discovered in 1963)

13. Arrhythmias generally arises due to

1. Abnormal impulse generation
2. Alternation in automaticity
3. Alteration in conductivity
4. Combination of 2 and 3.

14. Causes of arrhythmias in general are:

1. Ischemia/infarction (e.g. MI, ischemia, post-infarct, etc.) fibrosis in the endocardium or myocardium causes conduction disturbance
2. Inflammation (endocarditis, myocarditis)
3. Metabolic: Hyper or hypokalemia, acidosis, etc. alters the automaticity
4. Drugs: Especially digitalis and many proarrhythmic drugs.

15. There are 4 inherent heart rates.

1. SA node	70–80 min
2. Atrial	75 min
3. AV node	60 min
4. Ventricle	30–40 min

SA node is the normal cardiac pacemaker. It is in the posterior wall of the right atrium. SA node normally sets the rate of the heart. If the SA node does not function as a normal pacemaker, the potential pacemakers will take over the pace setting activity. These potential pacemakers are often referred to as 'ectopic pacemakers'. They are present within all parts of the heart including atria, AV node, and ventricles. Under normal conditions, these pacemakers are electrically quiet and do not function. Therefore, they are called as 'potential or ectopic pacemakers'.
In an emergency or pathological conditions an ectopic atrial or nodal or ventricle ectopic focus may suddenly begin to fire at a fast rate 150–250 bpm.

16. There are 4 conduction pathways in the atria.

1. Anterior internodal tract— Bachmann's bundle
2. Middle internodal tract— Wenckebach's bundle
3. Posterior internodal tract— Thorel's pathway
4. An accessory pathway called— Bundle of Kent

Sometimes, connects atria directly to the ventricle (cause of WPW syndrome).

17. The ventricular systole can be described into 4 stages.

1. *Period of isometric contraction:* The tension increases in the muscle but no shortening of the muscle fibers occur.

2. *Period of ejection:* Left ventricular pressure rises slightly above 80 mm Hg and right ventricular pressure rises slightly above 8 mm Hg; Ventricular pressure now pushes the semilunar valves to open, ventricular emptying occurs.
3. *Protodiastolic:* No blood flows from the ventricles into the large arteries. Ventricular pressure falls slightly below that in aorta though the ventricles are still contracting.
4. *Period of isometric relaxation:* Ventricular relaxation begins suddenly. Intraventricular pressures fall rapidly. Elevated pressure in large arteries push blood towards ventricles, which snaps aortic and pulmonary valves.

18. Action potential is caused by sequence of changes in the membrane permeability for sodium and potassium.

Normally there is negative potential of –80 to –90 mV in the resting cardiac muscle cell called as membrane resting potential (MRP). Inside of the cell is negative with respect to the outside (i.e. –90 mV), but the cells are electrically active and a sufficient stimulus is able to initiate a depolarization. Potassium is inside and sodium is outside the cell under resting state. Ionic gradients are maintained across the cardiac cell membrane. The extracellular concentration of sodium is about 10 to 15 times the intracellular concentration, and the intracellular concentration of potassium is 30 to 35 times its extracellular concentration. The potassium gradient is responsible for the transmembrane resting potential.

The sequence of changes are described in 0 to 4 phases.

The sequence of changes are described in 0 to 4 phases.

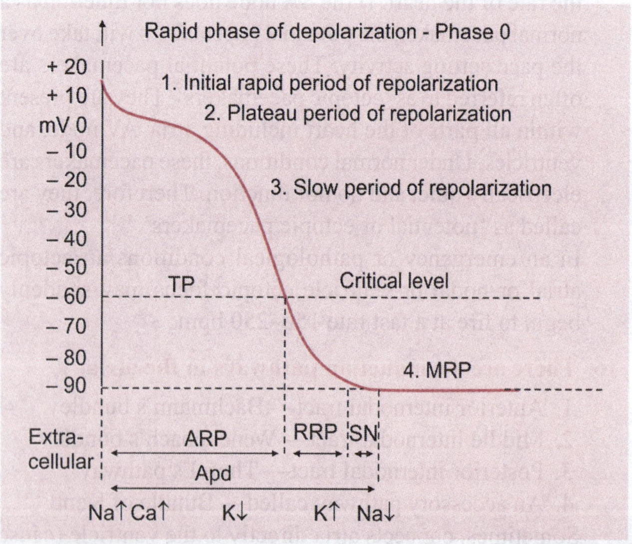

Fig. D-2: Action potential of a ventricular muscle cell

O = Rapid phase of depolarization; 1, 2, 3 = Phase of repolarization; 4 = diastolic phase = MRP membrane resting potential; Apd = duration of action potential; TP = Threshold potential; ARP = Absolute refractory period; RRP = Relative refractory period; SN = Supernormal period

RAPID PHASE OF DEPOLARIZATION ALSO KNOWN AS PHASE 0

There is a tremendous increase in sodium permeability as much as about 5000 fold increase. Since there is high concentration of sodium outside the cell, sodium ions diffuse rapidly carrying positive charges and changing the inside electrical potential from negativity to positivity. This results in overshooting of electrical deflection from –80 to –90 mV to +20 mV.

Phase I: An initial rapid period of repolarization.

Phase II: Plateau phase: Calcium ions enter the cell through slow calcium channels, whereas sodium enters fast in the phase 0.

Phase III: Potassium exist occurs with rapid repolarization. There is an increase of potassium permeability to outside coupled with a simultaneous decrease of sodium permeability back to normal. This allows large quantities of positively charged potassium ions to diffuse out of the cell.

Phase IV: Diastolic phase: Potassium gets in and sodium gets out of the cell. Reversal of phase III.

Phase IV is often considered as the resting phase but it is really a very active phase because at this phase adenosine triphosphate (ATP) is hydrolyzed to adenosine diphosphatase (ADP) by ATpase.

Sodium is pumped out and potassium reenters the cell.

The duration of action potential is longer in a Purkinje fiber than in any place. This is the cause of prolongation of phase II of repolarization.

19. There are 4 sequential events of sodium and potassium during the action potential.

1. First event is a tremendous increase in sodium permeability. Sodium ions from outside enter into the cell carrying positive charges, thus changing inside electrical potential from negativity to positivity.
2. Second event is an increase in potassium ions permeability coupled with simultaneous decrease of sodium ions permeability.
   Large quantities of positively charged potassium ions diffuse out of the cell due to which the inside membrane potential returns to its negative resting level.
3. Third event is the decrease of potassium permeability to normal.
4. Fourth event is active transport of sodium back out of the cell and simultaneously diffusion of potassium back into the cell, thus re-establishing the original state of the cell.

Some factors that can elicit action potential are

i. Electrical stimulation
ii. Application of chemicals of the membrane to cause increased permeability to sodium

iii. Mechanical damage to the membrane, e.g. heat, cold, ischemia, injury or infarction
iv. Drugs and electrolytes.

20. There are 4 points to know about plateau in action potential.

This type of action potential occurs in the heart where the plateau lasts for as long as two to three tenths of a second and causes contraction of the heart during the entire period.

1. First there is delay in inactivation of sodium channels. This allows sodium ions to flow continuously into the fiber for a long time after the onset of action potential.
2. Small amount of calcium ions also flow into the fibers along with sodium ions at the same time, and these two currents sodium and calcium ions together maintain the positivity inside the membrane that causes the plateau.
3. Probably, permeability of potassium channels decreases about five fold at the onset of action potential in excitable membrane that exhibits plateau and this prevents rapid outflow of potassium ions to the outside of the membrane and therefore delays the repolarization process.
4. When inactivation of sodium channels begins, the inactivation process continues combated simultaneously potassium permeability of the membrane increases a hundred-fold or more.
   This means, sodium and calcium ions stop diffusing into the cell while potassium ions diffuse outward extremely rapidly.

Influx of sodium ions in phase 0 of rapid depolarization records QRS complex.

Phase II – Plateau phase where calcium ions enter the cell via the slow calcium channels gives raise to ST segment which is a repolarization wave. The relatively slow and long duration of this even explain the slow channel calcium ions causing long straight ST segment. The T wave correlates with the potassium ions existing in the cells via potassium channels. This is why hypo-or hyperkalemia affects the T wave morphology and hypo- or hypercalcemia affects the ST segment. Hyperkalemia causes tall T waves. Hypokalemia causes flat T wave. Hypercalcemia causes shortening of ST segment. Hypocalcemia causes lengthening of ST segment.

Changes in sodium ion concentration does not alter the QRS morphology, because clinical hypo- or hypernitremia are not significant enough to alter the QRS morphology. Considering the availability of high levels of extracellular sodium ion concentration. Blood levels of both calcium and potassium are relatively low compared to the sodium ions hence the changes in calcium and potassium ions causes significant effect on ECG.

Possible role of calcium ions in closing the sodium gates: When calcium ions are deficient in the extracellular fluids, the sodium gates will not close fully between action potentials and membrane remains very leaky to sodium ion—sometimes, so much so, that membrane remains depolarized continuously or fires repetitively causing arrhythmias. Because of this effect it is believed that calcium ions in some way play a significant role in closure of sodium gates.

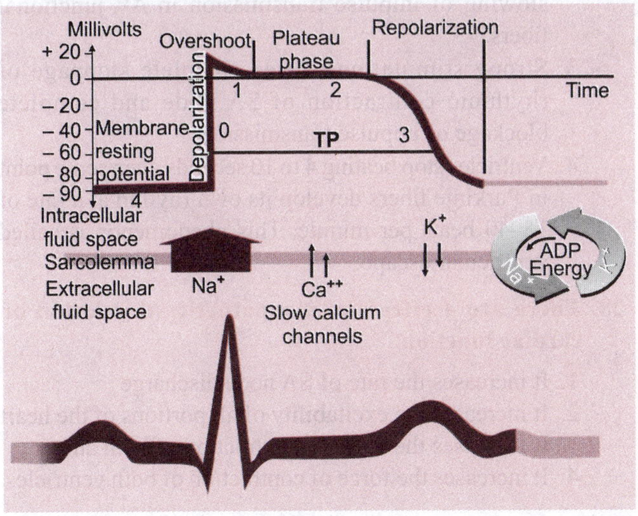

Fig. D-3: Relation of action potential with surface ECG

21. The monophasic action potential curve of a cell in the sinoatrial (SA) node is markedly different from ventricular and atrial muscle cells in the following 4 ways.

Action potential curve of an atrial muscle cell is different from that of a ventricular muscle cell. Phase 0 (depolarization) and phase 4 (MRP) are similar, but the duration of repolarization is shorter and hence the duration of action potential. This is mainly due to shortening and steeping of the slope phase 2.

1. There is a lower membrane resting potential (MRP) of –60 to –70 mV at the onset of diastole.

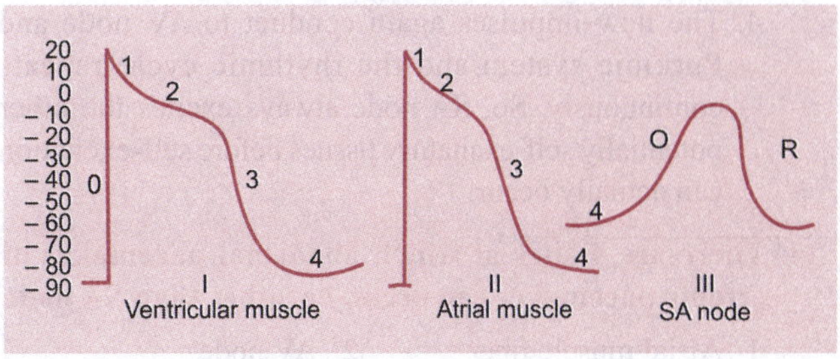

Fig. D-4: Action potential curves. I: Ventricular muscle cell II: Atrial muscle cell. III: SA node. *Note:* R-Repolarization phase of SA node is not divisible into phases 1, 2 and 3

2. There is a gradual raise of MRP instead of constant MRP during diastole. A prepotential is present in diastole which causes automatic function (automaticity) of SA node as a pacemaker.
3. Depolarization is slower and does not reach sufficient potential and so it could not be recorded on surface electrocardiogram.
4. The peak of action potential is rounded and repolarization is a single slow curve without definitive phases 1, 2 and 3.

22. The 4 inherent qualities that made the SA node to be the pacemaker are:

1. It has an inherent rate of 70–80 per minute.
2. It has low MRP (membrane resting potential) of only –55 to –60 mV in comparison to most of the other fibers which has –80 to –90 mV.
3. It has the more natural leakiness of the membrane to sodium ions.
4. Thus, the leakage of sodium ions causes the self-excitation of SA fibers.

23. There are 4 points to know why the SA node controls the heart's rhythmicity whereas AV node or Purkinje system cannot do it.

1. SA node has inherent rate greater than AV node or Purkinje fibers
   SA node: 70–80 min
   AV node: 40–60 min
   Purkinje fibers: 15–40 min
   SA node is the pacemaker because its rate of rhythmic discharge is greater than that of any other part of the heart.
2. Every time when SA node discharges its impulses, they are conducted to the AV node and Purkinje system discharging their excitable membrane. By that time, all these tissues recover from action potential and become greatly hyperpolarized.
3. SA node looses this hyperpolarization much earlier than others and discharges new impulses before others can reach of their own threshold for self-excitation.
4. The new impulses again conduct to AV node and Purkinje system and the rhythmic cycle repeats continuously. So, SA node always excites the other potentially self-excitatory tissues before self-excitation can actually occur.

24. There are 4 sites at which abnormal pacemaker or ectopic pacemaker can occur, i.e. other than SA node

1. Atrial muscle fiber
2. AV node
3. Ventricular muscle fiber
4. Purkinje fibers

25. There are 4 reasons for the ectopic focus to become irritable resulting in extrasystoles or ectopic beats. The cause is mostly an ectopic focus and not the SA node.

1. Local ischemia and change of ionic composition of the muscle
2. Calcified plaques irritating the adjacent muscle
3. Irritation of AV node or Purkinje system or myocardium due to drugs, nicotine, caffeine, etc.
4. During cardiac catheterization or cardiac surgery.

26. Since an extrasystole is a premature beat before it is due, the heart contracts from a smaller end-diastolic volume and has a smaller stroke volume. The pulse in such conditions may be too small to be palpable and is spoken as pulse deficit or missed beat. Normal rhythm of the heart may be changed due to several causes,

1. Changed rhythmicity of the SA node, i.e. sinus arrhythmia, sinus tachycardia or bradycardia.
2. Shift of the pacemaker from SA node to AV node, conducting tissue, or a focus in the myocardium (atrium or ventricle) which becomes more irritable than the SA node—Ectopic beats or extrasystoles.
3. Block to the transmission of cardiac impulse.
4. Abnormal pathway for transmission of cardiac impulse.

27. There are 4 effects of parasympathetic stimulation (Vagal) on cardiac function.

1. Release of acetylcholine increases the permeability of potassium which allows rapid leakage of potassium to the exterior. This results in greater negativity inside the fiber, an effect called hyperpolarization, which makes excitable tissue less excitable.
2. Results in decrease of rate of rhythm in SA node, slowing of impulse transmission in AV junctional fibers.
3. Strong stimulation causes complete stoppage of rhythmic contraction of SA node and complete blockage of impulse transmission.
4. Ventricles stop beating 4 to 10 seconds, then some point in Purkinje fibers develop its own rhythm at a rate of 15–40 beats per minute. This phenomenon is called ventricular escape.

28. There are 4 effects of sympathetic stimulation on cardiac function.

1. It increases the rate of SA node discharge
2. It increases the excitability of all portions of the heart
3. It increases the force of contraction of both atria
4. It increases the force of contraction of both ventricles.

29. There are 4 events that follow the sympathetic stimulation.

1. Norepinephrine is liberated at the nerve endings
2. It increases the permeability of the membrane to sodium and calcium at the SA node and AV nodal fibers.
3. Increased permeability to sodium causes the increased tendency for the resting membrane potential to delay the threshold for self-excitation at the SA node and decreases conduction time in the AV node.
4. Increased permeability of calcium is responsible for the increase in contractile strength of cardiac muscle fiber.

30. There are 4 causes of circus movement (causes reentry of the impulse).

1. *Hypertrophy:* A long pathway caused by dilated hearts.
2. *Ischemia:* Causes blockage of the Purkinje fibers resulting in decreased rate of conduction.
3. *Electrolyte imbalance:* Hyperkalemia causes delayed conduction.
4. *Drugs:* Causing shortening of refractory period, such as epinephrine, intense vagal stimulation, repetitive electrical stimulation. (Atrial flutter results from a circus pathway).

Figure D-5 illustrates several cardiac muscle strips cut in the form of circles. If such a strip is stimulated at 12 o' clock position, the impulse progressively travel in one direction around the circle until it returns to 12 o' clock position. If the originally stimulated fibers are still in a refractory state, the impulse then dies out because the refractory muscle cannot transmit a second impulse. However, there are some conditions that could cause this impulse to continue to travel around the circle, that is, to cause **'reentry'** of the impulse into muscle that has already been excited.

If the *length of the pathway around the circle is long,* by the time the impulse returns to the 12 o'clock position, the already stimulated muscle will no longer be refractory, and the impulse will continue around the circle again and again as seen in hypertrophy or dilatation (1).

In some, the length of the pathway remains constant, but the velocity of conduction becomes decreased enough; an increased interval of time will elapse before the impulse returns to the 12 o'clock position. Meanwhile, the originally stimulated muscle might be out of refractory state and the impulse can continue around and around the circle again and again. This is seen in blockage of the Purkinje system, ischemia, hyperkalemia, etc. (2 & 3).

In some, the *refractory period of the muscle might have become greatly shortened* by certain drugs or following repetitive electrical stimulation. In these conditions, the impulse could also continue around and around the circle (4).

Thus, in many different conditions, circus movements can cause abnormal cardiac rhythmicity that completely ignores the pacemaker effects of the SA node.

Circus movement results from the above causes in atrial flutter or fibrillation. The circus pathway is around and around in atrial flutter from top to bottom. In atrial fibrillation, many separate contractile waves spread in different directions over the cardiac muscle at the same time in either atrial or ventricular fibrillation. Obviously, these circus movement in fibrillation is entirely different from that in flutter.

Reentry is a simple concept, and is the mechanism of most clinically important arrhythmias. It describes the progression of a wave front of electrical activation through cardiac muscle over a pathway that leads back to its point of origin. This completes one circle of a reentrant circuit. In certain conditions as discussed above, the conduction will continue around circuit again and again to produce regular arrhythmias. The Wolff-Parkinson-White syndrome is a well-recognized tachycardia through reentry circuit of conduction from atria to ventricles via the atrioventricular node and then from ventricle to atrial via an accessory pathway of Kent which is a congenital anomaly.

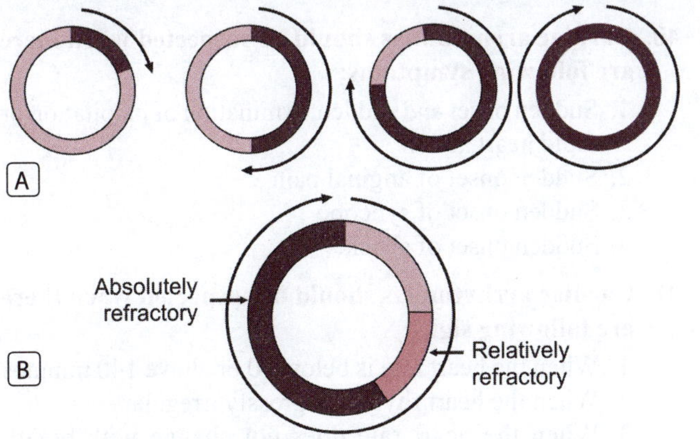

Fig. D-5: Circus movement. A. Normal pathway B. Long pathway. Illustrates annihilation of impulse in the short pathway and continued propagation of impulse in the long pathway

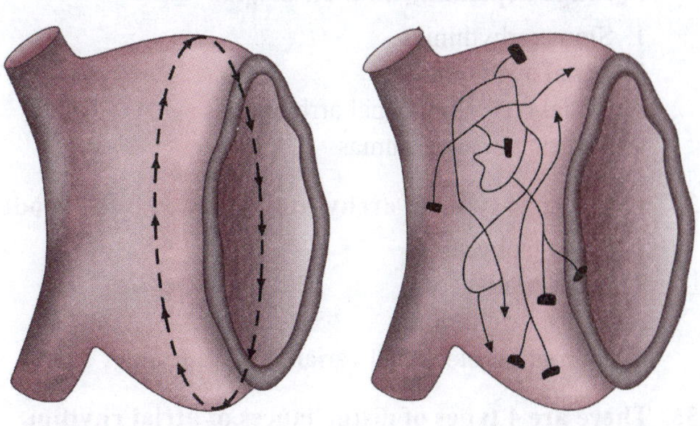

Fig. D-6: Pathways of impulses in atrial flutter and fibrillation

In any condition in which there is structural variation providing a similar circular conduction pathway—be it congenital (such as accessory pathway mediated tachycardia, AV nodal reentrant tachycardia and possibly atrial flutter) or acquired (such as ventricular tachycardia after myocardial infarction), there is potential for reentrant arrhythmias. By contrast, when reentrant wave fronts can pass aimlessly through the myocardium without following a fixed pathway, they lead to fibrillation. The mechanism underlying focal arrhythmias is abnormal, rapid, spontaneous electrical activity of a group of cells spreading to the rest of the myocardium.

31. Structural variant providing circular conduction can occur in:

1. Congenital – accessory pathway of Kent
2. AV nodal reentrant tachycardiac
3. Atrial flutter
4. Acquired ventricular tachycardiac after acute myocardial infarction.

In contrast, when there is severe generalized disruption of the electrical properties of the myocardium as occurs in many forms of structural heart disease (e.g. MS, after AMI) reentrant wavy fronts can occur aimlessly through the myocardium without following a fixed path resulting in fibrillation. The mechanism underlying focal arrhythmias is abnormal rapid, spontaneous electrical activity of a group of cells spreading to the rest of the myocardium.

32. The arrhythmias can be broadly classified into 4 groups:

Disturbances in impulse formation

1. Varying rhythm
2. Extra beats and skips
3. Rapid rhythm

Disturbances in impulse conduction

4. Heart blocks.

33. Arrhythmias can also be classified in a simple way into 4 groups depending on their origin.

1. Sinus arrhythmias
2. Atrial arrhythmias
3. Nodal (AV)/Junctional arrhythmias
4. Ventricular arrhythmias.

34. There are 4 types of arrhythmias caused by SA node.

1. Sinus tachycardia
2. Sinus bradycardia
3. Sinus arrhythmia
4. Sino-atrial block and variants.

35. There are 4 types of disturbances of atrial rhythm.

1. Atrial ectopics or extrasystoles or premature beats, Atrial premature contractions (APCs)
2. Atrial tachycardia—paroxysmal atrial tachycardia (PAT) with or without AV Block
3. Atrial flutter
4. Atrial fibrillation.

36. There are 4 types of arrhythmias of nodal origin.

1. AV junctional tachycardia
2. AV junctional escape beats
3. Nonparoxysmal AV junctional tachycardia
4. AV nodal reentry
   i. Reentry over a retrograde conduction (concealed accessory pathway)
   ii. Pre-excitation syndrome.

37. There are 4 types of ventricular arrhythmias.

1. Ventricular ectopic beats
2. Ventricular tachycardias
3. Ventricular flutter
4. Ventricular fibrillation.

38. Arrhythmias are:

1. Common (Seen even in anxiety)
2. Often benign (but may reflect underline heart disease often an incidental finding, e.g. PVBs)
3. Often intermittent causing difficulty in diagnosis (e.g. PVBs, PAT, WPW syndrome)
4. Occasionally severe causing cardiac compromise – severe AF, VT, VF.

39. Causes:

1. CAD/IHD (AMI)—common
2. Rheumatic heart disease
3. Cardiac muscle disease, e.g. DCM and HOCM/ myocarditis
4. Aberrant conduction pathways, e.g. WPW syndrome
5. Drugs–cardiac and noncardiac drugs
6. Electrolytes disturbances (K^+, Ca^{++}, Mg^{++})
7. Thyroid disease
8. Other noncardiac causes, such as acute respiratory infections, e.g. pneumonia.
   Smoking, alcohol, etc.

40. Cardiac arrhythmias should be suspected when there are following symptoms:

1. Sudden onset and sudden termination of palpitation or rapid heart action
2. Sudden onset of anginal pain
3. Sudden onset of syncope
4. Sudden onset of shock.

41. Cardiac arrhythmias should be suspected when there are following signs.

1. When the heart rate is below 40 or above 140 minutes
2. When the heart rhythm is grossly irregular
3. When the heart rate does not change with breath holding or exercise
4. When the heart rate suddenly slows by carotid sinus massage.

42. Arrhythmias are harmful to the patient because they cause:

1. Reduction in cardiac output
2. Lowering of BP
3. Reduce the perfusion of vital organs—brain, heart, kidney.
4. In the presence of heart disease, they precipitate acute heart failure or pulmonary edema, angina pectoris or myocardial infarction, syncope, poor cerebration with confusion or cerebral thrombosis. Therefore, arrhythmias should be treated to relieve symptoms or prevent sudden death.

43. Investigations: Routine blood test

1. Complete hemogram (e.g. anemia is very common-common cause of sinus tachycardia).
2. Urea and creatinine
3. Electrolytes – Na^+, K^+, Cl^-, $HCO3^-$, Ca^{++}, Mg^{++}
4. Blood sugar
5. Thyroid
6. ECG
7. Echocardiogram
8. Electrophysiological studies (EP) in rare conditions, e.g. arrhythmias may be stimulated and its therapeutic response to various medicines assessed.

44. There are 4 important points to be checked for rhythm in ECG.

1. *Check the P waves.* This is the single most important point in the diagnosis of arrhythmia.
   Verify:
   i. Morphology of the P waves. Whether P waves have the same morphology?
   ii. Rate of P wave?
   iii. Are the P waves regular?
   iv. Check for P waves before each QRS
   Do the P waves precede each QRS?
2. *Check for QRS waves*
   i. Morphology—is it constant or changing?
   ii. What are the duration of QRS?
   iii. Are the QRS regular?
   iv. Check for QRS after each P wave
3. *Check for PR interval* (i.e. atrioventricular conduction)
   i. Is it constant or changing?
   ii. Is there an RP-interval (i.e. ventriculoatrial conduction)
4. *Measure RR interval*
   i. Is it constant or changing?
   ii. Is it regularly irregular?
   iii. Or irregularly irregular?

SINUS ARRHYTHMIAS

The range of normal sinus rate is defined as 60 to 100 impulses per minute with regular rhythm.

45. Sinus node arrhythmias may be due to abnormal impulse generation, conduction, or propagation of the impulse inside the SA node or exit-blocks inside the SA node.

1. Sinus tachycardia
2. Sinus bradycardia
3. Sinus arrhythmia
4. SA block, arrest, sick sinus syndrome (SSS).

46. Sinus tachycardia is defined as an increase in sinus node depolarization with 'firing' of greater than 100 minutes. The upper limit in adults is 160–180 per minute having gradually decreased from infant rate of approximately 200–220 per minute. Its presence may represent hemostat response, e.g. need of increased cardiac output as in exercise or it may be caused by disease of the heart or other organs.

It is a normal finding with exercise and anxiety.

It is commonly seen in.

1. Fever and other hyperkinetic circulatory states. Heart rate increases approximately 10 beats/min per each degree of Fahrenheit rise in body temperature up to about 105°F. Beyond this the heart rate may actually decreases owing to progressive weakness of the heart muscle as a result of fever. Fever increases the rate of metabolism of SA node which in turn directly increases its excitability and rate of rhythm.
2. Peripheral circulatory failure, congestive heart failure: When the patient is in shock reflex stimulation of the heart increases its rate to as great as 150–180 beats/min.
3. Simple weakening of the myocardium: For example, toxins on the heart or cardiac failure. The weakened heart does not pump blood into arterial tree to a normal level, and this elicits reflexes to increase the rate of heart.
4. Hyperthyroidism.
5. Anxiety.
6. Anemia.
7. Pulmonary diseases including pulmonary embolism.
8. Drugs or toxins (e.g. atropine, catecholamines, caffeine, and nicotine).

The therapy is directed toward the underlying cause.

47. ECG diagnosis of sinus tachycardia depends on.

1. *Rate:* Greater than 100 per minute.
2. *Rhythm:* Regular sinus rhythm. (There may be slight irregularity, best demonstrated by caliper measurement over long continuous ECG rhythm strip.
3. *Morphology of P waves:* Normal. Most often PR interval is normal. Sometimes, a prolonged PR interval or rarely Wenckebach phenomenon may be seen in AV conduction problems.
4. *Ventricular response:* Carotid sinus pressure or Valsalva maneuver causes gradual slowing and then gradual speeding up of rate.

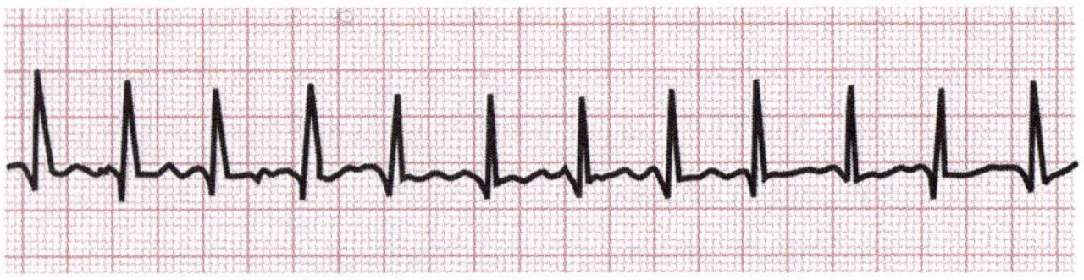

Fig. D-7: Sinus tachycardia: Regular sinus rhythm with a rate of approximately 150 beats per minute normally shaped and directed P waves, normal PR interval

In symptomatic patients with 'palpitations' and persistent incapacitating symptoms β-blockers are effective. Non-dihydropyridine calcium channel blockers like verapamil or diltiazem also may be useful. This should not be treated with digitalis unless it is a manifestation of underlying congestive heart failure. Treat the underlying process, metabolic state, or medication effect.

48. Sinus bradycardia is a normal finding in athletes. Heart rate less than 60 per minute. It does not usually cause symptoms until the rate is below 50 per minute.

It is commonly seen in

1. Myxedema
2. Obstructive jaundice
3. Increased intracranial tension
4. Immediately after myocardial infarction in some patients.

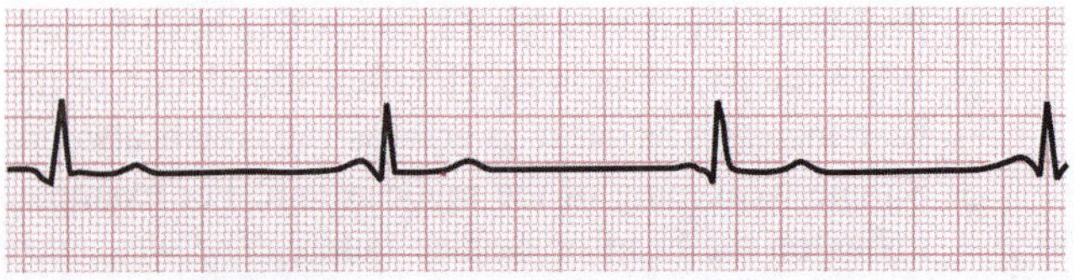

Fig. D-8: Sinus bradycardia: Regular sinus rhythm with a rate of approximately 42 bpm. Normally shaped and directed P waves, normal PR interval

49. Causes of sinus bradycardia may be broadly classified into 4 groups.

By convention, sinus bradycardia is said to be present when there is sinus rhythm at a rate of less than 60 per minute. Do not usually cause symptoms until the rate is below 50 per minute.

1. *Vagotonia:*
   a. Physiological: seen in highly trained athletes
   b. Faint or vasovagal attack
   c. Carotid sinus massage, eye ball compression, or Valsalva maneuver in which the subject voluntarily increases intrathoracic pressure by doing forced expiration against a closed glottis
   d. Raised intracranial pressure.
2. *Drugs:*
   a. Digitalis: Mainly due to vagotonia. It can cause direct depression of SA node in high doses.
   b. β-blockers: By reducing sympathetic drive to the heart
   c. Neostigmine by vagotonic/cholinergic effect.
3. *Cardiovascular causes:*
   a. Acute myocardial infarction: Either to vagotonia or ischemic dysfunction of the SA node. Reversible with atropine
   b. Sick sinus syndrome
   c. Acute hypertension
   d. Acute hypoxia and hypercarbia
   e. Congenital complete heart block
   f. Wandering pacemaker.
4. *Miscellaneous:*
   a. Severe jaundice
   b. Myxedema
   c. Hypothermia
   d. Infections like typhoid, brucellosis.

In asymptomatic patients who respond to exercise with an increase in heart rate, need no treatment.

With aging sinus node looses its excitable cells and an increase in fat, collagen and elastic tissue occurs. These changes of aging process probably play a role in sinus bradycardia with aging as well as in patients with sick sinus syndrome.

Rate increases during inspiration and decreases in expiration due to vagal effect.

Asymptomatic bradyarrhythmias in age individuals seldom requires treatment. Most of them disappear with exercise, e.g. sinus bradycardiac, congenital complete heart block, wandering pacemaker. Symptomatic patients will require an adrenergic or anticholinergic drug (orciprenaline, isoprenaline, atropine, etc.). In some rare cases where there is extreme bradycardiac and heart failure, a permanent pacemaker may be indicated to improve the heart rate so that the anti-congestive therapy including digitalis and β-blockers may be safely given.

50. Sinus arrhythmia: This normal variant is most common in children and decreases with advancing age. Sinus arrhythmia is set to be present when the variation between the longest and shortest cycle on a resting ECG is above 0.12 sec. It is defined as phasic sinus arrhythmia, if the cycle length shortens with inspiration and lengthens with expiration. The phasic respiratory sinus arrhythmia usually occurs in children between 5–12 years of age and does not need any treatment. It disappears with exercise or injection of atropine. The nonphasic sinus arrhythmia, if the condition is severe and symptomatic may need a pacemaker to maintain the heart rate and the treatment of organic condition that caused it. If unrelated to the respiratory cycle, it is referred to as nonphasic. It is frequently associated with sinus bradycardia. It usually disappears on exercise.

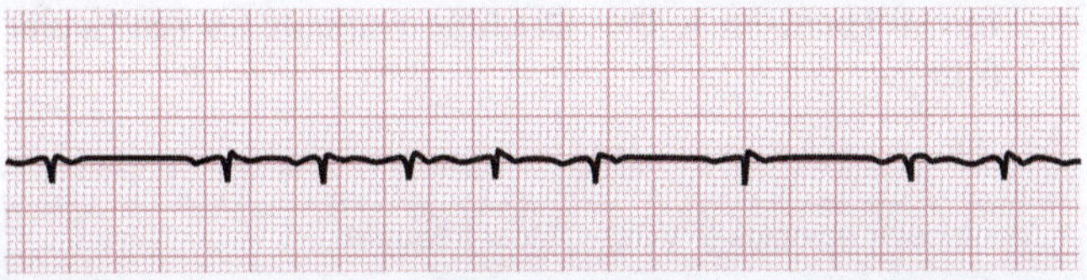

Fig. D-9: Sinus arrhythmia: PQRST normal but the RR interval between successive beats varies. One P wave per QRS complex. Constant PR interval

The 4 ECG findings of sinus arrhythmia are

1. Each QRS is preceded by P wave.
2. Normal PQRST—normally directed P wave with normal PR interval.
3. Interval between successive complexes varies. RR intervals irregular.
4. Variation between the longest and shortest cycle.

ATRIAL ARRHYTHMIAS

51. Atrial arrhythmias can be conveniently classified by considering the speed of the atrial waves they produce. The speed of the atrial waves in ascending order are.

Table D-1

Arrhythmias	*Speed of atrial waves (beats per minute)*
1. Atrial ectopics	moderate tachycardia
2. Paroxysmal supraventricular tachycardia (PSVT)	160–230 approximately
3. Atrial flutter	230–330 approximately
4. Atrial fibrillation (AF)	400–500 (F or fibrillary waves)

ATRIAL PREMATURE CONTRACTIONS (APCs)

Syn: ATRIAL PREMATURE BEATS (APBs)

APBs are caused by ectopic foci anywhere in either atrium.

52. The ECG diagnosis of Atrial Premature Beats (APBs)

1. *Rate:* May be normal. P waves are premature relative to sinus cycle length.
2. *Rhythm:* Irregular. Sinus beats present. Compensatory pause following premature beats are only partial. APCs

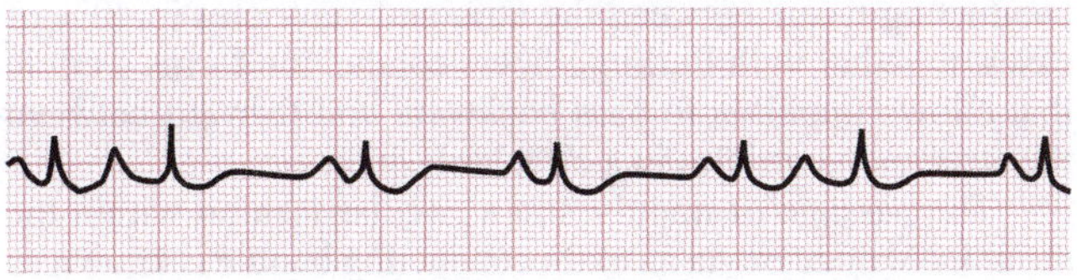

Fig. D-10: Atrial premature beat: Rhythm is irregular, QRS is preceded by P compensatory pause following QRS may be partial. QRS looks similar to normal beats

frequently reset the sinus node. PR interval of APC beat is usually more than that of sinus beat. Sometimes P waves are interpolated between two sinus P waves without pauses. If P waves come early, it may be obscured by superimposition on the T wave.
3. *Morphology of P wave:* P waves of APCs differ from sinus P waves. P waves contour varies. If the APCs are multiple with P waves of different shapes and varying PR intervals—it means that several ectopic foci are firing in the atria and resulting complexes are called multifocal APBs.
   QRS is narrow similar to sinus P wave.
4. *Ventricular response:* May be blocked at the AV node when the AV node is refractory to the atrial P wave. QRS will be absent—this is called 'locked APC.
   It may be conducted to the ventricles with normal QRS beat or one of the bundle branches may be refractory - partially or completely—resulting in prolongation and/or alteration of QRS complex.

53. Clinical factors responsible for premature beats.

1. May be no obvious heart disease.
2. Inflammatory diseases (Rheumatic fever, scarlet fever, diphtheria, etc. rheumatic mitral valve disease).
3. IHD/CAD, hypertension, cardiomyopathies.
4. Anoxic states like—cor pulmonale, during anesthesia and surgery on heart and blood vessels.
5. Reflexes from gastrointestinal, biliary, and genitourinary tracts.
6. During therapy, especially digitalis, calcium, potassium, and sympathomimetic.
7. Alternations in pH and hyperkalemia and hypocalcemic state.
8. During cardiac catheterization and cardiac surgery.

54. Treatment of atrial premature contractions (APCs).

1. Usually do not need any treatment, many normal individuals show APCs but they often do not complain of palpitations because often there is no full compensatory pause. Therapy is decided basing on other conditions rather than patient's symptoms alone.
2. When there is history of paroxysmal atrial tachycardia, APCs are controlled by β-blockers or digitalis to increase the AV nodal refractoriness so that APCs do not conduct to the ventricles. (APCs always initiate paroxysmal atrial tachycardia). Type I antiarrhythmic drugs may suppress APCs.
3. APCs in older patients may be a precursor of atrial fibrillation—digitalis therapy is initiated.
4. APCs in acute myocardial infarction: Indicate either paroxysmal atrial tachycardia or atrial fibrillation may follow shortly. Though either congestive heart failure,

AV block or premature ventricular contractions are absent APCs are best treated by careful observation only with type I antiarrhythmic drugs.

55. The 4 principle characters of ectopic beats or extrasystoles are:

1. They arise from an ectopic foci in the atria, the AV junction or ventricle–called as atrial ectopic; junctional or nodal ectopic, ventricular ectopics, respectively.
2. They cause irregularities of an otherwise regular pulse.
3. They are premature, weak or impalpable.
4. They are usually followed by compensatory pause.

Cardiac filling associated with them is usually incomplete. If the next sinus beat occurs during the refractory period of an ectopic beat it will fail to be propagated and there will be a compensatory pause followed by an unusually forceful beat due to the extra time available for ventricular filling.

56. The frequency of ectopics in ascending order are:

1. Ventricular ectopics (PVCs)	Most frequent
2. Atrial ectopics (APCs)	Frequent
3. AV nodal or Junctional ectopics	Less frequent
4. Sinus node ectopic	Rare (pacemaker can wander within the sinus node producing P waves of slightly different contour)

Ectopics are one of the most common causes of irregular pulse. Although ectopics arise in normal hearts, they are most often associated with structural heart disease and increase in frequency with age.

57. ECG abnormalities of different ectopics.

Table D-2

Features	*Atrial*	*Nodal*	*Ventricular*
1. Rate	May be normal	Normal, may be moderate tachycardia	Normal
2. Rhythm	Irregular, sinus beats present usually reset the sinus beat	Irregular	Irregular
3. P wave	Contour varies differing from sinus P waves; PR interval is usually greater than sinus beat. If the ectopics are multiple with P waves of different shapes and varying PR intervals, they are called multifocal APCs since they arise from several ectopic foci. P wave may be interposed between two normal QRS complexes; or preceded by a P wave that is early or even preceding T wave. Compensatory pause following ectopic beat is usually partial	Either no P wave before the QRS complex or if atrial contraction occurs by retrograde firing into the atrium, the P wave is inverted or occur red late after the QRS complex	P waves are absent because the ectopics arise from the ventricle rather than SA node or atrium
4. QRS complex	Normal	Normal	Appear as large, wide complexes of more than 0.12 sec. Usually associated with Compensatory pause. If the QRS complexes are of different shapes, they are called multifocal PVBs

PAROXYSMAL SUPRAVENTRICULAR TACHYCARDIAS (PSVT)

Paroxysmal tachycardia means sudden increase in heart rate which usually arises from an ectopic pacemaker.

This arrhythmia accounts for only around 10% of supraventricular tachycardias.

This arrhythmia is due to reentry in 20% of cases or an ectopic focus within the atrium. Repeated circulation of impulse within the AV node in 40% of cases. Second or extra bundle of conducting tissue between the atria and ventricles in 40% of cases, together with Purkinje fibers conduction forms a circle that allows impulses to pass backward and forward between the atria and ventricles in a circular fashion.

The passage of impulses in a circular fashion within the atrium, AV node or via an extra conducting bundle is known as reentry and occurs in conditions where there are two conduction pathways with different refractory periods and different conduction velocities.

The resulting tachyarrhythmia is regular with a rate of 150–250 beats per minute. Because the impulses come from atria or AV node the ECG looks normal but very fast unless there is bundle branch block in which case the QRS complexes are wide. P waves may or may not be seen.

Paroxysmal supraventricular tachycardia generally occurs in persons with abnormal circuits or reentry pathways without heart disease. The majority of patients have no organic heart disease. They may be symptomatic resulting in mild palpitation to hemodynamic collapse or may be asymptomatic. It is recurrent. It may last from seconds to days.

58. Paroxysmal supraventricular tachycardia (PSVT) is often associated with:

1. Nervous tension–anxiety, lack of sleep
2. Ingestion of coffee or alcohol
3. Consumption of cigarette
4. Thyrotoxicosis.

If paroxysmal atrial tachycardia is associated with block always suspect an underlying heart disease.

59. Documentation PSVT if possible is made by:

- 24-hour ambulatory monitoring: Holter's monitoring may not record because it may be sporadic
- Treadmill test is not useful because most of these episodes are not stimulated by exercise
- Electrocardiographic transmitting systems which allow the patients to transmit their rhythms over the telephone is useful. The transmitted signals are recorded on ECG in the physician's room
- ECG diagnosis of atrial tachycardia (Paroxysmal atrial tachycardia, PAT, supra ventricular tachycardia) depends upon:

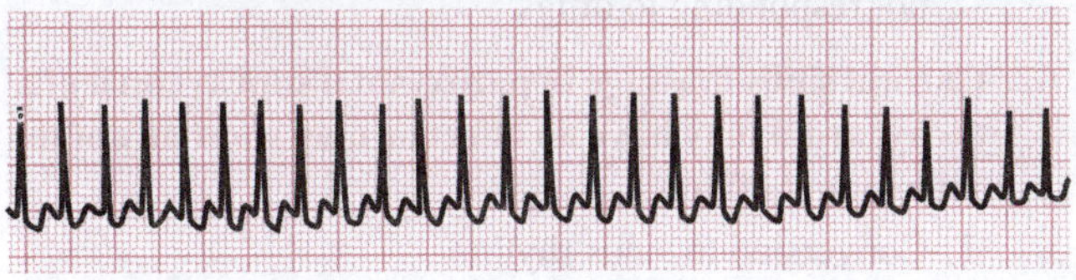

Fig. D-11: Paroxysmal atrial tachycardia: The rate is 190 per minute, QRS complexes are normal; P waves can be seen in superimposed on the T waves of the preceding beats.

1. *Rate:* 140–250/min. Lasts for few seconds to days when untreated. Coffee, alcohol, tobacco, anxiety, etc. can precipitate.
2. *Rhythm:* Regular. No saw-toothed appearance. Extrasystolic focus separates from atrioventricular node.
   If it is associated with AV block of varying degree it is seen by increased PR interval (1st degree) or irregular ventricular response (2nd or 3rd degree). The possibility of intrinsic disease in the AV node or digitalis intoxication should be suspected.
3. *Morphology:* P waves are abnormal depending on the origin. No saw-toothed appearance. Extrasystolic focus separate from AV node. Atrial activity is best seen in V1.
   QRS configuration is usually narrow unless conduction defect pre-exists.
   QRS is occasionally altered or prolonged resembling right bundle branch block (or, less commonly, left bundle branch block).
   It is important and difficult to differentiate it from ventricular tachycardia when the QRS is wide.
4. *Ventricular response:* Responds well in a regular one to one fashion producing the 'fluttering' sensation to which the patient seeks immediate medical attention.

60. There are 4 principles in the management of paroxysmal atrial tachycardias depending on sudden onset or long standing history.

Table D-3

Principles of management	Sudden onset (Transient)	Long-term (Chronic)
1. Physiological interventions	Rest, sedation, carotid sinus massage, Valsalva maneuver	Self-administered carotid sinus massage, or Valsalva maneuver, avoid inciting factors
2. Drugs	Vagomimetic or sympathomimetic drugs Direct effect on AVN or reentrant pathway Slow ventricular rate β-blockers, calcium channel blockers, digoxin help	Suppress triggering arrhythmias change properties of re-entrant pathways control ventricular rate
3. Electrical	DC shock-cardioversion or temporary pacing	Permanent pacemaker or antitachycardia pacing
4. Catheter ablation and surgery i. Direct current ii. Radiofrequency		Radiofrequency energy has been used successfully to ablate AV as well as accessory pathways. It does not produce barotrauma. It is now a treatment of choice for ablating PSVT

61. Treatment of atrial tachycardia (PAT, SVT): Aim is to restore sinus rhythm or to slow the ventricular rate to less than 100 per minute while waiting for the paroxysm to self terminate. Following treatment is tried in tachycardia with regular RR interval on ECG. Those who do not have hemodynamic deterioration can be treated with drugs.

1. *Vagal maneuvers:* These are effective in 10–30% of cases of supraventricular tachycardias.
   Unilateral carotid sinus massage: This should be performed after ascertaining that no carotid bruit is present. It should not be performed in elderly patients. It helps in both diagnostic and therapeutically. It may completely stop the attack or no response *'All or none'* phenomenon. It helps to differentiate it from sinus tachycardia, atrial flutter and fibrillation.
   Cardiac sinus massage technic: The patient should lie in the supine position turning the head away from the side in which massage is to the done. Confirm, that there should be no carotid bruit by auscultation. Massage with fingers over the carotids by locating the carotid bifurcation behind the angle of the jaw in the vertical direction. Gently massage for 5 seconds on one side at a time. Response may occur on one side but not on the other side. Usually response occur to the first massage or two.
2. *Drugs:*
   a. IV Verapamil: (Calcium channel blocker) Verapamil gives promising results. This drug is effective in 92% of patients. Acts by increasing the AV nodal refractoriness thereby slowing the ventricular rate. The dose is 1 mg IV followed by 2.5 mg every 5 to 10 min or AV block develops or a total of 15 to 20 mg have been given. Vagal maneuver should be performed prior to each dose. Contraindications: No recent β-blocker; patient of left ventricular dysfunction receiving β-blockers and WPW syndrome with atrial flutter or fibrillation; hypotension.
   b. IV Adenosine: This is the drug of choice in acute episode of supraventricular tachycardia. It binds to cardiac A1 receptors in SA and AV nodes. It has negative chronotropic effect in SA node, depresses conduction, increases refractoriness of AV node. It has no significant effect on most accessory pathways. Its half-life is 10 seconds. In therapeutic doses it does not have clinically significant negative inotropic effect. It is ineffective in terminating primary atrial arrhythmia like atrial flutter or fibrillation but slows the ventricular rate by inducing transient AV block. Dose is 6 mg bolus given IV in one or two seconds followed by rapid saline flush. If tachycardia does not terminate after one to two minutes then inject 12 mg. Adenosine is an excellent drug for termination of PSVT in 90% of cases and has almost replaced verapamil in patients where very rapid reconversion is required. Unlike verapamil, it does not cause problems if given in a patient with VT.
   c. Procainamide: If both verapamil and adenosine fail to control, try procainamide IV initially at a dose of 15 mg/kg followed by 2–4 mg/min. It terminates the arrhythmia by blocking retrograde conduction in the fast AV nodal pathway (β) or terminates reciprocal tachycardia by blocking conduction in the bypass tract.
   d. Amiodarone: This drug can be used in the treatment of SVTs, nodal or ventricular tachycardias, and the Wolf-Parkinson-White syndrome when other drugs cannot be used.
   Dose 200 mg/8 hourly po for at least one week.
   Maintenance dose 200 mg/24 hourly po.
   Side effects: Corneal micro-deposits (common but reversible after stopping the drugs, tremor, neuropathy, photosensitization, thyroid disorders.
   Other drugs like propranolol, digitalis can be tried alone or in combination.
   Maintenance therapy for long-term treatment is given by β-blockers, calcium channel blockers, and digoxin. These are effective in 30–50% of cases and have fewer side effects. Verapamil and magnesium may be helpful.
3. *DC shock:* Patients who are hypotensive or have severe angina or pulmonary edema should be promptly given synchronized DC shock.
4. Catheter ablation and surgery in long standing cases not responding to drugs.

62. Carotid sinus massage in paroxysmal supraventricular tachycardia may have no effect or may show any of the following 4 effects.

1. Conversion to sinus rhythm.
2. Slowing of tachycardia without conversion.
3. Increasing AV conduction ratio. (specially in SA reentrant or automatic atrial tachycardia)
4. Rarely it may convert into atrial flutter or fibrillation.

63. Treatment of atrial tachycardia with AV block.

It is more serious since it seldom occurs in normal hearts.

1. Stop digitalis, if the patient is on digitalis.
2. Supplement potassium: There is always intracellular hypokalemia even if serum potassium is normal.
3. Injection proctolol 5–15 mg over 2 min intravenously if the patient is in good condition and no β-blocker is given recently.

4. If it occurs in patients who are not on digitalis—it is paradoxical that digoxin is the treatment of choice if the ventricular rate is fast.

64. Atrioventricular reentrant tachycardia:

1. Structural heart disease is usually absent.
2. An accessory pathway remote from the AV node providing a second connection between the atria and ventricles is present.
3. The arrhythmia therefore results from the repeated circulation of an electrical impulse between the atria and ventricles.
4. The impulse usually conducts slowly from the atria to ventricles via the atrioventricular node and then rapidly reenters the atria via the additional pathway.

65. ECG diagnosis of atrioventricular reentrant tachycardia

1. *Rate:* 130–250/min
2. *Rhythm:* Regular
3. *Morphology:* Atrial activity is seen as inverted P wave in the ST segment after each QRS complex.
   P waves may be concealed by superimposed terminal portion of the QRS complex.
   QRS complexes are narrow and regular.
4. *Ventricular response:* Regular ventricular response.
   An accessory pathway may be evident as a short PR interval without a delta wave (as in the WPW syndrome or Lown-Ganong-Levine syndrome).

ATRIAL FLUTTER AND FIBRILLATION

Atrial flutter originates from a single atrial ectopic focus. P waves occur in rapid succession at a rate of 250–350/min and each P wave is identical to the other.

66. Pathogenesis of atrial flutter or fibrillation occurs in 4 ways.

1. Rise in right or left ventricular end-diastolic pressure (EDV) causing atrial distension, e.g. MR
2. Obstruction to either AV valves, e.g. MS
3. Infiltrative causes
4. Inflammatory causes.

67. The ECG diagnosis of atrial flutter depends upon

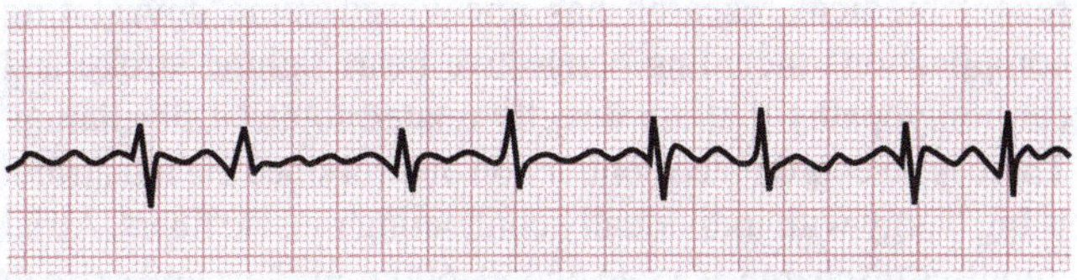

Fig. D-12: Atrial flutter: 2:1 and 3:1 rhythm. P waves look like edge of a saw (sawtoothed configuration)

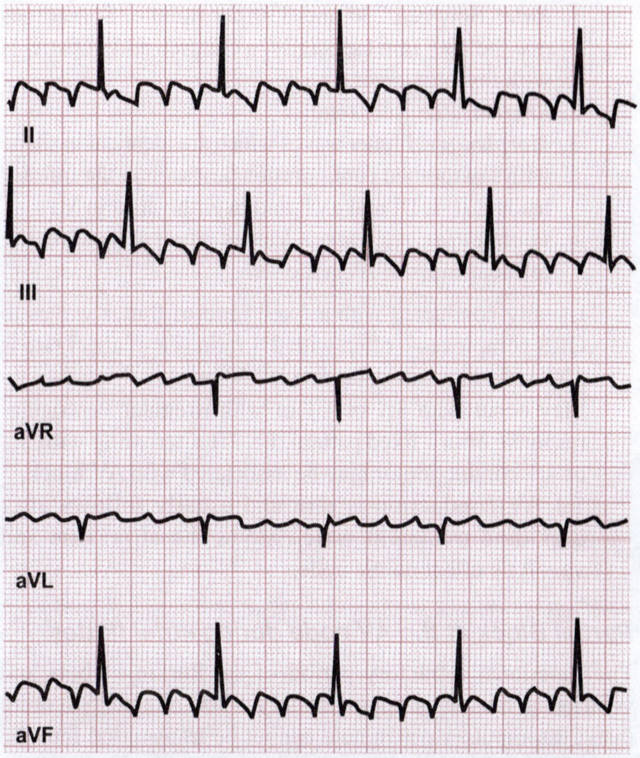

Fig. D-13: Atrial flutter with 4:1 AV block; There are 4 P waves per QRS complex and ventricular activation is regular

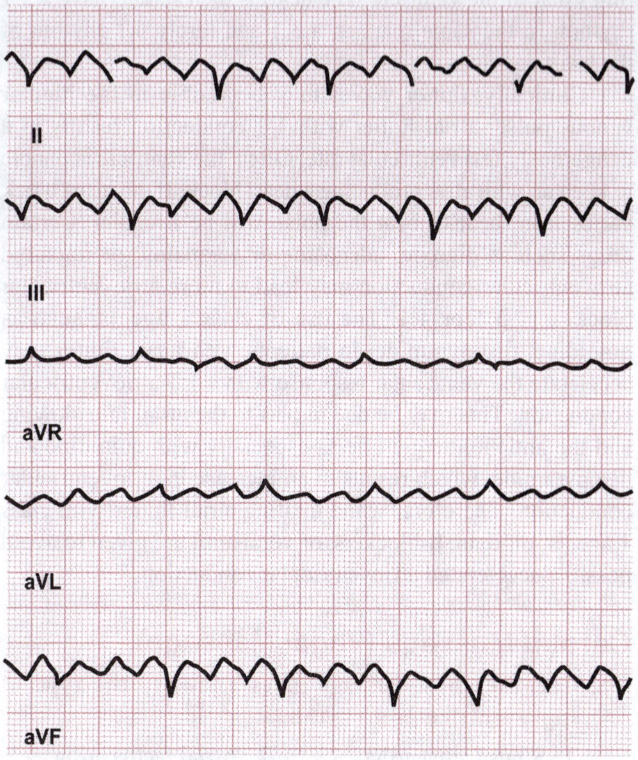

Fig. D-14: Atrial flutter at a rate of 250 bpm with varying AV block

1. *Rate:* Between 230 and 330 per minute. Sometimes may be 400/ min especially in children and in patients with thyrotoxicosis.
2. *Rhythm:* Precisely regular.
3. *Morphology*: Flutter waves which are identical in shape with sawtoothed configuration best seen in the inferior leads L II, L III and aVF and over the atria in V1.
4. *Ventricular response:* Varies inversely with the refractoriness of AV node.

Usually conducted with a fixed ratio of flutter waves to QRS complexes—often with 2:1 ratio (i.e. if atrial rate is 300/min, the ventricular rate is 150/min).

May occur with 3:1 or 4:1 or with irregular ventricular response or in a fixed pattern, i.e. 2:1 alternating with 3:1 or 4:1 conduction or may be associated with AV block.

1:1 AV conduction is rare and usually follows after quinidine treatment which slows the atrial rate and vagolytic effect on AV node.

Partial Block at the AV node during atrial flutter

The functional refractory period of the Purkinje fibers and ventricular muscle is approximately 1/200 minute. So, more than 200 impulses per minute cannot be transmitted into the ventricles. Therefore, when the atrium contracts as rapidly as 300 times per minute, only one out of every two impulses passes into the ventricles. Thus causing the atria to beat at a rate two times that of the ventricle. The heart is then said to have a 2:1 rhythm. In the same manner, a 3:1 and rarely 4:1 rhythm of the heart develops.

Clinically, flutter waves may be visible in the jugular venous pulse, atrial flutter with 1:1 conduction results in a dangerously fast ventricular rate. Often, the ventricle is unable to keep up with atria producing a heart block. If the heart block varies from beat to beat the pulse will be irregular. Certain drugs such as digoxin, adenosine or verapamil, or impaired atroventricular conduction may lead to more atrioventricular block, e.g. 3:1 or 4:1. The use of class 1 agents, such as quinidine, disopyramide, in patients with atrial flutter may accelerate the ventricular response with a 1:1 atrioventricular conduction. This may be due in part to the atrial rate slowing and the anticholinergic effects especially with quinidine and disopyramide, which results in an increase in atrioventricular conduction. Therefore, while treating atrial flutter with class 1 agents, digoxin, β-blockers, or verapamil are given to avoid possible accelerated atrioventricular conduction.

Carotid Massage (Vagal Massage)

68. Carotid sinus massage gives a clue to the type of supraventricular arrhythmia.

1. Sinus tachycardia
2. Atrial tachycardia
3. Atrial flutter
4. Atrial fibrillation.

1. How to do carotid sinus massage?

The massage is not on the carotid artery. The massage is meant for vagus nerve, which is behind the carotid (artery) body. The massage should be done vertically moving with slightly firm pressure for 1–3 min at a time, then on the other side. Should never be done on both sides at a time.

Carotid sinus massage (vagus nerve) is both diagnostic and therapeutic by its response.

1. *Sinus tachycardia:* After carotid massage rate comes down to 8–10 beats only, e.g. 150 to 140 bpm only.
2. *Atrial tachycardia:* The carotid massage has no response or rate comes to suddenly normally—all or none phenomenon, or goes to sinus tachycardia.
3. *Atrial flutter:* Rate 250–380 bpm (2:1, 4:1). Block is increased by 1–2; 1–3; 1–4. The carotid massage decreases the rate by arithmetical proportion.
4. No response in atrial fibrillation.

Sometimes, digitalis or Inderal is given and later massage is done. It may respond.

IV propanolol or IV Isoptin may give good response in supraventricular tachycardias. It stimulates vagus nerve and it prevents the reentry phenomenon.

Vagus stimulation, e.g. by applying pressure on the eyeballs by drinking very ice-cold water or by inducing vomiting does not achieve the same result as carotid massage. So, it is waste to try other methods except carotid sinus massage. It is both diagnostic as well as therapeutic.

ATRIAL FIBRILLATION

Atrial fibrillation is the most common form of arrhythmia affecting more than 2.2 million people annually in US and 4.5 million in Europe. Atrial fibrillation is the most sustained supraventricular tachyarrhythmia and is associated with increased cardiac morbidity and mortality and preventable cerebral stroke (emboli/thrombosis) accounting for approximately 1/3rd of cardiac arrhythmias, which needs hospitalization.

Atrial fibrillation is the most common of supraventricular tachyarrhythmias. Until just a few years ago, it was thought to be a "nuisance" arrhythmia with few consequences. However, recent medical research has uncovered some devastating complications including congestive heart failure, stroke and cardiomyopathy that are directly related to atrial fibrillation. There is no coordinated contraction of atria since the left atrium is big baggy with individually contracting muscle fibers. Atrial impulses discharge at a rate of 350–600/min. This gives rise to an irregular baseline of 'F' waves on ECG, which represent the sum at any one time of the action potentials produced by the haphazard contraction of dozens or hundreds of individually contracting atrial muscle fibers. Impulses are conducted haphazardly from the atria to the ventricles causing irregular ventricular contractions and irregular pulse.

Atrial fibrillation is common in the community, affecting up to 8% of people aged 80 years or over. The prevalence of the condition increases with age and affects men slightly more often than women. Atrial fibrillation will become increasingly common in the present day increasingly aged population. Thus, most physicians and general practitioners should know well about the management of this condition as it is a major cause of emergency admissions and cardiovascular deaths in developed countries. In the Framingham study, hypertension, cardiac failure, and rheumatic heart disease were the commonest precursors of atrial fibrillation. We see more number of cases of atrial fibrillation in rheumatic mitral valve disease in India in young and middle age, unlike the developed countries where rheumatic heart diseases are controlled. Atrial fibrillation due to hypertension, cardiac failure are seen in middle and old age in our practice. *Up to a third of patients with atrial fibrillation, however, may have idiopathic or 'lone' atrial fibrillation, where no precipitating cause is found and no structural heart disease evident.*

Atrial fibrillation is the commonest cardiac arrhythmia in general practice, though in many patients the condition remains unrecognized. In a single general practice population in Tamworth, screening a total of 819 patients aged over 65 years found 30 patients who were in atrial fibrillation (3.7%) (Hill et al, 1987). Hence, the general practitioner should know this condition well. The feasibility of diagnosing and managing these patients presents a clinical challenge for primary health care doctors.

Most important with atrial fibrillation is the risk of stroke. The risk of stroke increases with age, blood pressure, and other evidence of heart disease. Atrial fibrillation may also increase the risk of recurrent stroke. Patients with acute stroke with atrial fibrillation have significantly higher mortality than patient in sinus rhythm. It is found that nonrheumatic atrial fibrillation increases the risk of stroke by a factor of five.

Advantages of therapeutic benefits from treating atrial fibrillation have been proved. Control of hemodynamic effects of the poor cardiac output related to the arrhythmias and to reduce thromboembolic risks of atrial fibrillation are the main priorities. Electrical and pharmacological cardioversion to, and the maintenance of normal sinus rhythm remains the optimal strategy to enhance cardiac performance and reduce the thromboembolic risk. Cardioversion is increasingly considered now because of improvement in cardiac performance and exercise tolerance. The use of anticoagulants before and after cardioversion remains an option to the clinicians.

The advancements in the therapy with cardiac ablation and pacemker have raised new hope in the management. History of atrial fibrillation tells us the achievements for more than a century.

69. Atrial fibrillation is seen in

1. 87% of patients suffering from mitral valve disease
2. 30% of patients with cardiomyopathy
3. 25% of patients with chronic constrictive pericarditis
4. 15% of patients with acute myocardial infarction (AMI).

70. History.

1. Adams, 1827 is probably the first to recognize the condition clinically but as a 'sign of mitral stenosis'.
2. Bouillaud, 1835 found that digitalis reduced the ventricular rate even though irregularity of the pulse persisted.
3. Hope, 1839 identified irregular pulse in association with mitral stenosis—exercise worsened the total irregularity, whereas it abolished an intermittent pulse.
4. Marey, 1863 published a pulse tracing of atrial fibrillation from a patient with mitral stenosis.
5. Roberts, 1873 found that digitalis relieved the pulmonary symptoms of mitral disease especially in the presence of irregularity of the heart.
6. Lewis, 1909 recorded atrial fibrillation with electrocardiograph; studied mechanisms of the condition.
7. Rothberger and Winterberg, 1909 identified "arrhythmia perpetua" and "fibrillation of the auricles".
8. Lown, 1969 recommended cardioversion of atrial fibrillation.

The discovery of digitalis in 1785 by William Withering brought some relief to patient with severe heart failure. William Withering recorded a patient who had a weak, irregular pulse that became "more full and more regular" after five draughts containing Folx Digital Purp oz IV. In 1835 Jan Baptiste Bouillaud described digitalis to be a "a sort of opium to the heart". The main diagnostic breakthrough was resulted after the invention of electrocardiography by Willem Einthoven in 1900.

71. Importance of atrial fibrillation.

1. It is the commonest sustained cardiac arrhythmia
2. It is rarely directly fatal
3. It creates greater morbidity than probably all the other cardiac arrhythmias put together.
4. It becomes an increasingly common cause of stroke, thromboembolism and heart failure.

The mortality rate is about twice that of the patient with normal sinus rhythm.

The importance of atrioventricular node ablation and pacemaker therapy in refractory cases of atrial fibrillation is also increasingly recognized.

72. Atrial fibrillation may be classified under 4 types.

1. Lone or idiopathic AF – is described where there is no clinical or echocardiographic evidence of cardiopulmonary disease.
2. Recurrent – when a person has two or more episodes of AF if is considered as recurrent; when it is terminated it is referred to as paroxysmal AF. They are usually self-terminating and do not usually require direct current cardioversion.
3. Persistent atrial fibrillation – usually lasts longer than 7 days and usually requires cardioversion for its termination.
4. Permanent AF when chemical or electrical cardioversion is unsuccessful.

73. Causes of atrial fibrillation.

Table D-4

Common cardiac causes	*Common noncardiac causes*	*Less common causes*
1. Rheumatic heart disease, e.g. MS, MR, MVP	7. Thyrotoxicosis	13. Heart muscle disease, e.g. idiopathic dilated or hypertrophic cardiomyopathy, hemochromatosis
2. Hypertension	8. Acute infections especially pneumonia	14. Pericardial disease, including pericardial effusion, constrictive pericarditis
3. Ischemic heart disease/CAD	9. Alcohol abuse or smoking, etc.	15. Atrial septal defect
4. Congestive heart failure	10. Tumors: Carcinoma of bronchus involving pericardium	16. Atrial myxoma
5. Sick sinus syndrome	11. Other intrathoracic pathology (e.g. pleural effusion)	17. Pulmonary thromboembolism
6. Pre-excitation syndrome, e.g. WPW syndrome	12. Postoperative problems, especially after thoracotomy or coronary artery bypass/ any surgery with general anesthesia highest after mitral valve surgery (may be up to 35–50%)	18. Drugs commonly tricyclic (anti depressants) or amphetamine stimulants
		19. Physiological stress
		20. Obesity—seems to be mediated by left atrial dilation

Occurrence of atrial fibrillation in a normal healthy person is called "Lone Atrial Fibrillation"—occasionally inherited as an autosomal dominant in a familial form.

Surprisingly, atrial fibrillation is rare in congenital pulmonary heart disease and is an isolated disease of aortic valve.

Research has yet to uncover the definitive cause of atrial fibrillation.

Rheumatic heart disease is the common cause in India. Ischemic heart disease is probably the most common cause in Britain.

In hospital based studies, ischemic heart disease was the commonest cause, followed by hypertension and valve disease. By contrast, population studies of Framingham and the Manitoba follow-up studies revealed the hypertension was the most common cause. Many epidemiological studies have depended on electrocardiogram criteria or clinical history. Studies depending on ST-T wave changes only on the electrocardiogram may cause difficulties in interpretation, especially if the patient is taking digoxin or has left ventricular hypertrophy.

74. Atrial fibrillation and pulmonary disease: AF is commonly seen in COPD exacerbations general treatment include:

1. Treatment of underlying lung disease – COPD, pneumonia, bronchial asthma.
2. Correction of hypoxia.
3. Correction of acid-base imbalance.
4. Specific treatment.

Drugs that are commonly used to treat bronchospastic airway disease, such as theophylline and β-adrenergic agonists can precipitate AF.

Antiarrhythmic drugs with β-blocking properties such as sotalol, propafenone, and adenosine can worsen bronchospasm and are contraindicated in patients with severe bronchospasm airway disease. Ventricular rate control is usually achieved with a nondihydropyridine calcium channel blockers such as verapamil and diltiazem.

75. Several different terms are used to describe atrial fibrillation.

1. *Paroxysmal AF:* Occurs intermittently and varies in frequency and duration from a few seconds to more protracted episodes lasting several hours or even days. This is more often seen in younger people aged 30–50 years.
2. *Chronic atrial fibrillation:* It is persistent becoming the primary heart rhythm and it is usually unresponsive to medical therapy or other nonpharmacological interventions such as electrical cardioversion. This form of AF is typically seen in older population.

3. *Neurogenic atrial fibrillation:* It indicates an imbalance in the nervous system regulation of the heart.
   i. Vagal AF: Increased vagal tone causes the heart rate to slow down and the refractory period of the atria to shorten. Typically, vagal AF occurs more frequently at rest or following a meal, and is usually seen in men who are between 30 and 50 years of age. Often times, patients note the onset of this type of AF is preceded by a period of progressive bradycardia and in this case medications such as β-blockers or digitalis may actually worsen the atrial fibrillation.
   ii. Adrenergic AF: It occurs as a result of excessive adrenaline that comes from stimulation of the sympathetic portion of the nervous system. It causes increased rate and force of contraction. This type of AF is most likely to occur during the day and may be associated with emotional stress or physical exertion. Unlike the case of vagal AF, medical therapy with β-blockers may be quite helpful in controlling this form of atrial fibrillation.
4. *Familial atrial fibrillation:* It is a relatively uncommon type of AF often affecting younger people (< 20 years age). Early genetic research has identified a specific chromosomal defect that is responsible for this form of arrhythmia.

76. Rheumatic heart disease and atrial fibrillation

1. Rheumatic heart disease (mostly mitral valve disease) was present in 15% emergency admissions of patients with atrial fibrillation in a survey.
2. Rheumatic valve disease particularly mitral stenois is important as it increases the thromboembolic risk of patients with chronic atrial fibrillation about 18-fold.
3. The risk of stroke and thromboembolism for patients in atrial fibrillation is three to seven times that of patients with mitral stenosis in sinus rhythm.
4. Echocardiography in such cases may show left atrial thrombus. Transesophageal echocardiography (TEE) is ideal method of imaging left atrial thrombus.

77. Hypertension and atrial fibrillation: Hypertension accounted for about half of the cases of atrial fibrillation in the Framingham study. Hypertension contributes to stroke and thromboembolism if left ventricular hypertrophy is present. ECG shows LVH (SV1 + RV5 > 35 mm). If the ECG is abnormal, the echocardiogram will invariably show left ventricular hypertrophy. LVH is considered to be present if the left ventricular mass index is > 134 g/m² in men and > 110 g/m² in women.

1. Atrial fibrillation can be secondary to left atrial dilatation, which occurs in hypertensive patients, as a consequence of reduced left ventricular compliance.
2. May be associated with underlying coronary artery diseases, which itself is a risk for atrial fibrillation and thromboembolism.
3. Hypertension increases the risk of stroke in atrial fibrillation
4. Alcohol may contribute to both hypertension and atrial fibrillation.

78. Ischemic heart disease and atrial fibrillation: It is probably the most common cause of atrial fibrillation in Britain and other well-developed countries.

1. The fast ventricular rate due to atrial fibrillation may cause angina, leading to cardiac ischemia and heart failure.
2. Atrial fibrillation may complicate acute myocardial infarction in 10–15% of cases and is often a marker of extensive myocardial damage and a poor prognosis, with increased mortality.
3. Immediate DC cardioversion may be necessary in AMI complicating AF.
4. Atrial fibrillation is also a marker of underlying ventricular dysfunction and a compromised myocardium. Many years after MI, ventricular scarring and dilatation often predispose to atrial fibrillation and congestive heart failure.

79. Thyroid disease and atrial fibrillation: Thyrotoxicosis is an important curable cause of atrial fibrillation.

1. About 10–15% of patients with untreated thyrotoxicosis develop atrial fibrillation
2. Thyrotoxicosis may be underdiagnosed in whom clinical signs are not evident. Thyroid functions tests are often neglected particularly in old people in whom clinical signs are not seen.
3. One clinical clue is the failure of digoxin to control the ventricular rate without the addition of β-blocker.
4. Hyperthyroidism may also coexist with both ischemia and rheumatic heart disease.

It is advised to check the thyroid function tests routinely in atrial fibrillation of recent origin.

Hypothyroidism also may cause heart muscle disease and heart failure. Myxedema is also associated with hyperlipidemia and an increased risk of heart disease.

80. Alcohol abuse and atrial fibrillation:

1. Alcohol may account for a third of new cases of atrial fibrillation (up to two-thirds in patients aged under 65)
2. Often occurs during holidays or at weekends, giving rise to the term "holiday heart syndrome". It can precipitate atrial fibrillation in otherwise normal people.
3. Chronic alcoholics may have dilated heart (Dilated cardiomyopathy) and atrial fibrillation.

4. Most (about 90%) patients of atrial fibrillation convert spontaneously to sinus rhythm within 24 hours after stopping the alcohol ingestion.

81. There are 4 mechanisms of alcohol to cause atrial fibrillation.

1. Alcohol ingestion results in release of catecholamines from the adrenal medulla, especially noradrenaline
2. Alcohol causes release of cardiac stores of adrenaline
3. Plasma acetaldehyde, the main metabolite of ethanol, raises catecholamine concentrations systemically and in the myocardium
4. Alcohol directly affects the heart, with prolonged PR, QRS, and QT times, facilitating atrial arrhythmias.

Withdrawal of alcohol results in increased release of catecholamines.

Alcohol excess is associated with hypertension.

82. Brief note on some other causes of atrial fibrillation.

1. *Atrial septal defect:* ASD should be considered in a young patient with atrial fibrillation, especially if a pulmonary ejection systolic murmur in association with a split, second heart sound is heard.
2. *Wolff-Parkinson-White syndrome:* WPW syndrome is suspected in a young patient with fast atrial fibrillation. It is recognized by
   i. short PR interval (< 0.12 sec)
   ii. a delta wave
   iii. wide QRS (PR + QRS remains normal)
   iv. ST-T changes (T opposite of QRS).
3. *Cardiothoracic surgery:* Atrial fibrillation occurs in 20% of cases. Often requires treatment in the short term. Atrial fibrillation after noncardiothoracic surgery is usually self-limiting, often reverting spontaneously to sinus rhythm.
4. *Pneumonia:* It can precipitate atrial fibrillation predominantly in old patients. It is present in about 7% of cases admitted as medical emergencies. Often difficult to know whether the pneumonia is complicating pre-existing atrial fibrillation or is the precipitant of atrial fibrillation. The pneumonia should therefore be treated and cardioversion to sinus rhythm after treatment of the acute condition should be considered.

83. Primary or idiopathic or "lone" atrial fibrillation: No identifiable cause, no predisposing factor or associated abnormalities of the heart.

1. It can be either paroxysmal or persistent
2. It is present in between 3% and 11% of all patients with atrial fibrillation
3. Young patients (< 60 years age) are generally at a low thromboembolic risk and antithrombotic treatment may not be necessary.
4. Incidence of stroke is increased by five fold in elderly patients (> 65 years age) and anithrombotic treatment should be considered.

84. Diagnosis of "lone atrial fibrillation" is by exclusion.

1. No history of cardiovascular disease or hypertension
2. No clinical abnormalities
3. Normal chest X-ray, and ECG with no previous MI or LVH
4. Normal echocardiography.

85. The mechanism of reentry of multiple foci can be due to 4 main causes.

1. *Hypertrophy:* Caused by obstruction to either of atroiventricular valves, e.g. mitral stenosis.
2. *Distension or stretch:* Caused by increased right or left ventricular end-diastolic pressure, e.g. mitral regurgitation.
3. Infiltration.
4. Infective.

86. Pathophysiology: Atrial fibrillation is commonly associated with advanced age, hypertension, mitral valve disease, congestive heart failure, and coronary artery disease. These conditions result in hypertrophy, dilatation, etc.

1. Left atrial fibrosis.
2. Pulmonary vein dilation.
3. Reduced atrial contractility—which in turn results in abnormality in cellular level—which includes
   i. Intracellular handling of calcium.
   ii. Atrial myolysis.
   iii. Connexin down regulation.
   iv. Altered sympathetic innervation.

The cellular changes cause—atrial conduction abnormalities. Increased atrial activity, which causes the development of micro-reentrant circuits, which lead to the development of atrial fibrillation. The role of pulmonary veins has a source of triggers and/or drivers in AF is increasingly appreciated recently. Increased C-reactive protein levels in persistent AF rises the evidence of role of inflammation. The hormone atrial natriuretic peptile is found elevated in acute AF, this ANP remains normal in long standing AF.

87. There are 4 factors that predispose to long-term maintenance of the arrhythmia.

1. Atrial enlargement (e.g. secondary to mitral valve disease, hypertension)

2. Fibrosis of atrial tissue resulting in slowing of intra-atrial conduction
3. Altered autonomic tone, especially increased sympathetic activity
4. Homogeneity of atrial refractoriness and slow conduction times (allowing time for the myocardium to regain excitability between each wave front) help to perpetuate the process leading to long-term atrial fibrillation.

88. Atrial fibrillation (AF) impairs the circulation in the following 4 ways.

1. Loss of atrial contraction causes poor ventricular filling during diastole.
2. When left atrial pressure rises, stasis in the left atrium favors thrombus formation and can cause dangerous embolism.
3. Rapid ventricular rate in uncontrolled patient (100–200/min), which again impairs ventricular filling causes low cardiac output.
4. Irregular ventricular filling also impairs circulation.

Though the atria fail to act as primary pumps because of atrial fibrillation, the ventricle can still fill enough as the effectiveness of the heart as a pump is decreased only 25–30%, which is well within the "cardiac reserve"—of all even in severely weakened hearts. That is why, atrial fibrillation patients can continue for many years without profound cardiac disability.

89. Hemodynamic disturbances in atrial fibrillation: The hemodynamic disturbances of atrial fibrillation results mainly from the absence of atrial contraction ("atrial click") and from the rapid and irregular ventricular response, with a consequent loss of cardiac output (a loss of about 10% in normal individuals, with a greater loss at fast ventricular rates). Atrial fibrillation with fast ventricular rate gives rise to the following changes.

1. Atrial dilatation and loss of atrial systole (atrial click), leads to intra-atrial stasis, which results in the formation of thrombi
2. Reduced atrial transport (lack of organized atrial mechanical activity with a concomitant decrease in stroke volume and cardiac output)
3. Onset of a rapid ventricular response may also lead to some mitral incompetence, thus further reducing forward flow
4. Reduced diastolic filling period, especially with sudden changes to a very rapid heart rate, results in a further reduction in cardiac output (especially with valvar stenosis or reduced left ventricular compliance, e.g. in left ventricular hypertrophy).

90. Clinical features: Often the patient with atrial fibrillation have no symptom and is found during routine examination. Atrial fibrillation commonly presents as reduced exercise tolerance and heart failure.

There are 4 common presenting symptoms of atrial fibrillation.

1. Dyspnea—52%
2. Chest pain—34%
3. Palpitation—26%
4. Dizziness or syncope—19%

Many patients describe palpitation as an uncomfortable flopping sensation inside the chest with a sudden and keen awareness of every heart beat. The irregular, flopping sensation in the chest that is so uncomfortable and worrisome to patients with atrial fibrillation is not from the irregular atrial beat, but rather from the irregular ventricular beat in response to the AF. In fact, patients are not capable of feeling their atria beating, only the ventricles. So, the faster the ventricles beat, the more symptomatic patients usually become.

Syncope is rare with atrial fibrillation, unless associated with sick sinus syndrome or pre-excitation syndrome, such as the Wolff-Parkinson-White syndrome. The symptoms may be more pronounced on exercise, as a rapid ventricular response may substantially impair exercise tolerance.

91. Occasionally, patients may present as an emergency with a combination of 4 symptoms that include

1. Presyncope, syncope, fatigue—due to cerebral underperfusion
2. Dyspnea and lethargy—pulmonary edema due to heart failure
3. Angina—fall in stroke volume resulting in less coronary blood supply
4. Stroke—due to cerebral thromboembolism.

Heart failure is often precipitated by sudden onset of fast atrial fibrillation, particularly if left ventricular function is already compromised by coexisting heart disease, e.g. valvular or ischemic heart disease. Heart failure is associated with atrial fibrillation in about 35% of cases. In these patients, atrial fibrillation may be a marker of increased mortality and may also enhance the substantial risk of thromboembolism.

The risk of stroke in someone with atrial fibrillation is about 5% a year and epidemiological evidence suggests that this risk increases with age, increased blood pressure, diabetes and other evidence of heart disease. Risk of stroke is fivefold in nonrheumatic atrial fibrillation and is present in about 15% of patients presenting with acute stroke. Patients with atrial fibrillation may also have an increased risk of recurrent stroke and have often silent cerebral infarcts (multiple). In addition, patients with acute stroke and atrial fibrillation have a significantly higher mortality than patients in sinus rhythm.

The commonest site of thrombus is the left atrial appendage which may cause stroke and thromboembolism; right atrial thrombus with subsequent pulmonary thromboembolism is rare.

92. Physical findings include:

1. JVP shows rippling fibrillary waves with absence of 'a' wave and 'x' descent. Absence of 'a' wave result in a single positive wave form being discerned.
2. Pulse is irregular in rate, rhythm, and volume
3. First heart sound varies in intensity
   Irregularly irregular beats
   (Presystolic murmur of mitral stenosis disappears in AF)
4. Irregularly irregular pulse with pulse deficit.

With fast ventricular rates, an apex-radial pulse deficit appears. Impulses are conducted haphazardly from the atria to the ventricles causing irregular ventricular contractions and an irregular pulse. Since the pulse is irregular, the time available for ventricular filling varies causing a variable stroke volume. This results in both the rate and strength of the pulse vary continuously. Some beats are too weak to produce a perceptible peripheral pulse. This results in pulse deficit in the rate of radial pulse compared with the apical pulse. Because of this the apex rate should be always used during clinical assessment of heart rate in atrial fibrillation.

Atrial fibrillation is the common cause of irregularly irregular pulse with pulse deficit.

Rate varies from 100–200/min.

93. ECG diagnosis of atrial fibrillation depends on 4 factors.

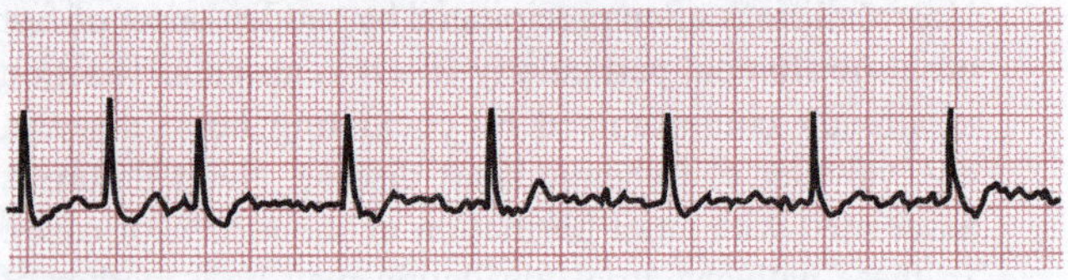

Fig. D-15: Atrial fibrillation: No P waves RR intervals are irregularly irregular, 'F' waves or fibrillary waves irregular coarse undulated, baseline is visible and irregular. Variation in RR interval is the important clue

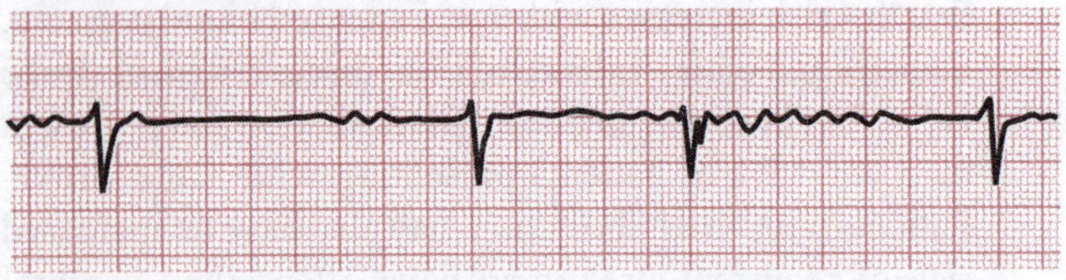

Fig. D-16: Atrial fibrillation: RR intervals irregular; No P waves; 'F' waves are of irregular line

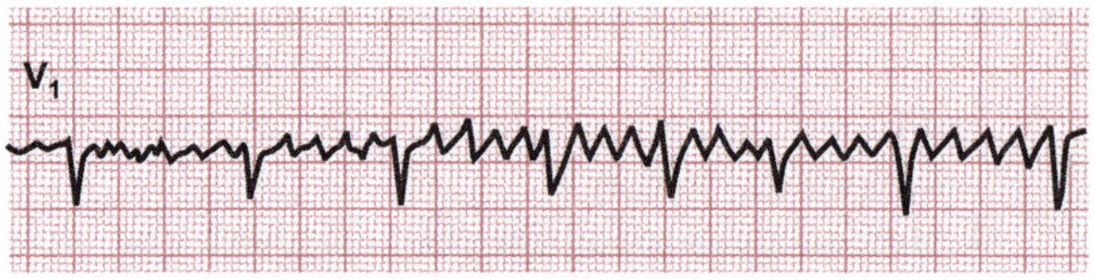

Fig. D-17: Atrial flutter/fibrillation

1. *Rate:* About 350 to 500 per minute.
2. *Rhythm:* Totally irregularly irregular—RR intervals.
3. *Morphology:* 'F' waves or fibrillary waves are irregularly undulated and the baseline is visible and irregular.
   QRS is wide only when there is BBB or aberrant pathway
4. *Ventricular response:* Totally irregular. As only occasional impulses penetrate the atrioventricular node, a totally irregular ventricular rhythm results which is characteristic of atrial fibrillation.

ECG of atrial fibrillation is characterized by an irregular baseline of f waves (and absence of proper P waves) and irregular QRS complexes of normal shape.

Fibrillary (F) waves about 400 per minute.

Varying RR interval.

Coarse F waves are seen in rheumatic and congenital origin.

Fine (straight lines) F waves are seen in hypertensive and ischemic origin.

V I is the best lead for identification

Next best are L II, L III, aVF

If AF is suspected with a regular ventricular response, then suspect either some form of heart block or junctional, or ventricular tachycardiac is present. Ventricular response is usually in the range of 120–180 per minute in the absence of drugs. Ventricular response of more than 180 per minute specifically if they are regular suggests the presence of an accessory pathway.

There can be combined flutter or fibrillation, which is called as atrial flutter fibrillation or impure flutter.

- In atrial fibrillation with a normal AV node, the ventricular rate is more than 150 per minute.
- or with AV block—irregular rate of 60/minute or less
- or with complete heart block—regular ventricular rate of less than 60 per minute.

12-lead ECG may provide a clue to the etiology or electrophysiological features that may cause arrhythmia, e.g. ischemic heart disease, previous myocardial infarction, left ventricular hypertrophy, or a pre-excitation syndrome if it is in sinus rhythm.

A 24-hour Holter monitor may be necessary to document paroxysmal atrial fibrillation or the sick sinus syndrome. This investigation also may not work out in patients who have only intermittent and infrequent symptoms, such as palpitations. In such patients, a "cardiomemo" (or "transtelephonic event monitor") may be preferred. This device transmits ECG trace via a telephone; the patient may thus "record" ECG during the episode of palpitations. Cardiomemo is fairly cheap, simple to use, and may even be used by general practitioners.

94. Chest X-ray is useful in most patients with atrial fibrillation as follows.

1. Left atrial hypertrophy in mitral stenosis shows straight left heart border with prominent left atrial appendage and dilated left atrium resulting in a "double contour" next to the right heart border.
2. In congenital heart disease, such as atrial septal defect shows cardiomegaly, prominent hila, and pulmonary plethora.
3. Left ventricular hypertrophy is evidenced by boot-shaped heart in hypertensive patients.
4. In older patients, it may give information on the size of the heart and whether the patient has heart failure.

95. Echocardiography in atrial fibrillation is useful in 4 ways.

1. To diagnose structural heart diseases, e.g. ASD, MS, etc. absence of any structural heart disease helps to classify "lone atrial fibrillation".
2. To document left ventricular function so that suitable patients are identified for successful cardioversion to sinus rhythm, e.g. poor ventricular function is an unfavorable sign.
3. To identify pulmonary hypertension.
4. To refine the thromboembolic risk stratification in patients unsuitable for cardioversion. It identifies the thrombus in left atrial appendage especially if a mitral prosthetic valve is in situ. It also helps to determine which patients need warfarin or aspirin. Transesophageal echocardiogram is particularly useful in these cases.

96. Echocardiac predictors of increased thromboembolic risk include:

1. Mitral valve disease—MS, MR, MVP, mitral prostatic valve.
2. Left atrial enlargement—evidence of thrombus in left atrium.
3. Decreased LV systolic function.
4. Decreased left atrial appendage emptying velocities—evidence of thrombus in left atrial appendage.

97. There are 4 standard investigations in atrial fibrillation.

1. Blood tests:
   - Full blood count—especially when anticoagulants are being considered—BT, CT, PTT.
     Thyroid, renal, and hepatic function tests.
   - Urea and electrolytes—to establish baseline and if the patient is on digoxin (dose of digoxin is to be reduced in renal impairment)
   - Thyroid function tests.
2. Electrocardiography including ambulatory ECG
   - 12-lead ECG
   - 24-hour Holter monitor—if patients present with syncope, and paroxysmal atrial fibrillation or when the sick sinus syndrome is suspected.
   - Possible use of "cardiomemo" – if symptoms are only intermittent and infrequent
3. Chest radiography
4. Echocardiography
   - Transthoracic echocardiography and Doppler echo examination
   - Possibly transesophageal echocardiography if a prosthetic mitral valve is in situ or if endocarditis or atrial thrombi are suspected.

98. Atria fibrillation should be differentiated from the following arrhythmias.

Variation in the RR interval is the important clue.

1. *Sinus tachycardia:* Sinus rhythm of more than 100 per minute. It has a gradual onset and offset. Each QRS is preceded by a P wave. These waves may be difficult to discern in a fast heart rate, and the rhythm may be mistaken for atrial fibrillation. Atrial fibrillation has distinction of irregular ventricular rate.
2. *Atrial ectopics:* Atrial extrasystoles occur commonly and may be a cause of irregular pulse. Morphology of ectopic P waves differ from sinus P waves. P wave contour varies. Long pause may follow as sinus node automaticity is depressed by the extrasystoles. If the P waves are multiple with different contours, it means that several ectopic foci are firing in the atria resulting in multifocal atrial ectopics. These are particularly common in pulmonary disease.
3. *Atrial tachycardia:* The main difference of paroxysmal atrial tachycardia is that the atrial rate is slower, at 140–250 beats/minute. Variation in the RR interval is the important clue for atrial fibrillation. At very high rates, with a short RR interval, beat to beat variation may be subtle. The difference becomes more obvious if the carotid sinus massage helps to terminate PAT or the speed of the electrocardiogram trace increased. Paroxysmal atrial tachycardia with block is commonly associated with digoxin toxicity which may have been given originally to control atrial fibrillation.
4. *Atrial flutter:* Characteristic saw-toothed F (flutter) waves are seen. AV node ability to conduct waves determines the ventricular response. Most commonly, alternate atrial impulses are conducted to the ventricles,

resulting in a ventricular rate close to 150 beats/minute—that is, atrial flutter with 2:1 block. Atrial flutter with variable atrioventricular block is commonly confused with arial fibrillation.

5. *Wolff-Parkinson-White syndrome:* In an young patient with fast atrial fibrillation, it is important to consider an underlying pre-excitation syndrome, as traditional drugs such as digoxin or verapamil will accelerate the ventricular response by blocking atrioventricular node impulses and increasing conduction through the accessory pathway. WPW syndrome is differentiated from atrial fibrillation by short PR interval, delta wave, wide QRS, T opposite of QRS.
6. *Atrioventricular nodal reentrant tachycardia:* This requires the presence of a micro reentrant circuit within the AV node, commonly with a slow antegrade limb and a fast retrograde limb. A typical ECG shows the P waves are buried in the QRS complex unlike the "F" waves of atria fibrillation.
7. *Sick sinus syndrome:* This syndrome is associated with various atrial tachyarrhythmias, including atrial fibrillation, atrial flutter, and atrial tachycardia. It is commonly known as tachy-brady syndrome. There can be inappropriate sinus bradycardia, sinus pauses or arrest, or sinus exit block. Bradycardia may alternate with tachyarrhythmia. This condition should be thought of before antiarrhythmic drug treatment or general anesthesia is given to any patient with atrial fibrillation and a history of syncope or dizziness. If an underlying sick sinus syndrome exists then direct current cardioversion of atrial fibrillation may result in asystole and should be covered by a temporary pacemaker. Permanent pacemaker therapy (using an atrial or dual chamber system, depending on atrioventricular conduction) may be successful in such patients, reducing arrhythmias and heart failure and improving prognosis.
8. *Ventricular tachycardia:* Ventricular tachycardia with a bundle branch block pattern on the QRS complex may be difficult to differentiate. The important difference again is the irregular RR interval present in atrial fibrillation. Broad QRS is suggestive of ventricular tachycardia or supraventricular tachycardia with aberrant conduction or pre-existing BBB. Broad QRS with left axis deviation is in favor of ventricular tachycardia. If QRS is wide and RR intervals are irregular, first consider atrial fibrillation. Even with broad QRS tachycardia, if it could be terminated by carotid sinus massage—it is supraventricular though it is broad probably of aberrant pathway.

99. Diagnosing and assessing atrial fibrillation.

1. Recording of patients history and clinical features—whether the symptoms are sustained or intermittent and whether any complications such as heart failure, stroke or thromboembolism present—Basic blood tests should be done.
2. Documentation of the arrhythmia—with a 24-hour Holter monitor in paroxysmal atrial fibrillation—with cardiomemo machine for monitoring intermittent and infrequent symptoms.
3. Echocardiography, especially in young patients
4. Exercise testing if ischemic heart disease is present—caution is needed in interpreting results with patients on digoxin.

100. Importance of treating atrial fibrillation.

1. To relieve symptoms of congestive heart failure, hypotension, or angina that can be directly attributed to a rapid heart rate.
2. To improve overall cardiac function
3. To improve exercise tolerance
4. To reduce the risk of thromboembolism and stroke.

101. The treatment of atrial fibrillation is determined by analyzing the following 4 points.

1. Nature and degree of underlying etiologically or predisposing factors should be sought.
2. Duration: Recent or long duration.
   Recurrent—if so, paroxysm or established. Paroxysmal arrhythmias may last only for few minutes or few hours or few days. When it lasts for more than 6 weeks, it becomes permanent arrhythmia. It is important to distinguish between chronic and paroxysmal atrial fibrillation as the two conditions have to be managed differently. In acute presentation of atrial fibrillation, the presence of any acute precipitating factors, such as infection should be considered.
3. Rate of ventricular response. It is also important to distinguish between atria fibrillation and atria flutter as important differences exist in the management of these two conditions.
   Results of previous treatment should be noted.
4. Associated complications such as congestive heart failure or embolism.

102. Restoration of sinus rhythm: Sinus rhythm is often restored with medications by

1. Slowing the conduction of electrical impulses
2. Decreasing the excitability
3. Decreasing the automaticity of cardiac cells
4. Prolonging the refractory period (rest period) of cardiac tissue.

AV node is located between the atria and the ventricles and has a protective "gatekeeper" mechanism that only allows so many impulses to travel through to the ventricles. Therefore, the goal is to reduce the ventricular rate to 70–90 beats per minute via the AV node during an episode of atria fibrillation. The idea is that even though the heartbeat is irregular, it is better to be irregular at 79–80 beats per minute than to be irregular at 140–150 beats per minute. This rate control in turn, decreases the workload of the heart and the symptoms of discomfort associated with a fast irregular heart beat. Some of the medications used to produce this effect include propafenone, propranolol, diltiazem, verapamil and digoxin.

103. General measures:

1. Avoidance of precipitating factors like alcohol or caffeine should always be considered in cases of paroxysmal atrial fibrillation.
2. Acute infections, such as pneumonia: It can be a complication of pre-existing arial fibrillation or it can precipitate atrial fibrillation.
3. In postoperative atrial fibrillation –hypoxia should be considered.
4. Electrolyte abnormalities should be excluded.

104. Therapy of atrial fibrillation should be considered in 4 areas.

1. Control of ventricular response—the present data is strong enough to promote rate control approach as the initial strategy for the vast majority of patients with persistent atrial fibrillation.
2. Minimization of thromboembolic risk.
3. Restoration and maintenance of sinus rhythm.
4. Highly symptomatic patients with chest pain, pulmonary edema, who are hemodynamically "unstable" who needs immediate direct current cardioversion (DCC).

105. Antiarrhythmic drugs for atrial fibrillation are used for:

1. Control of symptoms
2. Control of chronic atrial fibrillation.
3. Cardioversion of atrial fibrillation to sinus rhythm
4. Maintenance of sinus rhythm after cardioversion.

These drugs may be used as prophylaxis in paroxysmal atrial fibrillation. The ventricular response is generally controlled through the drugs that acts on AV node to slow the conduction. AF in WPW syndrome is treated in a different way from AF conduction down the AV node alone.

106. The following IV drugs are contraindicated in AF associated with WPW syndrome.

1. Intravenous calcium channel blockers.
2. Intravenous β-blockers.
3. Intravenous adenosine.
4. Intravenous Xylocaine/lidocaine.

These drugs are contraindicated in patients with AF and WPW syndrome because they facilitate conduction down accessory pathway thereby causing acceleration of the ventricular rate, hypotension, and ventricular fibrillation.

107. Digoxin in atrial fibrillation (see Chapter C-Heart Failure 93–106)

1. Digoxin is the most commonly prescribed antiarrhythmic drug in patients with atrial fibrillation. It is useful in controlling the resting ventricular rate in chronic atrial fibrillation. Though it does effective treatment in chronic atrial fibrillation, it may be detrimental in paroxysmal atrial fibrillation.
2. There is also no evidence that digoxin is useful for cardioversion of atrial fibrillation to sinus rhythm or maintaining sinus rhythm after cardioversion.
3. It has limited value in patients with an accessory pathway and it may even accelerate the ventricular response.
4. It poorly controls the ventricular response in exercise and in conditions of high sympathetic drive. In such cases, additional use of β-blockers or calcium blockers with actions at AV node such as verapamil or diltiazem is of value to control the ventricular rate.

Digoxin increases vagal tone, moderating the speed of AV conduction, and also reduces the atrial refractory period. This later property may paradoxically render the atrium more susceptible to fibrillation and may reduce or even prevent the chance of reversion to sinus rhythm.

108. Digoxin is usually used:

1. In controlling resting heart rate; however, it is less effective lowering the ventricular response.
2. Ideal in patients with decreased LV function.
3. In patient where there is contraindication for β-blockers or calcium channel blockers, e.g. asthma, COPD, and hemodynamic instability.
4. It may be combined with other drugs like β-blockers, amiodarone in rhythm control.

When digoxin alone is used in rate control, the patient should undergo monitored exercise and the exertional heart rate should be verified to be less than 110 bpm.

Digoxin is given intravenously or orally. The onset of action is slow (1–4 hours) those 0.25 mg IV every 6h for a total of 1 mg every 24 hours then a maintenance dose is given.

Digoxin is generally well tolerated although it is associated with adverse effects.

109. Conditions for refractory of atrial fibrillation to digoxin.

1. Not taking digoxin tablets properly.
2. Presence of accessory pathway (e.g. WPW syndrome)
3. Thyrotoxicosis
4. Poor left ventricular function
5. Respiratory diseases, such as cor pulmonale, plural effusion, lung cancer, etc.
6. Metabolic abnormalities
7. Electrolytic abnormalities
8. Hypoxia.

110. There are 4 points to consider while giving drug treatment for paroxysmal atrial fibrillation.

1. Avoid digoxin. Clinical evidence has shown that paroxysms of atrial fibrillation occur more frequently and appreciably longer in patients receiving digoxin.
2. Try sotalol, if no contraindication
3. Alternatively, try propafenone or other class 1 drug (but not if cardiac impairment is present)
4. Use amiodarone as first choice if left ventricular function is poor.

111. Flecainide—Class IC antiarrhythmic drug/may be used with caution in patients with atrial fibrillation especially to control paroxysmal atrial fibrillation in structurally normal hearts.

1. Without evidence of ischemic heart disease
2. Without ventricular dysfunction
3. To achieve pharmacological cardioversion—flecainide may be more effective than propafenone in converting to sinus rhythm (90% vs 55% conversion rate respectively)
4. To control atrial fibrillation associated with Wolff-Parkinson-White syndrome.

Treatment with these drugs should be started in hospital under supervision as per the current recommendations in the British National Formulary.

112. Sotalol, another commonly prescribed drug, combines the antiarrhythmic effects of drugs in both Class II (blockade) and Class III (prolongation of repolarization). Prolongation of repolarization is thought to be mainly due to the dextro (D) isomer of the sotalol compound. Sotalol is effective in paroxysmal atrial fibrillation.

1. in maintaining sinus rhythm post-cardioversion
2. in controlling the ventricular response in atrial fibrillation, thus permitting rate control, without the need for other drugs such as digoxin.
3. in patients with concomitant hypertension and
4. in patients with ischemic heart disease as it has β-blocker activity.

113. Amiodarone is a very effective drug for treating atrial fibrillation, but its use has to be moderated because of its common side effects. The side effects are more common with higher doses of amiodarone and with prolonged treatment; some of the side effects are reversible on withdrawal of the drug. Low doses of 200 mg/day (often much less than doses needed for controlling ventricular arrhythmias, which require 400 mg/day or more) may be effective with little risk of side effects (see - point 212).

1. It is particularly useful in atrial fibrillation which is refractory to other measures.
2. It is highly effective in converting atrial fibrillation to sinus rhythm.
3. It is also capable of maintaining sinus rhythm for longer periods.
4. It is highly effective in controlling symptoms more than either verapamil or quinidine, possibly moderating the ventricular response even if an attack occurs.
5. It is particularly useful in atrial fibrillation with poor left ventricular function.
6. It is useful in paroxysmal atrial fibrillation (intravenous amiodarone is seldom indicated to suppress paroxysmal atria fibrillation).
7. It can increase the plasma concentration of digoxin, thus leading to its toxicity.
8. It can lead to over anticoagulation in patients taking warfarin, perhaps by a hepatic interaction.

114. β-blockers in atrial fibrillation.

1. They have rapid onset of action as well as short half-life in both the oral intravenous forms.
2. These should be used cautiously in decreased systolic function or in heart failure.
3. IV preparations of metoprolol, esmolol and propranolol starts action approximately in 5 minutes.
4. Commonly used oral preparation include metoprolol, atenolol, propranolol and nadolol.

115. Verapamil and diltiazem in atrial fibrillation:

1. Verapamil controls the ventricular response in atrial fibrillation by increasing the atrioventricular block and the effective refractory period of the atroventricular node. This results in increased exercise capacity. It is therefore useful in controlling ventricular response both at rest and with exercise. Diltiazem acts in similar way and is popular in USA.
2. Verapamil is associated with a much lower rate of conversion to sinus rhythm than drugs in Class III (e.g. amiodarone, sotalol) or Class I (e.g. flecainide, propafenone).
3. Verapamil is ineffective in controlling paroxysmal atrial fibrillation.

4. Verapamil gives rise to serious side effects in patients with underlying Wolff-Parkinson-White syndrome including ventricular fibrillation and severe hemodynamic impairment. This is due to poor control of very fast ventricular rates in response to electrical impulses passing down the accessory pathway, as the atrioventricular node is blocked by verapamil.

116. Angiotensin-converting enzyme inhibitors (ACEI) and angiotension receptor blockers (ARBs) in atrial fibrillation.

1. They decrease the incidence of atrial fibrillation by decreasing the left atrial pressure thereby reducing the atrial premature beats.
2. They also reduces atrial fibrosis thereby decreasing the incidence of recurrent AF.
3. Withdrawal of ACEI is associated with postoperative atrial fibrillation in patients undergoing CABG surgery.
4. Concurrent therapy with ACEI and antiarrhythmic agents enhances the maintenance of sinus rhythm.

117. 4 useful drug options in various clinical situations.

1. Atrial fibrillation with heart failure and poor cardiac function—Digoxin or possibly amiodarone
2. Atrial fibrillation in hypertensive patients—Digoxin and calcium antagonsit (e.g. Verapamil, diltiazem)
3. Atrial fibrillation and thyrotoxicosis—Digoxin and nonspecific β-blocker (e.g. propranolol)
4. Atrial fibrillation and ischemic heart disease/ hypertrophic cardiomyopathy—β-blockers or calcium antagonists.

118. There are 4 steps in approach to drugs for rate control in chronic atrial fibrillation.

1. Try digoxin
2. If no response—add or substitute verapamil, diltiazem, or β-blocker
3. If still no response—consider adding or substituting propafenone, flecainide, or amiodarone
4. In resistant cases—refer to specialist may be needed in difficult case.

119. Treatment of atrial fibrillation is followed in the following 4 ways depending on the duration of onset, associated complications.

Digitalis remains the drug of choice for treating atrial fibrillation.

1. *Treatment of Paroxysmal or recent onset atrial fibrillation with recognizable cause without any hemodynamic failure:*
   (If BP fall is not below 90 mm Hg)
   Treat the underlying cause such as congestive heart failure, hypertension.
   If the digitalization is not done early, start digoxin and maintain until the ventricular rate is 70–80/min.
   If atrial fibrillation still persists:
   quinidine alone or with procainamide will help to convert to sinus rhythm.
2. *Chronic atrial fibrillation without hemodynamic failure:* Digoxin 0.25 mg/24 h po (0.125 mg in older patients). Aim at controlling ventricular rate than sinus rhythm. If ventricular rate is too fast, reassess the cause, increase the dose of digoxin if necessary.
   If no response:
   Cautiously add β-blockers—Propranolol 10–20 mg 8 hrly po. Propranolol is added when cardiac rate is unacceptably high in spite of adequate digitalization. Add β-blockers only in patients without heart failure and does not have features of bradycardia/tachycardia syndrome.
3. *Recent atrial fibrillation with hemodynamic failure:* Electrical counter shock is the immediate treatment of choice. If counter shock fails—Propranolol IV may be tried even in the presence of heart failure or pulmonary edema.
4. *Atrial fibrillation with Wolff-Parkinson-White (WPW) syndrome:*
   Ventricular rate more than 200/min
   Withhold digoxin.
   DC cardioversion
   Disopyramide: 2 mg/kg to maximum 150 mg IV slowly.
   Or give amiodarone.

Antithrombotic Treatment for Atrial Fibrillation

Only in the past few years, antithrombotic treatment has been proved by prospective clinical studies to be effective against strokes in atrial fibrillation. About 15–20% of patients who have an acute stroke, have atrial fibrillation at the time of their stroke.

120. American Heart Association (AHA) recommends individualized selection of antithrombotic agents depending on the patients risk for stroke and bleeding.

Factors associated with higher risk of stroke include:

1. History of previous thromboembolism (stroke, TIA, systemic embolism.
2. Rheumatic mitral valve.
3. Prosthetic heart valve.

Moderate risk include:

4. Coronary artery disease (CAD)/IHD
5. Congestive heart failure (CHF)
6. Hypertension (HTN)
7. Diabetes mellitus (DM)
8. Renal insufficiency (RI)

9. LV ejection fraction < 35%
10. Thyrotoxicosis
11. Age > 65 years
12. Female gender.

Presence of more than one moderate risk factor suggests the use of vitamin K antagonist. The goal of International Normalized Ratio (INR) of 2.0–3.0 is maintained. Aspirin 75 to 300 mg po, od is recommended in patients with low risk or in those who have contraindication for oral anticoagulation.

121. Nonrheumatic atrial fibrillation and stroke

1. Nonrheumatic atrial fibrillation has been associated with a five-fold increase in the risk of ischemic stroke.
2. The yearly risk is 5–7%, increase with age.
3. CT scan studies have shown that silent ischemic cerebral infarction is present in 26% of patients with nonrheumatic atrial fibrillation.
4. Mortality is one and a half to three times higher in those patients than in patients with sinus rhythm at the time of stroke.

122. There are 4 contributing risk factors of underlying heart disease for stroke and thromboembolism in atrial fibrillation.

1. Valvular disease
2. Hypertension
3. Enlarged left atrium
4. Poor left ventricular function.

The risk of thromboembolism in atrial fibrillation is 18 times greater when rheumatic heart disease is present. It is observed thromboembolism is a common cause of death in patients with congestive heart failure, occurring in up to 30% of patients, which is partly preventable by anticoagulation.

123. There are 4 major indications for anticoagulation therapy in atrial fibrillation.

1. *Atrial fibrillation combined with mitral stenosis:* The risk of arterial embolization is particularly high in this situation because of increased stasis of blood in the left atrium produced by the combination of atrial fibrillation and the large baggy left atrium associated with mitral stenosis. Trial have shown that the benefits of long-term anticoagulation, for instance with warfarin outweigh the risk of hemorrhage. All patients of atrial fibrillation with mitral stenosis should therefore be anticoagulated unless there is contraindication.
2. *Atrial fibrillation combined with mitral regurgitation:* Long-term anticoagulation is indicated in this situation where there is mitral regurgitation resulting in left atrium enlarging to more than 4 cm diameter. Anticoagulation is reserved in lesser form of mitral regurgitation with atrial fibrillation.
   Anticoagulants should be given before elective cardioversion in atrial fibrillation with mitral valvular disease.
3. *Atrial fibrillation without mitral valve disease:* It is undoubtedly wise to anticoagulate any patient with atrial fibrillation in whom there is suspicion of arterial emboli, e.g. dilated cardiomyopathy, coronary artery disease or hypertensive heart disease where there is previous history of embolic events related to atrial fibrillation. Anticoagulation is usually advized in these situation if the left atrium is larger than 4 cm diameter on echocardiogram. Computerized tomographic (CT) brain scan should be taken in suspected cerebral emboli to exclude hemorrhage as anticoagulants are contraindicated in the presence of cerebral hemorrhage.
4. Prosthetic valves.

124. Larger than 4 cm diameter of left atrium is indicated for anticoagulation therapy by some authorities.

125. Left atrial enlargement in atrial fibrillation and thromboembolism.

1. Left atrial enlargement has been associated with "spontaneous echo contrast" on transesophageal echocardiography (TEE)—a smoke-like appearance of blood in the atria, suggesting sluggish flow.
2. It is associated with intracardiac thrombi, thromboembolism, stroke.
3. It is associated with abnormal rheology.
4. It is associated with abnormal coagulation.

TEE is highly effective in the detection of thrombus in the atria and left atrial appendage and is more sensitive in this regard than transthoracic echocardiography (TTE).

126. Prophylactic anticoagulation for 1 to 3 weeks is indicated before cardioversion in 4 conditions.

1. Atrial flutter
2. Atrial fibrillation
3. History of thromboembolic disease
4. Mitral valve disease.

Thrombus formation occurs particularly in the atrial appendage because the atria do not contract or empty normally in atrial fibrillation, leading to blood stasis. As a consequence, there is a risk of systemic arterial emboli from the fibrillating left atrium and occasionally from the fibrillating right atrium.

127. The analysis of five primary intervention trials showed that antithrombotic agent, warfarin has shown the following 4 results:

1. It reduced the annual rate of stroke
2. It led to a similar risk reduction in stroke with residual deficit
3. It reduced the mortality by a third
4. It reduced the rate of the combined adverse outcome (stroke, systemic embolism, or death) by half.

The efficacy of warfarin was underestimated because most strokes in patients allocated to warfarin occurred while the patient was not taking the warfarin.

(Some important stroke prevention trials: AFASAK—Copenhagen Atrial Fibrillation, Aspirin, Anticoagulation Study; BAATAF—Boston Area Anticoagulation Trial for Atrial Fibrillation; CAFA—Canadian Atrial Fibrillation Anticoagulation Study; EAFT—European Atrial Fibrillation Trial; SPAF—Stroke Prevention in Atrial Fibrillation Trial; SPNAF—Stroke Prevention in Nonrheumatic Arial Fibrillation Study).

128. The five primary trials have shown the following observations while using warfarin.

1. The target range in all studies was 1.5 to 4.5 International Normalized ratio (INR) of prothrombin time.
2. Optimum therapeutic range in most patients for warfarin is 2.0 to 3.0, which seemed to have minimum risk of stroke.
3. A range of 3.0 to 4.5 is needed in patients with mechanical prosthetic valve.
4. In older patients and with recurrent thromboembolism also need higher intensity of warfarin (range of 3.0 to 4.5).

At present, a target range of 2.0 to 3.0 can be recommended in most patients for high intensity warfarin.

The efficacy of warfarin in clinical trials may not be reproduced in practice. This is due to the high selection of patients in these studies.

129. Risk of bleeding with anticoagulation treatment: Intracranial hemorrhage is the most feared complication of warfarin prophylaxis.

1. Bleeding is most common in patients with unstable anticoagulation control.
2. Patients with a history of thromboembolism ranges from 11–40%.
3. The risk of bleeding with warfarin increases exponentially with an increase in anticoagulation effect, rising from an annual risk of 0.2% with an International Normalized Ratio of 2.0–3.0% with a ratio of 4.0
4. However, the bleeding and its related complications often may occur even when the International Normalized Ratio is within the therapeutic range.

130. Aspirin (75–300 mg/day) is simpler to monitor and has a lower risk of bleeding. Aspirin has been evaluated as primary prophylaxis of systemic thromboembolism – in two randomized trials compared with no antithrombotic treatment and in one compared with warfarin. The following observations are made.

1. Aspirin was only about half as effective as warfarin. However, it may be given as secondary prophylactic in patients with previous stroke or transient ischemic attack, who have a higher risk of thromboembolism.
2. It has 36% decrease in risk of stroke
3. It has no significant effect on stroke with residual deficit or mortality
4. It has 28% decrease in the rate of the combined outcome of stroke, systemic embolism, or death.

131. Following factors may increase the risk of bleeding with warfarin

1. Age
2. Uncontrolled hypertension (SBP >180 mm Hg or DBP > 100 mm Hg)
3. Alcohol excess
4. Liver disease
5. Poor drug or clinical compliance
6. Bleeding lesions (GI bleeding and previous cerebral hemorrhage)
7. Tendency to bleeding (including coagulation defects, thrombocytopenia)
8. Concomitant use of aspirin with oral anticoagulants.

Before starting antithrombotic prophylaxis with warfarin or aspirin, it is important to consider the risk versus bleeding. To minimize the risk of intracranial bleeding with prophylactic warfarin, hypertension should be adequately controlled, and the risks and benefits of warfarin reviewed annually, especially in patients aged over 80 years.

132. A lower risk of stroke, annual risk of 1% exists in people with

1. Nonrheumatic atrial fibrillation
2. < 65 years age with no history of embolism
3. No history of hypertension
4. No history of diabetes mellitus

Aspirin or warfarin does not seem to be necessary unless some other indication coexists.

133. Moderate risk of stroke, annual risk of 4% exists in people with

1. Nonrheumatic atrial fibrillation without previous history of embolism
2. Aged under 65 years with a history of hypertension or diabetes

3. Aged 65–74 years with or without a history of hypertension or diabetes
4. Aged 75 years or above with no history of hypertension or diabetes

Aspirin seems to be as effective as warfarin in this group (reducing the annual risk of stroke to 1 to 3%)

134. Highest risk of stroke, annual risk of 12% exists in people with

1. Previous history of thromboembolic stroke, transient ischemic attack, or other atrial thromboembolism
2. Age > 75 years
3. History of hypertension
4. History of diabetes
5. Valvular disease or prosthesis
6. Heart failure
7. Thyrotoxicosis
8. Cardioversion.

These high-risk patients are considered for anticoagulation with warfarin.

135. Identifying patients in a community with atrial fibrillation at high risk of stroke and thromboembolism is needed as many such patients may be unrecognized and undiagnosed with few or no symptoms.

1. Formal screening for atrial fibrillation in primary care centers should be considered
2. Careful clinical history is needed to identify those with important risk factors
3. Echocardiography may be a further tool in thromboembolic risk stratification.
4. Recent studies suggest that a " hypercoagulable" state exists in patients with atrial fibrillation.

136. Following are considered to start anticoagulation after acute thromboembolic stroke

1. Patients with small or moderate thromboembolic strokes in whom an intracranial bleed is excluded by CT scan at > 48 hours
   Heparin followed by warfarin (International Normalized Ratio 2.0–3.0).
2. Patients with large embolic strokes or uncontrolled hypertensioon.
   No anticoagulation for 5–14 days because of the increased risk of hemorrhagic transformation.
3. Patients with nonvalvar atrial fibrillation as the presumed cause of thromboembolism.
   Warfarin only (after CT scan at 48 hours) owing to the low risk of early recurrent thromboembolism.
4. Patients with valvar atrial fibrillation causing thromboembolism (exclude hemorrhage by CT scan).

In patients with acute stroke and atrial fibrillation, intracranial hemorrhage should be excluded by CT scan before starting warfarin. This is important as 11% of patients with hemorrhagic stroke have atrial fibrillation compared with 18% with stroke due to cerebral infarction. It is important to start anticoagulation at the proper time after an acute stroke as there is the risk of hemorrhagic transformation of the cerebral infarct, by bleeding into the infarcted, softened brain.

Cardioversion of Atrial Fibrillation

Cardioversion from atrial fibrillation to sinus rhythm should be considered for suitable patients instead of leaving the patient in arrhythmia and treating with drugs.

137. There are 4 potential benefits of a return to sinus rhythm.

1. Improvement in well-being
2. Increase in exercise capacity
3. Avoidance of potentially dangerous drugs
4. Reduction in thromboembolic risk.

138. Cardioversion to restore sinus rhythm in atrial fibrillation is indicated in 4 conditions.

1. When anticipated that the sinus rhythm can be maintained as in atrial fibrillation of short duration (or paroxysmal atrial tachycardia, atrial flutter, persistent paroxysmal atrial tachycardia and atrial flutter should generally be converted to sinus rhythm because they eventually result in cardiac failure).
2. When anticipated that sinus rhythm can be maintained for long time when there is reversible cause such as thyrotoxicosis, pulmonary embolism, infections, etc. or after the surgical correction of valvular or congenital heart disease to restore persistent atrial fibrillation to sinus rhythm.
3. In younger persons in whom no obvious cause is apparent, a condition known as 'lone atrial fibrillation' to restore persistent atrial fibrillation to sinus rhythm.
4. In any other cause of established atrial fibrillation in the absence of marked atrial enlargement, significant mitral stenosis, mitral regurgitation, left ventricular or right ventricular failure.

Atrial flutter can be frequently terminated by low energy synchronized direct current cardioversion (100 W sec) but atrial fibrillation usually needs high energy up to 100–400 W sec.

Prophylactic anticoagulation for 1 to 3 weeks is indicated before cardioversion in atrial flutter or fibrillation in patients with history of thromboembolic disease and in patients with mitral valve disease.

Atrial fibrillation in the middle-aged and elderly persons aged over about 60 years is usually accepted because of its tendency to recur. They are generally given digitalis to control fast ventricular rate.

139. There are 4 methods of cardioversion.

Electrical

1. Synchronized external direct current shock
2. Transesophageal
3. Internal

Pharmacological

4. Drugs—class I and III drugs.

Electrical cadioversion works by permitting uniform repolarization and restoring ordered conduction. After the initial asytolic period, the sinoatrial node rapidly resumes its role as cardiac pacemaker, permitting synchronized atrial electrical activity. Effectiveness of external electrical cardioversion ranges from 20–90%, highest success rates are seen in patients with atrial fibrillation secondary to hyperthyroidism, while the lowest rates are seen in patients with severe mitral regurgitation.

140. Energy requirement and success of external cardioversion are directly related to the

1. Duration of atrial fibrillation
2. Size of the 'f' (fibrillation) wave
3. Presence of mitral valve disease (especially if there has been previous valve surgery)
4. Other factors like poor left ventricular function, cardiomyopathy, etc. predict refractoriness to successful cardioversion or unsuccessful maintenance of sinus rhythm.

Transesophageal cardioversion and internal cardioversion are alternative methods used less often in specialist centers.

141. Preparation for cardioversion

1. Admit the patient in a coronary care unit
2. Ensure electrolytes (especially potassium) are normal
3. Ensure anticoagulation is adequate, with an International Normalized Ratio of 2.0 to 3.0
4. If the patient is on digoxin and there is no digoxin toxicity, the drug may be taken up to the day before cardioversion; if digoxin toxicity is suspected, serum digoxin concentration should be checked and cardioversion delayed.

142. Electrical cardioversion

1. Patient should be in fasting
2. Short general anesthesia is needed to eliminate discomfort associated with transthoracic shock
3. Give synchronized direct current shock; start at 100 J, with intermediate "step-ups", eventually to 360 J
4. Monitor the patient after the procedure at least one hour to ensure stability of rhythm and blood pressure.

143. Direct current shock acts by depolarizing the myocardial cells and allowing the normal impulse to take over control of the heart beat.

The indications of direct current (DC) shock in supraventricular tachycardias are:

1. Failure of response to drug therapy
2. Patients who are actually ill with arrhythmia
3. Cardiac failure
4. Hypotension.

The DC shock is often the first choice of antiarrhythmia treatment in these conditions. Partly for reasons of speed but also because many antiarrhythmic drugs have negative inotropic effects, i.e. they decrease the force of contraction of the cardiac muscle.

About 25 to 100 joules is usually required to convert supraventricular tachycardias (up to 200 joules is often required for ventricular tachyarrhythmias).

Elective cardioversion is performed with the help of diazepam or with light anesthesia.

The energy necessary for cardioversion varies from 100 to 400 W sec depending on the nature of arrhythmia.

Emergent cardioversion is needed in ventricular fibrillation.

144. There are 4 precautions to be taken before giving direct current shock in a digitalised patient because

1. Digitalis increases the excitability of cardiac muscle, as a sequence there is danger of ventricular fibrillation.
2. Digitalis toxicity may be present. If possible, digitalis should be stopped for one or two days before cardioversion.
3. Digitalis competes with potassium for binding sites on cardiac muscle. As a result hypokalemia is associated with increased binding of digitalis on the heart. This results in increased danger of DC shock causing ventricular fibrillation.
4. If digitalis toxicity is present, then serum digoxin concentrations should be checked and cardioversion delayed.

Deliver the shock on the R wave at the time of ventricular depolarization.

Now, the defibrillators available are synchronized to deliver the shock on R wave.

145. Pharmacological cardioversion: The most commonly used Class I drugs are quinidine, flecainide, and propafenone, and class III drug is amiodarone.

1. *Quinidine:* It is effective in cardioversion of atrial fibrillation and in maintaining sinus rhythm, but side effects can occur in a fifth of patients, two-thirds of whom have to discontinue the drug.

2. *Flecainide:* It has 92% success rate when given intravenously. However, it has adverse effects in 74% of patients.
3. *Propafenone:* It may be more useful than flecainamide in view of its inherent rate limiting properties (as a β-blocker). Permitting potentially greater ventricular rate control.
   Class IA agents—quinidine, procainamide, disopyramide use have been come down due to high incidence of intolerance, toxicity and increased mortality in structural heart disease. Dofetilide, Azimilide class III agents are not approved by FDA.
4. *Amiodarone:* It has been shown to be highly effective in the cardioversion of atrial fibrillation, even in the previously refractory cases and in maintaining sinus rhythm. IV Amiodarone acts relatively rapidly, restoring sinus rhythm in up to 75% of patients, making it as effective as electrical cardioversion. In cases of resistant atrial fibrillation, a four week loading dose of amiodarone 600 mg od before cardioversion and a low dose of 200 mg od maintenance dose after successful cardioversion was effective in obtaining cardioversion and maintenance of sinus rhythm.

Although, verapamil is used occasionally, it has a much lower success rate of conversion.

Digoxin is no better than placebo for restoring sinus rhythm. It is not effective as prophylaxis against recurring atrial fibrillation after cardioversion. In addition, in patients with recurrent atrial fibrillation, paroxysms of atrial fibrillation occur more frequently, at a faster rate, and for longer in patients receiving digoxin.

146. 4 Intravenous medication used for cardioversion of atrial fibrillation.

Table D-5

Drug	Vaughn Williams class	Dose	Adverse effect
1. Amiodarone	III	5–7 mg/kg over 30–60 min followed by 1.2–1.8 g/day until 10 g then 200–400 mg daily for maintenance	Hypotension bradycardia, hypothyroidism, hepatitis, skin discoloration, phlebitis
2. Ibutilide	III	1 mg over 10 min, repeat as needed	Torsades de pointes, increased QTc
3. Propafenone	Ic	1.5–2.0 mg/kg over 20 min	Hypotension, atrial flutter with RVR
4. Flecainide	Ic	1.5–3 mg/kg over 10 to 20 min	Hypotension, atral flutter with RVR

147. Oral drugs for rhythm control in atrial fibrillation.

Table D-6

Drug	Vaughn Williams class	Cardioversion dose	Daily maintenance dose
1. Amiodarone	III	600–800 mg bid or (tid / day) until 10 g, then	200–400 mg
2. Sotalol	III	160–320 mg	Same
3. Propafenone	Ic	600 mg	450–900 mg
4. Flecainide	Ic	200–300 mg	Same

148. Amiodarone is commonly used drug.

1. It is unique in having properties of all four Vaughn-Williams classes
2. It is distinct with regards to its very long half-life (up to 120 days).
3. It is usually reserved for patients in whom other antiarrhythmic drugs are ineffective because it has potential organ toxicity that may occur mostly to the liver, lung, thyroid and eyes.
4. It is essential that patients treated with amiodarone should have regulars screening ophthalmologic examination, pulmonary function test, chest X-ray and blood test for liver and thyroid function.

149. Mechanisms and factors contributing to thromboembolism in cardioversion

1. Mechanical.
   – Embolization of any pre-existing clot can occur due to dislodgment by the mechanical effect of a change in cardiac rhythm during cardioversion.
   – The return of atrial systole and effective atrial contraction after cardioversion may take up to 3 weeks
   – Cardioversion may promote the formation of new thrombi due to transient atrial dysfunction ("stunning")
2. Duration of atrial fibrillation
   – It is affected by hemodynamic status, atrial size, underlying atrial pathology, and effectiveness of anticoagulation
   – A recently formed, poorly adherent thrombus is more likely to dislodge at the time of cardioversion.
3. Left atrial size
   – Formation of thrombi is more likely in dilated left atrium, particularly when it is > 4.0 cm.
4. Abnormalities in hemorheological function and prothrombotic markers
   – Clotting factor levels
   – Atrial natriuretic peptide, leading to hemoconcentration, and a raised packed cell volume.

150. The following 4 recommendations are made by American Association of Chest Physicians for anticoagulation before and after cardioversion.

1. Warfarin for 3 weeks before non-emergency cardioversion of atrial fibrillation of > 24–48 hours duration
2. Warfarin for 4 weeks after cardioversion
3. Intravenous heparin followed by warfarin if cardioversion cannot be postsponed for 3 weeks
4. Anticoagulants may not be needed for atrial fibrillation of < 2 days duration or for cardioversion of supraventricular tachycardia. Consideration should be given to managing atrial flutter similarly to atrial fibrillation.

The use of these drugs after cardioversion is to maintain sinus rhythm and prevent recurrence of arrhythmia. The optimal duration of anticoagulation is still unclear, although the American Association of Chest Physicians has drawn up recommendations including the suggestion that warfarin should be continued for 4 weeks after cardioversion. It may be worth to continue anticoagulation for longer than 4 weeks in patients with a high risk of recurrent atrial fibrillation.

151. Predictors of refractoriness of cardioversion or unsuccessful maintenance of sinus rhythm.

1. Age > 50 years
2. Arrhythmia for > 1 year
3. Hypertension
4. Valvular heart disease—mitral valve disease, aortic stenosis, etc.
5. Previous valve surgery or prosthesis
6. Poor left ventricular function
7. Structural heart disease such as cardiomyopathy or infarction
8. No correctable precipitating factors—for example, thyroid disease, infection.

Recent studies suggest that left atrial size does not influence the outcome after cardioversion but that the duration of atrial fibrillation is the most important predictor for outcome. Long-term sinus rhythm (about 80% at 12 months) is possible even with a dilated left atrium with the use of antiarrhythmic drugs.

152. Without antiarrhythmic drugs there is a high risk of relapse of atrial fibrillation, with the proportion of patient remaining in sinus rhythm ranging from:

1. 69% at 1 month
2. 58% at 6 months
3. 23% at 1 year
4. 16% at 2 years

153. Changes after cardioversion of atrial fibrillation.

Short-term changes

1. Hypotension.
2. Bradycardia—more common in patients with sick sinus syndrome and after myocardial infarction.
3. Arrhythmias, usually due to either inadequate synchronization or digoxin toxicity: ventricular arrhythmias are less common but more serious (ventricular fibrillation is the most common in about 1% of cases, but is usually reverted by repeat shock).
4. Premature beats and conduction disturbances (first degree or second degree atrioventricular block) are also common.
5. Small rises in creatine kinase concentration may occur, usually from skeletal muscle, and myocardial damage is unlikely.
6. Raised transient ST segment after cardioversion, usually associated with previous pericardiotomy, age, and diminished long-term maintenance of sinus rhythm.

Long-term changes

7. Reduction in left atrial size.
8. Improvement in ventricular function and also in some cases cardiac output and exercise or functional capacity due to a combination of a reduction in heart rate and the restoration of atrial systole.

Cardiac output may be decreased after cardioversion in up to one-third of patients and may persist for about a week. Rarely pulmonary edema occurs within 3 hours of cardioversion.

Atrial function declines, even after that occurring spontaneously or pharmacologically. Cardiac output should return to baseline within 4 weeks so that anti-coagulation is recommended for a minimum of 4 weeks after cardioversion.

After 4 weeks, the decision to continue anticoagulation or not depend on the individual risk for recurrence of atrial fibrillation.

Patients who are not responded to cardioversion should be anticoagulated for long-term.

154. Summary of cardioversion in atrial fibrillation.

1. Cardioversion to sinus rhythm should be considered for all suitable patients
2. In the short-term both pharmacological and electrical cardioversion restore sinus rhythm
3. Prophylactic treatment with antiarrhythmic drugs advisable after cardioversion in high-risk patients in view of the high relapse rate
4. Anticoagulants should be started before non-emergency cardioversion—ideally two to three weeks before—and continued for at least for 4 weeks after cardioversion in patients with atrial fibrillation of > 48 hours.

155. There are 4 methods of nondrug treatment

1. Electrical cardioversion
2. Pacemaker for sick sinus syndrome should be considered
3. Ablation of an accessory pathway—for example, the Wolff-Parkinson-White syndrome.
   Ablation of the atrioventricular node and insertion of a permanent pacemaker.
4. Surgery—for example, the "Maze" and "Corridor" procedures.

156. Ablations for specific arrhythmias. Several types of arrhythmias are amenable to ablation therapy including:

1. Wolff-Parkinson-White (WPW) syndrome
2. AV nodal reentrant tachycardia (AVNRT)
3. Certain types of atrial flutter
4. Some cases of ventricular tachycardia.

An electrophysiology (EP) study is performed to discover the characteristics of conduction from atria to ventricles and the presence of accessory pathways. Once the specific location is mapped, then the special catheters are precisely placed, radiofrequency (RF) energy is passed down the catheter to the heart tissue and the tissue is destroyed. The tissue is no longer able to initiate or to conduct any type of electrical impulse. This leads to a "cure" of the condition by transcatheter ablation of the accessory pathway.

157. Therapeutic approach to control of arrhythmias and maintenance of sinus rhythm (Adopted from American College of Cardiology/American Heart Association (ACC/AHA) practice guidelines.

Flow chart D-1

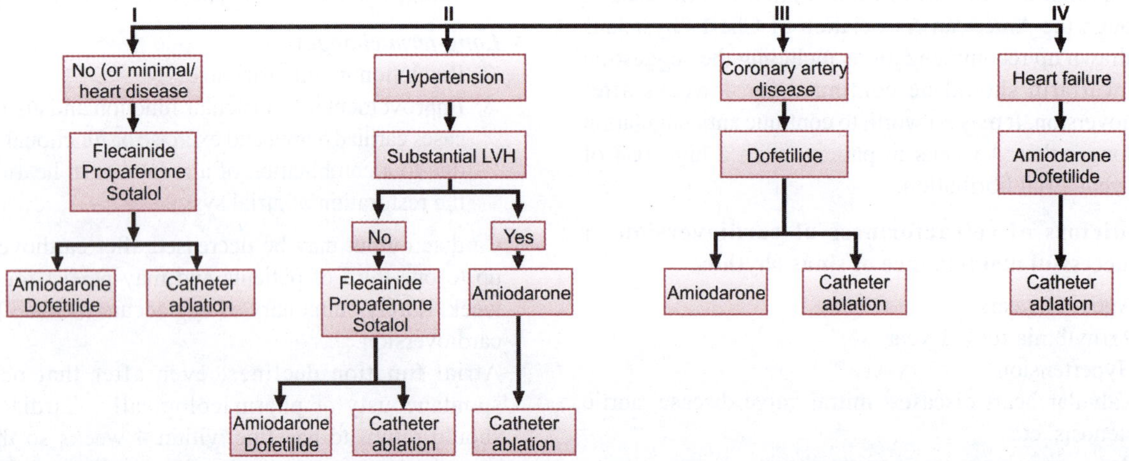

158. Indications of ablation and implantation of pacemaker.

1. In rapid ventricular response in atrial tachycardia
2. In atrial fibrillation with rapid ventricular rate
3. In sick sinus syndrome where paroxysmal atrial fibrillation is a complication
4. In some cases of ventricular tachycardia.

Electrical ablation of the AV node and His bundle with a transvenous catheter and insertion of a permanent pacemaker was first described by Scheinman and colleagues in 1982. This treatment is reserved for patients with rapid ventricular rates that are not well-controlled by medications and present with symptoms related to the uncontrolled heart rate. The procedure destroys the tissue at the AV node and His bundle and stops the conduction of all electrical impulses from the atria to the ventricles (complete heart block). Ablation of the AV node requires the placement of permanent pacemaker at the time of the procedure. The pacemaker then provides a steady and regular heart beat (i.e. ventricular beat). This often diminishes the symptoms associated with atrial fibrillation, even though the atria continue to fibrillate. This procedure does not cure atrial fibrillation nor does it diminish the risk of stroke and therefore, anticoagulation should be continued after the procedure. However, some patients are able to reduce or discontinue medications, such as β-blockers or antiarrhythmics following the AV nodal ablation because the ventricular rate is now controlled by the pacemaker.

Catheter ablation of AF with pulmonary vein isolation (PVI) was described in 1998 by Haissaguerre and colleagues described the presence of isolated foci in the left atrium and pulmonary veins and their role in the initiation of AF. Ablation of this foci could terminate AF. Anatomic ablation technique developed three-dimensional mapping systems to demonstrate the anatomy of left atrium and pulmonary veins.

The detection of the pulmonary veins as the source of ectopic foci that trigger the AF has led to catheter-based ablation strategies to electrically isolate the pulmonary veins by delivering the radiofrequency energy at their ostium. Their procedure is giving better results now.

Atrial defibrillators are investigational devices that are currently being studied at several centers in the USA. [This device utilizes specialized technology to accurately recognize AF and electrically converts the arrhythmia by delivering a small electrical shock via leads placed in the heart. It is too early in the research process to predict the reliability and efficacy of this device. It may yet offer another choice of therapy for selected patients with AF.]

Surgery for atrial fibrillation: Research and continuous mapping techniques have provided greater insight into the mechanism of atrial fibrillation. There are at least six different locations in the left and right atria where relatively large circular waves can occur, creating a pattern of continuous electrical activity, i.e. characteristic of complex atrial fibrillation. This important discovery paved the way for the development of the Maze procedure, a surgical intervention that extinguishes atrial fibrillation by interrupting the circular electrical patterns or wavelets that are responsible for this arrhythmia.

159. Maze procedure:

Both atrial appendages are excised and the pulmonary; veins are isolated. Appropriately placed atrial incisions not only interrupt the conduction routes of the most common reentrant circuits, but they also direct the sinus impulse from the SA node to the AV node along a specified route. The entire atrial myocardium (except for the atrial appendages and pulmonary veins) is electrically activated by providing for multiple blind alleys off the main conduction route between the SA node and the AV

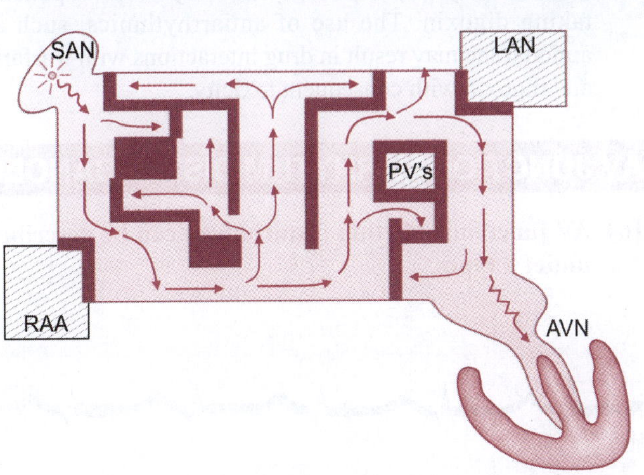

Fig. D-18: Conceptual diagram of the Maze procedure for atrial fibrillation

node, thereby preserving atrial transport function post-operatively.

1. Strategic placement of incisions in both atria stops the formation and the conduction of errant electrical impulses and channels the normal electrical impulses in one direction from the top of the heart to the bottom. Scar tissue generated by the incisions permanently blocks the abnormal paths of the electrical impulses that cause atrial fibrillation, thus eradicating the arrhythmia.

   Advantages of this procedure:

2. Ablates the arrhythmia.
3. Restores synchrony between the atria and the ventricles.
4. Preserves organized atrial contraction.

The name of this procedure is based on the concept of a puzzle. The incisions create barriers and several blind alleys allowing for only one major route for an electrical impulse to travel from the top to the bottom of the heart.

Dr James L Cox, Washington DC, USA, the inventor of the original Maze procedure has developed a new minimally invasive approach for the Maze, using a "key hole" incision on the right side of the chest. If other procedures such as valve replacement or coronary bypass are to be performed concurrently with the Maze procedure, then the standard open chest approach is likely to be used. The first successful human Maze operation was performed on September 25, 1987. The initial steps were modified in 1990 (Maze II) and again in 1992 (Maze III). In its current form, this procedure entails extensive surgical incisions combined with localized ablations with a cryoprobe.

To date over 300 cases have been performed by Dr James L Cox. Several thousand cases have also been done in Japan, as well. The Maze procedure has resulted in 100% cure of atrial fibrillation, with 97% of patients on no medications and only 3% of patients taking medication to maintain normal sinus rhythm.

In India, the first successful classical Maze III procedure (combined with mitral valve surgery) was performed at GB Pant Hospital, New Delhi in 1994. A modified version, where the cryolesions were replaced by radiofrequency (RF current catheter ablation was carried out at the Escorts Heart Institute and Research Centre, New Delhi around the same time.

"Corridor" procedure effectively isolates both the left and right atrium, leaving a strip of myocardium connecting the sinus node of the atrioventricular node. This procedure does not prevent atrial fibrillation but isolates the fibrillating atria. Although a 70% cure rate is reported, sequential atrioventricular contraction is not restored (with the consequent hemodynamic effects), and the risk of thromboembolism remains.

160. Atrial fibrillation in pregnancy: It occurs infrequently in pregnancy, it usually has an underlying identifiable cause such as mitral valve disease, thyroid, or pulmonary disease.

Treatment

1. Ventricular rate can be controlled by digoxin, β-blockers, or a nondihydropyridine calcium channel blockers.

Rhythm control

2. Quinidine is the agent of choice in pregnancy. It has the longest record of any antiarrhythmic drug for pharmacologic conversion of AF. Currently available antiarrhythmic drugs cross the placenta and are excreted in breast milk and should be avoided if possible in pregnant and lactating women but amiodarone, sotalol, and flecainide have all been used successfully during pregnancy in selected cases.
3. In the hemodynamically unstable patient, direct current cardioversion (DCC) can be done without any concern of fetal damage.
4. Anticoagulation should be given high priority. Patients with "lone atrial fibrillation" and low risk for thromboembolic complications should not receive anticoagulants.

Warfarin is generally avoided during first trimester of pregnancy because of its teratogenic factors and also during the last month pregnancy of bleeding concern during delivery.

Injection Heparin SC 100,00–200,00 every 12 hours adjusted to maintain PTT to 1.5 to 2 times control is given. Low molecular weight Heparin may also be considered during first trimester and last month of the pregnancy, there is limited data available to its use.

161. Role of general practitioner/family practitioner in dealing AF.

1. To identify patients with new onset atrial fibrillation
2. To assess thromboembolic risk and to start early treatment with antithrombotic drugs—warfarin will be needed for most patients, while aspirin may be suitable for patients aged < 65 years with no cardiac risk factors or structural heart disease
3. To be aware of potential drug interactions and toxicity with antiarrhythmic drugs and anticoagulants
4. To refer appropriate patients to a cardiologist for further assessment including echocardiography and consideration of cardioversion.

The general population is aging – that is, the proportion of elderly people is increasing. A survey in Britain, showed that at the end of the year 2000 the proportion of people over 70 years age constituted 20–25% of the total population. Atria fibrillation therefore will be an increasingly common cause of stroke, thromboembolism, and heart failure, emphasizing that atrial fibrillation is an important public health problem. Many patients will also be taking antiarrhythmic drugs and anticoagulation. The same situation may be seen in India after some years when the life expectancy is increased. Epidemiological and hospital statistics are not of much informative in developing countries like India. Of course, the priorities may be different in developing and underdeveloped countries.

162. When to refer patients with atrial fibrillation to a cardiologist

1. Age < 30 years
2. Atrial fibrillation resistant to "usual" drugs for rate control
3. Patients suitable for cardioversion
4. Further assessment needed—for example, valvular heart disease
5. Patients with moderate to severe heart failure
6. Patients with resistant heart failure
7. Frequent attacks of paroxysmal atria fibrillation
8. Syncopal attacks due to atrial fibrillation.

163. Whom to screen for atrial fibrillation in general practice?

1. Patients complaining of palpitations or syncope
2. Patients with stroke or transient ischemic attacks
3. Patients with heart failure taking diuretics regularly or digoxin
4. Patients with thyroid disease.

Hypokalemia secondary to the use of high doses of loop diuretics may result in dangerous arrhythmias in patients taking digoxin. The use of antiarrhythmics, such as amiodarone may result in drug interactions with warfarin and digoxin with consequent toxicity.

AV JUNCTIONAL RHYTHM DISTURBANCES

164. AV junctional rhythm disturbances can be described under 4 types.

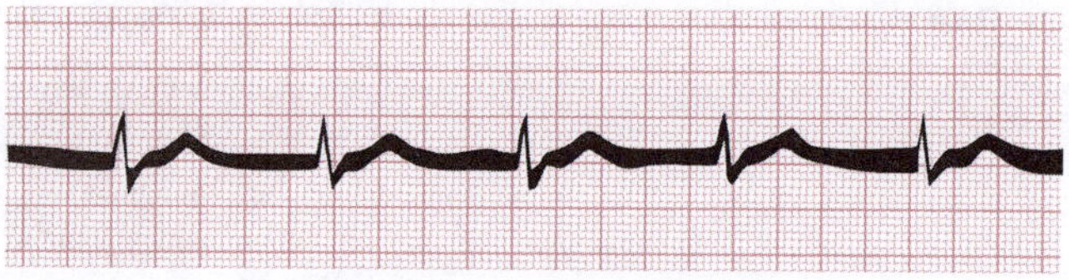

Fig. D-19: AV nodal rhythm

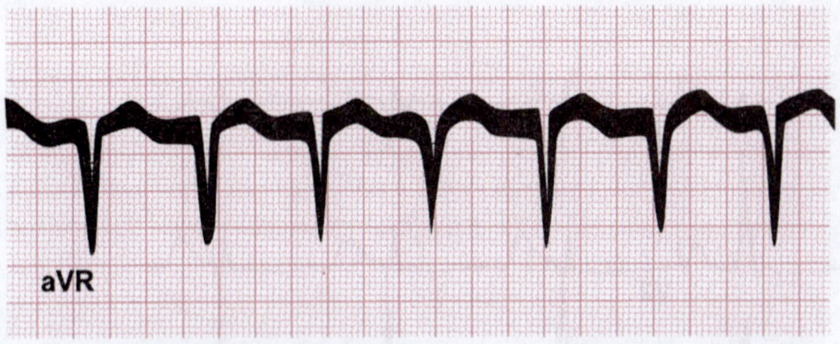

Fig. D-20: Nodal tachycardia; Note: Absence of P waves

1. AV junctional rhythm
2. AV junctional escape beats/premature AV junctional complexes
3. Nonparoxysmal AV junctional tachycardia
4. AV nodal reentry
   a. Reentry over a retrogradely conducting (concealed) accessory pathway
   b. Pre-excitation syndrome.

NONPAROXYSMAL JUNCTIONAL TACHYCARDIA

165. There are 4 common causes of nonparoxysmal junctional tachycardia.

It is due to increased automaticity of AV junctional tissue, i.e. AV node and bundle of His. It may persist for hours or days since its onset and termination are usually gradual. It is called as nonparoxysmal. It is manifested in:

1. Digitalis intoxication
2. Acute ischemia: Common with diaphragmatic infarction
3. Acute myocarditis
4. Chronic obstructive lung disease with respiratory failure.

It may also occur after cardiac surgery, electrolyte imbalance and rarely without any apparent cause.

166. ECG diagnosis of nonparoxysmal junctional tachycardia consists of.

1. *Rate:* 60–140/min—moderate tachycardia.
2. *Rhythm:* Junctional rhythm. Narrow regular QRS complexes, may occur with exit block resulting in irregularity of QRS complexes.
3. P waves absent or show variable morphology.
4. *Ventricular response:* Retrograde conduction is blocked so that there is AV dissociation. Usually the AV dissociation is incomplete so P waves may capture the ventricles in appropriate time causing early QRS during tachycardia. His bundle electrogram reveals that a His bundle potential precedes each QRS with a normal or prolonged AV interval.

167. Treatment of nonparoxysmal junctional tachycardia .

Generally does not require specific therapy. Hemodynamic effects are relatively minor because of relatively moderate ventricular tachycardia. However, loss of atrial contribution to ventricular filling may be deleterious hemodynamically in a compromised patient.

1. Digitalis intoxication: Should be suspected when the ventricular rate becomes regular in a patient with atrial fibrillation—stop the drug.
2. Diaphragmatic infarction—Treat the infarction. This arrhythmia is usually self-limited and subsides in 24 to 48 hours.
3. Correct electrolyte abnormalities.
4. Correct hypoxemia.

OTHER SUPRAVENTRICULAR ARRHYTHMIAS

WOLFF-PARKINSON-WHITE (WPW) SYNDROME.

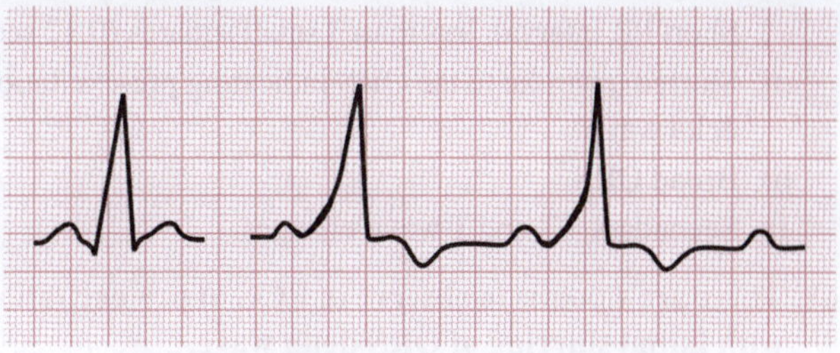

Fig. D-21: Wolff-Parkinson-White syndrome

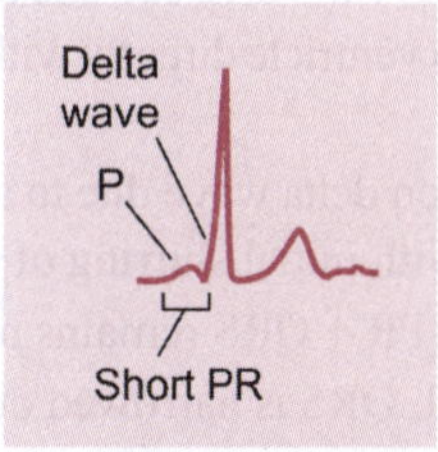

Fig. D-22: Wolff-Parkinson-White syndrome. Short PR interval with initial slurring of QRS delta wave

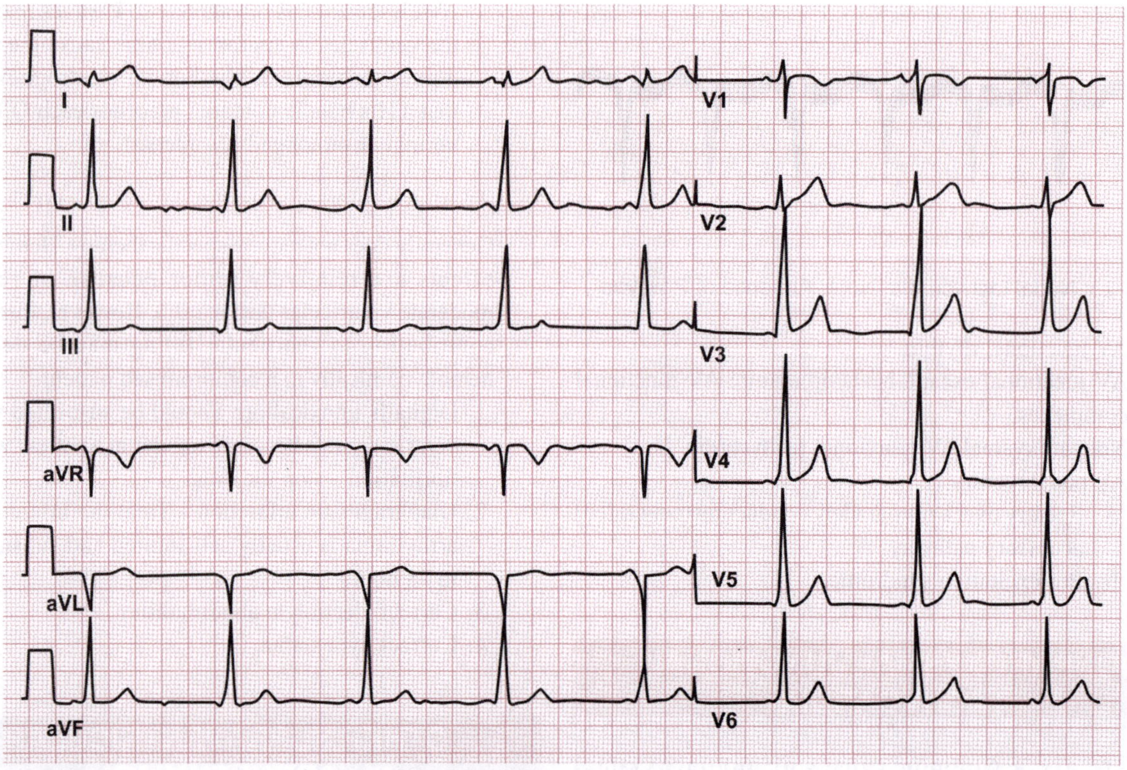

Fig. D-23: WPW syndrome

(See Fig. D-23 WPW syndrome (See Figs Q-57, 58, 59)

i. Short PR interval, less than 3 small squares (0.12 sec)
ii. Slurred upstroke to the QRS indicating pre-excitation delta wave
iii. Broad QRS
iv. Secondary ST and T wave changes.

168. There are 4 points to observe in ECG of pre-excitation with initial slurring of QRS delta wave.

(This is due to impulse conduction through abnormal pathway of Kent).

1. Short PR interval < 0.12 sec due to bypass of impulses from atria to ventricle directly without passing through AV node.
2. Pre-excitation delta wave due to abnormal ventricular activation with initial slurring of QRS.
3. Wide QRS (PR + QRS remains normal). PJ is normal, QRS is narrowed during tachycardia)
4. ST-T change as a result of abnormal repolarization. ST-T opposite of QRS.

This is a congenital disorder due to an accessory or abnormal conducting pathway of Kent between the atria and ventricles. It allows electrical impulses to bypass the AV node and its delaying effect on conduction results in abnormally fast conduction between the atria and ventricles.

PR interval appears to be short because the abnormal delta wave occurs before the R wave, although the interval from the top of P wave to the top of R wave is in fact normal.

The pre-excitation delta wave is due to the abnormally fast spread of the impulse through the ventricle from the accessory pathway and the normal R wave is due to spread of impulse from the normal conducting tissue.

The WPW syndrome is known to be associated with re-entrant form of paroxysmal supraventricular tachycardia and paroxysms of atrial fibrillation.

The fast conduction between the atria and ventricles may cause the ventricular rate to be dangerously fast with atrial fibrillation associated with the WPW syndrome.

Traditional drugs, such as digoxin or verapamil will accelerate the ventricular response by blocking atrioventricular node impulses and increasing conduction through the accessory pathway.

169. WPW syndrome — 4 facts.

1. It is relatively benign.
2. It affects males more and is found in all age groups. In younger people, it occurs mainly in individuals with no sign of heart disease.

3. It is found in patients with idiopathic hypertrophic subaortic stenosis.
4. Seen in 25% of patients with Ebstein's anomaly.

In many of the older patients, it results from serious heart disease and is therefore not always associated with a benign prognosis.

170. In most patients with WPW syndrome, have a tendency to develop atrial arrhythmias. The following 4 atrial arrhythmias are found.

1. Proxysmal atrial tachycardia	10%
2. Atrial fibrillation	16%
3. Atrial flutter	4%
4. Unidentified supraventricular tachycardia	10%

The mechanism appears to be circulating (or reentering) wave using both accessory (or bypass) bundle and the AV junction, going down one and up the other. When the QRS is wide and bizarre, it may mimic ventricular tachycardia.

171. Short PR interval can occur in

1. Wolff-Parkinson-White syndrome (WPW)
2. Lown-Ganong-Levine syndrome (LGG)
3. Low atrial rhythm, nonsinus (coronary) rhythm, nodal rhythm
4. Some hypertensive patients
5. Hypertrophic obstructive cardiomyopathy
6. Normally seen in infants and children
7. Glycogen storage disease (Type II)
8. Duchenne muscular dystrophy.

172. The presence of pre-excitation delta wave of WPW syndrome and ST-T changes can interfere with the diagnosis of

1. Ischemia
2. Ventricular hypertrophy
3. Bundle branch block
4. Infarction

173. Pre-excitation may be associated with

1. Ebstein anomaly
2. Hypertrophic cardiomyopathy
3. Mitral valve prolapse
4. Thyrotoxicosis.

It is familial in few patients.

174. Lown-Ganong-Levine syndrome has the following 4 features.

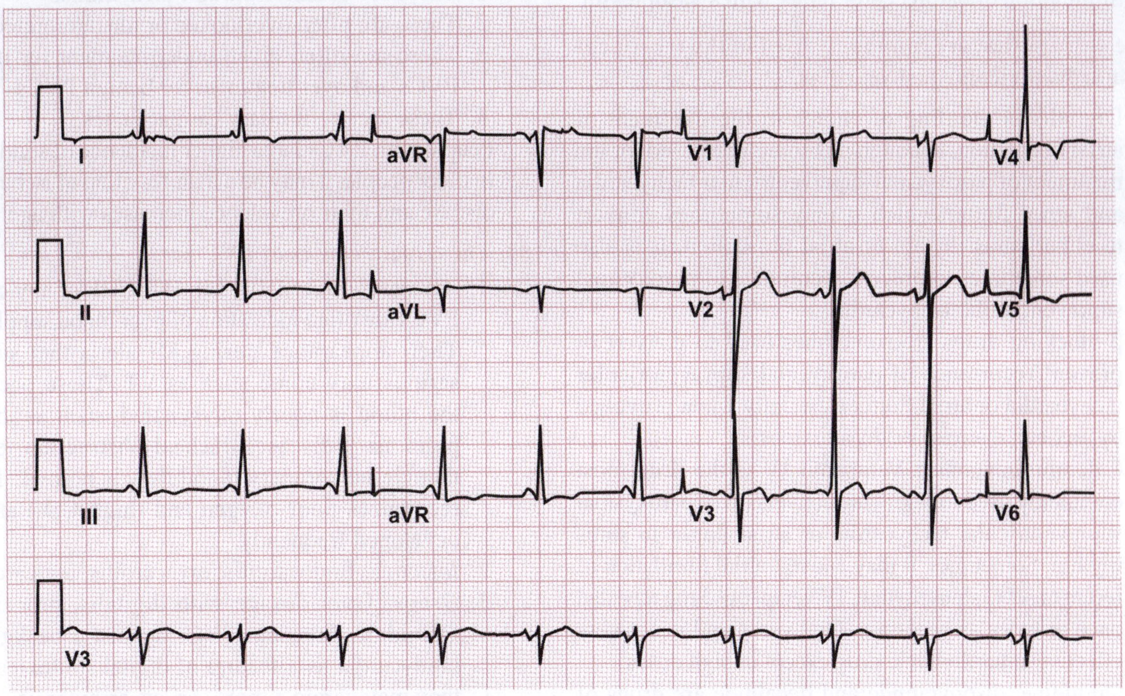

Fig. D-24: Lown-Ganong-Levine syndrome: short PR interval, less than 3 small squares (< 0.12 sec), no delta wave. In this ECG there is also nonspecific inferolateral ST-T changes and voltage criteria for left ventricular hypertrophy

1. Short PR interval (0.12 sec)
2. Narrow QRS complex
3. Reentrant tachycardia
4. Propensity to AV nodal reentry.

175. There are 4 supraventricular arrhythmias where carotid sinus massage can be used as both diagnostic and therapeutic measure.

1. Sinus tachycardia
   The rate comes down by 8–12 beats/min.
2. Paroxysmal atrial tachycardia
   "All or None" Phenomenon
   No response at all or comes to normal.
3. Atrial flutter: The ventricular rate may slow temporarily. The rate is decreased by arithmetical proportion from 2:1 to 3:1 block then to 4:1 block.
4. Atrial fibrillation
   No response to carotid massage.

176. There are 4 types of maneuvers to produce potent vagotonic effect.

1. Carotid sinus massage
2. Ocular pressure (not recommended because it involves the risk of retinal detachment)
3. Valsalva maneuver—forceful expiration against a closed glottis. Performing this in the supine position, up to 20% of PSVT may be converted to sinus rhythm
4. Stimulation of baroreceptor reflex with a vasopressor.

177. The 4 drugs that are commonly used in the treatment of supraventricular tachycardias.

1. Digitalis is the drug of choice in the treatment of atrial fibrillation, although it is sometimes used for the treatment of paroxysmal supraventricular tachycardia and atrial flutter which it may sometimes convert to either sinus rhythm or atrial fibrillation. It is also used sometimes to prevent recurrence of paroxysmal supraventricular tachycardia.
2. β-blocking drugs are sometimes used to convert or prevent recurrence of paroxysmal supraventricular tachycardia or atrial flutter especially when provoked by anxiety, exercise or thyrotoxicosis.
3. Calcium antagonist: Verapamil IV is the drug most commonly used for the acute conversion of paroxysmal supraventricular tachycardia or atrial flutter to sinus rhythm. Sometimes, it may convert atrial fibrillation of recent onset to sinus rhythm. IV verapamil 5 mg repeated once or twice as necessary. Oral verapamil is not very effective antiarrhythmic drug except in high doses.
4. Quinidine, disopyramide and flecainide are drugs of choice for the prevention of recurrent or intermittent supraventricular tachyarrhythmias, such as recurrent atrial fibrillation. They are also used in the treatment of ventricular tachyarrhythmias. Amiodarone is a class III antiarrhythmic drug and is used to treat recurrent arrhythmias not controlled by other drugs.

VENTRICULAR ARRHYTHMIAS

178. Ventricular rhythm disturbances can be described into 4 types.

1. Premature ventricular contractions (PVCs)
2. Ventricular tachycardia
3. Ventricular flutter and fibrillation
4. Miscellaneous
   i. Arrhythmogenic right ventricular dysplasia
   ii. Accelerated idioventricular rhythm
   iii. Torsades de pointes
   iv. Long QT syndrome.

PREMATURE VENTRICULAR CONTRACTIONS

179. Premature ventricular contractions (PVCs)—Synonyms are:

Ventricular premature contractions or
Ventricular premature beats (VPBs) or
Premature ventricular beats (PVBs).

They are to be recognized readily and correctly because:

1. These are common cardiac arrhythmias
2. These are often overlooked or misinterpreted
3. These are often given undertreatment for malignant PVCs and over treatment for benign PVCs
4. These are prefibrillary cardiac states.

People with PVCs have higher incidence of sudden death. In older people, it may be a manifestation of ischemic heart disease and their prevalence increases with age.

180. The 4 main causes of PVC are:

1. *Atherosclerotic:* IHD, MI, HT, CHF of any cause. PVCs are often indication of poor blood supply (CAD) Their appearance during MI alerts that something serious may come such as VT. These occur when the blood is poorly oxygenated, such as drowning, pulmonary disease, tracheal obstruction, etc. even though the coronary blood flow is normal. The heart recognizes poor oxygen and (high CO_2) and PVCs developed frequently.
2. *Infective:* Endocarditis, myocarditis, pericarditis.
3. *Drugs:* Over dosage with digitalis, procainamide, Quinidine. Frequent PVCs against a background of bradycardia as a feature of digitalis intoxication and they may herald a more serious arrhythmia.
4. *Electrolyte disturbance:* Hypercalcemia, hypo- or hyperkalemia. Hypokalemia may cause PVCs on its own and will potentiate other causes.

There are several other cardiac causes like secondary or primary myocardial or pericardial malignancy, cardiomyopathy, valvular disease, nutritional heart disease, glycogen storage disease, chronic or acute cor pulmonale, cardiac trauma, etc. PVCs are sometimes a feature of mitral valve prolapse and occasionally they may occur as escape beats in the presence of an underlying bradycardia.

In Cardiac Arrythmias, MRI Heart is advised in some

If it shows mediastinal lymphadenitis with inflammatory myocarditis - advise - PET CT Scan chest after giving FDG (Fluoro Deoxy Glucose) IV.

If the FDG uptake is increased by the lymph nodes, advise biopsy.

We should think of

1. Tuberculosis
2. Sarcoidosis
3. Atypical mycobacteria
4. Opportunistic mycobacteria which is resistant to routine ATT.

There are several other noncardiac causes like hypoxia, encephalopathy, encaphalitis, meningitis, pancreatitis, peritonitis, uremia, abdominal surgery, fever, pregnancy nervous tension, fatigue, excessive smoking or caffeine. Many patients come with recurrent PVCs without any known cause.

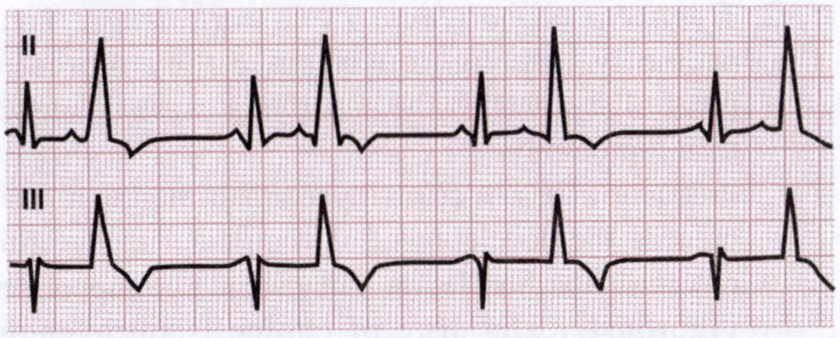

Fig. D-25: Premature ventricular beats; QRS > 0.12 sec, bizarre contour, compensatory pause: T is opposite of QRS

181. There are 4 characteristic features of PVCs.

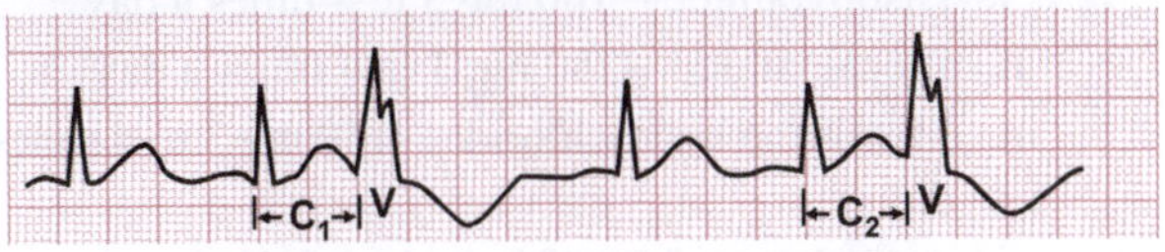

Fig. D-26: Unifocal PVCs fixed coupling

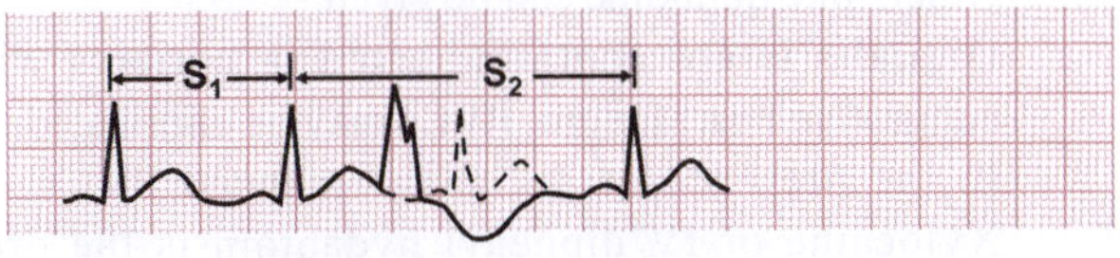

Fig. D-27: Compensatory pause

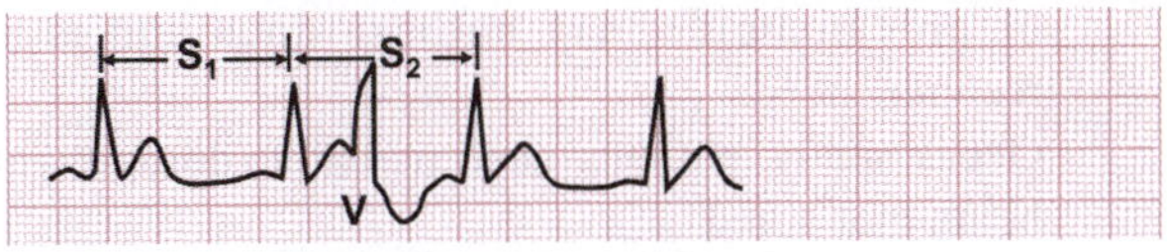

Fig. D-28: Interpolated PVC

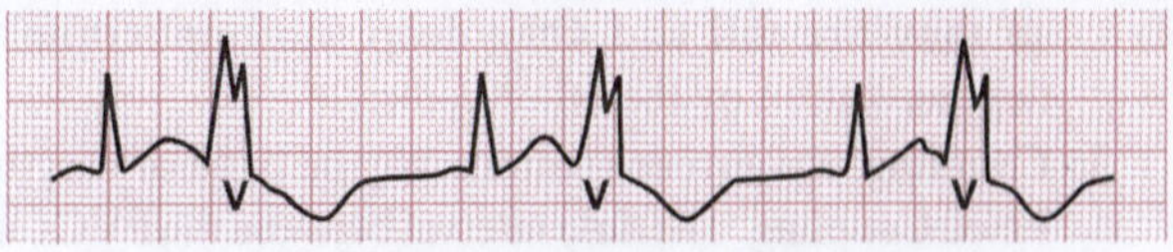

Fig. D-29: Bigeminy unifocal

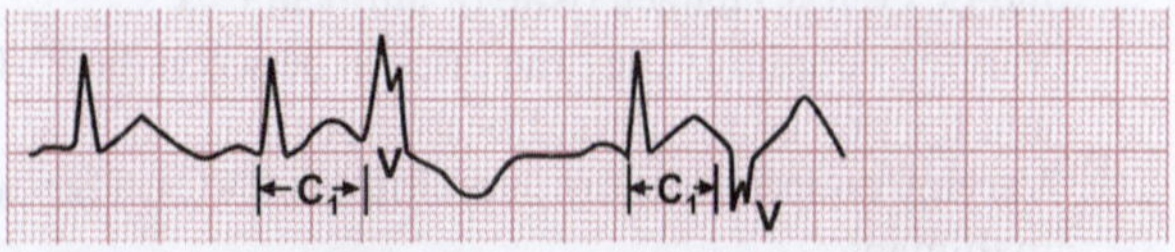

Fig. D-30: Multifocal PVCs fixed coupling

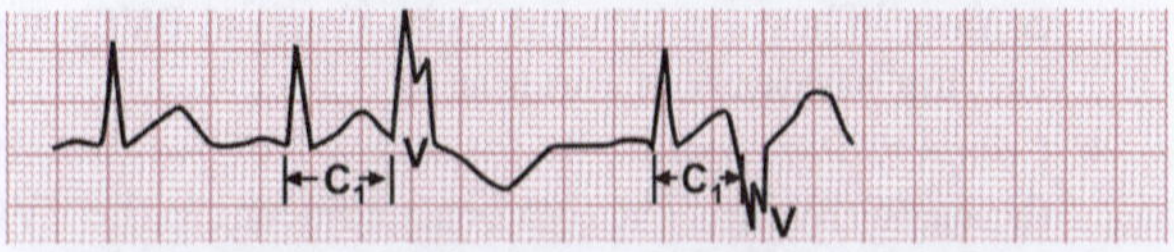

Fig. D-31: Multifocal PVCs varying coupling

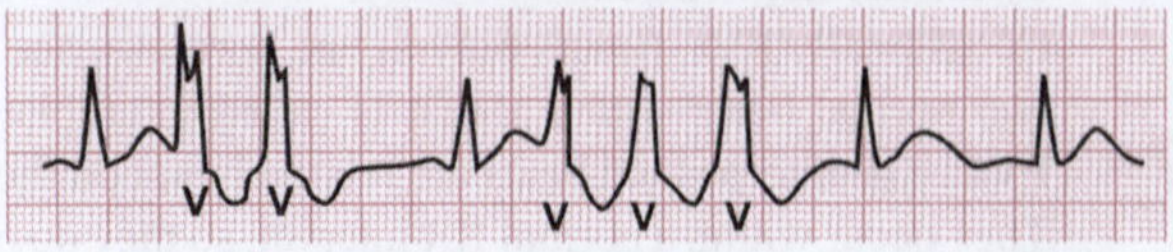

Fig. D-32: PVCs in pairs or runs

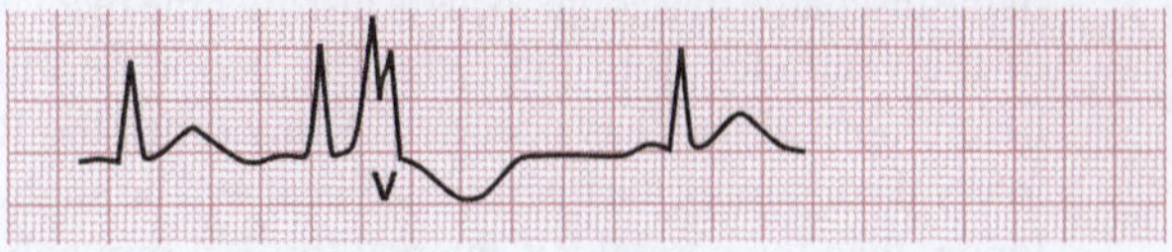

Fig. D-33: PVC on preceding T wave

1. *Prematurity:* They are premature to the normally conducted beats. They are not preceded by premature 'P'wave.
2. *Contour:* Bizarre contour; T wave points toward the opposite of QRS. QRS is more than 0.12 sec usually high voltage.

   Note, whether they arise from a single or multiple ventricular focus.

   Unifocal PVCs look identical in a given lead.

   Multifocal PVCs generally vary in contour.

   The PVCs do not follow the normal bundle branch conduction system. Therefore conduction is slow. That is why the QRS is very wide. The nervous conduction system transmits impulses rapidly at a rate of 2–4 meters per second. Whereas myocardium transmits impulses at a rate of only one meter per second. So QRS is narrow when conducted by the nerve impulses, whereas QRS is wide when conducted by the myocardium.

   Why high voltage?: Normally RV and LV depolarize simultaneously as a result, depolarization of LV going toward the left is somewhat opposed by RV and so relatively small (normal QRS results). But the PVC originate in one ventricle without any opposition so they are tall and very deep (no opposition of depolarization by the other ventricle.

3. *Coupling:* Recurrence pattern may be fixed or varying.
   Fixed Coupling: The time interval between the PVCs and the preceding normal beat remains constant throughout the ECG. It is characteristic of unifocal PVCs.
   Varying coupling: The time interval between the PVCs and the preceding normal beat varies.
   Varying coupling occurs in multifocal PVCs. They are malignant.
   Occasionally fixed coupling occurs with varying contour. They are thought to be unifocal PVCs with varying pathways of conduction.
4. *Compensatory pause:* It follows a PVC to preserve the basic rhythm. The two beats adjacent to the PVCs encloses a space equivalent to the usual time taken up by the normal two beats.
   Occasionally PVC occurs only in one normal space of two normal beats—such a beat is called interpolated PVC. The interpolated beats are relatively uncommon. They occur within a normal RR interval, so they do not have compensatory pause. They occur when the timing of the discharge of ectopic focus is just after the recovery of the ventricles from the refractory period and just before normal beat has occurred. Many times the RR interval containing the interpolated beat will be slightly longer than the normal RR interval (by 3–4 mm only).
   Absence of a compensatory pause is not a strong point to differentiate between a PVC and supraventricular beat conducted aberrantly.
   As showing in Figure D-27, ventricular bigeminy is common with (anticongestive therapy) digitalis which is one of the very common causes of ventricular bigeminy.

182. There are 4 points to differentiate between malignant and benign PVCs.

Table D-7

Malignant	Benign
1. Multifocal origin	Always unifocal
2. Unifocal or multifocal occur either in pairs or in runs. More than 6 per minute	Never occur in successive pairs or runs. They may occur frequently even to the point of bigeminy, PVC every alternate beat. (Trigeminy—every third beat is PVC. Quadrigeminy—every 4th beat is PVC)
3. PVCs of varying coupling	PVCs with fixed coupling
4. PVCs that occur early in the cardiac cycle to be superimposed on a preceding T wave. R on T phenomenon result in ventricular fibrillation	Never occur so early in the cardiac cycle to be superimposed on a preceding T wave. Never result in ventricular fibrillation

Any one or in combination of these malignant PVCs can result in ventricular fibrillation—consider them as cardiac emergency.

Benign PVCs never result in ventricular fibrillation.

183. PVCs can be investigated by

1. ECG
   i. at rest
   ii. Exercise ECG
   iii. 24 hours Holter's monitoring
2. Echocardiography
3. Radionucleide studies
4. Late potential studies.

184. Treatment of PVCs consists of:

1. *Treatment of underlying cause:* The best way to control them is to eliminate the underlying cause. Correction of congestive heart failure, infections, drug toxicity, electrolyte disturbances can eliminate all PVCs without further treatment. Thrombolysis during acute myocardial infarction decreases the incidence of ventricular arrhythmias.
   Simple control of fatigue, nervous tension, excessive smoking, excessive coffee or tea, are important in benign PVCs.
2. *Treatment of malignant PVCs with drugs:* Treat promptly and vigorously since they represent prefibrillary state. If the underlying cause is known, treat it promptly.
   Frequent PVCs in acute myocardial infarction often precede the development of ventricular tachycardia or ventricular fibrillation. They should be suppressed vigorously. The drug of choice is intravenous xylocaine. This can be followed by oral antiarrhythmic drugs.
   Any of the following antiarrhythmic drugs can be used.
   i. Disopyramide—100 mg 3 to 4 times a day.
   ii. Procainamide—250 mg 3 to 4 times a day
   iii. Mexilitine hydrochloride—150 mg 3 to 4 times a day
   iv. Amiodarone 200–400 mg 3 or 4 times a day
   Others like quinidine can be given.
   Digitalis is not contraindicated in patients with congestive heart failure, PVCs may be eliminated.
   In the presence of digitalis—induced PVCs IV. Xylocaine or IV diphenyl hydantoin is the drug of choice. Attempting suppression with quinidine or procainamide may be hazardous and is not recommended.
   Occasionally, patients need parentral dosage while being monitored.

3. *Counter shock treatment:* Occasionally, counter shock is necessary to treat runs of malignant PVCs or ventricular tachycardia or fibrillation. This is more commonly seen in acute myocardial infarction.
4. *Benign PVCs need no treatment:* Treatment is needed if the patient is severely nervous over 'Palpitation'.

When they are symptomatic, i.e. the beat following after compensatory pause will be more forceful and produces 'Palpitation'. The decision to suppress them is easily made even if there is no underlying pathology. If PVCs are asymptomatic, the decision is more difficult, and when they do not represent any underlying cause. Each case must be considered on its particulars.

See, whether PVCs increase or decrease with exercise. If they increase, it is likely to consider suppression with antiarrhythmic drugs.

Procainamide, disopyramide, mexilitine hydrochloride are useful. Quinidine and propranolol are less effective. Oral diphenyl hydantoin is not particularly useful.

185. Management of PVCs consists of:

The presence of PVCs in the absence of heart disease has no impact on longevity or limitation of activity. Therefore no drug treatment is necessary in asymptomatic isolated PVCs. Reassure the patient.

PVCs after myocardial infarction should not be routinely treated with antiarrhythmic drugs. They should be treated only:

i. When they are symptomatic and/or
ii. When there is risk of sudden death.

In symptomatic PVCs, irrespective of presence or absence of structural heart disease, the line of management should be as

1. Reassure the patient
   ↓ if no response
2. β-blockers—β-blockers decrease post infarct sudden death.
   ↓ if no response
3. Antiarrhythmic drugs—Amiodarone 200 to 300 mg/day. Risk of antiarrhythmic therapy may outweigh the benefit.
   ↓ if no response
4. Other methods like surgery or ablation therapy — Thrombolytic therapy during AMI decreases the incidence of ventricular arrhythmias.

VENTRICULAR TACHYARRHYTHMIAS

186. Ventricular tachyarrhythmias consists of idioventricular rhythm, ventricular tachycardia, ventricular flutter and fibrillation. The 4 common causes are:

1. Myocardial infarction
2. Severe ischemic heart disease
3. Digitalis toxicity especially in the presence of hypocalcemia
4. Cardiomyopathy.

The ventricular tachyarrhythmias occur most commonly after acute myocardial infarction. They are the commonest cause of sudden death, often occurring in the presence of severe ischemic heart disease without infarction. Ventricular tachycardia may precipitate cardiac failure and is frequently a harbinger of ventricular fibrillation immediately after acute myocardial infarction within hours or days. For these reasons, it requires immediate treatment.

187. Markers for dangerous postinfarct arrhythmic events are:

1. Anterior infarct
2. Reduced left ventricular function
3. Left ventricular aneurysm
4. More than 6 PVBs
5. Malignant PVBs, nonsustained ventricular tachycardia, and ventricular tachycardia on programmed ventricular stimulation
6. Presence of late potentials
7. New conduction defects
8. Residual myocardial ischemia.

188. Increased automaticity and reentrance are the main mechanisms in the causation of ventricular tachyarrhythmias.

Automaticity can be increased by the following 4 conditions.

1. Ischemia causing hypoxia of the cardiac tissue
2. Electrolyte imbalance
3. Abnormal catecholamine release
4. Stretch (Hypertrophy or dilatation).

189. Severity of the ventricular arrhythmias is strongly related to the severity of heart disease as observed in

1. High rate of ventricular ectopic activity in acute MI
2. Arrhythmias in obstruction of two major coronary arteries
3. Arrhythmias associated with high mortality rate in congestive cardiac failure
4. Arrhythmias in cardiomyopathies.

190. There are 4 electrolytes which may be responsible in the pathogenesis of cardiac arrhythmias and sudden death.

(More sudden deaths are reported in the people drinking soft water containing low calcium and magnesium)

1. Sodium
2. Potassium
3. Calcium
4. Magnesium.

Low potassium or magnesium diet or lower ratio of potassium to sodium increases cardiac arrhythmia.
It is important to estimate calcium and magnesium also along with sodium and potassium.

191. Ventricular arrhythmias due to hypokalemia occurs in (due to electrical irritability) the following 4 conditions.

1. Drugs—Digitalis—Hypokalemia during digitalis therapy causing ventricular tachyarrhythmias is mainly due to digitalis toxicity.
   Diuretics—Potassium loosing diuretics
   β-blockers.
2. In acute myocardial infarction—VF occurs in potassium depletion
3. Heart failure
4. Renal failure—Potassium balance is regulated mainly by kidneys.

Hypokalemia is commonly encounter metabolic consequences of chronic thiazide therapy for hypertension. The occurrence of PVBs has been associated with hypokalemia. In a patient of hypertension who is taking a diuretic, if arrhythmias are noted, one may be able to make arrhythmias disappear just by adding a potassium sparing diuretic like spirolactone, triamterene, or amiloride to the antihypertensive regime.
Kidney sometimes does not respond quickly to deal with sudden increase in potassium loads, e.g. potassium moves into skeletal muscles during exercise, which is facilitated by adrenergic mechanism. Rapid flow of potassium from plasma into tissues occurs during high adrenergic activity causing hypokalemia.

VENTRICULAR TACHYCARDIA

192. The approach to the diagnosis and treatment of ventricular tachycardia has been changed over the past decade by new tools for its treatment. They include:

1. Development of second and thrid generation anti-arrhythmic agents
2. Antitachycardia pacemakers
3. Implantable defibrillators
4. Several new surgical techniques.

The term VT is used when three or more ventricular ectopic beats occur consecutively at a rate of more than 100–120/min. VT develops almost always in a diseased heart, although rarely it may be observed in apparently normal hearts.

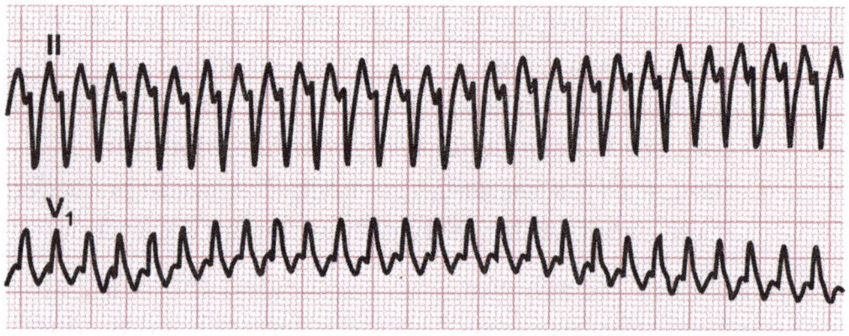

Fig. D-34: Ventricular tachycardia at the rate of 200 bpm

Wide QRS complexes: QRS complexes slightly irregular and vary slightly in shape.

193. Ventricular tachycardia has the following 4 ECG features.

1. Wide and bizarre QRS complexes occurring almost at a rate of 150 to 250 beats per minute.
   RR intervals are usually regular though slight irregularity may be observed. Gross irregularity is extremely rare.
   Rate is usually between 150–200 bpm. Rate more than 200 is uncommon. Occasionally, the rate may be slower (70–130 bpm).
2. Presence of AV dissociation :
   Independent 'P' waves may be seen in 20% of cases of VT resulting in AV dissociation.
   Occasionally VT may result in retrograde conduction of impulse and therefore retrograde 'P' waves.
3. Ventricular fusion beats are helpful in diagnosis but these are seen only with slow rates. These are due to partial depolarization of the ventricules by an opportunist sinus impulse. Such beats are always on time or slightly premature, but never late.
4. Sinus capture beats.

194. VT can be classified into 4 types based upon the morphology of QRS complexes.

1. *Monophasic VT:* Defines as VT with the same QRS morphology in a given lead. It may have a LBBB or RBBB pattern.
2. *Bidirectional VT:* Terms used when the QRS complexes alternate in polarity. They are often associated with digitalis toxicity.
3. *Alternating VT:* When QRS complexes alternate in height but have the same polarity.
4. *Polymorphous/multi form VT:* When QRS complex during VT, changes its morphology, it is termed as polymorphous VT.

Torsades de pointes is a type of polymorphous VT where the QRS keeps on changing its axis around an imaginary line.

It is associated with prolonged QT (0.6 sec).

VT is described as sustained or nonsustained VT based on its duration.

Sustained VT lasts for 30 sec or more requires termination by pacing or electrical cardioversion. Nonsustained VT lasting 6 beats, but terminating spontaneously within 3 sec.

195. Ventricular tachycardia (VT) should be differentiated from supraventricular tachycardia (SVT) with aberrant conduction.

Table D-8

VT	SVT
1. RR intervals regular, broad QRS (more than 0.14 even up to 0.2 sec) Border the QRS, it is more likely of VT	RR interval is 'Caliper hairline' regular in PAT
2. AV dissociation exists Atria and ventricles contract at different rates P wave when seen they are at different rates to the QRS	RR intervals irregularly irregular first diagnosis atrial fibrillation even QRS is wide—SVT with aberrant pathway QRS may be wide P wave is seen
3. No fusion beats are capture beats	Capture beat or fusion beats
4. An axis deviation of more than 30°	
5. A Concordant pattern of the QRS complexes in the precordial leads in which QRS complexes or entirely inverted from V1 to V6	
6. The identical QRS complex morphology in the same leads as seen in previously documented PVBs	
7. Intensity of S1 changes due to varying ventricular volumes from the dissociated atrial contractions. Cannon waves may be seen in JVP as at times the right atrium contracts against closed tricuspid valve	
8. No change in rhythm with carotid sinus massage	Change in rhythm with carotid sinus massage is seen 'All or none' phenomenon in PAT

196. Ventricular tachycardia should be differentiated from supraventricular tachycardia with left bundle branch block. It is sometimes difficult to differentiate because both of them cause wide QRS complexes. It is very important to differentiate them because intravenous verapamil which is usually given in supraventricular tachycardia is dangerous in ventricular tachycardia often causing cardiac arrest or hypotension. Whether the patient appears well or ill, it cannot be used to differentiate between the two. However, the followings signs are useful to differentiate them.

1. Atria and ventricles contract at different rates in ventricular tachycardia.
2. Intensity of the first sound varies because of atrio ventricular valves close intermittently against atrial contraction.
3. Cannon waves may be seen intermittently in jugular venous pulse as at times the right atrium contracts against closed tricuspid valve.
4. More wide the QRS > 0.14 sec, more in favor of ventricular tachycardia.

197. Broad complex tachycardia: The commonest cause of broad complex tachycardia is ventricular tachycardia (VT) wide complex should be differentiated from supraventricular tachycardia (SVT) with an aberrant conduction.

Findings in favor of SVT with aberrant conduction include:

1. The presence of P—waves associated with QRS complex.
2. QRS < 0.14 sec (more wide the QRS more in favor of VT).
3. Fusion beats or capture beats may be present.
4. Same QRS morphology as in sinus rhythm.
5. Normal axis.
6. Classical LBB or QRS morphology.
7. Response to adenosine in SVT.
8. History of MI or IHD increases the likelihood of ventricular arrhythmia over SVT with aberrant conductions.

If all complexes have similar polarities in the epicardial leads 'concordance' suspect VT.

198. Ventricular tachycardia in patients with structurally normal heart can occur as repetitive monomorphic VT or paroxysmal VT. Its clinical features are:

1. It occurs in young patients with frequent runs of sustained or nonsustained VT.
2. VT with only short interval periods of sinus rhythm.
3. Warm up phenomenon is present.
4. They respond to β-blockers or calcium channel blockers.

Paroxysmal VT usually occurs sporadically and patients are symptomatic. They respond to calcium channel blockers.

199. Ventricular arrhythmias—which ones to treat?

Ventricular premature beats occur in about half of the general population about the age of 50 years and even more frequently among people with underlying structural heart disease. The perception of significance of ventricular arrhythmias and their symptoms by both physicians and the public ranges from total ignorance to fear of sudden death. PVBs and short runs of ventricular tachycardia (VT) can be identified and quantified. Yet their significance mainly which should be treated and who is still under investigation. Consequently differentiating ventricular arrhythmic of serious consequence from one the lesser significance is a major clinical problem.

The following 4 guidelines are followed while selecting the patients of VT for drug treatment.

1. Nonsustained ventricular tachycardia (NSVT):
   Mostly it occurs in patients with structural heart disease. In structurally normal hearts, it occurs as paroxysmal monomorphic VT (LBBB with RAD).
   If no symptoms—No drugs, only reassure the patient.
   If symptoms are present—Give β-blockers.
2. NSVT with left ventricular dysfunction - due to non-coronary heart disease like hypertrophic obstructive cardiomyopathy (HOCM) and dilated cardiomyopathy (DCM), asymptomatic patients need no treatment.
3. NSVT with coronary artery disease (CAD) and ejection fraction (EF) more than 40% do not die suddenly and so do not require treatment. NSVT with CAD and EF less than 40% are at increased risk of sudden death. They should be subjected to programmed stimulation test. If sustained VT cannot be provoked, do not treat. If sustained VT is provoked, then treat. NSVT with symptoms such as syncope, dizziness should also be treated.
4. Sustained ventricular tachycardia :
   70% due to CAD
   10–15% due to HOCM/DCM.

Other causes are mitral valve prolapse (MVP), myocarditis, right ventricular dysplasia, prolonged QT and antiarrhythmic drugs. Rarely sustained VT can occur in structurally normal hearts.

200. There are 4 general measures in the treatment of ventricular tachycardia (VT) (usually occurs in myocardial infarction)

1. Rest and reassurance
2. Relief of pain
3. Oxygen
4. Correction of acid-base balance.

201. There are 4 steps of drug treatment of sustained ventricular tachycardia when the patient is in good condition without hypotension or angina, or congestive heart failure.

1. Give xylocaine 75–100 mg IV bolus dose slowly over 2–5 minutes followed by IV xylocaine drip 4 mg per minute reducing the dose to 2 mg per minute after 36 to 48 hours (IV 2–3 mg/kg).
   If no response to xylocaine
2. Try inj procainamide IV bolus 15 mg/kg, rate 25–50 mg/min IV to maximum of 1 g. If BP falls, reduce the rate to 25 mg/min.
   If no response to procainamide
3. Try disopyramide 2 mg/kg to a maximum of 150 mg IV slowly. Maintain 400 mg/kg/h IV drip (to a maximum of 800 mg/day) or inj amiodarone IV 5–6 mg/kg.
   If no response to disopyramide
4. DC shock.

202. There are 4 steps in the acute drug treatment of sustained ventricular tachycardia when the patient is in poor condition with hypotension, or angina or congestive heart failure. When the above usual drugs are ineffective,

1. Inj proctolol 5–15 mg IV slowly over 2 minutes
   If no response
2. Inj mexilitene: 100–250 mg IV slowly for 5–10 minutes followed by 0.1% solution IV drip, 250 mg in the first hour, 125 mg/for 2 hours followed by 500 mg/min.
   If still no response
3. Try synchronized cardioversion
   If there is response to cardioversion, it should be followed by disopyramide 300 mg po loading dose followed by 100–150 mg 6 h po or procainamide 250–500 mg po 6th hourly.
   Repeat the cardioversion if necessary
   If the cardioversion is also not effective
4. Consider overpacing with temporary wire.

203. Following 4 steps are observed for long-term treatment for prevention of sustained ventricular tachycardia.

1. Drugs	i. Empirical ii. EPS guided
2. Electrical	i. Antitachycardia pacemakers ii. Antitachycardia pacemakers with internal cardiac defibrillators
3. Ablative	i. Catheter ablation ii. Radiofrequency ablation
4. Surgery	

204. There are 4 electrophysiological studies (EPS) which may be conducted before considering surgical treatment in patient with resistant and recurrent sustained ventricular tachycardias.

1. Induction of VT in the laboratory and in operating room.
2. Endocardial mapping using electrode catheters to delineate the site of origin of VT in the laboratory.

3. Epicardial mapping by probe electrodes in the operating room.
4. Endocardial mapping in the operating room through a ventriculotomy.

205. Any of the following 4 surgical procedures is indicated in drug resistant and recurrent sustained ventricular tachycardias (VT) most of whom have coronary atherosclerotic disease or with previous myocardial infarction.

1. Simple aneurysmectomy.
2. Aneurysmectomy with resection of residual endocardial scar. It is the operation of choice because many tachycardias are due to ectopic activity of the endocardium surrounding the ventricular aneurysm.
3. Encircling ventriculotomy to isolate the origin of VT from the remainder of the heart.
4. Surgical ablation of areas of slow conduction in right ventricular epicardium in recurrent VT in arrhythmogenic right ventricular dysplasia.

The very high mortality associated with the development of sustained VT during the first few months after acute myocardial infarction has been significantly decreased by aggressive use of early electrophysiologically guided surgery with an operative mortality of 8–12%.

206. FLOW CHART

Electrophysiology Testing for Cardiac Arrhythmias.
Patients presenting with sustained VT or cardiac arrest.

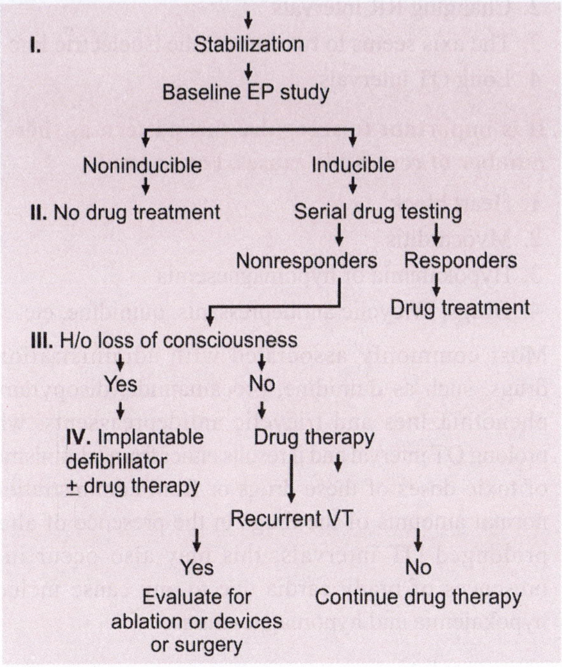

This is a guideline for treatment strategy for patients with life-threatening tachyarrhythmias.

VENTRICULAR FLUTTER AND FIBRILLATION (VF)

Ventricular fibrillation is probably due to multiple circular currents within the ventricle. There is no coordinated contraction of the muscle fibers of the ventricles. They are shimmering bags of individually contracting muscle fibers. As a consequence the VF is associated with lack of any coordinated pumping action of the heart. It leads to death immediately unless it is corrected quickly. On the ECG it shows an irregular uncoordinated wavy lines without any proper complexes.

207. 1/4th (25%) of persons die of ventricular fibrillation in acute myocardial infarction (AMI). So it is very important to know about ventricular fibrillation.

208. There are 4 basic causes of ventricular fibrillation.

(There is possibility of circus movement in the ventricles—ischemia, electrolyte imbalance, catecholamines, dilatation)

1. VF is more when the ventricles are dilated
2. When there is block in the Purkinje system
3. Ectopic foci initiating VF
4. Electric current—particularly with 60 cycle electric current causing electrical shock.

(See myocardial infarction for VF details)

209. The 4 ECG features of ventricular flutter.

1. Regularly occurring wide QRS complexes at a rate usually between 180–250 bpm.
2. Distinction between QRS complexes and T waves is not possible.
3. No P waves.
4. The amplitude of undulation may be large or smaller depending on the myocardial status. The amplitude is generally large when flutter occurs in apparently healthy individuals, while it is small in a severely damaged heart.

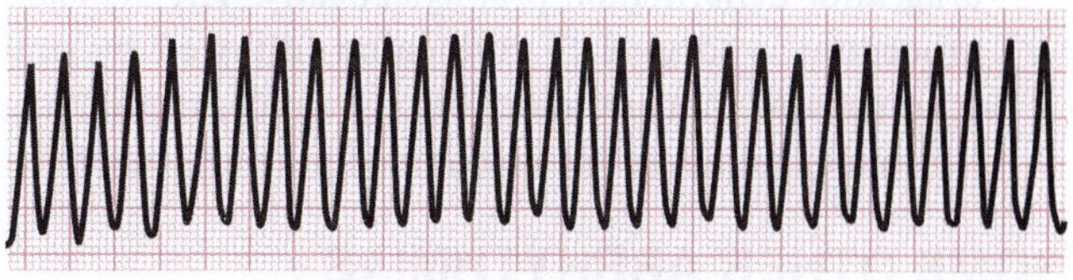

Fig. D-35: Ventricular flutter

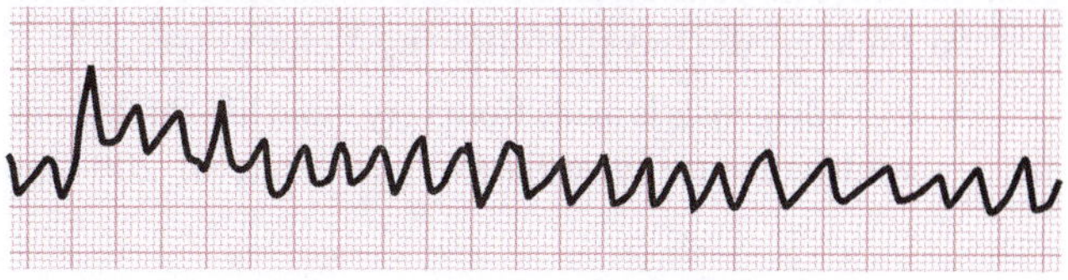

Fig. D-36: Coarse ventricular fibrillation

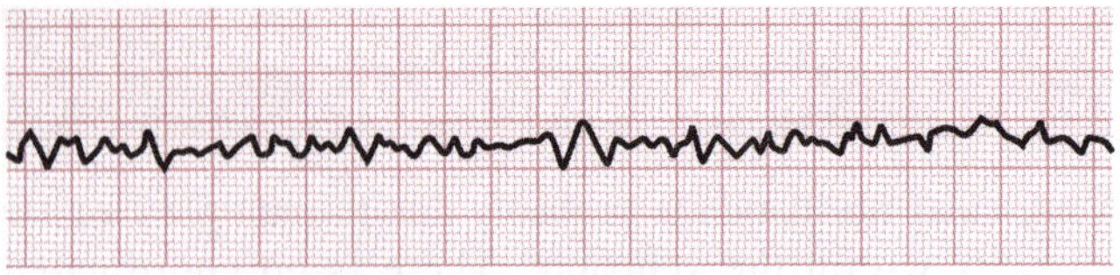

Fig. D-37: Fine ventricular fibrillation

210. ECG changes in ventricular fibrillation.

1. Characteristic irregularly irregular rhythm of varying configurations.
2. QRS, ST, T waves are replaced by fibrillary waves with sharp or round upper and lower ends at their contour and amplitude vary.
3. Ventricular rate may be as slow as 150 bpm or as fast as 500 bpm.
4. The amplitude of fibrillary waves progressively deteriorates (fine VF) immediately before asystole.

211. The incidence, types and treatment of ventricular fibrillation.

1. One-fourth of persons who die of acute myocardial infarction after hospital admission are due to ventricular fibrillation. Its incidence is greater in the hours immediately after the infarction, hence the importance of hospitalizing those patients who are seen early in the course of the illness.
   Traditionally, ventricular fibrillation is divided into two types.
2. *Primary VF:* This occurs in patient in whom there is no preceding heart failure or shock. This type has a relatively good prognosis if treated properly.
3. *Secondary VF:* This occurs in a patient who is ill with heart failure or shock. The prognosis is usually poor.
4. *Treatment of VF:* DC defibrillation with 200–400 joules.

Since there is a tendency of recurrence of this arrhythmia in 10–15% of cases, it is usual to give antiarrhythmic drug after defibrillation prophylactically. The standard procedure is to give IV xylocaine followed by oral drug such as procainamide, disopyramide, mexiletine, flecainide, quinidine or amiodarone for up to 3 months.

SOME OTHER ARRHYTHMIAS

212. Torsades de pointes, also called polymorphic ventricular tachycardia has the following 4 characters.

1. ECG diagnosis is made from very rapid life-threatening ventricular tachycardia (VT) at a rate of 200–250 beats/min with gradually changing QRS morphology in a sinusoidal fashion. QRS complexes seem to "twist" – that is, changes in QRS axis occur repeatedly.
2. It may be self-limiting but repetitive, leading to recurrent syncope; occasionally it may progress to ventricular fibrillation and sudden death.
3. This arrhythmia is often induced or worsened by antiarrhythmic agents (especially class I and III) –particularly if the QT interval is prolonged and there are electrolyte disturbances—or by drugs like phenothiazines, tricyclic antidepressants, some antihistamines that further prolong the QT interval.
4. Combination of torsades de pointes and prolongation of QT interval is known as QT syndrome. Most of them have prolongation of QT interval during sinus rhythm.

213. This is a form of ventricular tachycardia where there is no difficulty in recognizing its ventricular origin.

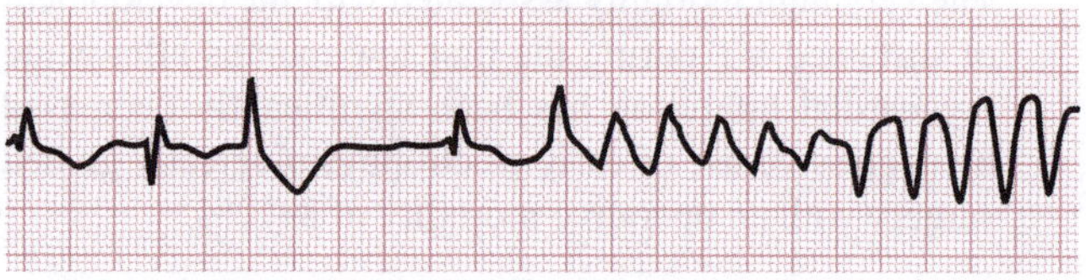

Fig. D-38: Torsades de pointes

1. Wide QRS complexes with multiple morphologies
2. Changing RR intervals
3. The axis seems to twist about the isoelectric line
4. Long QT intervals.

214. It is important to recognize this pattern as there are number of reversible causes. For example,

1. Heart block
2. Myocarditis
3. Hypokalemia or hypomagnesemia
4. Drugs: Tricyclic antidepressants, quinidine, etc.

Most commonly associated with administration of drugs, such as quinidine, procainamide, disopyramide, phenothiazines and tricyclic antidepreassents, which prolong QT interval and it results either from administration of toxic doses of these drugs or from administration of normal amounts of the drugs in the presence of already prolonged QT intervals; this may also occur in the presences of brady cardia due to any cause including hypokalemia and hypomagnesemia.

215. Long QT syndrome

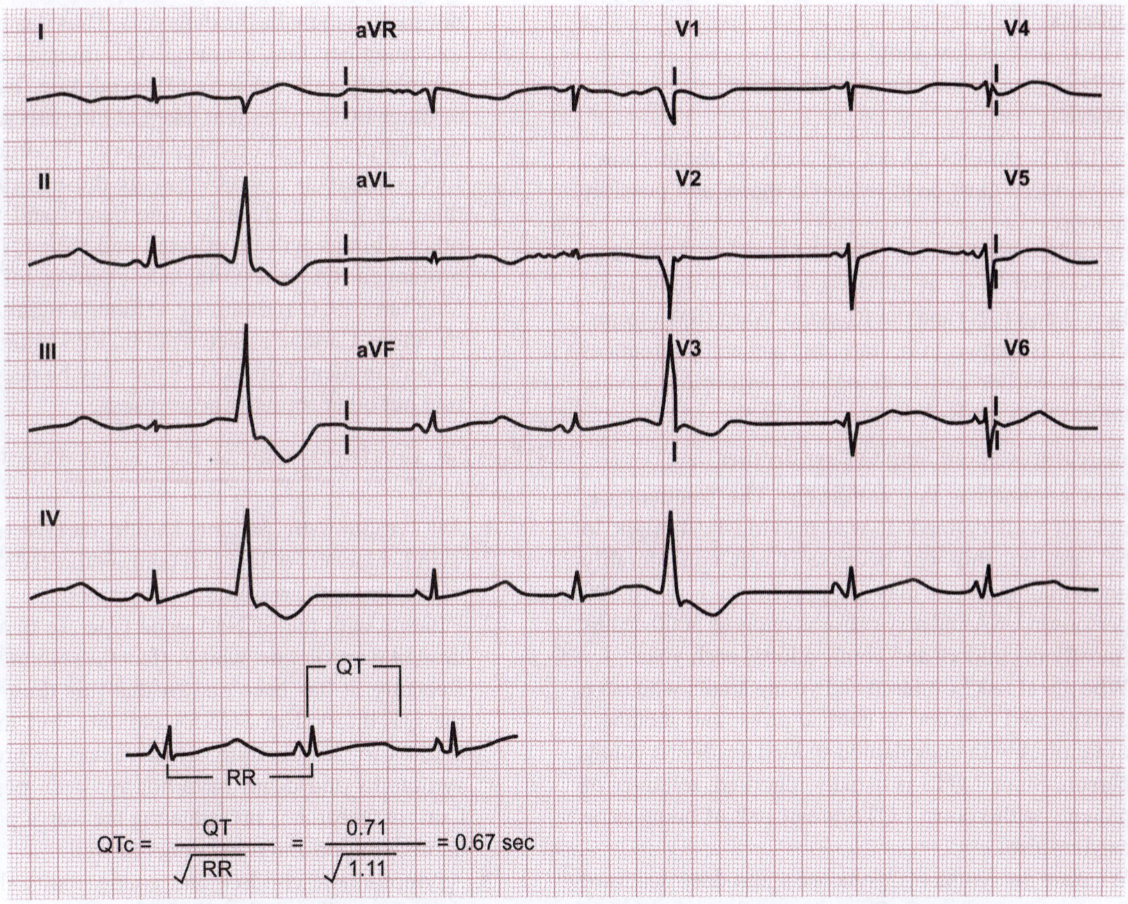

Fig. D-39: Romano-Ward syndrome is an autosomal dominantly inherited form of long QT interval and there is a risk of recurrent ventricular tachycardia, particularly torsades de pointes

Long QT interval normally varies with heart rate—becoming shorter at faster rates. It is usually corrected using the cycle length (RR interval) as shown above. Normal QTc = 0.42 seconds.

The figure also shows 2 ventricular premature beats. They are broad, premature, and have a full compensatory pause.

It involves the repolarization resulting in prolongation of QT interval. It is caused by dysfunction of protein structures in the heart cells called ion channels. Abnormalities of these channels can be acquired or inherited. The acquired form is caused by certain drugs and disease conditions. The inherited form occurs when a mutation develops in one of the genes which makes a channel. The mutations of the genes cause abnormal channels to be formed, resulting in impaired function. The abnormal function leads to the prolonged QT interval and the vulnerability to the abnormal fast heart rhythm, which causes the syncope and sudden death. The slow electrical recovery of the heart renders it vulnerable to fast, abnormal heart rhythms. Inherited long QT syndrome (LQTS) can be caused by mutations of at least 6 genes. Four different genes have so far been found. The location of a fifth gene is known, but the actual gene has not been found.

The 4 genes known at the present time include three, which form potassium channels and one which forms the sodium channel.

1. The SCN5A gene is a sodium channel gene on chromosome 3.
2. The HERG gene is a potassium channel gene on chromosome 7.
3. The KVLQT1 gene is a potassium channel gene on chromosome 11.
4. The mink or KCNE1 gene is a potassium channel gene on chromosome 21.

216. There is some variation of the ECG findings and the patient symptoms and frequency depending upon which gene and which mutations are involved.

1. The KVLQT1 gene appears to be the most frequent, being present in approximately 50% of genotyped patients
2. HERG gene is next about 45%
3. SCN5A gene is infrequent at about 5%
4. KCNE1.

Some LQTS families do not have any of these known genes, so there must be at least one more, and possibly many more.

Historically, two different clinical forms of LQTS have been described. They are known as the Jervell and Lange-Nielsen (J and L-N) and the Romano-Ward (RW) forms. J and L-N is known to be rare, but generally produces symptoms earlier and is associated with more severe symptoms than the R-W form.

217. Some features about long QT syndrome.

1. How common is this condition? The frequency is not yet well defined. It was previously thought to be rare, but this was because it was considerably underdiagnosed. It may be present in 1 in 50,000 persons in USA and may cause as many as 3000 deaths (mostly in children and young adults) each year.
2. Who are at risk? Children and young adults who have unexplained syncope or cardiac arrest and members of families with unexplained sudden death in a young person. Since LQTS is usually inherited, relatives of patients with known LQTS are at risk of being gene carriers also.
3. What are the symptoms? Syncope and sudden death are the common symptoms. Syncope usually occurs during physical exertion or emotional excitement like anger, fear or startle. The heart rhythm reverts spontaneously to normal and the patient regains consciousness within a minute or two. When the abnormal rhythm persists, however, the outcome is death. It is not uncommon for the syncope or sudden death to occur when the person is awake and at rest. About one-third never develop any symptoms. In the other two-thirds, some have just one or two syncopal spells as children, and none thereafter. Others have many episodes over a number of years. The symptoms may begin as early as first days or weeks of life, or as late as middle age. The symptoms start earlier in males than females, beginning on average at approximately 8 years in males and 14 years in females. The absence of any syncope or sudden death in a family does not at all guarantee the absence of this condition in the family.
4. How is the syndrome diagnosed? The primary finding is a prolonged QT interval on ECG which is present in 60–70% of affected persons. Sometimes QT prolongation is overlooked by doctors even when present. About 12% have a normal QT interval and 30% may have just borderline prolonged, which is not enough to make the diagnosis. Thus it is important to remember that a normal QT interval does not completely rule out long QT syndrome. Evaluation of other ECGs of patient taken at intervals where QT may be prolonged on other records. Examination of ECG on parents and siblings, are most helpful, since this is a genetic disorder, one parent and typically other siblings will be affected and their QT may be prolonged. Other tests include exercise ECG's, and long-term ECG monitoring –Holter's monitor, event monitors. Cardiac catheterization, EPS testing are not helpful in identifying LQTS but may be necessary to rule out other forms of heart disease.

218. What about treatment of LQTS and who should be treated?

1. All symptomatic patients should receive treatment with β-blockers unless it is contraindicated. The goal of therapy is the resolution of symptoms.
2. Patients with the SCN5A gene type are treated with drug like mexiletine, which affect the sodium channel. Recently, it has been shown that this drug shortens the QT interval in SCN5A patients, but long-term studies to demonstrate effectiveness in preventing symptoms and death have not yet been performed. Current research is investigating the use of potassium administration and other drugs as well.
3. Asymptomatic children and young adults should be treated as well, usually with β-blockers. Unfortunately, we cannot predict with any accuracy which LQTS patient will subsequently have sudden death or syncope. So, it is better to treat all the patients as sudden death is the first sign of LQTS in about 30–40% of patients.
4. When a person is 40–45 years or older, and has been asymptomatic lifelong or for many, many years, it may not be necessary to treat them, as their risk of developing symptoms at these later ages is quiet low, though not zero. They do need to avoid low blood potassium (caused by diuretics, vomiting or diarrhea) and the many drugs which lengthen the QT interval and which can cause LQTS themselves.

Once treated, it is important to continue the medication every day and not missed or omitted. The medications are not curative, they only provide protection while being taken and the protecting effect is gone within a day or two of stopping the medication. After that the risk of syncope or sudden death is the same as if the patient has not taken the medication at all. Parents should teach their children about the importance of daily medication, and should make sure each daily dose is taken.

Research is currently underway to try to identify those patients, perhaps those with a particular gene type, who are not as likely to respond to β-blockers. For them other drugs, the implantable defibrillator, pacemaker therapy, or left cervicothoracic surgical sympathectomy and are all options.

219. There are 4 causes of acquired QT syndrome.

1. Usually by common antiarrhythmic drugs like quinidine, procainamide, disopyramide and some phenothiazines (particularly thioridazine) and tricyclic antidepressant drugs.
2. Acute myocardial infarction.
3. Bradycardia particularly AV block.
4. Cardiomyopathies and myocarditis.
(Cardiomyopathy of amyloidosis, liquid protein diet, mitral valve prolapse, CNS disease can cause).

220. The 4 points to be followed in the treatment of QT syndrome.

1. β-blockers in congenital QT syndrome
(Transection of left stellate ganglion is done in resistant cases)
Acquired QT syndrome
2. Discontinue the drugs like quinidine, procainamide, disopyramide, etc.
3. Correct the electrolyte abnormalities like hypokalemia, hypocalcemia, hypomagnesemia.
4. Managed by (Torsade de pointes is prevented) ventricular pacing or isoproterenol infusion.

221. Jervell and Lange-Nielsen syndrome is also a dangerous arrhythmia which can cause syncope and sudden death. It has 4 characteristics.

1. Autosomal recessive transmission
2. Nerve deafness
3. QT prolongation
4. Torsades de pointes
(Romano-Ward syndrome is similar but it has autosomal dominant transmission without nerve deafness).

222. There are 4 important causes of prolongation of QT interval.

1. Electrolyte disturbances–hypokalemia, hypocalcemia, hypomagnesemia
2. Myocardial infarction
3. Antiarrhythmic drugs
4. Idiopathic prolonged QT interval syndrome.

223. Prolongation of QT interval is associated with

1. Increased sympathetic activity
2. Ventricular tachycardia (VT)
3. Ventricular fibrillation (VF)
4. Sudden death.

224. Differential diagnosis of some tachycardias (Ventricular rate over 100/min).

Table D-9

	Atrial rate	Ventricular rate	Atrial complexes (P wave)	Ventricular complexes (QRS)	AV relationship	Carotid massage
1. Sinus tachycardia	Seldom over 130	Seldom over 130 (= atrial rate)	Normal	Unchanged	Normal 1:1	8–10 beats less
2. Atrial tachycardia	140–250	140–220	Abnormal	Unchanged	Normal 1:1	'All or None' phenomenon. Normal sinus rhythm or no effect at all
3. Atrial tachycardia with block	140–250	Usually 1/2 of atrial rate (2:1 block)	Abnormal	Unchanged	Long PR (1:1) or dropped beats (2 or more:1)	—
4. Nodal tachycardia	140–220	140–220	Abnormal	Unchanged	Short PR	
5. Atrial flutter	260–350	Usually 140–160 (2:1 AV block)	'Saw-edge' shape flutter waves	Unchanged	2:1, 3:1	Reduction in arithmetic proportion
6. Atrial fibrillation	350–600	100–150 Irregular	Irregular fibrillary waves, low voltage	Unchanged	No relationship	No response
7. Ventricular tachycardia	60–100	140–220 Nearly regular	Normal	Broadened abnormal	AV dissociation (Usually)	—
8. Accelerated idioventricular rhythm	60–100	60–100	Normal	Broadened abnormal	AV dissociation	—

225. The antiarrhythmic drugs are classified into 4 groups.

Vaughan Williams classification of antiarrhythmic drugs This has been derived to a great extent from the in-vitro effect of various drugs upon the action potential of normal cardiac muscle. It's main disadvantage is that it does not include digitalis as an antiarrhythmic drug.

The rapid phase of depolarization is caused by the fast entry of sodium ions into the myocardial cells. The plateau of the action potential is maintained by the slow entry of calcium ions into the cells. Keeping this in view, the actions of the drugs in class I, II, III and IV may be summarized.

Class I. Sodium channel blockers: These drugs cause slowing of the fast entry of sodium ions into the cell and reduce the maximum rate of depolarization. Slow the fast rising phase of ventricular action potential by inhibiting fast sodium current. These drugs cause moderate depression of depolarization and prolongation of repolarization.

Class II. β-adrenergic blockers: These drugs act by diminishing the effects of catecholamines on the heart. These drugs have no effect on the duration of action potential.

Class III. Drugs of antithyroid like effect: These drugs prolong the duration of action potential and hence the effective refractory period without altering the rate of depolarization. They delay the repolarization, prolong plateau of ventricular action potential.

Class IV. Calcium channel blockers: These drugs slow the influx of calcium ions into the cell thereby maintaining the plateau of the action potential.

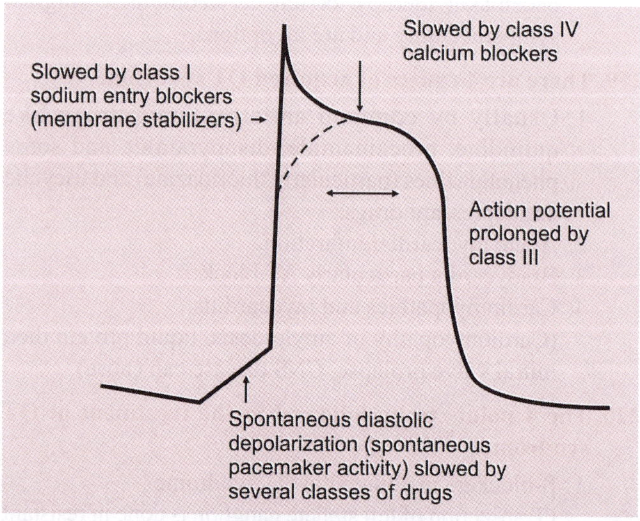

Fig. D-40: Action of antiarrhythmic drugs at various sites of action potential

Table D-10: Table of antiarrhythmic drugs

Class	*Depolarization*	*Repolarization*	*Responsive target tissue.*	*Indications*
I. Sodium channel blockers (Membrane stabilizers)	Depresses phase 0 depolarization			
A. Quinidine, Procainamide, Disopyramide, Moricizine	Moderate depression	Prolonged	Atrium, ventricle, Purkinje system, accessory pathway	SVT, VT prevention of VF symptomatic PVBs
B. Lidocaine, Tocainamide, Mexiletine, Phenytoin	Limited depression	No effect or shortened	Ventricle	Prevention of VT, VF symptomatic PVBS
C. Flecainide, Propafenone	Marked depression slows conduction	Minimal effect	Ventricle	life-threatening VT, VF Refractory SVT
II. β-blockers: Propranolol, Atenolol, Metoprolol, Esmolol, Acebutolol	No effect	Prolonged	SA node, AV node slows AV conduction	SVT, prevention of VF
III. Drugs of antithyroid-like effect: Amiodarone, Ibutilide, Bretylium, Dofetilide, Tosylate, Bethanidine, Sotalol (also has Class II effect)	Delay	Prolonged	Atrium, ventricle accessory pathway	Refractory VT prevention of VT, VF, SVT atrial flutter
IV. Calcium channel blockers: Verapamil, Diltiazem, Tepanil, Adenosine	Effect on plateau	Prolonged	AV node	SVT prevention of VF

226. Drug treatment for specific arrhythmias.

Table D-11

Arrhythmias	First line drugs	Alternative drugs	Drugs to be avoided
1. Sinus tachycardia	Usually does not require treatment	Small dose of β-blockers or CCB – Verapamil/ diltiazem	Class I agents
2. Sinus bradycardia	If symptomatic – Adrenergic or anticholinergic – orciprenaline, Isoprenaline, Atropine		Class I agents
3. PSVT/PAT	Adenosine	Verapamil, diltiazem, β-blockers, digoxin	Class I agents
4. Atrial flutter	Ibutilide		Class I agents
5. Atrial fibrillation	Paroxysmal AF Ibutilide Dofetilide Propafenone Flecainide Sotalol	Chronic AF β-blockers Verapamil Diltiazem Digoxin Amiodarone	Class I agents
6. AVNRT AV nodal Reentrant tachycardia	Quinidine Procainamide Flecainide Propafenone	Amiodarone Sotalol Ibutilide Dofetilide	Digoxin Verapamil Diltiazem β-blockers
7. Ventricular tachycardia	Lidocaine Procainamide Amiodarone	β-blockers Magnesium sulfate, bretylium	
8. Ventricular fibrillation	Lidocaine Procainamide Amiodarone	β-blockers Magnesium sulfate, bretylium	

227. Type I antiarrhythmic drugs act in 4 ways.

1. Reduces automaticity—depresses contractility
2. Reduces the speed of conduction velocity
3. Prolongs the duration of action potential
4. Prolongs the effective refractory period.

228. The three commonly used type I antiarrhythmic drugs - quinidine, procainamide and disopyramide phosphate have the following 4 similar effects.

1. Antifibrillatory effects on the atria
2. Depression of conduction in the retrograde limb in reentrant paroxysmal atrial tachycardias and in anomalous pathways (in paroxysmal supraventricular tachycardias).
3. Interference with circus movements within the ventricles
4. Reduction of automaticity of atrial or ventricular ectopic foci.

229. Antiarrhythmic drugs are potentially dangerous.

They are proarrhythmic also.

Percentage of proarrhythmias with some drugs

1. Amiodarone 30%
2. Mexiletine 19%
3. Quinidine 15%
4. Procainamide 11%
   (Procainamide + Mexiletine 22%)

These drugs have potential for prolongation of QT interval, which may result in ventricular tachyarrhythmias. They have potential of exerting vagolytic effect on AV node facilitating AV nodal conduction and increasing the ventricular rate.

Some of the commonly used drugs are to be understood in relation to their important side effects.

230. Quinidine: Class IA group

Dose. 200–600 mg × 6th hourly po—long acting.

1. Indicated in atrial fibrillation, atrial flutter, paroxysmal atrial tachycardia, premature ventricular contractions, etc.
   Absolutely contraindicated in complete heart block. It has vagolytic effect.
2. Long-term use causes side effects like nausea, vomiting, tinnitus, blurring of vision, vertigo, dizziness, headache, tremors, etc. The side effects come down once the drug is stopped. It crosses the placental barrier, so fetal arrhythmias can occur.
3. It has the risk of dislodging thrombus when used in long standing atrial fibrillation to convert to normal sinus rhythm. Antivagal activity may decrease the refractory

period of AV node and increases ventricular rate before conversion to sinus rhythm.
4. It increases the effects of coumarin anticoagulants and skeletal muscle relaxants.

231. Quinidine is used often, especially in North America, for reducing the frequency of paroxysmal atrial fibrillation and for maintaining sinus rhythm after cardioversion. Meta-analysis of six controlled trials have shown that patients treated with quinidine were less likely to have a recurrence of atrial fibrillation. Importantly, however, this analysis also revealed an excess of mortality for the treated group. Quinidine also interacts with digoxin and is associated with the following 4 serious effects.

1. Torsades de pointes – polymorphic ventricular tachycardia
2. Quinidine syncope
3. Blood dyscrasiasis
4. Cinchonism.

232. Procainamide of class IA group—250 mg tablet. Total 50 mg/kg at 3 to 4 hr interval.

IV 10–15 mg/kg at 25 mg/min then 1–6 mg/min.

Caution:

1. It can produce systemic lupus erythematosis (SLE) -like syndrome
2. Can cause agranulocytosis. Keep a check on leukocyte count
3. Can produce depressive psychosis
4. Should be more cautious while using in patients with myasthenia gravis as it may enhance the effects of skeletal muscle relaxants.

233. Disopyramide phosphate of class IA group: 100 mg. 150 mg capsule.

100–200 mg 6th or 8th hourly po
400–800 mg daily in 4 divided doses.

1. It has greater anticholinergic effect.
   Causes dryness of mouth, blurred vision, glaucoma, retention of urine, constipation
2. Should not be given in old people with enlarged prostate as it may cause acute retention urine.
3. It has negative inotropic effect. Can cause serious complications like bradycardia, heart block, torsades de pointes, cardiac arrest. Should not be used in complete heart block.
   Not recommended in children.
4. Do not give in heart failure as it may cause congestive cardiac failure.

234. Class IB group drugs used are

1. **Lidocaine (xylocaine)** of Class IB has—wide range of safety.
   It is very useful in the treatment or prophylaxis of ventricular arrhythmias or ventricular tachycardias following acute myocardial infarction. Useful in ventricular arrhythmias of diverse etiology by only intravenous infusion in the hospital setting.
   It depresses the automaticity of Purkinje fibers and counteracts the irritable focus in the ventricles.
   50 to 100 mg IV bolus followed by IV infusion of 2 to 4 mg/min.
   Dose is reduced in congestive heart failure or cardiogenic shock.
2. *Mexiletine:* Class IB group dose 200–400 mg × 8th hrly po
   It is a more useful oral antiarrhythmic drug
   It does not cause hemodynamic effect
   It can be used in combination with quinidine
   It is safe in long QT syndromes
   It requires careful titration.
3. *Phenytoin sodium:* Class IB group 100 mg capsule × 6 to 8th hourly po
   Drug of choice in arrhythmias caused by digitalis toxicity (Digitoxicity). It is useful in arrhythmias that occur during general anesthesia, cardiac surgery.
   100 mg IV every 5 minutes until the arrhythmias is abolished until 1000 mg given, or until drowsiness, nystagmus, vertigo, or nausea occur.
4. *Tocainamide:* 400–600 mg, 8–12 h .

235. Class 1C group of antiarrhythmic drugs:

Flecainide and Propafenone have been well investigated.

1. They have potent effects on conduction within cardiac cell membranes and lengthen the PR interval and QRS complex.
2. Flecainide has been shown to be effective in preventing recurrences of atrial fibrillation in up to 60% patients but does not limit the ventricular response.
3. Adverse effects have been reported in up to 74% of patients, but these effects are mostly tolerable.
4. Safety of flecainide has been raised by the cardiac arrhythmia suppression trial in which patients with old myocardial infarction given for ventricular arrhythmias had a worsened prognosis (with about three-fold increase in mortality).

236. β-blockers are Class II antiarrhythmic agents. β-blockers have negative inotropic effect. They mainly block the adrenergic activity. Prolongs the refractory period, decreases conduction through atrial and nodal tissue.

They should be used cautiously in patients with latent or overt heart failure.

β-blockers are useful in the following 4 types of cardiac arrhythmias.

1. Useful in supraventricular tachyarrhythmias
   - Sinus tachycardia, paroxysmal atrial tachycardia, extra systoles (atrial or ventricular). Atrial flutter and atrial fibrillation.
   - Acts by reducing rate of depolarization of SA node cells and junctional pacemakers. Slows conduction in the atria and AV node.
   - They can abolish PSVT when AV node is in reentrant pathway.
     – Useful in combination with digitalis to slow the ventricular rate in atrial flutter or fibrillation in which arrhythmia is not controlled by digitalis alone.
     – Useful in digitalis induced tachyarrhythmias.
2. Useful in ventricular arrhythmias that occur while recovering from acute myocardial infarction. Useful in premature ventricular contractions associated with stress or anxiety and in persistent PVCs.
   See the heart rate, left ventricular function and ejection fraction.
   Do not use in left ventricular dysfunction.
3. Useful in arrhythmias associated with thyrotoxicosis, pheochromocytoma, cardiac surgery where excess catecholamines are released.
4. Useful in prevention of recurrent ventricular tachycardias in congenital QT syndrome.

237. Commonly used β-adrenergic blocking agents: Class II group

Nonselective

Dose

i. Propranolol 10–100 mg × 6th hourly po
   IV 0.1 mg/kg in divided doses
   Cardioselective
ii. Atenolol: 50–100 mg/day po
iii. Metaprolol—50, 100 mg tab
   100–400 mg/day
iv. Esmolol—Intravenous only
   500 mg/kg/min × 1 min
   followed by 50 mg/kg/min × 4 min
   repeated with 50 mg increment to a maintenance dose of 200 mg/kg/min.

238. Intravenous propranolol is used in the emergency treatment of

1. Cardiac arrhythmias associated with heart disease
2. Digitalis intoxication
3. Arrhythmias during anesthesia
4. Thyrotoxic crisis.

A dose of 1 mg IV over a period of 1 minute, repeated if necessary every 2 minutes until a maximum total of 10 mg is given in conscious patients and 5 mg in patients under anesthesia. Similar doses have been used in thyrotoxic crisis. Atropine, 1 to 2 mg, given IV has been recommended before propranolol is injected in order to prevent excessive bradycardia. Propranolol is not suitable for the emergency treatment of hypertension, it should not be given intravenously in hypertension.

239. Adverse effects of β-blockers are:

1. Can precipitate cardiac failure see for LV function. Do not use in LV dysfunction.
2. Can precipitate air way obstruction ask for history of asthma.
3. Can precipitate hypoglycemia; be cautions while using in diabetes mellitus.
4. Can precipitate gangrene in peripheral vascular disorders.

240. Amiodarone—Class III group—is useful in supraventricular and ventricular tachyarrhythmias and in recurrent arrhythmias not controlled by other drugs.

1. Paroxysmal supraventricular tachycardia
2. Nodal tachycardia
3. Ventricular tachycardias
4. Wolff-Parkinson-White syndrome.

241. Amiodarone is useful in ventricular tachycardia, ventricular fibrillation. It is better than procainamide, disopyramide, mexiletine but should be cautious about its side effects.

800–1600 mg/day—1 to 3 weeks—po then
600–800 mg/day—2 to 4 weeks—oral then
200–400 mg/day

Amiodarone is very dangerous if not properly used. It is dose dependent and time dependent.

1. It can cause irreversible pulmonary interstitial fibrosis and death
   X-ray chest should be taken every 3 months for one year, then once a year.
   Less pulmonary toxicity if given less than 300 mg per day.
2. It can cause hypo- or hyperthyroidism as it contains lot of iodine. Check the thyroid function.
3. It can cause skin pigmentation (discoloration) which is not reversible—Photosensitivity and skin rashes
4. Hepatotoxic on long-term use—Liver function tests should be done every 3 months. Seventy-five percent side effects are over 5 years.
   Prolonged half-life may be 40–50 days.
   Needs discontinuation in 18–37% of cases.

It takes about a week to become active.

Verify: Maintenance dose of 200–400 mg/day/po. Reduce the dose of digoxin, warfarin and other antiarrhythmic drugs. It has synergistic action with β-blockers.

Bretylium: Class III group: IV 5–10 mg/kg min 1–2 mg/kg then 0.5–2.0 mg/min.

Used in refractory ventricular tachyarrhythmias when others have failed. Only intravenous route. IV 5–10 mg/kg at 1–2 mg/kg/min then 0.5–2.0 mg/min. It has many complications.

242. Calcium channel blockers: Class IV group.

Verapamil: Dose 80–120 mg 6th or 8th hrly po IV 5–10 mg in 1–2 min.

Diltiazem: IV 0.25 mg/kg over 2 min, if response is inadequate wait 15 min, then 0.35 mg/kg over 2 min, maintenance 10–15 mg/h.

1. Act by blocking the slow inward calcium channels.
2. Depolarization is delayed so conduction velocity in the AV node is depressed and its functional refractory period is increased making it unresponsive to reentrant rhythm.
3. Useful in supraventricular arrhythmias especially in reentrant type.
4. It is not useful in supraventricular arrhythmias caused by accessory pathway. It worsens the WPW syndrome. Verapamil given with digoxin increases the digitalis toxicity.

Other Drugs

Digoxin 1.25–1.5 mg po in divided doses over 24h followed by 0.125–0.375 mg/day.

IV approximately 70% of oral dose

Adenosine IV 6 mg rapidly, if unsuccessful within 1–2 min, 12 mg rapidly.

243. Direct current shock (DC shock—Cardioversion) is useful in

1. Atrial tachycardia (PAT)
2. Atrial flutter or fibrillation (AF)
3. Ventricular tachycardia (VT)
4. Ventricular fibrillation (VF).

HEART BLOCKS

244. Heart blocks may be broadly classified into 4 groups

1. Sinoatrial (SA) block and variants: Disturbance of sinus impulse formation.
2. AV block: Disturbance of sinus impulse conduction to the atria, AV node or ventricles.
   1st degree block—PR > 0.2 sec
   2nd degree block
   Dropped beats
   Fixed PR (Mobitz)
   Varying PR (Wenckebach)
   Fixed AV relationship (2:1, 3:1)
   3rd degree block
3. Bundle branch block (BBB)
4. Intermittent block.

245. The blocks are described depending on the site of block.

1. Sinoatrial heart block—at the SA node
2. First degree heart block—at AV node
3. Second degree heart block or incomplete heart block at bundle of His.
4. Third degree heart block or complete heart block at His Purkinje system.

246. Sinoatrial block and variants may be described in 4 variants.

1. *Sinoatrial block:* Sinus node does not conduct impulse into atrium. It results in sudden loss of P wave and QRS complex and a gap in otherwise regular sinus rhythm. This also represents as a slow P wave rate and is differentiated from sinus pauses by the fact that the long PP intervals are exact multiples of the shortest PP intervals. It should be differentiated from Mobitz Type II heart block in which a P wave occurs without a following QRS complex.
   i. Sinus beat is followed by a wide gap, then again a sinus beat.

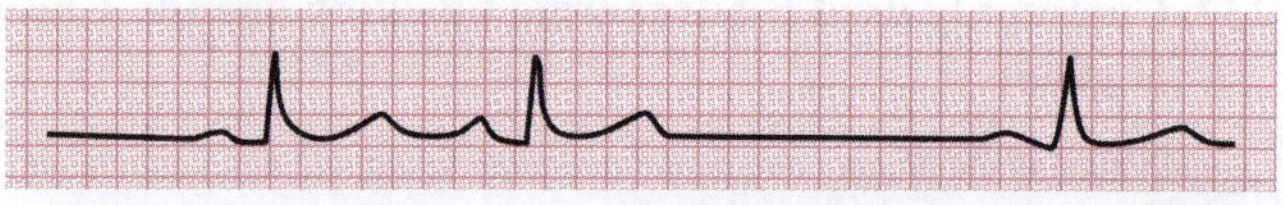

Fig. D-41: SA block. A complete PQRST is omitted in a regular sinus rhythm; and the PP interval is double the normal length

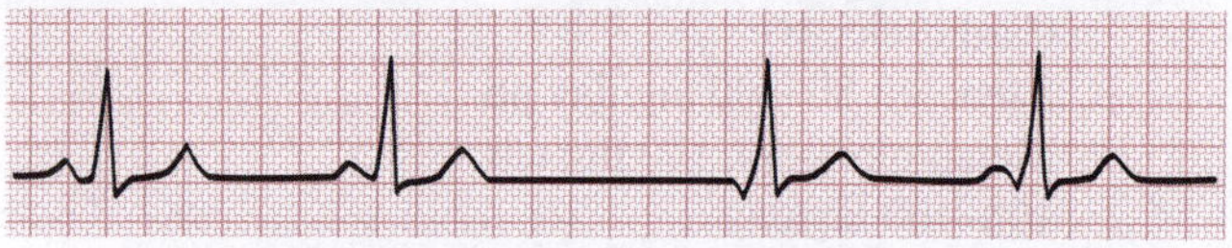

Fig. D-42: Sinus arrest. Absent PQRST is followed by a junctional (nodal) escape beat

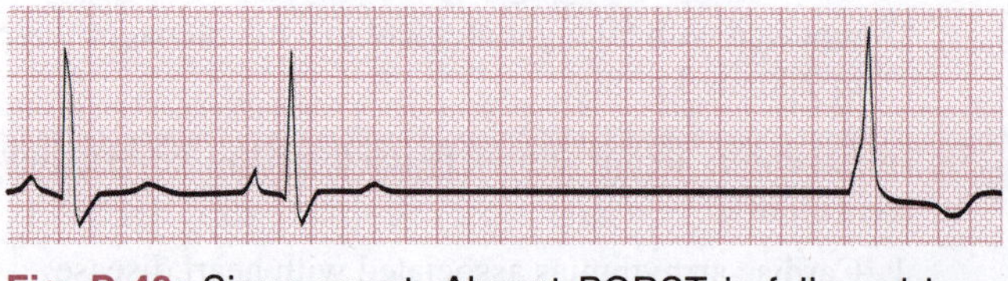

Fig. D-43: Sinus arrest. Absent PQRST is followed by a ventricular escape beat. An abnormal QRS complex without a preceding P wave

ii. RR interval of these two beats is double that of RR interval of normal sinus beat.
iii. Absent PQRST—misses a complete cycle.
iv. Followed by normal sinus conducted beats.

This arrhythmia is most often ischemic, degenerative and drug induced origin.

2. *Sinus arrest:* SA node cannot originate impulse, so no activity at SA node which results in slow heart rate without any P waves. This is followed by either a junctional (nodal beat) or ventricular beat. There is also a gap but the differentiating points are
   i. Preceding beat of the gap is a sinus beat.
   ii. Following beat of the gap may be atrial beat.
   iii. Following beat of the gap may be junctional beat.
   iv. Following beat of the gap may be a ventricular beat.

   RR interval are equal normal beats. It has to be differentiated from third degree heart block in which there is AV dissociation with P waves independent of QRS complexes. If the atrium is electrically unstable, it may lead to atrial fibrillation.

   Sinus arrest refers to arrest of the pacemaking activity of the SA node, resulting in temporary electrical inactivity. So pacemaking activity is taken over by another area of ectopic focus at atria, AV node, or ventricle resulting in atrial escape, nodal escape, or ventricular escape beat.

   Absence of JVP during an attack is the characteristic feature due to sinus arrest.

3. *Stokes-Adams syndrome:* It is mainly a clinical diagnosis. Prolonged sinus arrest without escape beats may result in Stokes-Adams attack.

   JVP continues to pulsate in Stokes-Adams attack due to AV block. There is a sudden loss of consciousness due to ventricular standstill caused for instance by Mobitz type II or third degree heart block or transient ventricular fibrillation. The patient is pulseless, pale and falls unconscious. Recovery occurs after one or two minutes. It may give rise to a full blown epileptic seizure due to cerebral anoxia. Unlike epilepsy, the recovery is usually sudden and may be accompanied by flushing of the skin as the circulation starts up again.

4. *Sick sinus syndrome (SSS): Tachy-brady-arrhythmia-asystole.* It is usually a degenerative condition of the SA node associated with old age, ischemic heart disease, diabetes, etc. The patient presents with palpitations, giddiness, or syncope.

   The arrhythmias consist of tachycardia, alternating with bradycardia, SA block, etc. Many-a-times, it is associated with atrial arrhythmias as a result of SA node dysfunction (hence palpitation).

   It is supraventricular in nature, i.e. sinus tachycardia, supraventricular tachycardia following or preceding SA block, SA arrest and nodal beats.

   Thirty percent of SSS are complicated by intermittent 1st, 2nd or 3rd degree AV block.

   SA node dysfunction is said to be due to ischemic or rheumatic heart disease, drugs, such as digitalis or quinidine, infiltration with amyloid or tumor or cardiomyopathies.

   During the spell of sinus bradycardia, IV atropine fails to increase the sinus rate. Clinically, SSS is manifested by palpitations, dizziness and syncope. Drug treatment may worsen. Cardiac pacing is indicated in symptomatic patients.

   In SA block, the impulse is formed but gets blocked inside the SA Node, whereas the rhythm is maintained inside the SA node. Hence, the long pause is usually a multiple of a normal sinus interval (twice or thrice of the normal sinus interval depending on whether it is 2:1 or 3:1 SA block).

   In SA arrest, the long pause not a multiple of the abnormal sinus interval. This is because impulse is not generated in the SA node for that particular period. Therefore important to measure the long pause to see whether it is multiple of a normal sinus interval or not. In many cases, there may be escape nodal beat or ventricular beat after the long pause.

   These patients usually present with giddiness, or syncope. Many a time, the arrhythmias form a part of the sick sinus syndrome (SSS).

   SA block, SA arrest and SA Wenckeback are associated with SSS that requires a permanent pacemaker, unless it is drug induced, when discontinuing the inciting drug would be sufficient.

247. Sick sinus syndrome: As the name implies, the sinus node is sick:

1. It is common especially in elderly, diabetics, etc. due to idiopathic degeneration of SA nodal cells
2. It is caused by SA node dysfunction due to ischemic or rheumatic heart disease, drugs such as digoxin or quinidine or infiltration with amyloid or tumor or cardiomyopathies.
3. Main problem is the development of sinus bradycardia or episodes of sinus arrest.
4. This is often associated with various atrial tachyarrhythmias, such as atrial tachycardia, atrial flutter or atrial fibrillation.

   It may be associated with coronary artery disease particularly that involving the right coronary artery although many of these patients show normal coronary angiogram.

248. The ECG findings in SSS are:

1. Inappropriate sinus bradycardia
2. Sinus pauses or arrest
3. Sinus exit block
4. Bradycardias may alternate with tachyarrhythmias, especially slow and fast atrial fibrillation, atrial flutter, atrial tachycardia (resulting in tachy-brady syndrome).

249. Symptomatology of SSS: It may be asymptomatic or may have nonspecific symptoms, such as:

1. Dizziness/syncope
2. Palpitations
3. Fatigue
4. Sudden death.

250. Management of sick sinus syndrome: Permanent pacing is indicated in the presence of symptomatic bradyarrhythmias. Regular atrial pacing, either alone or combined with ventricular pacing is indicated because:

1. It is often effective in preventing paroxysmal atrial fibrillation associated with the "tachy-brady syndrome".
2. It stabilizes the atrium electrically
3. It preserves the normal sequence of cardiac chamber activation
4. It improves the overall prognosis

   Patients with tachy-brady syndrome seem to be at greater risk of thromboembolism. Such patients, therefore, need formal anticoagulation.

251. Simple ventricular pacing system is contraindicated because

1. It may result in an increase in the incidence of permanent and paroxysmal atrial fibrillation.
2. It may cause hypotension with a fall of cardiac output of up to one-third
3. It may increase thromboembolic events (stroke or peripheral artery embolus)
4. It may precipitate congestive heart failure.

252. The blocks are also named after their site of origin.

1. Sino atrial block—at SA node
2. Atrioventricular block—at AV node
3. His bundle block—at bundle of His
4. Bundle branch block (BBB) at bundle branches—LBBB, RBBB.

253. The causes of heart block which decrease the rate of conduction or totally block the impulses at AV node are

(The damage or depression can be at AV junctional fibers or at the AV bundle).

1. Myocardial infarction/Ischemic heart disease. Coronary insufficiency can delay or block the conduction from atria to ventricles.
2. Inflammatory process, such as sarcoidosis or collagenosis.
3. Infection such as diphtheria, rheumatic fever, etc. can cause various types of myocarditis.
4. Idiopathic fibrosis—the commonest cause in old age.

   2, 3, 4 can result in scar formation or calcified portion which can delay or block the conduction from atria to ventricles.
5. Aortic valve disease: especially aortic stenosis.
6. Congenital.
7. Cardiac surgery.
8. Extreme stimulation of the vagus: Vagal excitation sometimes result from strong stimulation of baroreceptors in persons with carotid sinus syndrome.

254. There are 4 points to know about congenital heart block:

1. It is due to lack of connection between atria and junctional fibers; the block is at the AV junctional fibers
2. Ventricular rate is high
3. Ventricular rate goes up with exercise
4. No need of pacemaker.

In general, heart block means block at AV node. It is due to delay or obstruction in conduction of the electrical impulse from the atria to the ventricles.

255. AV blocks can be described under 4 types.

Heart block is due to delay or obstruction in conduction of the electrical impulse from the atria to the ventricles. (Actually AV blocks are described into 3; but for rhythmic convenience to fit into 4, it is described here into 4 types—as second degree block has Mobitz type I and Mobitz type II).

1. *First degree heart block:* It is defined as a prolonged PR interval with intact AV conduction. Every impulse from atria goes to ventricles, i.e. every P is followed by QRS but the conduction at the AV node is delayed. PR interval is more than 0.2 seconds. The first degree heart block in young people may be due to increased vagal tone.

   Second degree AV block: It is defined as incomplete AV block with blocked P waves. Some impulses from atria go to ventricles and some do not go. The sinus rate is normal. It is the harbinger of higher grade blocks and is therefore important to recognize. It does not cause bradycardia by itself. It is further described into Mobitz type I (Wenckebach) and Mobitz type II.
2. *Mobitz type I heart block or Wenckebach phenomenon:* Some Ps have QRS and some do not have. PR interval is progressively lengthened in successive beats till the beat is dropped at which point the AV node is sufficient to obstruct the conduction completely. This results

in absence of QRS following P wave in ECG. In the pulse, there is a gap of one beat. Typically the AV node recovers and the process is repeated. First degree and Mobitz type I block do not cause symptoms but may progress to complete heart block. Symptomless first and second degree blocks do not require pacemaker.

3. *Mobitz type II:* PR interval is fixed but there is intermittent failure of conduction of the atrial impulse to the ventricle. A P wave occurs without a following QRS. This may effect single beat or multiple beats. The ventricular response is in some mathematical ratio with atrial stimulation as 2:1, 3:1 heart block, i.e. for 2 or 3 consecutive atrial contractions the ventricle responds once. If it is multiple there will be marked gaps in the pulse and syncope may occur.
   This may occur as infranodal block or bundle branches. There is no gradual prolongation of PR intervals as seen in Mobitz type I. P may sit on top of T. Some Ps have QRS and some do not have and prepare for the absence of QRS. This is more dangerous as it goes into third degree block without warning.
   First and second degree blocks are known as partial or incomplete heart blocks.
4. *Third degree or complete heart block:* It is defined by the total lack of conduction between atria and ventricles nothing is conducted from atria to ventricles. There is total failure of conduction of atrial impulse to the ventricles; so, it is more dangerous. Atria and ventricles beat independently but at different rates. Ventricular rate depends on the site of pacemaker within it. Usually it is slow at a rate of 30–40 beats per minute.
   Mobitz type II with multiple pulse gaps and third degree block may be asymptomatic or cause dizziness, syncope or heart failure. Symptomatic Mobitz type II block and complete heart block whether it is asymptomatic or symptomatic should be treated with a pacemaker because pacing considerably prolongs the life.

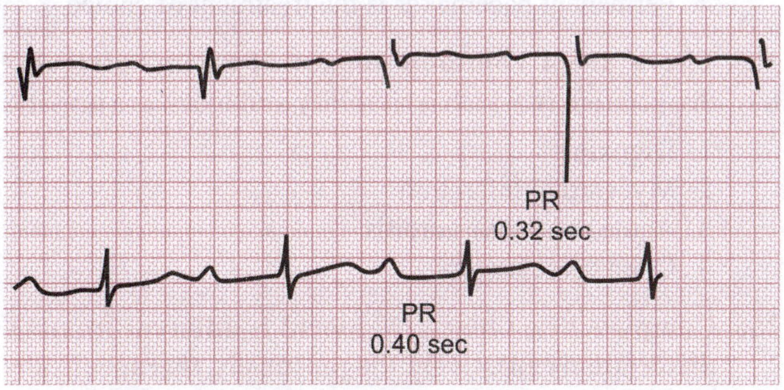

Fig. D-44: First degree AV block PR interval is prolonged above 0.2 sec. Each P is followed by a QRS complex

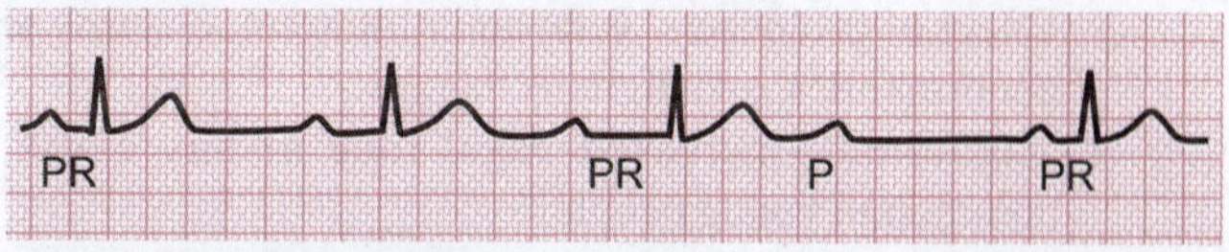

Fig. D-45: Wenckebach (Mobitz type I) second degree AV block: PR interval lengthens progressively with successive beats until one P wave is dropped

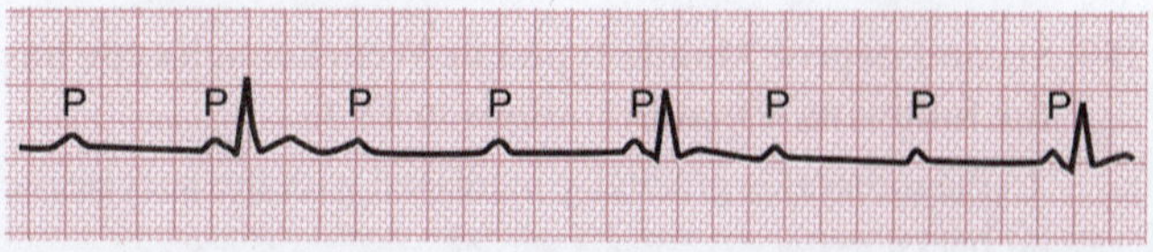

Fig. D-46: Mobitz type II second degree AV block: There are nonconducted P waves, but the PR interval in conducted beats is constant

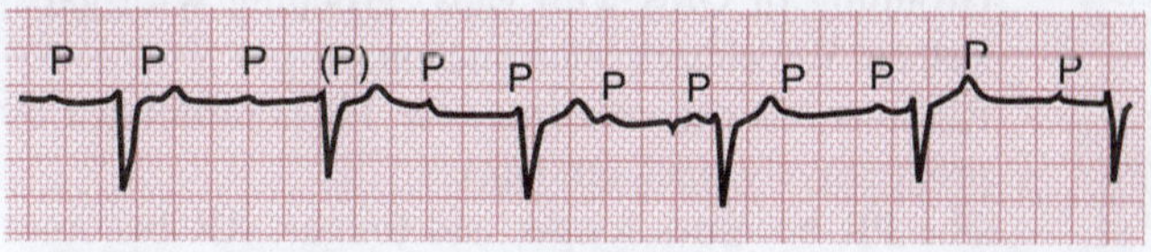

Fig. D-47: Third degree (complete) AV block: Atrial and ventricular activity are independent of each other and PR intervals are independent of each other

256. Causes of complete heart block:

1. Ischemia
2. Infarction—common with inferior valve MI, but can occur with anterior valve MI also
3. Drug toxicity
4. Infiltrative diseases of AV node like sarcoidoses, scleroderma, etc.
5. Degenerative diseases like amyloidosis
6. Calcific aortic sclerosis
7. Infective endocarditis
8. Electrolyte imbalance.

257. AV blocks are not uncommon in the day-to-day general practice.

These are briefly considered because

1. Often no treatment is required.
2. When indicated, treatment is often stoppage of digitalis.
3. Use of atropine or isoproterenol is needed.
4. Use of temporary or permanent pacemakers is needed.

258. There are 4 common causes of first degree heart block, where PR interval is prolonged > 0.2 sec.

1. Rheumatic carditis.
2. Ischemic sclerotic (atherosclerotic) coronary artery disease.

3. Effect of β-blockers, verapamil/diltiazem, electrolyte abnormalities, and digitalis therapy.
4. Vagotonia—increased vagal tone of any cause, common in young people.
   No treatment is needed in asymptomatic patients. In symptomatic patients, the inciting cause is controlled and if still not responded dual chamber pacing may be needed.

259. Second degree Mobitz type I or Wenckebach type has the following 4 manifestations in ECG.

1. PR interval is gradually increased with the successive beats.
2. Gradual increase in PR interval is reached until a P wave is not conducted, i.e. "Dropped beat" and then succession of cycles are repeated.
   Grouping of QRS with gaps 'grouping with gaps' suspect Wenchback phenomenon.
3. RR intervals decrease since the PR is prolonged by progressively small amounts.
   The PR becomes longer and longer; RR becomes shorter and shorter (decremental increment).
4. PP intervals are equal: (Wenckebach described this phenomenon in 1899 by observing neck veins when there was no ECG. AC wave in JVP becoming longer and longer with a dropped beat. ECG came in 1903. Mobitz described it in 1924 with ECG).

260. Second degree Mobitz block is:

1. Commonly seen with inferoposterior MI.
2. Inflammation.
3. Drugs and electrolyte imbalance.
4. Degenerative—conductive tissue.
   It is usually a benign and do not go to complete heart block. In symptomatic patients, IV atropine or temporary pacemaker may be needed. If symptoms are still persistent a permanent pacemaker may be needed.

261. Second degree Mobitz type II block has the following 4 features.

1. It is an infranodal block. It occurs in the common His bundle or in the bundle branches.
2. PR interval is constant in the conducted beat (No gradual prolongation of PR interval)
3. One or more P waves are blocked
4. More serious because it goes into third degree block without warning signs. Mobitz type II in myocardial infarction is more dangerous.
   It is potentially serious as it usually leads to 3° or complete block. It is seen in MI or severe degenerative disease, drug intoxication. In hemodynamically unstable patients, a temporary transvenous pacemaker followed by permanent pacemaker may be needed.
   The presence of BBB with Mobitz type II is ominous sign of impending complete heart block. Atropine may be contraindicated because it may aggravate the degree of AV block by the atrial tachycardia that it produces.

262. Third degree or complete heart block has the following 4 manifestations.

1. Pacemaker is from His-Purkinje system.
   Nothing is conducted from atria to ventricles.
2. More proximal the site of pacemaker higher the spontaneous rate of firing (< 50)
   Shorter QRS duration
3. Long-term management with sublingual isoproterenol is no longer preferred.
4. A permanent transvenous pacemaker is advised.

263. Third degree or complete heart block has the following 4 ECG features.

1. P and QRS are independent—P waves are not conducted to the ventricles because of the block at the AV node and show no relation to the QRS complex. They probe every part of the ventricular cycle but are never conducted. Ventricles are depolarized by a ventricular rhythm.
2. Ps are irregular and show no relation to the QRS complexes. They 'probe' every part of the ventricular cycle but are never conducted.
3. PR intervals are irregular.
4. Ventricular rate is slow—idioventricular rhythm. The ventricles are depolarized by a ventricular escape rhythm.

264. Treatment of complete heart block consists of

1. Atropine 0.6–1.2 mg IV or IM unless given previously
2. Isoprenaline 0.2 mg IV unless given previously
3. Hydrocortisone 300 mg IV stat
4. Permanent pacemaker is the treatment of choice.

265. There are 4 common causes of atrioventricular dissociation in which irritability and block are present.

1. Digoxin
2. Myocardial infarction
3. Acute rheumatic carditis
4. Open heart surgery.

266. Complete heart block (3° block) is different from AV dissociation causatively, diagnostically, therapeutically and prognostically.

Table D-12

Complete heart block	*AV Dissociation*
1. **Cause**	
AV node is incapable of conducting organically	AV node is incapable of conducting functionally
Conduction can never go through AV node	Can conduct but the AV node is refractory—slow
2. **Diagnosis**	
AV node is organically blocked	AV node is refractory
Ventricular rate < 40/min	Ventricular rate 90/min
Atrial rate > ventricular rate	Ventricular rate > atrial rate
No impulse can pass through	Some beats can pass through
AV node	AV node
So, no captured beat	Captured beats are possible (take a long ECG strip)
PP intervals irregular RR intervals irregular	Fixed PP intervals which are different from RR intervals which are also fixed
P need not be upright	P is upright P is marching through 'Captured beat'. Narrow QRS
3. **Treatment**	
Difficult to treat	Do not treat at all or treat the cause
Needs permanent pacemaker	Only medical
4. **Prognosis**	
Serious condition	Benign condition
Bad prognosis	Excellent prognosis

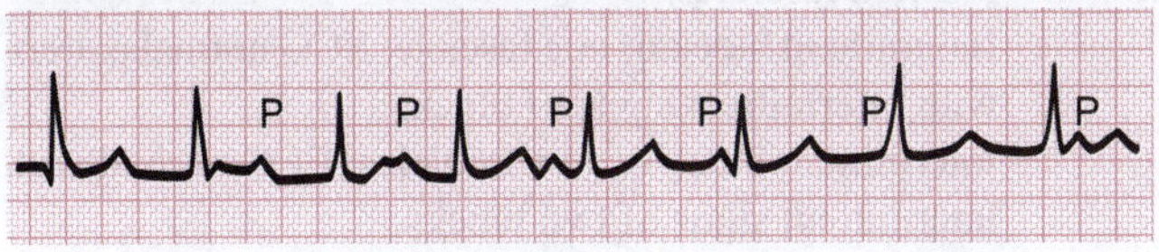

Fig. D-48: AV dissociation: The ventricular rate is slightly faster than atria and the PR interval gets shorter and shorter. The last P wave can be seen to have 'marched through' QRS

267. AV dissociation is a condition where there is irritability around the AV node due to

1. Ischemia
2. Inflammation
3. Digitalis toxicity
4. Functional unidirectional retrograde block in the AV node.

Capture beats are present in AV dissociation. The AV node can conduct antigrade (proved by capture beats) but functionally prevented from conducting because the high ventricular rate or nodal rate makes the junctional tissues refractory.

This is different from acquired complete heart block where the AV node junction cannot conduct due to organic disease of the AV node.

268. Congenital complete heart block:

This is a congenital condition leading to a complete heart block pattern. The important future is narrow QRS complexes, and the heart rate is usually faster than acquired congenital heart block. The block is at the upper part of the AV node (Atrionodal block) and so the escape rhythm arises from the AV junction, which has a relatively higher rate of rhythmicity. Since the impulses pass through the AV node and His bundle, the QRS complexes are relatively narrow and not as wide as in acquired complete heart block. It may be associated with some congenital heart disease, which have to be excluded by complete cardiac evaluation.

The 4 differences between congenital heart block and acquired heart block.

Table D-13

Congenital heart block	*Acquired heart block*
1. ECG shows normal heart rate (60–90 bpm) with narrow QRS complexes (< 0.25 mm or 0.1 sec)	ECG shows bradycardia and broad QRS complexes
2. Heart rate increases with exercise	Heart rate does not increase with exercise
3. Often benign condition	Serious condition
4. Usually does not need a permanent pacemaker Rarely needs a pacemaker if associated with attacks of syncope	Permanent pacemaker implantation is the treatment of choice

269. Diagnosis of bradycardia may be made by the following 4 factors.

1. P wave rate, regularity and morphology
2. QRS rate, regularity and morphology
3. P and QRS relationship, i.e. AV relationship
4. Additional clues.

270. The following 4 features help to differentiate some of the bradyarrhythmias.

1. Atiral rate
2. Ventricular rate
3. AV relationship
4. Some additional clues.

Table D-14

	Atrial rate	Ventricular rate	AV relationship	Some additional clues
Sinus bradycardia	Less than 60	Less than 60 (= atrial rate)	Normal 1:1 P always follows QRS	May be arrhythmia
Sinus arrest	Less than 60 abrupt halving of atrial rate	Less than 60	May be nodal or ventricular escape	Preceding beat is a sinus beat. Following beat is either nodal or ventricular
Nodal rhythm	Less than 60	Less than 60	Short PR or P waves buried in QRS or superimposed on ST segment	Normal QRS complexes P waves may be hard to see or P waves absent
Wenckebach Block second degree Mobitz type I	Normal usually above 60	Less than atrial rate	PR interval lengthens with successive beats until QRS is dropped The cycle is repeated	QRS complexes often in pairs or triplets
Second degree block Mobitz type II	Normal usually above 60	Usually 30–50. A fraction (1/2, 1/3) of atrial rate	2:1 AV block or greater (3:1,4:1 etc.)	P waves never occur in QRS complexes
Third degree or complete block	Normal usually above 60	Regular 30–50	AV dissociation No P follows QRS No PQRS relationship	P waves from time to time in QRS complexes No captured beat PP, RR intervals irregular

271. Bundle of His is divided into two fascicles. One for the right ventricle and one for the left ventricle, the later is again divided into anterior (superior) and posterior (inferior).

Blocks can occur at one place or many.

Fascicular blocks can be divided into 4.

1. Monofascicular block—block at one place
   Right bundle branch block (RBBB)
   Left bundle branch block (LBBB)
   Main bundle of His itself.
   (Congenital block is also a monofascicular block).
2. Bifascicular block: When two fascicles are blocked at two places.

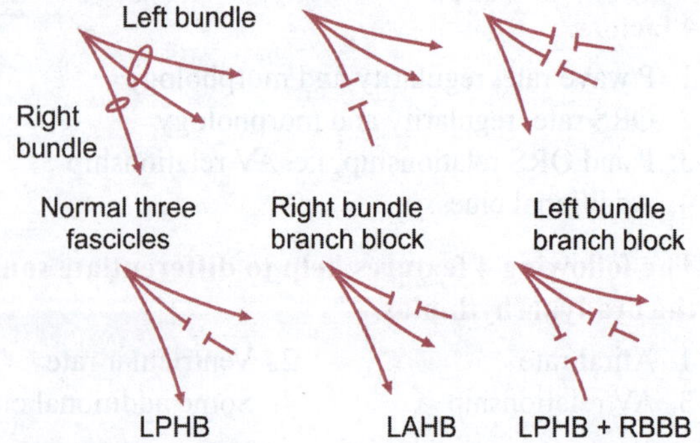

Fig. D-49: Purkinje conducting system and bundle branch block

   RBBB + left anterior hemiblock, i.e. anterior division of left bundle.
   RBBB + left posterior hemiblock, i.e. posterior division of left bundle.
   (Anterior hemiblock + posterior hemiblock = LBBB)
3. Trifascicular block: When all the three fascicles are blocked—namely right bundle, left anterior and left posterior divisions.
   or bifascicular block with prolonged PR interval.
4. Intermittent blocks with at least one normal non-blocked fascicles.
   Intermittent block of one fascicle: ECG normal pattern with intermittent signs of block.
   Intermittent block of two fascicles: ECG normal with intermittent signs of two blocks.
   Intermittent block:
   One intermittent block + one permanent block. ECG shows signs of one permanent block and intermittent signs of another block.

272. The incidence of bundle branch block (BBB) is as follows:

1. RBBB is more common even in normal people because it is thinner, and in same direction of bundle of His continuation.
2. LBBB is more common but less common than RBBB because left bundle is more thicker than right bundle.
3. Left anterior hemiblock is less common than RBBB or LBBB but more common than posterior hemiblock because it is thicker.

4. Left posterior hemiblock is very less common because it is thickest branch. Pure isolated posterior hemiblock is rare because posterior division is thickest, short and commonly has dual blood supply.

273. The 4 common causes of RBBB (can occur normally in young people) are:

1. Right ventricular strain (especially pulmonary embolism)
2. Atrial septal defect (ASD) (especially ostium secondum)
3. Ischemic heart disease
4. Myocarditis.

274. The 4 common causes of LBBB are:

1. Ischemic heart disease
2. Hypertension
3. Aortic valve disease
4. Cardiomyopathy or myocarditis.

275. Right bundle branch block (RBBB) has the following 4 clinical features.

1. Abnormal splitting of second sound due to delayed activation of right ventricle—may be physiological.
2. Usually associated with diabetes mellitus, coronary heart disease, pulmonary hypertension or in conditions producing right ventricular hypertrophy.
3. Incomplete RBBB is seen with atrial septal deful (ASD).
4. RBBB in mitral stenosis suggests tricuspid valve disease.

276. Left bundle branch block (LBBB) has the following 4 manifestations.

Fascicle in the left ventricles is blocked. It is considered as a serious disease.

1. Paradoxical splitting of S_2
2. Leads to left ventricular dysfunction or failure
3. May go into complete heart block
4. May develop Adams-Stokes attack.

277. Bundle Branch Block is due to lack of conduction of electrical impulse along only one or two of the three fascicles of the bundle of His beneath the AV node.

Table of differences between the right bundle branch block (RBBB) and left branch block (LBBB):

Table D-15

	RBBB	LBBB
I. Significance BBB after myocardial infarction may be a harbinger of threatening complete heart block with all its complications	Isolated RBBB may signify disease but may occur in normals. More common because it is thinner and continued in same direction of bundle of His	Always signifies disease of the conducting system. Less common than right bundle because it is thicker
II. Causes	Usually in right ventricular hypertrophy or dilatation, e.g. ASD (incomplete RBBB) Pulmonary stenosis Pulmonary embolism	Usually in left ventricular hypertrophy or dilatation, e.g. aortic stenosis, hypertension, Cardiomyopathy, ischemic heart disease, acute myocardial infarction
III. Clinical features By itself BBB does not produce symptoms and is associated with sinus rhythm. The signs are mainly of the underlying heart disease	Pulmonary valve closure is delayed in right ventricular hypertrophy and increased right ventricular stroke volume which causes increase in systolic time of right ventricle Wide fixed split of S2 occurs in ASD due to delayed closure of pulmonary valve	Aortic valve closure is delayed due to delayed left ventricular systole. Aortic valve closure occurs after pulmonary valve closure—reversed splitting of S2. Closure of the aortic valve delayed leading to narrowing of the split of the S2 during inspiration
IV. ECG changes QRS > 0.12 sec Depolarization in ventricles does not occur simultaneously and is delayed on one side	RSR' pattern is better seen in right chest leads V1, V2	RSR' pattern is better seen in left chest leads V5, V6 and lateral leads L1 and VL. Since the left ventricle dominates ECG changes, wide QRS complexes are seen throughout

278. Left anterior hemiblock (LAHB) has the following 4 characters.

(No impulse passes in the anterior division of left bundle, so more impulses travel in the posterior division—therefore, left axis deviation occurs. It is usually associated with myocardial infarction or other heart disease)

1. Left axis deviation—30° to 60°
2. L I QRS positive
   L II QRS is either equiphasic or negative
3. Q I S3 pattern
4. QRS slightly widened; more when it is associated with other blocks—bundle branch system.

Exclude left ventricular hypertrophy, myocardial infarction, horizontal heart, etc.

Note: LBBB and RBBB do not shift the axis

Only hemiblocks shift the axis—LAHB or LPHB.

279. Left posterior hemiblock (LPHB) has the following 4 characters.

(No current passes through posterior division; more current passes to right side, so RAD)

1. RAD + 120°
2. L I QRS negative LII QRS may be positive
3. S1 Q3
4. Wide QRS
   (Exclude right ventricular hypertrophy, extreme rotation of the heart).

280. Treatment of bradycardias in general are:

1. Treat only symptomatic bradyarrhythmias
2. Sinus bradycardia after acute myocardial infarction is common. Give injection atropine 0.6 mg IV slowly. Repeat up to 3 mg in 24 hours.
3. Bradycardia with heart block—is treated by pacing.
4. Bradycardia caused by drugs.
   β-blockers, calcium blockers–verapamil, dilitazan, digoxin—is treated by stopping the drugs.

281. Indications of pacemaker in general are:

1. Bradycardias—only in symptomatic patients
2. AV blocks
   Trifascicular with symptoms
   Complete heart block
   Mobitz type II
3. Supraventricular tachyarrhythmias—over driving
4. Ventricular tachyarrhythmias—over driving.

282. There are 4 indications for temporary pacing in bradycardia.

1. Sick sinus syndrome (SSS) symptomatic Stokes-Adams syndrome
2. Complete heart block with heart rate below 50 or with hemodynamic disturbances due to slow heart rate
3. Mobitz type II
4. All cases of anterior wall infarctions with heart block.

283. The 4 indications for pacing with normal heart rate in fascicular block are

1. Bilateral bundle branch block (BBBB)
2. RBBB with left axis deviation with history of repeated Stokes-Adams syndrome
3. RBBB with first degree heart block
4. LBBB with first degree heart block.

CLINICAL APPROACH TO BRADYARRHYTHMIAS

284. Bradycardia is defined as a heart rate of < 60 bpm. Such a rate may be physiological (which is acceptable) in athletes, young people or during sleep. It has clinical significant when it results from:

1. Acute myocardial infarction
2. Sick sinus syndrome (SSS) (sinus node disease)
3. Drugs, e.g. β-blockers and digoxin
4. Noncardiac conditions such as hypothyroidism, hypothermia, jaundice, increased intracranial tension.

Bradycardia can either result from failure of initiation of the heart beat (at SA node) or failure of passage of electrical current through the heart (at AV node).

Sinus node "Spark plug" activity is disturbed to initiate the heart beat or interruption or blockage of current pathway at AV node.

285. Symptoms of bradycardia can be varied from

1. Sudden death
2. Recurrent syncope
3. Milder symptoms such as lethargy, breathlessness, etc.
4. Epileptic fits (rare).

The history can be very revealing, but can be very unreliable especially in those who lose consciousness. Some bradycardias have only intermittent problems like blackouts but no abnormality found after many years of investigation, evidence for intermittent problem can be very difficult.

286. Recognizing the different types of bradycardia is sometimes relatively straightforward and are considered in them.

1. Sinoatrial disease (SSS)
2. Carotid sinus hypersensitivity
3. Vasovagal syndrome
4. AV block.

1, 2, 3 conditions are predominantly problems with SA node or its innervation.

SSS patients may be completely asymptomatic for whom no treatment is required. They can present with symptomatic bradycardia, dizziness, and syncope. These patients may need 24 hours ambulatory ECG to demonstrate correlation between periods of bradycardia or sinus pause and symptoms. It is accepted that a pause of over 3 seconds is significant.

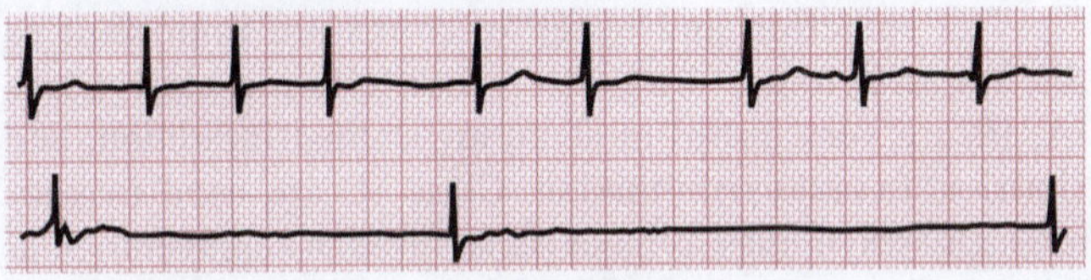

Fig. D-50

The pause is more than 3 sec.

Normal PR interval because this is an SA node, but not AV node problem. Every P is followed by a normal QRS complex (unless dual pathology), but there are periods when interval between P wave (PP internal) is prolonged.

Treatment is to remove extrinsic causes of bradycardia and/or permanent pacemaker (PPM). In brady-tachy syndrome, once a PPM has been implanted, medications which would normally slow the intrinsic cardiac rate can then be used to control SVT—for example, β-blockers.

Carotid sinus hypersensitivity: Similar symptoms can occur in hypersensitive carotid sinus reflex. It is diagnosed by finding either a sinus pause or of AV block greater than 3 seconds in response to 5 seconds of carotid sinus massage. PPM is indicated whom there is an association is made between symptoms and ECG. The carotid sinus massage affects both SA and AV node (supraventricular tachycardia). Therefore, it can cause sinus bradycardia as well. The PR interval can also be prolonged resulting in AV block (see Fig. D-45).

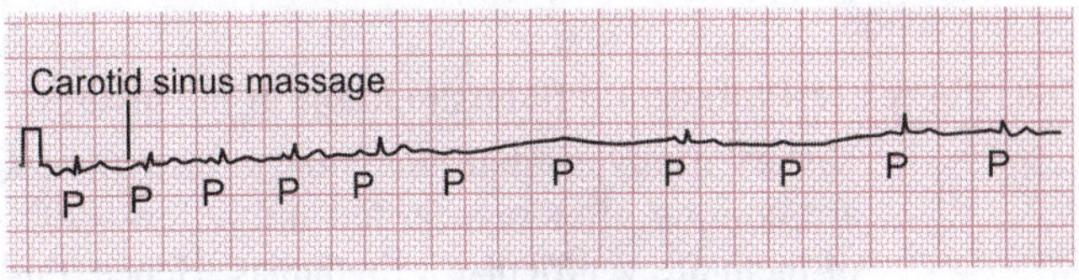

Fig. D-51

Vasovagal syndrome: This is a common condition in younger people and a more malignant variety is seen in the more elderly. This vagally mediated bradycardia can be treated by PPM.

287. AV Blocks: (see D 255–268)

First, second and third degree block suggest the problem at the AV node. All three variants involve the associatlon between the P wave and the QRS complex. Since the problem is not with the SA node or the ventricular polarization itself, then both the P wave and QRS complex commonly looks normal. The association between sinus node and ventricles are seen to be different, and this is because they are connected via the AV node.

Causes of AV Block:

1. Acute myocardial infarction/ischemia due to degeneration or idiopathic fibrosis of conducting system.
2. Drugs: β-blockers, verapamil, digoxin, Class I antiarrhythmic drugs.
3. Infection: Diphtheria, rheumatic fever, endocarditis, Lyme disease.
4. Infiltration: Sarcoidosis, syphilis, scleroderma, tumor, calcific aortic stenosis.

First degree block does not require any active treatment.

Second degree Mobitz type I (Wenckebach) has a lower chance of progressing to thrid degree block. Pacemaker implantation is not mandatory without evidence of correlated symptoms or undue bradycardia.

Mobitz type II second degree block usually indicates an extensive infranodal abnormality and therefore, except in there context of an acutely reversible condition, requires a permanent pacemaker.

Third degree AV block: P waves cannot conduct the impulses through "broken" AV node. The lonely ventricle are electrically separated from the atrium usually produces its own slow heart rhythm. Often this starts from the beginning of His-Purkinje system leading to a narrow QRS complex. If the QRS complex arises more distally, then the complex cannot be propagated in the normal manner. Therefore, it takes longer time to transmit across the ventricle and therefore the QRS looks wider.

(see Fig. D 46–49)

A permanent pacemaker is essential even if asymptomatic, as there is risk of sudden death.

Agonal rhythm: This is a slow irregular rhythm with wide and bizarre QRS complexes of varying morphology which is often seen at the end stage of unsuccessful resuscitation attempts as the heart dies. The complexes become progressively border before the end stage, there is no mechanical activity (EMD electromechanical dissociation); this is also a rate pre-terminal arrhythmia.

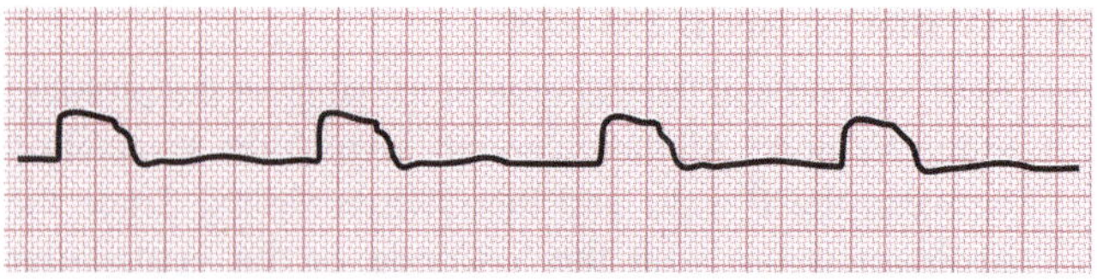

Fig. D-52

Cardiac asystole or arrest not really a bradycardia, rather complete absence of both atrial and ventricular activity with a straight line in the ECG. It most commonly follows ventricular fibrillation or prolonged episodes of electromechanical dissociation (EMD) and always signifies cardiac death. This fatal arrhythmia requires immediate cardiopulmonary resuscitation (CPR), and intravenous epinephrine/atropine are the only drugs that might rarely revive the patient.

If the ECG shows straight line of asystole and the patient is speaking to you then one has to check that your leads are properly attached. If P waves are persisting but no ventricular activity then it is called ventricular standstill.

The emergency treatment of most bradycardias is atropine, pacemaker or sympathomimetic drugs such as adrenaline or isoprenaline. Immediate treatment needs when there is a hemodynamic consequence of arrhythmias, which is significant when the rate drops below 40 per minute.

Bradycardia can occur just because someone is fit, many professional athletes have a heart rate around 40 bpm.

Bradycardia is also a major cause of blackouts and it is very difficult to diagnose when it occurs rarely and is intermittent. Patients who have blackout will not always be aware of truly losing consciousness and many 'remember' tripping over.

Rarely ever the occasional case of epilepsy can be cured with a pacemaker.

CLINICAL APPROACH TO CARDIAC TACHYARRHYTHMIAS

Two distinct cardiac entities are frightening to the physician—they are acute myocardial infarction and arrhythmias more; so if the former is associated with the latter. The arrhythmias are broadly classified into bradyarrhythmias and tachyarrhythmias. The tachyarrhythmias at bedside are described into supraventricular (above the bundle of His) and ventricular. The supraventricular are not life-threatening, while the ventricular ones are life-threatening by virtue of their low cardiac output. Usually supraventricular arrhythmias patient comes for check-up routinely, whereas the patient with dangerous ventricular arrhythmias who may be sweating, breathless and anxious is brought by the attendees.

There can be an error of overtreating benign arrhythmias and less treating malignant or dangerous arrhythmias. Usual impression is that ventricular arrhythmias cannot be tolerated by the patient. This error is common with premature ventricular contractions (PVCs).

The selection and usage of drugs are important as the antiarrhythmic drugs are proarrhythmic also. Class IA, IB are very useful in acute myocardial infarction, and ventricular tachyarrhythmias. Class IC are used in very resistant arrhythmias. β-blockers are used in supraventricular tachycardias and in some ventricular arrhythmias when the left ventricular ejection fraction is good. Although Class III amiodarone has efficacy in a wide range of arrhythmias. The food and drug administration (FDA) in USA has recommended it only as oral therapy for life-threatening ventricular arrhythmias refractory to all other forms of treatment. Class IV calcium blockers are useful only in supraventricular tachyarrhythmias but it worsens the WPW syndrome as it has no action on arrhythmias caused by accessory pathways. Caution is taken when they are used with other drugs like digoxin, anticoagulants in conditions like atrial fibrillation.

All arrhythmias do not need drug treatment. Almost all antiarrhythmic drugs depress left ventricular function limiting their use in LV dysfunction except amiodarone. This is also given in tachyarrhythmias with LV dysfunction but restricted in bradyarrhythmias. Most drugs cause new arrhythmias or aggravate old ones especially in patients with structural heart disease and EF $< 40\%$ and these are sometimes difficult to diagnosis making the management troublesome.

When a patient is brought with a dangerous arrhythmia in collapsed condition, immediately assess the airway, breathing, circulation (follow the ABC of cardiac arrest) and first start immediate treatment administer oxygen do quick physical examination, get 12 lead ECG and with single long lead if required, start IV lifeline. Hemodynamically unstable patient may need immediate external cardiac massage and electrical cardioversion.

288. There are 4 important points to know in the history.

1. i. History of myocardial infarction: If arrhythmias are coming after myocardial infarction—90% of them are ventricular arrhythmias. Hence, this group needs immediate treatment.
   ii. Is it associated with chest pain? Ischemic heart diseases are associated with chest pain.
   iii. Is it associated with sudden thumping in the chest or palpitation?
   iv. Any previous history of arrhythmias.

2. Relation to precipitating factors:
   i. Are they precipitated by exertion
   Even little exertion precipitates in some especially in older people.
   ii. Is there any particular posture that increases arrhythmia? If a patient can tell at what position it produces – this usually a benign PVC.
   iii. Too much of alcohol during holidays can cause arrhythmias—'Holiday Heart'.
   iv. Coffee, tea, anxiety, etc. can cause arrhythmias. For some patients, however, one has to try to reduce or stop their ectopic activity by eliminating 'trigger' factors, such as caffeine, smoking, alcohol, stress, fatigue, or unnecessary antiarrhythmic drugs.
3. How are the previous episodes terminated?
   Sudden onset and sudden termination is suggestive of paroxysmal tachycardia. Paroxysmal atrial tachycardias rarely cause death but they are nuisance arrhythmias. Paroxysmal atrial tachycardias occasionally terminated by simple holding of breath, cough, drinking sips of water.
   Is he on digitalis or any other drug?
4. History of sudden syncope or blackouts.
   Mostly suggestive of ventricular arrhythmias.

289. Also note in the history.

1. Past history of rheumatic fever in childhood.
2. History of severe illness or other infections that might predispose to viral myocarditis or cardiomyopathy.
3. Past history of MI.
4. Family history of premature sudden deaths since this may rise the suspicion of long QT syndrome, which is hereditary.

290. Clinical examination of tachyarrhythmias:

One can only suspect arrhythmias by clinical examination but the confirmation has to be done by ECG.

General examination and CVS examination should be done thoroughly to establish the arrhythmia and as well as their underlying cause. Patient who is pallor sweating, anxious, with fall of BP is more in favor of dangerous ventricular tachyarrhythmia. Patient's general condition is less serious in supraventricular tachycardias.

Do the routine examination of anemia, jaundice, cyanosis, clubbing, edema, JVP, etc.

Special attention is paid to the following 4 features in CVS examination for tachyarrhythmias.

1. Rate: Atrial and ventricular rate.
   Ventricular rate more than 150/min is usually ventricular tachycardia.
2. Rhythm: Regularly irregular or irregularly irregular.
   Irregularly irregular with pulse deficit is atrial fibrillation.
   Occasional ectopics or frequent ectopics.
3. Response to carotid sinus pressure:
   If there is response to carotid sinus pressure it is supraventricular tachyarrhythmia—even though ECG shows broad QRS, which probably is caused by aberrant pathway or pre-existing BBB.
4. Signs of AV dissociation.

291. The following 4 signs are to be looked for AV dissociation.

1. JVP: If irregular cannon 'a' waves are seen. It is suggestive of AV dissociation—Atria and ventricles beat on their own way. Atria contracts against closed atrioventricular valve. It is suggestive of ventricular tachycardia.
   Regular cannon 'a' waves are seen in junctional rhythm. 'a' waves are absent in atrial fibrillation.
   Progressive delay between the 'a' wave and carotid pulse with a missed beat is called Wenckebach phenomenon—Mobitz type I block.
2. Varying volume of pulse: Some beats have good contraction and some with less contraction. So, ventricular filling is affected.
3. Varying intensity of S1: It is in favor of AV dissociation. Sometimes—AV valves widely open and closes narrowly—full proof of AV dissociation so, it is ventricular tachycardia. Listen for clicks and murmurs in left lateral position for gallop. Mild systolic click identify the presence of mitral valve prolapse (MVP), which is commonly associated with ventricular tachyarrhythmias. See for anything that suggests severe valvular heart disease or left ventricular aneurysm. If cardiomegaly is apparent on clinical examination or X-ray needs thorough investigation.
4. Fusion beats or capture beats in ECG are in favor of AV dissociation.
   AV node is refractory, incapable of conducting functionally. Some beats can pass through AV node. P wave is upright, marching through captured beat.

The 4 common causes of irregular pulse.
(See Chapter A-69)
The 4 methods that help to differentiate the irregular pulse clinically at the bed side (assuming that you do not have ECG) (See Chapter A-70)
The 4 common causes of a regular pulse of 170–190 beats per minute in a person at rest.
(See Chapter A-71)

292. There are 4 findings to be studied systematically in ECG for diagnosing the arrhythmias.

ECG findings correlated: Routine ECG is sufficient to make an accurate diagnosis of rhythm and conduction disturbances.

ECG helps to distinguish the two rhythm disturbances which are considered as

- 'Triggering arrhythmias', such as premature atrial or ventricular contractions.
- 'Sustained or potentially lethal arrhythmias', such as supraventricular or ventricular tachycardias ventricular fibrillation, bradyarrhythmias.

Sir Thomas Lewis used the electrocardiographic findings in ladder diagrams freely for analyzing the cardiac arrhythmias. They are sometimes called as Lewis lines.

Study the information of:

1. P wave
2. QRS wave
3. PR interval
4. RR interval.

1. **P wave:** This is the single most important element in the diagnosis of arrhythmias P wave is caused by depolarization of atria.

   Know the P wave for

   i. Rate and rhythm
   ii. Morphology
   iii. Axis
   iv. Preceding of QRS (relation to QRS).
   First recognize P wave. Absence of P wave is suggestive of ventricular or junctional arrhythmia

   P wave is better seen in inferior leads L II, L III, aVF

   Superoinferior—L II

   Inferosuperior—L III, aVF

   Height of P wave—more than 2.5 mm is suggestive of—(amplitude) right atrial hypertrophy

   Width of P wave—more than 2.5 mm is suggestive of—(duration) left atrial hypertrophy

   If both height and width of P wave are more than 2.5 mm, it is suggestive of biatrial hypertrophy. Hypertrophy predisposes to arrhythmias. Atrial ectopics are first activated in left atrium.

   Morphology—note whether

   monomorphic—unifocal origin

   polymorphic—multifocal origin.

   Ectopic rhythms may have P waves with polarity similar to that of sinus P waves but different in shape or they may be difficult to differentiate from retrograde P waves of atrioventricular origin. P waves of atrial tachycardia in digitalis toxicity look as normal direction but of small amplitude and 'P' intervals are slightly irregular.

   Multifocal atrial tachycardia or also called chaotic atrial tachycardia is diagnosed when ectopic P waves vary in shape and P 'P' intervals: Sawtooth in atrial flutter 'F' waves—Fibrillary waves in atrial fibrillation.

   Axis—denotes the direction of activation

   If P is inverted in L II, L III, aVF means atria are activated in the retrograde fashion.

   Occasionally, P is inverted in L I it means the left atrium is activated first and later right atrium.

   Note: P inversion in L I, is seen in dextrocardia.

   Atrial ectopics are first activated in left atrium.

   Sometimes, in difficult cases of atrial tachyarrhythmias, e.g. atrial fibrillation with rapid ventricular rate and in atrial flutter with fixed 2:1 block—increase the AV nodal refractoriness either by carotid sinus massage or giving edrophonium to slow the ventricular rate thereby seeing the atrial activity—'P' waves in ECG.

   Use the calipers for measuring the intervals and "marching out" the waves—especially P waves are invaluable.

   If more than one arrhythmia is present, consider one at a time. If two independent pacemakers are firing, either parasystole or AV conduction disorder is present.

2. **QRS complex**: QRS is caused by ventricular depolarization.

   Measure the QRS duration.

   Simultaneous: Narrow QRS less than 0.12 sec means both ventricles are simultaneously depolarized.

   Sequential: Broad QRS—more than 0.12 sec

   One ventricle is activated later.

   Narrow QRS tachycardia is suggestive of supraventricular tachycardia.

   Broad QRS tachycardia is suggestive of ventricular tachycardia or supraventricular tachycardia with aberrant conduction or pre-exiting BBB.

   In ventricular tachycardia: QRS is broad and the RR intervals are regular.

   If QRS is broad and RR interval is irregular first diagnose atrial fibrillation.

   Broad QRS can exist in supraventricular arrhythmias also.

   QRS is 0.14 sec ventricular tachycardia or supraventricular with aberrant conduction.

   Broader the QRS, it is more likely to be ventricular.

   Broad QRS with left axis deviation of more than 30° is in favor of ventricular tachycardia.

   Even in broad QRS tachycardias, if it could be terminated by carotid sinus pressure—it is supraventricular though it is broad–probably of aberrant pathway.

   Observe QRS morphology:

   Monomorphic—unifocal ectopics

   Polymorphic—multifocal ectopics

   Wide QRS—RSR pattern seen with blocks.

   PVBs couplets with a short run of VT are quiet evident.

3. **PR interval**—atrioventricular conduction

   If more than 0.2 sec—it can be AV block or AV dissociation

   If less than 0.12 sec—there can be an accessory pathway.

Observe whether the interval is constant or changing? Is there any RP interval, i.e. ventriculoatrial conduction>

4. **RR intervals**: Regular in ventricular tachycardia though QRS is broad.
If RR intervals are irregularly irregular, first think of atrial fibrillation even though QRS is wide. Broad QRS can be supraventricular tachycardia also.
So, see for QRS and RR interval.
If R-on-T phenomenon is seen in the presence of symptoms, always consider the possibility of torsades de points, so QT interval should be carefully measured. Torsades de pointes is an important arrhythmia, but it is very rare in ambulatory patients except in patients with a congenitally long QT interval. It is usually due to type I antiarrhythmic agents such as quinidine, procinonide, disopyramide, or to electrolyte abnormality.

293. There are 4 special methods to know about P waves.

1. Lewis lead—modified lead I: Left atrial ECG by esophageal electrode: lead in esophagus behind the atrium or lead in the coronary sinus.
2. Right atrial ECG is taken by transvenous catheter in the right atrium. Intra-atrial—pacing wire directly in the atrium.
3. Intracardiac electrography—within the cavity of the atrium.
4. Direct atrial—suturing the wires to the atria for both diagnostic and therapeutic information.
By utilizing these leads, one can recognize the total disorganization as in atrial fibrillation or regular rhythm in atrial flutter.

294. A simple plan for diagnosing common tachyarrhythmias on an ECG.

The common tachyarrhythmias which need immediate treatment are six—Paroxysmal supraventricular tachycardia, atrial flutter, atrial fibrillation, junctional tachycardia, ventricular tachycardia, and ventricular fibrillation.

A. Normal looking thin and tall QRS complexes are supraventricular.
   1. Regular: Paroxysmal supraventricular arrhythmia tachycardia or atrial flutter within regular block or junctional tachycardia.
   Look for P wave to differentiate, if present its relationship to the QRS complex.
   2. Irregular: Atrial fibrillation or atrial flutter with variable block.

B. Large wide 'ugly' QRS complexes are ventricular or supraventricular with aberrant pathway or LBBB.
   3. Regular: Ventricular tachycardia or paroxysmal supraventricular tachycardia with left bundle branch block.
   4. Irregular: Ventricular fibrillation or atrial fibrillation with left bundle branch block or the Wolff-Parkinson-White syndrome.

295. The 4 common narrow QRS supraventricular tachycardias which are automatic.

1. Sinus tachycardia
2. Ectopic atrial tachycardia
   a. Unifocal b. Multifocal
3. Ectopic junctional tachycardia
4. Idiojunctional tachycardia.

296. The 4 common narrow QRS supraventricular tachycardias which are reentrant.

1. Sinus tachycardia
2. Atrial tachycardia
3. Atrial flutter
4. AV nodal tachycardia
   a. slow-fast b. fast-slow.

Others like atrial fibrillation, sinus rhythm with simultaneous conduction via both slow and fast pathways.

Any of the above 'narrow QRS' tachycardias may show wide QRS when it is associated with aberration or pre-existing BBB.

297. There are 4 wide QRS tachycardias of ventricular origin.

1. Monomorphous ventricular tachycardia
   a. automatic b. reentrant
2. Dimorphous ventricular tachycardia
   a. alternating b. bidirectional
3. Polymorphous ventricular tachycardia
   Torsades de pointes
   Jervell and Lange-Neil son syndrome
4. Ventricular flutter
   Any supraventricular tachycardias with aberration or pre-exiting BBB can cause wide QRS tachycardias.

298. There are 4 common causes of error in the diagnosis of ventricular tachycardia while studying ECG.

Primarily the physician is under the belief that ventricular tachycardias cannot be tolerated.

1. Depending on a single lead reading especially L II
2. Ignorance or neglect of studying QRS morphology
3. Depending on the study of independent atrial activity
4. Putting more faith in irregularity.

299. Follow the 4 steps in unknown supraventricular tachyarrhythmia tracing.

1. Look for any failure of AV conduction
2. Look for QRS alternation
3. Note the position of P wave in cardiac cycle
4. Note the P wave axis in frontal plane.
   P wave polarity in horizontal plane.

300. There are 4 points to distinguish supraventricular ectopic tachycardia from reentrant supraventricular tachycardia.

Table D-16

Supraventricular ectopic tachycardia	Supraventricular re-entrant tachycardia
1. Shows 'warm-up' Progressive acceleration for the first few beats	Do not show 'warm-up'
2. Similar P waves in all including the first	P waves differ from subsequent (retrograde) P waves
3. 'Resetting' of the tachycardia by a premature stimulus just as an atrial extrasystole resets the sinus	Premature stimulus does not 'reset' but it may terminate even the tachycardia
4. Prolongation of the first PR interval is not the rule	Prolongation of the first PR interval is the rule

301. The following investigations are done to evaluate cardiac arrhythmias.

1. Routine 12-lead resting ECG is sufficient to diagnose cardiac arrhythmias but special investigations are needed when difficulty arises, especially to know the organic lesion and in cases not responding to treatment. These are specially useful in conditions like PVBs where 12 lead ECG may reveal only 10–40% of cases.
2. *Exercise test:* It may be important to know if exercise makes an arrhythmia worse. During exercise test, the patient will walk and run on a treadmill—or ride a stationary bicycle—while the heart rate and rhythm are monitored. This is painless but requires patient's cooperation. It is done for 15–20 minutes. It reveals 50–60% PVBs. Exercise lowers the vagal tone and PVBs increase sympathetic tone. This test will unfold the ischemic zone to give a clue to the organic problem which can also be treated. It unfolds some of the arrhythmias. PVBs which come on exercise testing respond well to the β-blockers.
3. *Continuous ambulatory electrocardiographic monitor (Holter's 24 hour monitoring):*
Sometimes an ordinary ECG shows no abnormality, even when it is repeated several times. Continuous electrocardiographic monitoring is used to make long ECG tracings. Holter's monitoring is named after the person who devised it.
The ECG is a sort of a "snap shot" of the heart's electrical activity. It records about 12 seconds of the heart's electrical activity. Holter's monitor in contrast, is more like a "movie" of the heart's electrical activity. It records for a long period of time.
In Holter monitoring, electrodes are placed on the chest and taped to the body. The wires are connected to a portable, battery-operated recorder that can run for 24 to 48 hours. The patient can do most normal activities while being tested. Then the tape is analyzed on a computer that can rapidly identify rhythm disturbances. It reveals about 80–90% of PVBs. It is useful in determining the range of ventricular rate in atrial flutter and fibrillation and helps in knowing the adequacy of treatment. Inappropriate rapid ventricular response during activity is significant of inadequate treatment. Useful in cases where sudden transitory attacks of palpitation or blockouts are complained, of which clinical examination and routine ECG are normal. This test will bring out abnormalities which are missed by routine ECG.
4. *Transtelephonic monitor/Event recorder:* Sometimes the symptoms of arrhythmia happen infrequently, or do not last enough for you to get to a doctor or hospital. In these cases, a " transient event monitor" may be used. These small recorders are sent home with a patient for one to two months. When the patient has symptoms, the recorder is attached with bracelets, finger clips or patches under the arms, and the ECG is recorded and stored in the device. When it is convenient patient can transmit the ECG by telephone to his cardiologist to be analyzed.
5. *Echocardiogram:* It is a simple, painless test that often provides valuable information about the heart of a person with arrhythmia (See point 269).
6. *Tilt test:* A tilt test may be recommended for some patients who had recurrent fainting spells (syncope). This test shows how the patient's heart rate and blood pressure respond to a change in position from lying down to standing up. To perform this test, an IV line is usually started. A catheter also may be placed in the artery to monitor blood pressure. In some cases, medications will be given through the intravenous route. If a cause of the fainting spell is found, medications can be given through the IV line to help to prevent the episodes. This information will help to find the best way to treat these patients.
7. *Esophageal electrophysiologic procedure:* In this procedure, a thin, soft, flexible plastic tube is inserted and positioned in the esophagus. Since the esophagus is close to the atria, an ECG recording there gives more precise information than a regular ECG. An electrical stimulator may be used to make the heartbeat faster to try to restart the patient's arrhythmia.
During this procedure certain medications may be tested to find the one that will be most effective.

The esophageal electrophysiologic procedure also may be performed to temporarily stop certain types of arrhythmias.

8. *Electrophysiological studies by intracardiac electrography:* It is invasive. In this one or more long catheters are placed into the large blood vessels in the legs, arms or both. Then the tips of the catheters are moved into the heart. Once in the heart, the catheters are placed in different chambers of the heart and arrhythmias are induced, analyzed, and drugs tried. Their efficacy is also noted. By using these intracardiac leads in atrial fibrillation, it is distinguished from regular rhythm in atrial flutter by its total disorganization.
If late potentials (having high frequency) are recorded, a recurrent ventricular tachycardia can be predicted and care is taken before hand.

302. Reasons for Holter monitoring.

1. To correlated symptoms with arrhythmia. Frequently palpitations occur in the absence of arrhythmia establishing the absence of relationship indicates, that trying to treat palpitations with antiarrhythmic drugs is not appropriate. Sometimes, cause of ventricular arrhythmia has not been established despite many symptoms.
2. To document mode of onset and termination of arrhythmia—whether drugs are reducing or aggravating the arrhythmia.
3. To determine whether AV block is an initiating factor.
4. To determine whether ischemia initiates or accompanies arrhythmia, i.e. ST depression or elevation precedes arrhythmia.
Presence of CAD, PVBs or complex ventricular ectopies has shown to be a marker of sudden death. LV dysfunction, especially LV ejection fraction of < 30%, is the strongest independent predictor of mortality.

303. Exercise test: Indications

1. The first indication is a history that suggests exertion as a precipitating factor.
2. Second is to know if there is any likelihood of ischemic heart disease—ST segment changes—if present to know whether it is related to arrhythmia or independent.
3. Third in some needlessly worried patients should be reassured that exercise will not harm them, and worried parents should be assured that exercise will not harm their children. This is especially important for young active people who have occasional ectopy and PVBs on routine examination.
4. Fourth is to assess the effects of therapy.

304. Four types of patients should be thought of:

1. Patients whose quality of life is compromised by palpitations whether they have heart disease or not and who simply cannot function because of their symptoms.
2. Patients who have been resuscitated from sudden death.
3. Patients with ventricular tachycardia with possible exceptions of teenagers with benign tachycardia.
4. Patients with PVBs in the presence of CAD, especially those with history of MI or evidence of myocardial impairment such as poor LV function (EF < 30%).

305. Intracardiac electrography gives the final judgment in difficult cases of arrhythmias.

It can differentiate.

1. Origin of wide QRS complex—ventricular tachycardia from supraventricular tachycardia with aberrant pathway.
2. Site of accessory pathway in Wolff-Parkinson-White syndrome.
3. The level of AV block—above or below the bundle of His and to distinguish genuine AV block from pseudo-block caused by concealed junctional extrasystoles.
4. To evaluate sinus node function.

306. Electrophysiological studies (EPS) are indicated in the following settings.

1. Frequent drug intolerance or drug refractory arrhythmia
2. In some patients prior to initiating with type IC drug treatment
3. Severe hemodynamic symptoms with PSVT
4. WPW syndrome with symptomatic SVT
5. WPW syndrome with AF or syncope
6. High-risk professionals
7. Patients who desire nonpharmacological therapy
8. Young age
9. Documented sudden death episode of without MI, i.e. ventricular fibrillation
10. Symptomatic VT with runs spaced too far apart in ambulatory monitoring or selected patients with recurrent sustained VT
11. Patients before and after initiation of experimental drug therapy, unless their tachycardia is frequent enough to establish response
12. Patients with neurological symptoms (e.g. syncope) but no evidence of neurologic cause.
At this point, we have seen VT on ECG/or Holter monitor and aggravated or not aggravated with exercise test. Now, should we treat the patient empirically or send him to EP studies?
Any patient with sustained VT should have an EP test. An exception is the patient with torsades de

pointes secondary to a known treatable cause, such as hypokalemia.

307. Echocardiography is useful to know the organic lesions in the heart that cause arrhythmias and left ventricular function to help the treatment. Following are few examples.

1. Mitral stenosis—cause of atrial fibrillation.
   Left atrial size is noted before planning for cardioversion.
2. Mitral valve prolapse—premature ventricular contractions are frequent in this condition.
3. Cardiomyopathies—dilated, hypertrophic, restrictive, endomyocardial fibrosis—give rise to arrhythmias.
4. Left ventricular aneurysm—aneurysmal dilatation can give rise to arrhythmias.
   Congenital heart diseases, valvular heart diseases, ischemic heart diseases, pericaridal diseases that can cause arrhythmias can be identified by echocardiography.
   It is also useful in evaluating functional status of the heart.
   Hypokinesis, akinesis, dyskinesis, left ventricular end-diastolic pressure (LVEDP), ejection fraction (EF), etc. are all helpful in the treatment of arrhythmias. Premature ventricular contractions are frequent in chronic ischemic heart diseases, cardiomyopathies accompanied by reduced ejection fraction.

308. Assessment of cardiac tachyarrhythmias is done by following 4 steps before planning the treatment.

1. *Where is the site and type of disorder?*
   a. Anatomical site–SA node, Atria, AV node, ventricle
   b. Rate disorder or rhythm disorder
   Tachycardia or bradycardia
   Tachyarrhythmia or bradyarrhythmia.
2. *What is the form of arrhythmia?*
   a. Triggering arrhythmias,
      e.g. premature atrial contractions
      Premature ventricular contractions
      Unifocal or multifocal
      Benign or malignant.
   b. Sustained or potentially lethal arrhythmias:
      Supraventricular tachycardia
      Ventricular tachycardia ventricular flutter
      Majority of the sustained arrhythmias are re-entrants.
3. *When does the arrhythmias occur in the clinical setting?*
   a. Acute, transient
      During acute myocardial infarction—more dangerous
      Arrhythmias during cardiac catheterization; Cardiac surgery or reperfusion after thrombolytic therapy are transient—respond well to treatment
      Metabolic disorders
   b. Chronic persistent, recurrent arrhythmias
      Chronic ischemic heart diseases
      Cardiomyopathy
      Atrial tachycardias seen after myocardial infarction or myocarditis may be distressing and resistant to treatment.
4. *Do they have cardiac origin or noncardiac origin?*
   a. Cardiac origin, e.g. acute myocardial infarction
      Ischemic heart disease
      Cardiomyopathy, myocarditis, cardiac failure
      Hypertensive heart disease
      Coronary heart disease
      Mitral valve prolapse—PVBs are frequent
      Mitral stenosis—Atrial fibrillation
      Pericardial diseases.
   b. Noncardiac origin:
      For example, Pulmonary: Pulmonary embolism
      Chronic obstructive lung disease.

   Endocrinal:
   Hyperthyroidism—Premature atrial contractions
   Paroxysmal atrial tachycardia.
   Atrial flutter
   Patients of thyrotoxicosis may have atrial fibrillation in 10–25%
   Hypothyroidism: Pericardial effusion, increased incidence of coronary heart disease.
   Diabetes mellitus: Coronary atherosclerosis, cardiomyopathy
   Cardiac autonomic neuropathy—causes silent myocardial infarction.
   Primary aldosteronism—hypertensive heart disease
   Pheochromocytoma
   Oral contraceptives—cause increased incidence of coronary artery disease.
   Electrolyte disturbance:
   Hypercalcemia—shortening of ST segment and QT interval
   Hypocalcemia—prolongation of ST segment and QT interval
   Hyperkalemia—various bradyarrhythmias
   Hypokalemia—supraventricular tachycardias, ventricular ectopics.

309. Where is the origin of arrhythmia?

There are 4 sites to look for the origin.

1. SA node
   - Sinus tachycardias
   - Sinus bradytachyarrhythmias

2. Atrium
   - Atrial premature contractions (APCs)
   - Paroxysmal atrial tachycardia
   - Atrial flutter
   - Atrial fibrillation.
3. AV node
   - Junctional—junctional paroxysmal tachycardia or
   - Nonparoxysmal tachycardia
   - They cause nuisance to the patient. They rarely cause death.
4. Ventricular
   - Nonsustained
   - Premature ventricular contractions (PVCs)
   - Sustained—ventricular tachycardia
   - Ventricular flutter
   - Ventricular fibrillation.

310. There are 4 methods of treating cardiac arrhythmias.

1. Drugs
2. Electrical therapy of cardiac arrhythmias
   a. Direct current cardioversion
   b. Antitachycardia pacemakers
   c. Automatic Implantable cardioverter/defibrillator (ICD).
3. Catheter ablation using
   i. Direct current
   ii. Radiofrequency.
4. Surgery

   The question of drug versus electrical therapy.

   Direct current (DC shock) and/or pacemakers often arises in institutions.

   The drug therapy is chosen in most of our hospital settings.

   Pacing in tachyarrhythmias is by overdrive suppression.

311. There are 4 most important principles of using antiarrhythmic drugs for controlling any arrhythmia. Treat those patients who are

1. Symptomatic
2. Having malignant arrhythmias such as ventricular tachycardia or fibrillation
3. Hemodynamically compromised—for example with hypertension
4. In heart failure
5. Palpitations that compromised quality of patient's life
6. Sudden deaths survivor
7. Propensity for sustained VT
8. PVBs or nonsustained VT + CAD + MI or other myocardial impairment.

   Reassurance often improves the quality of patient's life. Many antiarrhythmic drugs depress cardiac function and may precipitate heart failure. Most of the antiarrhythmic drugs especially Class I agents are proarrhythmic, can aggravate or cause an arrhythmia. Therefore, treatment with antiarrhythmic drugs should be avoided when a patient has only mild and infrequent symptoms. This strategy is justified by evidence of substantial morbidity and worsened by long-term prognosis.

312. Aims of treatment of tachyarrhythmias depend upon clinical setting and mechanism of arrhythmias.

1. Control of ventricular rate:

   Antitachycardiac, antifibrillatory or heart rate supporting treatment in which the aim is prevention or reversion of sustained or potentially lethal arrhythmias whether they are well-tolerated, symptomatic or life-threatening.
2. Converting into normal sinus rhythm:

   Antidysrhythmic treatment targeted to the suppression of triggering arrhythmias or events of acute episode.
3. Correction of precipitating factors:

   Which interact with the underlying etiology, e.g. hemodynamic, metabolic and respiratory abnormalities. Drug induced.
4. Management of specific underlying cardiac disease, e.g. acute myocardial infarction

   Chronic ischemic heart diseases

   Cardiomyopathies, myocarditis

   Pericarditis

   Valvular diseases

   WPW syndrome.

   The goals are to prevent ventricular fibrillation, prevent or suppress tachycardia or at least slow it to a tolerable rate, and prevent arrhythmias, PVBs.

   Also consider the individualized approach according to age, life expectancy, temperament, and lifestyle, and regardless of the arrhythmia.

313. The 4 principles to be followed in the treatment of cardiac arrhythmias are:

1. *To treat or not to treat.*

   There is a tendency of the physicians to expose patients to a proarrhythmic risk by drugs (all the antiarrhythmic drugs are proarrythmic also) unnecessarily, which may be having higher risk than the arrhythmia being treated. There often exists a conflict between the need to treat and the urge to treat. This often happens in premature ventricular contractions (PVC); PVCs do not need any treatment in the vast majority of patients, e.g. benign PVCs do not need treatment.

   Run's of PVCs, multiple PVCs, multifocal—malignant—need treatment especially in post-myocardial infarction.

2. *Symptomatic:* Palpitation/Hemodynamic collapse. Sudden thumping or palpitation of paroxysmal ventricular tachycardias are not serious. Whereas ventricular arrhythmias occurring after acute myocardial infarction are dangerous. They should be promptly treated. PVCs occurring in acute myocardial infarction are 'warning arrhythmias' of more serious ventricular tachycardias and ventricular fibrillation.
3. *Risk:* Disability/Death.
   Arrhythmias that cause disabilities should be analyzed in regard to specific etiology.
   For example, PVCs that occur frequently with mitral valve prolapse are of low risk than PVCs that occur with dilated cardiomyopathy. In general, supraventricular arrhythmias are less risk than ventricular arrhythmias.
   Deaths that occur in first hour to 24 hours in acute myocardial infarction are maxim due to ventricular tachyarrhythmias—ventricular tachycardia, ventricular flutter and fibrillation.
4. *Underlying heart disease and left ventricular dysfunction:* Arrhythmias that occur in acute myocardial infarction are dangerous and should be promptly treated. Underlying cause of atrial fibrillation such as mitral stenosis should be surgically corrected. Arrhythmias of aberrant pathways respond well to ablation or surgical correction, e.g. WPW syndrome.

314. Following basics or to be followed while managing all cases of arrhythmias.

1. Continues cardiac monitoring done and defibrillator should be at hand.
2. Start IV line and give oxygen.
3. Send the blood for electrolytes and blood gas analysis in severe cases.
4. If pulse is not felt, start cardiac arrest protocols.

315. Drug selection and dosage details of administration in cardiac arrhythmias vary depending mostly upon.

1. Clinical situation:
   Acute episode—in first 24–48 hours of acute myocardial infarction—life-threatening arrhythmias.
   Late myocardial infarction arrhythmias.
   Chromic recurrent, persistent arrhythmias.
   Electrolyte status of the patient.
2. Concomitant drug therapy, e.g. digitalis, certain drugs increases digitoxicity.
   Complication with anticoagulants.
   Synergistic actions.
3. Existence of renal or hepatic dysfunction.
   Excretion and metabolization are interfered.
   Dose has to be adjusted.
4. Patient's acceptance and tolerance of the medication. Long duration of medication is needed in chronic persistent arrhythmias.

316. Arrhythmias should be treated since they are harmful to the patient because they cause:

1. Reduction in cardiac output
2. Lower the blood pressure
3. Reduces the perfusion of vital organs, e.g. brain, heart, kidney, etc.
4. In the presence of heart disease they precipitate acute heart failure, pulmonary edema, angina pectoris or myocardial infarction.
   Syncope or poor cerebration with confusion.
   Pulmonary embolism or cerebral embolism.

317. Table of arrhythmias and drugs recommended.

Table D-17

Arrhythmias	*Recommended drugs*
1. Supraventricular	Usually nil
2. Chronic heart disease	Mexiletine, quinidine, disopyramide, procainamide, consider amiodarone in refractory cases
3. Supraventricular tachycardia	Carotid sinus massage, adenosine, verapamil, β-blockers, DC cardioversion
4. Atrial flutter or atrial fibrillation	Digoxin, quinidine, amiodarone, disopyramide, DC cardioversion consider anticoagulants
5. Premature ventricular contractions—Normal heart PVCs in the acute MI PVCs in post-MI	Usually nil Symptomatic – Anxiolytics, β-blockers, lidocaine, disopyramide, procainamide
6. Ventricular tachycardia in acute myocardial infarction	Lidocaine, procainamide, amiodarone, β-blockers IV, bretylium DC shock, pacing
7. Chronic ventricular tachycardia or ventricular flutter or fibrillation	Mexiletine, procainamide, disopyramide consider DC defibrillation
8. Arrhythmias after myocardial infarction	Mexiletine, procainamide, disopyramide
9. Cardiomyopathy (obstructive or nonobstructive)	Verapamil or β-blocker, type I drugs
10. QT prolongation	Stop all type I drug, ventricular overdrive pacing, correct electrolytes, correct bradycardia, β-blockers may shorten QT interval

Contd...

Contd...

Arrhythmias	*Recommended drugs*
11. Prolapsed mitral valve	β-blockers specific therapy of underlying infection or infiltrative disease
12. Idiopathic VT	Type I drugs, or amiodarone, mexiletine, tocainide

In case of suspected arrhythmia due to drugs– (digitalis, psychotropics) – stop causal drugs. In patients with digitalis use potassium, phenytoin, or β-blocking agents.

318. A simple plan for treating most of the tachyarrhythmias.

Table D-18

	Acute	*Long-term*
Supraventricular I. PSVT	Adenosine Verapamil IV	Disopyramide Quinidine
Atrial Flutter	? DC shock	Flecaimide β-blockers—associate with hypertension Thyrotoxisis— Amiodarone when resistant to other drugs
II. Atrial fibrillation	Digitalis (Recent onset)? ? DC shock	Digitalis
Ventricular III. Ventricular tachycardia	Xylocaine IV DC shock—overdrive pacing for recurrent cases	Flecainide Disopyramide Quinidine
Ventricular fibrillation	Blow on chest defibrillation	Amiodarone

319. Indications of cardiac pacemakers in arrhythmias can be classified into 4 broad groups.

I. *Pacing for bradycardias*
1. Sick sinus syndrome (SSS)
   a. Sinus bradycardia
   b. Sinoatrial block and sinus arrest
   c. Brady-tachy arrhythmias or sick sinus syndrome.
2. Acquired complete atrioventricular block.
   a. Complete AV block with Stokes-Adams seizures
   b. Asymptomatic complete heart block.
3. Congenital complete atrioventricular block
4. Atrial fibrillation with slow ventricular rates.

Although AF is usually not an indication for a pacemaker, some underlying conditions, such as sick sinus syndrome could necessitate the placement of a pacemaker.

II. *Pacing with normal heart rates*
1. Intermittent complete heart block
   a. "Bilateral bundle branch block"
   b. RBBB with axis deviation
   c. RBBB with first degree block
   d. LBBB with first degree block
2. Prevention of recurrent tachycardias
   a. Supraventricular tachycardia
   b. Ventricular tachycardia

III. *Pacing for conversion of tachycardias (overdrive pacing)*
1. Supraventricular
2. Wolff-Parkinson-White syndrome
3. Ventricular tachycardias

IV. *Special situations*
1. Acute myocardial infarction
   a. AV block
   b. Bundle branch block
   c. Sinus bradycardia
   d. Ventricular irritability
2. Pacemakers in cardiac surgery
3. Pacing during cardiac catheterization.

The first pacemaker inserted nearly 40 years ago was limited to pacing only one chamber at a fixed rate. Today's pacemakers consist of two major parts; a generator that houses a battery and electronic sensors, and the leads that connect into the heart. The generator provides a small electrical current that stimulates the heart to pump via the leads. Sophisticated electronic sensors provide continuous feedback and information from the heart instructing the pacemaker to compensate according to the bodies requirement.

There are two common types of pacemakers namely AV synchronous type and demand pacemaker.

In the AV synchronous type, one electrode is in the right atrium to stimulate the right atrial contraction and these after a small cause, the second electrode in the right ventricle stimulates the right ventricular contraction. The whole AV conduction takes place in a synchronized fashion.

In the demand pacemaker, it stimulates the ventricle regularly at a fixed rate that can be changed externally using another device. This has the advantage that the pacemaker gets switched off when the patients inherent rate is higher than has prefixed pacemaker rate. The demand pacemaker has two basic functions.

i. Sensing (sensing the patients own rhythm through the same pacing electrode) and
ii. Pacing ('capturing' function)—there are many new innovative types of pacemakers in the last four decades, which are beyond the scope of this book.

320. Complications of pacemaker:

1. Infection
2. Lead displacement
3. Myocardial perforation (more common in the past with stiff temporary leads)
4. Subclavian or superior vena caval thrombosis (rare).

321. Precautions for pacemaker.

1. Avoid direct blows on the pacemaker site
2. Avoid working with cellular phones and areas with pronounced electromagnetic interference
3. Avoid working with unipolar cautery machines during surgery
4. In case of any emergency for DC cardioversion, the paddles should be kept well away from the pacemaker pocket in a line perpendicular to the intracardiac axis of the electrodes.

322. Automatic implantable cardioverter-defibrillator: Often called an AICD includes a pulse generator and one or more leads that are surgically implanted in the body (below the left or right clavicle or on the abdomen (tummy area). The pulse generator, which constantly watches the heart beat, is like a small computer. It runs on a battery. The lead is a wire from the pulse generator that connects to the inside of the heart. The lead takes signals from the heart to the AICD and then takes energy from the pulse generator to the heart. How does the AICD work?

1. The AICD constantly "watches" the heart rhythm. If it "sees" any arrhythmia, it delivers the treatment programmed by the doctor.
2. Pacing: If there is ventricular tachycardia, the AICD can deliver several pacing signals in a row. When those signals stop, the heart may go back to a normal rhythm. No other treatment is needed.
3. Cardioversion: If the pacing does not work, cardioversion can be used. In cardioversion, a mild shock is sent to the heart to stop the tachycardia.
4. Defibrillation: If ventricular fibrillation is detected, a defibrillation shock is sent. This stronger shock can stop the fast rhythm and help the heartbeat go back to normal. The AICD can also "identify" bradycardia. It can act like a pacemaker and bring the heart rate up to normal.

323. What does the patient feel like with an AICD treatment?

1. Pacing a bradycardia uses very little energy. Patient may not feel this treatment at all.
2. Some people may not feel anything when the AICD delivers pacing therapy for ventricular tachycardia. Other people feel a fluttering in their chest. They usually say that it does not feel uncomfortable or painful.
3. Cardioversion is stronger than a pacing pulse. It feels like being thumped in the chest.
4. The defibrillator shock is the strongest treatment. Many people say it feels like being kicked in the chest. It usually comes suddenly and lasts only a second. Some people are upset for a short time after a defibrillation shock, but other people feel reassured that the AICD is treating their heart rhythm problem.

324. The advantages of automatic implantable cardioverter-defibrillator (AICD) are:

1. Therapeutic
   – Recurrent ventricular tachycardias/ventricular fibrillation
2. Supportive
   – Drugs/surgery
   – Concomitant drug therapy
3. Minimize
   – Frequency of ventricular tachycardia/ventricular fibrillation
4. Concomitant
   – Pacemaker and defibrillator in single unit.

325. Catheter ablation is a safe and curative option for most arrhythmias with 85–98% cure rates among the arrhythmias treated most frequently. The results have been born out by a recent large prospective multicenter study of 1050 patients, which provide further evidence of the benefit of catheter ablation. (Circulation 1999; 99:262-70). The study found overall cure rate of 95% and that a second procedure was required in 4% of patients. The rate of important complications related to the procedure was < 3%. The aim of catheter ablation is to eliminate the arrhythmias by locating and ablating the safest and most accessible point that will either transect and interrupt a reentrant circuit or eliminate a focus.

The catheter ablation that can reliably cure arrhythmias are:

1. Atrioventricular junctional reentrant tachycardia
2. Paroxysmal atrial tachycardias
3. Atrial flutter
4. WPW syndrome and some ventricular arrhythmias.

326. The only randomized trial comparing catheter ablation with drugs in the treatment of recurrent atrial flutter showed the following 4 advantages (Circulation 1998;98:315-22)

1. Better success rate
2. Greater impact on improving quality of life
3. Lower incidence of atrial fibrillation
4. Lower incidence of rehospitalization.

327. The patients that should be referred for catheter ablation includes:

1. Patients with indefinite drug treatment for arrhythmias particularly younger patients.
   (The older patients with long standing atrial fibrillation can be managed by controlling the ventricular rate and with anticoagulation treatment.)
2. Any patient with potentially life-threatening arrhythmias such as ventricular tachycardia.
3. WPW syndrome.
4. Those who have survived cardiac arrest.
   As a safe treatment, performed under local anesthesia, which is usually effective as a single procedure, catheter ablation is first choice treatment for most cardiac arrhythmias. Many eligible patients may not be referred for definitive treatment because the principles, techniques and availability of this procedure are not widely known. The number of cardiac departments with the expertise and facilities for catheter ablation is expanding and their facility is now widely available in all parts of the developed world. This is a cure that is safe, efficacious, and cost-effective. Although the word 'cure' is not widely applicable in medicine, it can now justifiably be used for the treatment of cardiac arrhythmias.

328. Surgery in cardiac arrhythmias is indicated in 4 conditions.

1. Refractory to drug therapy
2. Disabling paroxysmal/incessant arrhythmias
3. Life-threatening arrhythmias
4. Aborted episodes of sudden death.

329. Surgery is benefited in 4 ways.

1. It is cost effective
2. It is curative
3. Risk is only 0.5% with experienced surgeons
4. Useful in aberrant conduction pathways, e.g. WPW syndrome.

E Coronary Artery Disease/Ischemic Heart Disease

One of the preventable diseases prevalent worldwide is coronary artery disease (CAD), which has assumed epidemic proportions in India and allover the world. Coronary artery disease is still the most common cause of death. Prevalence rate has increased from 1.05% in 1960 to about 8–9.6% in 1990 in the urban population of India. It has been estimated that in India there are over 30 million people suffering from ischemic heart disease (Exact statistics are not available in India). About 10% of patients with coronary artery disease (CAD) die every year with an estimated number of deaths of about 24 lakhs. Prevalence of CAD and hypertension is fast approaching the western trends. Very soon we may be seeing heart diseases as severe and frequent as being reported in the West.

The disease is extensive, premature, severe and has an alarming course. It is increasingly and particularly affecting the younger generation between 20 and 40 years age group, the most productive years. For the 30–39 age group, the incidence of heart attacks is ten times that of western population groups. Moreover, the first heart attack is often massive. 54% of Indians vs 21% of Whites have all three coronary arteries involved often diffusely diseased, making them unsuitable for even for angioplasty or bypass surgery.

Asian Indians living overseas have up to three times more frequent heart attacks and up to 8 times more deaths due to CAD. Immigrant Indian physicians in the US have prevalence rates of CAD 3–4 times higher than native-born US physicians. It is estimated that Indians have six times as much CAD as the Chinese and twenty times as much as the Japanese. CAD has been prevalent worldwide in such an alarming proportions that both higher and lower socioeconomic state groups are suffering. On the one hand, those without funds for health care are dying in enormous numbers, and on the other, those who have health insurance or funds to pay for balloon angioplasty or bypass surgery have no guarantee of living more than a further five years. This is because the root causes of coronary artery disease are not being attended by the present approach.

Ischemic heart disease implies that coronary blood supply to the myocardium is inadequate as compared to its demands.

Ischemic heart disease is defined as a spectrum of disease of varied etiology which results in imbalance between myocardial oxygen supply and demand. Ischemia means lack of oxygen resulting from reduced perfusion.

Angina pectoris is a term used to describe discomfort or pain in the chest or adjacent areas due to transient myocardial ischemia and is associated with disturbance of myocardial function but without myocardial necrosis. It is a syndrome rather than a disease. Since its description by Heberden in 1768, angina pectoris has been Cinderella of medicine for research in cardiology. Epidemiology, electrophysiology, molecular biology, coronary imaging, nuclear cardiology and coronary endoscopy have revolutionized the concepts regarding etiopathogenesis, diagnosis and therapeutics of this syndrome. Cardiac interventions such as percutaneous transluminal coronary angioplasty (PTCA) have become the fashion of the day for its treatment from its discovery in 1977. Interventional procedures have rapidly grown in these two decades and about one million PTCAs are done every year now. Coronary artery bypass graft (CABG) is the surgical procedure of choice. Hence, it becomes imperative to evaluate the present day status of management of angina pectoris in the light of recent advances.

1. The fatal 4 'C's of developed countries are:

1. Cardiac failures e.g. AMI, IHD, HT, etc. Approximately one-third of all deaths result from coronary artery disease and almost all the elderly persons have at least some impairment of coronary artery circulation.
2. Cancer

3. Cerebrovascular accidents
4. Catastrophes like **Car** accidents, industrial accidents, agricultural accidents, etc.

2. USA Statistical estimates made in 1995 show that 58 million Americans have one or more forms of the following cardiovascular disease:

1. Hypertension
2. Coronary artery disease (CAD)
3. Peripheral arterial occlusive disease (PAOD)
4. Rheumatic heart disease

3. Cardiovascular diseases killed nearly

1. More than one million have AMI in US in each year. More than three lakhs die of AMI before hospitalization. One American has AMI every 25 seconds and somebody dies of CVD every 36 seconds. Overall mortality rate is >30% although mortality has declined over the last 30 years with the advent of ICCU, fibrinolytic therapy, and primary PTCA.
2. Half a million deaths by cancer in 1995
3. 90,000 deaths by accidents
4. 44,000 deaths by AIDS

4. Incidence of angina can be arranged into 4 age groups.

1. 70% between 50–70 years of age
2. 15% between 40–50 years of age
3. 3% between 30–40 years of age
4. 0.3% below 30 years of age.

5. Average mortality rate is about 4% per annum after the development of symptoms of angina or myocardial infarction from which the patient has recovered.

6. There is a spectrum of 4 syndromes that may result from CAD:

1. Angina pectoris
2. Acute myocardial infarction
3. Chronic post-ischemic cardiac failure or arrhythmias
4. Sudden ischemic cardiac death

7. Ischemia of the myocardium may manifest as following alterations.

1. *Clinical picture:* Typical or atypical anginal pain
2. *Electrocardiography:* ST segment depression on rest, exercise and Holter monitoring
3. *Echocardiography:* Segmental hypokinesia/akinesia, diminished ejection fraction
4. *Nuclear cardiology:* Demonstrates disordered thallium metabolism on exercise

The above-mentioned complex abnormalities detected on investigative cardiology which are described later, have resulted in many additions to the original clinical syndrome described by Herbeden.

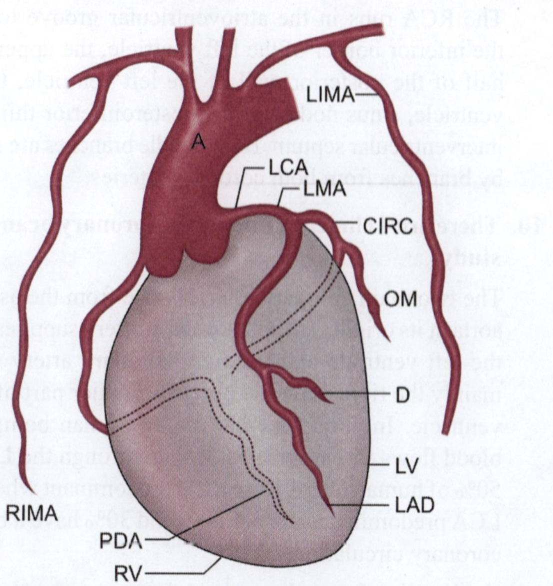

Fig. E-1: Coronary arteries and its branches. Mammary arteries are also shown

A. Aorta; CIRC = Circumflex artery; D. Diagonal artery LAD = Left anterior descending artery; LCA = Left coronary artery; LMA = Left main coronary artery; LIMA = Left internal mammary artery; LV = Left ventricle; OM = Obtuse marginal artery, PDA = Posterior descending artery; RIMA = Right internal mammary artery; RV = Right ventricle

Coronary arteries: The heart receives life-giving blood from vessels called coronary arteries. They are called coronary arteries because they form a 'crown' for the heart. There are two such main arteries. Left coronary artery (LCA) and right coronary artery (RCA) which arise from the left and right aortic sinuses, respectively.

8. Left coronary artery (LCA) has 4 important branches.

1. Left anterior descending branch supplies anterior surface of both ventricles, the lower third of the posterior surface of the right ventricle and apex.
2. Circumflex branch supplies lateral wall and the lower (apical) half of the posterior wall of the left ventricle
3. Obtuse marginal artery–a branch from circumflex artery
4. Diagonal artery–a branch from LAD

The LCA supplies the anterior, lateral and part of the posterior walls of the left ventricle and the anterosuperior two-thirds of the interventricular septum.

9. Right coronary artery (RCA) has 4 important branches:

1. Marginal branch supplies lateral and anteroposterior surface of the right ventricle
2. A branch to the AV node in 90%
3. A large branch forms a plexus around the superior vena cava which supplies the SA node in 60–75% of individuals.
4. Continues as posterior descending artery.

The RCA runs in the atrioventricular groove to supply the inferior border of the left ventricle, the upper (basal) half of the posterior wall of the left ventricle, the right ventricle, sinus node and the posteroinferior third of the interventricular septum. Both bundle branches are supplied by branches from both coronary arteries.

10. There are 4 clinically important coronary branches for study.

The two main coronary arteries arise from the ascending aorta at its origin. The left coronary artery supplies mainly the left ventricle and the right coronary artery supplies mainly the right ventricle but also a major part of the left ventricle. In about one-half of all human beings more blood flows through the RCA than through the LCA, i.e. 50% of human hearts have RCA predominant whereas the LCA predominates in only 20% and 30% have a balanced coronary circulation.

1. Anterior descending } LCA
2. Circumflex } LCA
3. Right main coronary artery } RCA
4. Posterior descending artery } RCA

11. Congenital anomalies of coronary arteries occur in 4% of patients.

12. The heart muscle is richly supplied by blood so that

1. There is one capillary for each muscle fiber.
2. About 0.8 ml of blood flows through the coronary arteries for every 1 g of heart muscle (i.e. 80 ml per 100 g).
3. The blood flow increases about 4 to 6 times during conditions of stress.
4. About 12 ml (12–14 ml) of oxygen is extracted from every 100 ml of blood and there is little change with increased activity.

13. 4 to 5% of total cardiac output goes to the coronary circulation.

14. Oxygen demand of the myocardium depends on 4 factors:

1. Contractile state
2. Heart rate
3. LV pressure
4. LV volume

LV pressure and ventricular volume together give rise to wall tension.

15. Oxygen supply of the myocardium depends on 4 factors.

1. AV oxygen difference
2. Regional myocardial distribution
3. Aortic pressure
4. Coronary vascular resistance

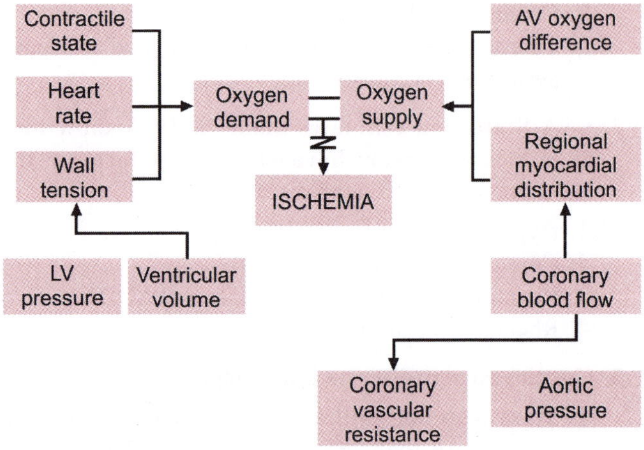

Fig. E-2

16. Acutely ischemic myocardium undergoes the following changes in 4 steps:

1. Biochemical
2. Functional
3. Morphologic
4. Electrical (ECG)

The changes occur depending on the severity and duration of blood flow deprivation.
(See Chapter AMI F-23)

17. The biochemical changes occur progressively in 4 steps.

1. The important first principal biochemical change is onset of anerobic glycolysis which leads to
↓
2. Inadequate production of ATP which in turn leads to
↓
3. Accumulation of potentially noxious breakdown products such as lactic acid which results in
↓
4. Glycogen depletion of mitochondrial cell and mitochondrial swelling

The result of oxygen deficiency leads to excitation of ischemic 'cascade', i.e. breakdown of high energy phosphate and phosphocreatinine leading to intracellular acidosis. Thus potassium ions, protons and lactic acid are released from the cell. These early changes are reversible and cell death is not immediate.

18. The 4 phasic changes in coronary blood flow during cardiac cycle—effects of cardiac compression.

The coronary blood flow like flow anywhere depends upon the pressure difference between the ascending aorta and the right atrium which obviously provides a safe margin for adequate flow. The phasic activity of the heart presents a peculiar situation to the coronary blood flow.

1. *During systole:* Blood flow through the capillaries of left ventricle falls during systole which is opposite to

the flow in all other vascular beds of the body. The reason being the strong compression of cardiac muscle around the intramuscular vessels during systole. Systolic contraction not only hinders the entry of blood flow into the capillaries, but it causes a little back flow into the epicardiac vessels. This matches well with the situation at the origin of coronary arteries which are lying behind the open cusps of the ascending aorta.

2. *During diastole:* Cardiac muscle relaxes completely and no longer obstructs the blood flow through the left ventricular capillaries. The coronary channels have low resistance. The mouths of the coronary arteries are opened due to closure of the aortic valve and the cusps lying flat. The pressure in the aorta is around 70–80 mm Hg which is much above the right atrial pressure. Thus maximum amount of blood flows into the coronary vessels during ventricular diastolic phase. On the contrary, most of the blood flows out of the coronary sinus and anterior cardiac veins during systole.

Epicardial versus subendocardial blood flow

3. *Effect of intramyocardial pressure:* Pressure gradient develops with the pressure in the subendocardial muscle having a pressure almost as great as the pressure inside the ventricle, while the pressure in the outer layer of the heart is only slightly above the atmospheric pressure, because the subendocardial vessels are compressed more than the outer vessels.
4. To compensate the lack of flow during systole, the subendocardial arteries are much larger than the nutrient arteries in the middle and outer layers of the heart. Therefore, the blood flow in the subendocardial arteries is considerably greater than blood low in the outer most arteries during diastole. This peculiar difference of blood flow in the subendocardial and epicardial arteries plays an important role in certain types of coronary ischemia.

Increased workload during stress and hypoxia are the two physiological dilators of coronary circulation.

19. There are 4 types of people in whom one has to suspect the future coronary attack or when presentation is with a typical chest pain.

1. When there is history of close relatives having suffered from ischemic heart disease.
2. When the person has acquired excess fat and the laboratory tests show high levels of serum cholesterol, triglycerides, uric acid, sugar, etc.
3. When the person is addicted to excessive smoking, living in sedentary habits, emotional reaction, etc.
4. When the person is mesomorphic somatotype personality with big bones and heavy musculature.

9 out of 10 heart attacks can be predicated on the basis of risk factors which are the same all over the world irrespective ethnic group or sex.

20. Coronary artery disease risk factors in Indians.

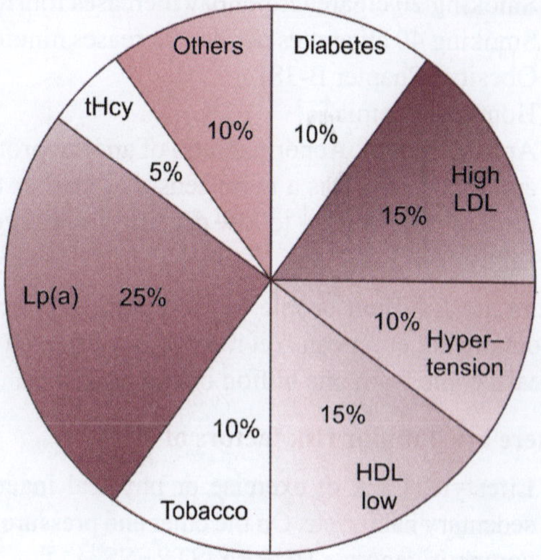

Fig. E-3

21. There are 4 nonmodifiable risk factors of IHD

1. *Old age:* The incidence of death from IHD increases every decade up to the age of about 85 years.
2. *Male sex:* It is common in males than females. IHD is less common in women prior to the menopause.
3. *Family history of IHD:* This factor results from the familial tendency to hyperlipidemia, hypertension and diabetes, although unrecognized factors operate in some families.
4. Mesomorphic somatotype personality.

22. The modifiable risk factors of IHD:

1. *Hypertension:* In men aged less than 45 years—The risk is related more to elevation of diastolic than systolic BP.

   In men aged between 45–60 years—The risk is same to elevation of either pressure.

   In men aged over 60 years—The risk is more to elevation of systolic pressure.

   The control of hypertension reduces the incidence of stroke, heart failure and renal failure. It has only a marginal effect on the mortality of myocardial infarction.
2. *Hyperlipidemia:* Decrease in high density lipoproteins (HDL) is more important than increase in low density lipoproteins (LDL) or total cholesterol.
3. *Hyperglycemia (DM):* The occurrence and mortality of IHD among diabetics is more than twice that of nondiabetics.

4. *Cigarette smoking:* There is a linear relationship between the number of cigarettes smoked per day and the risk of dying of IHD.
   Smoking 10 cigarettes per day doubles the risk of heart attack.
   Smoking 20 cigarettes per day increases fourfold risk.
   Smoking 40 cigarettes per day increases ninefold risk.
5. Obesity (Chapter B-38)
6. Homocystinemia↑.
7. Apo A1/Apo B. Abnormal ratio of apolipoprotein A to apolipoprotein B is a more sensitive marker than the ratio of high density to low density apolipoprotein.
8. Lp(a)↑.

There are 6 billion people in the world, 5 billion or of whom are not european. Yet most of our research of heart disease come from one billion of rich countries.

23. There are 4 minor risk factors of IHD.

1. Lifestyle: Lack of exercise or physical inactivity or sedentary habits, etc. On the other end pressure of time, competitiveness—HURRY/STRESS.
2. Psychological: Personality and behavior characteristics such as aggressiveness, anxiety, worry, tension, etc. for not achieving the desires—WORRY.
   The population can be divided into two groups on the basis of personalities, type A and type B. They have different risk of death from IHD. This has been suggested but disputed. Type A persons are at risk because of pressure of time, intense competitiveness, easily emotional. Type B persons are at lower risk because they are more contended or happy persons with what little they have.
3. Diet: Rich in total calories, total saturated fats, cholesterol and refined sugar, etc.—CURRY (here it means fats), daily low fruit and vegetable consumption.
4. Miscellaneous factors like softness of natural water, use of oral contraceptive pills in females (especially with smoking), intermittent claudication, gout (about 10% of patients with gout will develop ischemic heart symptoms within eight years), hyperuricemia, hypothyroidism, high levels of blood clotting factors, etc.

24. More than 75% of men who die suddenly without prior coronary artery disease (CAD) show at least two of the following 4 risk factors.

1. Hyperlipidemia: Hypercholesterolemia and/or hypertriglyceridemia—There is a direct relationship between the mean serum cholesterol and low density lipoproteins (on which most of the cholesterol in the plasma is carried) and the incidence of death from IHD. The role of plasma triglycerides and very low density lipoproteins (on which most of the triglycerides are carried) in the pathogenesis of IHD is not clear.
   The level of serum cholesterol and of the lipoproteins is determined by both genetic factors such as indigenous production and degradation and environmental factors such as the amount of fat in the diet. Intake of monounsaturated fat in the diet is the most important factor which determines the serum cholesterol and mortality from IHD.
   Therefore, the type of fat and amount of sugar eaten is important than quantity.
   Reduction in dietary intake of cholesterol and saturated fats and sugar reduces plasma lipids by about 10–20% on an average, which helps in reduction of mortality from IHD.
2. Hypertension
3. Hyperglycemia
4. Cigarette smoking.

Hypertension and smoking probably are effective in causing high mortality of IHD if the mean serum cholesterol is high.

25. Screening for hyperlipidemia is needed in 4 situations.

1. As a part of primary preventive care under 40 years of age.
2. If there is family history of ischemic heart disease.
3. If the individual is obese
4. If there are other risk factors such as smoking and/or diabetes and/or hypertension.
   Obesity is defined as weighing 120% or more of one's acceptable or standard weight.

Overweight is defined as weighing 110–119% of one's acceptable weight. Contribution of obesity makes the difference of incidence of death from IHD. It is now recognized that abdominal obesity giving the person an 'apple' shape is indicated by an increase in the ratio of abdominal/hip girth. It is an independent risk factor. Whereas obesity around the buttocks and thighs giving the person a `pear' shape is not a risk factor.

26. Following 4 tests should be done to assess the IHD risk factors by lipid disorders.

Blood sample is taken after 14 hours of fasting. The individual should not have heavy food or alcohol on the previous day.

There is no risk if the serum cholesterol is less than 200 mg/dL and serum triglycerides less than 150 mg/dL.

Hypertriglyceridemia may be associated with early atherosclerosis in some specific disorders.

(If the serum cholesterol is less than 110 mg/dl suspect hepatic damage).

If the levels exceed, test for LDL cholesterol, HDL cholesterol, VLDL cholesterol. Overnight refrigeration for 18 hr, for assessment of chylomicrons should also be undertaken along with total cholesterol and triglycerides.

Table E-1

Interpretation	High risk	Low risk
	Treatment required	No treatment required
1. Total cholesterol	> 275 mg/dL	< 200 mg/dL
2. LDL cholesterol	> 150 mg/dL	< 150 mg/dL
3. HDL cholesterol	< 35 mg/dL	> 35 mg/dL
4. VLDL cholesterol	> 30 mg/dL	< 30 mg/dL

This range varies with treating physicians

27. Cigarette smoking affects the CVS in 4 ways.

1. Causes elevation of circulating catecholamines
2. Causes elevation of circulating fatty acids
3. Causes elevation of circulating carboxyhemoglobin
4. Causes diminished oxygen carrying capacity of the blood.

In diabetic ketoacidosis, if the patient is seriously hypotensive, plasma or blood from a matched heavy smoker is preferable. In diabetic ketoacidosis, there is deficiency of 2, 3-DPG (diphosphoglycerate) in RBC which decreases the peripheral release of oxygen to the tissues. RBC in a heavy smoker contains 2, 3-DPG in large amounts.

Incidence of sudden deaths due to CVS collapse is higher in smokers than in non-smokers.

Smoking is a major risk factor for CHD.

28. Smoking causes any of the following 4 complications.

1. *Accelerated atherosclerosis:* It is due to multiple substances present within the tobacco rather than a single substance. Prevalence of CHD in smoker is 3–5 times than non-smokers. People who smoke 20 cigarettes a day are fourfold risk to have a heart attack than non-smoker. The risk is increased if 9–10 times if 40 cigarettes are smoked.
   Unanticipated sudden death is 4 times more common in smokers. With an increased prevalence of smokers, more and more young people are getting heart attack and dying suddenly.
   Studies revealed 3 out of 4 young victims of heart attacks are smokers.
   Smoking is the major or the only risk factor for CHD in people below 40 years age. Though men are more adversely affected by smoking, the risk of heart disease increased 10-fold in women taking birth control pills.
   Besides CHD, accelerated atherosclerosis increases the risk occlusion or aneurysm of the major arteries. This may lead to cerebrovascular accident (CVA) causing hemorrhage or thrombosis. Thromboangiitis obliterans of the lower limb may lead to amputation.
   Rupture of a major artery may lead to fatal bleeding in internal organs.
   1 out of 5 instances of stroke are attributed for smoking.
2. *Sudden death:* Reduction of oxygen content and rise of carboxyhemoglobin levels in the blood, increase in carbon monoxide predisposes to life-threatening arrhythmias. The stoppage of smoking rapidly reverses this risk.
3. *Carcinoma of the lung:* It is probably due to deposition of tars present in the tobacco smoke.
4. *The additive and psychological effects:* These are due to nicotine mimicking acetylcholine in the brain and the sympathetic and parasympathetic ganglia. Depending on the smokers environment, nicotine has either stimulating or depressing effect.

Tobacco contains about 4000 chemicals which fall in three categories.

Nicotine, carbon monoxide, and other organic chemicals.

Nicotine causes tachycardia, hypertension, and atherosclerosis.

Carbon monoxide has a better capacity to bind with hemoglobin resulting in carboxyhemoglobin which interferes with oxygen transport to the tissues. Majority of the chemicals in tobacco smoke, implicated in cancer are present in tobacco tar.

Passive smoking: Smokers, inadvertently expose others to the same risk who are in their close contact when they smoke. Passive inhalation of tobacco smoke is known as passive smoking. Studies showed that non-smoker-smoker equivalent of three cigarettes in a room where 40 cigarettes have been smoked. These patients who continued to smoke after myocardial infarction or heart surgery have a poor long-term prognosis. They are at increased risk of recurrent angina, MI, and sudden death. After CABG, grafts are more likely to block if smoking is resumed.

29. Pattern of coronary artery disease (CAD) in India is changing when compared to Western countries. It differs from north India to south India and even from state to state in some features like the following 4.

1. It is increasing in younger age groups.
2. It is increasing in vegetarians. Even the non-vegetarians take non-veg once or twice a week. They are also mostly vegetarians.
3. It is increasing in non-smokers and non-alcoholics
4. Coronary vessels are of small caliber and atherosclerosis is diffuse and the terminal branches may be hair thin and their occlusion need more endarterectomies and/ or transmyocardial reperfusion (ref Chapter U-21 Role of Surgery in Cardiology).

30. The narrowing of the coronary arteries by atherosclerosis may be 4-fold.

1. Mild
2. Moderate
3. Threatening
4. Total occlusion

Normal coronary flow at rest is 300 mL/min.

31. The clinical prognosis depends on the site of obstruction and number of vessels obstructed. The 4 varieties of obstruction are:

1. One artery obstruction
2. Two arteries obstruction
3. Three arteries obstruction
4. Multiple arteries obstruction

A proximal lesion is more serious than distal lesion because it threatens larger amount of myocardium.

A significant coronary artery disease is said to be present if the narrowing is more than 50%.

32. There are 4 precipitating factors.

1. Vascular hypertonus
2. Coronary endothelial dysfunction
3. Transient increase in obstructive atherosclerotic plaque
4. Tachycardia

Transient increase in obstruction is due to development of fissures and subintimal hemorrhage. In addition, platelet microaggregates or thrombi at the site of plaque, have been demonstrated on coronary endoscopy; in unstable angina. Tachycardia, increased contractility and myocardial wall tension as a result of cardiac or noncardiac pathologies may result in increased oxygen demand. This aggravates already existent oxygen insufficiency.

33. Vascular hypertonus: Vascular tone of coronary vessels is influenced by the neural and humoral factors. The epicardial coronary vessels have been shown to have various receptors e.g.

1. Adrenogenic receptors consisting of alpha, β-1, β-2, etc.
2. Glucagon
3. Dopamine
4. Histamine

Stimulation or depression of these receptors may result in variation in tonicity of coronary vessels.

34. Coronary endothelium plays an important role in vascular tonicity through paracrine secretion of vasoactive substances, i.e. both vasodilators and vasoconstrictors.

Vasodilator

1. Endothelial derived relaxing factor (EDRF) which is chemically nitric oxide
2. Prostacycline (PG)

Vasoconstrictors

3. Endothelins
4. Thromboxane A2 (TX A2)

Damaged endothelium may give rise to alteration in this balance and hence tonicity of coronary vessels.

35. The 4 types of cells involved in the pathogenesis of atherosclerotic lesion and their role.

1. *Arterial endothelial cells:* The atherosclerotic process is initiated as a result of injury to these cells by low density lipoproteins that bind to the cell membrane and pass into the subendothelial space. The other possibilities that may be thought are that endothelial cells are damaged by mechanical trauma, toxins or viruses.
2. *Leucocytes mainly monocyte:* It is well known that blood monocytes give rise to tissue macrophages or histocytes. In the atherosclerotic process, the chemotactic substances liberated by the injured endothelial cells attract the monocytes which then adhere before migrating subendothelially between the endothelial cells binding lipoprotein and becoming lipid laden macrophages (foam cells).
3. *Smooth muscle cells:* The chemotactic substances liberated by the injured endothelial cells influence the smooth muscle cells to proliferate and migrate from the media to the intima of the arterial wall.
4. *Platelets:* Platelets appear to be directly involved in the growth of atherosclerotic lesion. Firstly platelets become attached to lesions over injured epithelium exposing small areas of subendothelium. Secondly, by producing substances such as platelet derived growth factor (PDGF)—a small protein about 30000 daltons that affects the migration of other cells within the vessel wall.`

Exposure of the contents of the plaque produces a thrombogenic surface for interaction with platelets. Activated platelets release vasoconstrictive substances such as serotonin and thromboxane A2. Adenosine diphosphate is also released which also contributes to the activation and aggregation of platelets, ultimately leading to the formation of mural platelet thrombus. The rationale for the use of antiplatelet antithrombotic agents is to interrupt the cycle of platelet aggregation, platelet dysfunction and formation of mural platelet thrombus.

36. The above process results in fatty streaks and fibrous plaques. Fatty streaks are the earliest atherosclerotic lesion and are seen in young children. They are situated in the subendothelial area and consist of predominantly of lipid laden macrophages derived mainly from monocytes together with some smooth muscle cells which have migrated from the media.

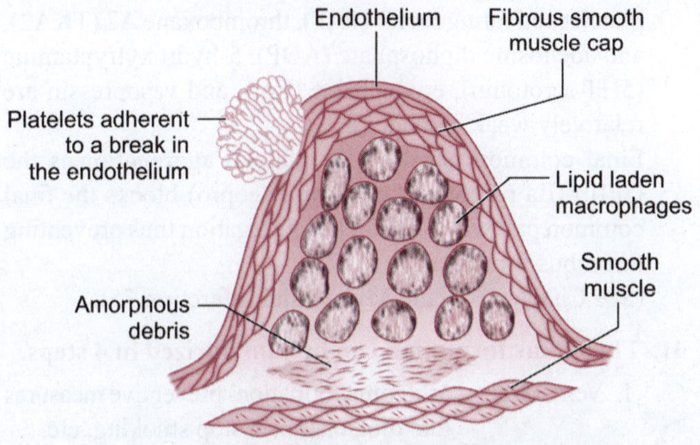

Fig. E-4: A fibrous plaque

Fibrous plaques consist of the following 4 changes.

1. Smooth muscle cells that have migrated to the intima
2. Lipid laden macrophages surrounded by a matrix of connective tissue and variable amounts of intra-and extracellular lipids.
3. Top of the lesion is a dense cap of smooth muscle cells and fibrous tissue.
4. Beneath the lesion may be an area of necrosis, cholesterol crystals and calcification. If the surface layer of endothelial cells has broken, there may be adhesion of platelets and thrombus formation.

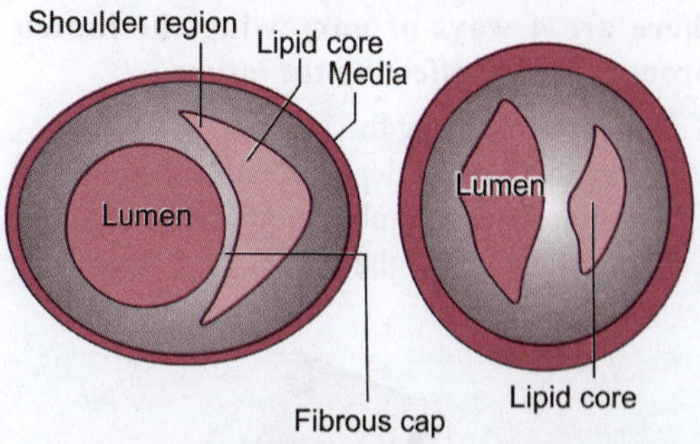

Fig. E-5: Lipid core with fibrous cap

37. Fibrous plaques are more advanced lesions and they may:

1. Protrude into the lumen of an artery
2. Rupture into pieces from a plaque with rough surfaces
3. Break off as a result of blood burrowing within the vessel wall beneath the plaques
4. Initiate aggregation of platelets and frank intra-arterial thrombosis on the roughened and broken surface of a plaque.

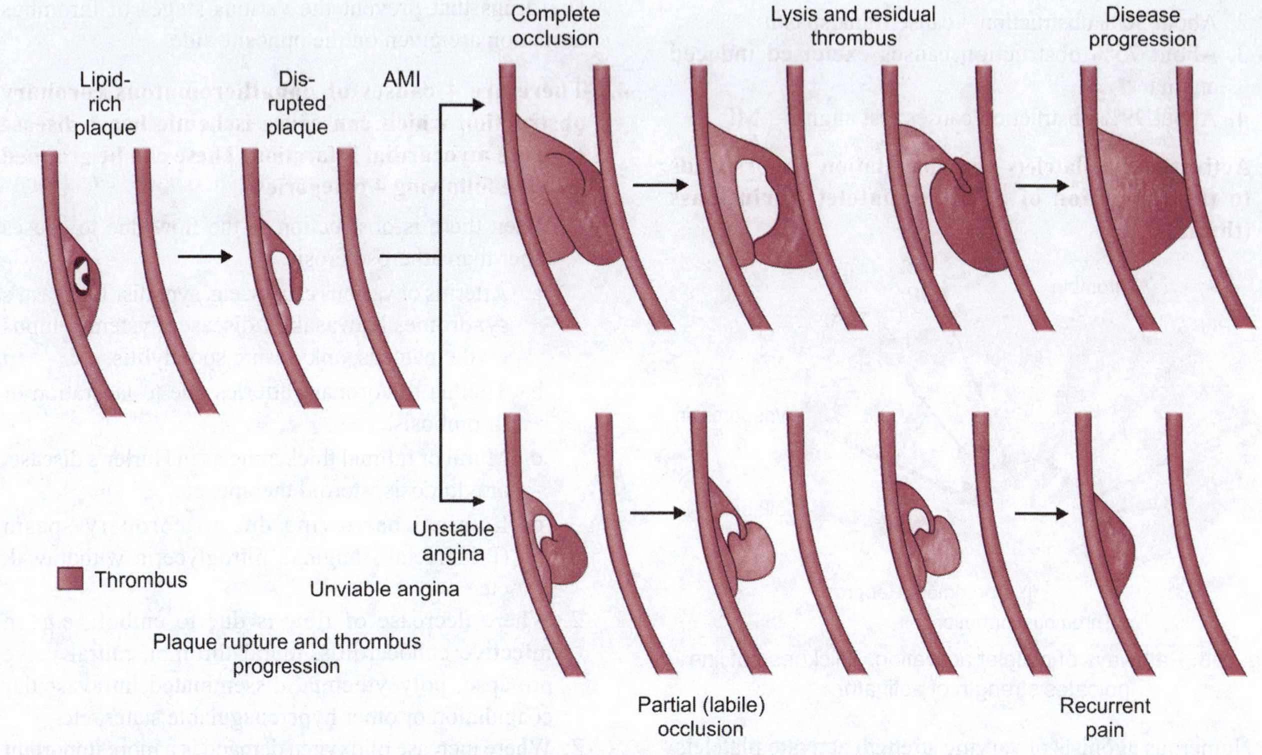

Fig. E-6: Thrombus progression and plaque rupture: Complete occlusion causes acute myocardial infarction (AMI). Partial occlusion causes angina, unstable angina. When a plaque ruptures and becomes thrombogenic, the result in thrombus can extend progressively from the lesion in either or both directions, antegrade or retrograde, within the coronary artery

38. There are 4 ways of narrowing the lumen of the coronary artery affecting the intima.

1. Atheroma affecting the intima
2. Fibrin and platelet deposition of the intima
3. Thrombosis or a combination of these factors
4. Hemorrhage under the intima.

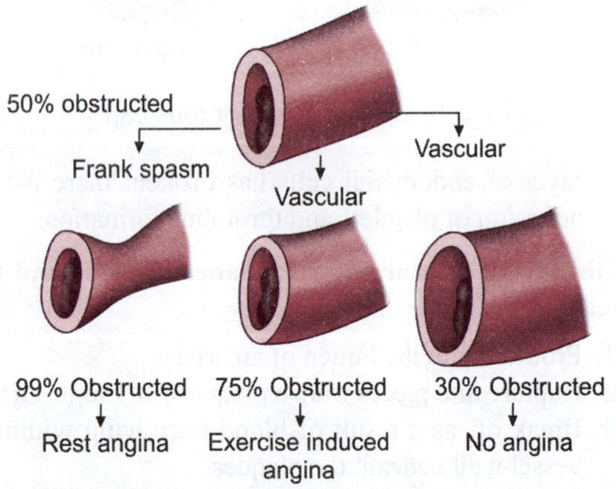

Fig. E-7:

39. Schematic diagram of the dynamic nature of an atherosclerotic coronary obstruction.

1. 30% obstruction—no angina
2. About 50% obstruction—cause frank spasm
3. About 75% obstruction causes exercised induced angina
4. About 99% obstruction causes rest angina—MI

40. Activation of platelets and coagulation factors leads to the formation of a stable platelet-fibrin mass (thrombus).

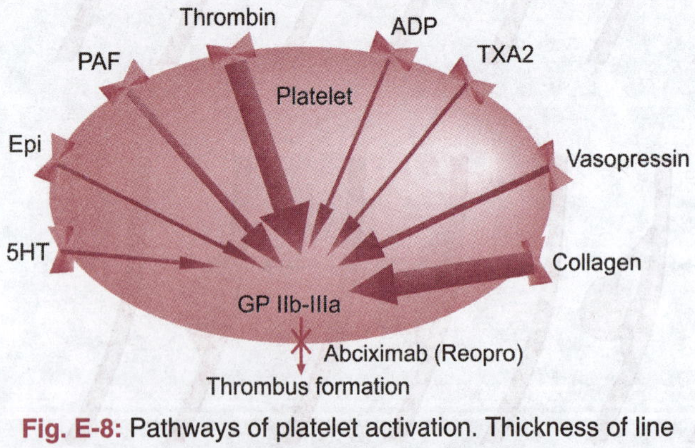

Fig. E-8: Pathways of platelet activation. Thickness of line indicates strength of activator

Numerous agonists of varying strength activate platelets. Thickness of the line indicates strength of the activator. Collagen and thrombin are strong activators followed by platelet activating factor (PAF), thromboxane A2 (TXA2), and adenosine diphosphate (ADP), 5-hydroxytryptamine (5HT-serotonin), epinephrine (Epi), and vasopressin are relatively weak activators.

Final common pathway for platelet aggregation is the GPIIb-IIIa receptor. Abciximb (Reopro) blocks the final common pathway for platelet aggregation thus preventing thrombus formation.

(See Chapter-F Acute Myocardial Infarction 75).

41. Thrombus formation can be summarized in 4 steps.

I. Vessel wall—Atheroma formation- preventive measures like diet, exercise, stop smoking, etc.
+ control of HT/DM, dyslipidemias

II. Platelets X—Aspirin, dipyridamole, ticlopidine act on TXA2
+ Abciximab (Reopro), Eptifibatide (Integralin) act on GPIIb-IIIa

III. Coagulation X Anticoagulants—Heparin, warfarin, acenocumerol, factors
↓

IV. Thrombus X—STK, UK, rt-PA, Reteplase

Thrombus formation starts with injury to the blood vessel wall, endothelium. Activation of platelets and coagulation factors leads to the formation of a stable platelet-fibrin mass—thrombus.

The drugs that prevent the various stages of thrombus formation are given on the opposite side.

42. There are 4 causes of nonatheromatous coronary obstruction which can cause ischemic heart disease or acute myocardial infarction. These can be grouped into the following 4 categories.

1. When there is obstruction to the flow due to causes other than atherosclerosis.
   a. Arteritis of various causes, e.g. syphilis, Takayasu's syndrome, Kawasaki's disease, systemic lupus erythematosus, ankylosing spondylitis, etc.
   b. Trauma to coronary arteries due to laceration or thrombosis.
   c. Mural or intimal thickening as in Hurler's disease, amyloidosis, steroid therapy, etc.
   d. Luminal narrowing due to coronary spasm (Prinzmetal's angina), nitroglycerin withdrawal, etc.
2. Where decrease of flow is due to emboli, e.g. in infective endocarditis, mural thrombi, mitral valve prolapse, polycythemia, disseminated intravascular coagulation or other hypercoagulable states, etc.
3. Where increase of oxygen demand is a more important factor, e.g. aortic stenosis, aortic regurgitation, thyrotoxicosis, etc.

There is ischemia without CAD where increase of oxygen demand is an important factor. For example,
Severe aortic stenosis
Hyperthyroidism
Hypothyroidism
Diabetes mellitus
Hypertension
Cardiomyopathy
Severe anemia (Hb < 4 g)
Hemoglobinopathies.
More than 50% coronary block only causes ischemia. 10%, 20%, 30%, and 40% block do not give ischemia. So, there can be coronary artery disease without ischemia.

4. Miscellaneous conditions such as ALCAPA (Anomalous Left Coronary Artery from Pulmonary Artery) and other congenital coronary abnormalities.

These form a very small number of patients of IHD or AMI.
These events result in narrowing of the lumen of the vessel and ischemia which may stimulate small nerve fibers with production of pain sensation.

43. Hypercoagulability of the blood is also recognized now as a risk factor. Some of the blood clotting factors are above average. The following 4 are important.

1. Rise in fibrinogen levels to some extent due to smoking.
2. Rise in factor VII } mainly due to dietary fat
3. Rise in factor VIII } mainly due to dietary fat
4. Rise in inhibitor of plasminogen activity (PAI).

Their rise in blood levels can cause intra-arterial thrombosis and death from IHD.

44. Coronary artery disease (CAD) causes ischemia which may manifest itself as any of the following:

1. Typical angina
2. Atypical angina (angina equivalent)
3. Silent myocardial ischemia (SMI)
   No subjective ischemia;
   There is objective ischemia documented by ECG stress test, thallium test, etc. SMI is common
4. Asymptomatic—Truly asymptomatic
   There may be no typical anginal pain in less than 50%.

45. The pathogenic mechanism of angina can be described into 4 types:

1. *Primary angina:* Decreased myocardial flow secondary to coronary artery spasm. It is the common mechanism of variant angina (Prinzmetal) and in some cases of unstable and effort angina, vasospastic angina.
2. *Secondary angina:* Angina on exertion beyond a fixed level due to increased myocardial oxygen demand.
3. *Mixed form:* Rest angina combined with angina on minor effort. It is the common form.
4. *Syndrome 'X':* Angina with normal coronaries and no evidence of spasm. Treadmill test is positive. Yet, the underlying mechanism is unexplained—probably due to inadequate vasodilatory reserve.

The total time a patient is ischemic each day is greater in many patients. A viable myocardium surrounding a fresh infarct may contract poorly for few days. This phenomenon is known as "Myocardial Stunning."

46. Angina with normal coronary arteries on angiography is probably due to the following 4 causes:

1. Intramyocardial vasculitis
2. Procoagulable states
3. Spontaneous thrombolysis
4. Inadequate vasodilatory response

This syndrome has got multiple etiologies. Some patients suffering from angina or myocardial infarction with demonstrable akinesia or hypokinesia of LV wall motion show normal coronary arteries on angiography. They are usually heavy smokers, young persons or women on oral contraceptives. Spontaneous lysis of thrombus in coronary vessels may explain normal coronary vessels on angiography.
Procoagulant states: Enhanced coagulability in incomplete or complete obstructive states.
Syndrome X: The syndrome shows intramyocardial vasculitis (in arterioles less than 100 μ diameter), while epicardial vessels are normal. As only epicardial segment can be visualized on coronary angiography and intramyocardial arterioles are not visualized, coronary vessels are thus reported to be normal in such patients. This entity usually occurs in middle-aged women. Intramyocardial vasculitis occurs not uncommonly in diabetes mellitus.

47. Reaven while describing the insulin resistance syndrome (IRS), he coined the term 'syndrome X' to denote a combination of risk factors for coronary heart disease which include:

1. Truncal obesity
2. Hypertension
3. Glucose intolerance
4. Hypertriglyceridemia

Kaplan described these 4 factors as 'deadly quartet' as they are often found together in association with severe premature coronary artery disease. All these have been currently grouped under one heading 'Insulin Resistance Syndrome' (IRS), or cardiovascular dysmetabolic syndrome (CDS) as the insulin resistance plays the key role in their pathogenic mechanism and their adverse effect mainly affects the cardiovascular system.

48. Dyslipidemia and hyperinsulinemia are closely related. An ideal lipid milieu for atherogenesis is created when insulin resistance syndrome (IRS) is associated with

1. Increase in small dense LDL
2. Increase in triglycerides
3. Increase in VLDL
4. Decrease in HDL

The procoagulant state of IRS is due to raised level of plasminogen activator inhibitor (PAI-1) contributed by increased hepatic synthesis in presence of hyperinsulinemia. Increased PAI-1 is not only associated with increased coronary heart disease but also renders thrombolytic therapy ineffective following myocardial infarction.

49. Thus the syndrome X has several components which is a coronary artery disease risk factor. It includes:

1. Insulin resistance/hyperinsulinemia/increased proinsulin
2. Central obesity
3. Hypertension
4. Impaired glucose tolerance (IGT)
5. Hypertriglyceridemia
6. Increase in small dense LDL
7. Increase in VLDL
8. Decrease in HDL-C
9. Microalbuminuria
10. Rise in C-reactive protein (CRP)
11. Rise in plasminogen activator inhibitor (PAI)
12. Endothelial dysfunction

Besides these, genetic, aging, lack of exercise are also contributory.

Central obesity specially in males, hypertriglyceridemia rise in homocystine levels seems to be genetic in Indians which are contributory to rise in CAD.

A rise in CRP levels appears to favor that atherosclerosis may be an inflammatory process.

Endothelial dysfunction gives rise to decrease in nitric oxide which is antiatherogenic and antihypertensive.

Platelet dysfunction gives rise to increase, plasminogen activator inhibitor (PAI) which is procoagulant and antifibrinolytic state.

Insulin resistance (IR) can cause endothelial dysfunction or vice versa.

IR ↔ endothelial dysfunction
↓ ↑
Hyperglycemia)
Hypertension) ——
Dyslipidemia)

All these components contribute each other for rise in CAD.

50. A patient of coronary artery disease may pass through the 4 stages:

1. Silent myocardial ischemia
2. Stable angina
3. Unstable angina
4. Myocardial infarction

51. The causes of angina pectoris can be arranged into 4 groups.

1. Coronary atherosclerosis—the commonest cause.
2. Syphilitic aortitis with coronary ostial stenosis, aortic stenosis, aortic regurgitation and other forms of aortitis.
3. Factors that increase ventricular preload which demand more myocardial oxygen, e.g. exercise, anemia, hyperthyroidism, chronic pulmonary disease, etc.
4. Factors that increase ventricular after load, which demand more coronary blood flow, e.g. hypertension, obstructive cardiomyopathy, dilatation or hypertrophy of the ventricle. Preload is the stretch produced within the myocardium at end-diastole. After load is the impedance to ejection of blood flow from the ventricle.

52. It is appropriate to mention in this context regarding the classification of functional capacity and objective assessment of patients with diseases of the heart by the New York Heart Association (NYHA).

In 1928, the New York Heart Association published a classification of patients with cardiac disease based on clinical severity and prognosis. This classification has been updated in seven subsequent editions of *Nomenclature and Criteria for Diagnosis of Diseases of the Heart and Great Vessels* (Little Brown & Co). The ninth edition, revised by the Criteria Committee of the American Heart Association, New York City Affiliate, was released March 4, 1994. The new classifications are summarized below for the many physicians and scientists who use them to describe the status of individual patients.

Four classes of functional capacity.

Class I. Patients with cardiac disease but without resulting limitation of physical activity. Ordinary physical activity does not cause undue fatigue, palpitation, dyspnea, or anginal pain.

Class II. Patients with cardiac disease resulting in slight limitation of physical activity. They are comfortable at rest. Ordinary physical activity results in fatigue, palpitation, dyspnea, or anginal pain.

Class III. Patients with cardiac disease resulting in marked limitation of physical activity. They are comfortable at rest. Less than ordinary activity causes fatigue, palpitation, dyspnea or anginal pain.

Class IV. Patients with cardiac disease resulting in inability to carry on any physical activity without discomfort. Symptoms of heart failure or the anginal syndrome may be present even at rest. If any physical activity is undertaken, discomfort is increased.

53. Objective Assessment

A. No objective evidence of cardiovascular disease
B. Objective evidence of minimal cardiovascular disease
C. Objective evidence of moderately severe cardiovascular disease
D. Objective evidence of severe cardiovascular disease.

Examples

A patient with minimal or no symptoms but a large pressure gradient across the aortic valve or severe obstruction of the left main coronary artery is classified.

Functional Capacity I. Objective Assessment D

A patient with severe anginal syndrome but angiographically normal coronary arteries is classified:

Functional Capacity IV. Objective Assessment A

54. Myocardial oxygen consumption is determined by 4 parameters.

1. Heart rate
2. Left ventricular pressure.
3. Left ventricular diameter (LV volume)
4. Contractility.

55. The 4 common clinical situations that precipitate anginal attack in the presence of coronary heart disease (CHD) are:

1. Tachycardia—caused by physical exertion, cold environment, anemia, hyperthyroidism, etc.
2. Intense emotions—anxiety, sexual intercourse
3. Heavy meals/hypoglycemia
4. Vivid dreams (nocturnal angina)

ANGINA

The name angina pectoris is derived from the Greek "*Ankhon*"(Strangling) and the latin "*pectus*" (chest). This term is used to describe the syndrome of chest discomfort resulting from myocardial ischemia. Angina pectoris is a term used to describe discomfort due to transient myocardial ischemias and constitutes a clinical syndrome rather than a disease, it may occur whenever there is an imbalance between myocardial oxygen supply and demand.

56. Angina pectoris can be clinically classified into 4 types.

1. Stable angina pectoris
2. Unstable angina pectoris
3. Variant or Prinzmetal's angina pectoris
4. Post-infarction angina pectoris

57. Stable angina pectoris is said to be present when the angina pectoris has been present for more than 60 days during which time the following 4 factors should be satisfied.

1. No change in the frequency of anginal attack
2. No change in the duration of angina
3. No change in the precipitating factors
4. No change with which the angina is relieved

These clinical manifestations indicate that the fault lies in the demand side of myocardial supply-demand system and the coronary arterial lesions are relatively stable.

Angina which occurs in a stable form over many years is also referred to as 'angina of effort' or 'stress angina.' The pathological substrate is usually fixed, e.g. atherosclerotic narrowing of an epicardial coronary artery. The precipitation circumstances tend to remain constant across episodes, therefore it is called "stable" angina. It is the commonest form of angina.

58. Chronic stable angina pectoris patients may have

1. Episodes of silent myocardial ischemia (SMI) – symptomless ischemia
2. Pain with typical distribution
3. Pain with atypical distribution
4. Pain in skip areas

In general, stable angina correlates with the stability or quiescence of an atherosclerotic plaque.

59. Unstable Angina Pectoris: It is said to be present when the stable angina pectoris has been present for less than 60 days and begins to show any one of the following 4 changes in clinical manifestations.

1. Occurring unpredictably or suddenly increasing in frequency of attacks
2. Increasing in severity of attacks (Crescendo angina) or duration of attacks
3. Precipitated without provocation, such as during sleep or rest
4. May not respond to nitroglycerin or others for which response was present earlier

These symptoms indicate the fault in the supply side of the myocardial oxygen supply-demand system. Its inference is that the obstructing abnormalities in the coronary arteries are increasing. Unstable aspect of the clinical symptoms differentiate from stable angina. These patients are in danger of having myocardial infarction or sudden death.

With the advent of coronary angiography, pathogenesis of unstable angina has been attributed to microthrombi consisting of activated platelets and increased vascular tone due to greater production of vasoconstrictors by platelets, while damaged endothelium fails to produce vasodilator substances to counter balance platelet derived vasoconstrictors. Thus underlying principle behind initial management of unstable angina consists of prevention of microthrombi formation and reversing coronary spasm.

In unstable angina pectoris, there is temporary ischemia because the blood supply is temporarily inadequate but there is no death of the tissue, whereas myocardial infarction by definition is characterized by the death of tissue. Some patients may develop manifestation of intermediary nature between these two extremes.

"It must be emphasized that ECG and cardiac enzyme alterations diagnostic of acute myocardial infarction are absent in unstable angina."

These patients should be admitted in the hospital without delay for coronary angiography unless there is definite contraindication. Patients with unstable angina usually should not undergo treadmill or radionuclide test. Coronary artery bypass graft (CABG) or angioplasty may be done, if needed.

In some patients with clear distinction between stable and unstable angina is not possible. These patients are considered to be an intermediate stage between unstable and stable angina.

60. The term 'Unstable angina' has replaced earlier 4 following nomenclatures given to this entity.

1. Crescendo angina
2. Acute coronary insufficiency
3. Intermediate coronary syndrome
4. Preinfarction angina

61. Following 4 clinical features have short-term risk or non-fatal myocardial infarction in patients with symptoms suggesting unstable angina.

1. Prolonged ongoing rest pain (>20 min)
2. Rest angina with dynamic ST changes > 1 mm
3. Angina with new or worsening mitral regurgitation murmurs, S3 or pulmonary rales
4. Angina with hypotension

62. Prinzmetal angina or variant angina:

This is thought to be due to epicardial coronary artery spasm in an already partially obstructed coronary artery but the spasm may occur in otherwise normal coronary arteries. It differs from others in the following 4 ways:

1. Episodes of severe pain occurring at rest or during ordinary activity and it does not follow a period of physical exertion or emotional stress. Attacks can be very painful and usually occur between midnight and 8 AM.
2. Transient angina with ECG abnormalities can be precipitated by triggering activity—e.g. smoking a cigarette.
3. ECG shows transient ST elevation rather than depression suggesting an acute myocardial infarction (vs No reciprocal ST depression as seen in AMI)
4. Relieved immediately on administration of rapid acting vasodilators.

It is a rare form of angina induced by spasm of epicardial component of coronary vessels associated with ST segment elevation. Spasm may be present in one, two or all the three vessels, and may affect main vessels or its major branches. About two-thirds of people with it have severe coronary atherosclerosis in at least one major vessel. The spasm usually occurs very close to the obstruction. In 75% cases, atherosclerosis of one or more vessels is demonstrated on coronary angiography and/ or autopsy studies. It is hypotheticated that the spasm of vascular segment adjacent to the atherosclerosis segment may be the trigger zone. The angina most often comes at night and depicts circadian rhythm, i.e. occurring mostly at midnight to 8 AM Pain is very severe and is associated with breathlessness and restlessness and may give rise to acute myocardial infarction, cardiac arrhythmias which may include ventricular tachycardia, ventricular fibrillation and sudden cardiac death.

It disappears immediately on administration of rapid acting vasodilators. ECG shows reversible elevated ST segment indicative of transmural ischemia leading to epicardial shift in ST vector. Enzymatic alterations typical of myocardial infarction are absent.

Many people who survive with Prinzmetal's angina go through an acute active phase. Anginal and cardiac events may occur frequently for six months or more during which time, nonfatal myocardial infarction occurs in up to 20% of patients; death occurs in up to 10%.

People who develop serious arrhythmias at this time are at greater risk of sudden death.

Most people who survive an infarction or this initial three- to six-month period stabilize, and symptoms and cardiac events tend to diminish over time. Long-term survival is excellent ranging from 89–97% at five years. Patients without significant obstructive coronary artery disease have an excellent long-term outlook.

The ergonovine test is the most sensitive and useful test for coronary spasm. In this, the drug ergonovine is administered to induce coronary spasm. Hyperventilation and coronary injections of acetylcholine are other means used to provoke variant angina.

Postinfarction angina pectoris: Some patients may have angina immediately following infarction and they are referred to as 'immediate postinfarction angina pectoris'. It is stated that dead myocardium does not produce pain. If pain is continued, it implies that more ischemia and more myocardium may be lost. Some patients may have angina after an interval of few days to weeks. It implies that myocardial ischemia is occurring in these patients and these are very serious forms of angina.

63. There are 4 variants of angina differing from classical types of angina.

1. Angina decubitus or recumbent angina' or nocturnal angina: It is a form of left ventricular failure—like paroxysmal nocturnal dyspnea increased venous return in the lying posture causes increase in myocardial oxygen demand and preload.
   Diuretics help in this type.
2. Angina precipitated by any triggering activity—e.g. smoking, taking heavy meal, lifting a child, sexual activity, exposure to cold weather, etc.
3. Air port angina—lifting a bag is an isometric exercise. Any act that lifts the arms above the head increases total body oxygen requirement associated with continuous contraction of antigravity muscles of the arms and shoulder girdle.
4. 'First hole angina'—a golfer will get angina for the first hole and will not get angina in the next seventeen holes.

64. Nocturnal or decubitus angina occurs due to various following causes:

1. Tachycardia as a result of dreams.
2. Increase in wall stress of left ventricle due to increase in end-diastolic volume on lying down.
3. Circadian variation in blood pressure.
4. Coronary vascular tone.

Patient gets relieved immediately on sitting up and /or on administration of rapid action vasodilators.
Digoxin is helpful in treating the syndrome nocturnal angina which is an expression of left ventricular failure.

65. There are 4 important questions to be asked in anginal pain:

1. Site and severity (intensity or nature of the pain).
2. Duration—usually lasts less than 5 min and rarely more than 30 min. Ischemic pain does not last more than 30 min. Chest pain that lasts < 1 min is unlikely to be of cardiac origin.
3. Radiation.
4. Precipitating and relieving factors.

66. Remember SAVE for anginal pain.

1. **S**– Sudden onset and short duration.
2. **A**–Anterior chest
3. **V**–Vague character like pressing, heaviness, tightness, squeezing, choking, etc.
4. **E**–Exertion precipitated—characteristically, pain appears after exertion and disappears after rest.

Chest pain triggered by emotional stress tends to last longer than that triggered by exertion.

67. There are 4 points to know about the distribution of anginal pain.

1. Anginal pain is felt in the center of the chest because the heart is a midline organ with mediastinal attachment.
2. Angina is felt in the arms.
3. Angina is felt across the chest.
4. Angina is sometimes felt in the neck.

1, 2 and 3—because embryologically the heart is supplied by the same dermatomes C7 to T4 as the inner sides of the arms and upper chest. The sensory nerves from the heart run back centrally along the sympathetic nerves that run out to the heart. Another explanation given for the heart pain that is felt across the chest and in the arms is that within the central nervous system, sensory nerves from the heart and the arms ascend in the same pathway to the brain.

68. The causes of angina-like pain felt in patients with normal coronary arteries are:

Some of the patients who have typical anginal pain on effort have shown normal coronary arteries on coronary arteriogram. The cause of pain in these patients is thought to be from any of the 4 factors:

1. Temporary spasm of a normal coronary artery.
2. Hyperventilation during exertion or other stressful conditions resulting in spasm of a normal coronary artery.
3. Reflex gastritis during exercise—similar to angina of effort.
4. Pain from musculoskeletal origin or some other organ.

A clue to the diagnosis of this type of angina is that often the pain is brought on by variable rather than fairly constant levels of exertion. Treatment is for the underlying cause. Diltizam helps in patients with coronary artery spasm.

69. The direct questions that should be asked about any chest pain are:

1. Where is it? i.e. site.
2. How long has it been present ? and how frequent does it occur?
3. Is there any relationship to any particular event such as fall or trauma, climbing up stairs, a previous heart attack?

4. How does it feel like? i.e. character.
5. Does it radiate and if so where?
6. How long does it last? i.e. duration.
7. What brings it on or make it worse?
8. What relieves it ?

Very often these questions were not asked. Correct diagnosis may be missed if these questions are not asked even though they are very simple and basic.

70. The additional questions that should be asked about a case of chest pain to differentiate the 4 important related systems.

Is it brought on by:

I. Walking, running, climbing stairs or hills, going out in the cold, excitement, anxiety, anger, worry or fear?	Suggesting angina or cardiac pain
II. Coughing, twisting, taking deep breath, pressure over the affected area?	Suggesting pleuritic pain
III. Eating, swallowing, bending forwards, lying flat?	Suggesting pain from esophagus or GI Tract.
IV. Bending, twisting, using the arms, lying on one side, taking a deep breath, coughing, pressure over the affected area?	Suggesting pain of musculoskeletal origin

71. What relieves it? The 4 questions.

Is it relieved by:

1. *Rest:* Suggestive of angina although musculoskeletal pain also be relieved by rest.
2. *Stoppage of movement:* Keeping the chest wall as still as possible—suggestive of both pleurisy and musculoskeletal pain.
3. *Nitroglycerin:* Suggestive of angina, nitroglycerin also relaxes esophageal smooth muscle thereby relieving pain due to esophageal spasm.
4. *Antacids:* Suggestive of pain from the upper GI tract such as peptic ulcer.

72. Test whether the pain is of musculoskeletal origin or not?

Test whether the pain is reproduced by any of the 4 actions.

1. Coughing.
2. Bending, twisting or stretching.
3. Pressing over the affected area.
4. Opposing various movements of the arms and shoulders abduction, adduction, extension and flexion of arms and shoulders.

73. There are 4 common causes of chest pain of CVS origin.

The pain originating from the heart is typically felt in the centre of the chest.

1. Coronary arteries: Angina pectoris: The pain is tight, crushing or constricting in nature. It is precipitated by exertion, emotion, meals, cold, etc. It radiates to one or both arms, the throat or lower jaw in half of the cases. It is relieved by rest or nitroglycerin. It lasts for 2–10 minutes.
   1. *Myocardial infarction:* It is angina—like pain, but generally very severe. It can occur during sleep or at rest and lasts for several hours or days. It is not relieved by rest.
   2. *Valvular diseases:* Aortic stenosis, aortic regurgitation mitral valve prolapse, mitral stenosis, pulmonary stenosis.
   3. *Pericarditis:* It is typically central pleuritic—like chest pain that is made worse by lying flat and eased by sitting up or adopting some other particular position.
   4. *From the aorta:* Dissecting aneurysm: It is a tearing pain that moves up to the neck and then down the front or back of the trunk as the dissection proceeds, generally of sudden onset, unrelenting.

74. There are 4 common causes of chest pain from respiratory system origin.

1. *Pleurisy:* The pain is unilateral, sharp that varies with coughing and breathing. The common causes of pleural pain are infection that may be within the pleura or secondary to pneumonia, pulmonary embolus with infarction or carcinoma of the bronchus involving the pleura.
2. *Spontaneous pneumothorax and pneumomediastinum:* Typically the pain is described as a tearing unilateral pain worsening with breathing.
3. *Pancoast tumor:* The pain is due to carcinoma at the apex of the lung invading the brachial plexus and the adjacent ribs. It is unremitting severe pain over the top of one shoulder and down the arm.
4. *Tracheobronchitis:* The pain is usually due to infection or inhalation of a noxious vapor. The pain is usually described as a central chest pain that is often made worse with coughing and breathing.

75. The common causes of chest pain relating to esophagus:

From the esophagus: The pain from the esophagus is described as a tight indigestion—like pain in the center of the chest. The main causes of esophageal pain are:

1. Esophageal spasm due to regurgitation of food or acid.
2. Esophagitis due to inflammation of the lower Esophagus caused by the regurgitation of food and acid.
3. Incoordinate tertiary muscle contraction: This occurs in the middle-aged and elderly and may be related to food or occur spontaneously.
4. Dysphagia: Difficulty in swallowing due to stricture of the esophagus.
5. Foreign body such as a bone.
6. Hiatus hernia.
7. Carcinoma of the esophagus or less commonly invasion of the esophagus by a carcinoma of the bronchus.
8. Esophageal rupture: Usually this occurs after vomiting and typically described as a deep severe pain.

76. The common causes of chest pain originating from the upper abdominal organs.

1. *From the stomach:* Reflux gastritis, peptic ulcer, carcinoma stomach.
   The pain may be at the lower end of the sternum, and epigastric areas. Sometimes radiates to the center of the chest. The pain is usually burning in nature, related to the food.
2. *From the liver:* Hepatitis, hepatic congestion and malignancy may cause chest pain. It is usually at the lower part of the right side of the chest.
3. *From the gallbladder:* Cholecystitis, stones in the gallbladder. It is usually colicky in nature and at the right hypochondrium radiating to lower part of right side of the chest and right shoulder.
4. *From the diaphragm:* The pain is felt in the abdomen and as well as in the shoulders since both areas are innervated from the same dermatome (C4). The diaphragmatic pain perceived in the shoulder is much the same way as that of angina felt in the arm.

77. The common causes of chest pain are from the musculoskeletal system. Pain of this type is usually localized and of a pleuritic nature.

1. Torn muscle fibers.
2. Cracked or fractured ribs: Due to trauma or spontaneous in association with osteoporosis or metastatic carcinoma.
3. Secondaries growing within a rib.
4. Osteoarthritis of the costosternal joints. Osteoarthritis of the synovial joints between the sternum and the rib cartilages.
5. Osteochondritis or Tietz's syndrome. It is a condition characterized by painful swelling of one or more of the upper costochondral joints. They are non-synovial joints between the ribs and rib cartilages.
6. Epidemic myalgia or Bornholm disease: This is characterized by fever and severe unilateral chest pain associated with focal necrosis of the muscles of the chest wall. This is caused by infection with coxsackie B virus.
7. Frozen shoulder: It is also known as adhesive capsulitis. The pain is in the area of shoulder on moving or lying on the arm and is due to inflammation with or without fibrotic thickening of the glenohumeral joint.
8. Referred pain from the cervical or thoracic spine or from a costovertebral angle.

78. Four common miscellaneous causes of chest pain are

From the skin

1. *Herpes zoster (Shingles):* The pain precedes the rash by a day or two and so it is possible to miss the diagnosis unless it is considered in the differential diagnosis of unilateral chest pain.
2. *Post-herpetic neuralgia:* It is characterized by chronic pain localized to a dermatome in which the sensory nerves have been damaged by a previous attack of herpes zoster

From the psyche

3. *Da Costa's syndrome:* The chest pain is of psychological origin in a patient with anxious personality. Patient may adopt a stooping or even apologestic posture. They complain of restlessness and breathlessness at rest or on minimal exertion. Palpitation and dizziness are common due to hyperventilation. The pain is usually over the left breast, and is of sharp or pricking in nature lasting from a few seconds to several hours.
4. *Hyperventilation:* It may give rise to typical angina -like pain and is usually overlooked as a cause of anginal pain unrelated to exertion. Dizziness and tingling of the fingers and feet are useful pointers to a diagnosis of hyperventilation.

79. Acute chest pain: table of differential diagnosis of some causes

Table E-2

Diagnosis	Site and radiation	Nature and Severity	Duration—precipitating and relieving factors	Associated findings	Important laboratory data	Pitfalls
1. Stable angina	Commonly substernal rather than over the heart, radiated to left axilla, arm, epigastrium, scapula, neck and lower jaw	Diffuse pressure or squeezing sensation, often vague	Usually lasts for 5–10 min. rarely more than 15 min. Exertion, meals, cold or emotional stress may precipitate the attack. Relieved by rest or nitroglycerin	The amount of exertion needed to produce pain is anticipated by the patient and takes nitroglycerin. Risk factors include increasing age, hypertension, obesity, diabetes, smoking	Resting ECG normal. ECG during pain typically shows ST depression. Enzymes normal	Variation of pain like increase in duration and frequency suggests unstable angina
2. Unstable angina	Same as above	Same as above	Pain has increased in severity, frequency	Occurs with less exertion. Nitroglycerin may not be much effective	ECG shows non-specific changes. Enzymes are normal. This is a clinical diagnosis	Decreased action of nitroglycerin may be due to ageing of pills. It is confirmed by asking about burning under tongue and light headedness or headache with each pill
3. Prinzmetal's angina	Same as above	Same as above	Not related to exertion. Lasts for less than 20 min Relieved by nitroglycerin, calcium blockers	Precipitating factors are absent. Often occurs at the same time during day or night, smoking may precipitate	ECG shows ST elevation instead of depression with no reciprocal changes during the attack. It is due to spasm of coronary artery	Change in pattern suggests unstable angina
4. Variant angina i. Angina decibutus or recumbent angina or nocturnal angina ii. Angina precipitated by triggering activity iii. Airport angina iv. First hole angina	Same as above	Often PND, LVF increase in venous return in lying posture, increase in O_2 demand and preload	Relieved by diuretics	Basal rales, S/S of LVF	ECG	Relieved by sitting with back rest
5. Myocardial infarction	Same as above	Same as above pain builds up flow peak over minutes of hours	Sudden onset at rest or with exertion. Lasts for more than 20 min. Up to several hours. It may be present for a day or two.	Pain does not respond to nitroglycerin Breathlessness, sweating, nausea occurs commonly	ECG shows ST elevation and T inversion with reciprocal changes initially. Q waves appear if necrosis occurs. ECG is occasionally normal in the initial stage. Enzymes show abnormality. Troponin↑	Painless or silent myocardial infraction may be present particularly in diabetic patients
6. Myocarditis	Same as above	Asymptomatic to severe chest pain, to sudden death	H/O fever, infections 1–2 weeks before the S/S pericarditis	ESR↑ CRP↑	ECG – arrhythmias, heart block/VT, sudden death or nonspecific changes	Depends on cardiac infection—noncardiac infection

Contd...

Contd...

Diagnosis	*Site and radiation*	*Nature and Severity*	*Duration—precipitating and relieving factors*	*Associated findings*	*Important laboratory data*	*Pitfalls*
7. Postmyocardial infarction syndrome	Same as above	consisting of fever, pneumonitis and painful pericarditis and pluritis	May occur 2 to 11 weeks after MI and is probably an autoimmune response to myocardial necrosis	Responds to nitroglyserin. Dangerous in the presence of anticoagulants, when it may produce a bloody effusion and tamponade	ECG changes present. No changes in cardiac enzymes	May resemble postcardiotomy syndrome and may be recurrent for as long as 2 years. Also called Dressler's syndrome
8. Hypertrophic cardiomyopathy	Substernal radiates to left and/or right axilla, shoulders arms, neck, lower jaw	Often pressure of squeezing pain. Virtually indistinguishable from coronary ischemia	Exertion may precipitate, resolves with rest. It may occur at rest occur at rest also	Systolic ejection Murmur indicates dynamic obstruction Valsalva maneuver or nitrogen provokes dynamic obstruction and worsen pain.	Echocardiography confirms the diagnosis	Atrial and ventricular arrhythmias are common, which are life-threatening
9. Mitral valve prolapse	Variable	Pain is atypical for angina, often varies greatly from episode to episode in the same individual	Variable, occasionally "whooping" or "honking" heard	Palpitation, breathlessness, weakness, light headedness, fatigue, may be present. Mid systolic click and mid-to-late systolic murmur	ECG shows non specific ST-T changes or arrhythmias. Echocardiography show systolic prolapse of mitral valve	Proper follow-up should be present. It is a benign condition. Reassured to avoid inducing cardiac neurosis
10. Aortic stenosis	Substernal pain gradually increases	Remains for hours, variable discomfort, or severe angina	Exertion precipitates	Fatigue, palpitation, exertional syncope due to reduction in cardiac output, arrhythmia, transient cerebral ischemia. Pulse pressure is less. Systolic thrill with mid-systolic diamond shaped murmur	X-ray chest will show if there is calcification of aortic valve. Echo, cardiac catheterization confirms the diagnosis	In rheumatic disease other valves (mitral) also involved
11. Pericarditis	Substernal, may radiate to upper abdomen, back, shoulder, scapula or neck	Sharp pleuritic pain, worsens with movement or dull pressure or ache. Relieved by leaning forward	Onset variable, may last days or weeks, may be recurrent	May be relieved by rest or bending forward. Pericardial rub may be present variably associated with pain. Rub disappears as effusion develops. Pulsus paradoxus may be accentuated with effusion	ECG shows diffuse or variable ST↑ with concave upwards. Saddle-shaped ST↑ throughout all or most of the leads. No reciprocal changes, no Q waves, Echocardiography shows effusion	Onset of accentuated pulsus paradoxus may warn Impending cardiac tamponade
12.Aortic dissection (Dissecting aortic aneurysm)	Anterior chest pain radiating into back between scapulae, sometimes into arms or neck. Hemiparesis (dissection of carotid artery) Paraplegia (spinal artery occlusion)	Severe tearing pain. Patient often writhing with pain. It may be minimal or absent in some cases. Pain occurs abruptly maximum intensity at the outside	Generally of sudden onset, not relieved by rest or nitroglycerin	Male > 40 years hypertension, Marfan's syndrome, pregnancy or postpartum, bicuspid aortic valve, coarctation of aorta. Unequal pulse or BP pulse deficit Hemiparesis (dissection of carotid A), paraplegia (spinal artery occlusion) pulses paradoxus. Murmurs of AR, S/S of pericardial effusion. Superficial catchy sound typically heard best at the lower left sternal edge	ECG shows non-specific changes may show LVH, X-ray chest shows mediastinal widening LVH, Aortography is required to confirm. CT scan is fairly sensitive. TEE, MRI are diagnostic	May be present with minimal or no pain and other clues such as neurological deficits may be the only clue

Contd...

Contd...

Diagnosis	*Site and radiation*	*Nature and Severity*	*Duration—precipitating and relieving factors*	*Associated findings*	*Important laboratory data*	*Pitfalls*
13. Pneumothorax and pneumomediastinum	Localized to the side involved	Sharp, tearing, uni lateral localized pain aggravated by breathing	Hours to days	Chest movements decreased on the affected side. VF,VR diminished with hypertympany. Breath sounds diminished. In pneumoperitoneum, a mediastinal crunch and subcutaneous air	Expiratory film may be necessary to show pneumothora Esophagogram will rule out the rupture of esophagus	Decompression of chest in severe tension pneumothorax
14. Pneumonia	Pleuritic pain on one side of the chest	Gradual onset. Pain with fever and productive cough. Breathlessness is a feature. Pyrexia and tachycardia are common	For days or weeks relieved by antibiotics, analgesics	Pyrexia and tachycardia common. Decrease chest movement on the affected side. Dullness on percussion, bronchial breathing over consolidation which is not always present. Coarse crepitations over the affected area are present	X-ray chest, blood counts	Chest wall pain in the early stages
15. Pulmonary embolism	Chest pain is substernal or diffuse, pleuritic pain may be localized over the involved segment. Small emboli cause pleuritic pain often with hemoptysis	Central crushing pain, pressure or squeezing pain. Pleuritic pain in some small emboli. Dyspnea and tachypnea	Pain may last hours or days. Pleuritic pain often develops with infarction. It may take 12–24 hr to become apparent. Large embolism can cause signs of acute RVF, JVP, parasternal heave can cause hemodynamic collapse	History of recent operation, prolonged bed rest, thrombophlebitis, pregnancy, birth control pills, HRT, malignancy treatment, palpitation and breathlessness usually present, fixed, wide S2 split, pleural rub may be present with infarction	In large embolus, ECG shows S1, Q3, T3, right axis deviation, tall P waves, ST-T abnormalities, new AF, blood gases show PO_2 < hypoxia 80 mm Hg. In about 90% of cases. Normal gases do not rule out small emboli perfusion scanning is gaining importance	Asthmatic breathing. Consider pulmonary emboli. Post-operatively with sudden onset of wheezing and dyspnea
16. Pleuritis	Usually confined to one area of the chest. Point of localization may be present	Severe sharp pain made worse with breathing or movements	Usually lasts hours to days	Fever is common. Shallow breathing. Bends towards the pain area. Friction rub may be heard and disappear with effusion	TWBC is raised in both pneumonia and epidemic plurodynia. X-ray shows pneumonic consolidation. Sputum for smear and culture may show pneumococci	X-ray may not show infiltration in pneumonia in course or due to dehydration
17. Esophageal rupture	Sudden chest pain radiating to back, epigastric area	Severe pain made worse by swallowing. May be in shock (pale, cold, clammy, hypotensive)	Provoked by recent esophageal instrumentation shock or prior vomiting (pale, cold, clammy, hypotension)	May be signs of left plural effusion	Chest X-ray will show mediastinal gas and evidence of plural effusion. A gastrograffin swallow confirms the diagnosis	May be thought as plurisy/plural effusion

Contd...

Contd...

Diagnosis	Site and radiation	Nature and Severity	Duration—precipitating and relieving factors	Associated findings	Important laboratory data	Pitfalls
18. Reflux esophagitis gastroesophageal reflux disease (GERD)	Subxiphoid or lower sternal area radiates to left or right arm, axillae, scapula, neck, jaw	Heart burn are discomfort, which arises from the stomach up into the chest. Burning sensation but may be of pressure or squeezing sensation. Occurs after meals made worse by bending over or lying	Pain remains for minutes to hours, most often after meals or in supine position. Relieved by standing or taking alkalis. The mouth fills with saliva (water brash)	Intolerance to acidic foods, chocolates, etc. Episodic sour taste in the mouth	Bernstein test acid perfusion reproduces patients pain. Fluoroscopy may confirm reflux. Manometry may confirm incompetent lower esophageal sphincter. 24 hr monitoring of esophageal pH is the best test to assess the correlation between symptoms and esophageal acidity.	Relief with antacids present, but it does not rule out ischemic heart disease. Proton pump inhibitor are used
19. Esophageal spasm	Substernal, radiating to the back, arms and jaw	Squeezing or pressure pain, often simulating cardiac ischemia	Sudden onset, often after taking meal or cool drinks. Lasts for minutes to hours	Rarely exertional. Sleep is disturbed	Esophagogram shows abnormal peristalsis. Manometry reveals specific disorder	Responds to calcium channel blockers. Response to nitroglycerin often stimulates cardiac ischemia
20. Acute reflex gastritis	Starts in epigastic area radiates to anterior chest wall	Burning pain related to food. History of 'gas' trouble. Radiating to substernal area	History of chronic alcoholism, taking NSAIDs. Previous history of dyspepsia	Sudden onset, often after taking alcohol, drugs. Tenderness may be in epigastric area	ECG normal, gastroscopy helps in diagnosis	Relieved by antacids, H2 blockers
21. Hepatitis	Mild or severe pain in right hypochondrium	Radiates to the anterior chest wall, epigastric area and right infrascapular area, right lower thoracic areas	Mild diffuse pain slowly increasing in severity pain may persist for 1–3 weeks. Relieved by rest	Jaundice may be present. History of amoebic dysentry may be present in acute amoebic hepatitis. Tenderness in right hypochondrium	Liver function tests, scanning abdomen	May be mistaken for plurisy. Presence of jaundice favors hepatitis
22. Cholecystitis	Mild or severe pain in right hypochondrium	Pain radiates to the back, epigastic area and right shoulder. Spasmodic pain	Movements may increase pain	Jaundice may be present. Tenderness in right hypochondrium	Plain X-ray abdomen, scanning abdomen helps in diagnosis	May be associated with hepatitis, pancreatitis
23.Acute pancreatitis	Excruciating pain upper abdomen sometimes radiating 'lower chest	Very severe, radiating to the back—not relieved by rest or NTG, or sedatives	Relieved by stopping alcohol, DM	Serum amylase↑, > 1000 IU/mL	ECG may be normal	
24. Perforation of peptic ulcer	Upper abdominal pain radiating to lower anterior chest, H/o peptic ulcer	Radiation to right hypochondrium, migrating to RIF	Obliteration of lever dullness		X-ray gas under right dome of diaphragm	

Contd...

Contd...

Diagnosis	*Site and radiation*	*Nature and Severity*	*Duration—precipitating and relieving factors*	*Associated findings*	*Important laboratory data*	*Pitfalls*
25. Herpes zoster	Dermatomal distribution. Usually one dermatome but may involve upto three adjacent segments	Deep unilateral pain usually worsen with movements, sometimes with breathing. Vesicles appear	Mostly typical pain for 1 to 4 days, later rash, vesiculating and crusting over 7 to 10 days. Pain may persist for 2 to 3 weeks. Sometimes persists for months as post-therapeutic neuralgia	Hypersensitivity to pain develops in affected area. Motor involvement is usually transient in small number of cases. Recurrence may occur	Clinical diagnosis. Tzanck smear may show giant cell inclusion bodies but also positive in herpes simplex infections	Immunocomp-romised patients are at increased risk for dissemination
26. Chest wall (Osteoarthritis of sterno costal joints/ Osteochondritis)	Usually localized well to the structure involved, which is also tender	Pain is generally sharp, worsening with some particular movement	Often fleeting, often resolves with rest osteochondritis/ costochondritis is very common reproduced by rotation of the trunk, deep breathing and direct pressure	History of recent heavy exercise or straining affected area. Pain is often triggered by weather changes or lack of sleep. Musculoskeletel pain in the back and neck after strenuous exercise	ECG is normal X-ray cervical spine may show arthritic changes in cervical outflow syndrome	Very common in old age, should be differentiated from simultaneous similar pains due to more serious cause, such as cardiac ischemia. Strenuous exercise also cause rise in total creatine-kinase which should be made by exclusion of other serious conditions
27. Thoracic spine (osteoporotic, metastatic carcinoma, infection (tuberculosis) collapse of osteoporotic or metastatic vertebrae	Starts at the back refers to the front of the anterior chest	Certain postural movements reproduce pain	Pain lost for hours or days	Tenderness over spine present may be dermotomal sensory loss. Response to NSAIDs	X-ray spine may show osteoarthritis metastatic carcinoma, infections (Tuberculosis)	Degenerative changes in the elderly people with vertebral collapse are not uncommon
28. Functional	Variable	Pain is commonly atypical. Typical pains are sharp fleeting, lasts for seconds or constant pain lasting for several days	Variable	History of general weakness, palpitation, hyperventilation with parasthesia is usually present. Pain is commonly triggered by emotional stress, often the patient is unaware of stress. Usually visits number of times for similar complaints with no cause found	ECG may show ST depression with T inversion with hyperventilation. Treadmill test, radionuclide scanning or angiography may be necessary to clarify the condition	This is a diagnosis by exclusion and can only be a presumptive diagnosis in the emergency setting. Importance of follow-up is stressed to avoid inducing cardiac neurosis

Acute myocardial infarction, acute aortic dissection, tension pneumothorax, pulmonary embolus, ruptured esophagus are potentially dangerous and so they should never be missed.

80. The patient of angina may show any of the 4 following clinical signs on auscultation during the attack. (The patient seldom shows any abnormality)

1. Transient apical systolic murmur from ischemic mitral regurgitation.
2. Ventricular or atrial gallop (S3 or S4).
3. Reverse splitting of S2—Paradoxical splitting of second sound.
4. Atrial or ventricular premature beats.

The auscultatory findings are due to dysfunction of the papillary muscles of left ventricle. They generally disappear with resolution of symptoms.

81. Physical findings include signs associated with high risk for coronary artery disease and occult cardiac abnormalities.

1. Hypertension—manifestations of hypertensive vascular disease such as retinal arteriopathy, left ventricular hypertrophy (LVH), etc.
2. Hyperlipidemia—includes corneal arcus or xanthelasma.
3. Diabetes mellitus—micro or macro angiopathy.
4. Carotid or peripheral vascular disease.

82. The patient of coronary artery disease (CAD) may present with or develop any of the following 4 complications:

1. Asymptomatic/presymptomatic coronary disease.
2. Angina or MI.
3. Cardiac arrhythmia.
4. Cardiac failure.

83. One out of every 4 IHD goes unrecognized or undiagnosed—silent myocardial ischemia (SMI)

84. There are 4 possible explanations for the so called silent coronary artery disease.

1. Unreliable history.
2. Witholding of alarming facts by the physician.
3. Lack of investigations.
4. Diagnostic errors.

85. The following 4 investigations are done normally in a case of angina.

The main purpose is to establish the diagnosis, severity of the condition and the line of treatment.

To identify any contributing factors such as anemia, hyperlipidemia or hypothyroidism, etc.

1. Hemoglobin for anemia or polycythemia.
2. Fasting lipids for hyperlipidemia. In familial hyperlipidemia, the younger members of the family should also be screened. It is not beneficial in persons over 65 years age.
3. Thyroid function tests if clinically indicated.
4. ECG.

86. The following laboratory evaluations are done in ischemic heart disease in the absence of history of documented infarction.

1. ECG.
2. X-ray.
3. 2D Echo.
4. Stress ECG.
5. Holtor's ECG.
6. Radionuclide studies.
7. Cardiac cathetarization.
8. Angiography—coronary arteriography and left ventriculography.

87. ECG changes can be noted in the following 4 ways:

1. During pain ECG may show ST depression, T inversion and left axis deviation (LAD).

   In Prinzmetal angina—ST elevation with upright coning may be seen which reverts to normal pattern after the relief of pain.
2. Master's two step test/double masters test.
3. Treadmill maximal exercise or submaximal exercise/bicycle ergometer.

   Exercise tests are useful means of assessing any inability of the coronary circulation to supply the heart muscle with the oxygen it needs during exercise.
4. 24 hours Holter's monitoring.

Other tests are echocardiography, coronary angiogram, LV catheterization with ventriculography.

88. Any of the following 4 changes seen in ECG indicate angina:

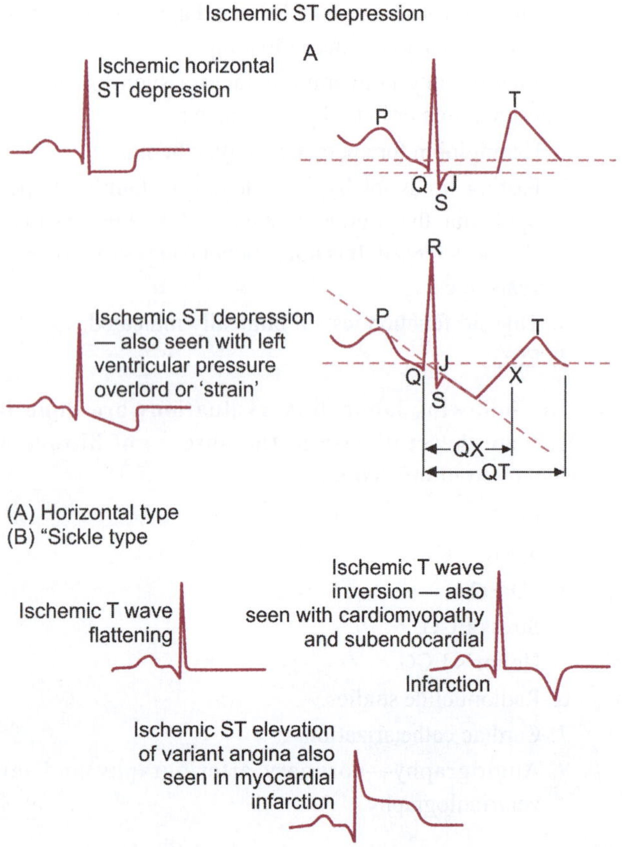

Fig. E-9: (See Fig. Q-144 also)

Cardiac ischemia causes changes in the ST segment and T wave.

ST depression, T wave flattening or inversion is due to endocardial ischemia and ST elevation due to epicardial or transmural ischemia.

1. ST depression: Horizontal depression or oblique depression.
   This is also seen with left ventricular pressure overload or strain or digitalis toxicity. ST depression of 2 mm or more after exercise is positive.
   ST segment can be horizontal, downgoing or upgoing from the J point (the point marking the end of QRS complex and the beginning of the ST segment). The horizontal and downgoing ST segment are relatively more specific than upgoing ones.
2. T wave flattening: This is also seen with hypokalemia, myxedema.
3. T wave symmetrical inversion. This is also seen with cardiomyopathy, subendocardial infarction.
   The resting ECG is normal in 60% of patients with history of angina. However, it becomes abnormal after exercise.
4. ST elevation of Prinzmetal's or variant angina: This is also seen with acute myocardial infarction, pericarditis, and ventricular aneurysm.

ECG may be normal even in three vessel disease. ECG is informative if it is abnormal. Therefore, clinico-electrocardiographic correlation is important.

ECG at the time of chest pain can help to identify the cause of chest pain. Transient changes in the ST segment, T wave or conduction abnormalities help to know the cardiac source of chest pain. A normal ECG does not exclude ischemia as a cause of chest pain.

89. Holter's monitoring: This comprises 24–48 hours continuous ECG monitoring. It has 4 advantages:

1. It identifies high-risk patients.
2. It identifies and quantifies silent ischemia.
3. It evaluates patients with atypical chest pain.
4. It quantifies arrhythmias.

This test is useful in diagnosing, evaluating the drug effects and follow-up of coronary artery disease (CAD) patients. This is now done routinely for risk stratification of post-MI cases. Causes of giddiness which is not identified by routine test may be revealed such as arrhythmias, sick sinus syndrome, etc.

90. 24 hours Holter's continuous recording of the ECG in patients with ischemic heart disease (IHD) has shown the following 4 observations:

1. About 3/4th (75%) of episodes of ischemic ST depression are associated with angina-like pain.
2. About 1/4th (25%) of episodes are painless or silent.
3. Most episodes occur during the daytime—early morning or early evening.
4. The peak number of episodes coincide with diurnal morning peak of catecholamine release, plasma cortisol, heart rate, blood pressure, onset of myocardial infarction and sudden cardiac death.

91. Exercise stress testing (see Q 167–196 for details).

Exercise stress testing provides useful information in patient with normal baseline ECG who are at high-risk for CAD. High-risk for CAD predicted with exercise ECG.

1. Early positive test results in $\leq$ 3 min.
2. Strongly positive result in $\geq$ 2 mm ST↓.
3. Inability to complete 6 minutes of Bruce protocol.
4. Sustained ST↓ $\geq$ 3 mm after stopping the exercise.
5. Down sloping of ST↓.
6. Ischemia at low heart rate of $\leq$ 120/min.
7. Flat or lowered blood pressure response.
8. Serious ventricular arrhythmias at heart rate $\leq$ 120/min.

92. An exercise test should not be done in the following 4 conditions:

1. When acute myocardial infarction is suspected.
2. In organic heart disease in the presence of normal resting ECG or abnormal resting ECG.
3. When the patient is on digitalis therapy or hypokalemia.
4. When ECG shows ventricular hypertrophy or WPW syndrome.

93. Standard maximal exercise test is not possible in the following 4 conditions:

1. Peripheral vascular disease of the lower limbs with severe claudication.
2. Lower limb orthopedic problem.
3. Poor physical condition, chronic airway obstructive disease, end-stage renal disease, etc.
4. Individuals unwilling to undertake exercise due to fear of exacerbation of their symptoms.
   Dipyridamole test is possible in these patients.

94. IV dipyridamole test has the following 4 advantages than treadmill test.

1. It acts as a pharmacological stress agent where the patient is unable to perform exercise.
   Whenever exercise is not possible, it can become a routine screening test for coronary artery disease.
2. It increases coronary flow five times as compared to two times increase by exercise.
   IV dipyridamole increases coronary blood flow similar to that of exercise but without physiological increase in myocardial oxygen demand.
3. When ischemia occurs with dipyridamole, it can be immediately reversed by IV aminophylline, providing rapid control and reversal of ischemia, whereas with exercise test, it takes time for heart rate and BP to come to normal with reversal of ischemia.
4. The drug may be used with other agents or in conjunction with other forms of stress in order to increase maximum coronary flow thereby getting better results.
   Dipyridamole is the most widely used agent because of its action for 20–30 minutes which allows vasodilatation that is sufficiently sustained for radio nuclide deposition. Dipyridamole is less frequently associated with complete heart block than adenosine.

95. A study with large doses of oral dipyridamole has been conducted on known cases of coronary artery disease. Cases are divided into 4 groups:

1. Angio-proven triple vessel disease.
2. Strongly positive treadmill test.
3. Mildly positive treadmill test.
4. Negative treadmill test.
   The results are consistently useful.

96. Utility of dipyridamole test in clinical practice.

In a developing country like India, most of the hospitals are community hospitals. Treadmill machines are not available in majority of the hospitals. Recently introduced computerized treadmill test machines and thallium scan are out of reach as they are very expensive and are not cost effective. In these circumstances, dipyridamole test is useful in our clinical setting as it is extremely cheap, useful and universally accepted test for early detection and assessment of coronary artery disease.

Dipyridamole test can be used as a screening method in coronary artery disease.

1. A negative resting test in an otherwise asymptomatic case will rule out any significant coronary artery disease. There are high chances of triple vessel disease if the resting dipyridamole test is positive.
2. False negative cases are seen only in severe tight single vessel disease. These patients are usually asymptomatic on mild exertion and dipyridamole test with submaximal stress is usually positive.
3. Less amount of exercise may be required to demonstrate ischemia in moderately stenosed vessels.
4. Useful in majority of cases of pre- and postoperative evaluation and helps in avoiding complications during major surgery.

97. Preparation of the patient for the test.

1. Should not eat or drink 4 to 6 hours prior to the test. A full stomach may interfere with the quality of the images. Foods like coffee and tea beverages (including caffeine-free), all forms of chocolate, soda (including caffeine-free and sugar-free).
2. Should not take certain medications (Prescription and Nonprescription): Anacin, cafergot (all forms), darvon compound, excedrin, etc.
3. Medications for asthma such as theophylline or aminophylline should be stopped for 36 to 48 hours before the test. Here is a partial list of medications that contain theophylline—Aerolat, Bronkodyl, Constant-T, ElixophyllineSR, Quibron-T/SR, Resbid, Slo-Bid Gyrocaps, Slo-Phyllin Gyrocaps, Teo-24, Theo Du Sprinkle, Sustaire, Theo Dur, Theobid Duracap, Theochron, Theoclear LA. Theolair-SR, Theophylline SR Theospan-Sr Theovent long acting, Uniphyl, etc.
4. Should wear clothing and footwear suitable for exercising—the test procedure requires hard work, and comfortable clothing will make it easier for the patient. Sometimes, exercise is combined with IV dipyridamole.

98. Dipyridamole can cause steel phenomenon.

The following are the contraindications for dipyridamole:
1. Unstable angina.
2. Acute myocardial infarction.
3. Critical AS—hypertrophic obstructive cardiomyopathy.
4. Asthma.

99. There are 4 points to suggest severe coronary artery disease after exercise test.

1. Low exercise tolerance.
2. Test end point of angina.
3. Fall or failure to rise in BP.
4. ECG changes such as ST depression, etc.

Doing treadmill test after dipyridamole test is complimentary and increases the sensitivity of detecting early cases of coronary artery disease.

100. The following 4 tests help in quantitative estimation of risk factors in angina.

1. Treadmill test—Horizontal ST depression, T flattening or inversion, ectopics, life-threatening, arrhythmias such as ventricular tachycardia, fall of BP are in favor of poor prognosis.
2. Holter's monitoring—ambulatory ECG—ST depression greater than 2 mm in more than 6 episodes is suggestive of poor prognosis.
3. Stress thallium—combined—stress MUGA fall in ejection fraction is in favor of poor prognosis.
4. Coronary angiogram: It gives the anatomical block. It does not give functional block. Angiogram does not reveal whether the perfusion is reversible or not reversible after treatment. It does not give final perfusion information.

101. Echocardiography in coronary artery disease (CAD)

(See R-68–76 for Echo in IHD)

It does not permit direct visualization of the coronary arterial tree. As such it is not useful in the primary diagnosis of coronary arterial disease. The effect of damage on the myocardium can be assessed providing information regarding coronary artery disease indirectly. It can obtain the following 4 information:

1. Abnormalities with left ventricular free wall and septal motion.
   - IHD may manifest as hypokinetic, dyskinetic or akinetic left ventricular free wall or septal motion. It can occur in both acute and chronic coronary artery diseases
   - Lesions involving the left anterior descending artery proximal to the septal perforating branches result in reduced, flat or paradoxical septal motion as well as abnormal left ventricular anterior wall motion
   - Lesion of left circumflex branch results in abnormal motion of left ventricular posterior wall
   - Abnormal motion of posterior wall can also result from lesion of right coronary artery
   - Abnormal motion is less marked and generally returns to normal in subendocardial infarction
   - Abnormal motion may sometimes disappear in inferior infarction
   - Abnormal motion generally does not return to normal in transmural anterior infarction
   - Presence of normal as well as abnormally moving myocardium in the same patient suggests coronary artery disease as against cardiomyopathy where there is global myocardial dysfunction
   - Reduced systolic thickening of the posterior left ventricular wall and/or the septum is also indicative of coronary artery disease
   - Some of the abnormal wall motions may disappear or revert to normal on giving nitroglycerin thus documenting the presence of coronary artery disease. This indicates that the myocardial damage is reversible thus indicating good prognosis while selecting the patients for coronary artery bypass surgery
2. Ventricular aneurysm: Sudden broadening of the ventricular cavity is indicative of aneurysm. In addition, paradoxical motion of the wall of the aneurysm, thinning of the wall and altered function of the myocardium can be identified.
3. Acute myocardial infarction (AMI): Clinical, ECG and enzyme studies clinch the diagnosis. Echo is not needed for the diagnosis of AMI. Presence or absence of left ventricular failure during AMI at times becomes difficult to make out clinically. It can be made out by echo.
   - Papillary muscle dysfunction or rupture can be picked up.
   - It is helpful in distinguishing postmyocardial infarction cardiac tamponade from right ventricular infarction.
4. Assessment of overall ventricular function: End-systolic size, end-diastolic size, percentage of shortening, left ventricular volume, ejection fraction and velocity of circumferential shortening can be calculated. The use of these parameters help in patients' care as well as selection of patients for coronary artery bypass surgery.

102. Stress echocardiography is an economical test with good specificity for recognizing the ischemia this is assessed by:

1. Regional wall motion abnormalities with stress.
2. Dilatation of left ventricle with stress which may be indicative of global ischemia.
3. To assess severity of valvular dysfunction.
4. To identity certain structural heart disease—such as hypertrophic obstructive cardiomyopathy (HOCM) or pulmonary hypertension.

Dipyridamole and adenosine stress echo are done at some special medical centers.

103. Nuclear studies are useful in evaluating the functional perfusion studies, which the angiography does not provide. Coronary angiography was once thought to be the final word before doing CABG. The myocardium may or may not be viable distal to the block. The CABG is benefited when the distal myocardium is viable. This can be assessed by nuclear studies. Since this is noninvasive, it may be preferred over the coronary arteriogram, when the facilities are available.

The following information can be obtained with nuclear studies:

1. Localization of myocardial injury; vascular territories can be defined.
2. Evaluation of functional viability before or after acute MI.
3. Evaluation before and after procedures like PTCA or CABG.
4. In difficult cases where there is small enzyme raise with equivocal ECG.
5. In uninterpretable ECG due to LBBB with equivocal enzyme.
6. Assessment of cardiac performance: LVEF, RVEF, ventricular volume, cardiac output, ejection fraction, regional ventricular function, quantification, etc.
7. Identification of shunts.
8. Identification of valvular diseases.

104. The following methods are used in nuclear cardiology:

Single-photon emission computerized tomography (SPECT) for assessment of myocardium perfusion.

1. *Thallium:* Quantitative thallium scintigraphy using exercise with late redistribution or reinjection at rest imaging as well as rest -redistribution imaging may provide most of the clinically relevant information regarding viable myocardium in patients with left ventricular dysfunction.
2. *(99^m Tc) Technetium:* 99^m Tc sestamibi is of value in measuring ventricular function and detecting ischemia but appears to be of lesser value in assessing myocardial viability (it is now available in India) Radionuclide ventriculography.
3. *Teboroxamine*
   Spatial resolution of SPECT is 1.5 mm. It is more sophisticated.
4. *Positron emission tomography (PET):* It has better spatial resolution of 0.5 mm. It is the 'gold standard' for the identification of myocardial viability but it is costly and generally not available.

Radionuclide angiographic studies are useful for prediction of long-term morbidity and mortality.

105. PET has the following 4 extra advantages besides perfusion studies:

1. Glucose utilization studies.
2. Fatty acid metabolism studies.
3. Oxygen consumption studies.
4. Neuronal control studies.

106. Exercise myocardial perfusion scintigraphy.

Thallium 201 is injected at the time of maximal stress during multistage treadmill test according to the Bruce protocol. Following 4 precautions should be taken.

1. The patient should not eat at least 4 hours before the test.
   This reduces the splanchnic uptake of the tracer to a minimum.
2. The drugs that protect the myocardium such as β blockers should be discontinued for a long enough time for the detection and evaluation of coronary artery disease. For drugs like propranolol, this would be approximately 48 hours before the test to allow the amount of drug in the blood to decrease to less than pharmacologically significant levels.
   On the other end, the drug dosage regimen should be maintained at the same levels prior to the test, if the protective affect of the specific drug is being studied.
3. A 12-lead ECG is taken prior to the test. An intravenous line is kept ready for rapid injection of the radiotracer and for the emergency use if necessary. ECG monitoring should be continued during and immediate post-test period.
4. Exercise should be graded and the injection is given at the time of maximal exercise, which should be maintained for at least 60–90 sec. This is to allow the tracer to be cleared from the blood.
   Exercise should be stopped as in the case of treadmill test, if there is any hypoxia, serious arrhythmia, etc.

107. Thallium scintigraphy of the heart shows 4 main patterns in coronary artery disease.

The specificity of the exercise testing is increased and further information about the state of coronary arteries is obtained. Thallium 201 when given IV is distributed in the tissues in a similar way to potassium. It is rapidly distributed to well-perfused normal myocardium, less well to areas of ischemia, not at all to areas of acute or postinfarcted areas. Scans are taken immediately and repeated after 2–4 hours.

1. *Normal:* Isotope is distributed to all areas of myocardium. It indicates that the blood flow is normal.
2. *Ischemia-reversible pattern:* Poor perfusion of isotope in ischemic areas immediately after the exercise. Reversal to normal perfusion of ischemic areas after 2–4 hours. It indicates some amount of blockage in one or more coronary arteries.
3. *Infarction:* Nonreversible pattern: Poor perfusion of isotope in necrosed area; and no change is seen after 2–4 hours.

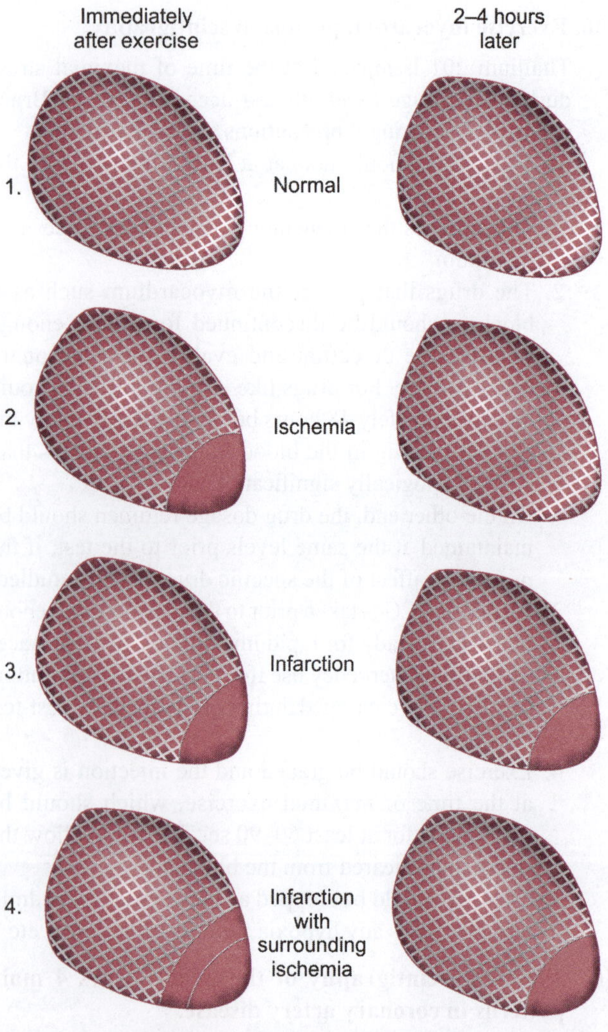

Fig. E-10: Thallium scintigraphy

4. *Infarction with surrounding ischemia:* Nonreversible in infarcted area and reversible pattern in ischemic areas is seen. An area of nonreversible poor perfusion of isotope is surrounded by an area with reversible perfusion.

108. The 4 disadvantages of thallium 201 are:

1. Low energy.
2. Relatively long half-life.
3. Artefacts with breast shadows, high diaphragm, etc.
4. Redistribution of tracer.

Technetium is now available and is cheap.

109. When the patient cannot do exercise, drugs like dipyridamole, adenosine, dobutamine can be used to increase the coronary blood flow. These have the advantage over the exercise. Patient can be reproducibly stressed to a predetermined end point and the method can be used in patients who cannot exercise to maximum level. An imaging test with technetium Tc99 sestamibi (Cardiolite) or thallium 201 (or other cardiac imaging agent) along with IV dipyridamole is performed to get still better results. The imaging test involves a small amount of radioactivity. The amount of radiation is comparable to that from an X-ray or CAT (CT) scan.

Precautionary measures include:

1. Have any allergy to dipyridamole or theophylline.
2. Have asthma, chronic lung disease or any known heart conditions.
3. Consumed foods or beverages containing caffeine within the past 4 to 6 hours.
4. Took any medications containing caffeine within the past 2 days.
5. Took any medications containing theophylline or aminophylline within the past 2 days.
6. Overnight fasting.
7. IV aminophylline 125 mg should be kept ready to reverse the adverse affects of dipyridamole.
8. In women—are pregnant, or suspect pregnancy, or are nursing (lactating), as this test may not be appropriate at this time.

Because the camera is outside the body and must 'see through' the chest into the heart, there is the potential for the left breast to partially cover the heart and cast 'shadows' or artifacts over the heart. If they have breast implants, they may also cause artifacts. Artifacts distort the actual look of the heart and increase the potential for an inaccurate (false positive) diagnosis.

If the patient is currently taking dipyridamole tablets, he can continue then as they will have no effect on the test IV dipyridamole is administered slowly. It takes up to 4 minutes for the full dose to be given. Low level exercise such as using a hand grip, walking in place, or some other small movements are advised.

This simple procedures will take the onset of stress more comfortable, possibly reduce side effects and improve the quality of the images. Once IV dipyridamole takes effect, technetium (99^m Tc) sestamibi or thallium 201 or any other cardiac imaging agent is administered. The pictures are taken at various positions. It takes about 15–30 minutes to obtain all the needed images.

One may notice a harmless metallic taste a few seconds after the administration of (99^m Tc) sestamibi. Side effects like severe hypersensitivity are rarely seen. Potential side effects include chest pain, headaches, dizziness, nausea and flushing may be seen. While this test may seem a bit complicated, it is very accurate in detecting coronary artery disease. These can substitute coronary angiogram. Dobutamine is used to assess the patients who are unable to exercise and tolerate dipyridamole. It is useful in evaluation of coronary artery disease in end stage renal disease. Echocardiogram and nuclear studies can be done before and after dobutamine.

110. Multi slice computed tomography angiography to detect coronary artery heart disease.

It can identify:

1. Left coronary artery stenosis (LCA).
2. Right coronary artery stenosis (RCA).
3. Aortic dissection.
4. Pulmonary embolus.

It is the latest noninvasive investigation. It has advantage over others and it may replace some cath labs and may act as a gate keeper to cath lab.

111. General preventive measures of angina are mainly 4.

1. Stoppage of smoking.
2. Attainment of normal weight.
3. Achievement of normal blood pressure.
4. Control of lipid levels by non-drug or drug treatment.

112. The treatable underlying conditions that may contribute to angina should be looked for:

Risk factors

1. Hypertension.
2. Hyperlipidemia.
3. Diabetes mellitus.

Cardiac conditions

4. Aortic valve disease particularly aortic stenosis, MS, MVP.
5. Arrhythmias particularly paroxysmal supraventricular or ventricular arrhythmia causing rapid pulse and hypotension.

Miscellaneous conditions.

6. Anemia
7. Hypothyroidism
8. Hyperthyroidism

113. Treatment of following 4 coexisting diseases should also be considered besides cardiac conditions.

1. Pulmonary disease.
2. Carotid artery disease.
3. Aortic disease.
4. Cerebral disease.

114. The 4 principles in the management of angina.

1. General measures
   - like reassurance, stoppage of smoking-designing protocol of daily activity—less stress and strain, yoga, meditation. Avoidance of precipitating factors for unfolding clinical angina syndrome
   - control of risk factors
   - exercise like walking if more exercise needed it should be done under the supervision of a physician.
2. Treatment or elimination of coexisting diseases—hypertension, dyslipidemia, diabetes, etc.
3. Drug therapy for angina itself: The aim of drug treatment is to relieve the pain and if possible improve the prognosis by reducing myocardial oxygen consumption or increasing blood supply along the coronary arteries.
4. End points to consider coronary bypass surgery or angioplasty.

115. The primary goal in the management of unstable angina is not acute reperfusion as it is in STEMI. But rather minimization of subsequent morbidity and mortality, i.e. death, nonfatal MI, and refractory angina.

Priority of medical therapy consists of:

I. Antiplatelet agents with aspirin and clopidogrel.
II. Antianginal therapy with nitrates and β blockers.
III. Anticoagulant with unfractionated heparin, low molecular weight heparin (LMWH), direct thrombin inhibitors or factor X inhibitor.
IV. Glycoprotein IIb/IIIa inhibitor in high patient or those undergoing PCI.

116. The 4 groups of drugs used in angina.

I. Nitrates:

For example, nitroglycerin sublingually—(0.4–0.6 mg) 0.5 mg tabs

Long acting nitrates—Isosorbide dinitrate 10–20 mg.

Causes dilatation of major or minor coronary arteries

Reduces BP, venous tone, ventricular volume, left ventricular diastolic pressure and reversal of ischemic changes.

II. β-blockers: Best in angina with hypertension.
Noncardioselective, e.g. Propranolol: 40 mg/day—may be increased to 160–320 mg/day.
Sotalol: 80–200 mg once daily
Oxyprenolol: Up to 320 mg daily in divided doses.
Cardioselective: Acts by blocking mainly B1 adrenoreceptors
Atenolol: 50–100 mg once a day.
Metaprolol: Up to about 400 mg daily in divided doses.
Nodolol: 40–160 mg once a day.

III. Calcium channel blockers
For example, nifedipine, verapamil, diltiazem, tiapamil, ildamen.
Chances of producing AV block is greater with verapamil than with other calcium blockers.
For example,
Nifedipine: 15 mg–60 mg per day in divided doses.
Verapamil: 120–360 mg per day in divided doses.
Diltiazem: 60–180 mg per day in divided doses occasionally up to 480 mg per day.
Combination Therapy
Nitrates form sheet anchor of treatment
β-blockers are given in all patients if there is no contraindication and if the patient is getting frequent attacks on effort inspite of nitrates.
Nifedipine can be combined with β-blocker.
β-blockers + Nifedipine may cause hypotension.
Do not combine β-blocker and verapamil which may even cause dangerous heart block.
Do not combine β-blocker and perhexiline.
In left ventricular failure (LVF)—Nitrates + Lidamine and Lidoflazine is good. Perhexiline is used only when refused for surgery, because it has serious effects on nervous system.

IV. Antiplatelet drugs—aspirin, dipyridamole, clopidogrel
Aspirin is a potent antiplatelet agent. Aspirin irreversibly blocks the enzyme cyclooxygenase which converts arachidonic acid to prostaglandin endoperoxide and ultimately to the formation of thromboxane A2, a powerful vasoconstrictor and platelet aggregating agent.

NITRATES

117. Organic nitrates which are polyesters of nitric acid are potent vasodilators and have been used successfully in the therapy of angina over 100 years. Although clinical efficacy of amylnitrate was described by Brunton in 1867, even today organic nitrates are the most commonly used drugs in angina.

Pharmacodynamics of nitrates: The exact mechanism of action in the relief of angina is not fully understood but appears to depend on their conversion to nitrate ion which is considered to generate oxide

1. Nitrate ion → nitric oxide (this is possibly the same as endothelium derived relaxant factor EDRF).
2. Nitric oxide combines with sulfhydryl radicals of the cells.
3. Stimulates the production of GMP (Cyclic gaunosine monophosphate).
4. Relaxes smooth muscle and hence vasodilatation

118. Action of nitrates can be summarized into 4 steps:

1. Redistribution of blood to ischemic regions in angina pectoris particularly subendocardial regions which are subjected to greatest amount of extravascular compression during systole. They do not increase the total coronary flow in angina. This is by direct vasodilatation of conductance or epicardial segment of coronary arteries . The atherosclerotic process probably prevents this in most of the cases. However, in some cases, collateral vessels may respond and dilate with benefit.
2. Reduction of preload: Predominant effect is vasodilatation of the venous capacitance vessels. This results in venous pooling of blood in veins such as those of the limbs and reduces venous return to the heart. This results in reduction of preload to the ventricles.
3. Reduction of after load by dilatation of arteriolar resistant vessels, so reduces the amount of work load on the hear. This is less prominent than venous dilatation with small doses of nitroglycerin.
4. Reduces wall tension and thereby reduces oxygen demand. Reduction of preload to the ventricles reduces wall tension.

In summary nitrates decrease cardiac work load and oxygen demand by reducing preload and after load (2, 3, 4). They also redistribute blood flow to the ischemic subendocardium by means of decreasing LV end diastolic pressure and vasodilation of epicardial vessels.

119. Remarkable effectiveness of nitroglycerin in angina pectoris is due to 4 advantages.

1. Relaxing effect on stenosed coronary arteries.
Increase in collateral flow to ischemic myocardium is also likely.
2. Reduction of BP.
3. Increase in vascular capacitance.
4. Consequent reduction of ventricular volume.

120. Nitrates are administered in 4 ways:

Table E-3

Route of administration	Generic name	Dose
1. Intravenous	Nitroglycerine (Glyceryl trinitrate)	5–10 μg/minute increased by 5–10 μg/every; 5–10 minutes
2. Oral	Isosorbide dinitrate	5–20 mg q 6 hr
	Isosorbide dinitrate SR	40–80 mg 8/12 hrs
	Isosorbide 5-mononitrate	20–40 mg/12 hrs
	Isosorbide 5-mononitrate SR	60 mg/day
	Erythrityl tetranitrate Spray in also available	10 mg/tid
3. Sublingual	Nitroglycerin	0.15–0.6 mg as needed
	NGR lingual spray	0.4 mg/spray as needed
	Isosorbide dinitrate	2.5–10 mg 2–3 hr
	Erythrityl tetranitrate	5–10 mg as needed
4. Transdermal	Nitroglycerin	1. disk 2.15–15 mg/24 hrs ointment 1.25–5 cm topically to skin 4–8 hr

Intravenous nitroglycerin preparations are used in conditions like acute myocardial infarction. Oral tablets and spray are available. Long-acting nitrates may be taken sublingually as a tablet placed at the side of buccal mucosa or below the tongue.

Transdermal nitroglycerin preparation acts by absorption through the skin via an impregnated patch or ointment. However, diminished efficacy develops in up to 40% of cases but may be overcome by omitting the medication overnight for about 10–12 hours.

121. Main side effects of nitroglycerine are:

1. Flushing.
2. Pulsating headache.
3. Dizziness.
4. Postural hypotension.

1 and 2 are due to vasodilatation of blood vessels supplying the head 3 and 4 are due to lowering of BP.

Headache is common and can be severe. Severity is more initially but decreases with continuous use and often can be controlled by decreasing dose.

Transient episodes of flushing, dizziness, postural hypotension are controlled by positoning and other procedures that facilitates venous return. Not only oral tablets, spray is also available.

122. Drugs interactions of nitrites.

1. Concurrent use of sildenafil (Viagra) and nitrates can cause severe hypotension and therefore absolute contraindication.
2. Use of direct vasodilator like hydralazine, prazosin can cause hypotension.
3. Use of ACEI, CCBs also can cause hypotension.

High doses of intravenous infusion (IVI) > 200 μg/min. Nitrate can displace heparin from antithrombin and cause relative heparin resistance. Frequent partial prothrombin time (PPT) is necessary when IV nitroglycerin infusion rate is high.

123. Nitrates should not be used in angina associated with following 4 conditions:

1. Old age with low BP
2. Stenotic lesions—aortic stenosis, hypertrophic subaortic stenosis.
3. Right ventricular infarction.
4. Hypertrophic cardiomyopathy.

β-adrenergic Blockers (See Chapter B β-blockers in Hypertension B-120–130)

124. β-blockers act by competitively inhibiting the actions of catecholamines on postsynaptic receptors. They are effective in reducing the severity and frequency of attacks of exertional angina. Their main action in angina is to reduce myocardial oxygen consumption, particularly with exercise by slowing the heart rate (negative chronotropic effect).

1. Reduction in BP and pulse rate.
2. Diminishing myocardial contractility—so oxygen consumption (negative chronotropic effect).
3. Decreasing stroke output.
4. Decreasing cardiac output.
5. Decreasing rate of rise of left ventricular pressure.
6. Increasing left ventricular end-diastolic volume.
7. Lengthening of systolic volume.
8. Quinidine like action.

125. β-blockers constitute a cornerstone in the therapy for effort-induced chronic stable angina. These drugs act through blockage of β-receptors both β1 and β2. Those which block β2 only are termed as selective β-blockers. Some of the compounds have an additional alpha-blocker activity. Difference in action of various compounds can be explained on the basis of

1. Lipid solubility.
2. Membrane stabilizing potential.
3. Selectivity of receptor blockade.
4. Intrinsic sympathomimetic activity.

These factors become essential while debating pharmacodynamic, pharmacokinetics and phamacologic action of these drugs. For the clinician, this variation in action is not of much significance. Hence, it is advised that the drug with which clinician is experienced should be adhered to.

126. Main side effects of β-blockers are:

1. *Bradycardia:* Pulse < 50 per minute or even heart block occasionally.
2. *Hypotension:* Due to reduction in cardiac output.
3. *Fatigue:* Possibly due to reduction of cardiac output.
4. *Precipitation of cardiac failure:* Due to their negative inotropic effect and the bradycardia. History of cardiac failure is usually a contraindication.
5. *Bronchial asthma:* Due to blockade of β-2 bronchodilator receptors in the lungs. They may precipitate severe asthma in known asthmatics and may also worsen chronic obstructive airway disease. Therefore, these drugs are contraindicated in these conditions.
6. Peripheral vascular disease/Raynaud's phenomenon due to reduction of cardiac output and blockade of vasodilator β-2 sympathetic receptors in the walls of arterioles.
7. *Impotence:* This is increased by about a third and should be enquired in all male patients on β- blockers.
8. *Bad dreams:* These occur mainly with those which are lipophilic that is highly fat soluble and thus more soluble in the brain than those that are hydrophilic, that is highly water soluble.

127. Dosing of β-blockers:

1. In patients with ongoing pain or persistent hypertension—initially IV metoprolol 5 mg with increments every 5–10 minutes until desired heart rate and blood pressure response.
2. For angina—maintains of:
   Metoprolol 25–125 mg od/bd po
   Atenolol 50–100 mg od/bd po
   And subsequently titrated as necessary
3. For stable angina
   Metoprolol 25–50 mg od/bd
   Atenolol 50–100 mg od/bd po
4. Hypertension
   Metoprolol 25–50 mg od/bd
   Atenolol 50–100 mg od/bd po

Calcium Channel Blockers

(See chapter B-Hypertension 134–140)

128. Calcium channel blockers show diverse physiologic effects like:

1. Vasodilation—both coronary and peripheral vessels.
2. Slowing of AV conduction.
3. Negative inotrophy.
4. Negative chromotrophy.

Calcium channel blockers in unstable angina showed no effect on death or nonfatal MI short acting nifedipine increased the risk for MI or recurrent angina.

129. Calcium channel blockers are indicated in unstable angina:

1. Only in patient with contraindication for β blocker.
2. When β blockers and nitrates fail to fully reveal the symptoms of ischemia.
3. Preferred in variant angina to relieve to spasm.
4. In cocaine induced vasospasm.

130. Contraindications of CCB are:

1. LV dysfunction.
2. Signs and symptoms of congestive cardiac failure.
3. Hypotension.
4. AV conduction abnormalities.

131. With the discovery of calcium channels regulating the entry and exit of calcium from cells to extracellular fluid and vice versa, a plethora of drugs which block these channels have been discovered.

The following are some of the channels:
1. Calcium channels.
2. Voltage dependent channels.
3. Receptor activated channels.
4. Stretch activated channels.

132. The heterogenicity of the chemical configuration of calcium channel blockers exhibit marked difference of action on 4 sites.

1. Cardiac muscle.
2. Vascular smooth muscle.
3. Pacemaker.
4. Conduction tissues of the heart.

133. Nifedipine is useful in the following 4 conditions because of its significant vasodilatation, reducing peripheral vascular resistance and cardiac after load.

1. Angina pectoris.
2. Hypertension.
3. LV dysfunction.
4. Congestive cardiac failure.

The main side effects of nifedipine are dizziness, flushing and headache due to arterial dilatation and also edema of the legs probably due to an increase in permeability of small blood vessels.

134. The calcium channel blockers block calcium entry into vascular smooth muscle cells and cardiac cells by inhibiting calcium channels but do not affect the regeneration of intracellular calcium release. This results in decreased contractions of muscle cells.

The 4 types of calcium channels are L, T, N, and P.

1. L-type channels contribute to entrance of calcium into the cell during phase III of the action potential.
2. T-type channels are located in the atria and sinoatrial node and affect the phase I of depolarization.
3. N and P-types of channels are present in the nervous system.

135. Nifedipine reduces the following 4:

1. LV systolic pressure by an average of 5–10%.
2. End-diastolic pressure by 15–25% (preload).
3. Mean arterial pressure by 5–17%.
4. Total peripheral and coronary vascular resistance by 30–40% (after load).

136. Nifedipine acts in 4 ways.

These drugs act by inhibiting the influx of calcium ions into the cardiac muscle and vascular smooth muscle cells. This results in reduced activity of the enzyme ATPase within the cells.

1. It dilates coronary as well as peripheral blood vessels.
2. It increases coronary flow to ischemic area by relaxation of coronary vascular smooth muscle of those coronary arteries that are not irreversibly stenosed. In this way these drugs are useful in angina due to coronary artery spasm.
3. It decreases cardiac after load by relaxation of arterial smooth muscles in the periphery.
4. It reduces myocardial oxygen demand by reducing contractility of the heart muscle cells resulting in reduction of cardiac work and output.

Increase mortality is noted by using short acting nifedipine among patients with coronary artery disease which was demonstrated in a retrospective study and meta analysis. Amlodipine is most likely to be tolerated by patients with compensation heart failure. In decompensated heart failure all calcium channel blockers should be avoided. Amlodipine is the only calcium channel blocker approved by FDA.

The above group of drugs can be administered alone or in combination. For rapid action, nitrates especially nitro-glycerine, or sublingual isosorbide are the ideal one. β-blocker and calcium channel blocker, especially verapamil and diltiazem group are indicated when tachycardia and hypertension are associated with angina pectoris.

Caution: Use of calcium blockers during acute myocardial infarction or postmyocardial infarction showed more deaths.

Diltiazem is useful in myocardial infarction with very high blood pressure only without Q wave.

137. ACE inhibitor.

1. They act by decreasing mainly the preload and to some extent after load.
2. Decrease myocardial oxygen demand and so helps in the management of chronic stable angina.
3. Ramipril has showed significant reduction in death in high risk population with MI, stroke, diabetes mellitus, and peripheral vascular disease.
4. The heart outcome prevention and evaluation (HOPE) trial showed usefulness in high-risk coronary artery disease, stroke, diabetes, peripheral vascular disease. They reduce risk even in patients with atherosclerosis who do not have evidence of systolic dysfunction.

138. ACEI in coronary artery disease.

1. Improves survival.
2. Helps in ventricular remodeling.
3. Helps in LV dysfunction.
4. Should be added to existing medical therapy in patients with unstable angina/non-STEMI/STEMI to improve overall favorable results in coronary artery disease.

139. Serious side effects of ACEI include:

1. Cough.
2. Hyperkalemia.
3. Decreased glomerular filtration rate.
4. Hypertension.
(See C/I of ACE –B129)

140. Antiplatelet drugs (Drugs modifying platelet function).

1. Aspirin 150–300 mg/day
2. Dipyridamole 25–100 mg/day
3. Ticlopidine 250 mg/day/clopidogrel
4. Synthetic glycoprotein IIb/IIIa antagonist, e.g. integretin, tirofiban, lamifiban seem promising.
(Dazoxiben and monoclonal antibody 7E3 are under evaluation).

ASPIRIN

141. Aspirin is the most commonly used drug in CVS and other disorders.

It is time to discuss about aspirin in the context of ischemic heart disease.

'An aspirin a day…..' just another cliché? Or should you take this advice to heart?

"Does not affect the heart". That assurance in the Bayer aspirin advertisement of the 1920 spoke to concern of the day that some drugs could damage the life-sustaining organ. Today it is clear that aspirin can affect the heart. Ironically, it turns out the effects are beneficial, so much so that some aspirin advertisement now carry the American Heart Association's seal to highlight the cardiovascular effects.

In fact, of the 80 million aspirin tablets Americans take each day, most are taken not for everyday aches and pains but to reduce the risk of heart disease, according to aspirin manufacturer Bayer Corporation.

Aspirin's ability to reduce the body's production of hormone "prostaglandins" is both the reason for its effectiveness in relieving pain and reducing inflammation and its protective effects against heart attacks and strokes. Prostaglandins cause platelets in the blood to stick together, which can eventually lead to blockage of the vessels. It is not the pain relieving quality of aspirin but it's major thrust on pharmacological effect on platelets with beneficial cardiovascular effects.

The name aspirin, wonder drug of 20th century was chosen on 23rd January 1899. It contained the root of aspiric acid from *Spirea* ulmaria. Chemically identical to salicylic acid together with A as an abbreviation for "acetyl". Aspirin was introduced into German pharmacopia on 1st February 1899.

Mode of antiplatelet action:

1. Phospholipid $\xrightarrow{\text{Phospholipase}}$ Arachidonic acid
2. Arachidonic acid $\xrightarrow{\text{Cyclo-oxygenase}}$ Prostaglandin (cyclic) endoperoxide
3. Cyclic endoperoxide ⟶ Thromboxane-A2
4. Thromboxane-A2 $\xrightarrow{\text{releases}}$ Proaggregatory ADP ⟶ Aggregation of platelets

In platelet, aspirin inhibits the cyclo-oxygenase enzyme which catalyzes the conversion of arachidonic acid into endoperoxides. In this way aspirin prevents the formation of thromboxane-A2 which is prothrombotic agent. Once platelets are inactivated by way of acetylation they remain throughout their life. Action of aspirin on the platelets is irreversible and thus will last for the life of the cell.

Platelet aggregation: Platelet synthesize PG E2, PG D2 and thromboxane A2(TX A2).

Thromboxane A2 is a potent stimulator of platelet aggregation in contrast to PGI2, formed by the endothelial cells of the blood vessel walls which is a potent antagonist of platelet aggregation. Since decrease in cAMP is associated with platelet aggregation, TXA2 and PGI2 may exert their opposing action by influencing platelet generation of cAMP.

Inhibitors of endogenous prostaglandin synthesis interfere with platelet aggregation, e.g. a single dose of aspirin can suppress normal platelet aggregation for 48 hours. This effect is presumed to be the result of suppression of cyclo-oxygenase mediated TXA2 synthesis. Cyclo-oxygenase inhibition by a single dose of aspirin is of longer duration in platelets than in other tissues, probably because the platelet in contrast to nucleated cells that can synthesize new proteins, does not have the necessary machinery to form new enzymes. Therefore, the effect of prostaglandin synthesis inhibitors persist until newly formed platelets have been released. Endothelial cells, on the other hand rapidly recover cyclo-oxygenase activity following discontinuation of treatment with inhibitors of prostaglandin synthesis, and PGI2 production is restored. This is one reason that patients taking these drugs are not predisposed to excessive formation of platelet thrombi. Another possible explanation is that platelet is more sensitive than endothelial cells to drugs that inhibit cyclo-oxygenase. Endothelial damage may lead to platelet aggregation along the blood vessels by causing a local decrease in PGI2 synthesis, thereby allowing platelet aggregation at the site of vessel wall damage. However by the same action, but in longer doses, it also probably reduces the production of prostacyclin by the cells of the vessel walls. This may explain why aspirin has been less effective in the production of thrombosis than was expected but the optimum dose of aspirin for this purpose has not yet been settled.

TXA2 levels are low in people eating seafood diet, e.g. Eskimos—in whom low incidence of thrombosis is observed.

(Prostaglandins were so named because they were originally identified in seminal fluid and thought to be secreted by the prostate)

142. Dosing of aspirin.

1. An initial dose of 162–325 mg on non-enteric coated aspirin (chewed and swallowed) should be given to all patients with suspected unstable angina/acute coronary syndrome.

The patients who are allergic to aspirin should receive clopidogrel as soon as possible.

2. Subsequently, daily aspirin dose can be reduced to 811–162 mg daily, with preferred dose for secondary prevention.
3. 162–325 mg/day for at least one month "after stenting" and three months thereafter.
4. After CABG 81–162 mg/day—indefinitely thereafter.

143. Other actions of aspirin unrelated to cyclo-oxygenase inhibition.

1. Acetylation of GTP binding protein
2. Acetylation of thrombin receptor
3. Inhibition of prothrombin
4. Inhibition of lipo-oxygenase pathway in platelet

144. The 100-plus-year-old drug, aspirin has shown to reduce the risk of the following cardiovascular diseases.

1. Aspirin and angina
   i. Randomized clinical trials in 333 male physicians with angina
   Aspirin 325 mg alternate day decreased the incidence of 1st myocardial infarction by 87%.
   ii. Sapat (Swedish angina pectoris aspirin trial) – Aspirin 75 mg/day + Sotalol.
   34% reduction in primary events—MI and sudden death.
   USA—50% decrease in MI and sudden death
   iii. Aspirin and primary prevention of CAD
   Physician health study—(22,071, healthy male physician aged 40–84 years)
   Aspirin 325 mg on alternate day—44% reduction in nonfatal myocardial infarction
2. Aspirin and myocardial infarction: 325 mg soluble/chewable aspirin—followed-up with 150 mg daily
   ISIS-2: 23% reduction in mortality in 35 days
   43% reduction in mortality with aspirin and ATK.
   ISIS-3: Aspirin + Heparin + STK/t-PA—significant reduction in mortality
3. Mitral valve prolapse and aspirin:
   Aspirin 325 mg/day reduce the incidence of thromboembolism
4. Aspirin and coronary bypass surgery should be started soon after surgery. At least for one year or for indefinite period.
   325 mg/day—92% patency rate 9 days; higher patency rate 1 year.
5. Aspirin and Stenting:
   Aspirin + Heparin recommended throughout during the procedure.
   Afterwards—Aspirin + Ticlopidine
6. Aspirin and pericarditis:
   i. Early post MI period—160–325 mg/day, 650 mg to 6 hourly.
   ii. Dresslers syndrome 160–325 mg/day.
   iii. Acute infective pericarditis 160–325 mg/day and steroids.
7. Aspirin and acute rheumatic fever
   100 mg/kg/day—fever and arthralgia disappear within 12–24 hours. Non-disappearance of symptoms should raise suspicion about the diagnosis of acute rheumatic fever.
8. Aspirin and thromboembolic phenomenon in atrial fibrillation, valvular diseases, prosthetic valve.
   SPAF: Stroke prevention and atrial fibrillation—325 mg/day—Ischemic stroke or septic embolization reduced by 42%.
   Primary embolic event and death reduced by 32%.
   AFASAK (Atrial Fibrillation and Aspirin Study)—14% reduction in risk.

145. Aspirin and pregnancy (See hypertension and pregnancy)

1. Prophylaxis against pre-eclampsia—50–75 mg/day
2. May cause premature closure of ductus.
3. May cause IUGR.
4. May cause Abortion.

In general aspirin should be advised unless strongly indicated.

146. Uses of aspirin in other arterial occlusive diseases.

1. CNS diseases: Transient ischemic attack, cerebrovascular occlusive disease, secondary prevention of cerebrovascular accident.
2. Renal disease: To slow the progression of glomerular disease, to maintain the patency of AV canula.
3. Blue toe.
4. Kawasaki disease.

147. Contraindications of aspirin.

1. Aspirin intolerance.
2. Congestive heart failure.
3. Hemophilia.
4. Hepatic cirrhosis.
5. Renal failure/stones.
6. Peptic ulcer.
7. Potential source of bleeding: Piles, GI bleeding.
8. History of bleeding.

148. Relative contraindication of aspirin.

1. Dyspepsia.
2. Iron deficiency anemia.
3. Gout.
4. Asthma.

149. Thienopyridines (Ticlopidine and Clopidogrel).

Ticlopidine and clopidogrel acts by inhibiting adenosine diphosphate (ADP) induced platelet aggregation.

Table E-4

	Ticlopidine	Clopidogrel
1. Pharmacokinetics	By inhibiting adenosine ADP induced platelet aggregation	By inhibiting ADP induced platelet aggregation
2. Onset of action	Delayed usually 2–3 days for maximum antiplatelet affect	Within 2 hours after administration
3. Dosing	Loading dose of 500 mg followed by 250 mg bd	Conventional loading dose of 300 mg maintenance dose of 75 mg od
4. Side effects	Neutropenia (1–5%) rarely thrombotic thrombocytopenic purpurea (TTP)	Rarely TTP also reported

Clopidogrel is preferred over ticlopidine because of its rapid onset of action, less frequent dosing, and fewer serious side effects. It is recommended in all patients with NSTE, ACS.

The benefit of treatment must be balanced against the bleeding risk in patients undergoing CABG. It should be stopped at least 5 days before CABG to decrease the risk of perioperative bleeding complications including reoperation for bleeding.

150. Anticoagulants the choice of anticoagulant therapy depends in unstable angina/NSTEMI depends on the risk and initial management strategy (invasive Vs conservative in NSTE/ACS).

The anticoagulant therapies available are:

1. Unfractionated heparin (UH).
2. Low molecular weight heparin (LMWH).
3. Direct thrombin inhibitors.
4. Factor X a inhibitor.

151. Mode of usage of heparin.

1. *Dosing:* heparin should be given as a weight adjusted bolus (60 μ/kg) followed by an infusion of 15 IV/kg/hour.
   Activated partial prothrombin time (aPPT) should be monitored every 6 hours until it stabilizes between 50–70 seconds, and monitored subsequently every 12–14 hours.
2. *During of therapy:* Unfractionated heparin should be continued at least 3–7 days to achieve clinical benefits.
3. *Rebound ischemia:* It is thought to result from the accumulation of thrombin during unfractionated heparin therapy and the ensuring platelet aggregation. This is prevented by concomitant use of aspirin.
4. *Recommendations:* IV unfractionated heparin used in patients with NSTE-ACS undergoing either invasive or conservation treatment unless contraindicated (For example, history of active bleeding, allergy to heparin, history of heparin induced thrombocytopenia)

152. Some advantage of low molecular weight heparin (LMWH) over unfractionated heparin (UH) are:

1. Increased bioavailability.
2. Fixed dosing (Enoxapen -1 mg/kg SC every 12 hours).
3. More effective thrombin inhibition.
4. Lower rates of heparin induced thrombocytopenia.

153. Direct thrombin inhibitors (DTIs).

1. They inhibit clot bound thrombin more effectively unfractionated heparin.
2. They are not inactivated by plasma protein or platelet factor 4.
3. They can be used in conjunction with thenopyridine or GP IIb/IIIa inhibitor.
4. Used in initial conservative therapy or before invasive angiography presenting with NSTE-ACS.

Bivalirudin (previously Hirulog) is a synthetic derivative of Hirudin.

154. Factor X a inhibitors: Fondaperimaux.

1. It selectively inhibits factor X a.
2. It has decreased binding to plasma proteins compared to unfractionated heparin.
3. It hase dose-independent clearance with longer half-life.
4. Fixed dose and once daily.

The dose of for UA/NSTEMI is 2.5 mg SA once daily.
Contraindicated when creatine clearance is < 30 mL/min.

155. Glycoprotein IIb/IIIa inhibitors.

1. Platelets aggregation needs the activation of glycoprotein IIb/IIIa receptors on the platelet surface (see Fig. E7). The glycoprotein IIb/IIIa receptors of adjacent platelets bind fibrogen molecules which subsequently initiates thrombus formation. Blocking of glycoprotein IIb/IIIa receptor prevent platelets aggregation there by reduces thrombus formation.
   There are 4 common IV glycoprotein IIb/IIIa inhibitor in use:
   1. Abciximab (approved by FDA).
   2. Tirofiban (approved by treatment of unstable angina).
   3. Eptifibatide (approved by FDA).
   4. Lamifiban.

156. Digoxin and diuretics are useful in "Nocturnal angina"

Angina → Impairment of LV systolic function → LVDV ↑ + ischemic myocardium suffer in diastole
↓
Pulmonary vascular pressure

Digitalis is useful in treating the syndrome nocturnal angina'. Agents used in congestive heart failure are also useful in angina.

Decrease in heart size → reduces wall tension → reduces myocardial oxygen requirement.

If heart is of normal size, digitalis aggravates angina by increasing contractility and hence oxygen requirement.

Diuretics are useful in nocturnal angina or angina at rest.

Diuretics are useful in 4 conditions by causing mild reduction in blood volume.

1. Ventricular dysfunction.
2. Hypertension.
3. Peak rise of BP.
4. 'Recumbent angina' or 'angina decubitus' or 'nocturnal angina'.

157. Management of asymptomatic IHD patient depends on 4 factors.

1. Age.
2. Occupation.
3. Degree of positivity of exercise test and duration and stage at which the ECG changes appear.
4. ECG leads in which the changes occur. (Changes in the anterior precordial leads indicate less favorable prognosis than in inferior wall chest leads)

158. Medical therapy for the 4 types of angina pectoris.

I. Stable angina pectoris
   - Sublingual nitroglycerin
   - Oral isosorbide dinitrate

   β-blocker if pain continues—the angina is due to deficiency in the demand end of myocardial oxygen supply-demand system.

   Calcium blockers if necessary.

   Aspirin 300 mg on alternate days.

II. Unstable angina pectoris

   Most patients should be admitted in ICCU.

   Sublingual nitroglycerin

   Oral isosorbide dinitrate.

   Nitroglycerin ointment should be used several times daily.

   IV Nitroglycerin in frequent and recurrent unstable angina.

   Diltiazem or nifedipine is added if discomfort continues.

   The unstable angina is due to decrease in the supply end of myocardial oxygen supply-demand system.

   β-blockers are given if the symptoms continue.

   IV heparin is given with increasing frequency in new onset angina and if the angina is increasing rapidly, aspirin is added.

   The US Food and Drug Administration approved in mid-may, 98 (6-10-98 HeartInfo), the use of tirofiban also known as Aggrastat for patients with unstable angina and for patients who have experienced minor heart attacks. The drug helps to prevent further heart attack that may precede the onset of full-fledged heart attack caused by total blockage of coronaries. Tirofiban can delay and may even prevent the need for angioplasty. About 10% of people who experience unstable angina or a limited heart attack go on to suffer a full heart attack or die within a month.

   According to one trial, tirofiban used intravenously with heparin and aspirin for seven days, reduced by 32% of the combined risk of death, heart attack or ischemia compared to patients who received heparin alone. But after a few months, researchers found that patients who received it were no better off than those on standard treatment.

   The most common side effects of tirofiban when used with heparin and aspirin is bleeding. It was developed from the poisonous venom of Africa's saw-scaled viper.

III. Prinzmetal's angina pectoris or variant angina

   Nitrates-Calcium blockers—Nifedipine–15–60 mg /6–8 hr

   Diltiazem 120–360 mg/8 hrly.

   Nifedipine or diltiazem—to relieve the coronary spasm and dilatation of the coronary vessels.

   Aspirin is added.

IV. Postinfarction angina pectoris

   Oxygen

   Intravenous drip of nitroglycerin

   Heparin

   Oral diltiazem

   β-blockers

   Aspirin, etc.

If the patient continues to suffer from disabling angina despite nitrates, β-blockers, calcium blockers and when angioplasty or surgery cannot be performed because of poor distal vessels or myocardial damage, it may be necessary to continue medical therapy with methamizole or radioactive iodine to reduce the metabolic state. Many of these patients are unable to work.

159. Four groups of drugs are commonly used in ICCU management of patients with unstable angina.

Table E-5: 4 Drugs in ICCU management of USA

Drug category	Clinical condition	Contraindication	Dose
1. Aspirin	Unstable angina	Hypersensitivity bleeding risk	324 mg (160–324) daily
2. Heparin	Unstable angina in high-risk patients	Active or severe bleeding risk H/o heparin-induced thrombocytopenia Recent stroke	80 units /kg IV bolus followed by infusion of 18 IU/kg/hr Titrated to maintain a 'P' 2.5 times control
3. Nitrates	Symptoms are not fully relieved with three sublingual nitroglycerin tablets and initiation of β-blocker therapy	Hypotension	5 to10 mg/min by continuous IV drip-Titrated up to 75–100 mg until relief of symptoms or (headache or hypotension, BP < 90 mm Hg or 30% below starting pressure level if significant is present) Topical, oral or buccal routes are acceptable alternatives
4. β-blockers	Unstable angina	2nd or 3rd degree AV block 5 min heart rate < 60	Metoprolol 5 mg increments by slow IV repeated every by dose of 15 mg followed in 1 to 2 hours by mouth BP < 90 mm Hg every 6 hours Shock Propranolol LV failure-0.5–1.0 mg IV followed in 1–2 hours by mouth every 6 to 8 h Severe reactive airway disease Esmolol Starting dose of 500 mcg/kg over 1 minute then 50–250 mcg/kg/min infusion Atenolol 5 mg over 5 minutes 2 doses followed orally 50 mg 12 to 48 hours then 100 mg daily

Calcium blockers in unstable angina are given only when the patient is unable to tolerate adequate doses of nitrates and β-blockers or in patients with variant angina.

When the pain is not relieved after 3 sublingual nitroglycerin tablets or whose symptoms recur with anti-ischemic therapy, injection morphine 2 to 5 mg IV dose may be given. They may be repeated every 5 minutes to relieve symptoms for patient comfort.

160. There are 4 factors to consider while advising coronary.

Artery bypass graft (CABG) operations.

1. Age: Indications are relatively stronger in younger age because of their longer expectation of active life. Upper age is generally agreed to be the early or middle seventies, although CABG is done successfully in many patients in their eighties with severe angina.
2. Symptomatic status.
3. Coronary arterial status as demonstrated by coronary arteriography, e.g. stenosis of main stem of the LCA, two vessels if one being due to left anterior descending artery, three or more vessels.

   It is generally agreed that surgery is indicated when there is marked occlusion of > 70% of a vessel's lumen. A proximal lesion is more serious threat to life than a distal lesion because it involves larger amount of myocardium.
4. Left ventricular function as determined by left ventricular angiography and hemodynamics: Operation is contraindicated in patients with frank left ventricular failure because operation does not improve the function of the previously damaged myocardium. Operation is justified in severe angina without cardiac failure but have very low ejection fraction for instance as low as 30%.

161. Angioplasty or bypass surgery is considered when the discomfort continues despite all the medical treatment.

There are 4 investigations—the results of which help to decide the procedure.

1. Exercise stress electrocardiogram, treadmill or computerized treadmill test or dipyridamole test.

2. Coronary arteriography.
3. Left ventriculography including the contractility of the myocardium, ejection fraction as well as the presence of other diseases.
4. Radionuclide thallium scan.

162. Indications of coronary arteriography are:

Arteriography demonstrates the anatomy of an artery by the injection of radiopaque contrast medium along its course. In the case of coronary arteriography, this is demonstrated through a catheter introduced into a coronary ostium via the femoral or brachial artery.

1. In patients in whom coronary artery bypass graft (CABG) is contemplated.
2. In whom angioplasty is contemplated.
3. For assessment of severity of the lesion in patients with severe symptoms.
4. When there is doubt about the diagnosis of coronary artery disease after clinical assessment and exercise testing.

One out of 4 suspected stable angina pectoris have normal or minimal disease when studied with coronary arteriography.

So, when the prediction value of history is 90%—the stable angina pectoris patients should have coronary arteriogram and left ventriculogram. When prediction value is less than 80–90% one should have exercise thallium or exercise electrocardiogram.

163. Left ventriculography may show any of the 4 abnormal dysfunctions in coronary artery disease.

1. *Anterior dyskinesia:* When left anterior descending artery is obstructed. It is generally seen in about 93% of ADA obstructions.
2. *Inferior dyskinesia:* When right coronary artery is obstructed, seen in about 83% of patients with severe obstruction.
   Anterior and inferior dyskinesias are described under local dyskinesias where inward systolic movement of the ventricular wall is reduced compared to the adjacent wall.
3. *General dyskinesia:* When all the three vessels are obstructed. (seen in cardiomyopathies also).
4. *Ventricular aneurysm:* When total occlusion of left anterior descending artery is seen. Local enlargement of ventricular wall is seen in systole and usually in diastole with total lack of inward systolic movement with or without paradoxical outward movement.
   Ventricular volumes and ejection fraction are calculated from ventriculogram and hemodynamic effect of the coronary artery disease is assessed.

164. The 4 indications of percutaneous transluminal coronary angioplasty (PTCA) in angina pectoris.

This involves dilatation of stenosed artery by passing a balloon catheter into the narrowed vessel and inflating the balloon to a predetermined size under controlled pressure. The dilatation is achieved by stretching the vessel, cracking the media and intima and by compression of soft plaques.

1. Stable angina pectoris depends on the Canadian Cardiovascular Society Functional Classification.
   Patients with class 1, 2, 3, 4 of stable angina who have proximal disease of a single coronary artery.
2. Unstable angina pectoris—patients with single coronary artery disease.
3. Prinzmetal's angina pectoris—In selected patients of coronary spasm who also have atheromatous obstruction of left anterior descending artery, right coronary artery or circumflex coronary artery. Great care is taken to manage any superimposed coronary spasm that might develop immediately following angioplasty.
4. Postinfarction angina pectoris—decided after coronary arteriogram and left ventriculogram. Angioplasty is indicated in a single vessel obstruction.

In stable angina of class 1, 2, 3, 4 who have triple vessel disease with positive treadmill or radionuclide scan, angioplasty results of randomized trials are still awaited. The disadvantage of PTCA by balloon are that in a few cases emergency bypass surgery becomes necessary during the procedure. Restenosis may occur in 25% of cases and angina may occur within a few months.

165. The 4 indications for bypass surgery in angina pectoris.

Prerequisite—Coronary artery must be suitable—proved by coronary arteriography.

1. Stable angina pectoris
   a. In class 3 or 4 patients with single vessel obstruction who are not ideal candidates for angioplasty.
   b. In class 1, 2, 3, 4 patients who have left main coronary artery obstruction.
   c. In triple vessel obstruction with positive exercise electrocardiogram and radionuclide scan.
   d. In class 1, 2, 3, 4 patients who have high grade obstruction of the proximal portion of the left anterior descending artery plus obstruction in one or other artery who have poor treadmill test.
2. Unstable angina pectoris: Left main coronary obstruction, triple vessel coronary obstruction especially when one of the obstructions is located in the proximal portion of the left anterior descending artery.

Angina is more reliably relieved when the ejection fraction is decreased.

3. Prinzmetal angina pectoris: Coronary spasm superimposed with coronary artery obstruction in patients with left coronary artery, triple coronary artery, double coronary artery diseases, single coronary artery obstruction.
4. Postinfarction angina pectoris should have coronary arteriogram and left ventriculogram to decide the feasibility of bypass surgery. If the coronary anatomy and left ventricular wall motion permit, revascularization with bypass surgery is performed in order to relieve angina and salvage the remaining jeopardized myocardium.

The combination of ischemic heart disease and systolic dysfunction (with or without overt clinical heart failure) carries a poor prognosis and this subset gain greatest benefit from revascularization. In some patients with coronary artery disease, left ventricular systolic dysfunction may reflect the reversible effects of intermittent or prolonged ischemia ("myocardial stunning" or "hibernation"). For example, survivors of myocardial infarction may have evidence of "hibernating" myocardium, that is, hypokinetic, hypoperfused myocardial areas that are still viable and improve after reperfusion. Even with ejection fraction < 15–20% show significant improvement in ejection fraction and functional state after revascularization of hybernating myocardium. Patients with angina and moderate to severe left ventricular systolic dysfunction, including those with congestive heart failure have been shown to have improved survival after CABG. Patients with prior myocardial infarction and congestive heart failure but without angina are commonly evaluated with noninvasive testing to detect ischemia or hibernating myocardium or with coronary arteriography to document the extent of coronary artery disease. However, CABG has not been shown to improve survival in patients with coronary artery disease and heart failure without angina, although regional ventricular function may improve. Potential benefit of coronary revascularization is directly proportional to the extent of ischemic but noninfarcted myocardium that can be revascularized.

166. Coronary artery bypass graft (CABG) surgery—current operative mortality is only 1–2% and perioperative myocardial injury is 2–5% because of the 4 factors.

1. Improved technical skills.
2. Better preoperative care.
3. Improved myocardial protection.
4. Improved postoperative care which results in decrease in myocardial injury and mortality.

Prognosis of CABG in IHD is best predicted by LV function and the extent of coronary obstruction but not severity of angina.

167. CABG can now be done with reasonable safety with a variety of serious and coexisting problems such as the following 4:

1. Renal failure.
2. Coagulopathies.
3. Pregnancy.
4. Hypothyroidism.

168. The 4 contraindications for CABG are:

1. Limited life span due to old age or associated illness.
2. No evidence of reversible ischemia—coronary arteries not technically suitable for grafting.
3. Ischemic cardiomyopathy states.
4. Severely elevated pulmonary arterial pressure (more than 70 mm Hg) with right heart failure.

169. Medical management after angioplasty or coronary artery bypass surgery (CABG—coronary artery bypass graft) is of utmost important.

Postangioplasty

The 4 drugs that are used

1. Calcium blockers.
2. Antiplatelet drugs—Aspirin 300 mg—od or on alternate days.

Post bypass surgery

3. β-blockers.
4. Antiplatelet drugs—Aspirin 300 mg od or on alternate days.

When angioplasty or bypass surgery cannot be performed because of poor risk and the patient continues to have disabling angina pectoris despite nitrates, β-blockers or calcium blockers, it may be necessary to use methimazole (Tapazole) or radioactive iodine to supress thyroid function and to reduce metabolic state.

170. Role of physician in the follow-up of these patients in 4-fold.

1. *Antiplatelet drugs:* All patients should be put on antiplatelet drugs like aspirin or clopidogrel. Aspirin 50/75/150/300 mg od or on alternate days (the dose is widely varied depending on physician/individual choice—number of articles are available)

   This should be continued for lifelong as per the present day of knowledge.
2. *Risk factor control:* Hypertension, obesity, dyslipidemia, diabetes, smoking, etc. should be kept under check as long-term results are significantly altered by these factors.
3. Identification of hypercoagulable states that may require sodium warfarin (coumarin).

4. *Rehabilitation:* All patients should be encouraged to get back to normal life in 6–12 weeks. More than 50% of these patients remain unemployed, not because they are physically unfit but because of misgiven faith that they should take rest. Cardiac rehabilitation program assumes added importance.

171. The 4 important protective factors from ischemic heart disease are

Lifestyle modification.

1. *Exercise:* Regular physical exercises have shown beneficial effect. Minimum requirement suggested is probably about 20 minutes × 3 per week, raising the pulse rate to more than 130 beats per minute. Exercise conditions the skeletal muscles, which decreases total body oxygen consumption for the same amount of workload. Exercise also lowers the heart rate for any level of exertion, which decreases the oxygen demand on the myocardium for any workload. Higher physical activity and exercise, lowers the cardiovascular morbidity and mortality.
2. *Diet:* A low fat diet lowers the incidence of IHD. Lowering fat content from 40–30% total calories is advisable.
   High density lipoprotein (HDL): This is thought to carry cholesterol away from the arterial wall to the liver. (The low density lipoprotein is associated with its deposition on the arterial wall). HDL is not cardio-protective in association with obesity or smoking.
   A strict vegetarian diet with less than 10% fat and dairy products has shown to be beneficial. Individual approach according to personal and cultural needs helps to decrease fat and caloric intake. Traditional food of that family is continued instead of changing to fast-food culture.
3. *Smoking cessation:* (See 27, 28)
   Cigarette smoking is associated with progression of atherosclerosis, increased myocardial oxygen demand due to an alpha-adrenergic increase in coronary tone, and adverse effects on hemostatic values, and elevation of circulating fatty acids, all of which can lead to worsening of stable angina. Smoking cessation has shown to decrease in risk among established CAD patients including who have undergone CABG. Adjunctive therapies include who nicotine replacement patches, gum or sprays or medications such as bupropion and varenicline.
4. *Psychological factors:* Anger, hostility, depression, and stress are shown adverse affect on CAD. Biofeedback and various relaxation exercises, "Dhyana", can alter these factors.
   Prophylactic aspirin: It has a definite beneficial effect in preventing the second attack. Regular aspirin intake in healthy middle-aged persons may have beneficial effect, but is not yet proven.

SILENT MYOCARDIAL ISCHEMIA (SMI)

Myocardial ischemia may also appear to be 'silent' symptomatically, electrocardiographically or echocardiographically. So named as silent myocardial ischemia. This is more dangerous as the intensity of damage is not detected in early stage and patient could present as a heart failure as his first sign.

172. Prevalence of silent myocardial ischemia:

There is substantial increase in the prevalence of coronary artery disease in the country. More number of cases are recognised now because of availability of more investigative facilities but no accurate statistics are available.

Therefore, the prevalence of silent myocardial ischemia is difficult to estimate but the prevalence is likely to be high. The probable prevalence is:

1. 2–4% in asymptomatic middle aged men.
2. 20–30% of asymptomatic postmyocardial infarction.
3. 80–90% of patients with angina.
4. About 25% of myocardial infarction (i.e. 1/4th) are silent.

In Framingham study, 12.5% patients with MI had an unrecognized 'Silent' infarction.

173. There is an objective evidence of myocardial ischemia in the absence of angina equivalent symptom at that time—unrecognized myocardial ischemia. It may be totally asymptomatic in normal persons and post-myocardial infarction or in intervals of angina episodes - but still demonstrates active ischemia. So, there can be any of the following 4:

1. Asymptomatic coronary artery disease with silent myocardial ischemia.
2. Postmyocardial infarction with silent myocardial ischemia
3. Stable angina with silent myocardial ischemia.
4. Unstable angina with silent myocardial ischemia.

These patients are normal at rest but exercise ECG shows heart rate increase and ST depression. Coronary arteriogram shows spasm or obstruction.

174. There are 4 main causes of SMI where the ischemia is silent.

1. Defective pain system:
   - Global deficiency of cardiac nociception, e.g. elderly patients with dementia or cerebrovascular disease
   - Higher pain threshold (somatic or visceral)
   - Autonomic changes in receptors
   - Parasympathetic and sympathetic neuropathy, e.g. diabetes mellitus, alcoholism.
2. Brief duration—protection by collaterals.
3. Prior myocardial infarction—pain innervation is lost in the scar tissue of myocardial infarction.
4. Mechanical or surgical denervation—during coronary artery bypass graft.

175. There are 4 minor causes of SMI.

1. In pulmonary edema when dyspnea is the prominent symptom.
2. ? β-blocker therapy.
3. Under general anesthesia.
4. Failure to recognize the symptoms by the patient/doctor.

1/4th of the patients with SMI do not have pain with no obvious cause.

176. Diagnosis: The 4 aids are:

1. ECG— exercise
   Treadmill exercise: ST depression is in more number of cases ST elevation is in less number of cases.
   Stress incidence: ST depression-demand side of myocardial oxygen supply-demand system.
   Ambulatory 24 hour Holter's monitoring—use minimum two channel.
2. Echocardiogram: Regional wall motion abnormality.
3. Perfusion studies: Decreased myocardial perfusion.
4. Coronary arteriogram.
   Left ventriculogram radionuclide ventriculography.

Radionuclide ventriculography shows abnormal left ventricular function with low ejection fraction with exercise.

177. Radionuclide thallium imaging in detection of silent myocardial ischemia. It has 4 advantages.

1. It is complimentary to other techniques.
2. High degree of sensitivity and specificity.
3. Perfusion abnormalities precede angina.
   Hence, it can detect ischemic changes at lower heart rate and blood pressure production.
4. Useful in risk stratification.
   Limitations are 4.
   a. Artifacts.
   b. False positive.
   c. False positive in LBBB.
   d. Exaggerated left ventricular thinning.

Radionuclide ventriculography showed similar global and regional abnormalities, left ventricular dysfunction abnormalities in silent ischemia. Ejection fraction is less with exercise.

178. Prognostic implications are 4.

1. Asymptomatic coronary disease—high risk versus low risk.
2. Silent myocardial ischemia in stable angina—worse.
3. Silent myocardial ischemia in unstable angina—still worse.
4. Silent myocardial ischemia in postmyocaridal infarction—worst.

179. The 4 principles of treatment are:

1. To abolish ischemia rather than merely eliminate symptoms.
   Demand form
   - Induced by risk in heart rate and BP.
   - β-blockers are useful.

   Supply form
   - Induced by spontaneous reduction of blood flow
   - Occurs at rest.
2. Drugs
   - Nitrates
   - β-blockers
   - Calcium blockers
   - Antiplatelet drugs.

   Long acting nitrates are useful.
   Transdermal nitroglycerin gives good results due to constant blood flow during sleep without side effects.
   Aspirin 300 mg—1/2 tablet a day or one tablet on alternate day.
3. Coronary angioplasty.
4. Bypass surgery in severe left main coronary artery stenosis, triple vessel coronary artery disease with resting left ventricular dysfunction, failure of angioplasty.

DYSLIPIDEMIAS AND CORONARY ARTERY DISEASE

It is appropriate to study the dyslipidemias in the context of ischemic/coronary heart disease. Pathogenesis of lipids is well established in the causation of coronary artery disease (CAD). South Asian people, Indians in particular, are more vulnerable to develop CAD as compared to Caucasians. There is abundant evidence (clinical, biochemical, epidemiological, experimental) of an established relationship between high plasma cholesterol and CAD all over the world. But recorded evidence of cases are available where CAD is present in Indians with normal or low cholesterol levels. Hence, it is not essential to have that every case of CAD has elevated cholesterol level.

180. Different chemical compounds in the food and in the body are classified as lipids. These include:

1. Triglyceride—they are neutral fats.
2. Phospholipids.
3. Cholesterol.
4. Few others of less importance.

The lipid moiety of both the triglyceride and phospholipids is fatty acids, they are single long chain hydrocarbon organic acids.

181. Physiological consideration of fats in the body.

1. Body fats are present in the form of phospholipids, triglycerides and cholesterol in combination with proteins.
2. Blood cholesterol is both exogenous and endogenous, whereas blood triglycerides in chylomicrons are entirely of dietary origin, and phospholipids are manufactured by all cells of the body.
3. Lipids in the plasma are those in transit from the intestines to the stores (adipose tissue and liver) or from stores to the tissue cells for providing the material for oxidation.
4. These lipids and some insoluble proteins for the basis of all cell membranes right from the central nervous system to the gastrointestinal tract. This is responsible for the selective permeability of these membranes.
5. Fat stores in the adipose tissue are the energy reserve as well as insulation against climatic variations.
6. Cholesterol form an impervious layer under the skin to prevent the entry of undesirable water soluble substances into the body as well as evaporation water from the surface.
7. Cholesterol provides the raw material for the manufacture of bile salts and these aid in the absorption of fat from the gut. Hormone synthesis in the testes, ovaries and adrenals is also dependent on adequate cholesterol supply.
8. Dietary intake, state of nutrition of the body, and physical activity, hormones like insulin adrenocorticoid, thyroxin, and growth hormone influence the plasma lipid levels.

182. Plasma cholesterol is affected by:

1. Increased dietary intake—compensated to a great extent for this by synthesizing smaller quantities of endogenous cholesterol.
2. Saturated fat diet—increase fat deposition in the liver. It provides increased quantities of acetyl Co-A in the liver cells for production of cholesterol.
3. Diet with highly unsaturated fatty acids decreases cholesterol.
4. Thyroid
   - Hypothyroidism—cholesterol↑.
   - Hyperthyroidism—cholesterol↓.
   - Believed to be increased metabolism of lipid substances under the influence of thyroxin.
5. Diabetes mellitus—cholesterol↑.
   Believe to result from general increase in lipid mobilization.
6. Estrogen—cholesterol↓.
7. Androgen—cholesterol↑.
   Higher cholesterol in the male is associated with higher incidence of heart attacks.
8. Renal retention disease—cholesterol↑.
   Along with ↑ in triglycerides and phospholipids this is believed to result from inhibition of lipoprotein lipase resulting in diminished removal of lipoprotein from the plasma.

183. Hyperlipidemia, mainly low-density lipoprotein (LDL cholesterol—the bad cholesterol) is a risk marker for atherosclerosis.

Arterial rigidity is caused by:

1. Endothelial dysfunction.
2. Cholesterol deposition.
3. Smooth muscle cell proliferation.
4. Platelet aggregation.

184. There are 4 early clinical manifestations of atherosclerosis

1. Hypertension
2. Ischemic/coronary heart disease—Chronic coronary insufficiency because of coronary arteries involvement.
3. Apoplexy—Brain ischemic attacks when carotid or vertebral systems are involved.
4. Peripheral vascular disease—atherosclerosis involving limb arteries.

185. It is the responsibility of the practising physician to recognize early the risk factors of coronary artery disease and to take appropriate measures to prevent. Screening of lipids is an important step in the prevention of CAD.

Screening for lipid profile is needed in 4 situations.

1. As a part of primary preventive care under 40 years of age.
2. If there is any family history of CAD.
3. If the individual is obese.
4. If there are other risk factors such as smoking, diabetes, hypertension, and others like hyperuricemia, chronic renal or hepatic disease.

186. Obesity (Body mass index (BMI) > 30) is a troublesome disease which predisposes to

1. Ischemic or coronary heart disease.
2. Hypertension.
3. Stroke.
4. Type II diabetes mellitus.
5. Osteoarthritis.
6. Obstructive sleep apnea.
7. Gallstones.
8. Some cancers sensitive to sex hormones (gynecological irregularities).

Overweight is defined as a BMI of 25–29, and obesity as a BMI of at least 30 kg/m^2. Overweight and obese patients may be maintaining a state of low-grade systemic inflammation thus increasing their risk for cardiovascular disease. The clue is their consistently above normal blood concentrations of C-reactive protein (CRP), a sensitive marker for systemic inflammation. The prevalence of CRP levels increased with increasing BMI in both men and women. Obese men were two times more likely and obese women six times more likely to have elevated CRP levels than their counterparts on normal weight. These findings remained clinically significant after adjusting for age, race, waist-to-hip ratio, inflammatory disease and other factors known to influence CRP concentrations (e.g. smoking).

187. Lipids in circulation are in the form of lipoproteins. The lipoproteins which carry the cholesterol and triglycerides are classified into 4 according to their density.

1. VLDL—very low-density lipoproteins.
2. IDL—intermediate density lipoproteins.
3. LDL—low-density lipoproteins.
4. HDL—high-density lipoproteins.

VLDL are covered by apoproteins B100, A and C. They chiefly contain endogenous triacylglycerol.

LDL are covered by B100 apoproteins and they chiefly contains cholesterol and its ester.

About 70% of the plasma total cholesterol (TC) is carried in the LDL fraction and 25% in the HDL fraction. HDL are the heaviest and smallest of the lipoproteins. These are covered by A, C, D and E. They are constituted with phospholipids as the major fraction. The apoprotein A1, A2, C and D activation of enzyme LCAT and help the clearing agents, C lipoproteins cause activation of another enzyme, lipoprotein lipase and causes clearance of IDL (Intermediate density lipoproteins). About 20% of total cholesterol (TC) is carried in the HDL fraction.

Chylomicrons are the largest and lightest and are covered by apoproteins A, B48, and C. They are composed mainly of exogenous triacylglycerol.

188. Atherogenic lipoprotein phenotype for Asians has been characterized by elevated:

1. Triglycerides
2. LDL
3. APO B-100
4. Lipoprotein a [(LP(a)]

Lp(a) levels above 30 mg/dL have been found to be an independent risk factor for CAD in Indians.

HDL-C and APO A1 levels are decreased.

189. Basing on serum cholesterol levels, National Cholesterol Education Program has indicated complete lipid profile evaluation. As per this complete lipid profile is indicated.

1. In all individuals with total cholesterol over 240 mg/L.
2. In individuals with total cholesterol levels between 200–240 mg/dL with at least two risk factors which include male sex, obesity, smoking, etc.
3. In individuals with previous history of coronary artery disease or family history of CAD without risk factors.
4. It is advisable to screen women who had undergone early hysterectomy (it is the observation made in certain areas where hysterectomy was done in early age for other indications but literature is not available). Women who had hysterectomy with bilateral oopharectomy are much prone for CAD. One of the reasons for this natural protection from ischemic heart disease is believed to be the female sex hormone, especially estrogen, secreted by the ovaries. This protection is lost after the menopause.

190. A simple test such as overnight refrigeration of serum at 4°C for 18 hr would indicate the type of hyperlipoproteinemia. Serum will be clear at the end of refrigeration in normal.

1. Thick layer of cream on top with clear serum below in type I.
2. It may have yellow tint in IIa; slightly turbid in type IIb.
3. Turbid to opaque with thin layer of cream on top in type III.
4. Turbid to opaque in type IV.
5. Thick layer of cream on top with turbid serum of bottom in type V.
6. The creamy top is an index of chylomicrons while the turbidity is an index of TG.

Electrophoresis separates lipoproteins as fastest moving alpha band (HDL). Pre and lipoprotein (VLDL), ad lipoprotein (LDL) and W band (Chylomicrons). Electrophoresis helps to distinguish type IIb, type III (Broad B) and type V.

The complete evaluation of lipid profile requires estimation of serum cholesterol, HDL cholesterol, VLDL cholesterol, LDL cholesterol, triglycerides (TG) and chylomicrons.

191. Tracing of cholesterol travels.

Cholesterol is an essential part of body cells. It has an important role in making hormones and bile salts, which help break up fats, and in transporting fats through the bloodstream. Too much of cholesterol can lead to atherosclerosis, coronary heart disease or strokes.

1. The small intestine absorbs fats and cholesterol from the food into the blood which carries them to the liver.
2. The liver manufactures most cholesterol from saturated fats. It distributes this and the cholesterol absorbed from food through bloodstream to body tissues.
3. Cholesterol and fats cannot dissolve in water. To travel in blood, they combine with proteins produced by the liver and intestine and form complexes called lipoproteins. There are two major types of lipoprotein. Low-density lipoprotein or LDL moves cholesterol from liver to tissues and deposit it throughout the body including the heart and blood vessels. So, LDL is known as 'bad' cholesterol. High-density lipoprotein, or HDL seems to gather cholesterol from body cells and transports it to the liver. So, HDL is known as 'good' cholesterol.
4. The liver also breaks down cholesterol, eliminating its products through the bile duct.

192. The goal should be to have a ratio of total cholesterol to HDL cholesterol below 4.5.

Specific example

1. Total cholesterol 200 mg /dL = 4.4 Ratio—near normal HDL cholesterol 45 mg/dL.
2. Total cholesterol 200 mg/dL = 4.0 Ratio—good HDL Cholesterol 55 mg/dL.
3. Total cholesterol 175 mg/dL = 3.0 Ratio—very good HDL cholesterol 55 mg/dL.
4. Total cholesterol 250 mg/dL = 6.0 Ratio—very bad HDL cholesterol 40 mg/dL.

193. What are the normal ranges of lipids in circulation in Indians?

The normal range of lipids in circulation in fasting condition, i.e. after 14 hr fasting are as follows.

1. Serum cholesterol—lower socioeconomic group-110–220 mg/dL.
2. Serum cholesterol—higher socioeconomic group-150–250 mg/dL.
3. Serum triglycerides up to 150 mg/dL (up to 200 mg/dL in Westerners).
4. Serum chylomicrons—nil.
5. Serum HDL cholesterol—greater than 45 mg/dL.
6. Serum LDL cholesterol—up to 150 mg/dL (upto 200 mg/dL in Westerners).
7. Serum VLDL cholesterol—up to 30 mg /dL (Up to 40 mg /dL in Westerners).
8. Serum IDL cholesterol (intermediate density lipoproteins).

Lipoprotein analysis: Total-cholesterol, total-triglycerides, HDL cholesterol

LDL levels can be calculated from Friedwald's equation:

LDC-C = TC (TG/ 2.19 + HDL-C)

194. How are lipoproteins metabolized?

1. Chylomicrons are synthesized as nascent chylomicrons in the intestine and combine with HDL formed from liver to form chylomicrons.
2. Chylomicrons in peripheral circulation in arteries are cleaved by lipoprotein lipase into HDL, glycerol, fatty acids and a remnant, which is taken up by the liver. Glycerol migrates to liver as it cannot be utilized by adipose tissue and whereas fatty acids enter adipose tissue.
3. VLDL is synthesized in liver as nascent VLDL. These, while circulating in peripheral arterioles are cleaved by lipoprotein lipase into glycerol, fatty acids, HDL and IDL. IDL are cleaved further to HDL, FA and glycerol. LDL so formed from VLDL enters into cells of various tissues including those of liver by passing through specific receptors and get metabolized. In liver they lead to formation of bile acids.
4. HDL is synthesized as nascent HDL. In both intestine and liver, nascent HDL scavengers cholesterol from peripheral tissues to form HDL3. HDL3 combines with nascent chylomicrons or VLDL and after cleavage is converted into HDL which unloads cholesterol into liver and get reconverted to HDL3 and takes up cholesterol from peripheral tissues. This cycle of HDL helps in shifting cholesterol in peripheral tissues and arterioles and prevents atherosclerosis. Hence, it is called as 'good' cholesterol. HDL is also helped in this venture by LCAT, which is associated with it.

195. Recent reports which have reviewed the problem of CAD among Indians and Indians settled abroad have stressed the alarming situation regarding its magnitude. It is emphasized that the following 4 causes in Indians replace smoking, hypertension and high cholesterol levels in Westerners as risk factors.

1. Diabetes
2. Insulin resistance
3. Low HDL
4. High triglycerides

Krishnaswamy, et al in their study of over 3000 patients who underwent coronary angiography, found that 2002 patients showed CAD and the remaining 1049 cases had normal coronary arteries. All those cases had lipid profile done. When percentile distribution was done, it was found that 50% of CAD occurred with total cholesterol levels below 152 mg/dL and 5% below 140 mg/dL. The levels in those with normal coronaries were even lower. The significant finding was elevated triglyceride levels and low HDL levels in CAD patients. TG levels were found to increase with age in statistically significant manner. Further analysis revealed that 95% of males and 100% females having high TG levels (> 96 mg/dL) and low HDL (< 19 mg/dL) had CAD. This is now considered as atherogenic phenotype for Indians with reference to Westerners. There are several reports supporting this view and it is claimed that over 75% Indians settled abroad belong to this group.

Indian context

Population is vast in India and there is heterogenicity in origin or race, geography and habitat, socio-economic status, dietary habits, methods of cooking and preservation besides known variables like sex, age which influence the lipid profile of individuals. The south Asian population particularly Indian race is now known to be at-risk for atherosclerosis. It is now observed that CAD can be seen in Indians with normal cholesterol levels. Hence, to measure only serum cholesterol (which is being practised by several Indian physicians) in cases of high-risk group and in cases of CAD does not give proper evaluation. Hence, it is strongly suggested to do complete lipid profile to know TG and HDL levels. The combination of high triglycerides and low HDL seem to be important for our Indian population. We do not have exact cut-off levels. We have to answer safe levels of lipids for Indians.

The next question is whether doing lipid profile alone is adequate and do they need still sensitive tests to correlate with presence of CAD. It is now found that APO A1, APO B100 and Lp(a) estimation is more sensitive. Higher values Lp(a) more than 30 mg/dL is an independent risk factor of CAD.

Lp(a) is a complex made of Apo B linked by disulfide bridge to Apo(a). Increased Lp(a) in serum is constantly and strongly associated with the presence of CAD.

196. Study of coronary artery disease among Indians in USA was commissioned by AAPI in 1990 with Dr Enas Enas, Indian physician, from Chicago as the principal investigator. This study involved collaboration with several prestigious medical centers, including the National Institute of Health and McMaster University in Canada. This study reported a 4-fold high rate of CAD among Indians in the US compared with whites, whereas other studies found a sixfold higher rate compared with Chinese-Americans. Currently, the CAD rates in urban areas in India are 4-fold higher than the overall US rates although these rates were similar 30 years ago. Among the one million Indians settled in the US, 30,000 are physicians, including 2,000 cardiologists. These physicians are not only aware of the major coronary risk factors, but appears to have made maximum modifications of lifestyle and have low prevalence of most of the conventional risk factors. Yet, they have the highest prevalence of CAD among all Americans. The CAD study, involving 1,688 physicians showed the following prevalence:

1. CAD—10%.
2. Obesity—2%.
3. Cigarette smoking—3%.
4. Saturated fat intake—8% (of the daily energy).
5. Hypertension—14%.
6. High cholesterol—17%.
7. Sedentary lifestyle—20%.
8. Diabetes.

Among the risk factors, only diabetes was more common. Interestingly, all minorities in the US, including Blacks, Hispanics, and American Indians (Red Indians) have high rates of diabetes but low rates of CAD. Blood cholesterol levels among Indians are similar to whites, but they have low levels of HDL, resulting in a high TC/HDL ratio, a powerful predictor of CAD risk in diverse populations.

197. Following are some of the observations made in Indians in US:

1. Individuals of Asian-Indian origin have a 3-to 4-fold increased risk of heart disease.
2. Many Asian-Indian individuals have a metabolic disorder(s) not detected by routine tests.
3. Each disorder has a specific treatment.
4. Much of the Heart disease risk appears to be inherited.

Additional scientific information is needed to fight heart disease in Asian-Indians in US.

198. The Asian Indian Heart Disease Registry is a National program designed to collect information on people of Asian-Indian origin in US and the characteristics that result in increased heart disease risk. Demographic data and the results of sophisticated blood tests will be used to clarify the causes(s) of heart disease risk. Blood tests may include:

1. Lipid profile.
2. LDL subclass pattern, LDL peak diameter, 7 LDL and 5 HDL subclasses.
3. Apo B, Apo E isoforms.
4. Lp(a).
5. Homocysteine.

6. Fibrinogen.
7. Insulin.
8. CRP.

199. Indians have elevated serum levels of lipoprotein(a) [(Lp(a)], which render them genetically susceptible to CAD. Following risk factors are noted among Indians:

1. Lp(a) increases the risk of CAD by a factor of 2 to 4. More importantly, the presence of Lp(a) > 40 mg/dL, associated with hypertension by a factor of 4.6.
2. High TC/HDL ratio by a factor 6.9.
3. High homocysteine by a factor of 9.3.
4. All three by a factor of 122.

At least about a third of the Indians have high levels Lp(a) and homocysteine. Certainly, the presence of diabetes, high triglycerides, or smoking can further double or triple his risk. These multiplicative effects of emerging risk factors appear to provide a possible explanation for the excess burden of CAD among Indians, many of whom are lean, non-smoking, vegetarian, *yoga guru*, and marathon athlete.

Safe and effective medications are now available to correct even the worst lipid profile and metabolic milieu. Medications to lower the cholesterol to 140–150 mg/dL (LDL goal of < 100 mg/dL) similar to that of treating patients with CAD seems justified in high-risk Asian-Indians.

200. The following levels are advised to bring down the risk of CAD among Indians in US.

1. Lp(a) < 15 mg/dL
2. Triglycerides < 100 mg/dL
3. LDL < 100 mg/dL
4. HDL > 50 mg/dL
   (Homocysteine < 10)

Higher the HDL, lower the heart risk. Lower the LDL, lower the heart risk.

201. From the above risk factors, the description of cholesterol types with the following names may be justifiable.

1. HDL cholesterol as good cholesterol.
2. LDL cholesterol as bad cholesterol.
3. Triglycerides as ugly cholesterol.
4. Lp(a) as deadly cholesterol.
   (Homocysteine is called as pseudocholesterol)

202. Dietary management—not all fats are equal.

The type of fat you eat is important.

Following are the different types of fats:

1. *Saturated fat:* Rises LDL and total cholesterol levels. Animal products, coconut oil, palm and palm kernel oil, cocoa butter, and hydrogenated oils contain saturated fat.
2. *Hydrogenated fat:* This chemical process hardens fat, makes it creamier and keeps it fresh longer. It also makes the fat more saturated.
3. *Polyunsaturated fat:* Substituting polyunsaturated fat for saturated fat can help to reduce LDL levels, which lower total cholesterol. These fats are found in most vegetable oils and fish oil.
4. *Mono unsaturated fat:* Substituting monounsaturated fat for saturated fats lower LDL and total cholesterol levels. Oil and kernel oils are high in unsaturated fat.

Fats are measured in grams. One gram of fat equals to 9 calories. If you eat 2000 calories per day, 30% fat would equal to no more than 65 grams of fat.

203. Possible mechanisms of action omega-3 fatty acids.

1. Antiarrhythmic
2. Antithrombotic
3. Antiatherosclerotic
4. Anti-inflammatory
5. Improves endothelial function
6. Lowers blood pressure
7. Lowers triglyceride concentrations
8. Lowers production of growth factor.

Arrhythmias: In animal models, fish oil protects against ventricular fibrillation after surgical exclusion of coronary artery. The addition of eicosapentaenoic acid or docosahexaenoic can prevent or terminate pharmacologically incudes arrhythmias in cultured cardiomyopathies from new born rats.

Thrombosis: Large doses reduces platelet aggregation but smaller doses have modest platelet inhibitory effects.

Atherosclerosis: Prevents the progression of atherosclerotic plaques in experimental animals these effects may be due to reduction in lipids, inflammation, production of growth factor, or suppression of smooth muscle cell proliferation.

Inflammation: Has a central role in the development and progression of coronary artery disease. Omega-6 fatty acids can be converted into arachidonic acid and then metabolized into the omega-6 eicosanoids. These are less active and can partly oppose or antagonize the proinflammatory actions of the omega-6 eicosanoids.

Independent of the effects on the metabolism eicosanoids, fish oil, suppress proinflammatory cytokines and reduce expression of cell adhesion molecules.

Endothelial function: They improve systemic arterial compliance and supplementation with docosahexaenoic acid increased vasodilator response in the human.

Blood pressure: They produce moderate reduction in blood pressure possibly through their effect on endothelial function.

Triglycerides lowering: Intake about 4 of omega-3 fatty acids lower triglycerides by 25–30%. Only a small reduction in triglycerides occurred at the lower doses used in (GISSI prevention trial).

Clinical implications: Omega-3 fatty acids from fish or fish oil supplements should be considered in the secondary prevention after myocardial infraction, patient should consume 1 g/day of eicosapentaenoic acid and docosahexanoic acid preferably by increasing their intake of oily fish to at least two servings per week. Some studies found that a higher consumption of omega-3 fatty acids was associated with a lower incidence of CAD and mortality in diabetic women.

204. Omega-3 fatty acids from fish and fish oils can protect against CAD. There is evidence to support fish and fish oil supplements after myocardial infarction, but the mechanism by which fish oils can help are not fully understood.

If the mechanism unfolded, they can guide the future therapeutic development in CAD.
Summary of fats available:

Fatty acids are saturated, monounsaturated and polyunsaturated 2 types of polyunsaturated fatty acids exist – omega 6-and omega-3. Omega-6 fatty acids are available mainly from vegetable oils. Three types of omega-3 fatty acids exist. α-linolenic acid is available from certain plants but eicosapentaenoic acid and docosahexaenoic acid must be obtain from marine sources.

Most studies have shown inverse association between fish consumption and coronary artery disease (Greenland Inumit-Danish investigators-Bang and Dyersburg-1970) and high concentrations of omega-3 fatty acids have associated with reduce risk of sudden death.

The EISSI myocardial prevention trial showed the benefit of 800 mg omega 3 capsule, 300 mg vitamin E both or either after MI.

205.

Flow chart E-2

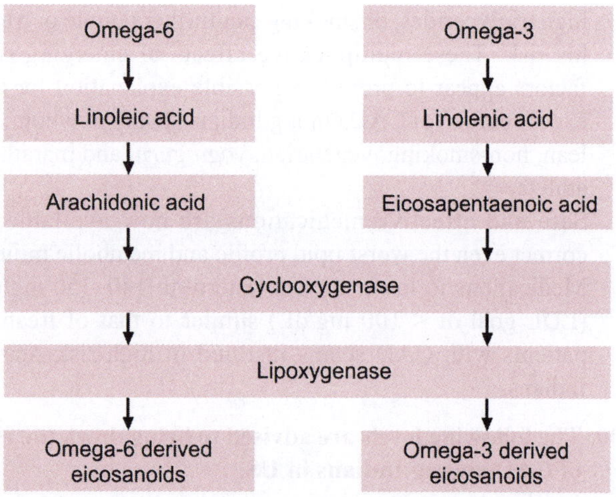

Flow chart E-1

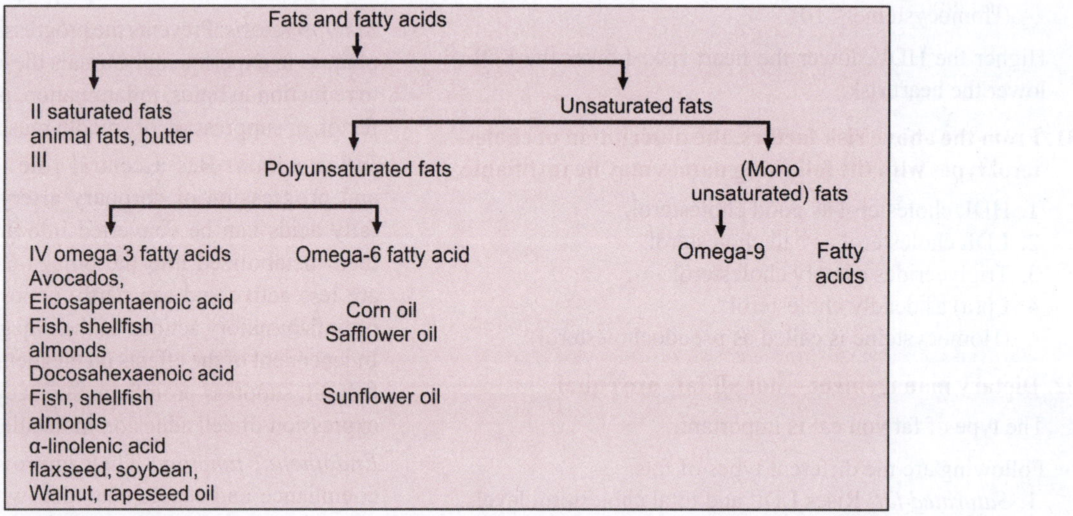

Synthesis of eicosanoids from omega-6 and omega-3 fatty acids.

Arachidonic acid and eicosapentaenoic acid compete for the cyclooxygenase enzymes for conversion into eicosanoids. Those derived from arachidonic acid are proinflammatory and proaggregatroy, whereas those derived from omega-3 fatty acids are anti-inflammatory and inhibit platelet aggregation.

206. It is now accepted that elevated plasma concentration of homocysteine (Pseudocholesterol) is a risk factor for atherosclerosis vascular disease affecting the coronary, cerebral and peripheral arteries. It is appropriate to mention about homocysteine with lipids because of its atherogenicity.

1. Homocysteine is a sulfur amino acid produced by demethylation of the essential amino acid methionine. It may be irreversibly degraded by cystathionine β-synthetase. This enzyme requires vitamin B_6 as a cofactor. Alternatively, homocysteine may be remethylated to conserve methionine, a process requiring several enzymes. Of these, methionine synthase requires methylcobalamin as a cofactor and methyltetrahydrofolate as a cosubstrate. Production of methyltetrahydrofolate requires both an adequate supply of folate and the enzyme methylene tetrahydrofolate reductase.
2. Dysfunction of enzymes or inadequate amount of nutrients may therefore lead to an elevated concentration of intracellular homocysteine, which is then exported to the plasma.
   Both genetic and nutritional factors influence homocysteine concentrations.
3. Patients at high-risk can be identified by stressing the methionine pathway by means of a methionine loading test, analogous to glucose tolerance test.
4. Simple nutrient supplementation with folic acid can reduce homocysteine concentrations in almost all subjects. These observations may have substantial public health implications.
   For high-risk patients in whom dietary measures fail to lower homocysteine, the American Heart Association (AHA) suggests a daily dose of 400 µg of folic acid, 2 mg of vitamin B_6 and 6 µg of vitamin B_{12}. Dietary supplementation with folic acid reduces plasma homocysteine concentrations by about 30% in almost all subjects. The effect of vitamin B_{12} is modest except in deficient subjects. Vitamin B_6 has more effect on lowering homocysteine concentrations unmasked by methionine loading than on basal concentraions, but the clinical importance of this observation is uncertain.

207. There is complex association between hypertriglyceridemia and the risk of CAD. The risk is more where there is family history of CAD combined with other risk factors but not in pure hypertriglyceridemia The chylomicrons remnants and the intermediate density lipoproteins are the main triglyceride rich atherogenic particles. One of the mechanisms suggested is that high triglycerides are associated with.

1. High plasma levels of tissue plasminogen activator inhibitor-1.
2. High levels of clotting factor VII.
3. High levels of clotting factor X thereby increasing the chances.
4. Thrombus/plaque formation in the coronary arteries.

It is observed, that many patients who come for routine executive check up show normal ECG, normal TMT but their HDL is normal or below normal and TGs are high normal or elevated.

208. Hyperlipoproteinemias are described into following types:

1. Type I (Uncommon): Hyperchylomicronemia is characterized by presence of chylomicrons, increased TG and cholesterol in serum, and lipoprotein lipase deficiency, which is not effected by heparin. Clinically it is characterized by eruptive xanthoma, abdominal colic, hepatosplenomegaly, lipemia retinalis. Primary type is rare, secondary type is observed in diabetes mellitus, alcoholism, pancreatitis, hypothyroidism and dysglobulinemia. The patient is generally a child and complains of bouts of abnormal pain (pancreatic) associated with fatty meal.
2. Type IIa (Common): It is characterized by increased cholesterol and normal triacyglycerol.
3. Type IIb is characterized by increased cholesterol and triacyglycerol.
   These are clinically seen with tuberous and tendon xanthelesma, juvenile arcas. This disease is characterized by LDL receptor defect, in primary type. Secondary type is associated with hypothyroidism and obstructive jaundice.
4. Type III (Uncommon): It is characterized by broad B lipoproteinemia, which is due to increased IDL. Hyperuricemia is associated with it. It is usually familial and transmitted as a recessive triat. Incidence of coronary artery disease is high at an early age specially in males.
5. Secondary type III is commonly associated with myxedema.
6. Type IV (Common): Hyper-pre-B-lipoproteinemia is characterized by increased triacyglycerol, xanthoma,

hyperuricemia. The patient is a young adult often suffering from diabetes mellitus and premature atherosclerosis. There is raise in endogenous triglycerides associated with abnormal glucose tolerance curve and raised blood urea. The condition is worsened if it is associated with obesity.

7. Secondary type IV is seen along with pancreatitis, myxedema, nephrotic syndrome, alcoholism and diabetes mellitus.
8. Type V (Uncommon): It is a mixed hyperlipidemia in which both chylomicrons, exogenous and endogenous glycerides are raised in the fasting plasma. It is familial and often secondary to acute metabolic disorders like diabetes, pancreatitis, alcoholism and nephrosis. Hepatosplenomegaly and pancreatic pain are present. Triglycerides rise to several thousand mg/100 mL. The patient shows symptoms at the young adult age.

209. Secondary causes of hyperlipoproteinemias include:

1. Diabetes mellitus.
2. Hypothyroidism—cholesterol ↑
3. Obesity
4. Chronic renal failure—TG↑
5. Nephrotic syndrome—CH↑, ±TG
6. Alcohol abuse—TG↑, HDL↑
7. Drugs—diuretics, β blockers, oral contraceptive, retinoids, corticosteroids, anabolic steroids or progesterone related to testosterone
8. Cholestasis—CH↑, biliary obstruction, biliary cirrhosis
9. Pancreatitis
10. Bulimia—TG↑
11. Anorexia neruosa—CH↑
12. Pregnancy—TG↑.

210. Relationship of risk factors with lipid fractions.

1. Hypertension is associated with increased triacylglycerol, and decreased HDL cholesterol in 10% of cases.
2. Diabetes mellitus patients show low HDL in 19.6% and high triacylglycerol in 9.8% .
3. Obese individuals show low HDL cholesterol in 56% and high triacylglycerol in 56%.
4. Coronary artery disease patients show increase in LDL and decrease in HDL cholesterol. Coronary angiographic studies suggest that HDL cholesterol is an important factor affecting the progression and regression of CAD.

Every 1 mg increase in HDL cholesterol decreases cardiovascular mortality by 4–5%.

Management of Hyperlipidemias

Treatment of high cholesterol is really worthwhile. Consider just these two simple but reliable rules.

- Every 1% reduction in your cholesterol level lowers your risk by 2%.
- Each increase of 1 mg/dL (not percent) of your good cholesterol (HDL) decreases your risk 2–3%.

211. Always first trial with non-drug treatment should be done unless the patient is first seen with high lipid profiles with other CAD risk factors. It consists of:

1. Exercise
2. Diet
3. Weight loss
4. Avoid smoking.

All patients with hyperlipidemia are advised to have regular dynamic (isotonic) exercise like walking, running, jogging, skipping, swimming, any racket game whichever is convenient for the patient. Isometric exercises like weight lifting, bull-works should be avoided because they increase the peripheral vascular resistance.

Both, exercise combined with diet regulation helps in weight reduction. Restriction of diet alone without exercise can cause muscles flabby with less strength followed by tiredness even for routine work. Hence, exercise and diet regulation should be practised combindly.

Stopping of smoking also improves lipid profile.

Dietary Management

Dietary management with reduction of refined carbohydrate, increase in fiber diet and increased use of oils containing monounsaturated fatty acids should be started if LDL cholesterol is greater than 160 mg/dL and HDL cholesterol is less than 40 mg/dL. In Indian population where triglycerides are raised, one should cut down free sugar, sweets, alcohol and saturated fat and should do regular exercise. Various important components of diet, e.g. linoleic acid and alpha-linolenic acid—when taken in optimum ratios are beneficial in management of hypertriglyceridemia and CAD. Diet rich in argenine protects from atherosclerosis.

Taking fish, which is rich in omega-3 fatty acids helps in lowering triglycerides. The benefits of eating fish may stem in part from eating less red meat and therefore less saturated fats. However, omega-3 polyunsaturated fatty acids (PUFAs) may lower other harmful fats in many cases.

PUFAs do make platelets less "sticky". However, they may depress the immune system as well. The amount of fish that is required to lead to substantial drops in cholesterol would require the ingestion of 1–3 pounds of fish per day, an amount the average person is unlikely to eat. Fish oil capsules can supply the 6–15 g of fish oil necessary to make a difference. It is not yet time to recommend fish oil capsules as a general measure for preventing arteriosclerosis, particularly with concerns regarding their effect on the immune system long-term. However, a diet rich in fish can clearly be very helpful, and is recommended.

212. Low fat, low cholesterol food chart

I. Free foods
- (a) Juices like lime juice, tomato juice; (b) Pepper water (rasam) and clear soup; (c) Plain soda; (d) diluted buttermilk.
- Green leafy vegetables fresh green salads and other vegetables except roots and tubers.
- Fat free pickles.

II. Foods permitted in limited quantities
- Refined oils suffola, sunflower, sesame and soyabean oil are better than other vegetable Allowance/day 34 tsp
- Mayonnaise and other sauces made in vegetable oils may be taken in limited amount
- Egg white can be taken
- Lean meat, chicken, fish in limited amount provided they are cooked without fat, i.e. boiled, steamed, raosted or baked. Chicken and fish (50 g) not more than 2 times a week and red meat not more than once in 15 days.
- Skimmed-milk intake per day not to exceed 500 mL.
- Fruits like guava, orange, papaya, watermelon, apple—100 g/day.

III. Food to be avoided
- Fats like butter, ghee, vanaspati, coconut oil.
- Fried food, e.g. chips, samosa, patties, pappad, pakora, etc.
- Puddings and cakes, pastries made in saturated fats (or butter), ice creams, etc.
- Ham, bacon, yolk of eggs, red meat, organ meats crab, shrimps, etc.
- Pickles made in oil.
- Milk products like cheese, khoa, cream, etc.
- Canned, tinned, preserved and processed foods to be avoided like tinned fruits processed cheese, etc.
- High calorie fruits like banana, mango, grapes, chiku.

IV. Foods recommended
- High fiber food items like green leafy vegetables and green salads should be an essential daily item.
- Inclusion of wheat flour with black chana flour or barley flour (4:1) is advisable.
- Whole grams and pulses are preferable to polished ones, may be included in at least one meal, in sprouted or raw form.
- Whole wheat bread is preferable to refined flour bread.

Note: golden rule "no feast, no fast"

Equal spacing of the three major meals per day is very important. Free food items should be taken between major meal and whenever hungry.

Omission of any food item from the list given above does not imply that they are freely allowed or prohibited. Keeping in mind the composition of the food and the food group it belongs to one may use ones own discretion.

213. The recommended dietary guidelines for management of hyperlipidemias are as follows:

1. Restrict total calories to reduce the weight to the expected normal for height, age and sex.
2. It is not advisable to restrict all forms of fats as severe restriction results in mental and physical depression.
3. The total ingestion of fats should be 30% of total calories.

   Step 1 diet: Total fat < 30% total calories, with no more than 10% as saturated fat.

   Step 2 diet: Total fat < 25% total calories, with no more than 7% as saturated fat.

   A ratio of 1:1 of saturated: monounsaturated fats should be allowed. One should also look at the relative ratio of omega-6 and omega-3 in a particular fat. Recent studies have shown that traditional cooking of fats like *desi ghee* and mustard oil are more healthy due to an ideal ratio of omega-6 to omega-3 fatty acids. In ghee, ratio is less than 3 and mustard oil ratio is 1:5. However, in polyunsaturated oils (safflower) the ratio of n-6 to n-3 is very high which leads to peroxidation and more oxidative stress. Hence, the recommendation is consume more of mustard oil, desi ghee, and groundnut oil and less of (< 10%) safflower oil as that would provide an optimum ratio of omega-6 to omega-3.
4. Proteins should substitute 20% of daily calories. Substitute fish and fowl instead of red meat.
5. Carbohydrates should substitute 40–50% of calories. Rice, rich in south Indian diet, wheat, rich in north Indian diet is to be continued. Wheat contains alpha-linolic acid. Complex carbohydrates rich in fiber should be taken. Refined carbohydrates, e.g. sugar should be avoided.
6. Increased intake of green vegetables, fruits and fibers is highly beneficial.

7. Some of the dietary items like garlic, onion, turmeric, fish, soybeans, fibers, gingers, sprouted vegetables which have been found to be beneficial in hyperlipidemia should be taken liberally.
8. Fast foods, fatty, refined and processed foods should be avoided.

   After 6 months of diet therapy combined with regular exercise, if the lipid profile do not show improvement, then drug management should be initiated. Obese persons should show weight loss.

For reducing weight, a useful rule of thumb to follow is that 3500 calories is equivalent to approximately 1 pound of body weight. Therefore, if your aim is to loose 1 pound a week, you must cut 3500 calorie or 2 pounds a week, you must cut 7000 calories. For example non-vegetarians can take 100 g of lean meat or fat free fish in place of whole day allowance of skimmed milk. Daily allowance of fat/oil should not exceed 10 g. Overweight persons with high blood cholesterol should avoid all foods, which are rich in cholesterol.

Coconut oil is used in Kerala State contains high saturated fat—a cause of high rate of coronary artery disease in Kerala.

Musturd oil contains erucic acid used in Bengal state is a cause of high rate of heart blocks by myocardial fibrosis—"Calcutta hearts" or "Bengalese hearts".

214. Weight loss is noticed by:

1. Reduction in glucose levels.
2. Reduction in insulin levels.
3. Reduction in glycosylated hemoglobin.
4. Reduction in triglycerides.
5. Reduction in LDL level.
6. Increase in HDL level.
7. Reduction in BP.
8. Reduction in uric acid level—starvation increases uric acid, so beware when uric acid is > 6 mg%

215. Cholesterol—lowering drugs are mainly 4 groups.

1. 3 hydroxyl, 3 methyl glutaryl coenzyme A reductase inhibitors (Hmg CoA reductase inhibitors), also called statins.
2. Fibric acid derivatives.
3. Bile acid sequestrants (cholestyramine, colestipol).
4. Nicotinic acid.

Others, probucol and psyllium hydrophilic mucilloid are not much used now. Probucol is not used in practice because along with lowering LDL, it decreases HDL by 25%. Psyllium hydrophilic mucilloid acts as a bulk laxative because of increased fiber content. It is not very effective and may have a place in the treatment of mild hypercholesterolemia.

216. Bile acid sequestrants are appealing because they are not absorbed, simply staying in the intestines and absorbing bile and not allowing it to be reabsorbed. By removing bile acids which are made from cholesterol, the liver is forced to use some of its cholesterol to make new bile acids. It is usually taken as a powder mixed with a beverage, such as water or juice.

Bile acid sequestrants are rarely used because of large dosages and side effects, with many patients reporting bloating, constipation, intestinal gas, and nausea. Depending on the dose and the patient's response, these drugs will lower LDL cholesterol by 15–30%. HDL levels often rise by 3–5%, which is also a benefit. These drugs can interfere with absorption of other drugs, including digoxin, warfarin, thiazide, thyroxine, β-blockers and others, so bile acid sequestrants may need to be taken at different intervals to avoid interactions.

You should also be aware that these agents, some of which are available over the counter, may also cause:

Table E-6

Low cholesterol diet (High in polyunsaturated fat)—1800 calories		
Early morning	Lime juice in cold or hot water, tea	
Breakfast	Skimmed milk	240 g
	Bread or porridge or corn flakes	30 g
	Honey	½ teaspoonful
	Fruit	1 serving
Lunch	Atta or rice	90 g
	Skimmed milk curd	120 g
	Cottage cheese or paneer	60 g
	Green mixed vegetables	100 g
	Salad	50 g
Evening	Skimmed milk, tea or coffee	150 g
	Bread	1 slice
	Honey	½ spoon
	Fruit	1 serving
Dinner	Atta or rice	90 g
	Green mixed vegetables	100 g
	Salad	50 g
Before bed	Skimmed milk	150 g
Total daily allowance	Vegetable oil	15 g
	Sugar	30 g
	Honey	5 g
	Skimmed milk	500 g

Table E-7

Weight reducing diet—1000 calories		
Early morning	Lime juice or tea without sugar (if desired)	—
Breakfast	Skimmed milk	225 mL
	Bread	25 g
Midmorning	Skimmed milk or fruit juice	150 mL
Lunch	Atta or rice	25 g
	Dal	15 g
	Skimmed milk curd	100 g
	Green vegetables	100 g
	Salad	50 g
Evening tea	Skimmed milk tea or coffee without sugar	150 mL
Dinner	Atta or Rice	25 g
	Skimmed milk cheese	50 g
	Skimmed milk curd	100 g
	Green mixed vegetables	100 g
	Fruit	1 serving
Before bed	Skimmed milk	150 mL

1. Increased levels of triglycerides, sometimes to dangerous levels.
2. Alterations in absorption of other medications.
3. Decreased absorption of fat-soluble vitamins.
4. Dangerous interactions with some drugs.

217. Nicotinic acid or niacin: has the appeal of being "natural". It is a vitamin which lowers cholesterol and triglycerides. It also raises the good cholesterol. However, its effect are only modest. The advantages of nicotinic acid are:

1. LDL reduction of 5–25%.
2. Triglycerides reduction of 20–25%.
3. HDL elevation of 15–30%.
4. Reduces Lp(a) up to 30%.

It is one of the only agent that reduces Lp(a) significantly up to 30% unfortunately compliance is poor because of frequent side effects. Flushing, pruritis, gastrointestinal discomfort, glucose intolerance, and hyperuricemia often accompany the use of niacin.

Nicotinic acid should not be used in patients with active liver disease or diabetes mellitus. It is best used in those with either elevated LDL or triglyceride levels.

218. Nicotinic acid derivatives.

1. Inhibit lipolysis in adipose tissue.
2. Decrease esterification of triglycerides in the liver.
3. Increase the activity of lipoprotein lipase.
4. Useful in type IIa, IV and V hyperlipoproteinemia.

219. Nicotinic acid is a useful drug but for proper effect, the daily dose has to be 2–10 tablets of 50 mg each. At such dosages flushing occurs and compliance becomes poor in 40% of patients and prevent them from taking on a long-term basis. Hence, this drug is used in combination or alone when other drugs fail.

Flushing can be minimized by using a gradually increasing schedule, and taking it with food. One aspirin or coated aspirin can be taken prior to taking niacin (as long as you have not been told not to take aspirin for other reasons). Antacids can be used if heartburn or indigestion occur.

After starting 50 mg three times a day for 1 week

A reasonable schedule for increasing the dosage of niacin is:

1. 100 mg three times a day for 1 week.
2. 250 mg three times a day for 1 week.
3. 500 mg three times a day for 1 week.
4. 1000 mg three times a day for 1 month.

Then repeat the blood test for cholesterol and triglyceride levels.

220. 4 other things to remember about niacin

1. Niacin can cause liver problems
2. Niacinamide, nicotinamide or long-acting niacin preparations should not be substituted without specific instructions.
3. These agents should not be continued if "statins" (see below) are prescribed, unless you are specifically instructed to do so.
4. Patients with active stomach ulcers, arthritis caused from gout, diabetes, or asthma need to be aware that niacin can worsen these conditions.

221. Isobutyric acid derivatives (Fibric acid derivatives). This group includes:

1. Clofibrate
2. Gemfibrozil
3. Fenofibrate
4. Benzafibrate

Initially clofibrate was used. Gemfibrozil has been a frontline drug after the Helsinki Heart Study trial. It reduces cholesterol, LDL-C and triglycerides and raises HDL cholesterol. It is most effective in lowering triglycerides. This is useful in Indian patients who have high triglycerides. It is given orally 600 mg twice a day half an hour before meals. They have been used less often now because they have not been shown to reduce deaths. Caution is needed to use this agent in addition to statins, since there is a significant increase in the incidence of muscle inflammation, which may be quite severe. This combination needs close medical supervision.

222. HMG CoA reductase inhibitors or statins. This group includes mainly 4.

1. Fluvastatin (Lescol)	2. Pravastatin (Pravachol)
3. Lovastatin (Mevacor)	4. Simvastatin (Zocor)
5. Pitvestatin	6. Orlistat (Xenical)
7. Atorvastatin (Atocor)	8. Rosuvastatin (Rosutac).

These are listed in order of increasing potency.

Statins are the best drugs for lowering cholesterol. All seems to be similar in their actions and none has emerged as being superior to others. At standard doses, statins reduce LDL by 20–25%, raise HDL by 5–10%, and lower triglycerides by 10–20%. They are generally safe and well-tolerated. They can be used in combination with other cholesterol-lowering drugs and are currently the most widely used of all. These are given as single daily dose of 10–80 mg daily. These are less effective than gemfibrozil and nicotinic acid in the treatment of hypertriglyceridemia alone.

Atorvastatin (Lipitor) is an addition to statin, which has lowering effect on triglycerides.

Orlistat (Xenical) is a newer statin drug. It was licensed at the end of 1998 in UK and the rest of the Europe, is a powerful inhibitor of pancreatic lipase, so some 30% of dietary fat is not digested is excreted in feces.

Dose: 120 mg capsule three times daily with each meal. Many patients on orlistat experienced fatty stools, increased defecation, and oily spotting (the test was not completely double blind) and after 2 years on orlistat up to 5.8% of them had abnormally low blood concentrations of β-carotene, vitamin D and vitamin E. A multivitamin tablet always advised 2 hours before or after taking statins such as at bedtime.

In practice, combination of gemfibrozil with statin are used when patient had both raised triglycerides and cholesterol. If there is raised cholesterol only, statins alone are advised and when there is only hypertriglyceridemia, gemfibrozil alone is the drug of choice. In few case, one may add nicotinic acid to gemfibrozil to lower triglycerides. The drugs should be stopped as soon as the lipid levels have come within normal range. But the patient is advised to follow diet and exercise program to keep his lipids within normal range. It is not uncommon in practice that patients indulge in dietary indiscretions and sedentary lifestyle resulting in recurrence of hyperlipidemia. They have to go back to drug therapy to correct hyperlipidemia.

Atorvastatin and rosuvastatin are now commonly used.

223. The results of several studies are impressive.

1. The Scandinavian Simvastatin Survival Study (SSSS)—investigated over 4000 patients who had a heart attack, showing a 40% reduction in deaths over about 5 years in patients treated with simvastatin (Zocor).
2. In patients who had undergone heart bypass surgery, lovastatin was shown to reduce blocked bypass grafts by about one-third.
3. The "West of Scotland" study showed a reduction in mortality in people who had no previous events such as heart attack or bypass surgery. These were just folks with modest elevations of cholesterol in the range of 250 mg/dL. The incidence of first heart attacks was reduced by about 31% death by 32%, and mortality from any cause by 22%.
4. Most recently, a study examining multiple published trials comprising approximately 29,000 patients showed a 29% risk of stroke, 28% reduction in cardiovascular deaths and 22% reduction in overall mortality. This confirms the decrease in the incidence of blockage of vessels to the brain as well as to the heart.

Severe studies done such as Mercury trial, Uranus, Andromeda, Corall, Natural Cholesterol Education Program (NCEP), Adult Treatment Panel (ATP III), to show different claims over one another. It seems that rosuvastatin has slight edge over Atorvastatin.

224. It is appropriate now to mention about diabetic dyslipidemia.

Raised plasma cholesterol in diabetes is associated with a disproportionately greater risk of coronary vascular disease with 4 time's higher mortality in diabetes than in non-diabetes with the same concentration of serum cholesterol.

225. The characteristic pattern of lipoproteins in diabetes included an:

1. Increase triglycerides ↑	2. Increase LDL ↑
3. Decrease HDL ↓	4. Postprandial lipemia.

The majority of type II diabetes mellitus, insulin resistance, or metabolic syndrome, exhibits the atherogenic lipoprotein phenotype.

This condition occurs due to disturbances in the production and clearance of plasma lipoproteins.

226. Various studies showed that rosuvastatin has slight edge over others.

1. Rosuvastatin 10 mg dose is equivalent to 20 mg atorvastatin, 40 mg of simvastatin.
2. Water soluble—can be administered at any time.
3. Low incidence of myopathy, rhabdomyolysis/or liver toxicity, lung toxicity, at a dose as high as 20 mg per day is negligible compared to other statins particularly the lipid soluble ones.
4. Cost-effective.

Ezetimibe combination with simvastatin and atorvastatin are also used.

The combination of statin plus ezetimibe has been studied in small studies and has proved to be highly safe and effective at lowering LDL-C levels. The combination should be reversed for the patients who fail to maximum statin doses or are intolerant of statins. Ezetimibe reduces cholesterol absorption by the enterocyte. Ezetimibe reduces cholesterol absorption from the small bowel by 23–50% and reduces serum LDL level by 14–20% when used in combination with statins.

227. Rosuvastatin has the pleiotropic effects.

1. Anti-inflammatory role.
2. Immunomodulatory activity.
3. Antioxidant action.
4. Plaque stability—it is known to improve by endothelial function, reducing platelet aggregation or limiting the inflammation.

228. Rosuvastatin (10–40 mg)

1. Lowers LDL-C up to 45–55%
2. Increases HDL
3. Lowers triglycerides
4. Lowers C-reactive protein independently.

229. HMG/CoA reductase inhibitors (statin) have the side effects.

1. Myopathy
2. Rhabdomyolysis
3. Acute renal failure secondary to myoglobinuria
4. Lung toxicity.

230. Treatment of hypercholesterolemia patients with statins reduce the incidence of fatal and nonfatal myocardial infarction by 30–35%. The benefits are accompanied by fewer coronary revascularization procedures and strokes. Other benefits, which have not yet been clearly shown include reduction in the incidence of:

1. Anginal symptoms
2. Congestive heart failure
3. Disability
4. Unemployment.

Quality of life is improved. Moreover, cost-effectiveness of statins in secondary prevention is comparable to or better than other standard preventive measures.

Statins may have produced additive or even synergistic effects in combination with non-lipid treatments like cessation of smoking, aspirin or β-blockers.

Annual sales of cholesterol-lowering drugs during 1997 in USA increased by a remarkable 29% to $3.7 billion (International Marketing Services). The great popularity of statins is due to their efficacy and tolerability.

231. Therapy for specific lipid disorders.

1. Very high LDL levels
2. Very high triglycerides levels
3. Low HDL cholesterol
4. Diabetic dyslipidemia.

1. *Very high LDL level:* Usually result from inherited disorders of lipoprotein metabolism and carries early atherosclerosis.

   Hypothyroidism may be associated with markedly elevated LDL and should be ruled out in many patients with elevated LDL level. Most of these patients respond to high dose statin therapy in addition to dietary restriction.

   Addition of bile acid sequestrant with an additional thrid agent (Niacin) is often warranted to achieve the target level. Ezetimibe is another agent that may improve in this group.

2. *Very high triglyceride levels:* Elevated triglyceride levels: is caused by many factors and more than one cause may be active in a given patient. Minor elevated triglyceride levels of 150–299 mg/dL commonly caused by sedentary lifestyle, obesity, smoking, alcohol, and high carbohydrate diet.

   In other patients—secondary causes, such as diabetes mellitus, renal failure, Cushing's disease, nephrotic syndrome, or some medications, such as protease inhibitors, corticosteroids, retinoids, oral estrogens may be responsible.

   Genetic causes in some patients.

   The patients are benefited by lifestyle changes, total calorie restriction, changing from high carbohydrate diet to a more balanced diet and treatment of secondary causes if present.

   Intermediate: Intermediate rise in triglycerides level—(200–499 mg/dL) these patients are more of heterogeneous group.

   Very high triglyceride levels (≥ 500 mg/dL): Usually results from genetic defect of lipoprotein metabolism.

   In some patients—combination of factors ≥ 1000 mg/dL–these patients are at high-risk for acute pancreatitis and treatment is directed to the prevention of this condition.

   These patients are benefited by very low fat diet, weight reduction, physical activity—initiation of fenofibrate or niacin therapy. Fibrates are especially effective and statins are not of much use.

   This often results of interaction of poor lifestyle, secondary causes, genetic factors. These patients may have other atherogenesis marker such as increased small LDL, low HDL, or elevated VLDL remnants.

The patient needs aggressive treatment to lower LDL to target level by statins.

After the LDL target has been achieved, the secondary goal is non-HDL-C (goal of 30 mg/dL higher than target LDL-C).

The choices are niacin or fibrates in addition to statin. These combination increases the risk of hepatotoxicity or myopathy and careful monitoring is necessary.

Refectory cases may benefit from fish oil supplements (> 3 mg/day) which reduces VLDL production, can lower the serum triglyceride concentration by as much as 50% or more. Fish oil supplements contain less than 50% of active omega-3 fatty acids.

3. *Low HDL cholesterol:* Often seen with minor or modest elevations in triglyceride levels.
   It is an independent risk factor of cardiovascular disease.
   Diet modification, lifestyle changes, weight reduction, medications, e.g. progestational agents, anabolic steroids.
   Fibrates or niacin therapy is a reasonable choice to rise HDL-C.
   Current guidelines specify rising HDL should be tertiary goal after LDL and non-HDL-C goals have been reached.
4. *Diabetic dyslipidemia:* It is often associated with an increase in small LDL particles and often is associated with high triglycerides and low HDL level. Hyperglycemia is an independent risk factor for coronary artery disease. Primary prevention is important in this group. All diabetic patients (irrespective of LDL-C level) should be considered for statin therapy. Secondary goals include improved non-HDL-C level and treatment of elevated triglycerides level and blood sugar control. Insulin therapy often facilitates former, but fibrates and low dose niacin may be necessary in some patients. Patients of diabetes mellitus often have coexisting hypertension, which should be controlled to reduce cardiovascular events.

232. Some newer observations in the treatment of dyslipidemias which are controversial:

1. *Machines to lower cholesterol:* There are some people with a specific metabolic disorder who just simply cannot reduce their cholesterol with diet, medication, etc. However, while in the 'average case' an agent such as statin can increase the activity of the enzymes and receptors in the liver. In patients who have no particular enzymes or receptors in the liver, require a machine to filter the blood and remove the offending cholesterol. The liposorber is the most current model in use for the approximately 7000 Americans with this particular disorder. This is complex, expensive, not without risk, and certainly not for most of the patients.
2. *'Gene therapy':* Some patients have undergone removal of part of their liver. Cells were then 'transfected' with the gene for normal reception and removal of LDL. The cells were put back in the patient's liver. Improved cholesterol levels were noted. Again this is not for the majority of patients who have such receptors, even if they are not quite perfect.
3. Chromium is a trace element that gained notoriety first with diabetes. It is a cofactor for insulin and there must be enough of it around for insulin to work. It has a similar but lesser role in cholesterol metabolism. If a patient has deficiency in chromium, which is unusual, there is no meaning in supplementing it. However, most of us have the chromium we need and that case taking more has never been shown to do any significant good.
4. *Daily regular use of alcohol:* It is true that modest alcohol ingestion raise the 'good' HDL cholesterol. It appears that the equivalent of 1 or 2 ounces can raise the level by 5–10%. Red wine may provide some additional benefit, as can some dark beers. Everyone knows that alcohol is the most abused drug worldwide. It will probably kill number of people from its multiple negative health effects (including traffic accidents) than it helps with this modest improvement in cholesterol.

Women and coronary artery disease:

Women have lower incidence of CAD than men. However, a striking increase in the incidence of CAD occurs in women after menopause. Women in their reproductive age have a favorable pattern of fat components in their blood, They have higher levels HDL and lower levels of LDL and total cholesterol than men under 50 years age. One of the reasons for this natural protection from ischemic heart disease/CAD is believed to be the female sex hormone, especially estrogen, secreted by the ovaries. This protection seems to disappear after the reproductive age. The use of hormone, especially estrogen, after menopause seems to afford protection against developing heart disease, although the point is still debated. One study done by the Harward Medical School involving 33,000 postmenopausal women showed that the hormone-users had a significantly lower incidence of CAD than non-hormone-users. An association between the use of oral contraceptives and nonfatal myocardial infarction in younger women has also been observed. Two prospective studies in UK confirmed an increase in nonfatal myocardial infarction in users of oral contraceptives.

One interesting point established by a German study was the fact that single or widowed women, and housewives who did not pursue a career of some sort were more at-risk of having a heart attack in postmenopausal stage. The stress factors affecting this group of women seem to be different and often suppressed in comparison to the day-to-day stresses faced by career-women and older women with spouses/family. Smoking in women in India is very much less compared to the Westerners. Staying away from smoking by Indian women is another protecting factor from CAD.

233. The protection from CAD in women consists of:

1. Diet regulation free of animal fat.
2. Keeping body weight under control.
3. Regular exercise.
4. Supportive environment free of stress.

Use of estrogen for CAD in postmenopausal women is debated unless it is associated with other diseases like menopausal syndrome or osteoporosis. Estrogen given alone or in combination with progestins improves lipid profile and lowers fibrinogen concentration in post-menopausal women.

Bibliography

1. Bhatia ML. Prevalence of coronary heart disease in India. A contemporary view. Indian Heart J. 1995;47:339-42.
2. Enase Ae Yusuf S. Mehta JL. Prevalence of coronary artery disease in Asian Indians. Am J Cardiology. 1992;70:945-9.
3. Gupta R. Prakash H. Majumdar S, et al. Prevalence of coronary heart diseases and coronary risk factors in an urban population of Rajasthan. Indian heart J. 1995;47:331-8.
4. Krishnaswami SA. A study of lipid levels in Indian patients with coronary arterial disease. Int J Cardiology. 1989;24:337-45.
5. Vardans, Mookerjee S, Awadh K, Sinha N. Special features of coronary heart disease in people of the Indian subcontinent. Indian Heart J. 1995;47:399-407.

CYTOPROTECTIVES

234. The newer cytoprotectives or cellular acting drugs like L-carnitine, trimetazidine, and nicorandil are now in use.

Before proceeding to discuss the cytoprotectives or cellular acting drugs, it is important to mention briefly the metabolism at the cellular level.

How cell produces energy: ATP cell produces energy from the diet we eat. Most of our energy comes from the mitochondria, the power producer of the cell. Mitochondria are like a power plant which burns fuel to produce the electricity that runs the machines. The food you eat is the fuel that is 'burned' inside the mitochondria. A product of this burning is a compound called adenosine triphosphate (ATP). ATP is the 'electricity' that runs the cell's activities. It supplies the energy, for example:

1. When a protein is made.
2. When a muscle cell contracts.
3. When a nerve cell sends an impulse.
4. When a gland cell produces a chemical, etc.

235. ATP molecule consists of three substances: (1) adenosine (2) Ribose (3) Three phosphate groups.

The bonds that attach the second and third phosphate groups are rich in energy. Energy is released when they are broken. Body cell produces ATP in a very complicated process.

1. First, our digestive system breaks down the food we eat. The digestive system breaks down.
   - Proteins into ammonia
   - Fats into fatty acids
   - Sugar and starches into simple sugars.
2. The blood carries these substance into all the cells in the body. In the cytoplasm sugars are broken down into pyruvic acid and a small amount of ATP is produced. The aminoacids, pyruvic acid, fatty acids enter into mitochondria.
3. Mitochondria: Enzymes in the mitochondria break down these substances further in a series of chemical reactions. Oxygen must also be present in the mitochondria for these reactions to take place. The reactions produce carbon dioxide, water and many molecules of ATP.
4. The ATP molecules then leave the mitochondria and provide power wherever it is needed in the cell.

For any job that is done the enzyme breaks the ATP phosphate bonds, release the energy.

The enzyme responsible for ATP (ultimate source of energy) are called sodium potassium dependent ATPase, which changes its chemical form in a way that shuttles sodium and potassium into and out of the cells. While doing this, enzyme uses up between 20–50% calories in the food we eat. Too little enzyme activity may mean that the calories an obese person receives from even a meagre diet are stored as fat instead of being burnt into fuel for cell operations. This causes insufficient metabolization of fatty acids which in turn increases triglycerides and accumulation of fat in the body.

236. Role of L-carnitine in the metabolism of the normal and ischemic heart disease.

1. L-carnitine is an essential cofactor of fatty acid metabolism. It is a cofactor of several enzymes necessary for transformation of long free chain fatty acid into mitochondrial matrix. β-oxidation of these compounds precedes their entry into krebs cycle where energy (ATP) production occurs. Energy produced by utilization of long free chain fatty acid is the major and preferred source of energy for cardiac muscle. In the absence of L-carnitine, the accumulation of fatty acids in the cytoplasm produces toxic effect in the cell besides deficiency in energy (ATP) production.
2. L-carnitine, by increasing the myocardial uptake of free fatty acid, increases the energy available for myocardial contractility without increasing the overall oxygen consumption of the myocardium. Thus, L-carnitine increases the tissue level of ATP.
3. Deficiency of L-carnitine decreases oxidative utilization of glucose leading to reduction of excess lactic acid which is highly toxic to the myocardium, contributing to ischemia.
4. L-carnitine has a positive inotropic effect, decreasing pre-ejection period (PEP), increasing left ventricular ejection time (LVET) and reduced PEP/LVET ratio baseline.

237. The beneficial effects of L-carnitine in ischemic heart disease are:

1. Improvement in systolic and diastolic arterial pressure.
2. Decrease in anginal attacks.
3. Decrease in rhythm disorders.
4. Improvement in lipid pattern.

238. L-carnitine is administered in the following dosage:

1. In ischemic heart disease for adults: 990 mg 2 or 3 times a day depending on clinical response.
   Other uses
2. Hypertension: 330 mg bd/tid.
3. To improve athletic performance: 990 mg before exercise.
4. My be used in valproate toxicity: 50 mg/kg per day in divided doses for 4 weeks or longer.

239. Trimetazidine.

1. It prevents the shift from aerobic to anaerobic metabolism: It exerts direct anti-ischemic effects on the heart by interfering with the metabolic shift, either at the pyruvate level or by reducing the betaoxidation. This may allow the heart to oxidize fatty acids preferentially during reperfusion, thereby removing possible toxic acyl esters. Moreover, trimetazidine demonstrates the protection of mitochondrial function and also exerts control in the calcium regulation of mitochondria.
2. It prevents the development of acidosis: It prevents the influx of Na^+ and Ca^+ ions concentration inside the cells and also prevents the efflux of K^+ ions outside the cells. This effect can be attributed to the restoration of Na^+-K^+ATPase pump functioning.
3. It prevents free oxygen radicals toxic effects by its potent antioxidant action.
4. Trimetazidine inhibits platelet aggregation. Reduces calcium influx (and hence intracellular calcium accumulation) in stimulated platelets.

240. Trimetazidine is useful as an additive agent in:

1. Stable angina.
2. Acute MI in combination with thrombolysis.
3. Severe ischemic cardiomyopathy.
4. Cardiac involvement in scleroderma.

241. Nicorandil: It is a selective ATP dependent potassium channel opener and nitric oxide donor.

1. It activates potassium channel.
2. Donates nitric oxide (NO).
3. Comprehensively corrects endothelial dysfunction.
4. Continuously protects myocardium.

FREE RADICALS AND VASCULAR DISEASE

They have a role in the function of the normal endothelium and in atherosclerosis.

The discussion of free radicals along with ischemic/coronary artery disease and dyslipidemias is worth it. How much we know about free radicals and their role in atherosclerosis is limited. It is better to adhere the discussion in the clinician point instead of going in details of chemistry, pharmacology, pharmacokinetics, etc.

242. Vascular endothelium is a selectively permeable barrier between the blood and the vessel walls. It is not a passive barrier. Endothelial cells play an important part in:

1. Controlling vessel tone
2. Vascular permeability
3. Platelet aggregation
4. Adherence of phagocytes, such as neutrophils and monocytes.

243. Vascular endothelium can release many products which include:

1. Adenosine
2. Prostacyclin
3. Endothelin
4. Platelet activating factor.

244. Endothelium secretes a free radical, nitric oxide (NO*), endothelium derived relaxing factor (EDRF)

A free radical, denoted by a superscript dot, is an atom or molecule with one or more unpaired electrons; an unpaired electron is a lone electron in an orbit. Endothelium secretes both vasodilators and vasoconstrictor.

Vasodilators

1. EDRF which is chemically nitric oxide, a free radical
2. Prostacyclin (PG).

Vasoconstrictors

3. Endothelins.
4. Thromboxane (TxA2).

There is always a balance between vasodilators and vasoconstrictors to maintain the vascular tone. Damaged endothelium may give rise to alterations in this balance and hence change in the tonicity of coronary vessels

245. Endothelial cells also generate another free radical, superoxide(O_2*). Whether endothelial cells release superoxide all the time *in vivo*, or only after an insult (such as ischemia and reperfusion) is unknown.

When two free radicals meet they can join their unpaired electrons and form a non-radical. Superoxide and NO* react quickly to form ONOO, peroxynitrite. As a result, superoxide antagonizes the vasodilatory action of NO*. Addition of superoxide dismutase, an enzyme that scavenges superoxide prolongs the life of NO*.

It has been suggested that vascular overproduction of superoxide might be one cause of hypertension. ONOO (peroxynitrite) produced by the reaction between superoxide and NO* is itself cytotoxic.

Vascular endothelial cells can be damaged by:

1. ONOO peroxynitrite produced by the reaction between superoxide and NO*, nitrous oxide.
2. Hydrogen peroxide by mechanisms that involve damage to DNA and protein caused by free radicals as well as an increased concentration of intracellular free calcium ions.
3. High concentrations of organic peroxides, such as the lipid peroxides are produced when free radicals attack polyunsaturated fatty acids side chains and cholesterol in membranes and lipoproteins.
4. Injury by chemical or mechanical or by infection with certain viruses.

Lipid peroxide concentrations are higher in hyperlipidemic patients, even during treatment with lipid-lowering drugs, although whether concentrations are high enough to injure the endothelium is unknown.

More evidence is now coming that reactions involving free radicals especially peroxidation of low-density lipoproteins in vessel walls, are major contribution to the development of atherosclerosis.

246. How does low-density lipoproteins (LDL) contribute to the development of early atherosclerosis?

1. LDL in the early stages of peroxidation promotes adherence of monocytes to endothelium.
2. Monocytes develop into macrophages within the vessel wall.
3. Both cell types, monocytes and macrophages can generate superoxide and hydrogen peroxide, and macrophage may also generate nitrous oxide, NO*.
4. Extensively peroxidized low density lipoprotein (LDL) can be taken up by macrophages to form "foam cells" laden with lipid, which are present even in early atherosclerotic lesions.

Smoking aggravates atherosclerosis by increasing free radicals. An adequate dietary intake of vitamin E seems to have protective action against vascular disease, perhaps because vitamin E inhibits peroxidation of lipids

PREVENTION OF CORONARY ARTERY DISEASE AMONG INDIANS

Coronary artery diseases (CAD) are increasing in an alarming rate and needs immediate call for preventive action.

Prospective cohort studies for evaluation of coronary risk factors such as the Framingham study, do not exist in India. Should we wait till such epidemiological scientific data is available in India before preventive efforts are initiated? No, we can learn from the available data. It may take long time to collect correct statistical data evidence at the present government where we do not have even social security number to every member of the population even after 50 years of independence and also with unaccountable government medical field in India, by which time the situation becomes endemic in several areas with surprising explosive situation.

Although CAD is a fatal disease with no known cure, it is also highly predictable, preventable and treatable. During the past three decades, CAD rates halved in US, Australia, Canada, France, Japan and Finland. The reductions in CAD are attributed to nation wide changes in specific risk factors addressed through population based interactions, rather than extensive use of expensive high tech investigations. Ironically the CAD rates doubled in India during the same period.

247. Epidemiological research in other parts of the world revealed the following ethnic differences with the world's largest populations namely Indians and Chinese occupying the opposite ends of CAD spectrum.

1. Indians in US have a 4-fold prevalence than White Americans.
2. Indians in US have a 6-fold higher hospitalization than Chinese-Americans. The mortality rates among

Chinese immigrants are 3- to 4-fold lower than Indian immigrants in many countries.

3. The excess risk of CAD is seen in both men and women, although tobacco abuse is virtually non-existent among Indian women. Among women, Indians have the highest CAD mortality in UK, South Africa, Canada and Singapore and also in Fiji, Mauritius, Uganda and Trinidad.
4. CAD is prematurely affecting the young Indians. Three vessel disease with extensive areas of infarction is more prevalent in Indians.

248. One recent cross-sectional survey in India revealed CAD prevalence rates as:

1. 10% in urban Delhi and 5 in rural Haryana. (This latest CAD rate from rural Haryana is 2.5-fold higher than the 2% rates reported by Dewan in 1974 from the same village).
2. 10% in urban India is about double that of 5% in rural India—4-fold higher than in US (2.5%).
3. The rates appear to be higher in South India with a major tertiary care center in Chennai, reporting an 8-fold increase from 4–33% over the past 30 years.
4. The rates appear to be highest in Kerala with Thiruvananthapuram having a prevalence rate of 13% in urban and 7% in rural areas. This is mostly due to the use of coconut oil for cooking, which is a saturated fat.

249. Cardinal features of coronary artery disease in Indians compared to other populations.

1. Higher rates
   - 2- to 4-fold higher prevalence, incidence, hospitalization, mortality.
2. Greater prematurity
   - 5–10 years earlier onset of first AMI.
   - 5-to 10-fold higher rate of AMI and death in the young (< 40 years of age).
3. Greater severity
   - Three vessel disease common even among young premenopausal women
   - Large MI with greater muscle damage.
4. Higher prevalence of glucose intolerance
   - Insulin resistance syndrome, diabetes, central obesity.
5. Lower prevalence of conventional risk factors
   - Hypertension, obesity, cigarette smoking
   - Cholesterol levels—similar to Whites but higher than other Asians
6. Higher prevalence of emerging (thrombogenic) risk factors
   - High levels of lipoprotein (a) homocysteine, Apo B
   - High levels of triglycerides, fibrinogen, plasminogen activator inhibitor
   - High levels of small dense LDL
   - Low levels of HDL
7. Higher rates of clinical events for a given degree of atherosclerosis
   - Double that of Whites
   - 4-fold higher than Chinese
   - Higher proportion of unstable or vulnerable plaques.
8. Adverse environmental or lifestyle factors include those associated with affluence, urbanization, and mechanization.

The excess burden of CAD in Indians is due to a combination of nature (genetic predisposition) and nurture (environmental or lifestyle factors), whereas the genetics load the gun, the environment pulls the trigger. The genetic predisposition appear to be mediated by elevated levels of lipoprotein(a) or Lp(a).

250. Population based strategy of prevention.

The experiences in the US and Finland have clearly demonstrated that lowering the mean population serum cholesterol level has far greater impact than treatment of all those with high levels of cholesterol. This needs lifestyle modification of entire population. Most importantly, this ensure that children adopt healthy eating habits, slowing the rise in cholesterol level with age, creating a new generation with lower risk factor levels. In order to achieve this, 4 elements are necessary for a successful strategy:

1. Public health policy custom tailored for different parts of the National Health Education.
2. An educated and dedicated medical profession.
3. Responsible and empowered public.
4. Supportive media.

Indian Medical Association should join hands with other medical societies to make reduction in CAD rates in India-a lasting reality rather than an elusive dream

251. Primary prevention for high-risk Indians.

Indians at high risk of developing CAD are identities by early determination of emerging and conventional risk factors. They are targeted for maximum lifestyle modification (preferably from childhood). Important lifestyle modifications include exercise, dietary changes, weight loss (watched by waist and caloric intake) and avoidance of smoking.

The cholesterol levels should be reduced to:

1. < 200 mg/dL in individuals without risk factors.
2. < 160 mg/dL in those with CAD risk factors (level typically seen in rural India).

3. LDL < 100 mg/dL
4. LDL < 80 mg/dL is desirable in patients with coronary angioplasty with or without stent.

There is an increasing evidence for the past ten years that the inexorable progress of atherosclerosis can be slowed, arrested and even reversed by aggressive lipid lowering therapy.

252. Prevention of other risk factors. They include.

1. Lowering of elevated levels of Lp(a) to < 15 mg/dL.
2. Lowering of elevated levels of homocysteine to < 10 mg/dL.
3. Lowering of elevated levels of triglycerides < 100 mg/dL.
4. Raising the low levels of HDL to > 50 mg/dL.

Niacin can substantially raise HDL, lower triglycerides and Lp(a).

Instead of testing for homocysteine which may give false-positive and false-negative results, vitamin preparations with adequate folic acid, B_6 and B_{12} can substantially reduce elevated levels of homocysteine. B_1+B_6+B_{12} with folic acid (B-complex) supplementation may be justifiable than testing for homocysteine.

Lifestyle modification by exercise, diet changes, avoidance of tobacco and treatment of hypertension and diabetes can help in the prevention of CAD.

Since CAD is a multifactorial disease involving both genetic and environmental factors a multipronged approach for prevention and treatment is essential.

PATIENT'S EDUCATION

253. Some common questions asked by the patients are answered to educate them.

1. Do you want to maintain cholesterol level at 250 mg/dL?
   Ans: No
   The ideal cholesterol level for adult is below 200 mg/dl 200–250 is considered borderline high and usually increases the risk of CAD. Lipid profile is advised to know HDL, LDL and triglycerides levels.
2. Should you stop eating meat altogether to lower your cholesterol?
   Ans: No.
   Red meat is an important source of protein, iron, and other vitamins and minerals. You need not stop eating it or any other single food although red meat is high in saturated fat and cholesterol. However, you can reduce the amount of saturated fat and cholesterol that you eat. One way to do this is by choosing lean cuts of meat with the fat trimmed or to reduce the amount of meat to six ounces a day.
3. Do you take fish oil supplements to lower your cholesterol?
   Ans: No.
   Fish is a good food choice because of its low saturated fat. Fish oils are a source of omega-3 fatty acids, which are polyunsaturated fats. Fish oil supplements generally do not reduce cholesterol levels. Long-term effect of fish oil is not known. Fish oils reduces triglyceride levels.
4. What do you do to lower your high cholesterol and to lose your overweight?
   Ans: Eating less fat especially saturated fat, total fat and cholesterol with less total calories and regular exercise is adviced. Lifestyle should be modified. Generally, blood cholesterol should begin to drop after starting on a cholesterol-lowering diet. The fall of cholesterol level depends on the amount of saturated fat and cholesterol used to eat, amount of weight loss if you are overweight, and the body response to the changes.
5. Saturated fats in your diet raise blood cholesterol than anything else. What do you do to prevent raise in cholesterol?
   Ans: It is true that saturated fats in the diet raise blood cholesterol level than anything else. So, the best way is to cut back on the amount of saturated fats that you eat. These fats are found in largest amounts in animal products such as butter, cheese, whole milk, ice cream, cream and fatty meats They are also present in some vegetable oils such as coconut, palm and palm kernel oils.
6. Do all vegetable oils help to lower blood cholesterol levels?
   Ans: No.
   Most vegetable, e.g. canola, corn, safflower, soybean, olive, sunflower oils, contain monounsaturated and polyunsaturated fats which help lower blood cholesterol when used in place of saturated fats. However, a few vegetable oils, e.g. coconut, palm, and palm kernel oils contain more saturate fat than unsaturated fat.
7. Does lowering blood cholesterol levels can help people who have already had a heart attack?
   Ans: Yes
   People who have had first heart attack are at much higher risk for a second attack. Lowering blood cholesterol levels can greatly slow down (and, in some people, even reverse) the deposition of cholesterol and fat in the wall of the coronary arteries and significantly reduce the chances of a second heart attack. If you have

had a heart attack or have coronary disease, your LDL level should be around 100 mg/dL, which is even lower than the recommended level of less than 130 mg/dL for the general population.

8. Do all children and young adults need to have their blood cholesterol levels checked.
   Children from high-risk families, in which a parent has high blood cholesterol (250 mg/dL or above) or in which a parent or grandparent has had heart disease at an early age (at 45–55 years or younger), should have their cholesterol levels tested. If a child from such a family has a cholesterol level that is high, it should be lowered under medical supervision, primarily with diet, to reduce the risk of developing heart disease as an adult. For most children, who are not from high-risk families, the best way to reduce the risk of adult heart disease is to follow a low saturated fat, low cholesterol eating pattern. All children over the age of two years and all adults should adopt a heart-healthy eating pattern as a principal way of reducing coronary heart disease.

F Acute Myocardial Infarction

Acute myocardial infarction (AMI) is defined as death of cardiac muscle, part or whole due to sudden reduction of blood supply along a coronary artery as a result of atheromatous narrowing, thrombosis, embolus, hemorrhage or a combination of them in the blood vessel supplying that part. Most cases of AMI are due to sudden occlusion of a coronary artery by a thrombus forming at the site of a ruptured atheromatous plaque.

1. **1/4th of deaths that occur in acute myocardial infarction (AMI) are within the first few minutes to hours before any medical aid is given, i.e. death is the first indication of this disorder.**
2. **3/4th of deaths that occur in acute myocardial infarction (AMI) are within 24 hours.**
3. **40% of deaths that occur in acute myocardial infarction (AMI) are within the first month.**

Therefore, every effort should be made to minimize the mortality during this crucial short period.

4. **The probable incidence of ischemic heart disease in a year can be ascertained into 4 groups.**
   1. 1% of the population above 30 years of age may have coronary artery atherosclerosis without symptoms.
   2. 0.2% of them may have sudden death with or without history of angina.
   3. 0.3% of them may have angina.
   4. 0.5% of them may develop acute myocardial infarction with or without history of angina.

   For example, in a city of 10 lakhs population, there may be 5 lakhs people above 30 years of age—

Asymptomatic ——— Symptomatic

1% (5,000) may have asymptomatic coronary artery disease in whom
- → 0.3% (1500) → Angina
- → 0.2% (1000) → Sudden death
- → 0.5% (2500) → Acute MI

Incidence of myocardial infarction is more in Indians living in USA, UK than in local population. The incidence is notably increasing in India from 1965. Whereas in other countries like USA, Finland, there is fall of 30% from 1965. Incidence is very less in Japan. Incidence is more in men than in women, but the incidence is same in women after menopause.

Heart attacks in India are nowadays seen in younger population also below the age of 30 years.

5. **Incidence of acute myocardial infarction in the United States.**
   1. 1.5 million Americans express a new or recurrent acute myocardial infarction (AMI) each year.
   2. One-third of those Americans, nearly 500,000—will die.
   3. 50% of those—250,000, will die within 1 hour of the onset of symptoms and before they reach hospital.
   4. One AMI occurs every 20 seconds in the United States and a death occurs about every minute.
   5. Costs exceeds $60 billions per year.
   6. 14 million Americans are at highest risk who have a history of AMI, angina or both.
   7. From 1983 to 1993 AMI deaths fell 29.7%.

8. Still show 6% to 9% early mortality from AMI and much higher rates in certain high-risk patients.

(*Heart and stroke facts. 1996 statistical supplement, Dallas,* TX: AHA:1996:1-23)

1998 Statistics showed that each year 9,00,000 people in the United States have acute MI. Of these, roughly 2,25,000, including 1,25,000 die 'in the field' before obtaining medical treatment. Most of these deaths are arrhythmic in origin.

6. The reduction of incidence of AMI in USA in a short span of time is due to:

1. Reduction in smoking.
2. Change in diet habits.
3. Change in lifestyle.
4. Health education and awareness of heart attacks among public.

7. Myocardial infarction occurs mainly due to imbalance between the demand and supply of blood. There are 4 factors which change the balance of demand and supply of blood:

1. Rate
2. Contractility
3. Preload } (wall tension)
4. Afterload }

Increase in demand without increase in blood supply is the common cause of myocardial infarction.

It can also occur even though the demand is low as in sleep when the blood supply becomes still low at a certain level. The venous return is more during sleep (horizontal position) which causes more compression of the myocardium. The compression of coronary arteries cause less oxygen supply to the myocardium.

Coronary arteries are the only arteries that fill during diastole. About 85% of coronary arteries fill during diastole whereas other arteries fill in systole.

The demand is more at 10.00 AM while going to the work after restful night. Incidence of AMI in some groups are more on Mondays around 10.00 AM because of much stress while starting the work after restful weekends. The increased frequency during morning hours points to a correlation between circadian rhythm and its associated physiological processes and the cardiovascular events that lead to AMI. This further bears out the importance of patient activities in triggering AMI in about 15% of cases. The triggering activities are thought to act by generating hemodynamic, vasoconstrictive and prothrombotic forces that disrupt a vulnerable plaque leading to occlusive coronary thrombosis.

8. Myocardial oxygen supply from coronary blood flow depends on 4 factors:

1. Heart rate.
2. Duration of diastole (85% of coronary arteries fill during diastole in contrast to other arteries).
3. Aortic pressure.
4. Right Atrial Pressure.

(The pressure difference between the ascending aorta and right atrium obviously provides a safe margin for adequate coronary blood flow. The right atrial pressure is just around atmospheric pressure and raises to about 10 mm Hg during contraction. Aortic pressure is around 120 mm Hg during systole and falls to 70–80 mm Hg during diastole.)

Demand		Supply	
1. Rate		Rate	
2. Contractility		Period of diastole	
3. Afterload LV pressure	Wall tension	Aortic pressure	Coronary blood flow
4. Preload Ventricular volume	Wall tension	Right atrial pressure	Coronary blood flow

9. Anatomy of plaque disruption: Atherosclerotic plaque rupture is the major cause of thrombosis of the coronary arteries that leads to acute ischemia and AMI (see Figs E-5 and 6).

1. Plaque can be described as vulnerable or stable depending on their structural characteristics.
2. Plaques prone to rupture are commonly composed of soft lipids with abundant cholesterol crystals separated from the vessel lumen by a thin fibrous cap.
3. Plaque instability is promoted by accumulation of foam cells and lipids. Plaque is particularly susceptible whenever the extracellular lipid core makes up more than 40% of overall plaque volume.
4. Rupture of the plaque usually occurs at the margin of fibrous cap near an adjacent plaque-free segment of the coronary artery wall (shoulder region of the plaque) by a combination of:
   i. Stresses from intraluminal pressure.
   ii. Coronary vasomotor tone.
   iii. Tachycardia (which increases cycling stretching and compression).
   iv. Rupture of small nutrient vessels (vasa vasorum) in the walls of large blood vessels.

10. There are 4 causes of acute coronary artery occlusion:

1. *Hemorrhage:* Common cause is sudden hemorrhage under the already existing atheromatous plaque, and the clot extends into the lumen resulting in complete block. A thrombus is formed when a plaque ruptures, spilling its core contents into the blood. The effaced surface of

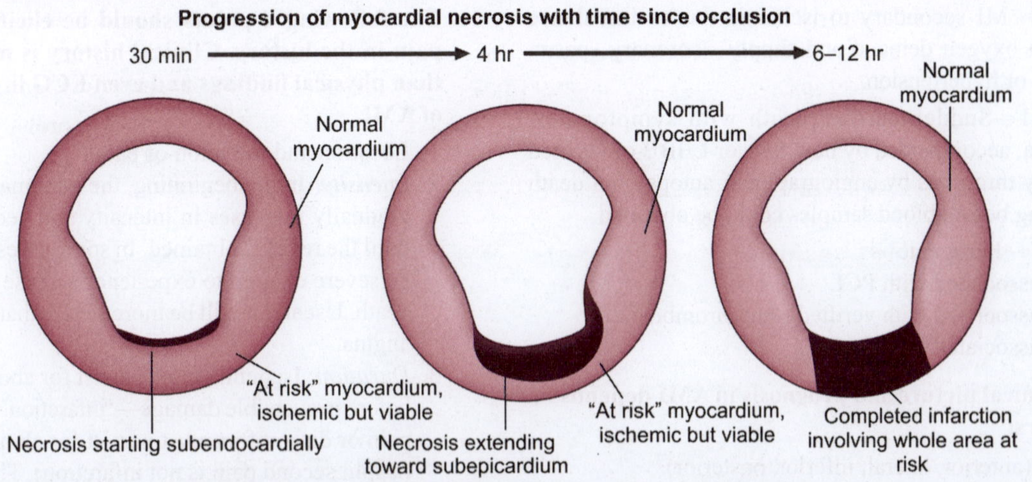

Fig. F-1: Complete infarction involving whole area at-risk

the plaque can become a site for thrombogenesis. Local factors such as lipid core composition also determine the thrombotic response.

2. *Thrombosis:* Recently formed clot causes complete obstruction on the already existing partially thickened atherosclerotic coronary arteries. Atherogenesis is prone for several injuries. Injury may be inflicted by lipid peroxidation, vasoactive amines, immunocomplexes, infection, and chemical irritants in tobacco smoke.
   The already existing atherosclerotic coronary artery will be completely blocked in acute myocardial infarction.
3. *Embolism:* Such a thrombus may break away from its original site and may embolize to block a distal artery.
4. *Spasm:* Irritation of the coronary artery can cause reflex spasm and temporary occlusion of the vessel.
   About 85–90% of cases of ischemic heart disease (IHD) are due to coronary artery disease (CAD). 10–15% are caused by aortic valve disease, anemia, etc. (See Chapter E - 42).
   Risk factors are same as for ishemic heart disease (See Chapter E 21-23).

11. Coronary artery occlusion: The evolution of infarction—

1. Infarction is not instantaneous following occlusion. Abnormalities of the affected myocardium caused by transient ischemia tend to be reversible. The longer the ischemic state lasts, more the myocardium progresses toward irreversible damage.
2. Necrosis spreads like an advancing wave front through the at-risk myocardial region supplied by the occluded coronary artery. Effective collaterals and/or endogenous fibrinolysis may help to delay the myocardial damage.
3. Myocardium is destined to die during the first 6 hours which can be salvaged by rapid restoration of coronary blood flow leading to smaller infarct size.
4. Early restoration of complete patency of coronary artery is the most effective way to restrict long-term damage, so that perfusion of the ischemic myocardium starts as soon as possible.

12. The symptoms of coronary artery occlusion can be described in 4 stages depending on the amount of narrowing from mild, moderate, severe to complete block. Common cause of the myocardial infarction is the complete blockage of an already existing atherosclerotic artery.

Stage I—Mild blockage—There may be no symptoms (silent) or the patient may have breathlessness or chest pain on unaccustomed exertion.

Stage II—Moderate blockage—There will be chest pain during accustomed exertion.

Stage III—Severe blockage—There will be chest pain even at rest or during light exertion. Spasm of the coronary arteries at the site of block can occur.

Stage IV—Complete blockage—Acute myocardial infarction—Severe chest pain at rest radiating to left arm, jaw or back, accompanied by breathlessness, sweating, giddiness, nausea or vomiting.

13. MI can be classified into four types:

Type I—Sponatenous MI related to ischemia due to primary coronary event such as plaque erosion or rupture, fissuring or dissection.

Type II—MI secondary to ischemia due to imbalance between oxygen demand and supply—coronary spasm, anemia, or hypertension.

Type III—Sudden cardiac death with symptoms of ischemia, accompanied by new ST↑ or LBBB or verified coronary thrombus by angiography or autopsy but death occurring before blood samples could be obtained.

Type IV—Iatrogenic—

a. MI associated with PCI.
b. MI associated with verified stent thrombosis.
c. MI associated with CABG.

14. The clinical picture and prognosis in AMI depends on 4 factors:

1. Site (anterior, lateral, inferior, posterior).
2. Size (vascular bed perfused by narrowed vessel—endocardium to epicardium).
3. Severity (atheromatous narrowing or coronary spasm).
4. Starting time and duration (development of collateral circulation of anastomosing vessels).

15. The cardinal symptoms of AMI (the ABCs).

1. A–**A** angina (chest pain or discomfort) deep aching radiating to back or left forearm.
2. B–**B**reathlessness or restlessness due to pulmonary edema.
3. C–**C**lammy perspiration.
4. D–**D**izziness—unexplained light-headedness even blackouts due to fall of BP particularly when the patient is upright.
5. E–**E**dema of ankles and/or lower legs (late stage).
6. F–**F**luttering (or) rapid tachyarrhythmias.
7. G–**G**iddiness or syncope due to fall of blood pressure particularly when the patient is upright. Arrhythmias and conduction defects may present with or without syncopal attacks.
   Gastric upset (or nausea) due to autonomic upset (injection morphine may also cause when given for relief of chest pain).
8. H–**H**eavy fullness—or pressure like chest pain between breast and radiating to the left shoulder or arm.

Atypical presentation—Dyspnea may be the only presenting symptoms in about 10% of patients with AMI. Other atypical presentations include fatigue, syncope, altered sensorium, stroke, nausea/vomiting or lethargy. Atypical presentation of acute MI is common in elderly, diabetics and women. (see Table A-3 for cardiac and noncardiac pain).

Hiccough is an unusual symptom of AMI

More than 50–70% of lumen will be blocked before getting symptoms.

Arrhythmias may present with or without syncopal attack.

16. The following 4 points should be elicited about the pain in the history. Clinical history is more valuable than physical findings and even ECG in the diagnosis of AMI.

1. Location and radiation of pain.
2. *Intensity:* In the beginning, the pain may be mild and gradually increases in intensity and becomes plateau until the relief is obtained. In some cases, the pain will be severe enough to experience a sense of impending death. Usually it will be more severe than any previous angina.
3. *Duration:* Ischemia must persist for about 20 minutes before irreversible damage—'infarction'—occurs. The pain or discomfort must persist for about 20 minutes. (a split second pain is not infarction). The pain occurs at rest or persists despite rest after exertion.
4. *Character:* It may be tightness, constriction, squeezing, sharp or heavy ranging from very mild to severe—causing a feeling of suffocation.

Pain in subendocardial infarction is seen when at least two thirds of the thickness of myocardium is involved. But in subendocardial infarction the pain is present for more than 30 minutes but usually less than an hour, otherwise patient has got all characteristics of acute myocardial infarction.

17. Location and radiation of the pain can be of 4 different types: (see Table E-2)

1. A central chest pressure, chest discomfort or pain or restrosternal pressure.
   Tightness, constriction, squeezing or heavy sensation ranging from mild to very severe causing a feeling of suffocation. Pallor conveys the seriousness of the situation. Pain may be mild or even unrecognized in some patients.
2. Pain radiating to the anterior precordium, medial side of the left arm and elbow where it may cause a sensation of weakness in the muscles.
3. Pain radiating up to the lower jaw and sometimes to the back.
4. An upper abdominal pain or discomfort which may be mistaken for acidity or indigestion.

The pain of myocardial infarction does not radiate above the maxilla or below the umbilicus.

18. Acute myocardial infarction is usually dominated by chest pain. Retrosternal pain is the most frequent presentation. However, it varies from patient to patient and the presenting symptom can be dominated by any one of the 4 following groups:

1. Cases dominated by chest pain present in 80–85% of cases. In the remaining 15–20%, infarction is painless particularly in diabetics and elderly.

2. Cases dominated by shock with or without syncopal attack (power failure).
3. Cases dominated by complications like arrhythmia (electric irritability).
4. Cases dominated by features of left ventricular failure (pump failure).

Majority fall in the first group.

History of anginal pain may be present before AMI which is called preinfarction angina.

Death may occur immediately after pain within the first few hours.

2, 3 and 4 can cause loss of consciousness particularly when the left ventricular dysfunction is due to the result of involvement of the main stem of the left coronary artery.

19. Cases dominated by chest pain should be differentiated from (see Chapter E-IHD/CAD Table E-2)

1. *Pericarditis:* Chest pain that is worsen when the person is supine and improves when the person sitting upright or slightly bending forward is typical of pericarditis. ECG shows diffuse ST elevation with concavity upwards in many leads as the pericardium, is present surrounding all over the heart (ST↑ with convexity upward in AMI). Reciprocal depression does not occur expect in aVL, and V_1. Q waves are absent. PR segment depression and peaked T waves are present. Echocardiogram is useful in evaluating pericardial effusion even in initial stage which may occur in either condition. In AMI lack of wall motion abnormality is present.
2. *Myocarditis:* H/o patient often tells a more insidious onset and associated viral syndrome. As in pericarditis, ECG may be similar to AMI. Echocardiography is less useful in differentiating the syndrome from AMI because diffuse LV dysfunction is in either condition.
3. *Acute aortic dissection:* Sharp, tearing chest pain, radiating to the back is typical. Proximal extension of the dissection into either coronary ostium can account for AMI. X-ray chest shows widened mediastinum. Echo may reveal a dissection flap in the proximal ascending aorta. Definitive diagnosis should be obtained from transesophageal echocardiography, CT or MRI.
4. *Pulmonary embolism:* Pleuritic chest pain with dyspnea but without evidence of pulmonary edema is suggesting of pulmonary embolism. ECG shows S1, Q3, RAD. PO_2 <80 mm Hg in 90% of patients. Echo rules out wall motion abnormalities and show RV strain, which is an indication of fibrinolytic therapy in pulmonary embolism.

Table F-1

ST elevation but no ischemia	*Chest pain but no ischemia*
Early repolarization	Pericarditis
LVH/LBBB	Myocarditis
Hyperkalemia	Pulmonary embolism
Brugada syndrome	Costochondritis

5. *Gastroesophageal disorders:* Reflux esophagitis, esophageal mobility disorders, gastritis (alcoholic gastritis, analgesic use, etc.) can all cause chest pain, the character of which is similar to cardiac chest pain. These disorders may coexist with CAD patients thereby confusing the diagnosis. These disorders do not show typical radiation of cardiac pain and are relieved by antacids. The only rare condition is esophageal rupture which is diagnosed by chest X-ray showing mediastinal gas, Gastrografin swallow confirms the diagnosis. No ST↑.
6. *Hepatobiliary disorders:* Hepatitis, cholecystitis can mimic symptoms and ECG may show signs of inferior MI. Tenderness in the right hypochondrium, fever, jaundice may be present. Pain is radiating to the right shoulder, right infrascapular and epigastrium which is not similar to pain in AMI. LFT ultrasound scanning abdomen help in the diagnosis.
7. *Chest wall disease:* Osteoarthritis of sternocostal joints, osteochondritis in which pain is localized, increased by rotation of the chest, deep breathing, and direct pressure. No typical radiation of pain of AMI. ECG is normal.
8. *Functional:* Last but not the least, it is seen mostly in neurotic people. Pain is variable nature, radiation variable, history of emotion, stress, other symptoms. ECG is normal. They go from one doctor to other for his atypical symptoms with apprehension cardiac neurosis.

20. 1/4th of the cases of myocardial infarction are painless.

The incidence of painless infarcts are greater in diabetes (autonomic neuropathy) and increases with age. The painless myocardial infarction in diabetics and elderly may present as:

1. Sudden onset of breathlessness which may result in pulmonary edema.
2. Sudden onset of confusion state or unconsciousness.
3. Sudden palpitation or arrhythmia.
4. Sudden unexplained fall of BP or profound weakness.

Nausea, vomiting and sweating may occur due to autonomic upset.

21. The clinical parameters that should be monitored are:

Assessing the patient as a whole should be the aim of good care in every situation and more important nowhere than in the coronary care unit. The following parameters should be assessed every time when the patient is seen:

1. *General appearance:* The patient may look ill or may be frightened, anxious, restless or sweating due to chest pain or may be normal.
   Note :
   a. Whether the patient looks well or ill?
   b. Whether the patient is frightened or anxious with pain?
   c. Whether the patient is short of breath due to left ventricular dysfunction?
   d. Whether the patient is sweating, cold or cyanosed due to cardiogenic shock or peripheral circulatory failure?
2. *Pulse:* Usually regular. May be irregular if there is arrhythmia, feeble if there is impaired pumping action.
3. *Temperature:* Pyrexia of 100–102° F may develop during the first 48 hours lasting up to 1 week. It is due to tissue necrosis.
4. *Respiration:* Note the rate, any irregularity like Cheyne-Stokes respiration, Kussmaul's breathing or orthopnea. Respiratory rate may rise due to anxiety itself even in the absence of left ventricular failure. In the presence of left ventricular failure, tachypnea is generally proportional to left ventricular failure and may be more than 40 per minute in patients with pulmonary edema.
5. *Blood pressure:* It may fall if there is pump failure or high if the patient is in pain or a known hypertensive.
6. *ECG and cardiac monitor:* For the diagnosis, prognosis and to identify the development of arrhythmias particularly the dangerous ventricular tachycardia or fibrillation as they occur during the course of AMI.
7. *Central venous pressure (CVP):* If it is being monitored, very useful particularly in infarction of right ventricle and helps as a guide to the fluid replacement.
8. *Fluid balance chart:* It is important to monitor the urinary output as it reflects the renal perfusion.

22. The 4 auscultatory signs in myocardial infarction due to ventricular dysfunction are:

1. *Sounds:* Decrease in intensity of S1 and S2 or may be quiet or muffled. Added sounds may be audible due to lack of compliance and stiffness of the ventricles.
   Ventricular gallop–S3: It generally reflects a large infarct or cardiac dilatation.
   Atrial gallop–S4 is usually audible.
2. *Split:* Paradoxical splitting of S2.
3. *Murmur:* Transient apical systolic murmur due to mitral regurgitation secondary to papillary muscle dysfunction or rupture of cardiac tendinae complication in AMI. It may be mid-systolic or late systolic. Most commonly this occurs with an inferior infarct involving the posterior cusp of the mitral valve.
4. Pericardial rub is often heard on the 2nd or 3rd day when there is transmural extent of infarct and is usually transitory. A rub occurring after a week or so is suggestive of Dressler's syndrome.

23. About 1/4th of the patients with acute myocardial infarction may develop an abnormal systolic pulsation in periapical area better heard in left lateral decubitus position in the first few days which may get resolved.

24. The order of changes immediately after AMI are:

1. Biochemical changes—enzyme changes.
2. Diastolic dysfunction.
3. Systolic dysfunction.
4. Electrical changes seen in ECG.

25. The biochemical changes occur progressively in 4 steps:

1. The important first principal biochemical change is onset of anaerobic glycolysis which leads to
   ↓
2. Inadequate production of ATP which in turn leads to
   ↓
3. Accumulation of potentially noxious breakdown products such as lactic acid which results in
   ↓
4. Glycogen depletion of mitochondrial cell and mitochondrial swelling.

The result of oxygen deficiency leads to excitation of ischemic "cascade", i.e. breakdown of high energy phosphate and phosphocreatinine leading to intracellular acidosis. Thus potassium ions, protons and lactic acid are released from the cell. These early changes are reversible and cell death is not immediate. If the patient is not attended in time, myocardial cell death occurs which is known as acute myocardial infarction.

26. The 4 pathophysiological effects of myocardial ischemia are:

1. *Biochemial changes:* Enzymes are normally confined within the cardiac cells but they are liberated when there is myocardial infarction. It is important to measure the enzymes at the time after the onset of symptoms at which they are at peak. It is generally accepted that a raise twice the normal levels is necessary for a positive diagnosis. Serial enzyme estimations are needed in doubtful cases because it is the change in enzyme level which is of diagnostic value.

Enzymatic diagnosis is perhaps the most sensitive. As little as 0.5 g of necrotic myocardium can be diagnosed.

2. *Electrical changes:* Seen in ECG

   Ischemia alters the electrical properties.

   Repolarization is altered early as evidenced by T inversion.

   Injury—ST segment shift in early MI—ST segment is elevated in two or more leads

   ST depression during the attack of angina.

   Infarction—Abnormal Q waves.

   The abnormal Q waves may or may not be present depending on the presence of necrosis.

   Electrical irritability or instability is another important change such as ventricular tachycardia, ventricular flutter or fibrillation.

   Most patients with AMI who die suddenly do so from these malignant ventricular arrhythmias.

   Sometimes ECG changes may not be seen in AMI in the early stages more so when circumflex artery alone is blocked, but the history of chest pain, etc. should be taken into consideration and patient is kept under observation. Serial ECGs help in the diagnosis.

3. *Mechanical changes with early uniform ischemia:*

   Ischemic zone may lead to necrosis or come back to normal.

   MI markedly reduces contractility and cardiac output.

   Myocardial ischemia also interferes with ventricular relaxation and filling—resulting in the elevation of diastolic pressure and thereby raising the pulmonary pressure and pulmonary congestion.

4. *Mechanical changes with nonuniform ischemia:*

   There is interference with symmetry and synchrony of ventricular contraction reducing the myocardial pump function.

   Ischemia of papillary muscles and other segments of myocardium may cause mitral regurgitation.

   Myocardium may bulge outward (myocardial dyskinesis) reducing the effectiveness of ventricular contraction; later, it may result in an aneurysmal dilatation also.

27. The 4 groups of laboratory tests to confirm myocardial infarction are:

1. Nonspecific tests for tissue necrosis and inflammation, e.g. TWBC, DC, ESR, etc. leukocytosis reaches peak on the first day. ESR is raised and may remain so for many days.
2. ECG.
3. Serum enzyme studies.
4. Radionuclide imaging tests such as acute infarct scintigraphy "hot spot" imaging with ^{99m}Tc stannous pyrophosphate, myocardial perfusion imaging with thallium 201 for defective "cold spot". These tests are available only at few centers.

The triad of symptoms and investigations in AMI is history of typical chest pain, typical or appropriate ECG changes, elevation of appropriate serum enzymes. The convention is that any two out of these three should be present.

28. Typical sequence of ECG changes during the evolution of acute myocardial infarction is described in 4 stages:

Normal, 1. Within hours—ST elevation, 2. After 6 to 8 hours to 1 to 3 days. Pathological Q wave, reductions in height of ST elevation, reduction in height of R wave, T wave inversion, 3. Within weeks: ST becomes isoelectric, Q wave, T wave inversion. 4. Within months—Reduction of R wave, T is upright, Q is present.

Several combinations of changes may occur but the typical sequence of changes are as follows:

1. Immediate or within first few hours: *Raise of ST segment.* This is the typical development of the so-called 'current of injury' and is due to failure of the ST relative to the normal surrounding tissue. Arrow-head symmetrical T inversion may occur along with ST segment to return to the isoelectric line as a result of incomplete repolarization of the damaged myocardium

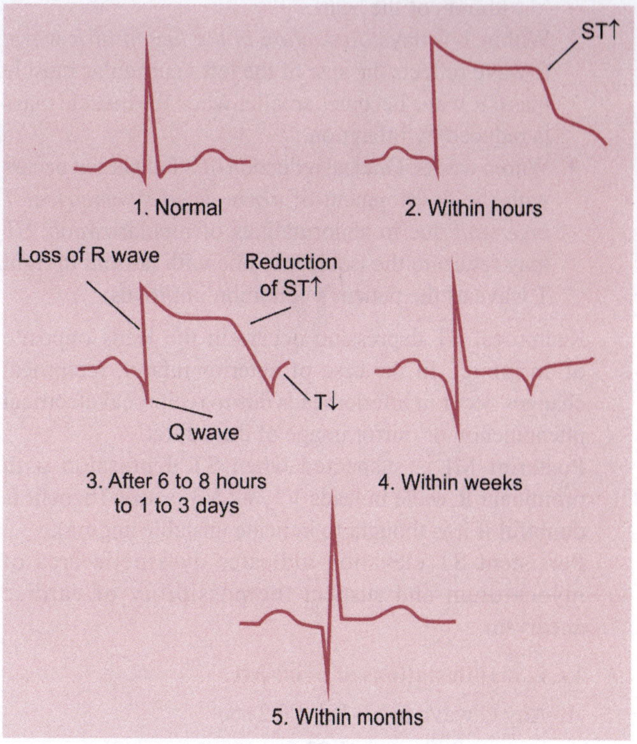

Fig. F-2: Sequence of ECG changes with time

elevation. Differential diagnosis of acute MI requires ST↑ of 1 mm or more in two or more contiguous leads, often with reciprocal ST↓ in the contralateral leads. In leads V2, V3, 2 mm of ST↑ in men and 1.5 mm in women is required for accurate diagnosis.

2. After 6–8 hours : *Development of Q waves*
   a. Q waves usually appear after 6–8 hours. This is indicative of necrosis. Due to this reason, thrombolytic therapy should be started within the first 4 to 6 hours after the onset of chest pain, i.e. before the development of Q waves. Infarction may be described as with Q waves or without Q waves depending on their presence.
   b. Q waves are due to the infarcted area of the ventricle under the electrode being unable to produce a large R wave. Therefore, the depolarization on the opposite side of the heart moving away from the electrode is reflected as negative or down wave, i.e. Q or QS wave.
   c. Q waves are considered to be significant if they are:
   more than 2 mm deep, more than 0.04 mm wide or 1/4th of the R wave that follows them.
   d. Q waves may persist for years signifying the old infarction. However, it is important to remember that they may occur with cardiomyopathies (HOCM) due to thick ventricular septum and tumors of the heart.
3. Within 1–3 days: *Reduction in the height of R wave.* R wave reflects the size of the left ventricular muscle mass. R wave becomes smaller when the muscle mass is reduced by infarction.
4. Within weeks: Gradual reduction of ST elevation occurs with the development of *arrow head symmetrical T inversion* due to abnormalities of repolarization. ST may return to the isoelectric line with normal upright T wave as the patient's condition improves.

Reciprocal ST depression occurs in the leads opposite of an infarct. In the case of anterior infarct, reciprocal changes occur in inferior leads due to reciprocal electrical phenomenon or mirror image of the infarct.

Posterior MI is suspected when ST depression with prominent R wave in leads V1, V2,V3 is seen (benefit is doubtful if it is thought to indicate unstable angina).

Persistent ST elevation indicates dyskinetic area of myocardium and suspect the possibility of cardiac aneurysm.

29. ECG manifestations of prior MI:

1. Any Q wave in V2-V3 ≥ 0.2 sec

   or

2. QS complex in V2-V3

   or

3. Q wave ≥ 0.03 sec and ≥ 0.1 mv deep

   or

4. QS complex in any two contiguous leads of LI, aVL, V4-V6, LII, LIII and aVF.

30. In general, ECG is far more valuable than physical findings in the diagnosis of AMI but of less value than clinical history.

ECG has certain limitations in diagnosing acute transmural MI due to the following 4 factors.

1. Delayed appearance of ECG changes sometimes occur due to its reduced sensitivity.
2. ECG changes will disappear when the new infarction occurs in a diagonally opposite of a previous infarction.
3. QRS changes are frequently absent when the infarction is isolated to the posterolateral or apical region.
4. Difficult in the presence of LBBB.

If the present symptoms persist, the patient should be considered to be in the manifestation stage of myocardial infarction despite the appearance of changes in ECG. Symptoms should take precedence.

The ECG should be interpreted in the light of the symptoms present at that time.

New LBBB in the setting of symptoms consistent with acute myocardial infarction may suggest a large anterior wall acute MI, involving the proximal left anterior descending coronary artery and should be managed in the same way as acute STEMI.

It is important to note that in as many as 15% of patients ECG may be initially normal. Initial ECGs may be diagnostic in 60% and abnormal but not diagnostic in 25% patients. Serial ECGs are a must as they are diagnostic in 95% cases.

Circumflex artery distribution is notoriously silent on an ECG as the posterolateral wall is under represented on a conventional 12-lead ECG. ECG cannot be used alone to exclude acute coronary syndrome (ACS). New LBBB suggest left anterior descending coronary artery lesion.

31. AMI may be described in 4 phases:

1. Early hyperactive phase—within hours—ST concavity is lost.
2. Fully evolved acute phase—within days.
3. Fully evolved subacute phase—within weeks.
4. Chronic stabilized phase—within months.

32. The following 4 points should be noted in ECG when describing acute myocardial infarction.

1. Site of infarction: For example, anterior, inferior, lateral, posterior, etc.

Site of infarction	*ECG leads*
1. Extensive Anterior	V1-V6
2. Anteroseptal	V1-V3 sometimes V4
3. Anterolateral	V4-V6, LI, aVL
4. Anteroapical	V5-V6
5. Inferior	LII, LIII, aVF
6. Inferolateral	LII, LIII, aVF, LI, aVL
7. Inferoanterior	LII, LIII, aVF, V1, V2
8. Inferoposterior	LII, LIII, aVF, V1, V2
9. Lateral	LI, aVL
10. Posterior	V1, V2
11. Anterior—extensive with LBBB	
12. Subendocardial without Q wave	

2. Age of the infarct (time): Is it recent (acute) or old ?
3. Thickness of the ventricular wall affected.
   Subepicardial—with or without Q wave.
   Subendocardial—with or without Q wave.
4. Transmural: ST elevation
   or subendocardial: ST depression.

33. ST segment elevation can also occur in the following 4 conditions besides AMI.

1. Ventricular aneurysm.
2. Pericarditis.
3. Coronary spasm (Prinzmetal angina).
4. Early repolarization.
   (See Electrocardiogram Chapter Q-41 for other conditions.)

34. ECG helps in localizing the myocardial infarction. Best seen in the leads which 'face' the infarction.

Infarcted areas

1. Anterior infarction

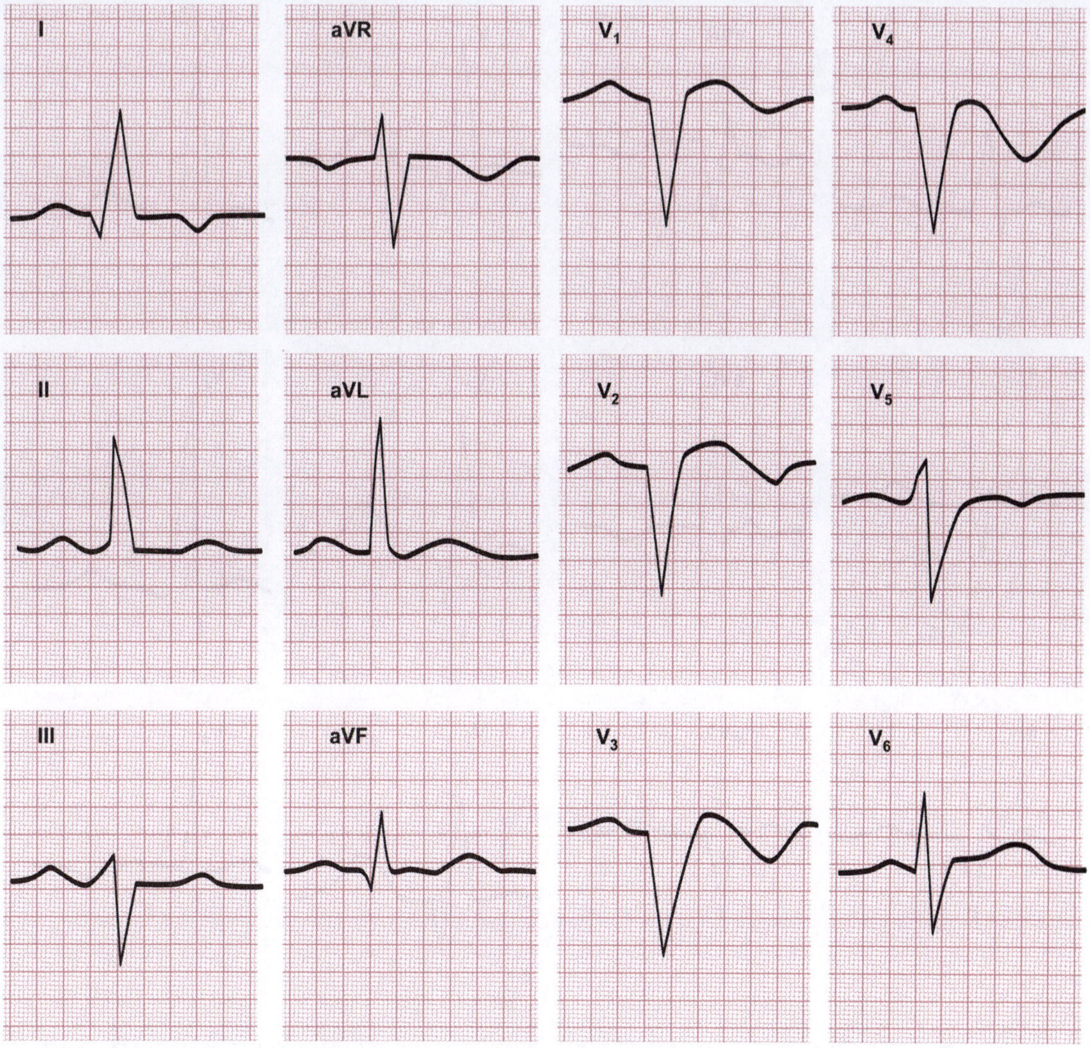

Fig. F-3: Acute anterior myocardial infarction: Significant Q waves and T inversions in LI, V1, V2, V3, V4. QS waves in V1-V4

2. Inferior or diaphragmatic infarction.
   Q and/or ST elevation and T inversion in L II, L III and aVF.
   In IWMI tall 'R' in V1 posterior MI.
   Take right sided chest leads V2R, V3R, and V4R in IWMI. Presence of ST elevation with coving is an indication of right ventricular MI. Carefully see for any bump in PR segment, this is due to an infarction in the atria causing upward deviation of the segment between the P wave and atrial repolarization wave. ECG may have signs of complete heart block also due to ischemia of AV node, which is supplied by the right coronary artery (RCA) in majority of the patients.
   Right ventricular MI and atrial MI are associated with extensive IWMI (RCA territory infarction). Circulatory failure and shock are common with right ventricular MI. Volume expansion by IV fluids form the baseline treatment in the early stages of MI apart from routine MI management. Extensive inferior wall MI always leads to suspicion of RVMI. Atrial MI, and AV nodal disturbance as all these tissues are supplied by the right coronary artery. Take V2R, V3R, and V4R to detect RVMI. RVMI comprises 20–25% of all MI and atrial MI comprises of 10% of all MI.
3. True posterior or posterolateral infarction.
   Tall R in V1 and V2, may be Q in V6, Mirror test.

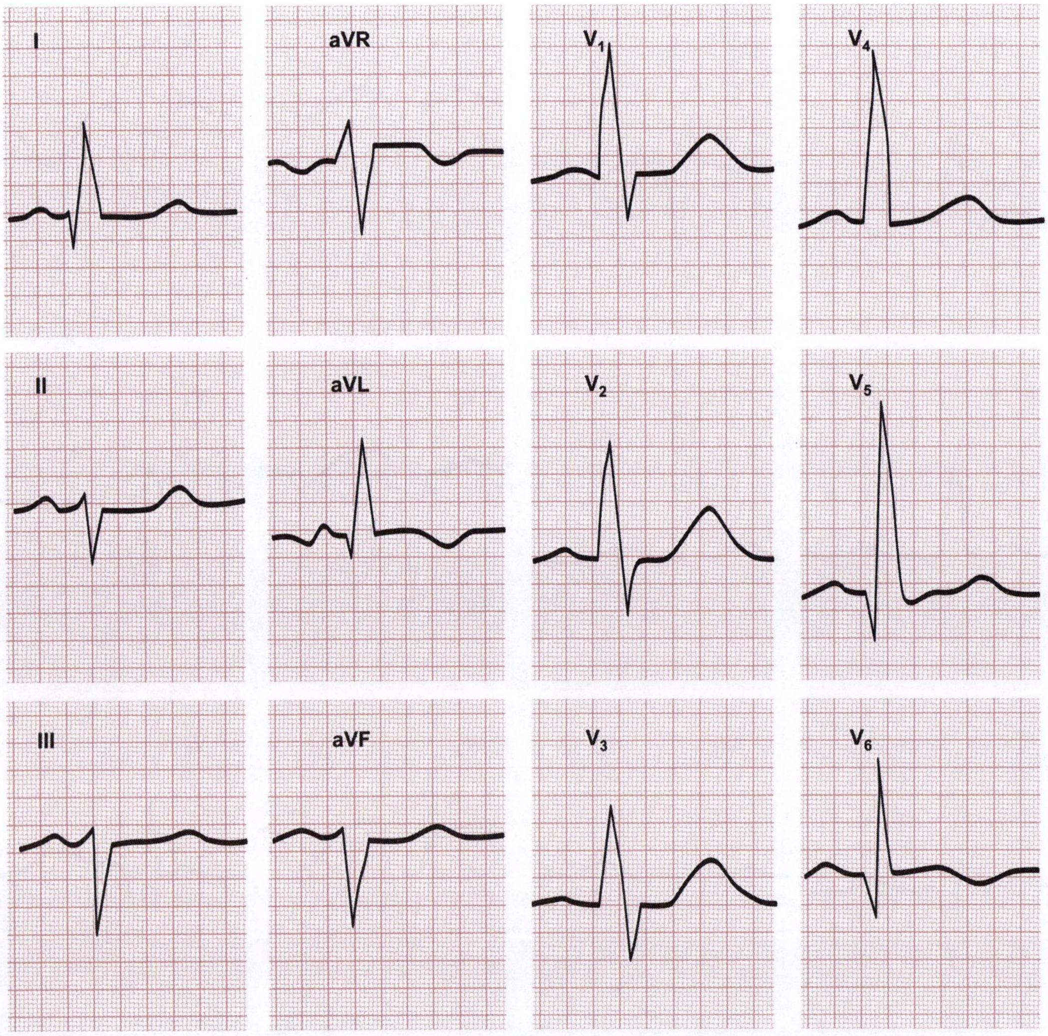

Fig. F-4: True posterior infarct: V1 shows unusually large R wave (reciprocal of posterior Q wave) and P wave reciprocal of posterior T wave inversion

Posterior or posterolateral infarction.

Posterior wall infarction of left ventricle is not recorded in the standard leads by ST elevation or Q waves. The reciprocal changes of ST depression and a tall R wave may be seen in leads V1-V4, i.e. opposite to those of anterior infarct.

The back of the infarcted heart is electrically inactive. So, the electrode picks up only the depolarization from the front of the heart as it passes from the endocardium to the epicardium. The result of the impulse traveling toward the electrode gives a positive wave that is an R wave. Posterior infarction is usually associated with inferior infarction.

Since the ST↑ is sometimes delayed in ECG, repeat ECG of after half an hour, one hour, etc. are necessary if symptoms are suspicious. It is common with circumflex artery block which goes to posterior side and supplies posterior part. So ECG picks up late.

ST elevation in LII, LIII and aVF with reciprocal ST depression in LI, aVL.

4. Subendocardial infarction or partial thickness infarction.

   About 1/4th (25%) of all infarctions are estimated to be subendocardial.

   Infarction involves the inner half of the total thickness of the ventricular wall. ST depression with T wave inversion is seen in the leads facing the epicardial surface of the ventricular wall overlying the infarcted area.

   Pathological Q waves do not develop with subendocardial infarction. Some nonischemic conditions also may show ST and T changes as seen in subendocardial infarction. If the changes appear for days, subendocardial infarction is to be suspected. Clinical diagnosis may be confirmed if they are accompanied by serial changes of the appropriate serum enzymes.

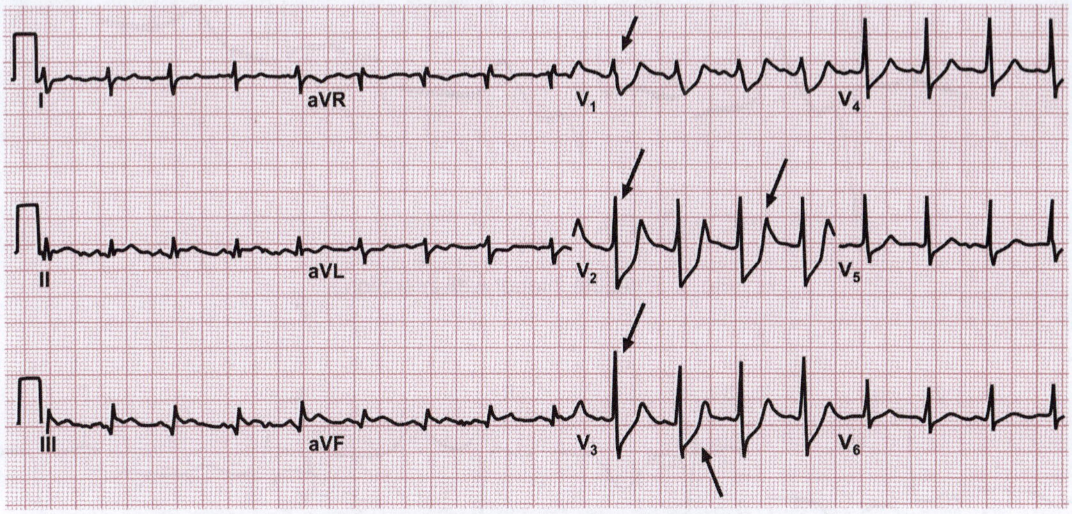

Fig. F-4(a): Acute posterior infarction

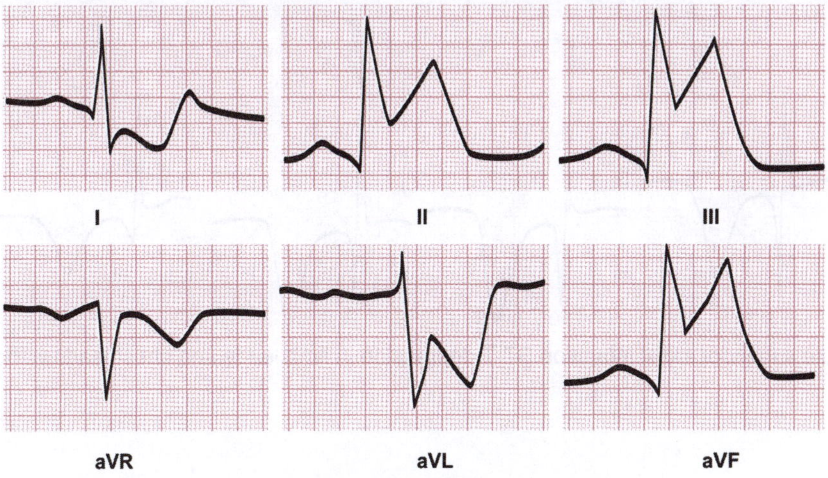

Fig. F-5: (Contd...)

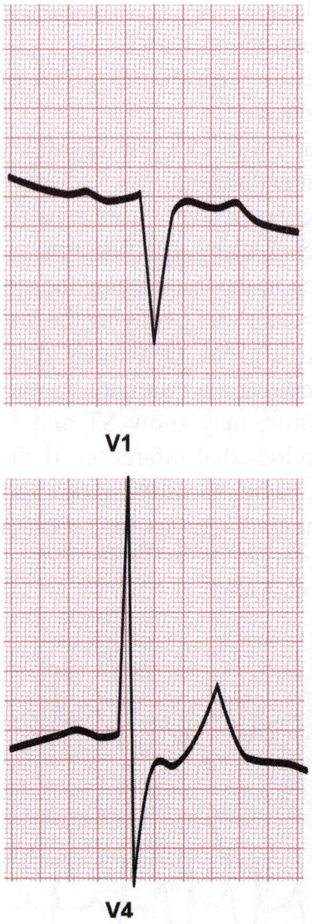

Fig. F-5: Acute inferior wall infarction

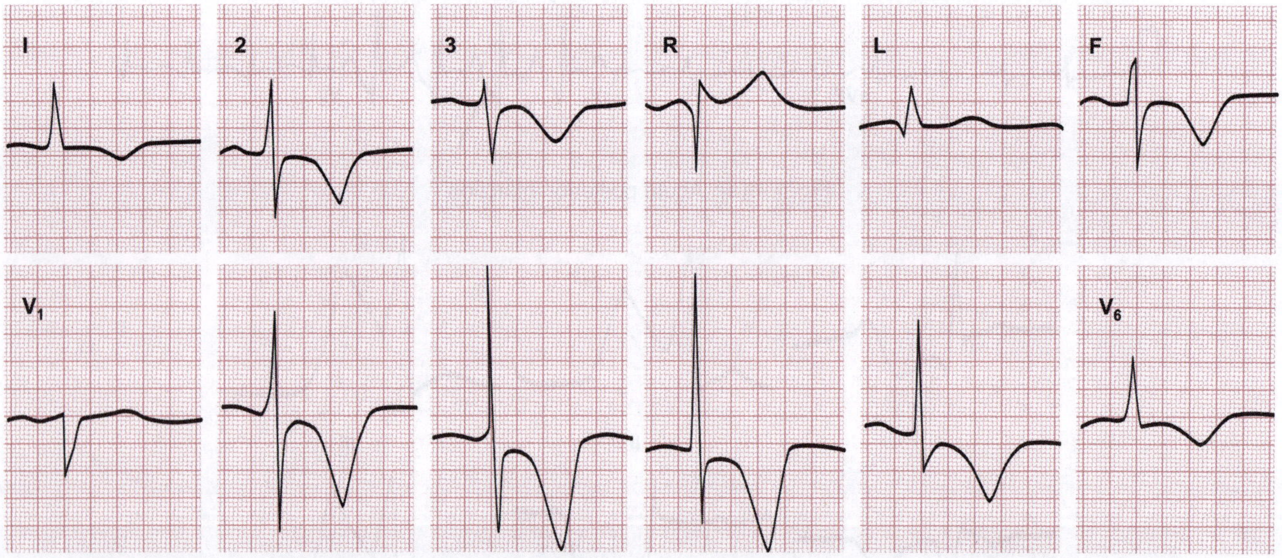

Fig. F-6: Acute subendocardial infarction ST-T depression in limb leads and chest leads without Q waves

ST elevation occurs in the leads overlying the infarction and reciprocal ST depression in the opposite leads. Suspect multiple infarcts if the ECG reverts to normal after the initial infarction, and a second infarct that occurs will produce a pattern as would be expected with initial infarction.

35. Anterior wall infarction can be further subdivided into 4 categories involving limited area:

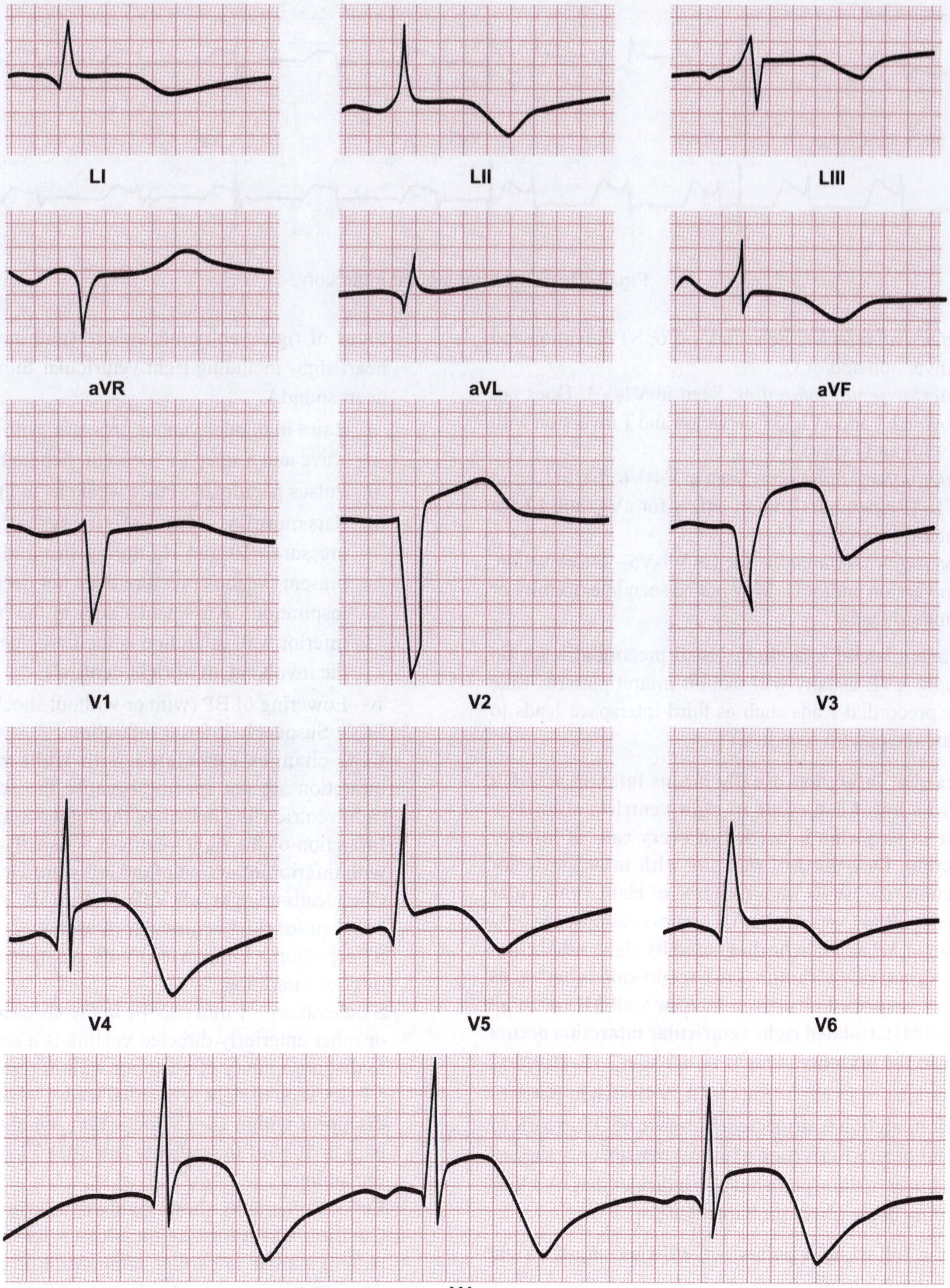

Fig. F-7: Acute anterior myocardial infarction; ST elevation VI, V2, V3, V4, V5, V6, with T inversion

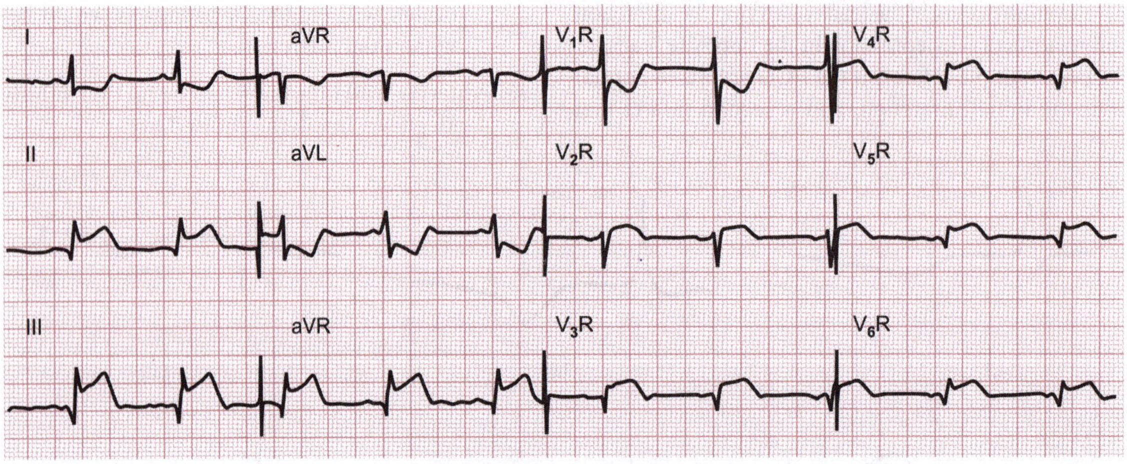

Fig. F-7(a): Right ventricular infarction

1. *Extensive Anterior:* Seen in V1-V6; ST elevation and T inversion and/or Q.
2. *Anterior septal infarction:* Seen in V1-V3. Does not show in L1 and aVL. ST elevation and T inversion with or without Q wave.
3. *Anterolateral infarction:* Seen in V4-V6 also in L1 and aVL. (Remember, Roman letters for aV**L** and L**I** for **L**ateral **I**nfarction.
4. *Anteroapical infarction:* Seen in V3-V5—ST elevation, T inversion and/or Q. May not be seen in extremity or standard leads.

High anterolateral infarction: Usual precordial leads do not show. aVL usually will exhibit infarct pattern. Take higher precordial leads such as third interspace leads to evaluate the pattern seen in aVL.

36. **Myocardial infarction usually means infarction of left ventricle, but it can occur in right ventricle also. High degree of suspicion is needed in every case of inferior infarction. One-third of patients with inferoposterior infarction may show minor degree of right ventricular infarction. Right ventricular MI occurs in almost 16–20% of cases of MI and can be diagnosed by right-sided chest leads. A good rule of thumb is to be right-sided chest leads in every suspected or proven inferior wall MI (or in all cases of MI). Isolated right ventricular infarction occurs rarely in the presence of right ventricular hypertrophy.**

Always take right chest leads V3R, V4R, when postero-inferior infarction is suspected. Presence of QS in V3R or V4R and/or an ST elevation of even 1 mm not only suggest involvement of the septum but also indicates that AV block of varying degress will probably develop.

Note the following 4 points while diagnosing the right ventricular infarction.

1. Signs of right ventricular failure (with no left sided heart signs including right ventricular third or fourth heart sound.)
   i. Raise in jugular venous pressure, with a large 'V' wave and a steep 'Y' descent, hepatomegaly.
   ii. Pulsus paradoxus: Pulse weakens in inspiration.
   iii. Kussmaul's sign: Fall in systolic arterial pressure >10 mm Hg during inspiration may be present (venous pressure does not decline during inspiration). Kussmaul's sign in the presence of inferior wall infarction is the first clue to suspect the involvement of right ventricle.
   iv. Lowering of BP (with or without shock).
2. ECG: Suspect in inferior infarction.
   ECG changes associated with right ventricular infarction are not specific because the artery to the right ventricle is a branch of the right coronary artery; Infarction of the right ventricle is usually associated with inferior infarction of the left ventricle.
   Chest leads on right side V3R, V4R, V5R, V6R, should be taken for right ventricular infarction.
   ST elevation > 1 mm in lead V4R in patients with acute inferior infarction.
   ST elevation > 1 mm in V4R in the absence of LBBB or other anteriorly directed vectors is a sensible way to diagnose injury of posterior wall of right ventricle.
   ST elevation of right pericardial leads is short lived and disappear within 10–18 hours after the onset of chest pain in 50% of the patients and after 72 hours in the remaining.
3. Echocardiography shows right ventricular dilatation.
4. Cardiac catheterization shows hemodynamic pattern similar to cardiac tamponade or constrictive pericarditis.

37. RV infarction:

1. In STEMI with RVMI is a high risk subject
2. Mortality rate in this subjects is 25–30%.
   In all cases of IWMI- RVMI should be suspected.
3. ECG recording in right sided precordial leads is a must. ST↑ in V4R is a powerful predictor.
4. Low cardiac output in IWMI is the key to RVMI.

38. Treatment objectives of RVMI are:

1. Aggressive treatment with reperfusion is a must to maintain preload.
2. Give inotropic support.
3. Reduce afterload.
4. Early perfusion by PCI, CABG or thrombolysis IV NS, no diuretics, nitrates, give ACEI, IABP.

39. The 4 enzymes most commonly measured in the diagnosis of myocardial infarction and their peak time of elevation are:

Table F-2

	Start to rise (hours)	Peak (days)	Duration of rise (days)
1. Creatinine kinase (total CK)	4–8	12–24 hr	3–5
2. Creatininekinase MB isoenzyme (CK-MB)	4–8	24 hr	3–5
3. Lactic dehydrogenase isoenzyme-1 (LDH)	24–48 hr	3–6 days	7–14
4. Troponin T	30 min		

Myoglobin is nonspecific. It goes up in one hour and comes down in 4 hours. Myoglobin levels should be done two times.

Creatinine kinase (CK) is also known as creatinine phosphokinase (CPK)

CPK and CPKMB rise in 4 to 8 hours and first to fall. CPK is present in skeletal muscle also and it is raised after an intramuscular injection or vigorous exercise. So, CPK-MB is more specific of myocardial necrosis.

If it remains normal for 48 hours after the event, AMI can safely be ruled out.

Lactic dehydrogenase isoenzyme-I (LDH) is also known as hydroxybutyric dehydrogenase (HBD).

LDH 1 isoenzyme is more specific for MI than total LDH Five enzymes of LDH are recognized. Heart muscle contains more of the isoenzyme LDH-I than liver or skeletal muscle.

LDH rises lately by and lasts longer. LDH is liberated from hemolyzed RBC also and therefore it is less specific. It rises 12–36 hours after, reaches peak after 3–4 days and may be elevated for a week or two. So, it is useful when the diagnosis is doubtful after several days of infarction. If CK-MB is raised but LDH levels are normal the diagnosis for AMI is less firm.

Troponin is the first to rise in 30 minutes after acute myocardial infarction.

Troponin T and I are regulatory proteins of action-tropomysin complex, and are highly sensitive indicator of myocyte necrosis. Blood levels of these proteins may also increase if the integrity of the myocyte cell membrane is impaired without myocyte necrosis. Cardiac-specific troponin T is more specific assay for AMI and is an important indicator of mortality risk and subsequent cardiac events. Reliable serial assays for troponin T can be done at the bedside very quickly and easily. Measurement of troponin T and I distinguished patients with chest pain who have ST elevation and those without in good numbers. The negative result of this test allows rapid safe discharge of patients who are admitted with acute chest pain. Troponin-T test should not be overestimated. It is primarily for the confirmation of a suspected AMI diagnosis. Enzyme confirmation may take up to 30 minutes after ischemia beginning.

Normal range

CPK	Up to 109 μ/L - >1000 UCK (severe infarct)
CPK-MB	Up to 20 μ/L - >150 UCK MB (severe infarct)
LDH	120–365 μ/L
Troponin T	Up to 0.2 ng/mL (some people take cut-off point at 0.1 ng/mL)

Initially, the diagnosis is made from history and ECG; Enzyme levels help later.

40. Cardiac enzyme kinetics

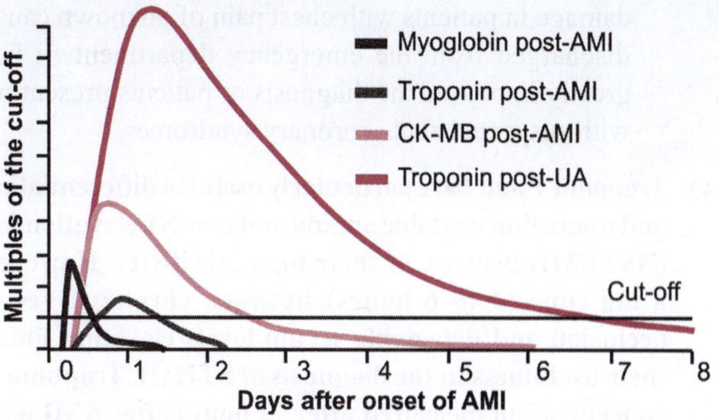

41. Cardiac biomarkers:

Table F-3

Top I to T	CK-MB	Myoglobin
1. Start 3–6 hours	• Start 2–6 hours	• Start 1–2 hours
2. Peak 24–36 hours	• Peak 12–18 hours	• Peak 6–8 hours
3. Lasts 5–14 day	• Lasts 1–2 days	• Lasts 12–24 hours
4. Very Specific	• Moderate specific	• Nonspecific

42. Measurement of cardiac troponin T and cardiac troponin I concentrations has greatly improved diagnosis of patients presenting with suspected acute coronary syndromes. The importance of troponin concentration estimation is increasing because:

1. Increase in concentrations of troponin T and troponin I are highly sensitive and cardiac specific markers for myocardial damage unlike increases in concentrations of creatine kinase and its MB isoenzyme, which can be due to noncardiac sources.
2. Troponin markers have 100% sensitivity for diagnosis of acute myocardial infarction. Its importance has greatly increased in patients with chest pain without electrocardiographic changes. A cut-off level of 0.1 µg/L is the optimal predictor of acute myocardial infarction. The amount of risk depends on how high the troponin concentration is. Data of 6.0 millions patients in USA attending the emergency department each year with chest pain, 5.7 millions have non-diagnostic electrocardiograms. 4.1 millions are sent home, of whom 75,000 (0.18%) have undiagnosed acute myocardial infarction. However, a recent study which measured cardiac troponin T and cardiac troponin I showed an incidence of prognostically important myocardial damage of 6% in patients without a diagnostic electrocardiogram on presentation (Ref: N Engl J Med.1997;337:1648-53).
3. The test is simple to do. Serum was analyzed for cardiac troponin T by enzyme-linked immunoabsorbent assay (ELISA - Roche Diagnostic, Lewes).
4. It is convenient diagnostic audit tool to assess the incidence of prognostically important myocardial damage in patients with chest pain of unknown cause discharged from the emergency department. It has greatly improved the diagnosis of patients presenting with suspected acute coronary syndromes.

43. Troponin T and I are particularly useful in differentiating and managing unstable angina and non-ST elevation MI (NSTEMI) because of their high sensitivity. However, a lag time (3 to 6 hours) between coronary vessel occlusion and detectable serum levels elevation limits their usefulness in the diagnosis of STEMI. Troponin T concentration measured after 72 hours after AMI may be predictive of MI size, independent of reperfusion.

Troponin is elevated in some other conditions also besides acute MI (STEMI).

1. Acute coronary syndrome such as unstable angina and MI without ST elevation/STEMI.
2. Congestive heart failure.
3. Aortic dissection.
4. Hypertrophic obstructive cardiomyopathy (HOCM).
5. Pulmonary embolism.
6. Acute neurologic disease.
7. Cardiac contusion.
8. Drug toxicity.

Since 1990, studies have repeatedly revealed that troponins are released by some patients with acute coronary syndrome and indicate a marker of risk for subsequent cardiac events. Some of these patients undergo early angiography and revascularization to reduce the risk of events. As a consequence management of acute coronary syndrome without ST elevation as changes dramatically in some countries like UK. In one hospital, a troponin positive patient with an acute coronary syndrome may be admitted for a few days and if asymptomatic, may be sent home whereas in another hospital, such a patient may be kept in hospital for early angiography and revascularization.

How can both strategies be correct?

Many centers in UK currently refer all patients with acute coronary syndrome who have elevated troponin concentrations for early angiography. Surely this represent a blunt tool in decision making. The second flaw is troponin measurement is eagerly perceived as a rule in or rule out test. The test has become a main compound of decision making for many clinicians. The final flaw is that troponin is elevated in many other clinical conditions that do not seem to be associated with myocardial ischemia. Troponin measurement in patients with acute chest pain is a mixed blessing; troponin measurement is a blunt screening tool for assessment of patient with acute coronary syndrome without ST elevation and you should avoid compounding this by ignoring clinical features. We need to refine our current strategy to provide optimal treatment for such patients.

44. The other groups of conditions that may show raise in serum enzyme levels are:

1. Isoenzyme CK-MB is the cardiospecific serum enzyme, because heart is the only organ to have it in large amounts. Small amounts are present in skeletal muscle, but it is raised in widespread and extensive damage of the skeletal muscle such as occurs in muscular dystrophy or crush injury.
2. Except CK-MB, other commonly measured enzymes are raised in conditions such as pulmonary infarction, liver congestion due to right heart failure, liver disease, pancreatitis, intestinal infarction, renal infarction, hemolytic anemia, muscular diseases such as muscular dystrophy, dermatomyositis.

3. Intramuscular injections may cause rise in total CK. DC shock generally causes rise in serum enzymes because of the trauma to the muscles of chest wall though effect on CK-MB is usually mild.
4. Aspartate transaminase (also known as SGOT) is present in many tissues including lung, liver, pancreas, gut, kidney and RBC. So, rise in SGOT is nonspecific marker in myocardial infarction.

All these changes may cause confusion when injections are given or in complications such as pulmonary infarction, hepatic congestion or when the DC shock is administered.

45. Echocardiography: 2D Echo provides valuable diagnostic findings on ventricular function and regional wall motion abnormalities.

1. AMI can cause abnormal segmental function of the myocardium manifested as impaired relaxation, hypokinesia, akinesia, or dyskinesia.
2. Useful in the assessment of the left ventricular function especially reperfusion therapy.
3. Test of choice in the evaluation of complication such as ventricular septal rupture, free wall rupture, papillary muscle rupture (MR), hemopericardium.
4. Normal Echo cannot be used reliably to rule out myocardial ischemia.

46. Echocardiography:

1. Detects wall motion abnormality—sensitivity moderate high.
2. Cannot distinguish old from new—many "false positives".
3. Many miss non-Q wave AMI—usually small infarcts.
4. Never compared to physician judgement or cardiac markers to assess incremental value.

47. The following 4 investigations may be useful but are not done routinely.

1. *Chest X-ray:* It can diagnose basically two problems. (i) Cardiomegaly and (ii) Left ventricular failure as evidenced by changes in pulmonary venous pattern. However, these changes may take 10–15 hours to appear in X-ray after symptoms appear (diagnostic lag) and may take similar duration to disappear after the treatment of pulmonary edema of left ventricular failure (therapeutic lag).
2. *Radionuclide perfusion scan:* They serve as "negative scans" and hence are difficult to quantify. Myocardial perfusion imaging with thallium 201, which is taken up and concentrated in the viable myocardium shows defect 'cold spot' during the first few hours of transmural infarct. It is difficult to quantify myocardial infarction using thallium 201 which is used in dynamic state. Tc ^{99} sestamibi scans are better and are used for the diagnosis of myocardial infarction.
3. *Radionuclide "hot spot" scanning (acute infarct scintigraphy):* 99^{m}Tc stannous pyrophosphate scan can be done. It is positive 24–120 hours after myocardial infarction but have no advantages over other methods. Antimyosin scans are quick, sensitive, specific and are now used.
4. *Radionucleide ventriculography with 99^{m}Tc labeled red blood cells:* It can be used in acute phase to see abnormal regional wall motion and reduction in ejection fraction that may help in the diagnosis.

48. The 4 goals of acute myocardial infarction therapy are:

1. Primary goal of therapy is to reduce the likelihood of mortality in the postinfarction period.
2. The second and equally important goal is to achieve AMI survivor with an improved outcome.
3. Limit the infarct size—Since large infarcts lead to deteriorating pump function and secondary arrhythmias, effective treatment consists of preserving left ventricular function, resolve ST-segment elevation and rapidly restore coronary flow to ischemic myocardium.
4. Very early initiation of thrombolytic therapy within 70–90 minutes after the onset of AMI symptoms is associated with significantly improved survival rates and better left ventricular function.

A key strategy to achieving all these goals is to shorten the time to perfusion.

49. Ischemic myocardium at risk can be immediately perfused by any of the 4 methods depending on the availability of facilities.

1. IVI thrombolytic therapy.
2. Intracoronary thrombolytic therapy.
3. Coronary angioplasty.
4. CABG.

50. Consider the following for initiating thrombolytic therapy:

1. Correct diagnosis: ST↑, or new LBBB.
2. Rule out contraindications.
3. Perform basic neurological examination.
4. Establish 2 or 3 IV lines.
   1st line for primary fluids and other medications.
   2nd line for heparin.
   3rd line for thrombolysis.

Reteplase can be administered through one of the existing lines following flushing of the line.

Blood should be drawn for: Coagulation profile, CBC, blood chemistry, cardiac enzymes, and ABG.

51. The 4 principles in the treatment of acute myocardial infarction are:

1. Relief of pain.
2. Prevention of electrical irritability, i.e. Arrhythmias. 65% male under 50 years who died within 1 hour. 85% died within 24 hours are due to life-threatening arrhythmias, such as ventricular fibrillation.
3. Prevention of 'pump failure', i.e. mechanical failure, or cardiac failure.
4. Prevention of 'power failure', i.e. cardiogenic shock.

52. The 4 aims of treatment in the recent advances of AMI management are:

1. Relief of pain.
2. Limitation of infarct size within 4 hours (2 to 6 hours is the time, average within 4 hours). Reduction of infarct size is the single most important factor in salvaging the ischemic myocardium to reduce mortality and morbidity.
3. Reduce the complications:
   Electrical irritability—arrhythmias
   Pump failure—cardiac failure
   Power failure—cardiogenic shock.
4. Prevention of further infarction and rehabilitation.

53. The following 4 drugs are used in order of preference for the relief of pain in AMI:

The pain and the accompanying anxiety contribute to each other to give excessive activity of autonomic nervous system resulting in restlessness. These in turn increase the metabolic demand of the myocardium. Physician assurance with affection and love increases the patient's confidence.

Narcotics remain the drugs of choice in alleviating pain and anxiety.

1. Inj morphine 5–10 mg IV for quick action repeated in small doses of 2 to 4 mg IV to achieve the required effect than giving larger quantities of 10–20 mg by subcutaneous route from which the absorption is not sure.
   Morphine blocks sympathetic efferent discharge at CNS level, resulting in peripheral venous and arterial dilatation reducing both preload and afterload and decreasing the myocardial oxygen demand. Relief of pain and anxiety reduces circulating catecholamines and possibly reduces arrhythmias.
   It can be supplemented by cyclizine 50 mg IV.
   It can be combined with phenergan.
   Watch for any respiratory depression.
   Morphine or diamorphine is given IV. They can be given subcutaneously or intramuscularly but less satisfactory because initial peripheral vasoconstriction after myocardial infarction delays absorption, while later vasodilatation leads to rapid absorption which may result in respiratory depression.
2. Second preference is diamorphine.
   Sublingual or injection is as good as morphine (5–10 mg SC or IV) or buprenorphine (IV 2.5–5 mg) 0.2 to 0.3 mg–available sublingually also.
3. Inj pethidine 50 to 100 mg IM.
4. Inj diazepam 5 to 10 mg IM or IV.
   30–50% nitrous oxide: If the pain is associated with anxiety, nitrous oxide may be administered with little or no depression of left ventricular function.
   Pentazocaine injection should not be given as it increases pulmonary wedge pressure leading to increase in preload and congestive cardiac failure.

54. Morphine acts as:

1. Analgesic.
2. Anxiolytic.
3. Antiarrhythmic.
4. Vasodilatory.

Morphine is given to anterior wall MI (AWMI), but not for posterior MI or inferior MI.

55. The 4 main side effects of both morphine and diamorphine are:

1. Nausea and vomiting due to stimulation of the brain stem. An antiemetic such as metoclopramide 10 mg or perphenazine 5 mg is to be given with the opiate.
2. Respiratory depression due to depression of the respiratory center with opiate. Therefore, should be avoided or given cautiously in small doses in patients with chronic bronchitis of the blue bloating type.
3. Hypotension can occur as a result of relaxation of vascular smooth muscle and should be differentiated from cardiogenic shock of myocardial infarction. It responds to elevation of legs and IV fluids.
4. Bradycardia due to vagotonic effect particularly in posterior infarction. It responds 4 mg IV atropine.

56. Early, 4 general measures are:

1. Bed rest with bedside commode privileges for initial 12 hours in hemodynamically stable patients free of ischemic-type chest discomfort.
2. Careful attention to maximum pain relief.
3. Selection of electrocardiographic monitoring based on infarct location and rhythm.
4. Avoidance of Valsalva.

57. Rest:

Rest is important immediately after acute myocardial infarction and strict bed rest is essential in the first few days. It helps in 4 ways to reduce mortality and morbidity:

1. It minimises the work of the heart.
2. It minimizes the oxygen requirement of ischemic myocardium surrounding the infarct area.
3. It minimizes or limits the infarct size
4. It minimizes the risk of arrhythmias.

58. General examination: The clinched fist pointing at the sternum indicates retrosternal pain suggesting acute MI before an ECG.

Check the vital signs:

1. *Pulse:* Anterior wall MI may be associated with sinus tachycardia and inferior wall MI may be associated with sinus bradycardia. Feeble and thready pulse is suggestive of shock (cardiogenic shock).
2. *Temperature:* Usually normal or may be 1°F rise. Profuse sweating can be due to apprehension of severe pain or cardiogenic shock.
3. *Respiration:* Respiratory rate is increased—see for any Kussmaul's (acidosis) or Cheyne-Stokes respiration (alkalosis).
4. *Blood pressure:* It is normal in uncomplicated cases. If the SBP is <90 mm Hg suspect cardiogenic shock, right ventricular MI, vagal response to inferior wall MI, or hemodynamically unstable.

59. Systemic examination:

1. *CVS:* JVP usually normal. It may be raised in left ventricular failure.
   Auscultate for S3 (left ventricular dysfunction).
   Auscultate for murmur (MR).
   Auscultate for pericardial rub.
   Usually sounds are feeble in cardiogenic shock.
2. *Respiratory system:* Auscultate for moist rales (left ventricular failure and pulmonary edema) Killip's classification of 4 groups of AMI with pump failure.
3. *Central nervous system (CNS):* For any neurological deficits.
4. *Abdomen:* Palpable for liver and spleen. For any signs of perforation.

60. Immediate management strategy and stabilization:

1. *Aspirin:* It is given immediately for antiplatelet activity in all cases of patients with acute MI unless there is clear history of true aspirin allergy (not intolerance) Immediate aspirin therapy provides as much mortality benefit as streptokinase/or urokinase. The dose should be 4 chewable tablets of 81 mg of each for more rapid absorption or one 325 mg nonchewable tablet. If it is not possible by oral route, a rectal suppository can be given. In aspirin allergy patient clopidogrel monotherapy is the best alternate.
2. *Thienopyridines:* Clopidogrel should be given in addition to aspirin in all STEMI patients regardless of whether they undergo primary percutaneous coronary intervention (PCI) or fibrinolysis. Loading dose of 300 mg per oral followed by 75 mg od.
3. *Nitroglycerin (See F 108–113):* Immediate sublingual glyceryl trinitrate 0.5 mg/or isosorbide dinitrate 5 mg/10 mg is given for coronary vasodilatation.
   The patient should be asked about recent use of sildenafil (Viagra) because administration of nitroglycerin within 24 hours of sildenafil may cause life threatening hypotension.
   Nitroglycerin is useful in acute MI complicated by ongoing symptoms of chest pain, hypertension, or congestive heart failure. A 30% reduction in systolic blood pressure can be expected with aggressive dosing of (10–20 µg/min with 5–10 µg/min increase every 5 to 10 minutes) intravenous nitroglycerin therapy can be continued for 24–48 hours followed by oral therapy.
4. *Oxygen:* It is given by nasal canula to all patients with suspected acute MI. Administration of oxygen by facemask or endotracheal tube may be necessary in patients with severe pulmonary edema or cardiogenic shock.

61. Oxygen: Hypoxemia is common in myocardial infarction and in itself may be a cause for chest pain and anxiety. The mechanism of hypoxemia is complex. It is likely that ventilation-perfusion mismatch plays a prominent role. Some patients are modestly hypoxemic initially even with uncomplicated myocardial infarction. Patients with associated congestive heart failure have more severe hypoxemia. There is growing concern about the routine use of oxygen.

The following are 4 guidelines for administering the oxygen:

1. Oxygen should be provided at least in the initial hours for all patients on arrival in the emergency department with suspected AMI.

2. Oxygen should not be withheld during transportation to the hospital especially if there is evidence of pulmonary disease.
3. In patients who are anxious with chest pain, who have obvious respiratory distress, administration of 2 to 4 liters of 100% oxygen/minute by mask or nasal prongs is mandatory.
4. Patients with severe congestive heart failure, pulmonary edema or a mechanical complication of acute myocardial infarction may fail to correct significant hypoxemia with supplemental oxygen alone. Endotracheal intubation and mechanical ventilation are often required in such cases and should not be unnecessarily delayed.

   Blood gas analysis is helpful before initiating the use of oxygen.

62. There are 4 recent advances in the management of myocardial infarction to reduce the infarct size:

Important advances have occurred in the treatment of myocardial infarction in the last two decades. Both conventional as well as new aggressive approaches are tried.

Main aim is to limit the infarct size. 'The open artery' principle is vital in improving the outcome in acute MI. The obstructed vessel should be unblocked as soon as possible and patency should be maintained to improve prognosis.

The GISSI-1 trial showed a 47% reduction in death if treatment with streptokinase was given within 1 hour of the onset of symptoms; GISSI-2 showed further reduction in mortality with the additional use of aspirin and a β-blocker. In fact, every major thrombolytic trial (Gusto-1, 'Fibrinolytic Therapy Trialists'(FTT) collaborative Group) has demonstrated that the greatest benefits are achieved when therapy begins earlier after the onset of symptoms.

Numerous trials support an inverse relation between time to treatment and survival benefit.

1. Thrombolytic therapy: It should be given in patients with ST-segment elevation (equal to or greater than 1 mV) in two or more contiguous leads provides strong evidence of thrombotic coronary arterial occlusion and makes the patient a candidate for immediate reperfusion therapy either by fibrinolysis or primary percutaneous transluminal coronary angioplasty (PTCA). Symptoms consistent with acute MI and left bundle branch block (obscuring ST-segment analysis) should be managed like ST-segment elevation. In contrast, the patient without ST-segment elevation should not receive thrombolytic therapy. The benefit of primary PTCA in these patients remains uncertain.

   Therapy should be more aggressive in the first few hours of infarction to reduce the size of infarct within 4 to 6 hours.

   Thrombosis within a coronary artery occurs in about 80% of myocardial infarcts.

   Streptokinase and urokinase digest fibrin, fibrinogen, prothrombin and clotting factors V and VII throughout the circulation. They lyse the thrombus immediately so as to restore the circulation sufficiently to prevent the infarction of ischemic areas surrounding the infarction. Thus, they limit the size of the infarct thereby reducing the mortality and morbidity.

   rt-PA, recombinant tissue plasminogen activator/ reteplase acts more specifically on the clot (clot specific) whereas streptokinase causes generalized fibrinolysis. Streptokinase, though it is not clot specific, it is widely used in India because of its less cost.
2. Protection of ischemic myocardium (see point 60)
3. Percutaneous transluminal coronary angioplasty (PTCA) (See Chapter T 8-12).

   If the patient still gets pain after thrombolytic therapy and the ECG still repeats ST elevation without Q wave, PTCA is tried particularly in young people with reocclusion or reinfarction.

   PTCA is invasive but nonsurgical technique, more economical and reduces hospital stay.

   Inflation of distensible balloon catheter is done during coronary angiography to compress the obstructive atheroma and subsequent disruption of atheromatous lesion.

   An immediate success rate of 80–90% revascularization is achieved in experts hands.

   There are 2–3% chances of aggravating infarction by displacing the emboli to the periphery. Therefore bypass team should be ready.

   PTCA is also indicated in resistant angina with localized single or double vessel disease.
4. Emergency coronary artery bypass grafting is done in patients who come after 6 hours not responding to the above treatment.

63. Primary PTCA: Only 18% of hospitals in US have angioplasty facilities. Primary PTCA is done immediately within few hours after the attack. Emergency surgical team should always be ready to attend if any complications occur. Primary PTCA is better in conditions:

1. When the patient is sicker
2. When there is extensive anterior infarction
3. When there is pulmonary edema
4. Elderly patient of > 75 years age
5. When there is cardiogenic shock
6. When the patient is seen later after 6 hours
7. When there is contraindication of thrombolysis
8. When there is increased risk of bleeding.

64. Primary PTCA is attempted only in advanced cardiac care centers. Give—

1. Aspirin
2. β-blocker
3. Inj heparin
4. Angiogram/angioplasty.

Patient is discharged in 72 hours.

65. If facilities for immediate coronary angiography and direct PCI are available, within 30 minutes of MI—this preferred to thrombolytic therapy—because it showed significant—

1. Reduction in the incidence of death.
2. Reduction in nonfatal MI.
3. Reduction in recurrent ischemia at long-term follow-up.
4. Reduction in the incidence of intracerebral hemorrhage.

Many large trials showed significant reduction of 22% in short-term mortality treated with primary angioplasty. Either PTCA or thrombolytic therapy is emphasized depending the facilities available.

66. For all practical purposes, thrombolytic therapy is preferred in Indian hospitals set-up where a general physician can do the treatment. It is preferred where the patient is in stable condition and in Inferior MI:

Presently used thrombolytic (fibrinolytic) agents are:

Agents not specific for fibrin—

1. Streptokinase
2. Urokinase
3. Anisolated plasminogen streptokinase activator complex (APSAC)
4. Arvin

Agents relatively clot-specific—

5. Staphylokinase (fibrin selective)
6. Recombinant single chain urokinase (fibrin selective) (pro-urokinase)
7. Recombinant tissue plasminogen activator (rt-PA) (Alteplase): It is a genetically engineered version of naturally occurring tissue plasminogen activator. Alteplase is a recombinant variant of natural t-PA, with certain segment deletions and local mutations. It differs from streptokinase and urokinase in preferentially converting fibrin bound plasminogen in the clot. This minimizes the risk of systemic bleeding.
8. Reteplase: Unlike alteplase, reteplase is a genetically engineered fragment of t-PA, a deletion mutation consisting of the second kringle and protease domains alone. Reteplase is produced in *E. coli* and is non-glycosylated.

Direct acting antithrombin drugs like hirudin, argatroban, efegatran are still under clinical trials.

Eptifibatide, lanoteplase, tirofiban (also known as aggrastat) are some newer drugs.

67. Indications for thrombolytic therapy:

Definitive indication:

1. ST ↑ >0.1 in V1, two or more contiguous leads. Time to therapy 12 hours or less. Golden time is < 4 hours (before the appearance of Q waves < 6 hours). Age < 75 years.
2. Newly identified bundle branch block (obscuring ST segment analysis) and history suggesting of AMI. Needs careful analysis.
3. Very early phase of AMI. Giant, hyperacute T waves without ST elevation in very early phase of AMI.
4. Direct posterior infarction with ST depression in V1-V4. Patients with anterior ST elevation MI and LBBB are at high risk from MI but they get greater benefit with thrombolytic therapy. Benefit is less with inferior MI but benefit is good in subgroup associated with right ventricular infarction. ST↑ in RV4, or anterior segment depression is indicative of a posterior current of injury as often occurs with occlusion of a large circumflex artery.

In patients older than 75 years the overall risk of mortality is high with or without therapy.

Blood pressure >180/110 mm Hg are associated with high risk of MI and intracranial hemorrhage, and in his situation, potential benefit of thrombolytic therapy must be weighed carefully against the risk of hemorrhagic stroke.

68. The ideal thrombolytic—

1. Thrombus specific: It should act preferentially on the fresh coronary thrombus so as to avoid undesirable systemic effects.
2. Rapid acting: It should act rapidly to minimize the duration of ischemia by recanalization.

3. High efficacy (60 to 90 minutes patency). It should be highly effective in establishing and maintaining perfusion.
4. Low incidence of side effects especially bleeding and ICH/stroke.
5. Its use should result in low incidence of reocclusion, rescue procedures, and serious adverse reactions.
6. It should be easy to administer (bolus vs infusion).
7. Good long-term effects on critical outcomes.
8. Cost-effective.

69. Considerations for initiating thrombolytic therapy:

1. Correct diagnosis is most important. It is indicated by ST elevation or new BBB. Patients without ST-segment elevation or new BBB should not receive thrombolysis.
2. Rule out contraindications for thrombolytic therapy
3. Establish 2 or 3 IV lines. First-line is for primary fluids and medications. Second line is for heparin. Third line is for thrombolytic.
   Reteplase can be administered through one of the existing lines following flushing of the line.
4. Draw the blood for laboratory tests—cardiac enzymes such as CPKMB, troponin-T, coagulation profile, complete blood count and chemistry. Should use existing lines for all blood draws whenever possible.
5. Perform basic neurologic examination.
6. Protect from trauma and optional interventional procedures.
7. Repeat evaluation q 15–20 min. Check vital signs. A 12-lead ECG should be repeated as potential fatal arrhythmias may occur as a result of perfusion after successful thrombolytic therapy. Continue cardiac monitoring.
8. Should be monitored for recurrent ischemia and/or thrombosis

70. Thrombolytic (fibrinolytic) therapy:

Therapy should be started within 4 to 6 hours before the appearance of Q waves. Thrombolytic therapy administered early after the onset of symptoms of myocardial infarction can restore:

i. Infarct related artery patency
ii. Preserve LV function
iii. Salvage myocardium and
iv. Reduce mortality

All thrombolytic agents currently in use act directly or indirectly as plaminogen activators. Experience from the five big trials of thrombolysis (GISSI-1, ISAM, ISIS, AIMS, ASSET) suggests that thrombolysis has reduced the mortality rate in AMI.

The Gruppo Italiano per lo Studio della Streptochinasi nell' Infarzto Miocardico (GISSI-1) was a milestone as the first large scale study to demonstrate a significant reduction in mortality achieved with streptokinase thrombolysis compared to placebo.

1. *Streptokinase:* Intravenous streptokinase 7,50,000 to 15,00,000 IU in over one hour in 100 mL of saline or 5% dextrose is given. Infusion continued till thrombolysis occurs or maximum of 15,00,000 IU.
   Intracoronary streptokinase: 10 or 30000 IU as bolus dose followed by continuous infusion of 2000 to 4000 IU per minute for 30–90 minutes.
   This is the first generation non-fibrin specific lytic. It is a reasonable alternative to 2nd and 3rd agents if new agents are not available or not be used because of high cost. Streptokinase should not be used in patients who have received in the past because of possible development of antibodies.
2. *Urokinase:* Available in 50,000 IU, 2,50,000 IU, 5,00,000 IU per vial inj 2,50,000 IU vial/5,00,000 IU vial to be dissolved in 10–20 mL saline or 5% dextrose. 2,50,000 IU (10 mL) IV bolus over 5–10 min followed by 2,50,000 IU (10 mL) in 50–100 mL drip over 30 minutes is given.
   Some patients may require another 2,50,000 IU (10 mL) in the next 30 minutes.
   Intracoronary urokinase: 6000 IU/min in saline or 5% dextrose. Therapy is continued until the coronary artery is opened maximum, usually 1/2 hour after initial opening. Total 10,000 IU per kg.
3. *Recombinant tissue plasminogen activator (rt-PA):* It is a second generation fast-acting agent. It is most effective even up to 7 hours after the onset of symptoms. Clot lysis is more. Available as 50 mg inj with 50 mL solvent water.
   Intravenous rt-PA 100 mg over 3 hours
   10 mg IV—initial bolus over 1–2min
   50 mg IV—over next 1 hour
   20 mg IV—over next 1 hour
   20 mg IV—over next 1 hour
   It has higher patency rate and a decreased incidence of reocclusion.
   (GUSTO Angiographic Investigators Study is a comparison of alteplase and streptokinase in which alteplase has shown more benefits—for every ten patients one extra patient is alive with rt-PA.)
4. *Reteplase:* A genetically engineered plasminogen activator in which a novel molecule not present in nature is engineered for desirable pharmacokinetic and fibrinolytic properties. It is a modification of

the tissue type plasminogen activator (t-PA) protein that maintains the kringle-2 and protease domains of t-PA, but lacks its kringle-1, finger, and growth factor domains. In contrast to t-PA, the reteplase molecule is nonglycosylated.

The first of these agents is a genetically engineered peptide. Fast, convenient double-bolus dosing. Administration is completed within two 10 IU bolus injections, each bolus is given over 2 minutes and 30 minutes apart.

2 × 10 U (10.8 U/18.8 mg) vials available.

71. Comparison of alteplase and reteplase:

Table F-4

	Alteplase	*Reteplase*
1. Molecular structure	Glycosylated	Non-glycosylated
2. Half-life	3 to 6 min	13 to 16 min
3. Administration	90 min from loaded infusion. Dosing requires adjustment based on weight	Double-blind—30 min. No dose adjustment regardless of weight
4. Fibrin affinity	High	Low

Fibrin specificity is high for both. They selectively activate thrombus-bound plasminogen on the surface of the clot, converting it plasmin, a proteolytic enzyme. Plasmin in turn degrades clot components and precursors—fibrin, fibrinogen and coagulation factors V and VII resulting in thrombolysis.

Glycosylation tends to increase clearance rates. Since, reteplase is non-glycosylate, half-life is longer than alteplase. Reteplase should be administered through IV line separately in which no other medication is being injected or infused simultaneously. Heparin and reteplase are incompatible when combined in solution.

Major clinical trial of reteplase, INJECT (International Joint Efficacy Comparison of Thrombolytics – is a double-blind randomized clinical trial comparison with Streptokinase in AMI has proved reteplase is a safe, effective therapy with better results.

RAPID-1 (Reteplase Angiographic Phase II International Dose-Finding Study) and RAPID-2 (Reteplase vs Alteplase Patency Investigation During Acute Myocardial Infarction Study) were not designed or powered to compare reteplase and alteplase with respect to outcomes of mortality or stroke, consequently comparison of these outcomes cannot be made.

72. Comparison of thrombolytics

Table F-5

Feature	*SK Streptokinase*	*tPA Alteplase*	*r-tPA Reteplase*	*TNK Tenectaplase*
1. Fibrin selective	No	Yes	Yes	Yes
2. Duration of Rx	60 min	90 min	10 mm	5–10 sec
3. Half-life in min	23	<5	13–16	20
4. Dosage	1.5 M IU in NS	15 + 50 + 35 mg	10 U + 10 U	0.5 mg/kg stat
5. BP⇓, Allergy	Yes	No	No	No
6. TIMI reflow 3	32%	45–54%	60%	60%
7. Major bleeds	6.3%	5.4%	5.9%	4.7%
8. 30 day mortality	7.4%	6.3%	6.2%	6.2%

73. Statistically, reteplase showed significant reduction in the incidence of mortality and morbidity in certain conditions like:

1. Congestive heart failure
2. Left ventricular function
3. Hypotension/shock
4. Atrial fibrillation.

Fewer acute coronary investigations (PTCA) are needed.

74. Eptifibatide, tirofiban, lanoteplase, are useful alternative drugs in AMI used before primary PCI tirofiban hydrochloride (aggribloc) is available 0.25 mg per mL infusion in 100 mL bottle.

Initially, bolus 20 mL added in 80 mL of normal saline given in 30 minutes followed by:

1. 20 mL + 80 mL of normal saline in 3 hours in pediatric drip set (PD set).
   Give 1 hour gap.
2. 20 mL + 80 mL of normal saline in 3 hours.
   Give 1 hour gap.
3. 20 mL + 80 mL of normal saline in 3 hours.
   Give 1 hour gap.
4. 20 mL + 80 mL of normal saline in 3 hours.

Total 100 mL of tirofiban is given in 15–16 hours of time

It is useful for prevention of evolving early MI in patients with unstable angina or non-Q wave MI with last episode of chest pain within 12 hr and with ECG changes and/or elevated cardiac enzymes. To be used with aspirin and heparin.

Total 100 mL of tirofiban is given in 15–16 hours of time. Tenecteplase (TNK) is another third generation fibrinolytic characterized by improved fibrin specificity, enhanced resistance to fibrinogen activator inhibitor (PAI-I) and decreased plasma clearance. These benefits are helpful in administering as a single bolus.

75. Thrombolytic therapy is definitely indicated in left main coronary artery, anterior descending branch thrombosis causing acute MI. It is indicated in inferior MI when it is associated with:

1. Block
2. Right ventricular MI
3. Anterior wall precordial MI
4. Complications like VT, pulmonary edema, cardiogenic shock, etc.

No contraindication for the use of streptokinase in unstable angina. Benefit is not clear. May be costing unnecessarily to the patient.

76. Patient monitoring before and during thrombolytic therapy should be done by:

1. Platelet count
2. Thrombin time (TT)
3. Activated partial thromboplastin time (APTT) or prothrombin time
4. Coagulation tests and/or measurement of fibrinolytic activity may be performed.

Following the infusion, before (re)instituting heparin, the TT or APTT should be less than twice the normal control value.

77. There are 4 other indications for thrombolytic therapy (Stk, Uk, rt-PA, Reteplase) besides AMI:

1. Pulmonary embolism
2. Deep vein thrombosis
3. Acute peripheral vascular thromboembolism (arterial thrombosis or embolism)
4. Occlusion of arteriovenous cannulae.

In deep vein thrombosis, patients blood pressure should not be taken in the lower extremities to avoid possible dislodgement of thrombus.

78. Only a minority of patients with myocardial infarction are treated by thrombolytic agents because of the following 4 reasons:

1. Patients presenting too late.
2. Presence of contraindications.
3. Misconceptions regarding age, etc.
4. Costly to bear the expenses.

79. The 4 advantages of early thrombolytic therapy (before 4–6 hours) are:

1. *Restores early patency of infarct related artery:* Early reperfusion may convert transmural infarction (Q waves) into subendocardial infarction (inverted T wave).
2. *Limits the infarct size:* Timely injection of fibrinolytic before 4 to 6 hours (or before the appearance of Q waves) will reduce the infarct size by reperfusion. Reduction of infarct size is the single most important factor in reducing the mortality rate.
3. *Preserves left ventricular function:* LV function is preserved by limiting the infarct size.
4. *Reduces mortality and morbidity rate by reducing the infarct size:* Early thrombolytic therapy within 6 hours reduces the mortality rate from fatal arrhythmias. Early rehabilitation is possible compared to control groups. Complications of myocardial infarction are less after thrombolytic therapy.

80. Physician should consider the following 4 points before starting the thrombolytic therapy:

1. Age: Younger the age, better the result–One should be very cautious in elderly over 70 years of age.
2. Duration of chest pain and the onset of chest pain. Therapy should be restricted to patients with chest pain of more than 30 minutes. Therapy should be started within 4 to 6 hours of onset of chest pain. Good results are obtained within 3 hours of onset of pain. Earlier the treatment, better the results. It improves the survival and preserve the left ventricular function if given within 3 hours of onset of pain.
3. Amount of myocardium involved. ST elevation in two contiguous limb leads, e.g. L III, aVF or chest leads V1, V2. These patients are more likely to have total or 80–85% occlusion than those with ST depression. Caution is needed in patients with only ST depression suspected of myocardial infarction since many of them have only incomplete coronary occlusion. Myocardial tissue is available for salvage for about 2 to 3 hours and possibly up to 6 hours. Therefore, thrombolytic therapy should be started before the appearance of Q waves. Benefit is less if started after 6–12 hours, diminished benefit but possibly still useful or continuous chest pain or stuttering pain course.
4. Other associated medical problems such as potential bleeding sites.

81. Response to thrombolytic therapy is assessed by the following 4 parameters:

1. Symptomatically by relief of chest pain.
2. Clinically by the onset of reperfusion arrhythmias.
3. ECG evidence of rapid resolution of ST elevation. Resolution of ST elevation is an excellent criteria of recanalization. ST becomes isoelectric within 1 hour.
4. Angiography.

82. The 4 advantages of intracoronary thrombolytic (urokinase or streptokinase) therapy are:

1. It directly delivers the fibrinolytic material to the thrombus in higher concentration.
2. Clot lysis needs only smaller doses.
3. Avoid systemic fibrinolysis.
4. Dissolution of thrombus by mechanical fragmentation with a soft guide wire is possible. (It needs very well-equipped catheterization laboratory and well-trained personal).

83. Comparison of intravenous versus intracoronary thrombolytic therapy in acute myocardial infarction:

Table F-6

	IV streptokinase	*Intracoronary streptokinase*
1. Logistics	Simple	Complex
2. Cost	Less	High
3. Applicability	Can be given at all hospitals	Possible only in specialized (cardiac) units
4. Clot lysis	35–50% (sk)	50–80% (sk)
	35–50% (uk)	50–80%
	60–70% rt-PA	

The delay caused by cardiac catheterization outweigh the therapeutic benefit and possible only in highly specialized cardiology department. So, intravenous thrombolytic therapy is preferred to intracoronary therapy because it is simple, less costly and can be given at all emergency centers.

84. The 4 main complications of thrombolytic therapy are:

1. Allergic reactions.
2. Hypotension.
3. Reperfusion arrhythmias, e.g. PVBs, VT, VF, accelerated idioventricular rhythm.
4. Bleeding-major or minor.

85. True allergic reactions can occur with thrombolytic therapy. There are 4 major and 4 minor allergic reactions with streptokinase (1 to 2%).

The 4 major allergic reactions are:

1. Anaphylactoid reaction.
2. Hypotension.
3. Angioneurotic edema.
4. Bronchospasm.

Therapy should be stopped immediately for anaphylactoid reaction.

86. The 4 minor allergic reactions are:

1. Rash
2. Urticaria
3. Flushing
4. Fever.

Milder reactions can be completely abolished by premedication with injection hydrocortisone 100 mg IV which is repeated at 6 to 12 hours interval.

Allergic reactions are more with streptokinase since it is a foreign protein derived from bacteria. Allergy to urokinase is extremely unusual since it is a human protein. Allergy to recombinant tissue plasminogen activator (rt-PA) and reteplase are extremely rare since they are made by genetic engineering.

Streptokinase therapy is ineffective in patients who have pre-existing high titers of streptokinase antibody. These neutralizing antibodies are present in patients with recent streptococcal infection or streptokinase exposure. These patients should be treated with urokinase or rt-PA or reteplase.

Fever occurs with streptokinase in 30% of cases whereas with urokinase in 1–2%.

Premedication with hydrocortisone injection effectively reduces the incidence of allergic reactions.

87. Bleeding is the major complication of thrombolytic therapy. Serious bleeding is defined as bleeding in such sites which necessitates transfusion or surgical intervention.

The 4 common sites of bleeding are:

1. Brain
2. GI tract
3. Urinary tract
4. Retroperitoneal space.

Most bleeding episodes are minor.

Nuisance bleeding such as venepuncture oozing is easily managed by local pressure.

Hemoptysis may be due to pulmonary edema. Hematemesis may be due to active peptic ulcer present earlier.

88. If a patient treated with fibrinolytic medication develops serious bleeding following steps are taken to control the bleeding:

Step 1: Cessation of fibrinolytic agent.
Cessation of any anticoagulation therapy.

Step 2: Supportive therapy—It includes volume repletion and transfusion of blood factors.
Fresh frozen plasma and/or cryoprecipitate may be used to replenish fibrin and clotting factors.

Step 3: When possible direct pressure should be used to control bleeding.

If the patients is receiving heparin, protamine sulfate may be used to reverse the heparin effect.

Step 4: Aminocaproic acid (Amicar) is a specific antidote for fibrinolytic agent. In adults, 4 to 5.0 g of aminocaproic acid is administered IV over the first hour then a continuous IVI of 1.0 g/hr is given for 8 hours or until the bleeding is controlled.

Aminocaproic acid should not be given unless hemorrhage is life-threatening because it inhibits intrinsic fibrinolytic activity and can precipitate runaway thrombosis with end organ damage at many sites.

89. Intracerebral bleeding is the most devastating of complications. The risk of intracranial bleeding is least with streptokinase and higher with rt-PA. The following 4 risk factors are identified:

1. Age beyond 70 years
2. Females
3. Uncontrolled hypertension at presentation (>200/110 mm Hg)
4. Less body weight.

90. The absolute contraindications for thrombolytic therapy (streptokinase, urokinase or recombinant tissue plasminogen activator or reteplase) are

1. History of recent stroke known to be hemorrhagic or transient ischemic attack, intracranial tumor, etc.
5. Chances of intracranial hemorrhage is high in older patients.
2. Uncontrolled severe hypertension > 180/110 mm Hg.
3. Active bleeding lesions (excluding menses).
   H/o recent GI bleeding within 3 months.
   H/o active peptic ulcer.
   H/o bleeding diathesis.
4. Major surgery or major trauma less than 10 days previously.
5. Suspected aortic dissection.
6. Pregnancy.
7. Diabetic hemorrhagic retinopathy or other hemorrhagic ophthalmic conditions.
8. Previous allergic reaction to the thrombolytic agent (streptokinase or APSAC).
9. Warfarin anticoagulation when INR may be >3.0.
10. Hemophilia.
11. Thrombocytopenia.
12. Severe liver disease (including varices).
13. Serious vaginal bleeding.
14. Tooth extraction (recently).
15. Tuberculosis with cavitation.
16. Endocarditis.

91. The 4 relative contraindications for thrombolytic therapy are:

1. Recent cardiopulmonary resuscitation including external cardiac massage.
2. Postpartum state.
3. Recent biopsy or needle puncture of poorly compressible areas.
4. Hypocoagulable state.

92. Limitations of thrombolytic therapy:

1. Thrombolysis takes an average of 45–70 minutes to occur (delayed recanalization reduces the magnitude of myocardial salvage).
2. Failure of thrombolysis occurs in 15–50% of cases (patients with failed thrombolysis have a several fold higher mortality).
3. Bleeding, particularly intracranial hemorrhage, in 0.3 to 1.5% of cases remains an uncommon but serious problem.
4. Reocclusion occurs in 5–15% of cases (reocclusion eliminates the benefits of initial thrombolytic reperfusion and is associated with increased mortality and morbidity).

Reocclusion and reinfarction rate is higher in patients who received thrombolytic therapy. Retreatment with thrombolysis can be given when reinfarction occurs. Streptokinase may be repeated within 1 week of its initial administration beyond which it becomes less effective by neutralizing antibodies. It is wise not to repeat streptokinase within 1 year of its initial use. In such a case, an alternate agent is preferred.

93. Magnitude of myocardial salvage is modest in some cases because of the following 4 reasons:

1. Delayed application of therapy
2. Slow lysis
3. Reocclusion
4. Reperfusion injury (controversial).

94. Failure of thrombolytic therapy or reocclusion can occur in:

1. Raised plasminogen activator inhibitor.
2. Recent streptococcal infection or streptokinase exposure where there is pre-existing high titers of streptokinase antibodies.
3. Displacement of thrombus to proximal or distal in the vessel.
4. When not followed by anticoagulants or antiplatelets.

95. The following 4 guidelines help while giving thrombolytic therapy in acute myocardial infarction:

1. Intravenous thrombolytic therapy is preferred over intracoronary therapy because it is simple and can be given at all emergency rooms.

At present rt-PA is the drug of choice but streptokinase is less expensive and alternative especially in patients who present in less than 2 hours after symptoms.

2. Give hydrocortisone 100 mg injection and chlorpheniramine maleate as premedication to abolish or prevent adverse allergic reactions. Repeat if necessary.
3. Start lidocaine (xylocaine) injection by bolus or infusion at 2 mg/min prior to thrombolytic agent and continued as an infusion following thrombolytic agent infusion. Many patients develop transient period of ventricular irritability at the time of coronary recanalization. Reperfusion arrhythmias are not usually proved to be a serious problem and have not limited the therapy.
4. Thrombolytic therapy should be followed by full dose of heparin for 3 to 5 days adjusted to maintain the partial thromboplastin time (PTT) at 1.5 to 2 times than that of control to prevent reinfarction. Aspirin (80–325 mg) is given during hospitalization and after discharge. Despite full dose of heparin, reocclusion or reinfarction can occur in 20–25% cases. Reinfarction during hospitalization within 7 days remain a major problem.

96. Fibrinolysis vs Primary PCI:

Table F-7

Fibrinolysis	Primary PCI
1. Early presentation < 3 hours from symptom of onset and potential delay to invasive strategy	Skilled PCI laboratory available with surgical backup. Medical contact to balloon time is < 90 min
2. Invasive strategy is not available	High risk patient, e.g. cardiogenic shock, Killip class ≥ 3, Age ≥75 years, anterior MI
3. Delay to invasive strategy > 90 min (including transfer time)	Contraindication to fibrinolysis
4. No contraindication to therapy	Late presentation Diagnosis of STEMI is in doubt

97. Fibrinolysis vs Primary PCI:

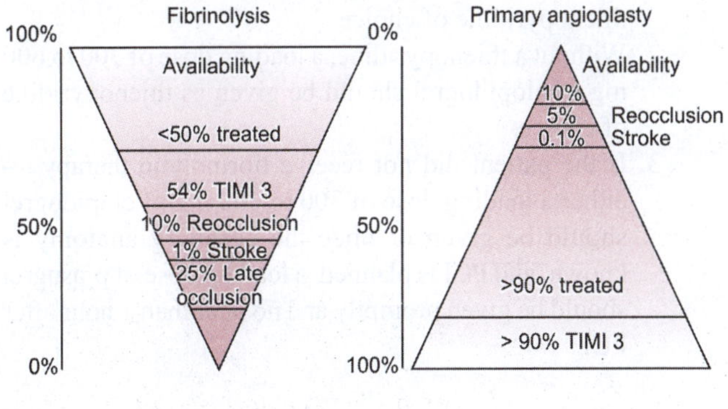

98. Anticoagulants—heparin:

Adjunctive anticoagulation: The activity of thrombolytic agents can be potentiated by the concurrent administration of heparin for its anticoagulant effect and aspirin for antiplatelet effect. Without heparin, ongoing coagulation may outpace thrombolysis and result in a lower patency rates.

Heparin is indicated in the following 4 conditions in acute myocardial infarction

1. In patients undergoing reperfusion therapy with thrombolytic agents either with nonselective fibrinolytic agent (streptokinase, urokinase, acylated streptokinase activator complex (APSAC) or clot specific recombinant tissue plasminogen activator, rt-PA, alteplase or reteplase).
   Routine intravenous heparin within 6 hours to patients receiving thrombolytic therapy followed by subcutaneous heparin helps in prevention of reocclusion.
2. Patients undergoing primary PTCA or surgical revascularization. When primary PTCA is performed, high dose heparin IV is recommended.
3. In patients who are at high risk for systemic emboli in large or anterior MI, atrial fibrillation, previous embolus, LV thrombus, arrhythmias, heart failure (Killip's class III or IV), cardiogenic shock, and continuous pain.
   Full dose of heparin IV or high dose SC is administered to prolong the activated partial thromboplastin time to 2 to 2.5 times the normal in patients with large anterior or apical infarction (CK more than 700 μ/L). This is an attempt to reduce the incidence of venous thromboemboli and left ventricular mural thrombi with peripheral arterial embolization. These patients should receive therapy with warfarin for 3 to 4 months to prolong prothrombin time to approximately 1.5 times the control.
   Warfarin can be discontinued if there is no persistent left ventricular dysfunction, particularly if atrial fibrillation is not present.
4. Subcutaneous heparin 7500 IU bd (IV heparin is an acceptable alternative) in all patients not treated with thrombolytic therapy who do not have contraindication to heparin. (Heparin is used as an alternative to thrombolytic agent in patients who could not afford. It is a poor man's thrombolytic agent.)
   Heparin is given for 10 to 14 days with and/or thrombolytic therapy.
   80 IU/kg as bolus followed by 18 IU/kg/hr
   10 to 15000 IU/day—5000 IU bd or tds.
   Heparin dose is adjusted to keep APTT between 60 sec and 80 sec, (with a control of 40 sec).

Heparin exerts an anticoagulent action by inhibiting a number of activated clotting factors including factors IX, X, XI, XII and II (thrombin)

Heparin is available in 5,000 IU in 5 mL and 25,000 IU in 5 mL vials.

Low molecular weight heparin (parnaparin) is available in:

0.3 mL subcutaneous prefilled-syringes (3,200 IU)
0.4 mL subcutaneous prefilled-syringes (4,250 IU)
0.6 mL subcutaneous prefilled-syringes (6,400 IU)
1.2 mL subcutaneous prefilled-syringes (12,800 IU)

Heparin antidose—Protamine zinc sulfate × should always be kept ready.

Oral anticoagulants for 3 to 4 months are to be given after heparin therapy, e.g. acenocoumerol, 1mg and 4 mg tablets are available.

99. Monitoring of Heparin.

1. Obtain an aPTT (activated partial thromboplastin time) 6 hours after initial therapy is started or any dosage change occurs and every 6 hours thereafter until a therapeutic level of 1.5 to 2.5 times control is obtained on two consecutive aPTTs.
2. Obtain an aPTT every 24 hours, once a therapeutic range is achieved.
3. Obtain an immediate aPTT if the patient's clinical condition changes significantly (e.g. recurrent definite ischemia, bleeding, hypotension).
4. Obtain an immediate hemoglobin/hematocrit and platelet count if any of the following occur:
   Clinically significant bleeding
   Recurrent symptoms
   Hemodynamic instability
   A drop in platelets necessitates close monitoring for heparin-induced thrombocytopenia.
   Obtain hemoglobin/hematocrit and platelet values daily for the first 3 days of heparin therapy.

100. Anticoagulants can be classified into 4 groups:

Fast acting

1. Heparin (including lower molecular weight heparin).

Slow acting

2. Coumarin derivatives—dicoumarol
3. Warfarin sodium.
4. Indanedione derivatives—phenindione and anisindione.
   Low molecular weight heparins are increasingly used now in place of heparin with satisfactory results.

101. Antiplatelet Drugs (drugs modifying platelet function) (See Chapter E Coronary artery disease 140 to 148).

1. Aspirin has been recommended for coadministration with thrombolytic therapy since the second International Study of Infarct Survival (ISIS-2), which showed benefit for aspirin when administered alone, as well as concurrently with streptokinase.
   Aspirin, 160–325 mg/day should be given on day 1 of acute MI and continued indefinitely on a daily basis thereafter. It is better given with antacids; it acts by inhibiting the production of thromboxane A2.
   Comparison of aspirin, streptokinase, aspirin + streptokinase was done in a survey.
   Aspirin alone showed—22% reduction in mortality
   Streptokinase alone showed—25% reduction in mortality.
   Aspirin + STK combinedly showed 45% reduction in mortality.
   So, aspirin is the most important and is the drug of choice.
   Other antiplatelet agents may be substituted if true aspirin allergy is present. Aspirin and ticlopidine combination complement each other.
   Aspirin is contraindicated in those who are hypersensitivity to salicylates and should be used with caution in patients with active ulcer disease.
   Aspirin suppositories (325 mg) can be used safely and are recommended root of administration for patients with severe nausea and vomiting or known upper gastrointestinal disorders.
   There is no current evidence that other antiplatelet agents such as dipyridamole, ticlopidine, or sulfinpyrazone have any advantage over aspirin for mortality reduction after MI.
2. Tablet clopidogrel 75 mg od/bd.
3. Ticlopidine 250 mg/day
4. Synthetic glycoprotein IIb/IIIa antagonist, e.g. integretin, tirofiban, lamifiban seem promising (dazoxiben and monoclonal antibody 7E3 are under evaluation).

102. Recommendation for the use of thienopyridines:

For STEMI patient undergoing non-primary PCI, the following regimes are recommended:

1. If the patient has received fibrinolytic therapy—and has been given clopidogrel, it should be continued as thienopyridine of choice.
2. Without a thienopyridine, a loading dose of 300 to 600 mg of clopidogrel should be given as thienopyridine of choice.
3. If the patient did not receive fibrinolytic therapy — either a loading dose of 300 to 600 mg of clopidogrel should be given or once the coronary anatomy is known, and PCI is planned, a loading dose of prasugrel should be given promptly and no later than 1 hour after PCI.

4. Prasugrel should be given as soon as possible for primary PCI.

The optimal loading dose of clopidogrel has not been established. Clopidogrel is a prodrug which must undergo hepatic conversion to its active metabolite for platelet inhibition, a process taking several hours. Clopidogrel at least 300 to 600 mg should be given as early as possible before or at the time of primary or nonprimary PCI .

103. Glycoprotein IIb-IIIa (See Chapter Fig. E-8)

The final common pathway of platelet aggregation is the GPIIb-IIIa receptor. Abciximab (ReoPro) blocks the final common pathway for platelet aggregation thus preventing thrombus formation. Abciximab—ReoPro—has been proven safe and effective in acute coronary syndrome patients undergoing percutaneous coronary intervention (PCI) including those with AMI and unstable angina (UA).

It is indicated in AMI patients undergoing percutaneous coronary intervention which include:

1. PTCA
2. Atherectomy
3. Stent placement and in
4. Unstable angina not responding to conventional medical therapy when PCI is planned within 24 hours.

This showed improved protection against ischemic cardiac complications compared to stenting alone.

Clinical trials (EPIC study, EPICLOG, EPISTEN, CAPTURE Trials) has only been studied with concomitant use of heparin and aspirin.

It is given as IV bolus + infusion

IV Bolus 0.25 mg/kg 18–24 hours before PCI followed by IV Infusion of 0.125 µg/kg/min (maximum of 10 µg/min) concluding 1 hour after PCI.

Anticoagulation is initiated with heparin to a target activated partial thromboplastin time (APTT) of 60–85 sec.

Oral aspirin 325 mg od.

The final common pathway to platelet aggregate is the crosslinking of platelet glycoprotein (GP) IIb-IIIa receptors by adhesive proteins fibrinogen and Willibrand's factor from the plasma. Climatric monoclonal antibody—abciximab (ReoPro) and cyclic peptide-eptifibatide (integrilin) are known GBIIa-IIIb receptor inhibitors (others, tirofiban, lamifiban). Both have been shown to reduce the incidence of ischemic episodes in patients undergoing angioplasty who have been at risk for abrupt closure.

Thrombolytic drugs lyse the existing clots but do not prevent the formation of new thrombi.

Antiplatelet drugs inhibit platelet aggregation in response to a limited set of agonists.

Anticoagulant drugs inhibit synthesis/function of clotting factors.

Standard antithrombotic management of patients with acute ischemic coronary syndrome and those undergoing coronary angioplasty includes anticoagulation with heparin and platelet inhibition with aspirin. Both heparin and aspirin prevent intravascular thrombosis, but they have also been associated with bleeding complications. Moreover, heparin does not inhibit platelet aggregation, a key event in coronary thrombosis leading to myocardial ischemia, whereas aspirin effect is mild and is limited to a single pathway. The discovery that the final common pathway of platelet aggregation involves activation and crosslinking of the platelet glycoprotein (GP) IIb-IIIa receptor has prompted the development of inhibitors of this receptor as a novel and potentially more effective class of antithrombotic agent.

Eptifibatide (integrilin) is a cyclic heptapeptide inhibitor of GPIIb-IIIa with an active pharmacophore, that is derived from the structure of barbourine, a GPIIb-IIIa inhibitor from the venom of the southeastern pigmy rattlesnake.

104. GPIIb-IIIa receptor is a member of the integrin family of receptors that is found in the membrane of platelets. When platelets are activated by a variety of stimuli including thrombin, collagen, EP, ADB, GPIIb/IIIa receptors changes confirmation to be receptive to one end of a fibrinogen dimer occupancy of a GPIIb/IIIa receptor by the other end of the dimer provides the basis for platelet aggregation. Thus, the GPIIb-IIIA is set to be final common pathway of platelet aggregation (Ref. Fig. E-8).

Following agents are available for clinical practice.

1. Abciximab (ReoPro) is a chimeric Fab fragment of a monoclonal antibody to the GPIIb/IIIa receptor.
2. Eptifibatide is a cyclical heptapeptide which binds the receptor with a short half-life.
3. Tirofiban is a small nonpeptide which binds the receptor with a short half-life.
4. Lamifiban.

Several clinical trials have documented nearly 50% reduction in death, MI, or urgent total vascular resistant (TVR) (RAPPORT—ReoPro and Primary PTCA Organization and Randomized trial) after primary PCI with or without stenting in patients of STEMI. Tirofiban may be equivalent abciximab in terms of infarct size and bleeding events. They increase the patency rates.

105. There are 4 other methods that can be tried to reduce the infarct size (These are not practised routinely—rarely used):

1. Dissolving atherosclerotic block by LASER therapy.
2. Intra-aortic balloon counter pulsations: It enhances the supply and reduces oxygen demand. Increases the coronary blood flow. Useful in cases of pump failure —cardiogenic shock.
3. Glucose-Insulin-Potassium therapy (GIK): It increases the anaerobic glycolysis by ischemic cells and reduces the concentration of fatty acids. Heart attack patients who receive a simple, inexpensive IV infusion of glucose, insulin and potassium are less likely to die in the hospital than those who do not receive the infusion (99, Nov 18th issue of Circulation journal, AHA). It is originally proposed by Sodi-Pallares in 1962, was recently evaluated in a pilot trial by the Estudios Cardiologicos LatinoAmerica (ELCA) collaborative group in South America. It is a metabolic modulation by increasing anaerobic glycolysis by ischemic cells and reduces the concentration of fatty acids in this recently reported study of 407 patients admitted within 24 hours of onset of symptoms of suspected MI regardless of age or ECG findings were randomly given GIK.
   High dose GIK:
   25% of glucose + 50 IU of soluble insulin + 80 mmol/L KCl at a rate of 1.5 mL × kg × 1 hour for 24 hours or
   Low dose infusion:
   10% glucose + 20 IU of soluble insulin + 50 mmol/L KCl at a rate of 1 mL × kg × 1 hour for 24 hours.
   A significant reduction in the composite end point of death, nonfatal severe heart failure (Killips Class 2) and nonfatal ventricular fibrillation (VF) was observed for the overall study population as well as the 252 (62%) who also treated with reperfusion strategies. This later group also showed statistically significant reduction in mortality rate. It is simple and inexpensive therapy.
4. Hyaluronidase to reduce the myocardial ischemic injury.

106. Protection of ischemic myocardium and limitation of extension of infarction is done by 4 means:

1. Oxygen: Every patient of myocardial infarction should receive oxygen because the oxygen uptake is less in myocardial infarction. It helps to limit the infarct size.
2. Nitroglycerin:
   Nitroglycerin 5 mg per mL—(5 mL and 10 mL ampoules)—IV.
   Glyceryl trinitrate—0.5 mg tablets.
   Isosorbide dinitrate—5 mg, 10 mg tablets.
   Start with small doses and increase the dosage.
   Reasonably begin nitroglycerin for any patient with chest pain lasting more than 15 minutes when it is thought to be due to acute myocardial infarction.
   Intravenous nitroglycerin is started with a dose of 5 to 10 μg/min and increase the dose depending on the response of blood pressure and heart rate with an average dose of 5 to 10 μg/min not to exceed 20 μg/min. Systolic pressure should not fall below 100 to 110 mm Hg. Heart rate should not increase by more than 10 beats per minute.
   Reduction in infarct size is noticed in inferior infarction and non-Q infarction.
   It can be given for 24–48 hours followed by sublingual or transdermal route.
   Continue with sublingual glyceryl trinitrate 0.5 mg or isosorbide dinitrate 5 mg 8th hourly and increase to 6th hourly and 4th hourly.
   Headache is controlled with mild analgesics.
   Sinus tachycardia and hypotension should be avoided by careful titration of the dose as both have potential for increasing the infarct size.
   Though potential benefit is not guaranteed, its low risk when the dose is carefully adjusted gives the drug a favorable 'risk-benefit ratio'.
3. β-blockers to reduce the infarct size.
   Can be given before 6 hours, i.e. before the appearance of Q waves.
   (Do not give calcium channel blockers in acute MI)
4. Injection xylocaine is given for arrhythmias as a prophylactic and curative.

107. Nitrates in acute myocardial infarction was believed to be contraindicated until the early 1970s. Today, with the exception of hypotensive patients, virtually all patients with acute ischemic syndrome will receive at least one sublingual nitroglycerin tablet before admission to the hospital.

Nitrates in acute myocardial infarction acts in the following 4 ways.

These effects of nitroglycerin produce reduction in the myocardial oxygen consumption or demand and thus a more favorable supply-demand ratio.

1. Control of pain by intravenous nitroglycerin in the early phase of evolving myocardial infarction is the result of reduction of myocardial oxygen demand. In the early hours of infarction nitroglycerin is relatively ineffective in relieving pain because ischemic pain sufficient to produce necrosis requires analgesic such as morphine whereas anginal pain occurring after few hours after the onset of infarction usually responds to nitroglycerin. If pain is severe and persistent intravenous nitroglycerin is preferred.
2. Nitroglycerin has the dilatory effect on the vascular smooth muscle in vessels throughout the body. Thus vasodilation of the coronary arteries themselves

(especially at or adjacent to sites of recent plaque disruption), the peripheral arteries and venous capacitance vessels are particularly beneficial to the patient with acute MI.

Nitrates dilate the coronary arteries including the capacitance vessels as well as collateral vessels. Therefore, it is likely to increase the blood flow into the ischemic area and reduce the infarct size. Reduction of predicted extent of infarct size is seen well in inferior and non-Q infarction. Relaxing effect on collateral vessels particularly coronary collaterals contribute to the beneficial effect in angina pectoris.

3. Intravenous nitroglycerin given within 10 hours of chest pain reduces the chance of congestive heart failure, infarct extension and cardiac death. It is the drug of choice for afterload reduction during the formation of myocardial infarction and in cardiac failure.
4. Nitrates have profound venodilating effect. They dilate the pulmonary vasculature and results in lowering of pulmonary vascular resistance. It lowers the preload, irrespective of pain or no pain nitrates reduce preload, help in remodelling of myocardium.

108. Intravenous nitroglycerin is indicated in the following 4 conditions:

1. For the first 24 to 48 hours in patients with acute myocardial infarction:
   a. With or without congestive cardiac failure.
   b. Large anterior infarction.
   c. Persistent ischemia and
   d. Hypertension.

   Continued use beyond 48 hours in patients with recurrent angina or persistent pulmonary congestion with large or complicated infarction.

   It is not effective or may be harmful in AMI patients with SBP < 90 mm Hg or severe bradycardia <50 beats/min or tachycardia.
2. Angina pectoris, including unstable angina, post-infarction angina in patients who have not responded to recommended doses of orgal nitrates and\or β-blockers.
3. Control of blood pressure in perioperative hypertension, especially hypertension associated with cardiovascular procedures such as hypertension seen during intra-tracheal intubation, anesthesia, skin incision, sternotomy, cardiac bypass and in the immediate postoperative period.
4. Production of controlled hypotension during surgical procedures and in certain cases of eclampsia.

   IV Nitroglycerin 5 mL and 10 mL ampoules are available. Each mL contains 5 mg of nitroglycerin.

109. Nitroglycerin is basically a vascular smooth muscle relaxant. It dilates both arterial and venous bed. However, it has preferential effect on postcapillary vessels including large veins. It decreases venous return to the heart leading to the reduction of left ventricular end diastolic volume (preload). Arterial relaxation leads to reduction in systemic vascular resistance and arterial pressure (afterload).

Thus, intravenous nitroglycerin therapy reduces:

1. Elevated central venous pressure.
2. Pulmonary capillary wedge pressure.
3. Pulmonary vascular resistance (preload).
4. Systemic vascular resistance (afterload).

110. Following are 4 advantages when intravenous nitroglycerin is given early in the course of acute MI:

1. Reduces mortality to 10–30% by reducing infarct size.
2. Decreases susceptibility of ventricular fibrillation both during ischemia and reperfusion.
3. Suppresses ongoing myocardial ischemic pain.
4. Beneficial when acute MI is complicated by congestive heart failure or pulmonary edema.

111. Nitroglycerin (NTG) is started with a pump-controlled infusion of 5–10 micrograms per minute and increased by 5–10 micrograms per minute every 5–10 minutes, while carefully monitoring hemodynamic and clinical response.

The titration end points are:

1. Control of clinical symptoms.
2. Decrease in mean arterial pressure of 10% in normotensive patients and of 30% in hypertensive patients but never a systolic pressure <90 mm Hg.
3. Increase in heart rate >10 beats per minute but not usually more than 110 beats per minute.
4. Decrease in pulmonary artery end-diastolic pressure of 10% to 30%.

Although there is no absolute upper dosage limit, doses more than 20 micrograms per minute are associated with an increased risk of hypotension and alternative therapy should be considered.

There is no fixed optimum dose of intravenous nitroglycerin and the dosage should be individualized on the basis of continuous monitoring of blood pressure, heart rate and pulmonary capillary wedge pressure. Adequate systemic blood pressure and the coronary perfusion pressure must be maintained. Once a partial blood pressure response is observed, the dose increase should be reduced and the interval between the increments should be lengthened.

112. It is reasonable to treat the patient with AMI without hypotension, bradycardia and excessive tachycardia with intravenous nitroglycerin.

The 4 precautions to be observed while administering the nitrates are:

1. BP and heart rate should be carefully watched. As long as hypotension is not present administration of nitrates may lessen the pain. Carefully observe the improvement in symptoms and change in hemodynamics.
2. If initial dose is well-tolerated, continue the nitrates by careful monitoring of the vital signs. Long-acting nitrates should be avoided in early stage of myocardial infarction. Intravenous nitroglycerin may be beneficial in prolonged period of waxing and waning chest pain, and in controlling symptoms of ischemia.
3. Should be used cautiously in inferior wall infarction because even small doses may produce fall in BP and bradycardia, a life-threatening complication which can easily be reversed by atropine if it is recognized early.
4. Should be used with extreme caution in right ventricular infarction since these patients are sensitive to venodilating effects of the drug, with sudden fall in BP resulting from inadequate right ventricular filling.

However, inadvertent systemic hypotension causing worsening of myocardial ischemia is the most serious potential complication of nitroglycerin therapy therefore above precautious are to be taken care while giving nitroglycerin.

Patients with right ventricular infarction are especially depending on adequate right ventricular preload to maintain cardiac output and can experience profound hypotension during administration of nitrates.

113. Contraindications of nitroglycerin.

1. Known hypersensitivity to nitroglycerin or other organic nitrates.
2. In acute myocardial infarction patients with systolic pressure less than 90 mm Hg or severe bradycardia of less than 50 bpm. It could produce severe hypotension or shock.
3. Increased intracranial pressure (e.g. head injury or cerebral hemorrhage).
4. Inadequate cerebral circulation, constrictive pericarditis and cardiac tamponade.

114. β-blockers are useful in acute myocardial infarction for the following 4 reasons:

1. To limit the infarct size by reducing the oxygen demand of myocardium.
2. To reduce the intensity of chest pain by anxiety thereby reducing the requirement of analgesics.
3. To lower the frequency of supraventricular arrhythmias but they do not prevent ventricular fibrillation.
4. To lower mortality and morbidity.

The reduction in mortality is probably due to a reduction in the incidence of rupture of the softened area of the infarct. Presumably this is due to its negative inotropic effect reducing the power of contractility of the myocardium.

β-blockers are beneficial if given by IV within 6 hours of chest pain in myocardial infarction to limit the infarct size especially in patients with increased sympathetic tone (either tachycardia or systemic hypertension). IV propranolol or metaprolol is given followed by oral preparation.

β-blockers are associated with greater prevalence of adverse effects particularly hypotension and bradyarrhythmias than nitroglycerin. Risk-benefit ratio is not favorable as that of nitroglycerin.

115. β-blockers in acute myocardial infarction are indicated in the following 4 conditions:

1. Patients without a contraindication to β-blocker therapy who can be treated within 12 hours of onset of infarction, irrespective of administration of concomitant thrombolytic therapy.
2. In patients with continuing pain with enzyme elevation with non-Q wave MI, thought to represent recurrent injury. It is safe and effective in relieving anxiety, pain and myocardial ischemia. It reduces the incidence of reinfarction following Q wave infarction with or without preceding thrombolytic therapy.
3. Patients with supraventricular tachyarrhythmias such as atrial fibrillation with a rapid ventricular response. It is recommended to reduce the increased heart rate whether it is associated with anxiety or supraventricular tachycardia.
4. Patients including those receiving thrombolytic therapy with reflex tachycardia or systolic hypertension or both without signs of congestive heart failure.

Patients with moderate or severe left ventricular failure or other contraindications with β-blocker therapy may be harmful. In general, there should be no left ventricular dysfunction.

116. The 4 β-blockers with membrane stabilizing activity (MSA) without intrinsic sympathetic activity (ISA) should only be used in myocardial infarction.

1. Propranolol
2. Atenolol
3. Metoprolol
4. Esmolol

(Atenolol, Metoprolol, Esmolol: Cardioselective)

ISA is now referred as partial agonistic activity (PAA).

β-blocker Heart Attack Trial (BHAT) has shown 20 – 25% reduction in post-MI incidence (second attack).

117. The following 4 β-blockers with intrinsic sympathetic activity (ISA) should not be used in acute MI. They reduce cardiac output and increase mortality.

1. Alprenolol
2. Oxprenolol
3. Acebutolol
4. Pindolol.

118. The 4 commonly used β-blockers and their doses are:

Table F-8

Agent	Intravenous	Oral
1. Propranolol	0.33 mg/kg over 2 minutes, 3 doses	20–80 mg q 6 h
2. Atenolol	5 mg over 5 minutes 2 doses	50 mg q 12 h for 48 hours then 100 mg daily
3. Metoprolol	5 mg over 2 minutes 3 doses 2 mg bolus every 5 min BP normal	50 mg q 6 h for 48 hours then 100 mg bid
4. Esmolol	500 mcg/kg over 1 minute then 50–250 mcg/kg/min infusion	

119. β-blockers in Q wave myocardial infarction have following 4 uses:

1. They are effective in relieving anxiety, pain in myocardial ischemia and reduces the incidence of reinfarction with or without preceding thrombolytic therapy. It is especially useful when myocardial infarction is associated with hypertension.
2. They reduce the incidence of PVBs, atrial fibrillation and nonfatal cardiac arrest.
3. They reduce the frequency of progression of threatened infarction to complete infarction.
4. They reduce recurrent ischemia and infarction during first 6 weeks after initial event.

120. β-blockers are contraindicated in myocardial infarction in the presence of:

1. Heart block of second or third degree.
2. Bradycardias below 50 bpm.
3. Systolic blood pressure below 90 mm Hg.
4. Pulmonary artery wedge pressure greater than 24 mm Hg.
5. Rales extending more than one-third of the way up the lung fields.
6. Bronchial asthma.
7. Moderate to severe chronic obstructive lung disease.
8. Cardiac failure.

In case, if the patient on β-blocker whose heart rate is maintained between 50–75 bpm and systolic blood pressure is above 90–100 mm Hg starts presenting with or developing severe pulmonary edema, suspect the β-blocker is aggravating or precipitating cardiac failure. Then administer intravenous non β-receptor dependent agonist, such as milrinone or increase the dose of dobutamine if the patient is already receiving, to overcome the β-blockade.

121. Monitoring β-blockers:

1. Monitor heart rate (target heart rate for β-blockade is 50 to 60 beats per minute).
2. Monitor blood pressure.
3. Monitor for congestive cardiac failure.
4. Monitor for bronchospasm.

Utilize continuous ECG monitoring.

122. Patients on β-blockers have less heart attacks compared to control groups due to the following 4 factors:

1. Less stress.
2. Less heart rate.
3. Less CPK-MB.
4. (Less) Heart size is not increased.

123. Angiotensin-converting enzyme inhibitors are indicated in:

1. Patients within the first 24 hours of a suspected acute MI with ST-segment elevation in two or more anterior precordial leads or with clinical heart failure in the absence of significant hypotension or known contraindications for ACE inhibitors.
2. Patients with MI and LV ejection fraction less than 40%.
3. Patients with clinical heart failure on the basis of systolic pump dysfunction during and after convalescence from acute MI.
4. All other patients within the first 24 hours of a suspected AMI provided there is no significant hypotension or renal failure or other clear contraindications are absent even without heart failure. Hence, started orally within the first 24 hours.

In patients with asymptomatic left ventricular dysfunction after myocardial infarction, long-term administration of ACE inhibitors is associated with an improvement in reduced mortality and morbidity.

124. Calcium channel blockers:

1. Nifedipine (short acting) calcium blocker is generally contraindicated in routine treatment of AMI because of its negative inotropic effects and the reflex sympathetic activation, tachycardia, and hypotension associated with its use.
2. Diltiazem and verapamil are contraindicated in AMI and associated LV dysfunction or CHF. They are indicated in the management of supraventricular

tachyarrhythmias, cocaine induced MI, or relief of postinfarction angina unresponsive to β-blockers. Amlodipine is an effective antianginal and may be safe to use in patient with MI with CHF.

3. Diltiazem may be given to patients in whom β-blockers are ineffective or contraindicated for relief of ongoing ischemia or control of a rapid ventricular response with AF after AMI in the absence of CHF, LV dysfunction or AV block.
4. In non-ST elevation MI, diltiazem may be given to patients without LV dysfunction, pulmonary congestion or CHF. It may be added to standard therapy after the first 24 hours.

Calcium channel blockers have not been shown to reduce mortality in patients with AMI and in certain persons with cardiovascular disease. They appear to be harmful. So, use of calcium channel blockers in the acute setting has come into question, with some randomized controlled trials and retrospective studies showing increased adverse effects.

125. Magnesium:

Magnesium ion has several cardiovascular effects. It has myocardial protective action by 4 effects:

1. It is a coronary vasodilator.
2. It is a systemic vasodilator.
3. It is antiarrhythmic.
4. It inhibits platelet function.

Magnesium sulfate is given as needed to replete magnesium deficits for 24 hours. It is viewed as a calcium antagonist.

126. The magnesium effect is independent of thrombolytic therapy in myocardial infarction. The 4 beneficial effects of intravenous magnesium in acute MI are:

1. It reduces coronary care unit deaths and causes of death.
2. It reduces congestive cardiac failure in coronary care unit.
3. It reduces ventricular arrhythmias.
4. It probably preserves myocardium by its myocardial protective action.

8 mmol in 4 mL injected over 5 min with 65 mmol infused over the next 24 hours. It is beneficial when used before 6 to 8 hours of starting pain of myocardial infarction. More confirmatory data about magnesium is awaited.

127. Magnesium is indicated in:

1. In correction of documented magnesium (and/or potassium) deficits, especially in patients receiving diuretics before the onset of infarction.
2. Episodes of 'torsades de pointes' type ventricular tachycardia associated with a prolonged QT interval should be treated with 1 or 2 g magnesium as IV bolus over 5 minutes.
3. Magnesium IV bolus in high-risk patients such as elderly.
4. In those patients for whom reperfusion therapy is not suitable.

128. The 4 indications of IV xylocaine in acute myocardial infarction are:

1. Benign PVBs as a prophylactic to prevent dangerous arrhythmias. Benign PVBs more than 6 per minute or and occurring in short bursts of three or more in succession.
2. Malignant PVBs.
3. Ventricular tachycardia
4. Ventricular fibrillation

(2–4: both in association with defibrillation and cardiopulmonary resuscitation as indicated.)

Antiarrhythmic drugs are not given routinely as a preventive measure unless arrhythmias are present.

129. Inotropic agents: In general, these agents should be avoided in AMI because:

1. They tend to increase myocardial oxygen demand.
2. Risk of tachycardia.
3. Risk of arrhythmias.

Given when

4. IABP counter pulsations proves inefficient, IV inotropic support may be given, but its use should be guided by means of pulmonary arterial catheter monitoring wherever possible.

130. The following 4 drugs are continued to prevent further extension of infarction.

1. Sublingual nitrate 5–10 mg 6th hourly. It is supposed to limit the infarct size.
2. Aspirin 300 mg OD to prevent platelet agglutination. Aspirin and ticlopidine complement each other
3. Clopidogrel 75 mg OD/BD.
4. Heparin Inj SC following thrombolytic therapy or depending on Killip's classification of 'pump failure' followed by oral anticoagulants.

131. The 4 points to consider the strategy for the treatment of acute myocardial infarction are:

There is no standard strategy but a reasonable plan is to be maneuvered.

1. Whenever acute myocardial infarction is diagnosed, immediately give:
   Oxygen
   Narcotics
   Intravenous nitroglycerin
   Intravenous β-blockers (see the discussion).
2. Thrombolytic therapy with streptokinase or urokinase or rt-PA or reteplase. Transfer the patient after he is

stabilized to a place where facilities are available for coronary arteriography. If the patient is pain free coronary arteriogram is performed within 3 to 7 days and decision is to be taken for coronary angioplasty or bypass graft.

If the pain occurs soon after thrombolytic therapy (rt-PA) coronary arteriogram is performed without delay and if necessary coronary angioplasty is done or decision is made for bypass graft.

3. If the patient is admitted within 1 hour of myocardial infarction where the facilities are available, coronary arteriography is performed within the first hour of onset of chest pain and a decision can be made regarding angioplasty with or without stent or bypass graft.
4. When the patient with stable or unstable angina is in the hospital waiting for bypass surgery develops infarction it may be possible to do bypass graft.

132. Myocardial infarction usually means infarction of left ventricle but it can occur in right ventricle also.

The following 4 points should be considered in the treatment of severe right ventricular myocardial infarction:

1. Hemodynamic monitoring—IV fluids.
2. Inotropic agents—dopamine, dobutamine.
3. Establishing normal rhythm—atropine.
4. Temporary pacing for AV block.

The 'bradycardia-hypotension syndrome' is the most frequent correctable cause that frequently occurs in inferior infarction and right ventricular infarction. Parasympathetic overactivity results in bradycardia and hypotension. Frequent occurrence of bradycardia in inferior infarction suggests that the receptors may be in the inferoposterior left ventricular wall. Reperfusion of the right coronary artery commonly produces bradycardia and hypotension. Establish the normal rhythm by atropine which reverses the bradycardia which in turn raises the blood pressure. If hypotension still persists, central venous blood volume should be raised by elevating the legs and fluid administration.

Hypotension is corrected by administering the colloidal solution. Hemodynamic monitoring is done by volume expansion and the fluids are continued until hypotension is corrected or the capillary wedge pressure reaches 15 to 20 mm Hg.

Inotropic agent: Dopamine is needed when hypotension persists. It may increase the cardiac index and right ventricular ejection fraction.

AV block is a common complication of right ventricular infarction and usually needs temporary pacing. AV sequential pacing may be needed in patients with AV block or AV junctional rhythm because a synchronous right atrial contraction may improve right sided forward flow and help to maintain systemic circulation.

134. Atrial infarction is related to extensive ventricular myocardial infarction. It is suspected when:

1. Atrial arrhythmia develops in a patient with large ventricular myocardial infarction.
2. Changes in morphology of sinus P wave but it is also nonspecific.
3. Elevation of PR segment in the left chest leads with reciprocal depression in right chest leads in the presence of atrial arrhythmia.

or

4. Elevation of PR segment in L I with reciprocal depression in L III.

135. Increased concentration of circulating free fatty acids in the first 24 hours of acute myocardial infarction are associated with the following 4 bad effects:

1. Cardiac arrhythmias.
2. Increased myocardial oxygen consumption.
3. Decreased contractility.
4. Increase in infarct size.

136. The following 4 dietic principles in acute myocardial infarction should be observed to prevent further rise in free fatty acids by the following measures.

1. Avoid fasting—adequate diet should be given.
2. Avoid diet rich in cholesterol and fat. Saturated fats and prolonged fasting further increases the circulating free fatty acids.
3. Prophylactic restriction of salt: Development of cardiac failure leads to retention of sodium and water.
4. Take diet rich in carbohydrates. Caution is taken in diabetic patients.

137. Criteria for good risk in acute myocardial infarction.

when there is ***no***

1. Previous myocardial infarction.
2. Intractable pain.
3. Extreme or persistent shock.
4. Arrhythmias.
5. Gallop rhythm
6. Congestive heart failure
7. Significant enlargement of the heart
8. Diabetic acidosis or other predisposing factors.

COMPLICATIONS OF MYOCARDIAL INFARCTION

138. The 4 immediate complications of myocardial infarction are:

1. Arrhythmias: PVBs, VT, VF, sinus tachycardia, AF, heart block, etc.
2. Heart failure
3. Cardiogenic shock
4. Death.

139. The 4 complications after a short period of myocardial infarction where medical management is indicated:

1. Embolism
   a. Pulmonary b. Cerebral
   c. Peripheral d. Visceral
2. Pericarditis
3. Congestive cardiac failure
4. Post-MI angina.

140. The 4 complications after a short period of myocardial infarction where surgery is indicated:

1. Post MI cardiac aneurysm.
2. Post MI ventricular septal defect.
3. Post MI mitral regurgitation.
4. Post MI free wall rupture (hemopericardium).

Allowing small ventricular septal defect to heal by medical management had shown higher mortality in the long run, than immediate surgical treatment.

141. Free wall rupture is very dangerous. Electro-mechanical dissociation occurs. Immediate death can occur if the surgery is not attempted. It is common:

1. After cardiogenic shock
2. In females
3. In elderly
4. Surprisingly, common with small areas of infarction than with extensive infarctions.

142. The 4 late complications of myocardial infarction are

1. Postmyocardial injury syndrome (also known as Dressler's syndrome).
2. Periarthritis of shoulder (shoulder hand syndrome).
3. Mental changes.
4. Addiction to narcotic drugs.

143. The 4 different percentages of patients dying with acute myocardial infarction are:

1. 25% of deaths within the first few minutes to hours before reaching the hospital.
2. 10–15% of deaths in the hospital.
3. 40% of deaths within the first month.
4. 10% of deaths during the first year after hospitalization.

More deaths occur within the first 2 hours. Therefore, efforts must be made to minimize mortality in this very short crucial period.

The age adjusted mortality is three and half times normal even after 10 years.

The percentage of deaths in the hospital or after hospitalization varies widely depending on the facilities and expertise available.

144. The 4 major causes of death immediately after acute myocardial infarction are:

1. Ventricular fibrillation → electrical irritability.
2. Cardiogenic shock → power failure.
3. Acute left ventricular failure→pump failure.
4. Rupture of the infarcted area.

145. Ventricular arrhythmias are common in acute myocardial infarction. Ventricular extrasystoles or premature ventricular beats are due to increased excitability of the heart. It is presumed that PVBs appearing in hours or days after AMI are indicative of impending life threatening ventricular fibrillation. However, it is now realised that ventricular fibrillation occurs as often in patients with sinus rhythm as in those with PVBs. Prevention of ventricular fibrillation is extremely important because 1/4th of deaths are due to ventricular fibrillation. If there are malignant PVBs, ventricular tachycardia, the following 4 medications are tried:

1. Inj xylocaine: One should start immediately IV lidocaine (xylocaine, xylocard or lidocard)
   Intravenous xylocaine 50–100 mg IV bolus followed by 50 cc of xylocaine in 5% glucose (bottle of 540 cc) at the rate of 15 drops per minute, i.e. 2 mg/min. Maximum dose is 4 mg/min continued for 2–3 days depending on PVBs.
   If there is no response—IV β-blocker.
2. Inj proctolol 5 mg IV slowly to a maximum of 25 mg or mexiletine or atenolol 5–10 mg or sotalol 10 mg.
   If there is no response or ventricular fibrillation develops.
3. DC shock is tried without cardiac massage or artificial ventilator.
   If there is no response,
4. Cardiac resuscitation is tried.

146. If PVBs are persistent after 72–96 hours even after Injection xylocaine IV drip, chronic antiarrhythmic therapy should be started with any of the following 4 drugs singly or in combination:

1. Procainamide hydrochloride—0.5–2 g IV followed by 250–500 mg po 6th hourly up to 1500 mg 3 hourly.
   Risk of systemic lupus erythematosus like syndrome which is reversible by withdrawing the drug is there.
2. Mexiletine—200 to 250 mg 8th hourly. It may supersede procainamide as it has fewer side effects. Ataxia can be a troublesome complication.
3. Disopyramide—100–300 mg 6th hrly po.
   Great care should be taken in left ventricular failure as it has a negative inotropic effect.
   It has weak atropine like effect which may cause retention of urine or precipitate glaucoma.
4. Quinidine—200–600 mg 6th hrly po.
   It is a myocardial depressant and should be avoided in poor left ventricular function.
   Causes abdominal discomfort and diarrhea.

Prevention of ventricular fibrillation is extremely important because 1/4th of deaths are due to ventricular fibrillation.

147. The 4 situations where ventricular fibrillation (VF) in acute myocardial infarction result as a response to

1. Acute myocardial infarction
   - Primary ventricular fibrillation as a primary response to myocardial infarction
   - survival rate is good.
2. Congestive cardiac failure
   Pump failure after MI
3. Cardiogenic shock
   Power failure after MI
4. Ventricular aneurysm after MI.

(2–4: Secondary cause following after myocardial infarction. Prognosis is not good.)

148. The 4 factors which contribute to the causation of ventricular fibrillation in AMI are:

1. Ischemia increases the membrane permeability to potassium causing rapid depletion of potassium from the ischemic musculature. Elevated extracellular potassium concentration increases the irritability of the myocardium.
2. Ischemia of the muscle causes an "Injury current" (seen as ST elevation in ECG). The Ischemic muscle is unable to repolarize following depolarization. Continuous state of depolarization maintains a difference of electrical potential between normal and injured muscle. This potential difference causes another focus of excitation.
3. Excessive release of catecholamines increase the irritability of the cardiac muscle and thereby predisposes to fibrillation.
4. Myocardial infarction itself can cause the ventricle to dilate excessively thereby increasing the pathway of conduction. It frequently causes abnormal conduction pathway around the infarcted area itself. Both of these predispose to circus movement.

Any prolongation of the conduction pathway allows an impulse to reenter the muscle that is already recovering from refractoriness thereby initiating another cycle of excitation and the process continues. Thus the ventricular contraction continues here and there in bundles of muscle fibers. This has two disadvantages. One is that the co-ordinated relaxation necessary for filling does not take place, secondly, the co-ordinated contraction essential for emptying also does not occur.

149. The 4 situations where circus movement in the ventricles initiating ventricular fibrillation is greatly increased:

1. When the ventricles are dilated.
2. When the rapidly conducting Purkinje system is blocked.
3. When ectopic foci are present—irritability is the usual cause. Infarct area is the irritable focus.
4. Electric shock.

150. There are 4 ECG findings in ventricular fibrillation that depend on the time after which it is taken:

ECG is extremely bizarre and show rhythm of any type. (See chapter- D- Cardiac arrhythmias - Fig. D-35, 36, 37) and (See chapter Q-ECG-Fig. Q-126-128)

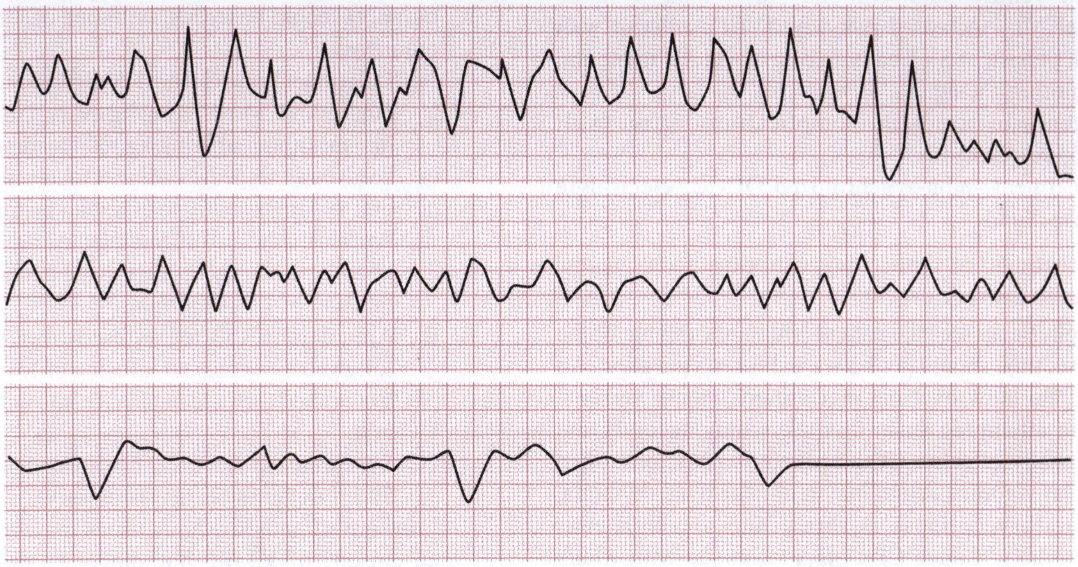

Fig. F-8: Ventricular fibrillation: Ventricular complexes are rapid, bizarre, irregular. Voltage is becoming low terminating with asystole. This tracing is from a patient dying of a myocardial infarct.

1. In the early stages the voltage of the fibrillary waves are usually about 0.5 mV since relatively large masses of muscle fibers contract simultaneously and this causes strong though irregular voltage in the ECG.
2. After about 20 seconds—the voltage may be only 0.2 to 0.3 mV. Large contractions of ventricles disappear and ECG changes to new pattern of low voltage 0.2–0.3 mV and very irregular waves.
3. Minute voltage of 0.1 mV or less may be recorded for 10 minutes or longer after ventricular fibrillation begins.
4. This is followed by a cardiac stand still.

151. The following 4 points are to be noted when the diagnosis of ventricular fibrillation is doubtful:

1. It is important to remember that ventricular fibrillation has a 'vector'.
2. ECG during ventricular fibrillation may appear to record ventricular asystole depending on the ECG lead and amplitude of the fibrillary wave.
3. The diagnosis of 'asystole' should always be confirmed in at least two ECG leads.
4. If the distinction between fine ventricular fibrillation and asystole is in doubt, delivery of a countershock to the unconscious patient will be appreciated.

152. Ventricular fibrillation is classified into four types depending on cause and timing.

1. Primary ventricular fibrillation—sudden event with no warning—10% of STEMI before thrombolytics. It is much less now.
2. Secondary ventricular fibrillation—occurring in setting of heart failure or shock.
3. Late ventricular fibrillation—more than 48 hours after MI—increased risk with IVCD, anterior wall MI, persistent SVT early in course and RV infarction requiring pacing.
4. Occurs in structural complications—(free wall rupture), ischemia.

   Treatment—non-synchronized DCCU, electrolyte correction.

153. The treatment of ventricular tachycardia/ventricular fibrillation is very urgent.

If the physician sees the patient within one minute of the collapse, time should not be wasted for oxygenation. An immediate blow over the precordium "thump version" may be attempted since this takes only seconds and occasionally effective. If the patient is conscious when first seen vigorous cough may terminate dysarrhythmia. (Circulatory collapse is rarely due to ventricular tachycardia.) "Cough CPR" is a technique with which a conscious patient can maintain cardiac output for brief intervals despite ventricular fibrillation. Repetitive coughing increases intrathoracic pressure stimulating the changes induced by conventional cardiac massage by chest compression.

Defibrillation of the ventricles is to be done if the facilities are available.

If a very strong electrical current is passed through the ventricles for a short interval of time, it can stop fibrillation by throwing all the ventricular muscle into refractoriness at the time. All the impulses stop and the heart remains silent for 3 to 5 seconds after which it starts beating again with SA node or often any other etopic foci becoming the pacemaker.

Occasionally the same irritable focus which originally caused ventricular fibrillation repeats immediately.

1. VF should be treated with an unsynchronized electric shock with an initial energy of 200 J: if unsuccessful, a second shock of 200 to 300 J should be given, and if still no response, a third shock of 360 J.
2. Sustained (more than 30 seconds or causing hemodynamic collapse) polymorphic ventricular tachycardia (VT) should be treated with an unsynchronized electric shock using an initial energy of 200 J; if no response, a second shock of 200 to 300 J should be given and if still no response, a third shock of 360 J.
3. Synchronized electric shock of 100 J initial energy is given for episodes of sustained monomorphic VT associated with angina, pulmonary edema or hypotension (blood pressure < 90 mm Hg). Increased energies may be used if not initially successful.
4. Sustained monomorphic VT not associated with angina, pulmonary edema or hypotension (BP < 90 mm mg) should be treated with one of the following regimens:
   i. Lidocaine: bolus 1.0 to 1.5 mg/kg. Supplemental boluses of 0.5 to 0.75 mg/kg every 5 to 10 minutes to a maximum of 3 mg/kg total loading dose may be given as needed. Loading is followed by infusion of 2 to 4 mg/min (30 to 50 µg/kg per minute).
   ii. Procainamide 20 to 30 mg/minute loading infusion, up to 12 to 17 mg/kg. This may be followed by an infusion of 1 to 4 mg/min.
   iii. Amiodarone 150 mg infused over 10 minutes followed by a constant infusion of 1.0 mg/min for 6 hours and then a maintenance infusion of 0.5 mg/min.
   iv. Synchronized electrical cardioversion starting at 50 J (brief anesthesia is necessary).

   Infusions of antiarrhythmic drugs may be used after an episode of VT/VF but should be doscontinued after 6 to 24 hours and the need for further arrhythima management assessed.

Electrolyte and acid-base disturbances should be corrected to prevent recurrent episodes of VF when an initial episode of ventricular fibrillation has been treated.

Prompt correction of acidosis increases the success of defibrillation. Soda bicarbonate IV initial dose of 1 mg/kg. Repeated once within 5–10 minutes.

Drug-refractory polymorphic VT should be managed by aggressive attempts to reduce myocardial ischemia, including therapies such as β-blockade, intra-aortic balloon pumping, and emergency PTCA/CABG. Amiodarone, 150 mg infused over 10 minutes followed by a constant infusion of 1.0 mg/min for up to 6 hours and then a maintenance infusion of 0.5 mg/min may also be helpful.

Prophylactic antiarrhythmic therapy when using thrombolytic agents are also advised.

154. Accelerated idioventricular rhythm (AIVR) may occur in 1/4th of the patients with acute myocardial infarction.

1. It is defined as a ventricular rhythm with a rate of 60–125 beats/min. Frequently called as "slow ventricular tachycardia".
2. Seen up to 20 % of patients with AMI.
3. Occurs during first 2 days.
4. Probably results from enhanced automaticity of the Purkinje fibers.
5. Often obscured shortly after successful reperfusion .
6. Frequent in inferoposterior infarction which is usually associated with sinus bradycardia.
7. It usually looks like sinus rhythm which precedes and follows it with very minor hemodynamic effects and it is difficult to detect by other means than cardiac monitoring.
8. May be benign or may go into fatal ventricular tachycardia or ventricular fibrillation.

155. Sinus bradycardia—

1. Common arrhythmias occurring during the early phases of AMI.
2. Frequent in patients with inferior and posterior MI.
3. Isolated sinus bradycardia is accompanied by hypertension or ventricular ectopy, should be observed rather than treated initially.
4. Atropine should be utilized if hypertension accompanies with any degree of sinus bradycardia.

156. Intraventricular blocks—

1°AV block

1. Occurs in <15 % of patients of AMI admitted in ICU, generally does not require treatment.
2. 2°AV block Mobitz type II or Wenckebach.
   - usually transient and does not present more than 72 hours after MI.
   - rarely progress to complete AV block.
3. Do not appear to effect survival caused by ischemia of the AV node
4. Does not require specific therapy.

157. The following 4 points should be considered in the treatment of sinus tachycardia after myocardial infarction:

1. It can be due to pain, fear or anxiety.
2. If the sinus tachycardia is due to increased catecholamines, β-blockers reduce the heart rate and oxygen requirement of the heart and help to preserve ischemic myocardium around the infarct.
3. If the sinus tachycardia is due to compensatory sympathetic drive to maintain the threatened cardiac output, β-blockers cause the heart to beat less hard due to its negative inotropic effect and may precipitate cardiac failure. Therefore, giving a β-blocker in this situation is potentially dangerous.
4. Because of the two opposite results of β-blockers the sinus tachycardia is probably best treated with an opiate or sedative like diazepam.

158. The following 4 points should be observed in the treatment of sinus bradycardia after acute myocardial infarction. It is the most common bradyarrhythmia. More common in inferior infarction. Whether it is a predisposing factor of ventricular fibrillation or not is controversial. It should be treated when it is associated with hypotension, cardiac failure or PVBs.

1. Sinus bradycardia will be seen within 1 hour after myocardial infarction (mostly noticed in MCCU) and is more consistently associated with PVBs than occurring in the later course of the disease.
2. Elevation of the legs or rising the foot end of the bed frequently helps.
3. Atropine injection 0.3–0.6 mg IV if the pulse rate is below 60 per minute, which may be repeated if necessary after 15 minutes, up to 2 mg total in divided doses.
4. Persistent bradycardia of less than 40 per minute even after atropine should be treated by pacing especially when it is causing hypotension or cardiac failure. Isoproterenol is better avoided.

159. AV blocks and intraventricular blocks—

1. 1st and 2nd degree AV block – Mobitz type II.
2. Rare conduction defect after AMI.
3. Often progress suddenly to complete AV block.

4. Treated with a temporary external or transvenous demand pacemaker.

160. Atropine is indicated in the following conditions of AMI:

By its parasympatholytic (anticholinergic) activity, it reduces the vagal tone, enhances the rate of discharge of the SA node and facilitates AV conduction. It may be given as an adjuvant to morphine when nausea and vomiting occurs.

Atropine is very much useful during the early hours of AMI particularly in treating sinus bradycardia associated with reduced cardiac output and signs of peripheral hypoperfusion including arterial hypotension, confusion, faintness or frequent PVBs.

In this setting, leg elevation, IV atropine may be life-saving.

1. Sinus bradycardia greater than 40 bpm with or without evidence of low cardiac output and peripheral hypoperfusion or frequent premature ventricular ectopics at onset of symptoms of AMI.
2. Acute inferior infarction with second degree type I, or third degree atrioventricular block associated with symptoms of hypotension, ischemic discomfort or ventricular arrhythmias with new wide QRS complex presumed due to acute MI.
3. Asymptomatic patients with inferior infarction and second degree type I, or third degree heart block.
4. Symptomatic patients with inferior infarction and second degree type I, or third degree heart block at the level of AV node with QRS complexes or with known existing BBB.
5. Ventricular asystole.
6. Sustained bradycardia and hypotension after administration of nitroglycerin.
7. For nausea and vomiting associated with (before or after) administration of morphine in the presence of sinus bradycardia.
8. Second or third-degree heart AV block of uncertain mechanism when pacing is not available.

161. The 4 common supraventricular arrhythmias that occur in acute myocardial infarction are:

1. Junctional rhythms and nodal tachycardias
2. Atrial tachycardia
3. Atrial flutter
4. Atrial fibrillation.

162. Atrial fibrillation after acute myocardial infarction: It occurs in about 10–15% of infarcts especially in the elderly. It indicates a large infarct and hence a relatively poor prognosis.

The treatment consists of:

1. Electrical cardioversion for patients with severe hemodynamic compromise or intractable ischemia.
2. Rapid digitalization to slow a rapid ventricular response and improve LV function.
3. Intravenous β-blockers to slow a rapid ventricular response in patients without clinical LV dysfunction, asthma or any bronchospastic disease or AV block.
4. Heparin should be given.

   When β-blockers are contraindicated or ineffective, either diltiazem or verapamil IV given to slow a rapid ventricular response.

163. Complication with heart block is commoner but less of a threat in inferior infarction. Therefore, it is reasonable to observe a patient well without complications. First and second degree blocks can be safely observed.

Electrical pacing in heart block is beneficial in acute inferoposterior infarcts when complicated with the following 4 conditions.

1. Heart failure
2. Low BP
3. Marked bradycardia
4. Significant ventricular ectopics.

164. The relationship between the site of myocardial infarction and complete heart block.

1. Complete heart block is more frequent with inferior infarction than with anterior infarction
2. In about 85% of persons, SA node and AV node receive their blood supply from the branches of right coronary artery which also supplies the inferior surface of the heart. So, the block is associated with sinus bradycardia.
3. Very large infarcts extending backwards into the interventricular septum to involve the conducting tissue may also cause complete heart block and they carry a poor prognosis due to their large size.
4. Large anterior infarct is a threat to stroke volume and carry poor prognosis. An adequate heart rate and cardiac output in the presence of complete heart block can be achieved only by pacing. Even first or second degree block and bundle branch block may be a harbinger of complete heart block in anterior infarction. Therefore, some authorities advise prophylactic pacing for anterior infarction complicated by first or second degree heart block or sinus rhythm with left anterior hemiblock and right bundle branch block.

   Complete heart block though commoner with inferior infarction, it is a less threat. Therefore, it is reasonable to observe and pacing should be done if there is hypotension or pulmonary edema.

165. Intraventricular blocks—

Isolated fascicular blocks.

1. LAFB
2. LPFB
3. RBBB
4. Bifasicular block.

Temporary Pacing

166. Placement of transcutaenous patches and active (demand) transcutaneous pacing is indicated in:

1. Sinus bradycardia (rate less than 50 bpm) with symptoms of hypotension (systolic pressure less than 80 mm Hg) unresponsive to drug therapy.
2. Mobitz type II second-degree AV block.
3. Third-degree heart block.
4. Bilateral BBB (alternating BBB, or RBBB and alternating left anterior fascicular block (LAFB), left posterior fascicular block (LPFB) (irrespective of time of onset).
5. Newly acquired or age indeterminate LBBB, LBBB and LAFBa, RBBBB, and LAFBa.
6. RBBB or LBBB and first-degree AV block.
7. Newly acquired or age-indeterminate RBBB.
8. Newly acquired or age-indeterminate first-degree AV block.

167. Indications for temporary transvenous pacing in acute myocardial infarction:

In patients with acute MI and symptomatic sinus bradycardia with atrioventricular block should receive atropine. Temporary pacing should be performed in patients with:

1. Symptomatic sinus bradycardia not responding to atropine.
2. Mobitz type II second degree A-V block.
3. Third degree (complete heart block) with a heart rate below 50 or with hemodynamic disturbance.
4. All cases of anterior wall infarction with complete heart block.
5. Sick sinus syndrome (SSS).
6. Stokes-Adams syndrome.
7. Bilateral bundle branch block (BBBB).
8. Newly acquired BBB.
9. Left bundle branch block in conjunction with first degree atrioventricular block.
10. Right bundle branch block in conjunction with first degree atrioventricular block.
11. Right bundle branch block with left anterior or posterior hemiblock, i.e. bifascicular block.
12. Asystole.

168. Permanent pacing after acute myocardial infarction is indicated in

1. Persistent second-degree AV block in the His-Purkinje system with bilateral BBB or complete heart block after acute MI.
2. Transient advanced (second-or third-degree) AV block and associated BBB.
3. Symptomatic AV block at any level.
4. Persistent advanced (second- or third-degree) block at the AV node level.

169. The degree of left ventricular dysfunction can be crudely assessed from the following 4 physical findings:

1. Tachycardia
2. Third heart sound—S3
3. Crackles at the lung bases
4. Elevated venous pressure.

X-ray chest, ECG, Echo findings supplement this.

170. The treatment of heart failure following acute myocardial infarction is same as heart failure secondary to other heart diseases with the following 4 exceptions:

1. Digoxin should not be used in heart failure after myocardial infarction. It does not improve the function of the infarcted tissue. Digoxin should be restricted to treat patients with atrial flutter or fibrillation or to treat patients with heart failure that persisted after appropriate therapy.
2. Diuretics are very effective in heart failure after myocardial infarction. They reduce the left ventricular filling pressure. Improvement in orthopnea, paroxysmal nocturnal dyspnea is seen.
3. Vasodilators (Nitrates): They lower the afterload, improve the left ventricular function and increase pulmonary venous pressure. They are indicated only to treat patients with adequate arterial pressure.
4. Newer drugs:

   Amrinone (noncatecholamine non-glycoside group) increases cardiac output, decreases peripheral vascular resistance.

   Captopril, enalapril, lisinopril, ramipril (ACE inhibitors) are also showing good prospects by decreasing the preload and afterload by reducing the peripheral vascular resistance. ACEI should not be given to patients with cardiogenic shock.

   Acute circulatory failure in AMI usually reflects extensive myocardial damage and indicates a bad prognosis.

171. Killip classified acute myocardial infarction with "pump failure" into 4 groups:

Class I: No signs of pulmonary or venous congestion, i.e. No rales over the lungs, S3 is not heard.

Class II: Moderate heart failure as evidenced by rales over 50% or less over the lung fields, S3 gallop, tachypnea, or signs of right heart failure including venous and hepatic congestion.

Class III: Severe heart failure, pulmonary edema—rales over more than 50% of lung fields.

Class IV: Shock, i.e. cardiogenic shock—'power failure', Systolic pressure of 90 mm Hg and evidence of peripheral vasoconstriction, diaphoresis, peripheral cyanosis, mental confusion, oliguria, etc.

172. The mortality rate is divided into 4 groups by Killip classification in myocardial infarction with pump failure.

Table F-9

Class I	0–5% mortality
Class II	10–20% mortality
Class III	35–45% mortality
Class IV	85–90% mortality

173. The need of anticoagulant therapy is described according to 4 classes of Killip in AMI. One should see for contraindications if any:

1. Class I: No pulmonary or venous congestion—There is no need for anticoagulants.
2. Class II: Moderate heart failure is present as evidenced by pulmonary rales, S3, etc. One should use anticoagulants if CHF persists for more than 3 to 4 days.
3. Class III: Severe heart failure is present, chances of venous thromboembolism are more—so great risk of pulmonary embolism. Anticoagulants are indicated prophylactically.
4. Class IV: Cardiogenic shock—Same as class-III anticoagulants are advised prophylactically.
   Heparin injection—7,500 IU SC 8th hourly for 2–3 days followed by 5,000 IU SC every 8–12 hour. It is given for 10–14 days. Later it should be followed by oral anticoagulants.

174. 30 day mortality based on Killip hemodynamic calcification:

Table F-10

Killip class	Characteristics	Patients (%)	Mortality rate (%)
I	No evidence of CHF	85	5.1
II	Rales, JVP↑, or S_3	13	13.6
III	Pulmonary edema	1	32.2
IV	Cardiogenic shock	1	57.8

CHF, congestive heart failure, JVP jugular venous pulsation, S3 third heart sound.

Results from an international trial 41,021 patients GUSTO-1 investigations. *Circulation* 1995;91:1659-1668.

175. Mortality rate is classified by forrester on the basis of pulmonary capillary wedge pressure (PCWP) and cardiac index.

There are 4 hemodynamic subsets:

Table F-11

Subset	PCWP	Cardiac index	Mortality rate
I	<18	>2.2	3
II	>18	>2.2	9
III	<18	<2.2	23
IV	>18	<2.2	51

Subset II represents congestive heart failure (CHF) without shock. Subset III patients may be hypovolemic and therefore respond to fluid replacement. Subset IV correlates to true cardiogenic shock and mortality is high >50%—however, this data is largely complied from the era before reperfusion.

176. Relative hypovolemia in acute myocardial infarction is due to one of the following 4 reasons:

1. It is very often due to reduction in ventricular contractility and compliance.
   It may be secondary to:
2. Previous use of diuretics.
3. Less fluid intake in the early stages of infarction.
4. Vomiting associated with pain or drugs.

Fluids are given until the left ventricular filling pressure rises to 18–20 mm Hg. Central venous pressure reflects the right ventricular pressure than left ventricular and is not reliable in this situation because left ventricular function is more adversely affected than right ventricular function.

177. The diuretics (mainly furosemide) can effect badly in 4 ways if it is not used cautiously in heart failure following myocardial infarction:

1. It reduces plasma volume.
2. It reduces cardiac output.
3. It reduces systemic blood pressure.
4. It reduces coronary perfusion.

178. The 4 criteria to be followed in defining the cardiogenic shock—power failure where 85–90% mortality can occur.

(Hypotension alone is not the basis of shock syndrome.)

1. Systolic pressure less than 90 mm Hg which declines by at least 30 mm Hg than previous normal BP.
2. Clinical signs of peripheral circulatory failure such as feeble and thready pulse, cold and moist skin, cyanosis, etc.
3. Oliguria—less than 20 cc per hour.
4. Failure of improvement following sedation and oxygen.

179. Causes of cardiogenic shock:

1. Extensive left ventricular infarction.
2. Extensive right ventricular infarction.
3. Ventricular septal rupture.
4. Acute severe mitral regurgitation/papillary muscle rupture.
5. Cardiac tamponade with or without free wall rupture.

Other conditions:

6. Aortic dissection.
7. Myocarditis.
8. Massive pulmonary embolism.
9. Critical valvular stenosis.
10. Acute mitral regurgitation.
11. Acute aortic regurgitation.
12. Over dosage of calcium channel blockers or β-blockers.

180. 40% of left ventricular infarction is affected in patients with cardiogenic shock (autopsy studies have shown) usually have triple vessel disease (TVD) and commonly have involvement of left anterior descending artery.

181. 40% of patients have prior MI. If the pervious MI was large, even a small acute MI may cause shock.

182. Hemodynamic effects medication used to manage heart failure.

Table F-12

Medication	*Preload* ↓	*After-load* ↓	*Contractility*	*Vasoconstriction*
1. Dopamine				
a. Medial dose	–	–	++	–
b. High dose	–	–	++	++
2. Dobutamine	+	++	+++	–
3. Milrinone	++	++	+++	–
4. Nitroglycerin	+++	+	–	–

-No effect; + little effect, ++ moderate effect, +++ great effect

183. The 4 other causes of hypotension are:

1. Vasovagal reaction
2. Arrhythmias
3. Drug reaction—morphine can cause hypotension
4. Hypovolemia—misuse of diuretics.

184. Low BP in AMI can occur by vasovagal reaction.

1. Vasovagal reaction
↓
2. Vasodilatation
↓
3. Profuse sweating
↓
4. Fall in BP.

This condition does not show S3 gallop or pulmonary rales. No hesitation in giving IV fluids in the absence of S3 gallop and pulmonary edema. 1 liter of normal saline (500 mL fast followed by 500 mL in 1 hour) is a simple treatment. If no improvement is seen with IV fluids then think of cardiogenic shock.

185. The 4 other complications that arise if the cardiogenic shock is persistent.

1. Life-threatening arrhythmias
2. Extension of the infarct
3. Pulmonary edema
4. Renal failure.

Cardiogenic Shock

Cardiogenic shock in AMI impairs myocardial function which causes reduction in arterial pressure and coronary blood flow which further decreases left ventricular function. Aim of the treatment is to increase the cardiac outflow.

If cardiogenic shock is not caused by a reparable lesion, or if the lesion is not repaired in efficient or effective manner, the mortality rate is ≥ 80%. Therefore, cardiogenic shock should be approached with diagnostic and therapeutic vigor in an attempt to identify a treatable lesion and to intervene in a definitive manner. Patients presenting with hypoperfusion but adequate blood pressure may be considered to be in near shock and should be approached in the same manner to prevent the progression to frank shock and death.

186. Clinical features—

1. Signs of hypoperfusion, oliguria, cold, clammy skin, especially hands and feet.
2. SBP < 90 mm Hg
3. LVEDP-(PCWP) ≥ 18 mm Hg
4. Cardiac index ≤ 18 L/m/m^2 (CO/BSA)

187. Cardiogenic shock in acute myocardial infarction is treated by the following 4 methods.

1. All patients with shock in myocardial infarction should receive 100% oxygen.
2. Vasopressors—Dopamine or Dobutamine IV drip to rise the BP for maintaining coronary blood flow.
   Dopamine IV infusion 2–5 µg/kg/min to start with, increased every 2–5 min up to a maximum of 20–50 µg/kg/min.
   Dobutamine IV infusion can be given instead of dopamine safely. 3 to 10 µg/kg/min IVI. It is a synthetic catecholamine with positive inotropic action and minimal peripheral vasoconstrictor effect. It is arrhythmogenic. (Dobutamine IV drip is given once a week for 24 hours in some cases of cardiomyopathy with good results).

Norepinephrine may be used as second-line therapy in desperate conditions.

Portable infusion pump sets are available.

Vasopressors act by reconditioning and resetting of β-receptors.

Use of phosphodiesterase such as milrinone is problematic because of their arrhythmogenicity and tendency to increase myocardial oxygen demand, because of their combined vasodilating and inotropic actions.

3. IV fluids to a level that brings left ventricular filling pressure to an optimum of 18–20 mm Hg.

   Patients with hypotension accompanied by a pulmonary capillary wedge pressure (PCWP) less than 15 mm Hg should be given rapid infusion of normal saline boluses, as in patients with inferior infarction who have concomitant right ventricular infarction.

   After replenishing IV volume and the PCWP is greater than 15 mm Hg, dopamine is indicated at doses up to 20 mcg/min if hypotension or signs of heart failure persist.
4. Intra-aortic balloon counter pulsations to improve the blood flow.

188. Intra-aortic balloon pump (IABP) in the treatment of cardiogenic shock.

IABP counter pulsations helps in the treatment of cardiogenic shock because

1. It increases the systolic blood pressure.
2. It decreases afterload.
3. It decreases oxygen requirement.
4. It increases diastolic coronary flow.

IABP is contraindicated in marked aortic regurgitation because it may worsen the regurgitation and cause rapid hemodynamic deterioration.

189. Investigations.

1. Biochemical changes: Lactic acidosis, raised creatinine levels and arterial hypoxemia are common.
2. X-ray chest shows pulmonary edema.
3. ECG in cardiogenic shock shows extensive abnormalities consistent with massive infarction, severe diffuse ischemia or evidence of large previous MI.

   Extensive ST depressions are also common.

   Rare abnormalities in the presence of shock suggest mechanical complications like free wall rupture, ventricular septal rupture (VSR), dynamic LVOT obstruction, very rarely aortic dissection.
4. Echo determines the extent of myocardial necrosis and the complications that contribute to the cardiogenic shock.

190. Diagnostic testing: Cardiac catheterization with an arterial line and pulmonary artery catheter helps in every minute to minute care. Hemodynamic changes help to identify—

1. Right ventricular infarction,
2. Free wall rupture,
3. Acute papillary muscle rupture (acute MR), and
4. Ventricular septal rupture, etc.

   which contribute to the cause of shock.

191. In patients with cardiogenic shock, a relative or absolute reduction in left ventricular filling pressure as the cause of hypotension must be excluded. This can occur in the following 4 conditions:

1. Prior diuretic therapy or acute interspace volume shifts, it is estimated that 10–15% of patients with acute myocardial infarction may be significantly volume depleted.
2. Right ventricular infarction
3. Pericardial tamponade
4. Certain instances of pulmonary embolization of acute heart failure.

Unless there are signs of left heart volume overload (e.g. S3 gallop, moist pulmonary rales, vascular or pulmonary congestion on chest radiograph), normal saline should be administered intravenously at a reasonably fast rate (≥ 500 mL bolus, followed by 500 mL/hr). Jugular venous pressure is not a consistently reliable indicator of left heart filling pressure and thus the elevation of jugular pressure does not obviate the need for intravenous fluids in a number of clinical situations (e.g. pericardial tamponade, right ventricular myocardial infarction).

192. In patients with acute myocardial infarction of inferior wall with shock, right ventricular infarction should be suspected, resulting in right ventricular failure and inadequate filling of the left heart system. Right sided precordial leads in addition to the standard leads should be taken in these patients. An injury pattern is often but not uniformly observed in V3R, V4R in patients with right ventricular infarction. The diagnosis of right ventricular infarction frequently can be made on the basis of clinical findings such as an increase in jugular venous pressure during inspiration. An echocardiogram or the insertion of a pulmonary artery balloon catheter, or both are helpful in patients in whom the diagnosis is unclear. Right sided cardiac pressure recordings generally show mean right atrial and right ventricular filling pressures equating or exceeding pulmonary artery occlusive (wedge) pressure with normal or low pulmonary artery pressure.

Echocardiogram can be used to establish or confirm the
1. Presence of right heart involvement
2. Assess tricuspid valve competence
3. Evaluate the extent of left heart damage and left ventricular function
4. Exclude pericardial tamponade which can have a similar presentation

193. Fluid volume administration is a major component of therapy for patients with right ventricular infarction to maintain the elevated right sided filling pressure necessary to maintain cardiac output. Fluid administration initially may be guided by the following 4 clinical variables.

1. Systemic blood pressure
2. Peripheral perfusion
3. Urinary output
4. Ventricular gallop sounds.

If facilities are available, hemodynamic monitoring by a pulmonary artery catheter is generally advised to optimize fluid volume administration. Failure of intravenous fluids to achieve clinical and hemodynamic improvement and stabilization in these patients requires additional therapeutic approaches (e.g. dobutamine, intra-aortic balloon counter pulsations or interventional procedures). The use of diuretics or vasodilators in patients with right ventricular infarction can result in severe hypotension.

Occasionally, vasodilator agents and diuretic drugs produce hypotension with AMI and pulmonary edema because the translocation of fluid into the lung reduces intravascular volume.

Severe hypotension, (systolic blood pressure ≤ 70 mm Hg) or clinical shock or both occurring in the presence of volume overload or persisting after bolus IV saline should be approached with moderate (4 to 5 μg/kg/min), then if necessary, increasing doses of dopamine.

If hypotension, clinical shock or near shock persists at dopamine doses of ≥ 15 μg/kg per minute, institution of intra-aortic balloon counter pulsation should be considered. If intra-aortic balloon counter pulsation is not available, nor-epinephrine can be added to increase systemic blood pressure to acceptable levels (SBP ≥ 80 mm Hg) and the patient transferred on an emergency basis to a more comprehensive medical facility.

Patients with volume overload (or after adequate volume loading) in near shock or with a lesser degree of systemic hypotension often respond favorably to dobutamine (2 to 3 μg/kg per minute initially) or low to moderate doses of dopamine (2 to5 μg/kg/minute initially).

194. Pharmacodynamics, dosage and administration of dobutamine.

1. It is an analog of dopamine. It is a β-adrenergic stimulating agent. It is a sympathomimetic amine which has a strong stimulating effect on cardiac β-1 receptors and a weak effect on β-2 receptors.
2. It does not directly release norepinephrine as does dopamine nor it effects dopamine receptors.
3. Major character is that it exerts a potent inotropic effect with only limited undesirable side effects on heart rate and blood pressure. The inotropic effect of dobutamine results from direct stimulation of cardiac β-1 receptors, unlike the effect of dopamine which is based on endogenous noradrenaline release.
4. Useful as an inotropic agent in heart failure to increase cardiac output while reducing ventricular filling pressures as an intravenous infusion 2.5 to 4.0 mcg/min, usually 2.5 to 10 mcg/min, the dosage should be adjusted at according to the patient's
   a. Heart rate b. Rhythm
   c. Blood pressure d. Diuresis

   Dobutamine is available in 5 mL ampoules each mL contains 50 mg. The dosage is determined as follows:

Table F-13

250 mg dobutamine in 1000 mL infusion	
Dose mcg/kg/min	Infusion rate mL/kg/min
2.5	0.01
5	0.02
7.5	0.03
10	0.04
12.5	0.05
15	0.06

The infusion rate values corresponding to each dosage are multiplied by the patient's weight. This gives the infusion rate as mL/min. Partial tolerance may develop if infusion time exceeds 72 hours, and such cases may call for an increase.

For infusion, the dobutamine is diluted in normal saline or 5% dextrose. Dobutamine should not be diluted in alkaline solutions.

Concomitant administration of dobutamine and sodium nitroprusside increases cardiac output and usually produces pulmonary capillary wedge pressure more than either of these drugs alone. Dobutamine may prove ineffective in patients recently treated with β-blockers.

195. Dobutamine is indicated in the following 4 conditions:

1. Cardiogenic shock after severe AMI, after cardiac surgery.
2. Refractory heart failure

3. Excess β-blockade
4. Perioperative spasm of internal thoracic artery

Dobutamine is contraindicated in obstructive cardiomyopathy, known hypersensitivity to dobutamine and in the presence of tachycardia. Dopamine should not be used in the presence of tachycardia because the patient may go into life-threatening tachyarrhythmias. Always prevent tachycardias while treating AMI.

196. During treatment of cardiogenic shock, attention should be focused on the following 4:

1. Status of the patient's intravascular volume
2. Condition of the patient's ventricular function
3. The presence of myocardial injury/infarction with or without cardiac failure
4. Whether correctable, mechanical lesion are present?

Status of intravascular volume: Best means of assessing and monitoring intravascular volume is by hemodynamic measurements through the pulmonary artery catheter. The optimal left ventricular diastolic filling pressure, as estimated by the pulmonary artery occlusive (wedge) pressure (or pulmonary artery diastolic pressure when comparable) for most patients with shock or near shock secondary to AMI resides between 14–18 mm Hg.

Status of patient's ventricular function: Two-dimensional echocardiogram is helpful. Segmental hypokinesia or akinesia suggests the presence of occlusive coronary artery disease. Similar findings may be seen in acute myocarditis, or idiopathic dilated cardiomyopathy. Global left ventricular enlargement and dysfunction generally indicates a more diffuse or chronic process.

Existence of myocardial injury/infarction with or without heart failure: Emergency cardiac catheterization is advised. Reperfusion by thrombolytic therapy, angioplasty has reduced mortality from 85% to 60% in those patients with shock not responding to fluid administration. The effect of thrombolytic therapy on mortality under these conditions is unclear.

Are correctable, mechanical lesions present? Two-dimensional echocardiogram is helpful in this situation.

197. The most commonly encountered potentially reversible defects in the clinical setting of cardiogenic shock which can be diagnosed by two-dimensional echocardiogram are:

1. Pericardial tamponade
2. Massive pulmonary embolism
3. Rupture of chordae tendinae, papillary muscle
4. Rupture of ventricular septum
5. Critical valvular stenosis or acute valvular regurgitation
6. Aortic dissection with complicating lesions (e.g. acute coronary occlusion, acute aortic valvular regurgitation)
7. Acute destruction or incompetence of a prosthetic heart valve
8. Cardiac tumors.

198. Summary of therapeutic management of cardiogenic shock or near shock.

1. Oxygen therapy
2. In the absence of obvious intravascular volume overload, brisk intravenous administration of fluid volume
3. In the presence of intravascular volume overload or adequate intravenous fluid therapy, intravenous administration of cardiovascular support drugs (e.g. dopamine, dobutamine, norepinephrine) to attain and maintain stable clinical hemodynamic status.
4. Urgent coronary angioplasty with or without stent or revascularization (CABG) for acute myocardial injury/infarction, if the facilities are readily available.

199. Summary of the management of 4 important complications that are to be attended in AMI.

1. Tachyarrhythmias
   PVBs, ventricular tachycardia, ventricular fibrillation, ventricular asystole, atrial fibrillation.
   In ventricular tachycardia, inj xylocaine bolus IV 100 mg is to be given followed by drip 15 drops/min—i.e. 2 mg/min (maximum dose 4 mg/min).
   If no response is found and causes hemodynamic disturbance—300–400 joules DC shock is to be given.
   In ventricular fibrillation—DC shock is to be given.
   Atrial fibrillation and flutter—Digoxin or quinidine is to be given.
   If no response—DC shock may be given.
   Paroxysmal atrial tachycardia (PAT)—IV verapamil or adenosine is to be given.
   If PVBs persistent after 3 or 4 days—give oral antiarrhythmic drugs like procainamide 250 mg 6th hourly is to be given depending on the condition.
2. Bradyarrhythmias
   Atropine IV 0.4–0.6 mg is to be given.
   If rate remains below 60/min, additional dose of 0.2 mg up to a total of 2.0 mg in divided doses is to be given.
   If less than 40 beats per minute persist in spite of atropine—may be treated with electrical pacing.
   Isoproterenol should be avoided if possible in this condition.
3. Cardiac failure.
   Furosemide 40 to 120 mg is to be given daily to reduce preload inj deriphylline or aminophylline IV.
   Digoxin should be used with caution
   Oxygen
   Antibiotics are to be given.
4. Cardiogenic shock or 'Power failure'

Start inj dopamine 200 mg IVI in 540 cc of 5% dextrose—8–10 drops/min are to be given.
Dobutamine IVI is more desirable since it has less effect on heart rate and systemic vascular resistance.
Oxygen is to be given to increase myocardial oxygen perfusion and to reduce the infarct size.

200. The 4 sequel of myocardial infarction are:

1. *Cardiac failure:*
   i. Low output failure. Overall pumping of the left ventricle is decreased. The ischemia of peripheral tissue and further damage of myocardium leads to gradual failure and death.
   ii. Congestive cardiac failure: The blood gets dammed in the venous system. The renal shut down in the acute attack of infarction increases the congestion resulting in congestive cardiac failure.
2. *Rupture of the heart:* Infarcted area does not contract during systole and on the other hand, it bulges outward due to raise in pressure. Repeated stretch leads to thinning and aneurysmal dilatation which ultimately may rupture causing hemorrhage and death.
3. *Pump failure:* It causes back pressure resulting in pulmonary edema. The pulmonary edema leads to respiratory failure and death unless treated promptly.
4. *Ventricular fibrillation:* It is the common cause of death immediately following myocardial infarction. More likely to occur at 2 stages.
   1. Within 10 minutes of infarction.
   2. About 5–6 hours after infarction to several days—next dangerous period.

201. Pathophysiology of heart failure due to dilatation in AMI differs from heart failure due to hypertrophy.

Table F-14

Dilatation due to MI	*Hypertrophy*
1. Full thickness in AMI is followed by thinning and stretching of the infarcted segment (infarct expansion)	Common with HT, AS.HOCMP Increase in muscle fibre bulk
2. Increase in wall stress with progressive dilatation and hypertrophy of the remaining ventricle (ventricular remodeling). Unable to deal with normal workload	Increase muscle mass is able to deal with increased pressure load
3. Further dilatation of infarcted segment	Further increase to maximum extent
4. Heart failure	Heart failure

202. The pathophysiology of 4 rare complications following myocardial infarction where surgery is indicated.

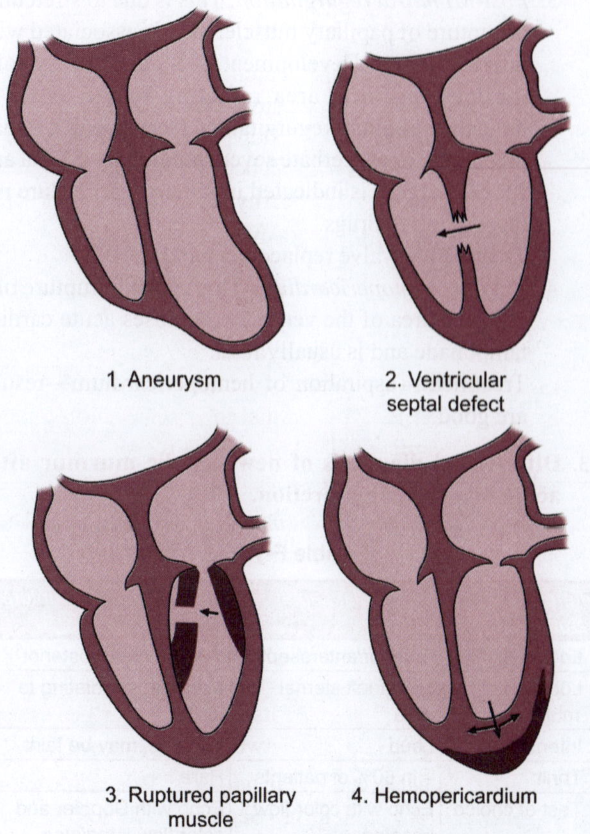

Fig. F-9: Mechanical complications of AMI where surgery is indicated

1. *Postmyocardial infarction aneurysm*: This is particularly common when there is persistent occlusion of the infarct related vessel. This causes ballooning of an area of damaged heart muscle during systole. It is usually symptomless.
   It is suspected when there is persistent ST elevation in ECG. Check the old ECGs. Treatment is aneurysmectomy.
2. *Postmyocardial infarction ventricular septal defect*: This is due to rupture of the softened part of the infarcted area in the septum causing left to right shunt through VSD. This occurs in about 1% of infarcts and is more common with anteroseptal than inferior infarction. Development of characteristic new systolic murmur at the lower left sternal edge indicates the VSD. It may result in severe hypotension, venous hypertension and fatal cardiac failure. There is dilemma about the timing of operation. Best results are achieved with surgery after about 2 weeks after infarction by which time some healing occurs. Meanwhile, some salvable patients die whilst waiting for surgery.
   Treatment—Repair of VSD and CABG

3. *Post-MI mitral regurgitation*: This is due to stretching or rupture of papillary muscle. This is associated with inferior infarct. Development of S3 and parasystolic murmur in mitral area radiating to the axilla is indicative of mitral regurgitation. Occasionally, it may precipitate or exacerbate severe pulmonary edema and shock. Surgery is indicated in severe heart failure not responding to drugs.
   Treatment—Valve replacement and CABG
4. *Post-MI hemopericardium*: This is due to rupture of a softened area of the ventricle. It causes acute cardiac tamponade and is usually fatal.
   Treatment—aspiration of hemopericardium—results are good.

203. Differential diagnosis of new systolic murmur after acute myocardial infarction.

Table F-15

Differentiating features	*Ventricular septal rupture*	*Papillary muscle rupture*
1. Location of MI	Anterior/anteroseptal	Inferior/inferoposterior
2. Location of murmur	Lower left sternal area	Mitral area radiating to axilla
3. Intensity	Loud	Variable, may be faint
4. Thrill	+ in 50% of patients	Rare
5. Test of choice	Echo with color flow imaging	Echo with Doppler and color flow imagining
6. V waves in PCWP	Present or absent	Always present
7. V waves in PA tracing	Absent	Present
8. Oxygen step-up in PA	Almost always present	Present or absent

PA: Pulmonary artery, PCWP: Pulmonary capillary wedge pressure

204. Post MI intraventricular septal rupture.

1. Occurs in 0.2% of patients with AMI.
2. Characterized by appearance of a new harsh loud holosystolic murmur:
   – Best heard at the lower left sternal border
   – Usually accompanied by a thrill.
3. Elevated features associated with increased risk of rupture:
   – Lack of development collected network
   – Advanced age
   – HT
   – Anterior location of infarction
   – Thrombolysis.
4. Higher 30 day mortality 74% compared to those patients who do not develop this complication
5. The size of the defect determines the:
   – Magnitude of the left to right shunt
   – Extent of hemodynamic deterioration
   – Likelihood of survival
6. Associated with heart block, RBBB, and atrial fibrillations in 20–30% of patients.
7. Can be recognised by 2D Echo
8. Catheter placement of umbrella-shaped device at the rupture septum.

205. Aneurysms are 4 times more common in anterior wall and apical infarctions than inferoposterior wall infarctions.

A left ventricular aneurysm develops sometimes in patients of AMI and is particularly common when there is persistent occlusion of the infarct related vessel.

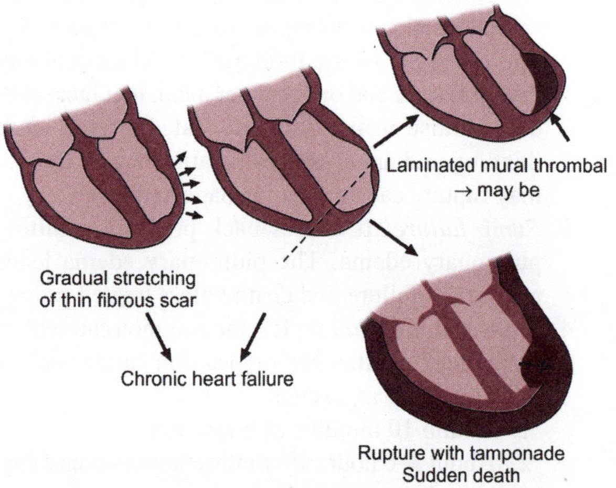

Fig. F-10: Cardiac aneurysm

206. Ventricular aneurysm following myocardial infarction is demonstrated by the following 4 investigations.

1. X-ray chest and cardiac screening: Shows abnormal bulge of the left border in anterior wall or aneurysm of the apex.
2. ECG shows persistent ST elevation at rest in precordial leads in 25% of patients.
3. Echocardiography reveals aneurysmal dilatation. Paradoxical lateral displacement of the cardiac apex during systole or abnormal outward movement of ventricular wall during systole. Mural thrombosis in anterior wall or apical aneurysm may be seen.
4. Left ventricular angiogram or isotope gated scanning of the heart demonstrates the aneurysm.

207. The 4 complications of left ventricular aneurysm are:

1. Congestive cardiac failure
2. Arterial embolism
3. Recurrent ventricular arrhythmias

4. Rupture of the heart causing hemorrhage/cardiac tamponade and death.

This is particularly common when there is persistent occlusion of the infarcted vessel.

208. The 4 conditions where recurrence of ST elevation occurs after the treatment of myocardial infarction are:

1. Reinfarction
2. Aneurysmal dilatation (after 3 to 6 weeks)
3. Local pericarditis
4. Prinzmetal angina

209. Pericarditis after acute myocardial infarction: This may occur at any stage of the illness but is particularly common on the 2nd or 3rd day of MI or as later as 6 weeks. It is suspected when the patient recognizes any of the following 4 symptoms.

1. A different type of pain after the first 12 hours even though at the same site
   Or
2. It is becoming worse
   Or
3. When the pain appears with inspiration
   Or
4. When the pain is altered by change in position pericarditis is to be suspected at the infarct site. The diagnosis is confirmed if pericardial rub is heard.

Treatment of pericardial discomfort consists of aspirin at doses as high as 650 mg at every 4–6 hours (corticosteroids should be avoided because they may interfere with myocardial scar formation).

210. Pericardial effusion.

1. More common in patients with anterior MI and with larger infarcts and when CHF is present
2. Generally detected by 2D echocardiography
3. Majority do not cause hemodynamic compromise
4. When tamponade occurs, it is usually due to ventricular rupture or hemorrhagic pericarditis.

211. Dressler syndrome/Postmyocardial syndrome.

1. Usually occurs 1–8 weeks after MI
2. Patient present with malaise, fever, pericardial discomfort, leukocytosis, elevated ESR and pericardial effusion
3. Cause of this syndrome is not clearly established (probably immunological process).
4. Treatment ASA 650 mg qd.

212. Management of recurrent chest pain/discomfort.

1. Aspirin, indomethacin, corticosteroids for pericarditis.
   The patient with recurrent chest pain believed due to pericarditis should receive high dose aspirin 650 mg every 4–6 hours
   β-blockers intravenously, then orally for ischemic-chest discomfort
2. (Re) administration of thrombolytic therapy (Stk, Urk, Alteplase, Reteplase)
3. Nitroglycerin intravenously for 24 hours, then topically or orally for ischemic type chest discomfort
4. Coronary arteriography for ischemic-type chest pain or discomfort recurring after hours to days of initial therapy and associated with objective evidence of ischemia in patients who are candidates for revascularization.

213. Balloon flotation right-heart catheter monitoring is indicated in:

1. Severe progressive congestive heart failure or pulmonary edema
2. Cardiogenic shock or progressive hypotension
3. Suspected mechanical complications of acute infarction, i.e. VSD, papillary muscle rupture or pericardial tamponade
4. Hypotension that does not respond promptly to intravenous fluids in a patient without pulmonary congestion.

214. Intra-arterial pressure monitoring is indicated in:

1. Patients with severe hypotension (systolic pressure less than 80 mm Hg) and/or cardiogenic shock
2. Patients receiving vasopressor agents
3. Patients receiving intravenous sodium nitroprusside or other potent vasodilators
4. Patients receiving intravenous inotropic agents.

215. Intra-aortic balloon counterpulsation.

A balloon is placed in the aorta and inflated in diastole causing increased flow of blood into the coronary arteries which normally receive blood in diastole. Each inflation of the balloon increases the cardiac flow by about 30 mL.

The 4 indications of intra-aortic balloon counterpulsation in myocardial infarction are:

1. Cardiogenic shock or pump failure not responding promptly to pharmacologic therapy as a stabilizing measure for angiography and prompt revascularization.
2. Acute mitral regurgitation or ventricular septal defect complicating acute MI as a stabilizing therapy for angiography and repair/revascularization.
3. Recurrent intractable ventricular arrhythmias in patients with hemodynamic instability.

4. Refractory post-infarction angina for stabilization before and during angiography/revascularization.

216. Coronary angiography in acute myocardial infarction is indicated in the following conditions.

1. Patients developing power failure, that is cardiogenic shock syndrome.
2. Patients developing severe pump failure, that is heart failure.
3. Patients suspected of having ruptured interventricular septum causing heart failure and shock.
4. Patients suspected of developing acute mitral regurgitation causing heart failure or shock.
5. Patients suspected of developing subacute cardiac rupture (pseudoaneurysm).
6. Persistent or recurrent ischemia or both despite thrombolytic therapy.
7. Patients with recurrent episodes of ischemic chest pain, particularly if accompanied by ECG changes or post-infarction angina pectoris.
8. Patients with evidence of myocardial ischemia or laboratory testing such as
   A. Exercise-induced ischemia (with or without angina pectoris) manifested by ST depression of 1mm or more.
   B. Exercise-induced reversible thallium perfusion defects, increased lung-thallium uptake.
   C. Exercise-induced reduction of ejection fraction
   D. Wall motion abnormalities on radionuclide ventriculography or two-dimensional echocardiography.

217. Primary percutaneous transluminal coronary Angioplasty (PTCA) with or without stent in acute myocardial infarction is indicated in the following 4 situations.

1. As an alternative to thrombolytic therapy in patients presenting within 6 hours of the onset of pain involving large amount of myocardium at risk and who meet the criteria for thrombolysis but in whom thrombolytic therapy is clearly contraindicated. It should be performed in a timely fashion by individuals skilled in the procedure and supported by experienced personnel in high-volume centers.
2. As a reperfusion strategy in patients who are candidates for reperfusion but who have a risk of bleeding contraindication to thrombolytic therapy.
3. Patients in cardiogenic shock
4. As a reperfusion strategy in patients who fail to qualify for thrombolysis therapy for reasons other than a risk of bleeding contraindication.

When the cholesterol plaque ruptures, clot is formed on the rough surface at a weak point. There are two components to consider—clot and ulcerated part. Thrombolysis dissolves the clot and has no action on the ulcerated part. Ulcerated part takes about a month to heal. In the mean time reinfarction can occur. In PTCA, once the balloon is dilated clot is washed off. Stent seals the ulcerated portion. Clot, as well as ulcerated portion is taken care of thereby the chances of reocclusion is very less. First hour is the 'golden hour'. Early open artery is achieved with PTCA. Angioplasty done after failure of thrombolysis is called sequential angioplasty.

Rescue angioplasty is done in case of thrombolytic failure, cardiogenic shock, recurrent angina/instability, etc.

218. Comparison of PTCA and thrombolysis in AMI.

Table F-16

PTCA	Thrombolysis
1. Maximum benefit—both clot as well as ulcerated part is taken care of	Less benefit. Only clot lysis occurs
2. Near normal flow—60% flow is Achieved	30–50% flow
3. Flow is sustained	Flow is not sustained
4. Costs around ₹ 60,000/-	About ₹ 4000/-

Though there are more benefits with primary PTCA, the procedure cost, etc. do not permit many patients to undergo and catheterization. Labs are available at few centers in big cities. Thrombolytic therapy can be given easily with less cost.

219. Delayed/elective PTCA with or without stent is indicated in:

1. Patients with evolving large or anterior infarcts treated with thrombolysis agents in whom it is believed that the artery is not patent.
2. Recurrent episodes of ischemic pain (postinfarction angina)
3. Patients with cardiogenic shock or persistent hemodynamic instability
4. Evidence of residual stenosis or myocardial ischemia on stress testing while on optimal medical therapy.

220. PTCA—4 benefits of reperfusion.

1. Many preserve a critical mass of myocardium
2. Lessen chances of infarct extension
3. Salvage subepicardial tissue of myocardium—prevents myocardial rupture
4. Prevents arrhythmias by restoring normal conduction

221. Limitations of stenting.

1. Diffuse disease
2. Small vessels < 2.5 mm
3. Excessive tortuosity
4. Lesions at the bifurcation.

222. Emergency or urgent coronary artery bypass graft (CABG) is indicated in the following 4 conditions.

1. Failed PTCA with persistent pain or hemodynamic instability in patients with coronary anatomy suitable for surgery. Failed PTCA and a small area of myocardium at risk; hemodynamically stable
2. Acute MI with persistent ischemia refractory to medical therapy in patients with coronary anatomy suitable for surgery who are not candidates for catheter intervention
3. At the time of surgical repair of postinfarction VSD or mitral insufficiency
4. Cardiogenic shock with coronary anatomy suitable for surgery.

223. Elective myocardial revascularization—coronary artery bypass graft (CABG)—is indicated in the following 4 conditions.

1. Patients with various subsets of angina not responding to medical treatment without severe left ventricular dysfunction, e.g. severe stable angina, unstable angina, Prinzmetal angina, postinfarction angina.
   - When obstruction is in more than one artery
   - When symptoms are severe even in single vessel obstruction—left main coronary artery
   - When left anterior coronary descending artery is obstructed the survival rate is lower than other single vessel obstruction.
2. In congestive heart failure secondary to AMI—may have acute intermittent failure from local ischemia.
3. Ancillary revascularization while doing other types of surgery especially in valvular heart disease when there is significant coronary artery obstruction with or without symptoms of angina or in failed angioplasty with persistent pain or hemodynamic instability.
4. Prophylactic—in asymptomatic patients with risk factors, e.g. young patient with positive exercise test, strong family history with certain risk factors of ischemic heart disease.

224. There are 4 indications of early coronary angiography and/or interventional therapy in non-ST segment elevation cohort.

1. Patients with persistent ischemic chest pain/discomfort despite medical therapy and an abnormal ECG or two or more risk factors for coronary artery disease.
2. Patients with ischemic type chest discomfort, hemodynamic instability and an abnormal ECG
3. Patients with recurrent (stuttering) episodes of spontaneous or induced ischemia or evidence of shock, pulmonary congestion, or left ventricular dysfunction
4. Patients with ischemic-type chest discomfort and a normal ECG and more than two risk factors for coronary artery disease.

225. The 4 indications for emergency cardiac repair are:

1. Papillary muscle rupture with acute mitral regurgitation resulting in intractable acute heart failure
2. Ventricular septal defect of free wall rupture
3. Aneurysmal infarction with intractable ventricular arrhythmias or pump failure or both.
4. Rupture with hemopericardium resulting in cardiac tamponade

226. Immediate surgical intervention is often required for the patient with

1. Failed PTCA with persistent chest pain or hemodynamic instability
2. Persistent or recurrent ischemic refractory to medical therapy who is not a candidate for catheter intervention
3. Cardiogenic shock and coronary anatomy not amenable to PTCA
4. Mechanical abnormality leading to severe pulmonary congestion or hypotension, such as papillary muscle rupture (with resultant mitral regurgitation) or ventricular septal defect.

227. Newer therapies.

1. Thrombus extraction catheter
2. Angiojet
3. Echoclysis—ultrasonic clot lysis
4. Intracoronary blocky therapy using radioactive stent or introducing radioactive wire in the stent for irradiation.

Future: Primary PTCA/Low dose thrombolytic therapy + Glycoprotein IIb-IIIa receptor blocker.

228. Summary of principles of management.

On arrival in the emergency department, the patient with suspected acute MI should immediately receive

1. Oxygen by nasal prongs
2. Sublingual nitroglycerin (unless systolic blood pressure less than 90 mm Hg or heart rate less than 50 bpm or more than 100 bpm)
3. Adequate analgesia (with morphine sulfate or meperidine)
4. Aspirin, 160 to 325 mg orally

   A 12-lead electrocardiogram is immediately taken. The patient with AMI should be continuously monitored and the diagnosis of AMI confirmed by serial ECGs and measurements of serum cardiac markers of myocyte necrosis, such as creatine kinase isoenzymes or cardiac specific troponin T or I. The patient should be monitored closely for adverse electrical or mechanical events because reinfarction and death occur most frequently within the first 24 hours. The patient's physical activities should be limited for at least 12–24 hours. ST-segment elevation, equal to or greater than 1 mV in two contiguous leads, provides strong evidence of thrombotic coronary artery occlusion and makes the patient a candidate for immediate reperfusion therapy, either by fibrinolysis or primary percutaneous transluminal coronary angioplasty (PTCA). Symptoms consistent with AMI and left bundle branch block (LBBB) or bilateral bundle branch block (BBB) obscuring ST segment analysis should be managed like ST-segment elevation. In contrast, without ST- segment elevation should not receive thrombolytic therapy. The benefit of primary PTCA in these patients remains uncertain.

5. Thrombolytic therapy as soon as possible-streptokinase, urokinase, rt-PA, Reteplase
6. Heparin should be administered
7. Angioplasty in selected patients at specialized centers
8. Continuous pain—IV nitrates and/or β-blockers: consider angiography
9. Consider indications for early β-blockade, ACE inhibition
10. Management of complications
    a. Left ventricular failure (after Swan-Ganz catheterization) – ACEI, diuretics, nitrates
    b. Ventricular arrhythmias—Lidocaine, if refractory, consider—procainamide, mexiletine disopyramide, bretylium, amiodarone
    c. Supraventricular arrhythmias – Vagal procedures, IV adenosine or verapamil, diltiazem or esmolol
    d. Cardiogenic shock—immediate angioplasty or intra-aortic balloon
    e. Bypass surgery (CABG)
    f. Right ventricular infarction—fluids, inotropic support—Avoid nitrates
11. Emergency cardiac surgery—for rupture of free wall, ventricular septal defect, failed PTCA, etc.
12. If the patient is non-insulin dependent diabetes mellitus—stop oral glycemic agents. Start insulin.

229. Acute MI associated with cocaine abuse (a brief note).

AMI caused by cocaine abuse differs from classic abuse.

1. Pathophysiology: The MI is caused by coronary spasm or thrombus formation occurring in a normal segment of an artery or superimposed on mild-to-moderate atherosclerotic segment of artery. This is caused by adrenergic stimulation in chronic cocaine use.
2. β-adrenergic stimulation causes increased heart rate → increased oxygen demand → increased contractility → onset of ischemia.
3. Chest pain caused by cocaine ingestion usually occurs within 3 hours (varies from minutes to days depending on the route of administration – in 30 minutes with intravenous cocaine, 90 minutes with crack smoking, 135 minutes with nasal inhalation.
4. More than 80% of patients with MI are smokers. Cigarette smoking has synergistic effect with cocaine use.

230. Therapy—4 stages in cocaine induced acute MI.

1. Initial management: in patients of MI with ST elevation with cocaine use includes routine treatment with aspirin, clopidogrel, oxygen, sublingual or intravenous nitroglycerin, or heparin.
   Intravenous calcium channel blockers or advised to relieve coronary spasm. There are no reciprocal ST depression changes if the ST elevation is caused by coronary spasm. This defers from classic MI with ST elevation and reciprocal ST depression in opposite leads.
2. Consider reperfusion therapy if vasodilator therapy is unsuccessful to relieve chest pain and ST changes. Many patients of cocaine users have contraindications to thrombolytic therapy because of severe hypertension or persistent coronary spasm (without thrombus which is not amenable to thrombolysis).
3. Immediate angiography and PTCA is more beneficial in cocaine induced MI.
4. β-blockers are contraindicated in patients with cocaine induced cocaine MI—though they block the undesirable β-adrenergic effects. These agents allow unopposed α-adrenergic stimulation and associated with increased mortality.

231. Postoperative acute MI following noncardiac operations:

1. Usually occurs on the 3rd or 4th postoperative day
2. Caused by combination of:
   Increased oxygen demand
   Increased adrenergic activity that accompanies pain and ambulation
   Increased arterial shear stress
3. Intravenous fluid volume shifts caused by redistribution of fluids, IV fluids
   Decreased enteral intake (orally)
4. Postoperative inflammatory state associated with hypercoagulability, known by fibrinogen content and acute-phase reactants.

232. Management of acute MI in postoperative noncardiac surgery.

1. It is complicated by limitation on the use of fibrinolyte and anticoagulant therapies because they can cause the postoperative bleeding
2. Treatment mainly depends on IV β-blockers
3. Urgent angiography
4. Mechanical revascularization.

233. It is relevant to discuss about acute coronary syndrome (ACS) at this juncture. It is an outpatient diagnosis of a patient with acute severe chest pain lasting for nearly 20 min. It may be unstable angina or acute MI.

The final diagnosis depends on the clinical, ECG, cardiac enzyme markers and echo. The ECG differentiate mainly with STEMI, and non-STEMI.

Table of differentiation between STEMI and non-STEMI (ACS)

Table F-17

STEMI	Non-STEMI
1. Total occlusion of epicardial coronary artery Subepicardial ST ↑	1. Subtotal critical occlusion of epicardial coronary artery. Subendocardial ST ↓
2. The thrombosis is fibrin rich, hence called red thrombus. So, fibrinolytic therapy	2. The thrombus is platelet rich, hence called white thrombus—only heparin is needed. Do not thrombolyze
3. There is macro infarction	3. There is micro infarction, coronary spasm may present
4. There is time bound necrosis of the myocardium "TIME IS MUSCLE"(door to needle time 30 min)	4. The myocardium is still viable with high probability of developing necrosis – if the occlusion becomes total
5. Sudden substernal pain, lasting more than 30 min, may radiate, not relieved by rest or sublingual nitrate	5. Pain is similar to anginal pain, may become worse, usually lasting up to 20 min. Pain is present at rest, there may be decreasing tolerance for exertion
6. There may be associated dyspnea, sweating, weakness, vomiting, along with features of heart failure	6. Transient cardiac failure may occur
7. Clinical findings of S3, S4 or murmur of papillary muscle dysfunction may present	7. S3 , S4 usually not present
8. ST ↑ present, ultimately Q wave, new onset LBBB with classical chest pain is also considered with STEMI	8. ST ↓ with T inversion No Q waves
9. Fibrinolytics are the drugs of choice –along with anti-platelets and anticoagulants	9. Antiplatelets and anticoagulants are the drugs of choice. UFH, LMWH, or fondara parmux are the drugs of choice
10. Serum cardiac markers CPKMB/troponin show elevation. Myoglobin is more sensitive	10. No changes in cardiac enzyme markers
11. Echo shows hypokinesia	11. May show regional wall motion abnormality
12. Fibrinolysis or /PTCA is the treatment of choice	12. Anticoagulants are the drugs of choice

Other cardiac medicines are same—Aspirin, clopidogrel, nitrate, pain relievers, etc.

Take the history of usage of Sildenafil within 24 hours or Tedalfen within 48 hours.

234. Post MI.

1. No smoking
2. Aspirin 150 mg lifelong
3. Clopidogel 75 mg at least 9–12 months
4. Statins –Atorvostatin 40 mg od (not 10 or 20 mg) or Rosuvastatin 10 mg od
5. β-blockers in maximum tolerated dose if no contraindication
6. ACEI and spironolactone if LV dysfunction present.
7. Diet—low fat diet, red meat, chicken and fish preferable
8. Optimal control of diabetes and hypertension.

235. Post MI quadruple therapy.

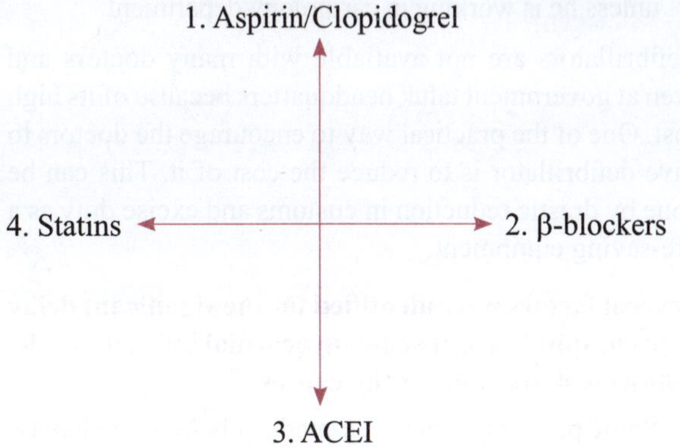

236. Advised post MI lipid profile desirable.

Total cholesterol < 200 mg
LDL < 70 mg
HDL > 50 mg
Triglycerides < 120 mg

MOBILE CORONARY CARE UNIT (MCCU)

The major mortalities of acute myocardial infarction occur in the first 4 hours after the onset of acute symptoms. Primary ventricular fibrillation is maximum during the first 4 hours and deaths occur outside the hospital. Immediate treatment is essential to save many lives.

MCCU units are started to provide immediate treatment before the arrival of patient to the Intensive Coronary Care Unit (ICCU). MCCUs are uncommon in India because of financial involvement. MCCU in New Delhi reported that average time they were able to bring the patient to the hospital is about 14 hours. Precious time is lost which costs many lives. Special telephone number should be allotted and known to the public. Public awareness is needed to reduce this delay. The MCCU has become an important tool in the prehospital management of myocardial infarction.

237. Pre-hospital issues of MCCU.

1. Emergency medical services (EMS) should be staffed by persons trained to treat AMI, cardiac arrest with defibrillation if indicated
2. Twelve lead telemetry
3. Prehospital thrombolysis in special circumstances during the transport itself if transport time is greater than 90 minutes
4. Paramedical or health care providers educate patients families about signs and symptoms of AMI, accessing EMS and medications, so that door-to-needle time can be drastically cut down. Paramedical staff are trained in giving thrombolytic treatment and defibrillation in MCCU in USA. Here, in India, even the qualified doctor is not trained in thrombolytic treatment and defibrillation unless he is working in cardiology department.

Defibrillators are not available with many doctors and even at government taluk headquarters because of its high cost. One of the practical way to encourage the doctors to have defibrillator is to reduce the cost of it. This can be done by drastic reduction in customs and excise duty as a life-saving equipment.

238. Several factors were identified for the significant delay in prehospital care of acute myocardial infarction. The following 4 are some of the causes.

1. Some patients do not seek medical help immediately.
2. Some patients are unable to contact their family doctor.
3. The ambulance service may not always be readily available.
4. There may be unnecessary delay in the casualty department.

In advanced countries, the average delay in admission has reduced to 1 hour 40 minutes after the introduction of MCCUs. Even the delay up to 1/2 an hour is considered to be due to administrative formalities which could be further eliminated. Emergency Medical Service should follow AMI protocol with targeted clinical examination and a 12-lead ECG within 10 minutes and a door-to-needle time within 30 minutes should be done.

239. Always advise the patients with known IHD, that chest pain that last more than 15 min is probably a heart attack. Known IHD patients are advised to use the glyceryl trinitrate (GTN) spray three times at 5 min interval before calling an ambulance.

Pharmaceutical companies of GTN spray give varying and sometimes nonspecific instructions regarding the dose, such as "no more than three metered doses at any one time" and a minimum of 15 min between consecutive treatment. Therefore, the responsibility lies on the attending doctor. Necrosis of viable myocardium predominantly occurs between 30–90 min after coronary artery occlusion this the "golden hour" during which time prompt perfusion strategies (thrombolysis or primary angioplasty) are performed to prevent ventricular dysfunction and worse prognosis.

This needs prehospital treatment we are far away to reach this assistance

1. Do not waste time to call your near relative or friend.
2. Immediately call the ambulance (it should be provided with equipment and experienced person.
3. Give GTN spray three times at 5 min interval before reaching the hospital.
4. Should have paramedical team with a life-saving equipment-defibrillator.

Successful defibrillation declines 7–10% each minute after cardiac arrest. Some studies show that median time from the onset of symptoms to cardiac was 10 min

Now, we can understand, how long we have to proceed to achieve these targets.

Because the government priorities are many to basic needs to control infectious diseases, anemia, malnutrition, and to reduce infant mortality, maternal mortality rates and others.

240. The success of the MCCU and ICCU program depends on the following 4 active steps.

1. Active community education—to minimize the delay between the onset of symptoms and starting of treatment. Public education in various aspects of the disease is necessary.
2. Ready availability and arrival of the MCCU to help the patient.
3. Properly organized and adequately staffed MCCU to initiate treatment and suppression of arrhythmias if possible.
4. Acceptance of patients into coronary care units at their own request.

241. Mobile coronary care unit (MCCU) is not a simple vehicle but consists of specially equipped ambulance manned by highly trained medical personnel. It should be equipped with the following 4 facilities.

1. Oxygen
2. Battery powered continuous cardiac monitoring with defibrillator.
3. Pulmonary resuscitation equipment—ventilator, ambu bag, suction, etc.
4. Temporary pacing facilities.

With all cardiac drugs and intravenous infusion facilities. Ventricular fibrillation occurrence in the immediate myocardial infarction period can best be corrected with the availability of MCCU. Long-term prognosis of these survivors from ventricular fibrillation managed at home is similar to that of patients with uncomplicated myocardial infarction. Long-term prognosis was also not affected by the number of episodes of ventricular fibrillation. Sophisticated units in advanced countries are equipped with a modulator and de-modulator. It enables the ECG and voice signals to be transmitted on a line of sight communication systems to the central station at the hospital.

Should be accompanied by a doctor familiar with its use.

242. The advantages and disadvantages of intensive coronary care unit (ICCU).

1. Provides facilities for continuous monitoring so that immediate detection of life-threatening arrhythmias especially the ventricular fibrillation can be detected and treated.
2. Provides facilities for administering the drugs such as thrombolytic drugs to reduce the immediate mortality of myocardial infarction and to allow immediate treatment of complications like heart failure or cardiogenic shock.
3. Provides facilities for intubation, ventilation or cardiac pacing, etc.
4. The disadvantage is the fear that may develop by the unnatural surroundings and high technology and fear that may be caused by the death of other patients in the unit.

The fear stimulates the release of excessive catecholamines to cause arrhythmias or sinus tachycardia which increases the oxygen requirement that causes the infarct to extend.

243. Intensive coronary care unit (ICCU) should have the following facilities.

1. Round the clock doctor and nursing service. The doctor is trained to handle cardiac emergencies.
2. Heart rate, rhythm, blood pressure and other vital functions are monitored round the clock.
3. Emergency drugs such as thrombolytic drugs.
4. Senior cardiologist should be easily contactable.
5. A battery operated portable DC defibrillator with a built in monitor, heart rate meter and a recorder.
6. Respirators including Ambu bag with face mask, endotracheal tubes and ventilator, etc.
7. Pacing catheters and flow directed balloon-tipped catheters.
8. Mechanical suction apparatus.

244. Rehabilitation program for the acute myocardial infarction patients are described in relation to the 4 phases of the illness.

Table F-18

Phase I	Acute illness	3–5 days	ICCU
Phase II	Acute illness	Remaining hospital stay 2–3 weeks	General ward
Phase III	Convalescence	3–8 weeks	Home
Phase IV	Recovery maintenance	After 8 weeks	Return to work or prior activity

Strict bed rest is essential during the first 48–72 hours after the chest pain to limit the infarct size. After this time he is allowed to sit up for short periods of time, and by 4th or 5th day he may be allowed to sit in a bedside chair and use a bedside commode.

He is mobilized gradually over a period of 2 weeks during which time he is allowed short distance walks in the hospital premises, 3–4 times a day.

Evaluation

Noninvasive evaluation of low-risk patients

245. Patients of AMI are to be examined daily during the rehabilitative activity for any evidence of:

1. Heart failure
2. Pericarditis with or without effusion
3. Arrhythmias
4. Calf vein thrombosis

A note is made if any dyspnea or angina develops during the rehabilitative activity.

246. The 4 specific tests to evaluate heart functions after myocardial infarction are:

(Laboratory investigations and chest X-ray—FBC, ESR, VDRL, BUN, creatinine, uric acid, serum calcium, serum electrolytes, serum cholesterol/triglycerides, GTT help to detect the presence of infection, risk factors, heart failure).

Table F-19

Tests	What the test detects
1. ECG including stress test (computerized Treadmill) Exercise ECG 24 hours Holter's ECG test	Position and axis of the heart Disturbance of rate and rhythm Hypertrophy Presence of myocardial infarction Strain on the heart Changes when put under stress ST - changes Rate changes Rhythm changes Abnormal response of BP
2. 2D - echocardiography/ color Doppler echocardiography	Anatomical and physiological (structural and functional) abnormalities of the heart
3. Stress thallium-201 imaging radionuclide perfusion studies	Which area of the heart gets less amount of blood during exercise
4. Coronary angiography	Complete occlusion or narrowing of the coronary arteries

247. Noninvasive evaluation of low-risk patients before or early after discharge from the hospital.

1. Stress ECG
   a. Submaximal at 4 to 6 days or symptom limited at 10–14 days before discharge for prognostic assessment or functional capacity
   b. 14–21 days – Early after discharge for prognostic assessment and functional capacity
   c. 3–6 weeks – Late after discharge for functional capacity and prognosis if early stress was submaximal

   When the baseline abnormalities of the ECG compromise interpretation.
2. Exercise two-dimensional echocardiography or nuclear scintigraphy (before or early after discharge for prognostic assessment)
3. Dipyridamole or adenosine stress perfusion nuclear scintigraphy or dobutamine echocardiography before discharge for prognostic assessment in patients judged to be unable to exercise.

   Assessment of ventricular arrhythmias
4. Ambulatory (Holter) monitoring, signal-averaged ECG, heart rate variability, baroreflex sensitivity monitoring, alone or in combination with two or other tests, including functional tests (ejection fraction, treadmill testing) for risk assessment.

248. Following 4 marked abnormalities in the resting ECG renders a displacement of ST-segment virtually uninterpretable

1. LBBB
2. LV hypertrophy with strain
3. Ventricular pre-excitation
4. Ventricular paced-rhythm

249. Exercise test: 3 to 6 weeks after recovery from myocardial infarction; the long-term prognosis can be evaluated by exercise test.

1. Major ST depression of more than 2 mm.
2. Development of typical angina or dyspnea at low levels of exercise with heart rate < 120 per minute or exercise duration < 6 minutes on the Bruce protocol.
3. Stress induced fall of BP at low level of exercise
4. Development of arrhythmias.

A maximal stress test performed 4 to 6 weeks later may identify a greater number of patients with residual myocardial ischemia. In contrast, the ability to complete the exercise test in the absence of prior pulmonary congestion indicates a low-risk subset. This low group comprises 70–80% of the total group.

250. The 4 contraindications for stress test are:

1. Heart failure or under digoxin therapy
2. Arrhythmias—specially ventricular tachyarrhythmia and bundle branch block
3. Unstable angina
4. Urea and electrolyte imbalance.

   Physically handicapped person could not perform the stress test.

   If the stress test is negative—prognosis is good.

   If the stress test is positive—prognosis is bad.

251. Exercise test should be stopped in the middle if the patient exhibits any one of the 4 following conditions.

1. If the patient experiences chest pain
2. If the heart rate goes above 200/min
3. If BP falls
4. If ST is depressed more than 2 mm.

252. It is well established that left ventricular function is an important early determinant of survival. 4 major hemodynamic subsets of patients have been identified depending upon their pulmonary capillary wedge (PCW) pressure and cardiac index.

Hemodynamic subsets in acute myocardial infarction.

Table F-20

Clinical subset	Cardiac index	PCW	Mortality
1. No pulmonary congestion or peripheral hypoperfusion	Normal	Normal	2.2%
2. Isolated pulmonary congestion	Normal	Normal	10.1%
3. Isolated peripheral hypoperfusion	Low	Normal	22.4%
4. Both pulmonary congestion and peripheral hypoperfusion	Low	High	55.5%

253. The 4 factors that affect the prognosis are:

1. BP: Isolated elevation of systolic BP and combined systolic and diastolic hypertension are unfavorable prognostic factors. Patients whose BP falls after the myocardial infarction have a worse prognosis than those whose BP remains the same.
2. Site of infarction: There is greater mortality after anterior wall infarction than inferior MI.
3. Post infarction angina generally has a less favorable prognosis because it indicates the presence of jeopardized myocardium.
4. Diabetic patients who survive, experience a more complicated postinfarction course than nondiabetic cases, including a higher incidence of postinfarction angina, infarct extension and heart failure. The long-term prognosis from unrecognized infarction appears to be similar to that following recognized infarction.

254. The 4 ECG findings that indicate poor prognosis besides life-threatening ventricular arrhythmias are:

1. Persistent advanced heart block, e.g. Mobitz type II second degree or third degree AV block or new bifascicular or trifascicular blocks in the course of an acute myocardial infarction.
2. Persistent horizontal or downsloping of ST-segment depression and Q waves in multiple leads.
3. Atrial arrhythmias like atrial fibrillation.
4. ST-segment depression in leads other than those with new Q waves.

255. Ventricular arrhythmias: 24 hours Holters ambulatory ECG recording has now become a useful tool. The following 4 are guidelines.

1. Early onset of ventricular tachycardia and ventricular fibrillation treated adequately do not influence long-term prognosis.
2. Late-onset ventricular arrhythmias carry an independent risk leading to death.
3. Cardiac mortality increases with increasing PVBs frequency. PVBs of more than 6/min is considered to be of high risk.
4. Repetitive PVBs are associated with increased mortality that is independent of PVBs frequency.

In exercise-induced ventricular arrhythmias isolated PVBs do not independently contribute to mortality; on the other hand, repetitive PVBs do contribute independently to mortality.

The PVBs risk stratification model was considerably less than that of left ventricular dysfunction.

256. Non-Q wave infarction versus Q wave infarction. The following 4 are comparisons.

1. Early hospital mortality is approximately 1 1/2 to 2 times more in patients with Q waves.
2. Patients with non-Q wave infarction tend to have smaller infarcts initially and only infrequently have total occlusion of the infarct related vessel when compared with patients with Q wave infarction.
3. Non-Q wave patients have lower incidence of heart failure after infarction, as a consequence lesser degree of left ventricular impairment.
4. Non-Q wave patients have more frequent angina related to the presence of preserved myocardium with marginal blood supply.

However, uncomplicated non-Q wave infarction is not a benign condition. Sixty percent of these patients have 2 or 3 vessel disease and frequently go on developing an acute Q wave infarction. In one series almost 50% patients with non-Q wave infarction developed unstable angina during follow-up. Extension of non-Q wave infarction appears to increase long-term risk with a doubling of one year mortality in one study. Thus it is known that patients with non-Q wave infarction may be considered as a relatively unstable condition with a lower initial mortality rate but a higher risk of later infarction. When overall long-term mortality is considered, both Q wave and non-Q wave patients have similar morbidity and mortality. Early search for ischemia by coronary arteriography justifies in some of the patients who need coronary angioplasty or CABG even in selected asymptomatic patients.

257. There are 4 points to observe in echocardiography to know the prognosis after infarction.

1. Area of myocardial infarction—hypokinesia, thinning of the walls at the infarcted area.
2. Left ventricular ejection fraction
3. Left ventricular function
4. Aneurysm.

If left ventricular ejection fraction is > 50%, no need of surgery but only medical treatment.

If left ventricular ejection fraction is < 30%, surgery is not useful.

The surgery is to be considered if the left ventricular ejection fraction is in between 30–50%.

(Coronary perfusion studies, nuclear studies facilities are available in very highly specialized units).

258. Echocardiogram is useful for both during acute myocardial infarction and postmyocardial infarction for diagnosis and therapy and during post myocardial infarction management for risk stratification, etc.

The following are the uses. It can identify:

1. Etiology of chest pain
2. Pathophysiology of ischemia

3. Extension of jeopardized myocardium
4. Functional disability of the lesion
5. Presence of infarction
6. Complication of infarct—MR, VSD, aneurysm, pericardial effusion, thrombus, rupture, etc.
7. Postmyocardial infarction risk area
   Echocardiography can assess
8. Myocardial perfusion
9. Tissue characterization
10. LV systolic/diastolic function
11. LV global/regional dyskinesia
12. Myocardial viability
13. Coronary anatomy (Transesophageal Echo is useful in assessing the proximal portion of the coronary anatomy to a certain extent).
14. Efficacy of revascularization
15. Exercise Echo—is useful to assess with physical, pharmacological and pacing methods.
16. Tissue color encoding—useful in assessing infarcted
17. Tissue Doppler imaging—area viability, etc.
18. Myocaridal contrast Echo—different color encoding.
19. Ultrasound clot lysis—by introducing catheter attached to Echo probe.
20. Ultrasound angioplasty.
    Ultrasound clot lysis and ultrasound angioplasty is not yet routinely done now. It may come into practice in future. The noninvasive Echo has several uses. In some patients coronary arteriography may show block in the coronary artery but still the myocardium supplied by those vessels may be viable which can be demonstrated by echocardiogram.

259. The 4 criteria for predicting poor prognosis after acute myocardial infarction by an abnormal exercise radionuclide perfusion scan are:

Exercise thallium-201 scintigraphy shows:
1. Multiple perfusion defects in more than one vascular region.
2. Presence of thallium-201 redistribution.
3. Increased thallium-201 uptake by the lung.
4. Exercise induced left ventricular cavity dilatation.

Other radionucleide imaging tests MUGA, MRI, electron beam CT (EBCT) are also useful.

Invasive Evaluation

Coronary Angiography and possible PTCA without Stent

260. Invasive procedure is considered in any patient with a positive exercise test in postmyocardial infarction phase.

However, coronary angiography and possible PTCA in postmyocardial infarction patients is indicated in:

1. Patients with signs and symptoms of spontaneous episodes of myocardial ischemia provoked at a low workload during recovery from infarction
2. Patients with persistent hemodynamic instability such as exercise induced fall in blood pressure at lower workload
3. Large (or multiple) reversible defects on thallium-201 imaging
4. Marked fall in left ventricular ejection fraction with exercise radionuclide ventriculography (MUGA scan)
5. Before definitive therapy of a mechanical complication of infarction such as acute mitral regurgitation, ventricular septal defect, pseudoaneurysm or left ventricular aneurysm
6. When myocardial infarction is suspected to have occurred by a mechanism other than thrombotic occlusion at an atherosclerotic plaque. This would include coronary embolism, certain metabolic or hematological diseases or coronary artery spasm
7. In post-MI patients with depressed left ventricular systolic function (EF < 40%), congestive heart failure, prior revascularization or malignant ventricular arrhythmias
8. In AMI patients who had clinical heart failure during acute attack but subsequently demonstrated well-preserved left ventricular function
9. In all post-MI patients to find persistently occluded infarct-related arteries an attempt to revascularize the artery or to identify patients with three-vessel disease
10. All patients with non-Q wave MI
11. In patients who have recurrent ventricular tachycardia or ventricular fibrillation or both in spite of antiarrhythmic therapy without evidence of ongoing myocardial ischemia
12. Survivors of MI who are thought not fit candidates for coronary revascularization

261. Though the coronary angiography is the gold standard, it has some limitations.

1. It may not find out 20% of the lesions
2. Eccentric blocks can be missed
3. Identifies only epicardial coronaries—endocardial vessels are not seen
4. Q wave are seen in MI with smokers, myocardial fibrosis but coronary angiograms may be normal. Q waves may be seen with diastolic dysfunction with negative TMT with normal angiogram.

262. Intravascular ultrasound has some advantages over coronary angiography where it is normal. Ultrasound probe is passed into coronary arteries and studied. It is used to study after stent procedure. It is done in risky patients

1. It can identify the borderline lesions
2. It can see the real cross-sectional area of the vessel and length of the lesions
3. It can identify the lesion at a bend
4. It can study the morphological character.

Secondary Prevention

263. The 4 adjustments are required in myocardial infarction patients lifestyle.

1. *Controlling the risk factors:*
   Stop smoking—abstain from any form of tobacco. (cigarettes, bidis, pan, snuff, etc.)
   Control hypertension
   Control diabetes
   Reduce overweight
   Reduce cholesterol/triglycerides
   Estrogen replacement therapy (ERT) in all postmenopausal patients who have an MI should be carefully counseled about the potential beneficial effects of ERT and offered the option of ERT if they desire it.
2. *Exercise program:*
   A little exercise does good to ones heart.
   Practice relaxing exercises slowly.
   'Limit Exercise Tolerance Test'—a modified stress is done before discharging the myocardial infarction patients to identify the high-risk patients and formulate specialized program for his/her physical activity. At home he/she is permitted short outdoor walk in the early mornings or late evenings. Walking distance is slowly increased over a period of time.
   He should not drive vehicle himself or travel by air during the first 3 months. Special arrangements are available at the airports for the transport of patients and for handling of luggage if advance information is given.
   One should avoid traveling in rush hours or rush to catch a bus or train.
3. *Return to work:* It depends on many factors, particularly the type of job. Those with sedentary occupations can often return to work at the end of 2 months.
   Persons who have heavy manual work should completely abstain from work for at least 3 months. They need a change to lighter work.
4. *Yoga and meditation:* Physical and mental relaxation are important. It helps to avoid stress and tension. They bring change in mental attitude toward life leading a more peaceful and active (not hectic) life.
   It is now proved that in myocardial infarction patients who take good care, the blockage and narrowing of coronaries reverses and slowly the coronary arteries open up.

264. Management of lipids (See Dyslipidemias E 211–232)

1. The AHA Step II diet, which is low in saturated fat and cholesterol (less than 7% of total calories as saturated fat and less than 200 mg/day any cholesterol), should be given to all patients after recovery from AMI
2. Patients with LDL cholesterol levels greater than 125 mg/dL despite the AHA Step II diet should be given drug therapy to reduce LDL cholesterol levels to less than 100 mg/dL HMG CoA reductase (Statins) drugs help to lower the LDL cholesterol.
3. Patients with normal plasma cholesterol levels who have HDL levels less than 35 mg/dL should be given nonpharmacological therapy (exercise) to raise it. If no response, drugs such as niacin is given to raise HDL levels.
4. Drug therapy using either niacin or gemfibrozil may be added to diet regardless of LDL and HDL levels when triglyceride levels are greater than 200 mg/dL.

265. β-blockers and aspirin after myocardial infarction.

1. In all but low-risk patients aged less than 70 years who had an uncomplicated myocardial infarction, without a contraindication to β-blocker therapy. Treatment should begin within few days of the AMI and continue indefinitely. Daily β-blocker reduces mortality in the first year or so by about 20% that is from 10–8%, saving about two lives for every 100 patients treated.
2. The benefit of β-blockers is due to reduction in sudden death suggesting that the drug acts as antiarrhythmic caused by infarction as well as excessive release of catecholamines. These are given provided there is no contraindication for β-blockers. Treatment should ordinarily begin within the first few days of infarction and should be continued for at least two years.
3. Small doses of prophylactic aspirin has shown to reduce the long-term mortality by about one for every 100 patients treated. It also prevents recurrent nonfatal infarction.
4. The benefit of aspirin is by prevention of platelet agglutination. Aspirin should be taken for years, some say lifelong.

How many years aspirin should be taken for, and whether β-blockers and aspirin together have an added prophylactic advantage is not yet fully known.

ACE inhibitors are also found useful in postmyocardial infarction management in reducing mortality and morbidity.

266. Long-term anticoagulation after AMI—4 indications.

1. For secondary prevention of MI in post-MI patients unable to take aspirin
2. Post-MI patients with persistent or paroxysmal atrial fibrillation
3. Patients with left ventricular thrombus
4. Post-MI patients with extensive wall motion abnormalities.

267. The 4 points to be observed for sexual life in patients with myocardial infarction are:

Sex is often a taboo for majority of myocardial infarction patients.

The patient may begin his sex after 6–8 weeks of infarction provided his heart holds sufficient reserves which can be assessed by exercise stress test.

Patient with extensive infarction with poor heart function must avoid all exercises including sex till they get better by coronary angioplasty or bypass graft.

1. All previous medicines should have been taken in time.
2. Avoid heavy meals and alcohol just before sex
3. Have sex preferably in the early mornings or at such times when one is fresh and not tired.
4. Keep a tablet of nitrate at hand. If chest pain develops during or after sex use the tablet sublingually to alleviate the symptoms and contact the doctor immediately.

DOMICILIARY MANAGEMENT OF ACUTE MYOCARDIAL INFARCTION BY FAMILY PHYSICIAN

Most of the deaths that occur in the first one hour or in the first 24 hours after acute myocardial infarction are due to cardiac arrhythmias.

Thus, the responsibility of early diagnosis and management during the most critical period rests on the family doctor/general practitioner.

Early diagnosis and immediate management by attending family physician mean all the difference between life and death of the patient.

Diagnosis of acute myocardial infarction lies in checking clear history and physical examination, ECG and enzyme estimation.

The positive investigations may confirm the diagnosis but if negative does not rule out the diagnosis.

268. Domiciliary management of acute myocardial infarction in an uncomplicated case consists of:

1. Aspirin 325 mg (preferably chewable)
2. Sublingual nitroglycerin—5 mg, 6th or 8th hourly to start with and slowly increase the dose.
3. Oxygen by a mask or nasal catheter if available.
4. Morphine injection 2 mg IV at 5 minutes interval till it is effective.
   (Start IV drip slowly to administer IV medication promptly in case of an emergency).

269. The following 4 vital signs record should be maintained at least 4th hourly.

1. Pulse—particularly the cardiac rhythm by a person who should anticipate and recognize for the prompt treatment of arrhythmias
2. Temperature
3. Respiration
4. BP.

270. Management of the 4 important complications in acute myocardial infarction consists of:

1. Bradycardia below 50 per minute should be treated by injection atropine 0.5 mg IV.
2. Frequent ventricular ectopics or ventricular tachyarrhythmias should be given injection xylocaine IV both for prophylactic and therapeutic use.
   Injection xylocaine 50 to 100 mg IV as a bolus followed by 2 to 4 mg per minute by IV drip.
3. Cardiogenic shock should be treated by vasopressors like dopamine or dobutamine.
   Injection dopamine 200 mg in 540 cc of 5% dextrose, 8 to 10 drops per minute.
4. In case of cardiac arrest, which may be of ventricular fibrillation or standstill—immediate cardiopulmonary resuscitation with external cardiac massage should be done.

271. Patients who are free from the following 4 conditions can be treated safely at home.

1. Those who are seen at home 12 hours or more after the onset of symptoms, so long as they appear well.
2. Who are no longer have continuous pain
3. Who have no evidence of arrhythmia
4. Who have no heart failure.

G Cardiac Arrest

Cardiac arrest is (also known as cardiopulmonary arrest or circulatory arrest) the sudden and complete cessation of cardiac function. Medical personal can refer to an unexpected cardic arrest as a sudden cardiac arrest (SCA).

1. There are 4 mechanisms which may cause sudden cardiac arrest followed by death.

1. Arrhythmias:
   a. Commonly ventricular tachycardia or ventricular fibrillation, sometimes following bradyarrhythmias. —Electrical irritability
   b. 25% cases are ventricular asystole or severe bradycardia.
2. Marked reduction in cardiac output as in mechanical blockage, e.g. massive pulmonary thromboembolism, cardiac tamponade—power failure.
3. Sudden ventricular failure—'Pump failure' which may occur in critical acute myocardial infarction (non-arrhythmic cardiac death) with or without cardiac rupture.
4. Activation of vasodepressor reflexes.
   For example, primary pulmonary hypertension
   pulmonary thromboembolism
   hypersensitive carotid sinus syndrome.

2. The 4 arrhythmias likely to cause cardiac arrest are:

1. Ventricular fibrillation (VF)
2. Ventricular tachycardia (VT) going into fibrillation
3. Less often ventricular asystole
4. Occasionally, the rhythm may be sinus rhythm without any perceptible cardiac output—a terminal condition known as electromechanical dissociation.

These can usually be known by an ECG or during cardiac surgery when the heart is visible. Resuscitation must be started before ECG is available.

3. The 4 cardinal signs of cardiac arrest are:

1. Sudden absence of pulsations in the major vessels—carotid or femoral
2. Loss of consciousness
3. Pupils dilated and not reacting to light
4. Arrest of respiration.

The last three signs are due to loss of brain activity. Lack of oxygen to the brain causes loss of consciousness, which then results in abnormal or absent breathing. Brain injury is likely if cardiac arrest goes untreated for more than 5 minutes. Therefore, immediate treatment is imperative for the best of survival and neurological recovery. Sudden stoppage of bleeding during surgery is another important sign of cardiac arrest.

The specific sign of cardiac arrest is pulselessness. If the pulse is present, the cause of unconsciousness may be due to some other condition such as faint, hypoglycemic shock or an epileptic seizure.

The diagnosis of cardiac arrest is established by unconsciousness and absence of the carotid or femoral pulse.

4. If the pulse is present and the patient is not breathing the cause of unconsciousness is respiratory arrest due to conditions, such as:

1. Asthma
2. Carbon dioxide narcosis in a blue bloating chronic bronchitis.
3. Chronic obstructive pulmonary disease (COPD)
4. Large dose of sedative.

5. The indication for resuscitation is clear when the cardiac arrest has occurred as a result of an accident, such as:

1. Electrocution

2. Drowning
During procedures, such as
3. Cardiac catheterization
4. Anesthesia (general/intravenous injection).
Resuscitation is most likely to be successful in these situations.

6. Resuscitation is nearly always unsuccessful if the acute circulatory failure is due to any of the following causes.

1. Acute myocardial infarction with severe heart failure
2. Aneurysmal rupture following myocardial infarction
3. Cardiac tamponade
4. Massive pulmonary embolism.

7. The 4 points to be known about the cardiac arrest team:

1. The number of persons in cardiac arrest team
2. The staff who are preferred in the cardiac arrest team
3. The role of each member of the team
4. The person who is an overall incharge.

Every doctor, nurse and member of staff who works in the clinical set-up should be proficient in cardiac resuscitation. In a hospital, the resuscitation team should consists of at least two or preferably three doctors of whom one should be a physician and another anesthetist. One senior nurse from a coronary care unit or intensive care unit or an operation theater assistant is preferred. Another nurse and a hospital porter to bring the emergency trolley.

In general, the anesthetist and the senior nurse from the operation theater should attend to the airway and intubation, if necessary, the other nurse attends to the cardiac massage. Physician should attend to defibrillator and recording the heart rhythm.

One of the doctors should be overall incharge. Although he helps the resuscitation, he should be looking after the overall view of what is happening.

One should note the time of resuscitation call given. A nurse or other member of the ward staff should be instructed to keep written timed record of events and treatment. All idle onlookers should be sent out.

8. Treatment of cardiac arrest must start immediately as soon as the diagnosis is confirmed before the arrival of the trained staff or cardiac arrest team. Treatment is given by the ward nurse or member of the staff who happens to be present. All nurses, other ward staff, ambulance drivers and attendants should receive training in this vitally important form of first aid and following treatment should start immediately within 2 or 3 minutes before the brain suffers from irreversible damage unless some circulation of oxygenated blood is achieved.

The 4 most important steps are:

1. A smart single blow should be given to the left of the sternum with the side of the clenched fist from a height of about 15–20 cm. It should be tried in all cases because sometimes this will convert ventricular fibrillation, ventricular tachycardia or asystole to sinus rhythm. This is known as 'thump version'.
2. Both legs should be elevated to 90°.
If the pulse is not immediately returned and if the patient does not immediately show signs of regaining consciousness.
3. Closed-chest cardiac massage.
4. Mouth-to-mouth breathing (expired air resuscitation) should be commenced along the lines indicated by the letters ABCD below.

The exception is that if a defibrillator is immediately available or if the arrest has occurred in ICCU, the rhythm of the heart is quickly ascertained and ventricular fibrillation or tachycardia is cardioverted without wasting time for cardiac massage.

If the patient is conscious when first seen he should be encouraged to cough vigorously (Cough CPR-See F-153). This may terminate a potentially fatal ventricular tachycardia.

Cardiopulmonary resuscitation is most easily organized according to the letters ABCD...

9. A for

1. Airway
2. Assess
3. Acidosis
4. Asystole.

10. B for

1. Breathing
2. Blow on the chest
3. Brook airway
4. Bag valve mask.

11. C for

1. Circulation
2. Closed-chest cardiac massage
3. Counter shock
4. Coronary care unit (CCU).

12. D for

1. Drugs
2. Drip
3. Defibrillation
4. DC Shock

13. E for

1. ECG
2. Endotracheal tube
3. Electrical pacing/defibrillation
4. Electrolytes.

14. F for

1. Fibrillation
2. Fluids
3. Floor
4. First aid.

15. G H I J

G for gauge.
H for hypothermia, severe hypoxia, hypovolemia hypo- or hyperkalemia.
I for ICCU, infusion.
J for joules.

Hs and Ts is the mnemonic used to aid in remembering possible treatable or reversible causes of cardiac arrest.

Hs: i. Hypovolemia
ii. Hypoxia
iii. Hydrogen ions (acidosis)
iv. Hyperkalemia
v. Hypokalemia
vi. Hypothermia
vii. Hypoglycemia
viii. Hyperglycemia.

Ts: i. Tablets
ii. Toxins
iii. Tamponade—cardiac tamponade (fluid around the heart)
iv. Tension pneumothorax (a collapsed lung)
v. Thrombosis (AMI)
vi. Thromboembolism
vii. Trauma.

16. Life support must be provided along the lines indicated by the letters ABCD... below.

If a thump on the chest is ineffective and the cardiac resuscitation is necessary follow the letters ABCDEFGH as below.

1. *A. Airway, Assess, Acidosis, Asystole.* Assess the cardinal signs to confirm the diagnosis. Unconsciousness should be checked by gentle shaking and shouting at the patient, 'You are alright'.
   Airway keep the airway clear, clear the vomitus debris, secretions in the mouth and pharynx. Dentures should be taken care. Tilt the patient's head backwards fully extending the neck, (if there is no cervical injury) rise the chin by pushing the lower jaw forward. Extending the neck this way lifts the tongue off the posterior wall of the pharynx.
   Assess the rhythm.
   Is he or she is in acidotic breathing, Kussmaul's respiration?
2. *B. Breathing, Brook airway, Bag valve mask, Blow on the chest.*
   Breathing directly by mouth-to-mouth, mouth-to-nose or mouth-to-airway. Ventilation is given until a face mask and bag are available. This is given by taking a deep breath, pinching the patient's nose and blowing forcefully into the mouth.
   Indirectly by Brook airway: This has a tube with a one way valve, a flange to fit over the patient's lips and a tongue depressor. It facilitates ventilation in an esthetic way than mouth-to-mouth ventilation.
   Bag valve mask Ambu bag: It allows the delivery of the oxygen and also allows the operator to stand back.
   An endotracheal tube should be introduced if the early attempts to restore the heartbeat is not successful.
   In each instance an airtight seal must be ensured; one must see that the chest should rise and fall for adequate ventilation. There should be at least 12 inflations per minute. Lungs should be inflated after every fifth compression of the sternum. If only one operator is present, the compression should be interrupted every ten cycles and the lungs ventilated twice.
   (presently 15 chest compression and 2 breathings are recommended).
   Practice with a dummy or mannequin is very useful. Attending the anesthesia session is very helpful. If a ventilator is available, 100% oxygen is administered under intermittent positive pressure.
3. *C. Circulation, closed-chest-cardiac compression, counter shock, coronary care unit (CCU)*
   Cardiac massage or circulation: The patient is laid on the back on the floor or any other firm surface. The surface should be hard, remove pillows. Hard board may be slipped under the back of the patient if necessary. If sitting in a chair put the patient immediately down. Attempting cardiac massage on a spring cot with cushion mattress does not serve the purpose.
   External cardiac massage is done by placing the heal of one hand at the junction of upper 2/3rds and lower 1/3rd of the sternum and covering with the other hand and press downward for about 4 cm or 1/3rd of anteroposterior diameter of the chest. Keeping the arms straight, the sternum is compressed with a pressure of 25–32 kg at a rate of 80 compressions per minute. Each compression and relaxation should be of the same time. The intrathoracic pressure changes caused by the compression alternately squeeze and relax the heart simulating a heartbeat and propels the blood into the circulation. The result should be checked by carotid or femoral pulse.

4. *D. Drugs, Drip, Defibrillation, DC shock.*
   Defibrillation: Before applying gel pads—ask every one to stand clear of the patient and check the anesthetist has removed the oxygen from the patient. Paddles should be smeared with paddle jelly, which has the property of electrical conductivity (not echocardiogram jelly). Peddles are named apex and base. Apply apex paddle at the apex and the other at right upper sternal border. After DC shock is given, it should be off and recharge again for repeating the shock.
   The possible rhythm encountered during cardiac arrest or "shockable" versus "nonshockable". The two shockable rhythms are now divided into ventricular fibrillation (VF) or pulseless ventricular tachycardia (VT) and non-VF/VT. These later rhythms include asystole and (pulseless) electromechanical dissociation (QRS complex visible with no discernible cardiac output). This refers to whether a particular class of dysrhythmia is treatable using a defibrillation. Often it is difficult to decide—if a rhythm is asystole or VF. If this occurs, treat the rhythm as VF and defibrillation given. Cardioversion is done in AF, VT or asystole. Shock is given on QRS wave, i.e. synchronized shock. There is a separate button in defibrillator machine—keep the synchronizing button 'ON' and perform the shock.
   For VF/pulseless VT—Initial
   Defibrillation—should be 200 joules followed by 200 joules, and then third shock 360 joules.
   If VF persists 1 minute cardiopulmonary resuscitation should be given.
   Give 1 mg adrenaline IV and the patient is intubated. If there is still VF, then further shock of 360 joules should be given. Give adrenaline IV after 3 minutes.
   If VF persists after 12 shocks, consider administration of antiarrhythmic drugs—Injection xylocaine 100 mg or bretylium.
   Non-VF/VT, asystole—in case of asystole, basic life support is given for 3 minutes followed by 3 mg of IV atropine. Endotracheal intubation is done in the meantime. If the cardiac monitor shows any atrial activity, temporary cardiac pacing is done by an external cardiac pacemaker. If no response, CPR should be continued with adrenaline given every 3 minutes. If no changes in rhythm, 5 mg adrenaline is given.
   Drugs for resistant VF/VT
   Injection xylocaine 100 mg can repeat once, then give 2.4 mg/min IVI. Bretylium torsylate (tosylate) 5 mg/kg IV. You should continue CPR for 20 minutes, procainamide 100 mg IV over 2 minutes is an alternative.
   Intracardiac injection of 5 mL of 1 in 10,000 adrenaline hydrochloride and 5 mL of 10% calcium chloride greatly improves myocardial tone and may be repeated after 2 to 5 minutes. Isoprenaline sulfate 0.1 to 0.2 mg IV given according to the BP.
   Adrenaline: Only vasopressor drug accepted uniformly for CPR since 1890 is still the choice drug in modern CPR. It increases peripheral vasoconstriction, leads to increase in aortic diastolic pressure (critical for coronaries) causing increased coronary perfusion pressure and myocardial blood flow.
   With invasive monitoring, one can know whether compression to be altered or more epinephrine to be given depending on whether aortic diastolic pressure is less than 40 mm Hg or if coronary perfusion pressure is less than 20 mm Hg. Empirical dose is 10 µg/kg body wt (0.5 mg) repeated every 5 minutes.
   Correct acidosis. Adequate ventilation reverses acidosis. However, a small quantity of sodium bicarbonate is given.
   The sodium bicarbonate at a concentration of 8.4% is used for cardiac arrest. The speciality of this concentration is that 1 mL = 1 mmol. About 50 mL, i.e. 50 mmol is usually given. Usually 7.5% sodium bicarbonate is available. 50 mL of it, i.e. 1 to 2 mg/kg is given and repeated after 10 minutes till spontaneous heartbeat returns).
   If external cardiac massage does not restore heart rhythm and is found due to asystole, 10 mL of 10% calcium gluconate or calcium chloride should be given intravenously together with 5 to 10 mL of 1 in 10,000 adrenaline either intravenously or via the endotracheal tube.
   Sodium bicarbonate has specific indication in prior metabolic acidosis, lengthy cardiopulmonary resuscitation and hyperkalemia.
   The side effect include
   a. Hyperosmolarity
   b. Hypernatremia
   c. Hypercapnia
   d. Paradoxical intracellular acidosis.
   Atropine is indicated in extreme bradycardia, heart block and asystole. Dose: Pediatric—0.1 to 0.002 mg/kg body weight. Maximum 2 mg. Adult—0.1 to 0.5 mg IV every 5 min. Maximum dose 2 mg by IV or endotracheal tube (ETT).

Drip: Intravenous dextrose/saline drip is to be started if the resuscitation continues for more than a minute or two. If the arm vein is not accessible, the subclavian or internal jugular vein should be cannulated.

Infusions:

Adrenaline: 0.1–1.0 µg/kg/min
Dopamine: 2–20 µg/kg body wt
Dobutamine: 5–20 µg/kg body wt
Isoproterenol: 0.1–1 µg/kg/min

Other drugs used in CPR:

Table G-1

Drug	Indication	Dose
Verapamil	AV nodal tachyarrhythmias Atrial fibrillation and flutter	0.075–0.15 mg/kg
Esmolol	AF, nodal tachycardia flutter, sinus tachycardia	0.1–0.5 mg
Amrinone	Low cardiac output—hypotension	loading dose: 0.75 mg/kg IV over 5 min.
Phenylephrine	Hypotension	50–200 µg/kg

5. E. *ECG, Endotracheal tube, Electrical pacing/defibrillation, Electrolytes, Electromechanical dissociation.*

ECG: Note whether there is ventricular fibrillation, asystole, bizarre complexes.

The paddles of a defibrillator may be used as ECG leads for quick assessment and when indicated should be used to cardiovert the patient immediately.

Electromechanical dissociation has a very poor prognosis. However, it can be treated if a underline cause is found. If the cause is found, then CPR is continued as before and adrenaline is given every 3 minutes.

Causes and association of electromechanical dissociation

Tension pneumothorax
Cardiac tamponade (fluid in pericardial sac)
Large pulmonary embolism (thromboembolic/mechanical obstruction)

Potentially reversible causes

Hypoxia
Hypovolemia
Hypokalemia, hyperkalemia
Hypothermia
Drug overdosage.

Do not intercept CPR >10 sec except to defibrillate.

Asystole with P waves: Start external pacing, use endocardial pacing if experienced. Use atropine 0.6 mg/5 min IV. Treat acidosis with good ventilation. Sodium bicarbonate may worsen intracellular acidosis and precipitate arrhythmia, so use it only in severe acidosis after prolonged resuscitation (e.g. 50 mL of 8.4% solution by IVI).

6. F. *Fibrillation, Fluids, Floor, First aid.*

Fibrillation: Ventricular fibrillation must be tackled immediately by defibrillation with a charge of 200 joules. If no response, defibrillation should be repeated with a charge of 400 joules (watt seconds). Sooner the shock is applied the more likely is to succeed.

If still there is no response:

Give injection xylocaine 100 mg IV bolus followed by IVI 2 to 4 mg per min or via endotracheal tube. Acidosis must be corrected. Bretylium tosylate 5–10 mg per kg given IV slowly followed by 1 to 4 mg per min in slow infusion. Both these drugs given intravenously not only treats ventricular fibrillation but also helps in effective cardioversion. Disopyramide or mexiletine may be tried. If ventricular fibrillation still persists, defibrillation may be successful after the administration of 5 to 10 mL of 1 in 10,000 adrenaline hydrochloride either IV or through endotracheal tube. β-blockers are tried in intractable ventricular fibrillation. In case of doubt whether the rhythm is fine ventricular fibrillation or asystole, it should be treated as ventricular fibrillation and the patient is defibrillated.

Transthoracic or transvenous electrical pacing should be the ideal procedure for the management of cardiac asystole. But still that facility is available one should give intracardiac adrenaline 1 mL of 1 in 1000 solution to stimulate the ventricular myocardium. An infusion of orciprenaline or isoprenaline can be started with the same purpose till facility for cardiac pacing is available.

7. G. *Gauge and evaluate the treatment, the cause of arrest. Maintain fluid and electrolyte balance.*

Transthoracic pacing is needed in asystole or extreme bradycardia.

8. H. *Hypothermia*

(Lastly I for IV infusion and Intensive Coronary Care Unit - ICCU).

17. Monitoring of the following is done:

1. ECG
2. Arterial line
3. Central venous line
4. Pulse oximeter
5. PCO_2, $PaCO_2$, PaO_2, pH
6. End-tidal CO_2
7. Temperature
8. EEG and evoked potentials

18. The following 4 points should be followed during the management after successful cardiac resuscitation.

This will depend upon the arrhythmia that caused the cardiac arrest and the condition of the patient after the resuscitation.

1. If the cardiac arrest is due to ventricular fibrillation or tachycardia, xylocaine or class I antiarrhythmic should be given.
2. If the arrest is due to asystole, a temporary pacemaker should be inserted unless it is caused by anoxia or some other readily reversible cause.
3. If the level of consciousness is impaired and cerebral edema is expected, parentral dexamethasone 4 mg twice a day should be given for 3 to 4 days to minimize the cerebral edema.
   Furosemide 40–80 mg IM/IV given for cerebral edema.
4. If the respiration is insufficient, the patient should be ventilated mechanically.

19. Following steps should be taken immediately in a non-hospital situation when the collapse is within minutes.

1. Give a thump over the left sternum
2. Ask your assistant or a member of the family to start external cardiac massage.
3. Give a few mouth-to-mouth respirations
4. Inject intracardiac adrenaline 1 mL of 1 in 1,000 and calcium chloride 10 mL if available.
5. Repeat the same procedure after 1–2 minutes and continue the massage and mouth-to-mouth breathing (one breathing for every 4 heartbeats)
   If the facilities are available.
6. Take ECG rhythm strip.
7. If the pulse is felt and there is change in rhythm, treat the arrhythmia accordingly.
   If nothing happens for 10–15 minutes, stop all the procedure.
8. If the patient recovers:
   Give intravenous Ringer lactate or sodium bicarbonate infusion to correct acidosis caused by anoxia.
   Give 8 mg of dexamethasone IV furosemide and 40–80 mg to relieve cerebral edema and repeated depending on the condition.
   Keep a check on heart rate for 24–48 hours and treat arrhythmias as and when necessary.
   Summary of CPR
   Cardio pulmonary resuscitation.

Cardiac arrest: 1997 UK adult advanced life-support algorithm

Each step assumes the previous one has been unsuccessful.

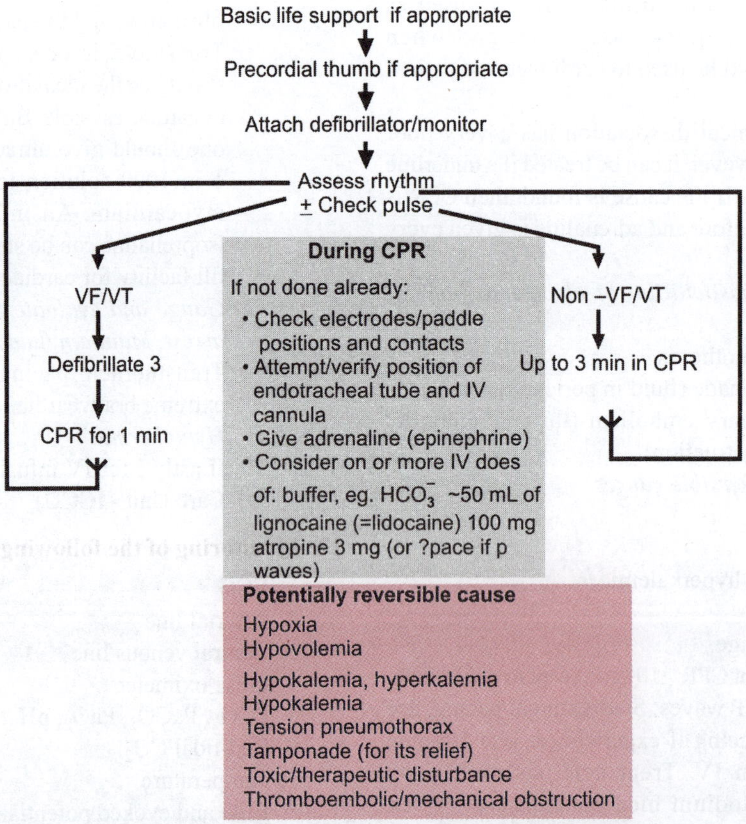

Do not interrupt CPR for > 10 sec, except to Defibrillate

Resistant VF/VT: consider: Lignocaine 100 mg IV, can repat once; then give 2–4 mg/min IVI

Different paddle position, e.g. anteroposterior

Bretylium tosylate 5 mg/kg IV; you must then continue CPR for 20 minutes.

Procainamide 100 mg IV over 2 minutes is an option

Seek expert advice from a cardiologist.

Asystole with P waves: Start external pacing (percutaneous transthoracic pacing through special paddles). Use endocardial pacing if experienced pacer avaliable. If unavaliable, use atropine 0.6 mg/5 min IV while awaiting further help.

Treat acidosis with good ventilation: Sodium bicarbonate may worsen interacellular acidosis after prolonged resuscitation (e.g. 50 mL of 8.4% solution by IVI).

H Rheumatic Fever/Rheumatic Heart Disease

Acute rheumatic fever (ARF) is a multi-system disease due to an inflammatory condition of the connective tissue particularly the heart, its valves and the joints caused by hyperimmune or autoimmune reaction to Lancefield Group A β-hemolytic *Streptococcus* infecting the throat (Pharyngitis, tonsillitis). The initial infection may be sore throat, scarlet fever or otitis media. It is by nature recurrent and derives its importance from the fact that it can lead to chronic heart disease.

The incidence of rheumatic fever and rheumatic heart disease vary substantially among countries. In many developing countries the incidence of ARF approaches or exceeds 200 per 1 lakh, whereas in US, it is estimated to be less than 1 per lakh. It is estimated that more than 1 million suffer from RHD in India.

Rheumatic heart disease (RHD) is the cardiac sequel of acute rheumatic fever. Acute rheumatic carditis is the most serious form of acute rheumatic fever. Though the name acute rheumatic fever implies the involvement of joints, it owes its importance to the involvement of the heart.

Rheumatic fever (RF) and rheumatic heart disease (RHD) in India is still appreciably high and does not seem to have changed to any appreciable extent in the last two decades. It is estimated that more than one million children suffer from RHD. About 75,000 patients are waiting for valve replacement surgery in India.

The RF is specially important to the general practitioner/family physician who plays a greater role because he is the first person to see the children with acute streptococcal pharyngitis and ARF and its sequelae.

1. Rheumatic heart disease is the most common cause of mortality in the first 4 decades of life.
2. Rheumatic heart disease accounts for 40% (25–40%) of cardiovascular diseases in hospital based patients among all age groups and is the leading cause of cardiac death under 50 years of age.
3. **There are 4 predisposing factors of streptococcal throat infection.**
   1. *Age:* Children between 5–15 years are more susceptible and the susceptibility diminishes with age. In developing countries, it occurs earlier, often in infancy and are associated with a higher incidence of severe carditis and valvular disease, and higher morbidity and mortality.
   2. *Sensitivity:* Those who have an attack of RF tend to have recurrence more often than others in general population. It has a tendency to recur in up to 70% of cases unless adequate treatment is given and has propensity to smoulder on causing rheumatic heart disease later in life in about 50% of patients. Recurrences are most common in the first 3 years of initial attack. Incidence falls rapidly after 5 years. The older the patient at the time of recurrence, the more obvious is the arthritis and milder the carditis.
      The recurrence occurred only when patient defaulted from penicillin prophylaxis.
   3. *Familial tendency:* Genetic factors play a role. The monozygotic twins have a much concordance rate for rheumatic fever than dizygotic twins. Some HLA types are more susceptible to this disease than others.
   4. *Social and environmental factors:* Overcrowding, unhygienic conditions, inadequate medical care, etc. are the causes of high incidence in developing and underdeveloped countries. (Because of the improved living conditions, the disease is controlled in developed countries). Rheumatic fever follows seasonal variation of streptococcal infection.

4. 1 to 4 weeks is the usual time after tonsillitis or pharyngitis to cause acute RF by group A β-hemolytic streptococci.

5. Some facts to know about group A β-hemolytic streptococci, which can be divided into several groups on the basis of polysaccharide antigen on the cell wall.

1. Some serotypes of group A streptococci such as type 12 and 49 are 'nephrogenic' and are associated with acute glomerulonephritis.
2. Some serotypes of group A streptococci such as type 1, 3, 5, 6, 14, 18, 19, 24, 27 and 29 are 'Rheumatogenic'.
3. Streptococci, which produce throat infection may produce acute rheumatic fever or acute glomerulonephritis. Pharyngeal route of infection is necessary to initiate rheumatic process.
4. Streptococci, which produce skin infection never produce rheumatic fever but can produce acute glomerulonephritis.

   Facilities for bacteriological identification of streptococcal infection and various antistreptococcal antibodies are available in urban areas only. The definitive diagnosis of streptococcal infection in the rural area is not possible. The diagnosis of acute rheumatic fever in the absence of cardiac involvement is at best an intelligent guess. Night sweats are more common in rheumatic fever.

6. Pathology of RF: Pathogenesis of RF is an enigma. Following are the pathological features of RF.

1. The basic pathologic changes in RF is an exudative and proliferative lesion of inflammatory reaction, which occurs in mesenchymal tissue of heart, joints, blood vessels and subcutaneous tissue. The characteristic lesion in RF is Aschoff nodule.
2. Group A β-hemolytic *Streptococcus* and the patient's connective tissue share common antigens and that the immune reaction mounted by the body against the organism leads to a reaction against the patient's own connective tissue causing inflammation.
3. Some autoimmune mechanism: Antigen-antibody reaction is believed to be responsible for the various systemic manifestations. The abnormal immune reaction probably results from a biased antigenic presentation and/or a disordered immune reaction. The abnormal immune response to streptococcal antigen occurs in susceptible individual and are cross-reactive to human cardiac tissue. In about half the cases the condition slowly causes thickening and distortion of heart valves that manifest later in life as chronic RHD. (Moreover, continued infiltration even after surgically excised left atrial appendages and valves from the patients of chronic rheumatic heart disease (RHD) suggests a chronic ongoing immunoinflammatory process even in quiescent phase of the disease).

   Lesions of rheumatic fever are spread throughout the body with special to connective tissues. Focal inflammatory lesions occur particularly around the small blood vessels.
4. Cardiovascular system: It affects the endocardium, myocardium and pericardium termed as rheumatic pancarditis. Myocardial Aschoff body consists of areas of fibrinoid necrosis surrounded by epitheloid giant cells and an outer layer of lymphocytes. Focal inflammatory lesions occur particularly around small blood vessels.

   Aschoff body is a submiliary granuloma, later converted into a spindle-shaped or triangular scar lying between the muscle bundle and surrounding blood vessels.

   Rheumatic endocarditis produces valvulitis, which leads to the most serious permanent cardiac damage. Tiny translucent nodules are seen on the valves and on the auricular endocardium, the so-called 'McCallum patch'. It may heal with variable degree of valvular incompetence and stenosis.

   Rheumatic pericarditis produces serofibrinous effusion. The pericardium may show calcification but pericardial constriction does not occur.
5. Involvement of joints is characterized by exudative rather than proliferative lesion and healing occurs without any scar or deformity.
6. Subcutaneous nodules: They are localized areas of 'fibrinoid' swelling of subcutaneous collagen bundles.
7. Chorea: Does not show any characteristic lesion in the central nervous system. Cerebrospinal fluid shows normal findings. Cases who come to autopsy show lesions in the basal ganglia and also in other parts of the brain.
8. Pulmonary and pleural lesions are less definite and less characteristic. Fibrinous pleurisy and rheumatic pneumonitis may occur with exudative and proliferative lesions but without definite Aschoff body.

7. History of pharyngitis or acute rheumatic fever: The 4 points are—

1. 45% of patients give positive history of pharyngitis.
2. In 10% of patients more than one member of the family may be affected.
3. In 1/3rd of cases, rheumatic fever is well preceded by throat pain.
4. 1/4 of the rheumatic fever patients may consult a doctor in underdeveloped countries.

There may be no history of sore throat especially in younger children who are poor at localizing sites of illness or this symptom may not be mentioned by the patient.

8. The 4 clinical features of streptococcal throat infection.

A. In typical cases:

1. Moderate to high fever.
2. Throat pain: A fiery red pharynx with white patches of exudate.
3. Tender swollen anterior cervical lymph nodes or may have large infected tonsils with posterior cervical lymphadenopathy.

B. Mild cases:

4. Little or no fever: The mild sore throat may not bring the patient to the doctor and yet causes rheumatic fever. The so-called 'Scarlet fever' seen in Western countries does not occur in many tropical countries.

9. Acute rheumatic fever: The 4 points are—

1. Usually comes 1 to 4 weeks after sore throat, tonsillitis
2. There may be fever of remittent type without raise over 39°C and subsiding even without treatment within 2 to 3 weeks.
3. There may be abdominal pain, very often without obvious cause. Severe epistaxis may occur.
4. The initial attack may last from 6 weeks to 3 months. It may last longer in patients with severe disease, the so-called chronic rheumatic fever.

10. Acute rheumatic fever patients may also present with the following 4 symptoms.

1. Early fatigue with vague throat symptoms
2. Only arthralgia with slight temperature
3. Affecting only smaller joints (vs bigger joints)
4. Abdominal pain.

11. Rheumatic fever can be described into 4 phases.

Phase I—Streptococcal infection—sore throat

Phase II—Asymptomatic or latent period lasting for 1 to 4 weeks

Phase III—Clinically active rheumatic fever

Phase IV—Postrheumatic fever sequelae.

12. The 4 acceptable criteria for the diagnosis of ARF with polyarthritis are:

1. Polyarthritis should involve two or more joints. Large joints of the extremities are more frequently affected but no joint is an exception to the inflammatory process. As pain and swelling subside in one joint other tends to become affected. Fleeting or migratory nature is characteristic but need not always be present. Should have at least two minor manifestations for the diagnosis of acute RF.
   The mildest form is arthralgia-joint pains without swelling. The joints are usually very painful and exquisitely tender, unlike in rheumatoid arthritis where there may be severe swelling with little tenderness. Pain is more marked than swelling and fleets from joint-to-joint. Usually the knee joints and ankle are first affected followed by those of the elbow and wrist joints. The small joints of the hands are least affected. Even if treatment is given the individual joint manifestations last for 1 to 5 days and usually all joint symptoms subside within 2 to 4 weeks. Polyarthritis does not result in permanent joint deformity. Severe polyarthritis and severe cardiac involvement seldom occur in the same patient.
2. Fever may be of remittent type.
3. Raised ESR.
4. Should be associated with high titer of antistreptolysin O (ASO) titer or some other streptococcal antibody.

13. Involvement of the joints in ARF shows diffuse delayed inflammatory, nonsuppurative nature. It has 4 characteristics.

1. Synovitis is mild and nonspecific
2. Exudative rather than proliferative
3. Healing occurs without scarring or deformity
4. Joints become normal after the disease has subsided.

14. Joint pains and fever do not present as in the textbook description in our patients. They differ as follows:

1. They need not have swelling
2. They need not affect the bigger joints
3. It need not be fleeting in nature
4. Smaller joints may also be affected.

Initial illness may be mild or short-lived. Isolated arthritis may be the presenting symptom in 14–42% of patients. Examination of fauces and throat swab should therefore be routine for all children presenting with arthritis. **Think of rheumatic fever in all cases of acute childhood arthritis.**

15. Carditis: Myocarditis is said to be present if there is endocarditis or pericarditis. Carditis may vary from a low grade in apparent inflammation to a fatal course. Carditis may be silent in many patients and may not have symptoms referable to the heart.

Unless there is associated polyarthritis or chorea, the patients with acute rheumatic fever (ARF) manifest only by carditis are frequently not recognized and in later life are found to have rheumatic heart disease without definite history of rheumatic fever. Death may result from heart failure in acute stage or permanent valvular damage may result as a serious disability. Presence of congestive cardiac failure in ARF in association with carditis always lead to chronic RHD. Less activity of carditis is noted in pregnancy.

The presence of carditis is suggested by.

1. Tachycardia: Out of proportion to the degree of fever. That is more than 20 beats rise per 1°C fever. Sleeping pulse rate differentiates tachycardia from anxiety or excitement.
2. Intensity of SI is decreased, gallop rhythm is often heard and the heart sounds may become fetal or 'tic-tac' in quality.
3. Carey-Coombs murmur: This is a short mid-diastolic apical murmur due to acute inflammation and swelling of the mitral valve in the early stage of mitral stenosis. The murmur may disappear as the inflammation resolves or develops into a more typical murmur of mitral stenosis.
   Basal ejection systolic murmur may present.
4. Mitral regurgitation is the hallmark of rheumatic carditis. Aortic insufficiency is less common and always associated with mitral insufficiency.
   A new apical systolic murmur of mitral regurgitation is caused by the dilatation of the mitral valve ring. Sometimes, murmur of the aortic regurgitation may also be heard.
   Rheumatic carditis is almost always associated with a significant murmur.
5. Arrhythmias: Prolongation of PR interval or varying degrees of heart block with dropped beats are common findings in the ECG. But these findings in the absence of clinical manifestation of carditis, such as significant murmur or cardiac enlargement are not diagnostic of carditis and have a benign prognosis. RBBB, wandering atrial pacemaker, AF, transient bigeminy may be seen.
6. Pericarditis: This occurs in about 10% of cases. May cause precordial pain and a friction rub may be heard which lasts for a week or two. ST-segment elevation is an important sign of pericarditis in ECG.
7. Cardiac enlargement: Either clinical or on X-ray or fluoroscopic evidence due to either true enlargement of the heart or pericardial effusion.
8. Frank cardiac failure: This is present in about 10% of cases. All patients with congestive cardiac failure continued to have chronic rheumatic heart disease.

16. Definitive clinical diagnosis of carditis is made when one or more of the following 4 are present.

1. Presence of an organic murmur, changing murmur—due to involvement of endocardium valvular
2. Pericardial friction rub or effusion—due to involvement of pericardium
3. Signs of congestive heart failure
4. Increase in heart size demonstrated by X-ray, ECG or Echo—due to involvement of myocardium.
   Rheumatic carditis is almost always associated with a significant murmur.

17. Rheumatic valvular disease occurs in the following order of frequency.

1. Most commonly in mitral—70%
2. Frequently in aortic—40%
3. Less frequently tricuspid—10%
4. Never affects pulmonary valve—2%?
   Mitral stenosis is more common in females (F:M-3:1), while males have higher incidence of aortic regurgitation.

18. The following 4 observations are made about the interval of time for development of carditis in RF.

1. Approximately 70% develop in the first week.
2. Approximately 85% in the first 12 weeks.
3. Approximately 100% in 6 months from the onset of first attack.
4. The prognosis is excellent and recurrences are prevented if there is no significant murmur in 6 months.

19. The term malignant rheumatic fever has been used to denote severe heart disease with the following 4 complications.

1. Rapid progression
2. Multivalvular disease
3. Gross cardiac enlargement
4. Congestive heart failure.

20. Chorea also known as Sydenham's chorea, Saint Vitus' dance, chorea minor: It is due to the rheumatic process causing inflammation of extrapyramidal system of CNS characterized by purposeless involuntary movements of face and limbs, hypotonia, and emotional instability The following 4 manifestations are observed.

1. It is a delayed manifestation of rheumatic fever. May occur 3 to 4 months after acute illness and other manifestations may or may not still be present at the time when it appears. When polyarthritis is part of the same attack, it always subsides before chorea appears. Carditis may be recognized first time when the presenting feature of RF is chorea. The majority of children with chorea subsequently develop chronic

valvular disease. Death from acute chorea is rare unlike acute carditis.

2. It affects girls more often than boys and is often associated with emotional disturbances, such as:
   - Depression
   - Weeping
   - Hysteria
   - Uncontrolled laughter
   - Relapse of chorea is seen when they become pregnant.
3. Grimacing and irregular jerky movements are seen in contradistinction to the more writhing movements of athetosis. Chorea is of gradual onset. Initially there may be nervousness and fidgety and may notice difficulty in writing, drawing, handwork, talking, walking or dancing. When the symptoms become severe, spasmodic movements extend to all parts and the patient finds difficulty in walking. Generally it affects all the 4 limbs although occasionally affects one side when it is known as hemichorea.
4. Symptoms are exaggerated by emotional disturbances and may become violent that cribs and beds should be padded to prevent injury. Symptoms subside during sleep. CNS stimulants exacerbate and sedatives suppress choreiform activity. It is important to differentiate the symptoms of Sydenham's chorea from tics, athetosis, conversion reactions, hyperkinesia and behavioral abnormalities (treatment—haloperidol 0.5 mg/8h po).

21. Following 4 observations are made with carditis and chorea.

1. No activation of carditis in pregnancy.
2. Activation and relapse of chorea is seen in pregnancy.
3. Death is common with carditis.
4. Death is rare with active chorea.

22. Following 4 observations of chorea are made with other manifestations.

1. Chorea is a delayed manifestation of rheumatic fever.
2. Polyarthritis always subsides before chorea appears.
3. Carditis may be noticed first time when the patient presents with chorea.
4. When there are no other manifestations it is called as 'pure chorea'.

23. Following 4 observations are made about subcutaneous nodules/rheumatic nodules of rheumatic fever.

1. They are painless inflammatory collections usually about the size of a pea, freely mobile unattached to the underlying skin and are found on the extensor tendons of hands and feet, the elbows, patella, scalp, spinous processes of the vertebrae.
2. They are found in about 10% of cases.
3. They are usually found late in course of the illness and often seen in those patients with significant carditis.
4. They may remain for several weeks.
   Erythema marginatum is a rare rash consisting of irregular pink rings with sharp margin and central pale area; varies in size and shape. Occurs over the trunk and proximal part of the limbs. It is a late manifestation of acute hypersensitivity.

24. Special features of RHD in India:

Rheumatic manifestations:

The pattern of rheumatic heart disease in India may be different. The symptoms described in the textbook may not be seen in our clinical practice. Jones criteria may not be applicable fully in our patients. The 4 common manifestations are:

1. Arthritis
2. Carditis
3. Chorea
4. Subcutaneous nodules
5. Erythema marginatum was seldom seen probably because of dark skin.
   Subcutaneous nodules are rarely seen in our patients.
   Chorea is seen in very few patients.
   Polyarthritis is a very important manifestation and is only significant if accompanied either by raised ESR or ASO titer especially in the presence of rheumatic valvular disease.
   Therefore, there are 4 major criteria of Jones instead of five because erythema marginatum is not seen in our patients. The 4 are—1. Arthritis 2. Carditis 3. Chorea 4. Subcutaneous nodules.

25. The diagnosis of acute rheumatic fever (ARF) can be easily missed because of the following 4 reasons.

1. Pharyngitis: Which is usually not severe can be easily ignored.
2. Arthralgia: When only arthralgia is present without any joint swelling or fleeting nature. It can also be easily missed if it affects single joint or smaller joints.
3. When it does not show precordial pain or other symptoms and signs of rheumatic carditis.
4. Low incidence of chorea and subcutaneous nodules.

26. The presentation of ARF/RHD in India is different from Western countries. The following 4 differences could be made out from the literature.

1. Arthritis is comparatively less common when compared to arthralgia and often the diagnosis is missed. It has often been said that the incidence of acute rheumatic fever is very low compared to RHD in India.

Logically this is not possible. A patient cannot have RHD unless he has had ARF. Therefore, it is said that due to some reason or other, the ARF is not being recognized or diagnosed correctly.

The incidence of chorea and subcutaneous nodules is low and erythema marginatum is practically non-recognizable because of the dark complexion of the skin. Thus only one or two major criteria are available for diagnosis.

2. Occurrence of severe symptomatic mitral stenosis in early age. The reason for this is not yet clear. This however does not mean that rheumatic mitral stenosis becoming symptomatic at a later age of 30, 40, 50 years does not occur. Why the difference between the two groups; one presenting as severe stenosis at an early age and the other at a later age is also not clear.
3. Rheumatic mitral regurgitation is a more frequent presentation than stenosis and not infrequently presents with marked cardiac enlargement and congestive heart failure solely on the basis of severe mitral incompetence.
4. Occurrence of severe tricuspid regurgitation is fairly common in India. Not infrequently, it is so severe enough to mask all of the auscultatory features of mitral stenosis.

The prevalence of ischemic heart disease is only next to rheumatic heart disease in the hospital based cardiac population.

27. In 1944, Dr TD Jones published a set of guidelines for the diagnosis of acute rheumatic fever (ARF) which is known as Jones Criteria. It is subsequently modified in 1955 and later revised in 1965 by American Heart Association last updated in 2002. The criteria were developed to minimize the over diagnosis of ARF as there is no single laboratory test, sign/symptom pathognomonic of ARF. The presence of "Two Major criteria" or '1 major and 2 minor' criteria are diagnostic of ARF.

Major criteria:
1. Carditis
2. Polyarthritis
3. Chorea
4. Subcutaneous nodules
5. Erythema marginatum.

28. Minor criteria:

1. Fever: Usually ranges from 101° to 104° F and is of relapsing type or it may run as a low-grade fever. Chills are most unusual. Fever is nonspecific but important for the diagnosis.
2. Arthralgia: Pain without objective changes in a joint.
3. Elevation of erythrocyte sedimentation rate (ESR) or C-reactive protein (CRP) or a leuckocytosis.
4. Prolongation of PR interval > 0.2 sec indicating delay in conduction at AV node.
5. Past history of rheumatic fever (RF).
6. Past history of rheumatic heart disease (RHD).

PLUS

Supportive evidence of a preceding Lancefield group A β-hemolytic streptococcal infection.

7. Positive throat culture or
8. Raised antistreptolysin-O titer (ASOT).

No single symptom or sign or laboratory test is pathognomonic of RF, so several combinations help in the diagnosis.

29. GAS infection (group A streptococcus): No single symptom or sign or laboratory test is pathognomonic, so several combinations help in the diagnosis besides raised ASO titer.

1. Culture
2. Anti-DNase base
3. Other antistreptococcal antibiotics
4. Streptococcal antigens

A rise in ASO titer provides much evidence of recent GAS infection. A greater than twofold rise in ASO titer compared with convalescent titers is diagnostic.

30. Jones criteria is designed to establish the diagnosis during the acute stage of rheumatic fever but:

1. It does not measure the rheumatic activity.
2. It does not establish the diagnosis of inactive rheumatic fever.
3. It does not establish the diagnosis of chronic rheumatic heart disease.
4. It does not predict the course and severity of the disease.

31. INVESTIGATIONS.

There is no specific laboratory test for the diagnosis of ARF. Though they are nonspecific, they are of value since they may indicate continued rheumatic inflammatory activity when clinical features are not apparent. The 4 diagnostic criteria are:

1. Raise in ESR.
2. Raise in antistreptolysin O titer (ASOT) usually above 250 Todd units. Serological evidence of recent streptococcal infection is very essential to make the diagnosis of ARF. A single titer of at least 250 Todd units in adults and at least 333 units in children over 5 years of age is considered to be increased.

3. Raise in C-reactive protein.
These are always abnormal in patients presenting with polyarthritis or acute carditis unless the patient has received corticosteroids or salicylates. These indicate the presence of inflammatory process. Other findings which indicate inflammatory reaction are leukocytosis, and increase in serum complement, mucoproteins, α- and γ-globulins.
Anemia of normocytic normochromic type, due to erythropoiesis suppression is characteristic of chronic inflammatory process of rheumatic activity.
4. Throat swab culture may show positive for streptococcal infection.
Current tools for diagnosing streptococcal illness are imperfect. The throat swab will be positive in only a third of patients infected with group A streptococcus before antibiotic treatment and in only a tenth of patients afterwards.
One should not conclude the diagnosis of rheumatic fever in the absence of serological evidence of streptococcal infection.

32. About 20% of patients in the early stage of ARF and most patients with chorea have a low or borderline ASO titer. In these situations, it is better to obtain another streptococcal antibody, such as any of the following 4 titers.

1. Antihyaluronidase (AH)
2. Antideoxyribonucleotidase (anti-DNase B titer)
3. Antistreptokinase (ASK)
4. Antistreptozyme test (ASTZ).

ASTZ is a hemagglutination reaction to a concentrate of extracellular streptococcal antigens absorbed to RBC. It is a very sensitive indicator of recent streptococcal infection. All patients with ARF have titers more than 200 units per milliliter. The low titer ASTZ can rule out the ARF in patients with isolated polyarthritis.
The anti-DNase B test detects antibodies against the deoxyribonuclease B enzyme produced by most group A streptococci.
These tests are more time consuming and expensive than the antistreptolysin O test, and should be used if clinical suspicion is high, throat cultures are negative, and the antistreptolysin O test result is borderline or low.

33. The 4 ECG changes that may be seen in rheumatic carditis are:

1. Prolongation of PR interval due to conduction defect at AV node. Second degree AV block and AV dissociation are also known to occur.
2. Arrhythmias, such as wandering atrial pacemaker, atrial fibrillation PVCs, transient bigeminy and even torsades de pointes may occur.
3. ST elevation is seen in pericarditis
4. Prolonged QT interval is suggestive of myocarditis.

34. Echocardiography with color Doppler flow is the most sensitive technique for detecting cardiac involvement.

1. Progressive mitral valve thickening
2. Progressive chordal shortening
3. Mitral or aortic incompetence or both with cusp thickening
4. Pericardial effusion or reduced ejection fraction are nonspecific.
1,2,3 are specific for acute rheumatic fever.
These findings should lead to repeat echocardiograms over the next 3 weeks, as valvular involvement follow.
Thickening of mitral valve together with chordal elongation and valve incompetence can be difficult to distinguish from a congenital myxomatous valve. However, if these findings are associated with reduced ejection fraction, in serial echocardiograms show an evolving picture, the combined changes are also specific for rheumatic fever.

35. Summary of investigations in acute childhood arthritis.

1. Full blood counts and film
2. Erythrocyte sedimentation rate
3. C-reactive protein
4. Culture of throat swab, blood, aspirated fluid (if swollen joint is aspirated)
5. Antistreptolysin O test (ASO serial titers)
6. Antinuclear antibody (ASTZ)
7. Serial anti-DNase B titers if antistreptolysin O titers are low/borderline and high suspicion
8. Viral titers (parovirus, rubella, Epstein-Barr, cytomegalovirus, hepatitis)
9. Arthrocentesis (if septic arthritis suspected)
10. X-ray of joint (to exclude trauma, tumor and infection)
If streptococcal infection or systemic juvenile chronic arthritis is suspected and X-ray chest for cardiomegaly, heart failure, infection
11. Electrocardiograph (look for prolonged PR interval)
12. Echocardiogram (if there are cardiac signs or evidence of group A streptococcal infection).
All these tests are not done routinely and selection of these tests depend on clinical presentation and high suspicion in borderline cases.

36. Course and prognosis of carditis following ARF:

Carditis involvement ranges from an asymptomatic presentation to progressive congestive heart failure and death. Heart failure is rare in acute stage, if present, it is usually due to myocarditis. The most characteristic of rheumatic carditis is endocarditis (valvular) involving mitral and aortic valve.

1. Approximately 75% of ARF attacks subside within 6 weeks, 90% within 12 weeks and less than 5% persists even after 6 months.
2. Once ARF has subsided then the frequency and recurrence depend on the severity of streptococcal infection, the duration of freedom following the last attack, presence or absence of cardiac damage caused by the first or subsequent attack.

   Cardiac damage caused by the first or subsequent attack: If the first attack is earlier than 10 years age, chances of recurrence are more. Recurrence is infrequent after the age of 20 years. The child should be carefully watched after the initial attack for any evidence of recurrence and myocardial valvular function. Recurrence of rheumatic carditis is more difficult to diagnose. They are more common in the first year of the attack and relatively rare after 20 years of age.
3. Onset may be insidious without any prodromal features. Easy fatigue or muscular pains may be the only presenting feature. In many patients with mild-to-moderate carditis, the only clue to the diagnosis may be tachycardia, easy fatigue, muscular aches and dyspnea on exertion. Cardiac murmurs and pericardial rub may not be present earlier. Murmur and rub may disappear soon in mild cases especially with early treatment.
4. Appearance of significant murmur, which was not present earlier in the absence of anemia and other physiological or hemodynamic disturbance favors carditis.
5. Cardiomegaly is present either in recurrent carditis or in moderate to severe carditis. There are many mild cases which can be picked up by echocardiogram and treated at an early stage and saved from late complications. Early picked up cases of carditis may have normal sized heart.
6. ECG may be normal. Prolonged PR interval of AV conduction defect, other arrhythmias or ST elevation of pericarditis are indications of severe form of carditis. Normal PR interval does not exclude acute carditis.
7. Early and prompt treatment can save lot of children from the sequelae.
8. Once diagnosis of rheumatic carditis is made, it is essential to follow up the child and ensure penicillin prophylaxis. Every subsequent sore throat should be treated with 10 days course of procaine penicillin. Every subsequent streptococcal infection can cause recurrence of carditis.

37. Differential diagnosis: The 4 main points are—

1. RF must be distinguished from other joint conditions that simulate rheumatic arthritis, like 'growing pains', rheumatoid arthritis, gonococcal arthritis, infectious arthritis, reactive arthritis, serum sickness, viral infections with arthritis.

   In rheumatoid arthritis joint involvement will persist and characteristic joint deformities may appear. The deformities are not seen in RF. Rheumatoid factor is characteristic of rheumatoid arthritis, which is not present in RF. Antibodies against nuclear components and other autoantibodies are absent in RF.

   Gonococcal polyarthritis may be differentiated from RF by the dramatic response to the therapeutic trial of penicillin.
2. Polyarthritis due to infective endocarditis in a patient who has already have RHD may be easily mistaken for a recurrence of ARF. Blood cultures should be done to exclude bacteremia because such infections may be masked by penicillin given early for presumed ARF. If streptococcal antibodies, e.g. ASOT are not raised, the cause of polyarthritis is not of RF and should be attributed to some other cause.
3. Cardiac conditions, such as viral myocarditis cause murmurs which should be differentiated from rheumatic carditis. It must also be distinguished from hematological disorders, such as leukemia, sickle cell anemia and other hemoglobinopathies which may produce heart murmurs. Sickle cell crisis may also be associated with joint pains, enlargement of heart and cardiac murmurs. The immediate response of arthritis to salicylates is characteristic of ARF.
4. Drug sensitivity with fever and arthritis may be mistaken for RF. This may occur after the administration of penicillin for a previous pharyngitis. Urticaria, angioneurotic edema, if present helps to differentiate from rheumatic fever.

   A common mistake is the early administration of salicylates or corticosteroids before the signs and symptoms of rheumatic fever develops. In the absence of curative agent, it is not wise to suppress the signs and symptoms of rheumatic fever until they are apparent.

38. Treatment of RF/RHD can be divided into 4 stages.

1. Acute streptococcal infection
2. Acute rheumatic fever
3. Rheumatic recurrences
4. Chronic rheumatic heart disease.

There is no specific treatment for the cure of rheumatic fever. However, good supportive therapy can reduce the mortality and morbidity of the disease.

39. Primary prophylaxis poses several logistic problems. The following are some of the problems.

1. Streptococci are usually isolated in 20–25% of cases only.
2. 0.3% of streptococci in nonepidemic and up to 3% in epidemic streptococcal throat infections are identified.
3. Clinical score assessment for screening all sore throat patients may be promising but needs to be assessed in the community setting for feasibility and cost-effectiveness.
4. Sledge-hammer method of treating all streptococcal throat infections is not cost effective.
5. Seasonal prophylaxis also poses the same problem of sledge hammer approach as the cases of other seasons may be missed.
6. Culture facilities are not widely available, and involve delay in diagnosis.
7. Rapid identification of streptococcus from sore throat swab by nonculture methods (ELISA technique) has sensitivity of 70% and specificity of 98%. But the feasibility and cost-effectiveness do not allow this method as a routine procedure.
8. Genetic marker of high prediction value to be demonstrated. HLA-DQ locus is more closely associated with susceptibility to RHD than the DR locus on class I HLA. There is increased frequency of DQW and decreasing frequency of DR2 antigens.

   D8/17-B lymphocytes alloantigen has been reported as a marker of susceptibility to rheumatic fever with sensitivity of 100% in Caucasians.

   Monoclonal antibodies β-cells alloantigen (D8/17) is detected in almost all the patients with rheumatic fever, whereas the antibody is present in less than 14% of general population. Susceptibility to rheumatic fever has also being linked with D-related human leukocyte antigen (HLA-DR)—1, 2, 3 and 4 halotypes. These genetic markers may be useful in the future to identify the susceptible individuals to rheumatic fever.

   Health education about the dangers of sore throat promote self-referral for primary prophylaxis. Thus, health education through media is the keystone of national strategy.

40. Prompt treatment of acute streptococcal infection prevents rheumatic fever if done at the very first infection. This constitutes primary prophylaxis.

Treatment of acute streptococcal infection—primary prophylaxis.

1. Benzathine penicillin G (6 lakhs,12 lakhs, 24 lakhs available). 12,00,000 IU in a single injection (deep intramuscular injection), (6,00,000 and 9,00,000 IU in children).
2. Crystalline penicillin G 12,00,000 IU (Crystalline sodium penicillin G and procaine penicillin) single IM injection (6 lakhs to 9 lakhs IU in children).
3. Penicillin G pot—2 lakhs IU 4 times a day po for 10 days (2 lakhs, 4 lakhs, 8 lakhs tablets available).
4. Penicillin V, phenoxymethyl penicillin 125 mg 4 times a day for 10 days (tablet and suspension are available).

   Anyone of the above 4 can be given.

   In penicillin sensitive patients, erythromycin 250 mg. 4 times a day for 10 days (40 mg/kg/day in children) is given.

   Sulphademidine 1g daily for more than 26 kg weight and 0.5 g daily for less than 26 kg weight

   Primary prophylaxis reduces the rate of recurrence of ARF from 70–4%

   It is generally agreed that prophylaxis should be taken at least until the age of 18 years or for 5 years after an acute attack in older persons. Tetracyclines are not given.

41. Treatment of ARF depends on the presenting symptoms with polyarthritis, carditis or chorea.

The treatment of ARF with fever, fleeting polyarthritis consists of 4 stages.

1. Bed rest: To rest the joints and hopefully to prevent carditis. All the patients should be watched for carditis.
2. Support the painful joints by pillows. Cribs and beds should be padded to prevent injury to children with exaggerated symptoms of chorea when become violent.
3. Analgesic and anti-inflammatory treatment—Salicylates 100 mg/kg/day in divided doses for 2 weeks and 75 mg/kg/day in divided doses for 4–6 weeks. The arthritis is nonerosive, rarely lasts more than 4 weeks, and responds well to aspirin and nonsteroidal anti-inflammatory drugs.
4. Antimicrobial treatment: One of the drugs recommended for the treatment of acute streptococcal infection should be given at the very start for the cases of ARF. The objective is to eradicate streptococci from the nasopharynx.

42. Guidelines for bed rest and ambulation in patients with acute rheumatic fever (ARF) depends mainly on the cardiac status.

Table H-1

Cardiac status	*Management*
1. No carditis	Bed rest for 2 weeks and gradual ambulation for 2 weeks given
2. Carditis, no enlargement	Bed rest for 4 weeks and gradual ambulation for 4 weeks
3. Carditis, with gradual enlargement	Bed rest for 6 weeks and ambulation for 6 weeks
4. Carditis with heart failure	Strict bed rest for as long as heart failure is controlled and gradual ambulation for 3 months

43. Drug treatment of ARF with carditis and/or cardiac failure consists of 4 approaches.

1. *Steroids:* Prompt corticosteroid therapy should be started in patients with unequivocal diagnosis of acute rheumatic carditis or in those children of ARF who do not respond adequately to salicylate therapy. Prednisolone 2 mg/kg/day or equivalent dose of dexamethasone is started (0.75 mg of dexamethasone = 5 mg of prednisone). Dexamethasone is preferred to prednisone because of its lesser side effects.
   The dose can be increased if the response is poor. The dose is continued for 4 weeks, after which the dose is reduced by one-third for another period of 2–3 weeks and subsequently it is tapered completing a course of 12–15 weeks. If recurrence is noticed at any stage, the dose is increased and tapering is prolonged. Steroids are preferred to salicylates.
2. *Salicylates:* 75 mg/kg/day continued for 6 weeks. Salicylates are used in those patients who cannot tolerate steroids or where the diagnosis is not unequivocal. They act as analgesic and anti-inflammatory. Acetyl salicylic acid (Aspirin) is preferred to sodium salicylate because it is better tolerated and has greater analgesic effect. Aspirin avoids extra sodium to the patient who has risk of heart failure. Aspirin 50 mg/kg divided into 4th hourly doses is given with double dose at night to avoid waking the patient is given. The treatment is continued for over 2 weeks or until the symptoms are controlled and then gradually reduced.
   Salicylates relieve symptoms but do not influence the cardiac complications. Prednisone with salicylates in high doses is the most effective treatment for severe cases.
3. *Decongestive therapy:* Required only in severe cases. Digitalis and diuretics are given.
   Digitalis should be given with caution.
4. *Penicillin:* Procaine penicillin 4 lakhs units daily for 10 days is recommended for the treatment of streptococcal infection. Prophylactic benzathine penicillin in the dose of 12 lakhs IU every three weeks is continued throughout the childhood. Every subsequent sore throat is treated with procaine penicillin for 10 days.
   Patients who have isolated persistent (rather than migratory) arthritis and group A streptococcal infection are usually classed as having poststreptococcal reactive arthritis. The relation between poststreptococcal reactive arthritis and acute rheumatic fever is debated, but as these patients are prone to subsequent attacks of acute rheumatic fever and carditis, they are usually given the same advice about antibiotic prophylaxis patients with acute rheumatic fever.

44. Treatment of chorea in ARF consists of:

1. Diazepam - IM or po:
2. Phenothiazine such as chlorpromazine and steps taken to
3. Relieve symptoms of arthritis/arthralgia
4. Reduce the likelihood of carditis.

45. Treatment of rheumatic recurrence:

Secondary prophylaxis
This is necessary in every case of RF with or without carditis. The secondary prophylaxis is given by injection benzathine penicillin 12 lakhs (6–9 lakhs in children, once in 3 weeks).

1. The treatment should be continued for at least five years after the last attack.
2. In countries like India where RF occurs even later in life, secondary prophylaxis is given till later age of 40 or 45 years.
3. Injection of benzathine penicillin is more satisfactory than oral penicillin.
4. Erythromycin should be given to those sensitive to penicillin.

WHOs seven country study including India, provided evidence that even partial or irregular prophylaxis with long-acting benzathine penicillin is better than no prophylaxis for reducing the recurrence of RF/RHD. Secondary prophylaxis is therefore mandatory to prevent further damage to the patient.

46. The limitations of secondary prophylaxis are 4.

1. 50% of patients of RHD do not give past history of RF.
2. These 50% of patients of RHD without past history of RF could not have been prevented from developing RHD by secondary prophylaxis alone.
3. Secondary prophylaxis can prevent fresh episodes of RF but does not effect the hemodynamics of an established case of RHD.
4. 60% of patients with RF have carditis residual lesions depending on the severity of carditis.

Secondary prophylaxis alone thus cannot reduce the burden of the disease.
One must realize that RHD can be prevented only by preventing the first attack of RF.

47. There are 4 points to recommend periods of maintaining prophylaxis.

1. Five years as a rule for patients without carditis.
2. Until the age of 25 years if he has carditis with disappearance of cardiac murmurs by treatment and with no permanent heart disease. Adjustment is made to 25 years, 35 years, 40 years. At least 5 years

following the onset if the patient is of 15 years age or older at the time of onset.

3. At least till the patient is 30 years old if he has rheumatic valvulitis or indefinitely for life if possible with chronic RHD.
4. At least for 5 years after the surgery or indefinitely if possible.

If these measures are maintained, rheumatic valvulitis does not undergo further aggravation, and cardiac murmurs in patients with mitral incompetence gradually diminish and may totally disappear in many cases. According to Tompkins et al, that cardiac murmurs in 70% of patients with mitral incompetence disappeared in 9 years which indicates the importance of prophylactic measures to prevent recurrence.

Injection benzathine penicillin IM is given once in 3 weeks but not once in a month as in USA. The blood dilutions of the effective drug concentrations do not maintain more than three weeks in our temperate climate. Therefore, injection should be given once in three weeks.

CHRONIC RHEUMATIC HEART DISEASE

It coins the tertiary prophylaxis of RHD.

It includes valvotomy, balloon valvuloplasty and valve replacement.

48. The course of chronic RHD is variable and depends on several factors such as the following 4.

1. The variability of duration, severity, frequency of recurrence of rheumatic inflammation.
2. The degree of scarring of valves and myocardium during the acute attack.
3. The site and severity of valvular insufficiency or stenosis.
4. The amount of valvular calcification and scarring.

49. The common sequelae of ARF with carditis are 4.

1. Mitral valve: MR, MSMR, MS alone—80%
2. Combined mitral and aortic lesions—20%
3. Aortic valve: AS and AR—20%
4. Tricuspid valve—10%

Tricuspid regurgitation results either as a primary lesion or as a result of severe pulmonary hypertension from mitral or aortic lesion.

All valves first become regurgitant and this is later followed by stenosis.

50. Center of aim in the management of RHD is left ventricular function. Chronic left ventricular overload develops in 4 phases.

1. Phase I—Early left ventricular hypertrophy (LVH)
2. Phase II—Completed left ventricular hypertrophy
3. Phase III—Decompensated but reversible myocardial dysfunction
4. Phase IV—Irreversible myocardial dysfunction.

51. There are 4 methods to evaluate left ventricular function.

1. Echocardiogram
2. Radionucleide studies
} Noninvasive
3. Cardiac catheterization
4. Angiocardiography
} Invasive

1 and 2 are noninvasive. 3 and 4 are invasive.

Surgery should not be denied on the basis of left ventricular dysfunction. Since left ventricular function improves in majority after surgery.

Surgery is not advised for asymptomatic patients.

52. Left ventricular dysfunction in mitral regurgitation (MR) has the similar features as in aortic regurgitation (AR).

The 4 likelihood developments are:

1. LV dysfunction exists with or without symptoms
2. LV dysfunction develops insidiously
3. LV dysfunction is often marked by decreased after load
4. LV dysfunction often deteriorates postoperatively.

53. There are 4 optimal points to observe for surgery in RHD.

1. LV dysfunction may exist without symptoms in MR or AR.
2. LV function determines the optimal timing for surgery.
3. Congestive cardiac failure does not always indicate irreversible myocardial damage.
4. Ejection fraction and other LV function indicators are considered.

54. Following 4 points are helpful while treating the patient with chronic RHD.

1. In tight mitral stenosis without symptoms:
   Surgery is advised irrespective of symptomatology. Patient can develop pulmonary edema at any time. Digoxin is not mandatory. Digoxin is mandatory if atrial fibrillation is present. Since digoxin can cause arrhythmia—it is not advised in all cases of mitral stenosis.
2. Surgery for MS is adviced. Closed valvotomy, balloon valvotomy.
   Balloon valvotomy is useful especially in young and unmarried woman.

Presence of opening snap (OS) means mitral valve is pliable. It responds to closed or balloon valvotomy. Results are good with balloon valvotomy since the dilatation affects all around the valve, whereas with finger dilatation, it does not affect all round.

Percutaneous balloon valvotomy is the method of choice in the pliable mitral valve without significant involvement of submitral apparatus in rheumatic mitral stenosis.

Presence of left atrial clot should be excluded before valvotomy as there is risk of embolization.

3. Mitral regurgitation or aortic regurgitation separately or in combination:
   - Valve repair or valve replacement: Valve replacement is necessary in patients with severely deformed and calcified valves with damage to subvalvular apparatus.
   - Surgery should not be delayed.
4. Bioprosthesis have limited value in children and adolescents.

   Homografts valves in aortic position have reasonable durability.

   Most patients need mechanical prosthetic devices which requires the use of long-term anticoagulant therapy with associated morbidity and mortality. Antiplatelet agents such as aspirin, dipyridamole have few side effects.

   (See the relevant chapters for further details).

Prevention of Rheumatic Heart Disease

55. Prevention of rheumatic heart disease can be discussed under 4 stages:

1. Social prophylaxis :Improving nutrition, hygiene, housing, control of overcrowding/population, eradication of poverty
2. Primary prevention :Treatment of sore throat
3. Secondary prevention :Treatment of arthralgia/arthritis
4. Tertiary prevention :Treatment after valves are affected

56. Dilemmas in social prophylaxis: It is difficult to control RHD as there is no vaccine. School health services should act vigorously. Every child with throat infection should receive appropriate antibiotics. Following points should be considered when we conduct school health camps by Indian Medical Association, social or charitable institutions.

1. It is inappropriate to focus only on prevention of RHD while conducting the school health camps.
2. Most of the school going children should have other preventable ailments of which most common are – worm infestations (85%), caries (25%), skin infection (5%), eye problems (5%), ENT problems (5%), vitamin deficiency and anemia (10%), sore throat (5–10%).
3. Therefore, it is appropriate to have comprehensive health care program for children.
4. Therefore, preventive health care must be given in the schools especially for the poor. The schools should act as primary and preventive health care centers.

The camps should have follow-up by one or two trained teachers to give treatment for the common problems in the school itself and refer to the children to the doctor when necessary. It should be continuous process than conducting health camps for one day in a year like *mela* and forgetting afterwards.

57. Dilemmas in primary prevention:

Following problems are faced in relation to primary prevention.

1. Throat swab culture: Should we do throat swab culture for all children with sore throat?–Not possible

   Is this affordable?– No

   Is it practical?—No

   Should we have facilities for typing of *Streptococcus*, if it is grown?– No
2. Should we give oral penicillin G or penicillin V, should oral penicillin is given od, bd or tds?
3. Should we give parenteral penicillin with disposable syringes?
4. What can we do if stray anaphylactic reactions occur?

   By considering the above difficulties this is not practically possible at the present day set-up. Ideal academic approach is not possible because of cost and numbers involved. It is better to treat all children with throat infection with oral penicillin, given twice a day by the teacher. The children with chronic throat infection may require antibiotics for several weeks.

Table H-2: Rheumatic prophylaxis (up to 40 years)

Above 27 kg	*Below 27 kg*
1. Benzathene penicillin Penidure, longacillin 12 lac units IM 3 wkly	1. Benzathene penicillin 6 Lac units IM 3 wkly
2. or Penicillin V-250 mg-1bid	2. or PenicillinV-125 mg-1bid
3. or Sulfadiazine 1 g/day	3. or Sulfadiazine 500 mg/day
4. Allergic to penicillin - Erythromycin 250 mg bid	4. Allergic to penicillin - Erythromycin 125 mg bid

58. Dilemmas in secondary prevention (See point H 43–45). Next dilemma is to diagnose the joint phase of RHD.

1. Many children have arthralgia without antecedent or concurrent throat infection.
2. It is rare to encounter overt arthritis. Countless children have arthralgia. In Indian scenario, recurrent episodes of arthralgia justify secondary prevention. It is rare to elicit history of overt arthritis, even in patients undergoing surgery for RHD. Overt arthritis and overt carditis are uncommon. Jones Criteria was adopted and revised to help a clinician in the Western scenario to diagnose rheumatic fever. We need to revise the criteria to decide whether we should start secondary prophylaxis in the absence of overt rheumatic activity.
3. Erythema marginatum, chorea and subcutaneous nodules are rarely seen (See H 23, 24). Overt arthritis and overt carditis are uncommon.
4. How long should secondary prevention be pursued? The period ranges from 5 years from the last episode of arthralgia/arthritis to lifelong medication. We should aim at secondary prophylaxis at least until the child leaves the school or for 5 years after the last episode of arthralgia. We rarely see active rheumatic process in fifties.

59. Dilemmas in tertiary prevention.

1. After the heart valves have been damaged, perhaps tertiary prevention might minimize further damage.
2. Dilemma related to tertiary prevention is the question of etiology of mitral valve prolapse syndrome (MVPS). In the Western context, it is considered to be due to myxomatous degeneration of the valve which is not common in Indian patients.
3. In Indian scenario, an ejection click in mitral area with or without a systolic murmur is found in several poor children.
4. In patients undergoing surgery for MVPS or mitral incompetence, subjected to valve repair or replacement have no evidence of myxomatous degeneration. Hence it is suspected in India, MVPS is a *forme frustes of RHD*. Therefore, penicillin prophylaxis is preferable.

RHEUMATIC PROPHYLAXIS

1. All cases rheumatic heart disease
2. S/P PTMC (Percutaneous Transluminal Mitral Commissurotomy)
3. S/P valve replacement surgery for RHD—MVR, TVR, AVR
4. S/P valve repair surgery for RHD—MV repair, TV repair

Concluding the debate on prevention of RHD, it is suggested that RHD may be declared as an infectious disease in its throat phase and wages war against streptococcus. Every nation is spending more on warfare than welfare while almost half of the humanity is deprived of basic needs of life. Priorities are still prevailing over like prevention of water-born diseases (more than 2 lakhs villages are deprived of protected drinking water supply), tuberculosis, malaria, filaria, and implementation of immunization programs, etc. Eradication of poverty, ignorance can prevent not only RHD but other preventable diseases too. In India, where the health is remembered only when it is lost, prevention of RHD is a dream. Yet, it is surprising to note that the number of RHD is falling in comparison with growing population.

I Valvular Heart Disease

MITRAL STENOSIS

1. Introduction

1. Mitral valve apparatus consists of :
   i. Anterior and posterior leaflets
   ii. Mitral annulus
   iii. Chorda tendinea
   iv. Papillary muscles
2. Mitral stenosis (MS)—usually valvular and more rarely caused by fusion of subvalvular components.
3. Mitral regurgitation (MR) can occur due to malfunctioning of any of the four components.
4. Mitral valve prolapse (MVP) occurs when one or both mitral leaflets extend across the plane of the mitral valve annulus into the left atrium during systole.

2. 4–6 cm^2 is the normal size of mitral orifice in an adult. Mitral stenosis is caused by the fusion of two valve cusps along their margins extending from the valve ring to the periphery toward the center.

3. Reduction to 1/4 of mitral orifice, i.e. 1 cm^2 rises the left atrial pressure by 25 mm Hg to maintain normal cardiac output. Consequently, dyspnea, fatigue, pulmonary hypertension and right ventricular failure set in. Hemodynamic abnormalities develop even when the orifice is reduced to below 2 cm^2.

4. The 4 causes of mitral stenosis are:

1. Rheumatic: Most common cause.
2. Congenital: Rare parachute mitral valve—Single papillary muscle to which chordae to both leaflets attach, results in MS or MR. Systemic diseases can cause valvular fibrosis.
3. Connective tissue disease: SLE, RA.
4. Carcinoid, myxoma.
5. Mucopolysaccharidosis.
6. Healed endocarditis.
7. Severe annular calcification.
8. Prior anorectic drug use.

The patients with history of rheumatic fever between 5–12 years of age usually exhibit clinical features between 25–31 years. But we see rheumatic valve diseases still early in India.

Mitral stenosis is the most common valvular lesion due to rheumatic heart disease.

5. Rheumatic mitral stenosis is less common than mitral regurgitation in the pediatric age group.

Juvenile mitral stenosis constitutes 1/4th of all rheumatic mitral stenosis.

6. The 4 steps that gradually set in the development of dyspnea in mitral stenosis are:

1. Increase in left atrial pressure.
2. Increase in pulmonary venous pressure.
3. Increase in pulmonary capillary pressure.
4. Decrease in pulmonary compliance resulting in exertional dyspnea.

When dyspnea precipitates in early stages the blood flow increases across the mitral orifice which in turn increases left atrial pressure. Increase in heart rate shortens diastole proportional to the systole and so the time taken to the left atrium to push the blood across the mitral valve decreases. Any cause that increases heart rate further increases left atrial pressure. In general, once symptoms develop, there follows a period of about 10 years before they become debilitating. Once, significant limiting symptoms develop, the 10 years survival rate is < 15%.

7. The 4 stages that gradually set in, finally result in pulmonary arterial hypertension. The clinical features and hemodynamic changes of mitral stenosis depend on the level of pulmonary arterial pressure.

1. Increase in left atrial pressure causes increase in backward pressure which results in
   ↓
2. Increase in pulmonary venous pressure which causes
   ↓
3. Increase in pulmonary arteriolar constriction which causes
   ↓
4. Organic obliterative changes in the pulmonary vascular bed that results in the pulmonary arterial hypertension.

Mitral stenosis causes obstruction to the flow of blood across the mitral valve during left ventricular diastole, which results in increase in left atrial pressure. Since there are no valves between the left atrium and the pulmonary veins, the increased left atrial pressure is transmitted to pulmonary veins. The increased pulmonary venous pressure results in pulmonary capillary engorgement and pulmonary congestion which causes dyspnea, the most common symptom of mitral stenosis. The pulmonary arterial pressure increases to maintain the forward flow from the pulmonary artery to the left side of the heart. Clinically, the pulmonary arterial hypertension is recognized by accentuation of pulmonary second sound. When the pulmonary arterial pressure exceeds more than 50 mm Hg in mitral stenosis or with any valvular lesion, right ventricular pressure increases. Right ventricular end-diastolic pressure usually increases as a compensatory mechanism since it is the right ventricle, which has to maintain the pulmonary pressure as well as the flow.

8. The 4 features that results from severe pulmonary hypertension in mitral stenosis are:

1. Pulmonary incompetence.
2. Increase in the right ventricular pressure—RVH.
3. Tricuspid incompetence.
4. Increase in right atrial pressure.

All can result in right heart failure.

9. The 4 associated conditions of mitral stenosis where left ventricular diastolic pressure increases are:

1. Mitral regurgitation.
2. Aortic valve disease.
3. Systemic hypertension.
4. Ischemic heart disease.

Increase in left ventricular pressure results in impairment of left ventricular function and/or reduces left ventricular compliance.

Left ventricular diastolic pressure is normal in isolated mitral stenosis.

10. The 4 important general points to be noted in the history of mitral stenosis are:

1. It is generally rheumatic in origin.
   50% of mitral stenosis patients give history of one or two attacks of rheumatic fever.
2. 40% with rheumatic heart disease may show pure or predominant mitral stenosis.
3. 2/3rd of all mitral stenosis patients are females.
4. Most frequent complaints in symptomatic patients with mitral stenosis are:
   a. Dyspnea.
   b. Fatigue.
   c. Palpitation.
   d. Hemoptysis.

Rapid ventricular response aggravates pulmonary congestion and cause dyspnea and fatigue.
Fatigue sometimes may be more severe than dyspnea. Fatigue is common due to reduced cardiac output.
Atrial fibrillation causes palpitation, which can be paroxysmal or sustained.
Pulmonary venous hypertension causes hemoptysis due to rupture of small bronchial veins.

11. In case of hemoptysis ask whether it is:

1. Mixed or pure.
2. Quantity.
3. Color.
4. Frequency.

If the blood is dark it arises from the submucosal bronchial veins due to high left atrial pressure caused by mitral stenosis. If it is associated with dyspnea or pleuritic pain, one should consider pulmonary infarction.

12. The 4 less frequent symptoms in mitral stenosis are:

1. Chest pain—can be due to pulmonary hypertension, pulmonary embolus or underlying coronary disease or emboli in the coronaries.
2. Hoarseness—due to enlarged left atrium compressing the left recurrent laryngeal nerve.
3. Stroke
4. Seizure } from systemic emboli to the central nervous system.

13. Hoarseness without obvious upper respiratory infection: This is Ortner's syndrome or cardio-vocal syndrome.

1. It is due to pressure of dilated left atrium on
   ↓
2. Enlarged pulmonary artery which in turn cause
   ↓
3. Pressure on the peribronchial lymph nodes which in turn
   ↓
4. Compress the left recurrent laryngeal nerve

14. The 4 important signs in general examination of mitral stenosis are:

1. Cyanosis—peripheral and facial cyanosis in severe mitral stenosis. The patient may show mitral facies with malar flush. Face looks pinched and blue.
2. Jugular venous pulse—neck veins will be distended if right ventricular failure is present. Prominent 'A' wave suggests tricuspid stenosis or pulmonary hypertension with sinus rhythm.
   Systolic pulsation of deep jugular veins indicate tricuspid regurgitation. When atrial fibrillation develops 'A' wave is absent and shows a single expansion during systole. (CV wave)
3. Radial pulse—tachycardia, with low volume.
   Irregular pulse with pulse deficit suggests atrial fibrillation.
4. Blood pressure—either normal or slightly low.

15. The 4 important findings on inspection and palpation of precordium in mitral stenosis are:

1. Accentuated first heart sound, which may be palpable with severe mitral stenosis but with pliable valve leaflets.
   Pulmonary second sound may be palpable in the second and third left intercostal space just left to the sternal border when pulmonary hypertension is present.
2. Apex beat is tapping.
3. Left parasternal heave is present in right ventricular enlargement.
4. Diastolic thrill is present at the apex particularly in the left lateral recumbent position and has a quality that stimulates a purring cat.

16. The 4 cardinal signs of mitral stenosis on auscultation are:

1. *Loud first heart sound*: Normally mitral valve closes at the end of diastole when the ventricular filling is complete. Whereas in mitral stenosis the valve remains open at the end of diastole and it is forcibly shut by the raise of pressure during left ventricular systole. So it closes rapidly resulting in loud first heart sound.
2. *Opening snap*: It is a loud sound heard just after the second sound. It results from high left atrial pressure that forces the mitral valve to open rapidly when the ventricle relaxes. The left atrial pressure is only slightly raised in mild stenosis so the opening snap is late. The left atrial pressure is considerably high in severe stenosis, so opening snap occurs early.
   If the mitral valve is rigid or calcified, the first sound is not loud and the opening snap is absent. So, opening snap indicate mobile mitral valve.
3. *Mitral diastolic murmur*: It is a low pitched rumbling murmur heard at the apex. It is caused by blood

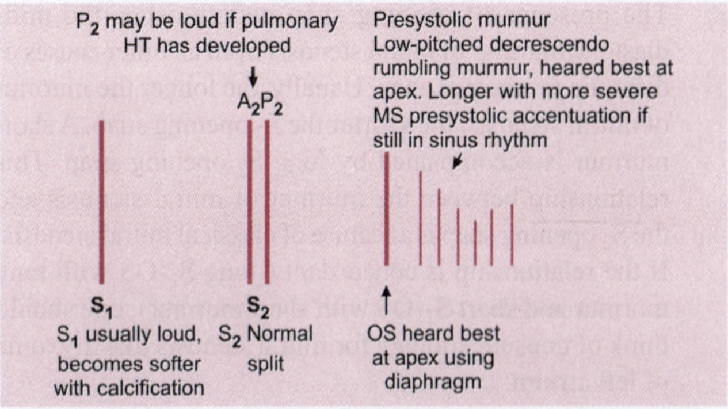

Fig. I-1: Auscultatory findings in mitral stenosis longer with more severe

passing through the stenosed mitral valve when there is pressure gradient between the left atrium and left ventricle. Diastolic murmur is short in mild stenosis and is long in severe stenosis. (No pressure gradient exists in the normal heart and pressure equalizes rapidly when the mitral valve is opened).
4. *Presystolic murmur*: It is caused by atrial systole and therefore immediately precede first sound. It is due to increased blood flow across the stenosed mitral valve during atrial contraction. If atrial fibrillation develops, there could be no effective contraction of atria, so there is no presystolic murmur but slight presystolic accentuation of diastolic murmur may be heard. The late diastolic accentuation is always present in the presence of mitral stenosis. Absence of late diastolic accentuation is against the diagnosis of dominant mitral stenosis.

17. The 4 points to be observed about the heart sounds in mitral stenosis are:

1. *Intensity*: The first sound is generally loud and snapping since the mitral valve does not close until the left ventricular pressure reaches the level of elevated left atrial pressure.
2. *Opening snap*: It is audible at just medial to the apex but may also be heard at the left sternal border or at the base, better heard during expiration in the left lateral recumbent position. It follows the pulmonary valve closure sound. It tends to be short 0.04–0.06 sec in severe stenosis and 0.10–0.12 sec in mild to moderate stenosis. The closer the opening snap to the second sound, the more sever the mitral stenosis. Intensity of the first sound and opening snap depends on the mobility of the mitral valve.
3. *Split*: In patients with pulmonary hypertension, pulmonary component of the second sound is often loud and both the components are closely split.
4. *Ejection sound*: Pulmonary ejection click is commonly heard with severe pulmonary hypertension and severe dilatation of pulmonary artery.

The presence of opening snap distinguishes the mid-diastolic murmur of mitral stenosis from all other causes of diastolic murmur at apex. Usually, the longer the murmur of mitral stenosis, the shorter the S_2 opening snap. A short murmur is accompanied by long S_2 opening snap. This relationship between the murmur of mitral stenosis and the S_2 opening snap is a feature of classical mitral stenosis. If the relationship is concordant (long S_2-OS with long murmur and short S_2-OS with short murmur), one should think of unusual etiology for mitral stenosis like myxoma of left atrium.

18. The loud first heart sound is usually caused by the mitral stenosis. Immediate attention is called to the loud first sound because this is the easiest physical sign to make out. Apart from this, it is often distinguishes mitral stenosis from other causes of mid-diastolic murmur at apex (Austin-Flint murmur) where the S_1 is diminished. A loud S_1 indicates a pliable, non-calcific valve. When the body of the anterior leaflet is mobile, loud S_1 is present in spite of calcification and immobility of posterior leaflet.

The following possibilities should be considered when the first heart sound is not loud in mitral stenosis.

1. Calcific mitral stenosis.
2. Mid-diastolic murmur due to Austin-Flint or severe pure mitral regurgitation.
3. Severe subvalvular fusion with fibrous immobile valve.
4. Associated mitral regurgitation.
5. Left atrial myxoma.
6. Associated severe aortic regurgitation.
7. Severe right ventricular hypertrophy with masked left ventricular events.
8. Associated aortic stenosis, coronary artery disease, cardiomyopathy with elevated LVEDP.

19. Observe the 4 features of the diastolic murmur in mitral stenosis.

1. The diastolic murmur is localized to a small area at or near the apex, better heard in left lateral recumbent position with 'bell' whereas the opening snap and loud first sound are widely distributed.
2. It is mid-diastolic/presystolic, rough and rumbling (low pitched).
3. Relation to physiological acts: Accentuated during expiration. Exercise accentuates it. In mild mitral stenosis, patient should be examined after exercise as it increases the cardiac output and so increases the pressure gradient and intensity of murmur.
4. Accompanying features:
   - Dyspnea/paroxysmal nocturnal dyspnea/orthopnea
   - Diastolic thrill
   - Loud S1
   - Opening snap
   - Right ventricular hypertrophy
   - Pulmonary hypertension
   - Atrial fibrillation
   - Absence of left ventricular hypertrophy.

All valvular lesions can sometimes be 'silent' with no murmur. The most common of these is mitral stenosis and in most of these, the bell of the stethoscope is not over the point of maximal impulse. It is always wise to palpate the maximal impulse first, a localized spot, which may be size of a 1/4 of an inch, use the bell where the diagnostic diastolic murmur is heard.

The murmur of mitral stenosis being low pitched is better heard with the bell than with the diaphragm. This feature is important because the high frequency murmur of aortic regurgitation, which is also heard at the apex is best heard with the diaphragm. It is inferred that the diastolic murmur better heard with the diaphragm means aortic regurgitation and the one better heard with the bell means mitral stenosis provided the diaphragm and bell are in good condition.

In a mild mitral stenosis why a mid-diastolic murmur occurs in some and presystolic murmur in other patients is not known. Probably, it is related to the health of left atrium, geometry of left ventricular inflow and the nature of subvalvular apparatus.

20. The normal flow across the mitral and tricuspid valves is noiseless. Any disturbance in the normal flow pattern across the atrioventricular valves can result in turbulence and there by a murmur.

Diastolic murmurs at apex are caused by various mechanisms. The following 4 mechanisms are examples:

1. By narrowing of mitral valve or left ventricular inflow.
2. Increased inflow across the AV valve.
3. Mechanisms that interfere with mitral valve opening. Austin-flint murmur with severe aortic regurgitation.
4. Ventricular aneurysm with narrow neck.

21. There are 4 causes of narrowing of mitral valve or left ventricular inflow.

1. Mitral stenosis.
2. Left atrial myxoma.
3. Hypertrophic cardiomyopathy (narrowing inflow cavity).
4. Constriction of AV groove as in constrictive pericarditis (A rare congenital anomaly—cor triatoma can also causes).

22. There are 4 causes, which increases flow across the AV valve giving rise to diastolic murmur.

1. Left to right shunt (ASD, VSD, PDA).
2. Severe mitral regurgitation.

3. Hyperkinetic circulatory states (Anemia, thyrotoxicosis, pregnancy).
4. Chronic complete heart block.

23. There are 4 causes of diastolic murmur arising some where else but heard at apex.

1. Aortic regurgitation.
2. Tricuspid stenosis.
3. Tricuspid flow murmur of ASD.
4. Ebstein's anomaly of tricuspid valve.

24. The presystolic murmur is usually absent after the onset of atrial fibrillation but is not a rule. The persistence of presystolic murmur in atrial fibrillation is surprising when it is realized that the genesis of presystolic murmur is not dependent on atrial contraction alone. It depends on atrial contraction, persistent AV gradient and left ventricular constriction in presystole reducing the mitral funnel.

There are 4 causes where presystolic murmur in mitral stenosis can be absent.

1. Atrial fibrillation.
2. Mild mitral stenosis.
3. Bradycardia with prolonged PR interval.
4. Elevated left ventricular end-diastolic pressure (left ventricular dysfunction).

25. There are 4 mechanisms which influence the length of murmur in mitral stenosis.

1. Cardiac output.
2. Heart rate and rhythm.
3. Left atrial pressure.
4. Left ventricular end-diastolic pressure (LVEDP).

With a normal heart rate, normal cardiac output and LVEDP, the longer the murmur the more severe the stenosis.

26. In the presence of severe aortic regurgitation, the apical diastolic murmur may be due to Austin-Flint murmur or mitral stenosis. The following accompanying features will help to distinguish one from the other.

Table I-1

Mitral stenosis	*Austin-Flint murmur*
1. Occurs with organic mitral stenosis with rheumatic heart disease	Occurs only with severe aortic regurgitation, Usually non-rheumatic. It is due to heavy jet of aortic regurgitation impinging on the anterior leaflet of mitral valve preventing adequate opening of the valve and creating turbulence of the flow from left atrium to left ventricle in diastole
2. History dyspnea is the presenting symptom	Asymptomatic for long time or palpitation is the presenting symptom
3. Localized to apex	Aortic regurgitation murmur is best heard along the left sternal border
4. Signs of pulmonary hypertension are common	
5. First sound is accentuated	
6. Opening snap is diagnostic	
7. Diastolic thrill is common	
8. Third heart sound of left ventricular origin never occurs	

27. The 4 commonly associated lesions seen with mitral stenosis are:

1. *Mitral regurgitation:* Apical systolic murmur is heard. Third heart sound at the apex often signifies mitral regurgitation. A presystolic murmur and a loud first sound are against mitral regurgitation. If the first heart sound and/or opening snap are soft or absent it is probable that mitral regurgitation and/or calcification of stenosed valve are present.
2. *Tricuspid regurgitation:* Functional tricuspid regurgitation may produce pansystolic murmur heard along the left sternal border accentuated by inspiration, diminished by expiration or valsalva maneuver.
3. *Pulmonary hypertension and pulmonary regurgitation:* Pulmonary component of the second sound is loud and closely split. Pulmonary ejection sound is heard in severe dilatation of pulmonary artery. When pulmonary regurgitation develops—Graham-Steel murmur—a high pitched diastolic decrescendo blowing murmur along the left sternal border is heard.
4. *Right ventricular failure:* Third heart sound heard along the left sternal border may originate from the right ventricle. Right ventricular enlargement may cause a clockwise rotation and form the cardiac apex, which may be mistaken for left ventricular enlargement. Left parasternal heave of right ventricular enlargement is seen.

28. The 4 main complications of mitral stenosis are:

1. Atrial fibrillation.
2. Embolism.
3. Hemoptysis.
4. Cardiac failure
   a. Acute pulmonary edema
   b. Chronic congestive cardiac failure.

29. The 4 other complications of mitral stenosis are:

1. Infection—Pulmonary infection: Recurrent bronchitis, bronchopneumonia, lobar pneumonia, etc.
   Infective endocarditis is rare in pure mitral stenosis but common with associated mitral regurgitation.
2. Pressure—dysphagia due to pressure on esophagus, hoarseness of voice due to compression of left recurrent laryngeal nerve.
3. Massive thrombus in left atrium.
4. Angina pectoris.

30. The 4 sequence of events result from increase in pulmonary vascular resistance which increases back pressure.

1. Pulmonary incompetence.
2. Increase in right ventricular pressure.
3. Tricuspid incompetence—pulmonary congestion temporarily reduces.
   Episodes of hemoptysis also decreases pulmonary congestion temporarily.
4. Right ventricular failure.

31. The following 4 signs are caused by right ventricular failure.

1. Edema feet.
2. Hepatomegaly.
3. Ascites.
4. Pleural effusion—particularly right sided pleural effusion.

32. Increase in pulmonary vascular resistance causes fibrous thickening of the walls of alveoli and pulmonary capillaries which result in:

1. Reduction of vital capacity.
2. Reduction of total lung capacity.
3. Reduction of maximal breathing capacity.
4. Reduction of oxygen uptake per unit of ventilation. In severe mitral stenosis oxygen uptake fails to rise during exertion causing severe dyspnea.

33. The 4 factors that cause hemoptysis in mitral stenosis are:

1. Mainly from rupture of pulmonary veins secondary to pulmonary venous hypertension. Frequently occurs in patients with increased left atrial pressure without increase in pulmonary vascular resistance and is never fatal.
2. Pulmonary edema in cardiac failure.
3. Pulmonary infarction from embolism.
4. Chronic bronchitis.

34. The 4 conditions where embolic complications are frequent in mitral stenosis are:

1. Atrial fibrillation.
2. Unstable rhythms.
3. Reduced cardiac output.
4. Older patients.

Systemic embolization may be the presenting complaint in an asymptomatic mild mitral stenosis patient. Freshly formed clots are usually dislodged as evidenced by absence of thrombi in left atrium during operation with history of embolization than in those without this complication. Chances of recurrent embolic episodes are frequent with history of one or more attacks of systemic emboli.

35. The 4 common sites of systemic emboli.

1. Brain.
2. Kidneys.
3. Spleen.
4. Extremities.

36. The 4 conditions when a large pedunculated thrombus or a free floating clot may rarely obstruct the stenotic mitral orifice as a 'ball-valve' thrombus which may produce:

1. Syncope.
2. Angina.
3. Intermittant auscultatory changes.
4. Changes in auscultatory signs with change in position as seen in left atrial myxoma.

37. The 4 causes of chest pain in mitral stenosis.

1. Pulmonary hypertension
2. Myocardial ischemia secondary to
3. Coronary embolization or coronary atherosclerosis
4. 'Ball-valve' thrombi
   Chest pain occurs in 10% of patients with severe mitral stenosis.

38. The 4 early roentgenographic signs in mitral stenosis.

1. Straightening of left border of cardiac silhouette.
2. Dilatation of upper lobe pulmonary veins.
3. Backward displacement of esophagus by the enlarged left atrium seen in right anterior oblique barium swallow.
4. Prominence of the main pulmonary arteries.

The left atrial hypertension, which results in left atrial enlargement brings about all these above changes. Since the left atrium occupies a position between pulmonary artery segment and left ventricle, left atrial enlargement causes straightening of left border on the standard postero-anterior view of chest X-ray.

(Ref. Fig. P-9). Left atrial enlargement is apparent with a double density along the right heart border.

39. The 4 roentgenographic signs in severe mitral stenosis: All chambers and vessels upstream to the stenosed valve are prominent including:

1. Two atria.
2. Pulmonary arteries and veins.

3. Right ventricle.
4. Superior venacava.

In mild to moderate stenosis, the overall heart size does not enlarge.

In long-standing severe mitral stenosis valves undergo calcification. In rare cases, left atrial calcification may be seen.

40. The 4 pulmonary changes that are seen in X-ray chest when chronic pulmonary venous hypertension develops in mitral stenosis are:

1. Kerley B lines: (Ref. Fig. P-10)
   a. They are fine dense opaque horizontal lines, which are perpendicular to the pleura at the base of the lungs.
   b. They are more prominent in the lower and mid-lung fields.
   c. They occur when resting left atrial pressure reaches 20 mm Hg or above which in turn increases the pulmonary capillary pressure. It exceeds oncotic pressure of plasma proteins which ranges from 20–25 mm Hg.
   d. It results in distension of interlobular septa and lymphatics with edema. Fluid will accumulate in the interstitial spaces of the lungs.
2. As the pulmonary arterial pressure rises, the smaller pulmonary arteries become thin and weaken first in the lower, later in the mid and finally in the upper lung fields. Rupture of them cause hemoptysis. Hemosiderin deposits occur in the lungs in those who have multiple hemoptysis.
3. Deposition of hemosiderin containing macrophages fill in the air spaces, coalesce resulting in a fine, diffuse nodulation most prominent in the lower lung fields.
4. Ossified nodules are prominent in the lower lung fields and are caused by true lamellar bone seen in the areas of chronic interstitial edema.
   The vessels become prominent and the blood redistributes from the bases to the apices of the lungs.

41. The 4 following abnormalities are to be identified in ECG of mitral stenosis.

1. P-wave becomes wide, well seen in LII, V1.
   Notched P 'mitral' in left atrial enlargement. P is more than 2.5 mm wide.
   When severe pulmonary hypertension or tricuspid stenosis complicates, P waves become tall and peaked in LII—P 'Pulmonale'—more than 2.5 mm height, when right atrium is enlarged.
   In severe cases when left atrium and right atrium are enlarged P is more than 2.5 mm tall and wide (biatrial enlargement).
2. Right axis deviation in severe pulmonary hypertension.
3. Right ventricular hypertrophy in severe pulmonary hypertension. R:S in V 1 > 1:1.
4. When atrial fibrillation develops, fibrillary F waves are seen. They are coarser and undulated in mitral stenosis than in coronary artery disease.
   'F' fibrillary waves are better seen in V 1.
   QRS may be normal or ventricular tachyarrhythmia may be seen.

When left ventricular enlargement is present in mitral stenosis, suspect an additional lesion, such as mitral regurgitation, aortic valve disease, hypertension, etc.

42. The 4 characteristic features in echocardiogram in mitral stenosis are:

1. The characteristic change is the decrease in E–F slope producing a square-wave configuration due to failure of anterior leaflet to float back to midposition in mid-diastole. This slope is related to the severity of mitral stenosis.
2. Anterior and posterior leaflets maintain a fixed position throughout diastole. They do not separate widely, i.e. less than 15 mm.
3. Multilayered echos or thickening of echo pattern is seen in calcification and thickening of mitral valve.
4. Mitral orifice area is best determined with two dimensional echocardiography.

Color Doppler provides estimation of diastolic gradient which helps to calculate mitral valve area. It also gives information on flow patterns.

Echocardiogram is the most sensitive, reliable and specific noninvasive method for diagnosing mitral stenosis. In isolated rheumatic mitral stenosis, the echocardiogram is so reliable that even cardiac catheterization is often not required in the evaluation of severity of stenosis. Serial echocardiograms help to follow the clinical course before and after surgery.

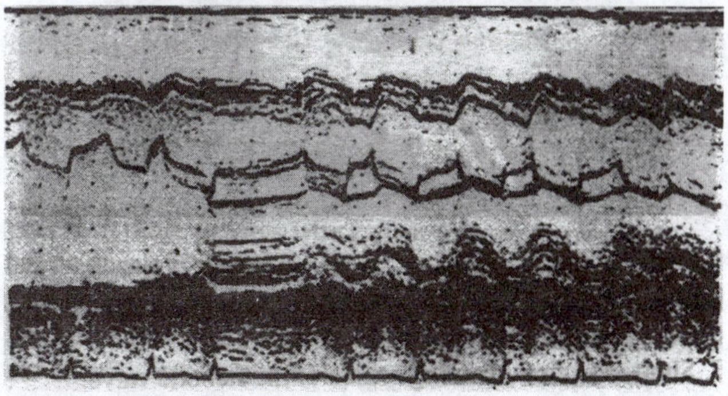

Fig. I-2: Mitral stenosis: M-mode echocardiogram of a patient showing decreased pliability of cusps (D-E amplitude). This type of mitral stenosis is benefited by valvotomy

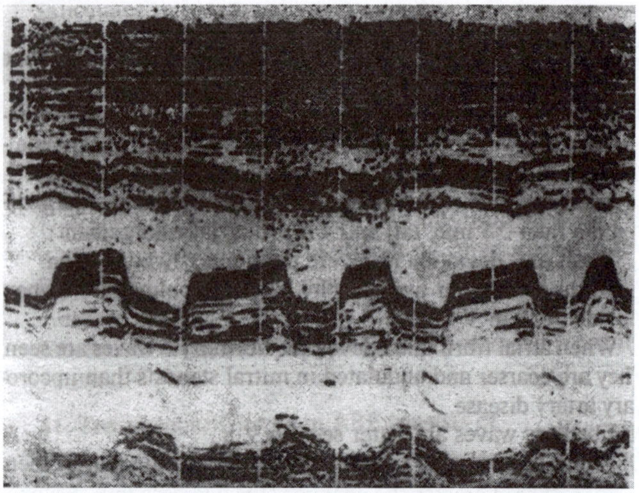

Fig. I-3: M-mode echocardiogram of a patient with mitral stenosis note the broadband of echoes moving parallel to the anterior mitral leaflet indicative of severe fibrosis or calcification. This type of mitral stenosis needs valve replacement

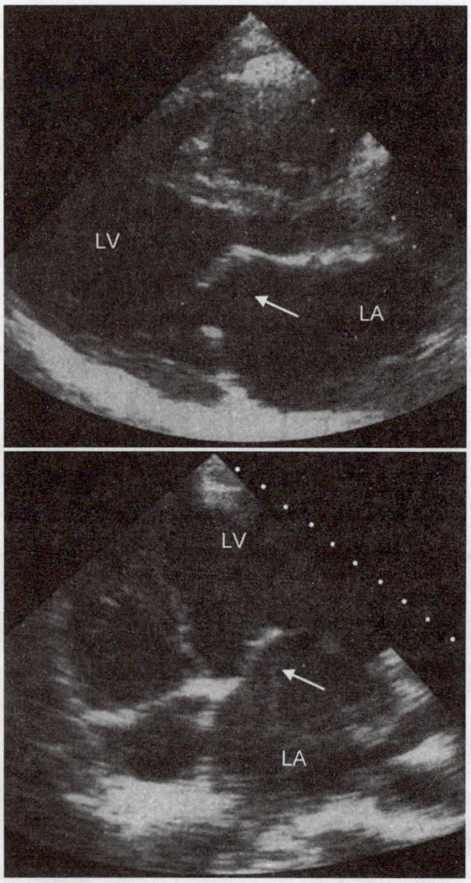

Fig. I-4: A. Two-dimensional echocardiogram; long-axis view showing domed mitral valve. B. Short-axis view showing orifice of the stenotic valve

43. The 4 following points are noted about the mitral valve in echocardiogram.

1. Thickening and restriction of diastolic movement of the leaflets.
2. Fusion of the commissuries and shortening. Fusion and thickening of chordae tendinae.
3. Size of the mitral orifice.
4. Mobility of the mitral valve—whether it is heavily calcified.

44. The following are noted in the 4 chamber view of echocardiogram.

1. Left atrial dimensions.
2. Right ventricular enlargement.
3. Right atrial enlargement.
4. Left ventricular enlargement.

45. One can identify the following 4 conditions of non-rheumatic mitral valve obstruction by echocardiogram.

1. Left atrial myxoma
2. Left atrial tumor.
3. Left atrial thrombi
4. Nidus of infection on mitral valve in bacterial endocarditis.

46. Determine the following 4 signs by cardiac catheterization in mitral stenosis.

1. Gradient across the mitral valve. It is obtained by simultaneous recording of:
   i. Pulmonary capillary wedge pressure.
   ii. Left atrial pressure.
   iii. Left ventricular pressure.
   iv. Cardiac output.

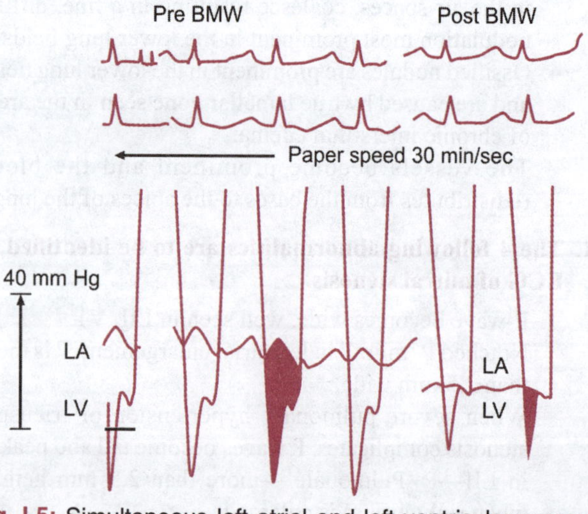

Fig. I-5: Simultaneous left atrial and left ventricular pressure recording in a patient showing significant transmitral gradient before valvuloplasty and complete disappearance of gradient after balloon valvuloplasty

2. Other valvular lesions.
3. Left ventricular function.
4. Status of the coronary arteries.

47. Left ventricular angiocardiography combined with aortography in mitral stenosis helps to determine the 4 associated lesions, such as:

1. Mitral regurgitation.
2. Aortic stenosis.
3. Aortic regurgitation.
4. Left ventricular dysfunction.

Left atrial thrombus and tumor can be detected by angiocardiography. Left sided catheterization and angiocardiography are indicated in patients who have redeveloped serious symptoms after mitral valvotomy.

48. Nuclear scan in mitral stenosis is useful to assess the left ventricular function by the following 4 measurements:

1. Ejection fraction (EF).
2. Left ventricular end-diastolic volume (LVEDV).
3. Stroke volume.
4. Diastolic filling rate before and after exercise.

An important contribution of nuclear scan in mitral stenosis is to obtain resting and exercise measurements before and after surgery during follow-up periods.

49. Differentiate the following 4 points of mitral regurgitation from mitral stenosis.

1. First heart sound is diminished in regurgitation.
2. Pansystolic murmur of at least grade III/VI.
3. Protodiastolic or ventricular gallop sound (third heart sound) is frequently audible at the apex.
4. Evidence of left ventricular enlargement on physical examination, X-ray and ECG.

50. The following 4 points of primary pulmonary hypertension differentiate it from mitral stenosis.

Frequent in young woman.

1. Opening snap is absent.
2. Diastolic, rough and rumbling murmur is absent.
3. No left atrial enlargement.
4. Pulmonary artery wedge pressure and left atrial pressure are normal.

51. The following 4 points of atrial septal defect differentiate from mitral stenosis.

Clinical, radiological, ECG evidence of right ventricular enlargement are mistaken for atrial septal defect—but it differs by:

1. Fixed and widely split second sound—it may be mistaken for opening snap.
2. Diastolic flow murmur of tricuspid valve—it may be mistaken for mitral diastolic murmur.
3. Absence of left atrial enlargement in X-ray, ECG and echo.
4. Absence of Kerley-B lines favor atrial septal defect.

52. One must look for the mitral stenosis in the following situations:

1. All patients with rheumatic heart disease, aortic valve or pulmonary valve disease.
2. All patients with atrial fibrillation.
3. All patients with loud first heart sound with normal heart rate and PR interval.
4. All patients with unexplained pulmonary hypertension.
5. All patients with peripheral embolism.
6. All patients with unexplained left atrial enlargement or right ventricular hypertrophy by ECG.
7. All patients with unexplained dyspnea.
8. All patients with bronchial asthma.

Exercise should be used routinely when mitral stenosis is suspected. Exercise brings in or increase the murmur by the increase in heart rate and blood flow secondary to the rise in cardiac output.

53. The 4 principles in the management of asymptomatic mitral valve disease in an adolescent are:

1. Rheumatic fever prophylaxis with penicillin should be continued until 35 years of age.
2. Prophylaxis for infective endocarditis, e.g. before dental procedures, bronchoscope, etc.
3. Detect and treat the accompanying anemia, infections, etc.
4. Strenuous occupation should be avoided to prevent premature retirement. Therefore, vocational counseling is needed.

54. The 4 principles in the management of symptomatic patients of mitral stenosis are:

1. Restriction of salt.
2. Oral diuretics.
3. Digitalis is useful for reducing the manifestations of right sided heart failure.
   Digitalis is not useful in pure stenosis with sinus rhythm. Digitalis is useful in slowing the ventricular rate in atrial fibrillation or flutter. Add propranolol 10 to 20 mg qid when digitalis could not control ventricular rate in atrial fibrillation in the absence of ventricular failure. β-blockers are useful in controlling heart rate than digoxin even there is heart failure. Digoxin is useful in atrial fibrillation.
4. Treatment of atrial fibrillation.
   If atrial fibrillation is of recent origin and mitral stenosis is not severe, reversion to sinus rhythm by electrical counter shock or quinidine is useful. Conversion to sinus rhythm is rarely helpful in severe mitral stenosis

particularly when the left atrial hypertrophy and atrial fibrillation are present for more than one year and it is impossible to maintain sinus rhythm and reversion to atrial fibrillation is common. β-blockers and digitalis are preferred drugs to achieve rate control. β-blockers blunt the chronotropic response to exercise and may improve excursive capacity. Atrial vasodilators should be avoided.

55. Four weeks of anticoagulation therapy is given before trying conversion to sinus rhythm. Anticoagulants are indicated for at least one year in patients with intermittent atrial fibrillation and patients who have systemic and/or pulmonary embolization.

56. The 4 indications for surgery in mitral stenosis are:

1. In symptomatic patients with pure mitral stenosis.
2. In mitral orifice less than 1.0 cm^2 per square meter of body surface area.
3. In asymptomatic patients with recurrent systemic embolization regardless of hemodynamic findings.
4. In pregnancy where pulmonary congestion occurs despite intensive medical treatment.

Operative mortality is less than 2%.

57. The 4 conditions where closed mitral valvotomy is preferable (with pump standby) are:

(Ref: T 23–27 percutaneous mitral balloon valvuloplasty)

1. Pure mitral stenosis.
2. Where no valvular or perivalvular calcification is detected by fluoroscopy or echocardiography.
3. No left atrial thrombosis.
4. In whom not operated previously.

(Ref: U 38–40)

58. The 4 conditions where open heart mitral valvotomy is indicated are (Ref: U-40):

1. Severe stenosis with significant associated mitral regurgitation.
2. Valvular calcification.
3. Left atrial thrombi.
4. Mitral valve distorted by previous operation.

Valve may have to be replaced by prosthesis, homograft or heterograft.

Operative mortality of valve replacement is about 5–8%.

59. When there are symptoms following immediately after valvotomy it is likely to be any of the following 4 conditions.

1. The operation was ineffective.
2. It induced mitral regurgitation.
3. It is associated with other valvular disease.
4. It is associated with myocardial disease.

60. When there is recurrence of symptoms after many years of surgery with initial satisfactory improvement it is usually suggestive of any of the following conditions.

1. Inadequate valvotomy.
2. Progression to other valvular disease.
3. Development of myocardial disease.
4. Restenosis of mitral valve.

or

Some combination of these conditions.

61. The 4 factors on which the result of valve replacement depends are (Ref: U 41–42):

1. Patient's myocardial function.
2. Level of pulmonary arterial pressure at the time of operation
3. Durability and long-term functioning of replaced valve.
4. Finally the technical skill of the operating team.

Patients with prosthesis should be given anticoagulants permanently.

62. The 4 late complications of valve replacement are:

1. Paravalvular leakage or mechanical dysfunction of the valve.
2. Infective endocarditis.
3. Thromboembolism.
4. Bleeding due to anticoagulants.

Overall 5 years survival following valve replacement is 70%.

63. Follow the 4 points in a pregnant women with mitral stenosis.

1. Pregnancy can be allowed in grade I and II A effort intolerance.
2. If symptoms develop, medical management followed by mitral valvotomy should be done in first trimester.
3. If patient with grade IIB effort intolerance wants pregnancy—valvotomy should be done first.
4. If she becomes pregnant, valvotomy should be done in first trimester or if she is not fit to continue pregnancy, MTP should be done.

If pregnancy is reached 5–6 months proceed to full-term under medical management.

MITRAL REGURGITATION (MR)

In mitral regurgitation blood flows backward into left atrium through the mitral valve during systole as a result of abnormalities in the mitral valve apparatus.

64. Mitral valve apparatus consists of 4 components:

1. Mitral annulus.
2. Mitral leaflets per se (both anterior and posterior).

3. Chordae tendinae.
4. Papillary muscles.

Abnormalities or dysfunction of anyone of these structures may cause mitral regurgitation.

65. Etiology—MR usually has a myxomatous or ischemic cause than a rheumatic cause.

The 4 common causes of chronic mitral regurgitation are:

1. Mitral leaflet prolapse (congenital, myxomatous degeneration).
2. Coronary artery disease.
3. Rheumatic fever.
4. Left ventricular dilatation of any cause which can alter the anatomy of mitral valve annulus, DCM, IHD, HTN.

For many years rheumatic etiology was considered as the most common cause of mitral regurgitation but after the advent of echocardiogram, mitral valve prolapse and coronary artery disease have become the predominant causes of mitral regurgitation. Mitral valve prolapse is one of the most common causes of mild mitral regurgitation and is probably the most common cause of mitral regurgitation in the adult population today. In contrast to mitral stenosis, pure rheumatic mitral regurgitation occurs frequently in males. Mitral regurgitation is the most common manifestation of acute as well as previous rheumatic carditis. Annular dilatation is the principal mechanism. The leaflets show edema with normal chordae. In chronic rheumatic heart disease progressive leaflet thickening with retraction of the cusps occurs. The posterior cusp is more involved, which becomes retracted and rolled with shortening of chordae or may elongate and rupture. The anterior chordae are frequently elongated, encouraging prolapse. Annular dilatation slowly increases and results in progressive mitral incompetence.

66. The 4 less common causes of mitral regurgitation are:

1. Calcification of the annulus: Massive calcification of the mitral annulus of unknown cause occurs most commonly in elderly women.
2. Papillary muscle dysfunction.
3. Congenital heart disease.
4. Prosthetic valve.

67. The 4 causes of calcification of mitral annulus which may give rise to mitral regurgitation are:

1. Idiopathic—more common in elderly women than in men
2. Rheumatic.
3. Degenerative: It is accelerated by systemic hypertension, aortic stenosis, diabetes, intrinsic defects of fibrous skeleton of the heart, such as Marfan's syndrome and Hurler syndrome.
4. Chronic renal failure with secondary hyperparathyroidism. It is probably secondary to hyperparathyroidism and elevated calcium-phosphorus product.

68. The 4 common causes of papillary muscle dysfunction are:

1. Coronary artery disease (acute myocardial infarction—rupture of papillary muscle: Complete rupture – typically not survived: Partial rupture—more typically encountered)
2. Infiltrative disease—amyloid, sarcoid.
3. Inflammatory conditions—rheumatic endocarditis, infective endocarditis of any cause.
4. Myocardial disease—cardiomyopathy.

Diseases of the left ventricular papillary muscle frequently give rise to mitral regurgitation. These are supplied by terminal portion of the coronary vascular bed and so are particularly vulnerable to ischemia and any disturbance of coronary artery disease can result in papillary muscle dysfunction. The posterior papillary muscle is supplied by the posterior descending branch of the right coronary artery, which becomes ischemic and infarcted more frequently than anterolateral papillary muscle, which is supplied by the diagonal branch of the left coronary artery and often by the marginal branches from the left circumflex artery also.

69. The 4 congenital heart diseases where mitral regurgitation occur.

1. Mitral valve prolapse.
2. Endocardial cushion defects—partial atrioventricular canal defects.
3. Corrected transposition of great arteries.
4. Endocardial fibroelastosis.

70. Mitral regurgitation can occur in prosthetic valve replacement due to:

1. Paravalvular leak.
2. Suture or pledget replacement.
3. Prosthetic valve endocarditis.
4. Degeneration of leaflets of tissue valve.
5. Deterioration of silastic disk.
6. Lodging of the ball or disk in the open position.
7. Dislodgment of the ball or disk.
8. Ring or strut fracture.

71. The 4 hereditary connective tissue disorders where mitral regurgitation occurs (Due to myxomatous degeneration):

1. Marfan's syndrome.
2. Ehlers-Donlos syndrome.
3. Osteogenesis imperfecta.
4. Pseudoxanthoma.

72. The 4 acquired connective tissue disorders where mitral regurgitation may occur.

1. Systemic lupus erythematosus.
2. Scleroderma.
3. Rheumatoid arthritis.
4. Ankylosing spondylitis.

73. The 4 causes of acute mitral regurgitation.

1. Rupture of the chordae tendineae.
2. Rupture of the papillary muscle (Myocardial infarction, trauma).
3. Perforation of the leaflet (Endocarditis).
4. Surgery—trauma during surgery/prosthetic valve.

74. The 4 causes of abnormalities or rupture of the chordae tendineae that may give rise to mitral regurgitation.

1. Spontaneous rupture (Primary) or secondary to myocardial infarction, trauma, mitral valve prolapse.
2. Infective endocarditis.
3. Rheumatic fever.
4. Myxomatous proliferation.

75. Rupture of posteromedial set of papillary muscle is 4 times greater than anterior set.

76. The 4 ways by which bacterial endocarditis cause mitral regurgitation.

1. Destructive effect of erosion.
2. Perforation of leaflets.
3. Rupture of chordae.
4. Less common cause is through healing of vegetation's in the angle between the posterior leaflet and the left ventricular wall resulting in immobilization of posterior leaflet.

77. The following 4 structural abnormalities are found with rheumatic origin. In rheumatic endocarditis the valve abnormalities that closes cause mitral stenosis whereas the abnormalities that cause valve to be held open cause mitral regurgitation.

1. *Calcification of commissures:* Calcification extends from one leaflet to another across one or both of the leaflets. This keeps the commissures apart.
2. *Fibrous contracture of the leaflets:* Fibrous contracture is usually dominant at one commissure but without fusion.
3. *Minor intrinsic shortening:* Shortening of the valvular tissue prevents the two leaflets to make complete contact.
4. *Distortion of the valve by left atrium:* The progressive dilatation of left atrium causes posterior leaflet to displace posteriorly, as a result of which the posterior leaflet looses its capacity to move. This results in a situation wherein "mitral regurgitation begets mitral regurgitation".

78. The 4 causes of coronary artery disease where mitral regurgitation can occur.

1. Dilatation of left ventricle in cases of extensively healed myocardial infarction.
2. Rupture of papillary muscle complicating acute myocardial infarction.
3. Infarction of a non-ruptured papillary muscle.
4. Left ventricular failure with dilatation or aneurysm.

79. There are numerous causes of left ventricular dilatation, which can give rise to mitral regurgitation. The following are 4 examples:

1. Left ventricular failure of any cause.
2. Dilated (Congestive) cardiomyopathy.
3. Primary form of dilated type of endocardial fibroelastosis.
4. Obstructive cardiomyopathy (hypertrophic subaortic stenosis).

80. The 4 points in hemodynamics of mitral regurgitation:

1. In mitral regurgitation, much of the blood that has flowed into the left ventricle leaks back into the left atrium rather than being pumped into the aorta. Since the regurgitant mitral orifice is in parallel with the aortic valve, the resistance to the left ventricular emptying also is reduced in mitral regurgitation. Almost half the regurgitant volume is ejected into the left atrium before aortic valve opens. Therefore, the effect is reduced 'net' movement of blood from the left atrium into left ventricle; the left ventricular volume declines. The volume of the mitral regurgitant flow depends on the size of the regurgitant orifice, and pressure gradient between the left ventricle and left atrium. There may be complete systolic emptying of the left ventricle in the beginning. Later, progressive increase in left ventricular diastolic volume occurs as the severity of the regurgitation increases and left ventricular function slowly deteriorates.
2. Enlargement of left atrium: The progressive increase in left atrial pressure causes progressive dilatation of the left atrium. The resultant left atrial dilatation increases the distance that cardiac impulse must travel in the atrial wall. Eventually, the pathway becomes so long that it predisposes to the circus movements. Therefore in late stages of the mitral valvular disease especially stenosis, atrial fibrillation usually occurs. This will still reduce the pumping effect of the heart and therefore causes still further cardiac disability.

The pressure-volume relationship of left atrium and pulmonary venous bed appears to effect much of hemodynamic and clinical picture.

Mitral regurgitation with normal or reduced compliance: Enlargement of the left atrium is little with marked elevation of mean left atrial pressure, particularly of the 'V' wave. This type occurs usually in acute severe mitral regurgitation in conditions like rupture of chordae tendineae, infarction or rupture of papillary muscle or tear of a mitral leaflet. Pulmonary vascular resistance is a frequent feature and therefore both right-sided heart failure and pulmonary edema are the clinical features with sinus rhythm.

Mitral regurgitation with increased compliance: In chronic mitral regurgitation there will be usually massive dilatation of left atrium and normal left atrial pressure. The pulmonary artery pressure and pulmonary vascular resistance are normal or slightly elevated. These patients show fatigue and exhaustion because of low cardiac output while symptoms from pulmonary congestion are less prominent. As the left ventricular dilatation occurs, atrial fibrillation is almost invariably present in long-standing cases. The association of normal left atrial pressure with a markedly enlarged thin wall of left atrium indicates that the left atrium is far more compliant than normal.

Mitral regurgitation with moderate increase in compliance; this group of patients are most commonly seen with hemodynamic and clinical features in between those other two groups with variable changes in the degree of left atrial enlargement and elevation of left atrial pressure.

3. Pulmonary edema in mitral valvular disease is caused by damping of blood in the pulmonary vasculature. Blood build up in the left atrium causes progressive dilatation of left atrium and increase in left atrial pressure which results in pulmonary edema. Ordinarily severe edema does not occur until the mean left atrial pressure rises at least above 30 mm Hg; more often it must rise to as high as 40 mm Hg, because the lymphatic vasculature enlarges many-fold and can carry fluid away from the lung tissue extremely rapidly. In left ventricular failure, the left ventricular diastolic pressure increases, the left atrial and pulmonary venous pressures increases and pulmonary congestion appears. There is an increase in pulmonary artery pressure and features of pulmonary arterial hypertension develops. Presence of features of pulmonary arterial hypertension in a patient having pure mitral regurgitation suggests severe MR or failing left ventricular myocardium or acute MR.
4. Compensatory changes in mitral valve disease: Blood volume increases in mitral valve disease. This increases venous return to the heart thereby helping to overcome the effect of cardiac debility to reduce cardiac output. Therefore, the cardiac output does not fall much until the late stages. As the left atrial pressure and pulmonary capillary pressure rise, blood begins to dam up in the pulmonary artery and the incipient edema of the lungs cause intensive pulmonary arteriolar constriction. These two effects together increases pulmonary arterial pressure sometimes to as high as 60 mm Hg. This in turn causes hypertrophy of the right heart which particularly compensates for its increased workload. There is another important adjustment that consists of decrease in the systemic vascular resistance to help increase the forward flow. The maximum ejection into the aorta takes place during early systole. The combination of these two factors results in an increased systolic and decreased diastolic pressure. Therefore, the pulse pressure is increased resulting in 'small water hammer pulse' of MR.

81. Mitral regurgitation patients who have reduction in cardiac reserve show the following 4 symptoms:

1. Fatigue: The forward output becomes insufficient during exertion. The decrease in systemic output results in fatigue—the most common symptom of significant MR.
2. Chronic weakness.
3. Exertional dyspnea.
4. Orthopnea.

82. Symptoms of right heart failure are characterized by 4 manifestations:

1. Raise in jugular venous pressure.
2. Hepatomegaly.
3. Ankle edema.
4. Ascites.

These symptoms are observed in patients with long standing mitral regurgitation or in acute mitral regurgitation with elevated pulmonary vascular resistance.

Angina is a rare symptom unless there is associated coronary artery disease.

Features of left ventricular failure are absent and appear late unless the MR is acute, severe or left ventricular myocardium is failing.

83. Mitral regurgitation patients develop symptoms depending on the 4 stages:

1. Severity of regurgitation.
2. Progression of regurgitation.

3. Level of pulmonary arterial pressure.
4. Presence of associated valvular or coronary artery disease.

Patients with mild mitral regurgitation may remain asymptomatic.

Majority of patients with mitral regurgitation of rheumatic origin will have mild disability unless regurgitation progresses as a result of rheumatic activity, intervening infective endocarditis or rupture of chordae tendineae. Mitral regurgitation tends to progress more rapidly in patients with connective tissue disorders, such as Marfan's syndrome than in those with rheumatic origin.

84. Comparison of 4 symptoms of mitral regurgitation with mitral stenosis.

Table I-2

Feature	MR	MS
1. Symptoms of pulmonary congestion	Less frequent because mean capillary pressure is less marked	More frequent because pulmonary capillary pressure is markedly elevated
2. Hemoptysis	Less common	Common
3. Systemic embolization	Less common	Common
4. Chronic weakness, fatigue	More prominent feature secondary to low cardiac output	Not prominent

85. Palpatory signs of MR are:

1. Tachycardia: The resting pulse rate is increased to maintain adequate cardiac output.
2. Pulse pressure is wide
3. The apex is displaced downward and outward with forcible apex and hyperkinetic precordium. The heart size is dependent on the severity and status of the left ventricular myocardium.
4. Systolic thrill: It is present in less than ten percent of patients. The cause of this is the direction of the regurgitant stream, which is backwards into the left atrium. Since the left atrium cannot be felt anteriorly over the precordium the murmur could not be felt as a thrill.

86. The auscultatory features of 4 heart sounds in mitral regurgitation are:

1. *First heart sound:* It is generally soft or buried in the systolic murmur and an accentuated first sound excludes severe mitral regurgitation. It is sometimes thought that the systolic murmur of mitral regurgitation 'obscures' or 'masks' the first sound. It is not so, because careful listening can detect the first heart sound. The murmur begins with the first sound.
2. *Second heart sound:* It is split normally but wide splitting resulting from early aortic closure indicates severe mitral regurgitation. With moderate or severe MR, the second sound is widely split but the width of the splitting varies with respiration becoming narrower during expiration and wider with inspiration.
3. *Third heart sound:* It is low pitched occurring 0.12–0.17 sec after aortic valve closure. It is produced by the large volume of blood in the left atrium filling the ventricles. It may be caused by the sudden tensing of the papillary muscle, chordae tendineae. Presence of third heart sound indicates severe mitral regurgitation and absence of it indicates that if mitral regurgitation exists it may not be severe.
4. *Fourth heart sound:* It is heard in acute mitral regurgitation with sinus rhythm.

87. The 4 adventitious sounds heard in mitral regurgitation are:

1. The classical diagnostic sign is the pansystolic murmur. It is the most prominent auscultatory finding in mitral regurgitation. A pansystolic murmur by definition begins with the first heart sound and occupies all of systole (holos = entire) up to the second sound on its side of origin. The configuration of murmur is plateau or even. A pansystolic murmur means a pansystolic pressure difference between two chambers. This pressure difference exists with left ventricle and left atrium as in mitral regurgitation, right ventricle and right atrium as in tricuspid regurgitation and between two ventricles as in ventricular septal defect. Nowhere else in the heart a pansystolic pressure difference exists to permit a pansystolic murmur. It must be differentiated from the systolic murmur of aortic stenosis, ventricular septal defect, and tricuspid regurgitation. In most cases, the systolic murmur starts immediately after the soft first sound and continues. It may obscure aortic second sound because of the persistence of the pressure difference between the left ventricle and left atrium. It is holosystolic, usually of grade III / VI of constant intensity, blowing, high-pitched and loudest at the apex. It radiates to the axilla and left infrascapular area. In few patients with primary abnormalities of posterior leaflet, the regurgitant jet strikes the atrial wall adjacent to the aortic root and the systolic murmur is radiated to the base of the heart and therefore may be mistaken with the murmur of aortic stenosis.
(Systolic murmur may have a 'cooing dove' or 'seagull' quality in ruptured chordae tendineae. It is not really typical of either birds call or cry. These descriptive terms should be considered as past).

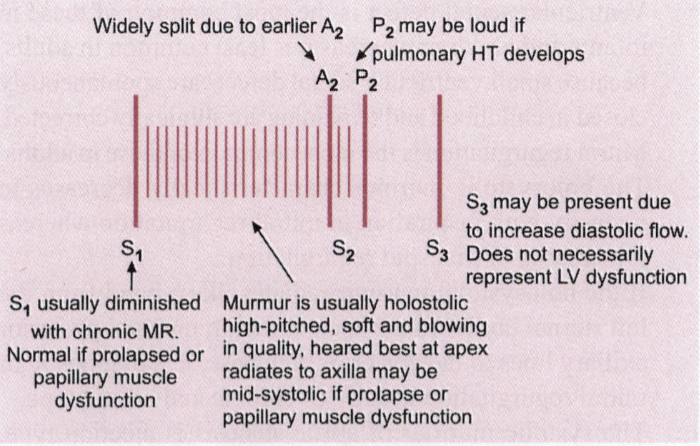

Fig. I-6: Auscultatory finding in MR

2. A diastolic murmur secondary to a large flow across the mitral valve during diastole may present. In pure MR, the delayed diastolic murmur always ends somewhere in mid-diastole and there is no late diastolic (presystolic) accentuation. This delayed diastolic murmur may be palpable as a short diastolic thrill. It may look unusual but a diastolic thrill in severe MR is more common than a systolic thrill.
3. Pulmonary ejection sound is heard in associated pulmonary hypertension.
4. An opening snap indicates associated mitral stenosis but does not exclude predominant regurgitation.

88. Summary of pansystolic murmur of mitral regurgitation

Table I-3

1. Timing	Pansystolic, late systolic, early systolic
2. Site of audibility and selective conduction	Apex, left sternal border, Left axilla, back Left sternal border/aortic area
3. Grading	Grade 3/6, thrill uncommon
4. Character	Soft, blowing, musical, honking

The murmur of rheumatic mitral regurgitation is classically pansystolic and this is true in most of the patients. Late systolic murmur occurs in mitral valve prolapse and papillary muscle dysfunction. The murmur of acute mitral regurgitation is early systolic as the pressure difference between left ventricle and left atrium gets obliterated by late systole.

Rheumatic mitral regurgitation murmur is usually best audible at the apex. In children, on the other hand, the murmur is sometimes best audible at the lower left sternal border. The murmur of mitral valve prolapse is occasionally best audible at the lower left sternal border and is possibly suggestive of posterior leaflet involvement. The selective of conduction of the murmur depends on direction of the jet, which is generally directed to the left and posteriorly in mitral regurgitation, so the murmur is commonly conducted to the left axilla and back. In some patients with mitral valve prolapse, the murmur is selectively conducted along the left sternal border and also to the aortic area. In this, the jet is directed medially along the aortic root. This type of jet is related to the dominant involvement of posterior leaflet of mitral valve in mitral valve prolapse. This is often confused with aortic stenosis. But the pansystolic murmur, the hyperkinetic apical impulse, and a normal upstroke of the arterial pulse favor mitral regurgitation. This variety of murmur in mitral valve prolapse with a posterior leaflet involvement is easily amenable to repair of the valve rather than replacement.

Mitral regurgitation murmur is characteristically soft and blowing. Musical murmurs occur when there is an unusual vibrating structure in the pathway of regurgitation as in ruptured chordae or the vegetations in infective endocarditis. The murmur of mitral valve prolapse is different in character from rheumatic mitral regurgitation and is usually rasping in quality. A musical honking murmur; is characteristic of mitral valve prolapse. A medium frequency or harsh murmurs of mitral regurgitation are usually non-rheumatic and are generally due to mitral valve prolapse. If the murmur is rough in quality it is better to rule out aortic stenosis or ventricular septal defect simulating mitral regurgitation.

89. Significance of presence or absence of thrill: The systolic thrill is less common due to the soft high frequency nature of the murmur. Presence of systolic thrill usually suggests:

1. Chordal rupture.
2. Infective endocarditis with vegetations.
3. Aortic stenosis.
4. Ventricular septal defect.

3 and 4 are mistaken for mitral regurgitation.

90. Relation of systolic murmur to physiological act and maneuvers:

Table I-4

1. Respiration	Fails to increase during inspiration
2. Posture	Standing: No change in rheumatic MR Increases in MVP
3.Valsalva straining	Decrease in rheumatic MR Increase in MVP
4. Phenylephrine	Decrease in MVP

Contrary to the general belief, the murmur of mitral regurgitation does not increases with expiration. Unlike the tricuspid regurgitation, it does not increase with inspiration. Rheumatic mitral regurgitation murmur may not change significantly with posture. The tricuspid regurgitation murmur decreases with standing and increases with supine position. The mitral regurgitation of mitral valve prolapse increases on standing (smaller left ventricle) and decreases with supine position (larger left ventricle).

The mitral regurgitation of mitral valve prolapse increases during straining of Valsalva maneuver whereas rheumatic mitral regurgitation decreases or disappears.

Phenylephrine decreases the mitral regurgitation of mitral valve prolapse due to reflex bradycardia and larger left ventricular cavity.

91. Associated features with systolic murmur in mitral regurgitation:

1. Hyperkinetic left ventricular impulse.
2. Diminished S_1.
3. Opening snap in associated mitral stenosis but does not exclude MR.
4. Wide, variable S_2.
5. S_3.
6. Mitral diastolic murmur in associated mitral stenosis.
7. Non-ejection clicks.
8. S_4.

92. There are 4 non-pansystolic murmurs in mitral regurgitation.

1. Mitral valve prolapse.
2. Papillary muscle dysfunction.
3. Acute mitral regurgitation (early systolic).
4. Trivial or mild mitral regurgitation (even rheumatic).

In acute myocardial infarction, the acute mitral regurgitation is due to papillary muscle dysfunction/rupture. The murmur may be faint or even silent.

93. Causes of silent mitral regurgitation are:

Acute MR

1. Acute myocardial infarction.
2. Infective endocarditis.
3. Postballoon valvuloplasty.
4. Postsurgical after closed or open commissurotomy.
5. Trauma.

Chronic

6. Paraprosthetic regurgitation.
7. Trivial MR due to any cause.
8. Trivial MVP.

94. Four conditions are to be differentiated when a holosystolic (or pansystolic) murmur is heard.

1. Mitral regurgitation.
2. Tricuspid regurgitation.
3. Ventricular septal defect.
4. Aortic stenosis.

Ventricular septal defect is the most common of these in infants and children whereas it is least common in adults, because small ventricular septal defects are spontaneously closed in childhood and remaining are surgically corrected. Mitral regurgitation is the most common of these in adults. The holosystolic murmur characteristically decreases in intensity with inspiration in mitral regurgitation whereas it increases in tricuspid regurgitation.

If the holosystolic murmur radiates like a band from the left sternal border to the apex, anterior, mid and posterior axillary lines to the posterior lung base, it is diagnostic of mitral regurgitation usually of chronic and severe type.

The systolic murmur of aortic stenosis is ejection type, rough and rumbling, diamond-shaped, radiating along carotids.

Whenever there is difficulty in differentiating murmur of aortic stenosis and that of mitral regurgitation, a valuable clue is to listen carefully to the murmur after a pause with a premature beat or listen to the beat after a pause with atrial fibrillation. The murmur of aortic stenosis increases in intensity whereas the murmur of mitral regurgitation shows little change.

Regarding which leaflet is more pathognomonic—anterior or posterior. If the radiation is more laterally and posteriorly directed—it is the anterior leaflet. If the murmur is directed more anteriorly and upwards over the precordium towards the aortic area, it is the posterior leaflet, which is adjacent to the aortic root. It should be remembered—if the anterior leaflet is affected the radiation is posterior, if the posterior leaflet is affected, the radiation of murmur is anteriorly directed—remember the opposite of terminology.

95. Chest roentgenography shows the following 4 changes:

1. Cardiomegaly with left atrium and left ventricular enlargement.

Fluroscopy reveals.

2. Hyperdynamic left ventricle.
3. Vigorous systolic expansion of left atrium
4. Marked calcification of the mitral leaflets occur in long-standing cases of mitral regurgitation, stenosis, and mixed lesions.

When a giant left atrium on X-ray examination is seen, even if a diastolic rumbling murmur is heard besides the typical holosystolic murmur of mitral regurgitation, no significant mitral stenosis exists.

Giant left atrium + Pansystolic murmur + Diastolic rumble = No significant mitral stenosis.

Cardiomegaly occurs in both MR, MS and combined MR and MS. It is often difficult to say which lesion is predominant to say from chest X-ray. Predominant mitral regurgitation is suggested when the heart is greatly enlarged and lung changes are inconspicuous. Extreme aneurysmally dilated left atrium usually signifies that mitral regurgitation is predominant and have existed for years. Predominant mitral stenosis is more likely in relatively mild cardiomegaly with straightening of left border with significant changes in the lung fields. Calcification of mitral annulus is seen in lateral and right anterior oblique views as a dense, coarse C-shaped opacity.

96. The structural changes of the 4 chambers of the heart are seen in the electrocardiogram:

1. Left atrial enlargement and atrial fibrillation.
2. Left ventricular enlargement in about 1/3rd of patients with severe regurgitation.
3. Right ventricular hypertrophy in about 15% caused by pulmonary hypertension.
4. Right atrial hypertrophy in severe pulmonary hypertension.

97. The following 4 abnormalities are seen in the echocardiogram:

1. Demonstrates the underlying cause of mitral regurgitation, e.g. rupture of chordae tendineae, mitral valve prolapse, a flail leaflet, vegetations, calcification of the mitral annulus, failure of the leaflets to close.
2. Enlargement of left atrium and left ventricle results in severe mitral regurgitation with increased systolic motion of both chambers.
3. Estimating two-dimensional echocardiography is useful in the hemodynamic consequences of mitral regurgitation with left ventricular dysfunction, increased left ventricular end-diastolic and end-systolic volumes.
4. Doppler echocardiography demonstrates high-velocity jet in the left atrium during systole.

98. Echocardiography with color Doppler plays a pivotal role in the evaluation of MR.

American College of Cardiology (ACC) and American Heart Association recommended 4 grades of MR depending on the severity and cause:

- 1+ for mild.
- 2+ for moderate.
- 3+ for moderately severe.
- 4+ for severe regurgitation.

The mechanism and severity of MR is determined by LA and LV size and function overtime.

Assess PA pressures and to revaluate periodically and after mitral surgery.

99. Table showing the differential diagnosis of mitral regurgitation (MR), ventricular septal defect (VSD), tricuspid regurgitation (TR), and aortic stenosis (AS):

Table I-5: Systolic murmur is the prominent physical finding

	MR	VSD	TR	AS
1. Systolic murmur	soft, blowing and pansystolic high pitched	Harsh and pansystolic combination of high and low frequency	Soft, blowing pansystolic high pitched	Ejection, crescendo-decrescendo Low pitch, rough and rumbling
2. Primary location of murmur	Apex	Diffusely heard left and right sternal border	Left sternal border	Base of the heart occasionally apex
3. Radiation of murmur	Axilla; occasionally base and neck	Diffusely heard in Left precordium and right of sternum	Little	Carotids
4. Murmur with respiration	Decreases with inspiration, increases with expiration	No change	Increases with inspiration	No change
5. Valsalva maneuver	May increase	Increase or No change	No change	Decrease
6. Pulmonary component of S_2	Normal , occasionally increased	Normal or loud usually delayed	Increased	Normal
7. Apical impulse	Hyperkinetic; occasionally heaving	Hyperkinetic	Weak or normal	Forceful and sustained
8. Jugular venous pressure	Often normal	Slightly Elevated with-prominent A and V waves	Elevated with prominent V waves	Usually normal

Contd...

Contd...

	MR	*VSD*	*TR*	*AS*
9. Thrill	Occasionally present at apex	Usually present at left sternal border	Rare	Occasionally present at base
10. Pulsatile liver	No	No	Yes	No
11. ECG	LVH and LAH	Biventricular hypertrophy	RVH, occasionally RAH	LVH with associated ST-T changes
12. Chest roentgenogram	Moderate cardiomegaly, marked LA enlargement	Cardiomegaly-both LV and RV enlargement	Enlarged RV	Often normal size or LVH

100. Other causes of differential diagnosis of MR in the pediatric age group include:

1. Atrial septal defect of primum type.
2. Coarctation of aorta with MR (congenital).
3. Left ventricular fibroelastosis.
4. Congenital corrected transposition of great arteries (I-TGA).
5. Papillary muscle dysfunction in dilatation of left ventricle from any cause including myocarditis.
6. ASD of the secundum type with floppy mitral valve.
7. Marfan and Hurler syndrome.
8. Anomalous origin of left coronary artery from pulmonary artery.

101. Cardiac catheterization and left ventricular angiography establish the diagnosis of mitral regurgitation.

1. The prompt appearance of contrast material in the left atrium following injection into left ventricle indicates mitral regurgitation.
2. The regurgitant volume can be determined from the difference between the total left ventricular stroke volume estimated angiographically and estimation of effective forward stroke volume by Fick's method. Cineangiography is helpful in estimating the quality and severity of mitral regurgitation.
3. Central regurgitant jet and reduced motion of thickened leaflets of mitral regurgitation is characteristic of rheumatic origin.
4. Eccentric regurgitant jet and excessive motion of thin valve filaments is suggestive of other causes, such as dilatation of mitral annulus, ruptured chordae tendineae or papillary muscle. The etiology of the regurgitation, e.g. prolapse of the mitral valve and a flial leaflet can be distinguished angiographically.

102. Left ventriculography helps in assessment of severity of MR. It is affected by multiple factors, such as adequate amount of contrast medium injected to fill the ventricle, the placement of catheter and by ventricular arrhythmia during injection.

The grading is done as follows:

1. *1+(mild):* Clears with each beat, whole LA is never opacified.
2. *2+ (moderate):* Does not clear with single beat. May faintly opacified the entire LA.
3. *3+ (moderate to sever):* Fills entire LA over 2 or 3 beats, complete opacification of LA: Equally in intensity to the LV.
4. *4+ (sever):* Complete opacification of LA in one beat: Contract material refluxes into the pulmonary veins.

Coronary angiography is useful to detect associated coronary heart disease in these patients.

103. Table of comparison of acute and chronic mitral regurgitation by 4 methods of investigations:

Table I-6

Acute mitral regurgitation	*Chronic mitral regurgitation*
1. ECG—commonly normal unless acute myocardial infarction is the cause	LAH—'P Mitrale' AF—common LVH—common with severe MR
2. X-ray chest and fluoroscopy heart size is normal. If regurgitation is severe there may be pulmonary congestion and interstitial edema	Cardiomegaly is common mainly due to LVH LA enlargement especially with rheumatic origin. Fluoroscopy may reveal calcification in rheumatic origin
3. Echocardiography LA normal LV usually of normal size may be vigorously hypercontractile. Cause may be demonstrated flail leaflets, rupture of chordae or papillary muscle, or vegetations in infective endocarditis, etc.	LA usually enlarged LV enlarged with signs of volume overload. Cause is demonstrated by rheumatic disease, mitral valve prolapse
4. Cineangiography eccentric regurgitant jet and excessive motion of thin valve filaments — ruptured chordae tendineae or papillary muscles	Central regurgitant jet and reduced motion of thickened leaflets of rheumatic origin, mitral valve prolapse can be demonstrated

104. Medical management of mitral regurgitation: Management includes all the measures used in the treatment of heart failure. Mild to moderate mitral regurgitation is well-tolerated for long periods. As a rule the severity of MR increases with time. Avoid all physical activities that produce fatigue and dyspnea.

1. Enhance the sodium excretion by diuretics.
2. Digitalis plays a more important role in MR than in MS. It increases the cardiac output of overburdened left ventricle. It is indicated in cardiomegaly and sinus rhythm. It can be used in patients with established atrial fibrillation.
3. Reduction of afterload is beneficial in both acute and chronic forms of mitral regurgitation. It reduces the impedance to ejection into aorta thereby regurgitant blood volume into the left atrium is reduced, which results in reduction of left atrial pressure and decline in V wave. The vasodilator therapy with an ACE inhibitor or oral hydralazine is particularly useful in relieving the physiological abnormality rather than simply dealing with its consequences. In addition, it reduces the left ventricular volume and reduces the size of mitral annulus and thereby regurgitant orifice. Afterload reduction with intravenous nitroprusside may be life saving in acute MR due to rupture of the head of a papillary muscle occurring in acute myocardial infarction. It may stabilize the patient's condition to allow the operation in an optimal condition. When surgery is contraindicated, chronic afterload reduction may improve the clinical state for months or years in patients with severe mitral regurgitation.
4. Prevention of infective endocarditis by prophylactic antibiotics.

   Treatment of atrial fibrillation in MR is same as for MS.

105. Mitral regurgitation caused by annular dilatation resulting in LV dysfunction is managed with the agents used to manage heart failure.

1. After load reduction by ACE inhibitors. They minimize the regurgitant volumes and maximize forward flow. These can be used in management of MR from primary valvular disease in patients with symptoms waiting for surgery.

For preload.

2. Diuretics and nitrates to reduce the pulmonary congestion.
3. β-blockers are also beneficial and added once after-load reduction has been initiated.
4. Ventricular rate-controlling agents and antiarrhythmics are used for atrial fibrillation. Digitalis and β-blockers are the mainstay of therapy in rate control.

106. Left-side cardiac catheterization, selective left ventricular angiocardiography and coronary arteriography are advised when the surgical treatment is contemplated.

There are 4 objectives of these studies:

1. To confirm the presence of regurgitation and estimate its severity.
2. To identify primary myocardial disease and relatively mild functional regurgitation secondary to ventricular dilatation who are not benefited by operation and the risk of operation is relatively high.
3. To detect and assess the severity of any associated valve lesion.
4. To determine the presence and extent of coronary artery disease.

107. When surgical treatment is considered, the chronic often slowly progressive nature of this disease must be balanced against the immediate risk and long-term uncertainties of surgical treatment. Following 4 points are to be considered while selecting the patients for surgical treatment.

1. Patients with MR who are asymptomatic.
2. Patients who develop symptoms only on strenuous exercise: 1 and 2 are not ideal for surgery since they may live long with little deterioration.
3. Patients who cannot do normal house hold activities inspite of good medical management.
4. Patients who have other associated cardiac lesions.

The results depend on the associated conditions, such as pulmonary, renal, hepatic disease as well as on the efficiency of the surgical team.

108. The 4 methods of surgical treatment.

Repair

1. Direct suture repair of the valve.
2. Elongation or shortening of chordae tendineae.

Replacement

3. Valve replacement with a mechanical prosthesis.
4. Valve replacement with a bioprosthesis.

1 and 2 are indicated in pure mitral regurgitation secondary to annular dilatation, papillary muscle dysfunction or rupture or chordal rupture.

3 and 4 are indicated in those patients who have thickened, severely deformed, calcified valves, vegetations on the valves and myxomatous degenerative changes, and partly stenotic are not fit for reconstruction.

MITRAL VALVE PROLAPSE (MVP)

109. Reid and Barlow et al. proposed in 1963 that mid to late systolic clicks and apical systolic murmurs were of mitral valve origin. Criley and colleagues after several years proposed the term 'Mitral valve prolapse' to describe posterior leaflet motion in systole. Since then many names have been given. They include:

1. Mitral valve prolapse syndrome.
2. Systolic click—murmur syndrome.
3. Barlow's syndrome.
4. Billowing mitral valve syndrome.
5. Floppy valve syndrome.
6. Ballooning mitral cusp syndrome.
7. Redundant cusp syndrome.
8. Prolapsing mitral valve leaflet syndrome.

110. High level of interest of this condition is due to one of the following 4 disorders:

1. Often asymptomatic and usually benign.
2. High prevalence rate (particularly in young people).
3. Non-specific clinical presentation.
4. Potential for various complications in otherwise normal healthy people.

111. It is the most common cardiac valvular abnormality in UK and USA next to aortic sclerosis. It is most common cause of mitral regurgitation in USA. Prevalence rate ranges from 8–12% in Western population. Prevalence rate falls in women with increasing age whereas it remains unchanged in men.

Wide disparity of prevalence among various studies are attributed to the following 4 causes:

1. Difference in age.
2. Difference in gender distribution.
3. Diagnostic criteria.
4. Diagnostic techniques.

During the past decade, lot of progress has been made in clarifying the diagnostic criteria and defining secondary causes and found more than 98% of cases are primary. Recently research has focused on the pathogenesis of 'nonspecific symptoms' and the natural history of this condition.

112. Mitral regurgitation occurs when there is billowing, floppy, frail leaflets resulting in mitral valve prolapse. Normally, mitral valve billows into the left atrium but an exaggeration is termed as 'billowing' of mitral valve.

1. 'Billowing' mitral leaflet with mitral valve prolapse: The exaggerated billowing causes MVP. The valve becomes incompetent. The billowing occurs due to excessive or redundant mitral leaflet tissue.
2. 'Floppy' valve with MVP: Floppy valve is an extreme form of billowing. MVP occurs when the leaflet edges do not come close resulting in mitral regurgitation.
3. Chordal rupture with MVP: The valve leaflets are 'flail' in chordal rupture and causes severe regurgitation. Ruptured minor chordae may cause MVP without detectable billowing of mitral leaflets.
4. Annular dilatation with MVP: Recent-onset annular dilatation causes MVP with minimal billowing of mitral leaflets.

The severity of mitral regurgitation depends on the extent of mitral valve prolapse.

The excessive or redundant mitral leaflet tissue is commonly involved with myxomatous degeneration and increased concentration of acid mucopolysaccharide. Posterior leaflet is usually more affected than anterior leaflet.

113. Etiology:

The etiology is unknown in majority of patients. But there are several conditions causing or associated with mitral valve prolapse. The following are some primary prolapse results from myxomatous proliferation of the leaflets. It appears to have a genetic predisposition. Higher prevalence is seen in some families affected, and an autosomal dominant mode of inheritance with variability is a possibility.

1. *Congenital heart disease:* ASD, VSD, PDA, AP window, membranous or supravalvular aortic stenosis, Ebstein's anomaly, corrected transposition of great vessels, infundibular pulmonary stenosis, Uhl's anomaly, congenital prolonged Q-T syndrome. It occurs in 20% of atrial septal defect patients.
2. *Rheumatic (infective):* Rheumatic endocarditis can coexist with mitral stenosis, following mitral commissurotomy. Rheumatic valvulitis is a proliferative process. It is unlikely that it causes myxomatous degeneration of the mitral valve. It is more likely that the relationship between these two common conditions is coincidental.

Bacterial endocarditis.

3. *Ischemic heart disease and MVP:* Both are common disorders and coexists frequently. It can also occur secondary to rupture of chordae, papillary muscle dysfunction, left ventricular aneurysm following myocardial infarction. It is proposed that MVP can cause coronary artery spasm as a reflex response which in them is responsible for angina, angina-like pain, infarction, arrhythmias and sudden death in this syndrome.
4. *Cardiomyopathy:* Dilated or congestive cardiomyopathy, hypertrophic cardiomyopathy. Usual anterior displacement of anterior mitral valve leaflet may accompany with prolapse of posterior valve leaflet in hypertrophic obstructive cardiomyopathy.

5. *Inherited connective tissue disorders and MVP :* Transmitted as autosomal dominant trait—Marfan's syndrome, cystic medial necrosis, Ehlers-Danlos syndrome, osteogenesis imperfecta, pseudoxanthoma elasticum, periarteritis nodosa, Duchenne muscular dystrophy, systemic lupus erythematosus, etc. MVP syndrome may represent one of the manifestations of many systemic connective tissue disorders.
6. *Inherited disorders of metabolizm and MVP.* Hunter-Hurler syndrome, Sanfilippo's syndrome, Fabry's disease, Sandhoff's disease.
7. *Endocrinal disorders and MVP:* Hyperthyroidism, Turner syndrome, Noonan syndrome.
8. *Miscellaneous causes:* Thoracic skeletal abnormalities, atrial myxoma, congenital prolonged Q – T interval, WPW syndrome, von Willebrand's syndrome, platelet abnormalities, migraine, hypomagnesemia, anxiety neurosis, neurocirculatory asthenia, autonomic dysfunction, etc.

   MVP syndrome may represent one manifestation of the systemic disorders or another manifestation of the same disorders which may frequently coexist.

114. There is evidence to suggest the presence of dysautonomia in many patients with MVP syndrome. The favorable points for this suggestion are:

1. Exaggerated heart rate and blood pressure response to stimuli. (Including vasodepressor response)
2. Postural hypotension.
3. High circulating catecholamine concentration.
4. Hyper responsiveness to infused catecholamines (with provocation of chest pain and other symptoms in some cases).
5. Abnormal catecholamine regulation.
6. Abnormal baroreflex modulation.
7. Decreased intraventricular and intravascular volume on standing.
8. Activation of atrial natriuretic peptide.

These findings have led the proposal that the syndrome may in part be a "neuroendocrinopathy".

115. MVP cases are detected incidentally when the patients come for evaluation for any of these 4 conditions:

1. Nonspecific symptoms referable to cardiac disease.
2. Nonspecific symptoms referable to neurological disease.
3. Symptoms referable to complications.
4. Some are detected incidentally during cardiac auscultation, or echocardiography for evaluation of systolic murmur or suspected unrelated cardiac disease.

116. There are 4 nonspecific symptoms that occur commonly associated with mitral valve prolapse:

1. *Chest pain:* Occurs in about 60% of patients. It may be typical of angina but most often atypical in that it is prolonged, not clearly related to exertion, sharp, sticking or lancinating.
2. *Palpitation:* In many patients otherwise asymptomatic suffer from undue anxiety once they are informed of the presence of heart disease. Palpitation occurs in half of the patients with this syndrome. Most often paroxysmal supraventricular tachycardia, premature ventricular contractions and ventricular tachycardias are accounted for it. In patients with supraventricular tachycardia, a left-sided atrioventricular bypass tract can often be discerned. There is often discordance between the symptoms and the timing of arrhythmias during ambulatory or patients activated electrocardiographic monitoring. Many report palpitation during acceleration of normal sinus rhythm suggesting that increased nociception may play a part.
3. *Presyncope and syncope:* It results from tachyarrhythmias. Postural hypotension, light-headedness and vasodepressor response occur commonly. Sudden death is a rare complication.
4. *Effort intolerance:* It is characterized by dyspnea and lassitude. The pathogenesis of effort intolerance in MVP is unknown. The discomfort may be secondary to tension on papillary muscles and may be associated with abnormalities of wall motion or indentations of the wall of left ventricle at the base of these muscles on angiography.

Many attempts to associate MVP with panic syndrome have produced conflicting information.

The term 'mitral valve prolapse syndrome' is now used to differentiate prolapse associated with non-specific symptoms from anatomical prolapse.

117. MVP occurs frequently in patients with various causes of chest pain such as the following 4:

1. Coronary artery spasm.
2. Esophageal spasm.
3. Chest wall pain.
4. Panic disorders.

Chest pain may coexist in patients with MVP syndrome. MVP syndrome and true angina pectoris may coexist secondary to coronary artery disease.

118. Physical examination: The 4 points to be noted are:

1. Inspection: There is higher incidence of pectus excavatum among patients with MVP. Straight back or scoliosis are also seen. The patient often have low body weight and relative hypotension.

2. Palpation of the precordium and carotid pulses reflects the severity of the existing mitral regurgitation, which may range from non-existent to severe.
3. Auscultation: The most important finding is one mid or late systolic click, which occurs 0.14 sec or more after the first sound and is thought to be produced by sudden tensing of slack, elongated tendineae or by the prolapsing mitral leaflet. In the mildest form valve bulges back into the left atrium during systole producing a mid-systolic click but remains competent and so does not produce murmur. The click is followed by a high-pitched late crescendo-decrescendo murmur, occasionally 'whooping' or 'honking', heard best at the apex in left lateral position.

   The combination of mid-systolic click and late systolic murmur is the clinical hallmark of mitral valve prolapse.
4. The maneuvers which decrease left ventricular volume such as standing, the Valsalva maneuvers or inhalation of amylnitrate cause the click and murmur to occur earlier. The maneuvers which increase left ventricular end-diastolic volume, such as squatting or isometric exercise diminishes the propensity for mitral valve leaflets to prolapse and so the click-murmur complex may be delayed or even disappear.

The presence of a click that responds to provocative maneuvers is sufficient for the diagnosis of prolapse even if an echocardiogram is not diagnostic.

The duration of the murmur is a function of the severity of regurgitation. If the murmur is confined to the later portion of the systole, regurgitation is usually not severe. Murmur comes earlier and becomes holosystolic in severe regurgitation. The findings are very variable in MVP. Some may have a mid-systolic click without a murmur; others have the murmur without a click. Some others may have only a click on one occasion and only a murmur on another; both on a third occasion.

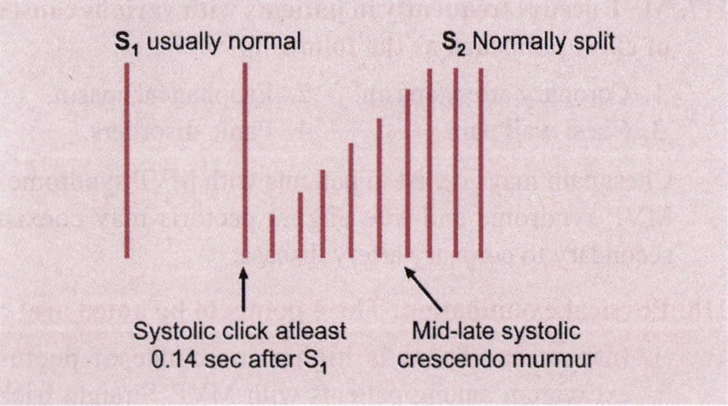

Fig. I-7: Auscultatory finding in mitral valve prolapse

Multiple clicks can be heard later in systole from snapping taut of chordae (heard best with diaphragm at lowest sternal border).

119. Electrocardiogram: It may be normal in asymptomatic patients or with typical clinical findings. It may show the following 4 characteristic findings:

1. Inverted or biphasic T wave.
2. Nonspecific ST-segment changes.

   1 and 2 are seen in LII, LIII and a VF; occasionally in the anterolateral leads. ST-T changes may become exaggerated by exercise or inhalation of amylnitrate. These changes may be related to the ischemia of the papillary muscles or of the left ventricle at their bases resulting from increased tension on these structures produced by the prolapsing mitral valve. It may reflect the underlying cardiomyopathy.
3. Arrhythmias: Atrial and ventricular premature contractions; supraventricular and ventricular tachyarrhythmias due to sinus node dysfunction or varying degrees of atrioventricular block. Serious ventricular arrhythmias more frequent in patients with ST-T changes on resting ECG. The incidence of paroxysmal atrial tachycardia is three times greater in MVP patients compared to general population.

   PAT may be related to the high incidence of atrioventricular bypass tracts in this syndrome. These bypass tracts are always left sided and may be associated with mitral valve abnormality. There is high incidence of MVP among patients with the Wolff-Parkinson-White syndrome. However, the absence of WPW syndrome should not be considered as evidence against the presence of bypass tracts in patients with MVP syndrome who exhibit supraventricular tachyarrhythmias. These patients should be subjected to the electrophysiological studies. These studies may be important because digitalis or propranolol, which may be useful in reentry tachycardias, may be hazardous in the presence of antegrade conduction over an atrioventricular bypass tract.
4. Association of prolonged QT interval: There is an increased association between MVP syndrome and prolongation of the QT interval. This may be a cause of ventricular arrhythmias.

120. Echocardiogram

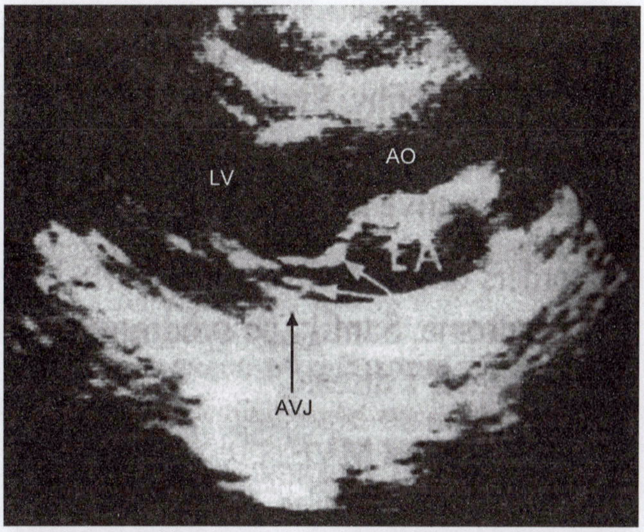

Fig. I-8: Two-dimensional echocardiogram; long-axis view of a patient with mitral valve prolapse. Both anterior and posterior mitral leaflets makes almost a hairpin turn as it moves to the atria side of the atrioventricular junction (AVJ). The anterior mitral leaflet makes a J-shaped angle with the posterior aortic root and the posterior left atrial valve. AO = aorta; LA = left atrium; LV = left ventricle

Echocardiography plays a most important role in the diagnosis of mitral valve prolapse. The 4 important findings are:

1. Most characteristic finding is the abrupt posterior movement of the posterior leaflet or both mitral leaflets in mid to late systole immediately after the click and during the systolic murmur. There may be considerable variation in the auscultatory and echo events.
2. A second finding is pansystolic posterior prolapse of one or both leaflets resulting in 'U' or 'hammock'—shaped configuration in the C-D segment. (It is the opposite of what is seen in obstructive cardiomyopathy in which the anterior leaflet of the mitral valve moves towards the ventricular septum in mid-systole)
3. Rarely there may be a sudden posterior collapse of the anterior mitral leaflet as it approaches the prolapsing posterior leaflet in early systole.
4. All the above three findings have in common the motion of the mitral valve posterior to the C-point.

While doing the echocardiogram, it is important to direct the echo beam to the junction of the posterior walls of the left atrium and ventricle in order to visualize the posterior leaflet adequately. Care is taken to angulate the transducer to record the valve motion from the free edge of the leaflet. M-mode echocardiography has missed MVP in some patients that was detected by two-dimensional echocardiography. The apical four chamber view is the single best technique to identify the syndrome in which the mitral valve leaflets lie in the left atrium rather than in the left ventricle during systole.

The echocardiographic findings of MVP has been recorded in large number of first-degree relatives of patients with established MVP. Some patients with systolic click with or without murmur may not show evidence of MVP on echocardiogram. Conversely, echocardiogram findings of MVP may be found in patients without click or murmur.

121. Angiography: The configuration of the left ventriculogram during systole is helpful. The right anterior oblique projection is useful in defining the posterior leaflet and left anterior oblique for studying the anterior leaflet of mitral valve. It reveals:

1. Prolapse of the posterior mitral leaflet.
2. Sometimes prolapse of both mitral valve leaflets.
3. Mitral regurgitation.
4. In some cases; bulging of the posteroinferior wall of the left ventricle into the left ventricular cavity, during systole and/or hypokinesis of the anterolateral left ventricular wall.
5. Extension of the mitral leaflet tissue inferiorly and posteriorly to the point of attachment of the mitral leaflets to the annular fibrosa.
6. Scallooped edges of the leaflets reflecting redundancy of tissue.
7. Dilatation and decreased systolic contraction of the mitral annulus.
8. Calcification of mitral annulus and/or leaflets.

122. Natural history: The 4 important points are:

1. The outlook for MVP in children is good, majority of them remaining asymptomatic for many years without any change in clinical or echocardiographic findings.
2. Incidence of mitral regurgitation is greater in patients with clicks and murmur than in those with isolated click.
3. Mitral regurgitation is progressive in 15% of patients over 10–15 years period.
4. Many of the complications occur most commonly in patients with thickened mitral valve leaflets and are more likely to occur in older men with prolapse.

123. Patients of mitral valve prolapse with mild symptoms often respond to reassurance. β-blockers may produce improvement in the following 4 situations:

1. *Chest pain:* Improvement is seen in 25–50% of patients.
2. *Palpitation:* Severe palpitation often respond well whether or not they are caused by arrhythmias.

3. *Presyncope or syncope:* Patients with vasodepressor syncope and mitral valve prolapse may respond to β-blockers. Patients with syncope that remain unexplained by noninvasive evaluation should be investigated for invasive electrophysiological studies.
4. *Effort intolerance:* It is difficult to treat. β-blockers may help in those patients in whom symptoms often occur in clusters during emotion or stress. β-blockers may be targeted at symptom peaks rather than given regularly.

124. There are 4 life-threatening complications of symptomatic mitral valve prolapse.

1. Congestive heart failure due to progressive mitral regurgitation.
2. Mitral regurgitation associated with ruptured chordae tendineae.
3. Infective endocarditis.
4. Cerebral embolism and sudden death.

125. Cerebral embolism occurs with high frequency in young people with MVP and probably in older people as well. Old age seems to be the main risk factor. Cerebral embolism occurs with equal frequency with normal or thickened mitral valve leaflets. It can give rise to any of the 4 complications.

1. Acute hemiplegia.
2. Transient ischemic attacks.
3. Cerebellar infarct.
4. Retinal arteriolar occlusion.

126. The pathogenesis of cerebral embolization complication in MVP patients may be attributed to the following 4 factors:

1. Loss of endothelial continuity over the myxomatous valve, which may initiate platelet aggregation and platelet fibrin complexes.
2. Paroxysmal arrhythmias that occur in MVP may contribute to embolization.
3. Shortened platelet survival time.
4. Increased coagulant activity.

It is possible that cerebral embolization secondary to MVP may be a cause of unexplained strokes and other cerebral and retinal complications in young people with undetected cerebrovascular disease. It is also possible that myocardial infarction in patients with MVP and normal coronary arteries may be secondary to embolization.

The efficacy of antiplatelet therapy in preventing thromboembolism is not proved as is often given empirically. Warfarin should be given in those who suffered previous thromboembolic episodes.

127. Infective endocarditis has been reported in 2–8% of known cases of MVP. Retrospective analysis indicate that MVP was present in one-third of cases of infective endocarditis. The 4 important risk factors for infective endocarditis in patients with MVP are:

1. Presence of mitral regurgitation.
2. Thickened valves.
3. Myxomatous degeneration of mitral leaflets.
4. Calcification of leaflets or mitral annulus.

The pathogenesis, clinical features, prognosis and therapeutic implications of infective endocarditis in MVP are similar to those associated with other forms of mitral valve disease.

128. The treatment of congestive heart failure due to severe mitral regurgitation associated with myxomatous degeneration and mitral valve prolapse is 4 fold.

Medical

1. Digoxin and diuretics.
2. Vasodilators.

Surgical

3. Mitral valve repair.
4. Mitral valve replacement.

Nitrates should be used with caution because of reduction of cardiac size induced by these drugs may intensify prolapse and cause ischemia of the papillary muscle.

Now, it is the most common indication for mitral valve replacement in elderly patients and for mitral valve annuloplasty at any age. Flail leaflets always require mitral valve replacement or repair.

AORTIC STENOSIS

(See Chapter L -Congenital Aortic Stenosis 42–58)

129. Aortic stenosis is obstruction to the left ventricular outflow across the valve.

The 4 etiological factors are:

1. Congenital: Congenital bicuspid valve stenosis is the most common cause; it may be stenotic from birth and slowly calcified during first three decades. Aortic stenosis may occur with unicuspid valve. Congenital aortic stenosis can occur as subvalvular or supravalvular stenosis. Rarely congenital papillary mass or flap of endocardial tissue may cause obstruction to an otherwise normal valve. Aortic stenosis before the age of 30 years is suggestive of congenital origin. Bicuspid aortic valve is associated with cooptation, aortic root dilation, and a propensity for aortic dissection.

2. Acquired or rheumatic: Rheumatic endocarditis causes fibrous contracture with shortening and fusion of the cusps at the commissaries.

   Aortic stenosis between 30 and 70 years age suggests rheumatic origin, but it can occur early also. Rheumatic aortic stenosis is almost always associated with rheumatic mitral valve disease.

   Rheumatic aortic stenosis has never been described in the pediatric age group.

3. Idiopathic calcification occurs in elderly—probably due to degeneration—a 'wear and tear' phenomenon. Aortic stenosis above the age of 70 years is suggestive of degenerative calcification.

4. Rare causes like extensive thrombosis at the valve site in diseases like systemic lupus erythematosus (SLE).

   Calcific degeneration of congenitally deformed bicuspid valve is a common cause of AS. Even in this country, isolated aortic stenosis is not rheumatic.

Age-related aortic stenosis and calcific stenosis are associated with traditional risk factors for atherosclerosis, such as smoking, hypertension, and hyperlipidemia. Age-related aortic sclerosis is associated with increased risk of MI and cardiovascular death and can progress to aortic stenosis. Other conditions associated with calcific aortic stenosis include Paget's disease and end-stage renal disease.

130. There are two etiologies of aortic stenosis for bicuspid state—congenital or rheumatic. In the calcific type of aortic stenosis, congenital bicuspid valve is 4 times more common than acquired bicuspid valve.

131. 1/4th of the patients among all the chronic valvular disease will show aortic stenosis.

132. Aortic stenosis is 4 times more common in males than females.

133. Incidence of bicuspid aortic valve is about 4 in 1000 live births.

134. Pathophysiology: The 4 important points are:

1. The primary abnormality is the left ventricular outflow obstruction. This results in pressure gradient between the left ventricle and aorta during systole. Because of the resistance to ejection by the stenosed valve, left ventricular pressure rises very high but rarely exceeds 300 mm Hg, while the pressure in the aorta still maintains normal.

   Aortic orifice of less than 0.5 cm^2 per square meter of body surface area, i.e. approximately less than 1/3rd of the normal or a systemic gradient exceeding 50 mm Hg. (The pressure difference during systole between the left ventricle and aorta) in a case with normal cardiac output is considered as critical obstruction to left ventricular outflow.

   The nozzle effect during systole with blood forcing through the stenosed valve at tremendous speed causes turbulence of blood impinging against aortic wall. This causes intense vibration and a loud murmur in aortic area and radiates to carotids. This sound is harsh and occasionally so loud that it can be heard without stethoscope. The sound vibration can be felt as a thrill in the aortic area.

2. The obstruction increases gradually over many years and the left ventricular output is maintained by the compensatory left ventricular hypertrophy. The elevated left ventricular end-diastolic pressure with severe stenosis does not necessarily represent the left ventricular failure or dilatation. It signifies the diminished compliance of the hypertrophied left ventricular wall. Aortic stenosis is a ventricular pressure overload condition whereas aortic regurgitation is a volume overload condition.

3. Because of the diminished left ventricular compliance, left atrial contraction increases, and the left atrial pressure rises resulting in a large 'A' wave in the jugular venous pulse.

   This left atrium works as a pump to maintain effective left ventricular contraction and to prevent the rise of pulmonary venous and capillary pressures. So occurrence of atrial fibrillation or atrioventricular dissociation may result in a rapid progression of symptoms. Though cardiac output is within normal limits in majority of patients, it does not show rise with exercise in severe stenosis.

4. Finally, when the cardiac output and left ventricular aortic pressure gradient decreases, the mean left atrial pressure, pulmonary wedge pressure, pulmonary arterial pressure and right atrial pressure rises resulting in pulmonary arterial hypertension.

135. Heart responds to the obstruction by hypertrophy. In the systemic circulation, the obstruction of the valve is associated with:

1. Small stroke volume.
2. A small slow rising pulse.
3. Low blood pressure.
4. Low cardiac output.

136. Left ventricular dilatation and impaired contractility at a late stage finally results in the following 4 altered parameters:

1. Raise in left ventricular end-diastolic pressure.
2. Reduction in ejection fraction.
3. Reduction in cardiac output.
4. Raise in pulmonary arterial pressure.

137. The 4 pathological complications of aortic stenosis are:

1. Systemic embolism.
2. Coronary occlusion in calcified aortic stenosis.
3. Aortic stenosis or aortic regurgitation causes downward enlargement of left ventricle which pulls the chordae tendineae resulting in secondary mitral insufficiency.
4. Dissecting or saccular aneurysm of the aorta can occur due to cystic medial necrosis of the aorta which accompanies aortic stenosis.

138. The 4 common causes of left ventricular outflow obstruction are:

1. Valvular stenosis.
2. Discrete congenital subvalvular aortic stenosis.
3. Supravalvular aortic stenosis.
4. Hypertrophic cardiomyopathy.

139. Symptoms: The patient may be asymptomatic until the aortic valve orifice has narrowed approximately to one-third of its normal size. It may be present for many years without discomfort because of the ability of left ventricle to compensatory hypertrophy and competent mitral valve behind the left ventricle. Whereas in mitral stenosis the symptoms appear as soon as the obstruction becomes severe because the left atrium being proximal to the mitral valve provides less compensatory dilatation when compared to left ventricle in aortic stenosis. The aortic stenosis gradually increases until third or fourth decade without showing any symptoms.

The 4 important symptoms are:

1. *Chest pain*: It is the most frequent symptom and occurs in 50–70% of patients with aortic stenosis. It usually occurs at a later stage. It is due to imbalance between the oxygen supply and demand. Hypertrophied left ventricle needs increased oxygen requirement. The pressure compression of the coronary vessels by hypertrophied left ventricle exceeds the coronary perfusion pressure. All this results in angina. This can also occur from accompanying coronary artery disease, which is not uncommon with aortic stenosis. Angina in aortic stenosis can occur with or without organic coronary artery obstruction. The absence of angina usually excludes severe coronary artery disease. Rare mechanism of angina is the complication of calcific emboli. Average life expectancy is about five years after the development of angina pectoris.
2. *Exertional syncope*: Mechanism of syncope following exertion is:
   a. Left ventricular failure with an abrupt reduction in cardiac output.
   b. Sudden fall of cardiac output in arrhythmias.
   c. Reduction in arterial pressure caused by vasodilatation in exercising muscles in the presence of fixed cardiac output.
   d. In elderly patients with calcific aortic stenosis.

   The syncope may be due to transient cerebral ischemia which is due to cerebrovascular disease. If the syncope is prolonged it may be accompanied by convulsions. Average life expectancy is about three to four years after the occurrence of syncope for the first time.
3. *Exertional dyspnea:* It is due to increase in pulmonary capillary pressure which in turn is caused by increase in left atrial or left ventricular end-diastolic pressure. Orthopnea, paroxysmal nocturnal dyspnea—the symptoms of left ventricular failure occurs in the late stage. Venous congestion, edema—the symptoms of right ventricular failure occur in preterminal stage. Average life expectancy after the development of symptoms of left ventricular failure is about two years.
4. *Sudden death*: Sudden death may occur in 15–20% of symptomatic patients and is attributed to arrhythmias and myocardial ischemia. Autopsy results revealed that approximately 15% of patients with aortic stenosis die suddenly without previous symptoms.

140. The 4 additional symptoms attributed to severe aortic stenosis are:

1. Fatigue—it is an early symptom in children.
2. Palpitation—is due to arrhythmias.
3. Central nervous system symptoms in the elderly—from associated carotid and cerebrovascular diseases.
4. Visual disturbances—visual field defects from calcific emboli originating from the stenosed valve. Rarely it is a presenting manifestation.

141. When aortic stenosis and mitral stenosis coexist, the features of aortic stenosis are masked by the mitral stenosis, the reduction of cardiac output is induced by mitral stenosis. This may have 4 advantages:

1. Lowers the pressure gradient across the aortic valve.
2. Reduces frequency of anginal attacks.
3. Delays the progress of aortic calcification.
4. Delays the left ventricular hypertrophy.

142. Physical findings.

1. Blood pressure: It is usually within normal limits; When the stroke volume falls, the systolic pressure may fall and the pulse pressure narrows. The more the severity of aortic stenosis, the more narrowing of pulse pressure. Systemic hypertension is rare and a basal systolic pressure exceeding 200 mm Hg practically excludes severe aortic stenosis.

2. Pulse: Is of small amplitude, with sloping upstroke, (plateau pulse) tidal wave well-developed and often higher than percussion wave. Anacrotic pulse is characteristic of aortic stenosis (See *Fig. A-1). The brachial artery is helpful in evaluating arterial wave abnormalities in aortic stenosis. The brachial artery can be occluded with a finger and gradual release of pressure permits recognition of an anacrotic notch. Delayed peak of the pulse, diminished amplitude and gradual downslope are described by the term pulsus parvus et tardus. A slow rising pulse helps to differentiate aortic stenosis from hypertrophic cardiomyopathy or mitral regurgitation. A palpable double systolic wave, the so called pulsus bisferiens excludes pure or predominant aortic stenosis and signifies dominant or pure aortic regurgitation or obstructive cardiomyopathy.
3. Jugular venous pulse (JVP) may be normal or 'A' wave may be prominent. This is caused by decreased distensibility of right ventricle caused by the hypertrophied interventricular septum (and/or pulmonary hypertension) and left ventricle. As a consequence the right atrium contracts against increased resistance producing 'A' wave.
4. Sustained, thrusting apex beat is characteristic of left ventricular hypertrophy. It is displaced laterally and inferiorly. A double apical impulse may be felt in the left lateral position. The first impulse is an outward expansion caused by atrial contraction to ventricular systole while the second impulse is forceful and sustained caused by ventricular systole. The left atrium may hypertrophy and dilate producing a palpable beat, which may be felt as second or double apex.
5. A systolic thrill is palpable in the right second inner space. The thrill may be transmitted to the carotids as the 'carotid shudder'. A thrill generally indicates a gradient across the valve exceeding 40 mm Hg.
6. An early systolic ejection sound, actually the opening snap of the aortic valve is heard with non-calcific aortic stenosis. This sound disappears when the valves become calcified and rigid. A_2 is usually reduced or absent.
   The sound of aortic valve closure is heard only in pliable, stenosed valves. The calcification of the valve diminishes the intensity of aortic sound. As the stenosis becomes severe, the left ventricular systole becomes prolonged, so that aortic valve closure sound may not precede the pulmonic valve closure sound and the two may become synchronous or aortic valve closure may still be delayed to occur later after pulmonic valve closure. This is called paradoxical splitting of the second heart sound. The delay of A_2 results in closely split, single or paradoxically split second sound according to the severity of the obstruction. In the absence of left ventricular conduction defect, presence of paradoxical splitting of second sound usually signifies severe aortic stenosis. The delay of A_2 results in closely split, single or paradoxically split S_2 according to severity of obstruction.
7. A fourth heart sound heard at the apex in severe aortic stenosis reflects the forceful atrial contraction in an elevated left ventricular end diastolic pressure.
   A third heart sound usually occurs when the left ventricle dilates and left ventricular failure occurs.
8. A characteristic harsh midsystolic diamond-shaped or crescendo-decrescendo murmur is heard in the aortic area and radiates along the carotid arteries. The murmur starts shortly after the first sound, increases in intensity to reach peak in the middle of the ejection period and diminishes thereafter to end just before the second sound. It is usually low pitched, rough and rumbling in character. The murmur is soft and brief when the stenosis is mild and in heart failure where the cardiac output is low. The murmur is at least III/VI grade in significant obstruction.
   Occasionally, the murmur may be transmitted downward towards the apex and it is confused with systolic murmur of mitral regurgitation. The systolic murmur of mitral regurgitation is holosystolic and radiates to axilla while the systolic murmur of aortic stenosis is of ejection type and is diamond-shaped, radiates towards carotids.
   A thrill is best felt and the murmur is best heard when the patient leans forward with breath held in expiration.

- S_1 intensity decreases as LV function worsens
- S_2 A_2 P_2 split. Intensity of A_2 decreases as progress; S_2 becomes soft as A_2 decreases in intensity
- May be paradoxically split as severity increases
- May become soft and single late in course
- S_3 may be present in the course
- S_4 often present due to LVH and poor LV complaisance

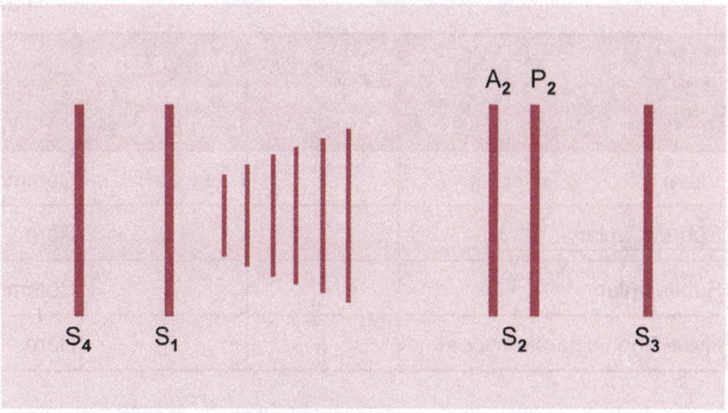

Fig. I-9: Auscultatory finding in aortic stenosis

- Murmur is systolic, harsh (rough and rumbling)
- Heard best at right upper sternal border
- Radiates to carotids
- Peaks in early to mid-systole until late in the course when it peaks later and is more intense.

143. Summary of the murmur of aortic stenosis.

Table I-7

1. Site of audibility and conduction	Aortic area—2nd right intercostal space Also heard at left sternal border, apex Along carotid artery
2. Timing	Ejection systolic
3. Character	Diamond shaped or crescendo-decrescendo murmur, low pitch, rough and rumbling Usually grade 3/6 in significant obstruction
4. Length of murmur	Short/medium/long

The murmur of valvular aortic stenosis is usually best heard at the right 2nd space but is also well heard at the left sternal border and apex. It is selectively conducted to the carotid vessels particularly to the right carotid. Any deviation has significance. When the murmur is heard only at the apex and nowhere else, a mistaken diagnosis of MR is often made but the lack of conduction to the axilla and back is helpful.

The presence of ejection systolic murmur localizes the lesion to the outflow of either ventricles. All other causes of ejection systolic murmur need to be differentiated from the murmur of aortic stenosis.

Any significant change in cardiac output makes changes in length of the murmur and so this sign is not reliable . Over estimation of the severity of aortic stenosis is a feature of high cardiac output such as anemia, thyrotoxicosis, pregnancy and under estimation is a feature of low cardiac output states such as heart failure myocardial infarction, hypothyroidism.

144. Four sites of audibility of aortic stenosis murmur and their significance.

Table I-8

Site of best audibility/selective conduction	*Significance*
1. Best audible at right 2nd ICS, conducted to right carotid	Valvular non-calcific aortic stenosis
2. Best audible at left sternal border, no carotid conduction	Subvalvular AS (fixed or dynamic) Calcific AS (loss of jet) Mistaken VSD Mistaken MR
3. Carotid murmur with or without right 2nd interspace murmur	Supravalvular AS Carotid stenosis
4. Audible only at apex	Calcific AS in elderly with emphysema, where apex is the only part of the heart coming into contact with chest wall Mistaken for MR

145. Physical findings and maneuvers useful in differentiating 4 forms of LV outflow tract obstruction.

Table I-9

	Pulse volume after PVC	*Valsalva effect on systolic murmur*	*AR*	*S_4*	***Carotid pulse***
Valve	↑	↓	Common	Common	Normal to anacrotic (parvus tardus)
Supravalvular	↑	↓	Rare	Uncommon	Unequal
Subvalvular	↑	↓	Common	Uncommon	Normal to anacrotic
Hypertrophic cardiomyopathy	↓	↑	Rare	Common	Rapid jerky upstroke

146. Aortic ejection sound is heard in aortic or mitral area and is not affected by respiration. It occurs in 4 conditions:

1. Aortic stenosis.
2. Aneurysm of ascending aorta.
3. Aortic insufficiency.
4. Occasionally in tetralogy of Fallot.

Ejection sounds can occur in the absence of valvular lesions of either aortic or pulmonary valve. A pulmonic ejection sound from a congenital pulmonary stenosis characteristically decrease or even disappear coincident with inspiration. A pulmonary ejection sound can occur in a patient with pulmonary hypertension, which in some (same as pulmonary stenosis) may decrease in intensity coincident with inspiration. An ejection sound may be present with aneurysm of aorta and in more advanced degree of aortic insufficiency.

147. Reversed splitting of second heart sound is due to delayed closure of the aortic valve. Aortic component closes after pulmonary component. It occurs in 4 conditions:

1. Severe aortic stenosis.
2. Left bundle branch block.
3. Severe ischemic heart disease.
4. Rarely in Wolff-Parkinson-White syndrome, right ventricular ectopics, patent ductus arteriosus with markedly increased left-to-right shunt.

148. There are 4 common conditions which simulate AS:

1. Aortic valve sclerosis
2. VSD
3. MR
4. PS.

149. There are 4 common associated defects in AS:

1. AR
2. Mitral valve disease
3. Coarctation of aorta
4. PDA.

150. Electrocardiogram: ECG abnormalities show the following 4 changes—

1. Left ventricular hypertrophy as evidenced by deep 'S' in right precordial leads and tall 'R' waves in left precordial leads.
2. In severe aortic stenosis, left ventricular strain pattern is noticed, ST depression and T inversion in LI, aVL, V5 and V6.
3. If calcification of the valve involves the conducting tissue, heart blocks are frequent and varies from first degree heart block to left bundle branch block.
4. Left atrial hypertrophy should suggest the presence of mitral valve disease.

A normal ECG does not exclude severe aortic stenosis.

151. Chest roentgenogram: There are 4 points to be checked in the X-ray chest:

1. Left ventricular hypertrophy suggests significant aortic stenosis. The heart size may be normal or show little enlargement for many years since the concentric hypertrophy is the initial response to obstruction.
2. Poststenotic dilatation of the aorta.
3. Aortic calcification is seen on fluoroscopy with an image intensifier. It is usually seen in patients over the age of 40 years. Absence of valvular calcification suggests that stenosis is not severe.
4. In late stages, progressive dilatation of left ventricle with decreased compliance causes left atrial enlargement. Left atrial enlargement is followed by pulmonary congestion, enlargement of pulmonary artery, right ventricle and right atrium. Excessive dilatation of left atrium rises the suspicion of other possibilities, such as mitral stenosis or idiopathic cardiomyopathy.

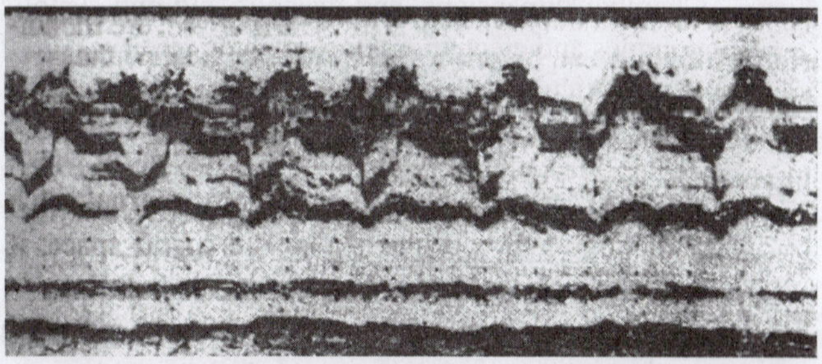

Fig. I-10: M-mode echocardiogram of a patient with aortic stenosis. Shows dense and multiple echoes within the aortic root, especially during diastole. These strong echoes are due to calcification and/or fibrosis of the cusps. If aortic cusps can be identified, they may appear thicker than the aortic wall

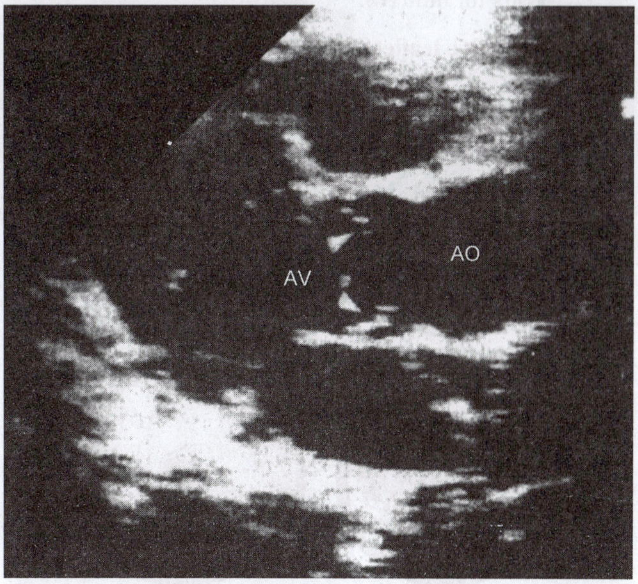

Fig. I-11: Two-dimensional echocardiogram of a patient with aortic stenosis. Absolute decrease in maximal leaflet separation and/or orifice size, systolic dome-like deformity. The leaflet tend to curve inward instead of lying parallel to the adjacent wall AV=aortic valve; AO=aorta

152. Echocardiogram: The 4 structures to be observed are:

1. *Valves*: Thickening, calcification and reduced mobility are the characteristic echo findings. Eccentric closure of the aortic valve cusps is characteristic of congenital bicuspid valve. Eccentricity index can be calculated by the asymmetry of the two leaflets. Aortic cusp separation of less than 8 mm is highly predictive of severe aortic stenosis. Echocardiogram distinguishes valvular stenosis from subvalvular or supravalvular stenosis.
2. *Left ventricle*: Septal wall thickness can estimate the extent of left ventricular hypertrophy and it can as well detect the asymmetrical hypertrophy in idiopathic subaortic stenosis.
   Chamber dimensions, end-diastolic and end-systolic volumes and ejection fraction provide information of left ventricular function.
3. *Aorta*: Poststenotic aortic dilatation can be visualized. The rate of blood flow across the aortic valve can estimate the systolic gradient by Echo Doppler technique. Stenotic area can be calculated from the pressure gradient by Echo Doppler.
4. Associated lesions-like mitral stenosis, mitral regurgitation can also be detected along with aortic stenosis with echo doppler technique.
   Echocardiography follow-up is done depending on the severity of the disease at least once a year for severe AS and more frequently as the severity increases.
   Every two years for moderate AS, every three to five years for mild AS.

153. Aortic valve leaflets.

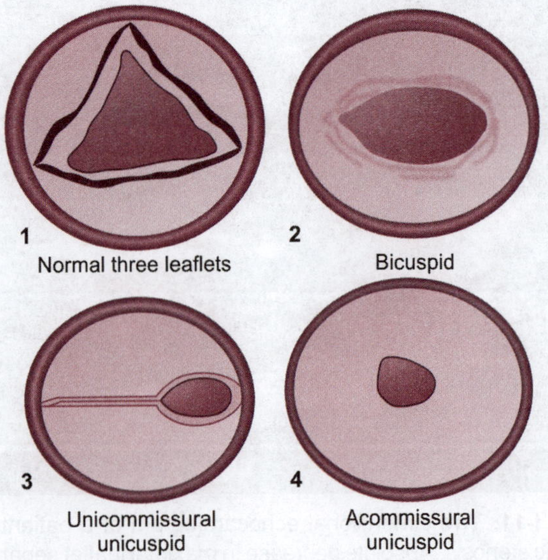

Fig. I-12: Morphology—its variations of aortic valve

Schematic representation of parasternal short axis of a congenitally aortic valve. This view is helpful in assessing the cause of congenital valve. The number of valves and the stage of valve orifice are assessed:

1. Normal three leaflets valve open as a triangle.
2. Bicuspid valve does elliptical opening.
3. In unicommisural valve—the opening is elliptical, but occurs across a radiance rather than diameter of the valve.
4. A commissural unicuspid valve.

154. Cardiac catheterization and angiocardiography:

Catheterization of the left side of the heart should be done in suspected cases of aortic stenosis particularly before operative decision is made. The indications are mainly 4.

1. *In young asymptomatic patient with non-calcific aortic stenosis:* To know the severity of obstruction, since operation is indicated even in the absence of symptoms with severe aortic stenosis.
2. *In whom the left ventricular outflow obstruction is suspected:* To know the level of obstructions at sub or supravalvular level.
3. *In patients with clinical signs of aortic stenosis and symptoms of myocardial ischemia:* To know whether aortic stenosis or coronary artery disease is the primary cause responsible for the symptoms. Coronary arteriography should be done along with catheterization of the left side of the heart.
4. *In patients with multivalvular disease:* To assess the affect of each valvular deformity before surgery.

155. Cardiac catheterization in aortic stenosis can record.

1. Severity of obstruction by estimating the stenotic area and gradient across the valve.
   Normal aortic valve area is 2–3 cm^2 and a reduction to less than 0.8 cm^2 significantly impedes systolic flow. A valvular gradient exceeding 50 mm Hg usually accompanies the stenosis.
2. Left ventricular function.
3. Location of the left ventricular outflow obstruction.
4. Other associated valve lesions and detect coronary artery disease by coronary arteriography at the same time.

156. Angiographic studies with left ventricular injection of contrast material are helpful to know 4 parameters.

1. Size of the left ventricular cavity. Thickness of the wall, site of obstruction to left ventricular outflow.
2. Degree of mobility and deformity of aortic cusps. When contrast substance is injected, the aortic valve cusps can be outlined and the associated aortic regurgitation can also be detected.

3. Diameter of the ascending aorta. A jet contrast substance passing through the stenotic aortic orifice is readily visualized.
4. Presence of other, valvular lesions like mitral regurgitation, etc.

157. Exercise studies should be performed cautiously observing the following points in patients with aortic stenosis, when there is a history of syncope. Assess the following 4 points:

1. Symptoms.
2. Exercise tolerance.
3. Blood pressure.
4. Ventricular function.

158. Analysis of several studies have showed the average duration of survival after various symptoms is as follows:

1. Angina pectoris—4–5 years.
2. Syncope—3–4 years.
3. Dyspnea—2 years.
4. Congestive heart failure—1.5–2 years.

159. In more than 80% of patients who died of aortic stenosis the symptoms existed for less than 4 years. Congestive cardiac failure is considered to be the cause of death in one-half to two-thirds of patients.

160. On an average, 4% (3–5%) of patients may die suddenly during an otherwise asymptomatic period presumably due to arrhythmias.

Symptoms in aortic stenosis indicate a much worse long term prognosis affecting the aortic or mitral valve. Aortic stenosis progresses more rapidly in elderly patients with congenital or rheumatic disease.

161. The clinical assessment of severity depends on the following:

1. Symptomatic patients have severe aortic stenosis. If the patient is asymptomatic, it does not exclude severe aortic stenosis.
2. Narrows the pulse pressure, the more severe the aortic stenosis.
3. Presence of a systolic thrill at the second intercostal space suggest at least moderately severe aortic stenosis. If the thrill is felt only in the suprasternal notch and not at the second right intercostal space, it favors mild or critical aortic stenosis in failure.
4. The later the peak of the ejection systolic murmur, the more severe the narrowing.
5. Delay in the A_2 is reasonably correlated with severity. Second sound is normally split with mild aortic stenosis. Closely split with moderate aortic stenosis. Single or paradoxically split with severe or critical aortic stenosis.
6. Presence of S_4 is an indirect evidence of severe aortic stenosis.
7. Presence of S_3 indicates severe aortic stenosis with congestive cardiac failure.
8. Evidence of left ventricular hypertrophy and ST and T changes in electrocardiogram favors severe aortic stenosis.

There is one problem which alters the clinical assessment is the presence of myocardial disease of ventricle which alters the physical findings to favor a more severe lesion. Aortic stenosis is a progressive disease becoming more and more severe with time. It is a serious disease because it is one the few lesions, which can cause sudden death.

162. Leaflets often thicken by the age of 40 years.

163. Calcium deposits are rarely detected before the age of 40 years.

164. The following 4 points are observed during:

Medical management: Strenuous physical activity should be avoided.

1. Rheumatic prophylaxis should be continued until 35 years of age when rheumatic etiology is suspected.
2. Prophylactic antibiotics should be given to prevent bacterial endocarditis before dental procedure, genitourinary procedure, etc. The same antibiotic coverage should be used as in mitral stenosis.
3. Exertional chest pain should be treated with nitroglycerine with caution. Patients are educated about complaints like orthostatic hypotension, syncope, etc.
4. Left ventricular failure should be treated with digitalis, diuretics. Vasodilators for heart failure in aortic stenosis are of little value.

165. Mechanical obstruction cannot be altered by medical treatment. There are 4 criteria for valve replacement:

1. Gradient across the valve more than 50 mm Hg.
2. Orifice size less than 0.8 cm^2 per square meter of body surface area.
3. Calcified aortic stenosis with symptoms
4. Patients with symptoms of angina, exertional syncope and congestive heart failure should undergo valve replacement promptly. Operation should be undertaken if possible before the symptoms of left ventricular failure supervene.

Surgical treatment of valve replacement in the severe AS is the mainstay.

166. Selection of surgical procedure: It depends on the age and nature of the valvular deformity. Patients with

aortic stenosis have the poorest prognosis. Following are the 4 guidelines for selection of the procedure:

1. For children and adolescents with congenital aortic stenosis with non-calcific valves: A simple commissurotomy by direct vision is usually be sufficient to relieve the obstruction. Simple commissurotomy can be performed by non-surgical percutaneous balloon dilatation also. The valve may deform and become stenotic again and most of them ultimately require valve replacement.
2. Calcified deformed valves with symptoms need valve replacement.
3. In patients with associated coronary artery stenosis: Coronary artery bypass graft should be done at the time of valve replacement. When concomitant bypass surgery is done, the distal graft anastomosis are performed prior to valve replacement so that cold cardioplegic solution can be infused via the grafts distal to the area of coronary obstruction. The proximal graft anastamosis are done after the valve replacement.
4. Restenosis of the valve and calcification: Valve replacement should be done in cases of restenosis and calcification. Repair of the associated anomalies should be done.

167. The 4 steps of operation: Surgery is performed under cardiopulmonary bypass, hypothermia and cardioplegia.

1. Median sternotomy incision.
2. Vent the left heart by a vent introduced into the left atrium or left ventricle via the right superior pulmonary vein.
3. Valve is excised and calcium is carefully debrided from the valve ring.
4. Prosthetic valve is then sutured.

Aortotomy is closed taking care to evacuate all the air from the heart before completing the closure. Aortic cross clamp is then released while suction is applied to a vent in the ascending aorta as a further precaution against air embolism.

168. Monitor the following 4 parameters in the immediate postoperative period. The patient is kept in the intensive coronary care unit for 24–48 hours.

1. Arterial pressure.
2. Left atrial pressure via a small catheter placed through the pulmonary vein at the time of operation.
3. Cardiac rhythm.
4. In patients with congestive heart failure and compromised left ventricular function, Swan-Ganz catheter is placed to measure the cardiac output.

169. Management of postoperative complications that are commonly met with aortic valve replacement surgery are mainly 4.

1. Hypertension which is frequently present should be treated with sodium nitroprusside infusion. Serum potassium is maintained at a level of about 4 mEq/L.
2. Ventricular arrhythmias are treated by xylocaine infusion. Digitalis is given only for the treatment of supraventricular arrhythmias.
3. Bradycardias are to be treated by an atrial pacing via small wire epicardial electrode placed at the time of surgery. It is initiated to augment cardiac output. It may also help to suppress ventricular ectopics in patients with a slow heart rate.
4. Warfarin is given to all patients to rapidly achieve a prothrombin deficiency approximately one and one-half to two times the normal. It is discontinued after six weeks in patients with tissue prosthesis but continued indefinitely in patients with mechanical prosthesis. Dipyridamole and warfarin combination decrease the incidence of thromboembolism—compared preoperatively and continued in patients with mechanical prosthesis.

170. Late deaths are most commonly due to 4 factors.

1. Heart failure.
2. Thromboembolism.
3. Myocardial infarction.
4. Cardiac arrhythmias.

Acute AR usually causes hemodynamic emergency because the LV does not have sufficient time to adjust to the rapid increase in LV volume. The fall in forward stroke volume and cardiac output results in hypotension and cardiogenic shock.

AORTIC REGURGITATION

Aortic regurgitation is the diastolic flow of blood from the aorta into the left ventricle due to incompetence of the aortic valve or any other cause of the valvular apparatus from the valve leaflets to the annulus of the aorta. (Aortic valve is the second most frequently affected valve, first being the mitral valve). Tricuspid and pulmonary valves are also frequently involved but much less frequently because the stress on the right side of the heart is less when compared with the left side.

171. There are 4 causes of aortic regurgitation.

1. Congenital-bicuspid valve, ventricular septal defect associated with sinus of Valsalva aneurysm. Prolapse of aortic valve in 15% of ventricular septal defect cases results in aortic regurgitation.
2. Specific infections: Rheumatic and syphilitic. Involvement of other valves is suggestive of rheumatic origin whereas isolated aortic regurgitation without

any stenosis is caused by syphilis. Acute aortic regurgitation may occur in infective endocarditis. Clinically pure aortic regurgitation without associated mitral valve disease is rare and occurs in 5–8% of patients. Pathologically pure rheumatic aortic valve disease is almost unknown.

3. Vascular disorders: Hypertension, atherosclerosis, aortic dissection non-specific aortitis like Takayasu's disease.
4. Connective tissue diseases which may be associated with aortic regurgitation: Marfan's syndrome, ankylosing spondylitis, Reiter's syndrome, rheumatoid arthritis, osteogenesis imperfecta, cystic medial necrosis.

Marked dilatation of aortic annulus without primary involvement of the valve leaflets results in aortic regurgitation in 3, 4 and syphilis. Any primary cause of aortic stenosis frequently results in aortic regurgitation of the fixed stenotic leaflets.

Rheumatic fever and syphilis were the major causes in the past but these have been diminished due to effective antibiotic therapy. Diseases of the connective tissue and congenital abnormalities have been recognized more frequently.

172. AR can develop from primary disease of the valve leaflet or from abnormalities of the aortic root or ascending aorta. The chronic and acute forms of AR different disease entities with variable causes. Clinical presentation, natural history and treatment strategies.

Major causes of chronic aortic regurgitation.

Table I-10

Leaflet abnormalities	*Aortic root or ascending aortal abnormalities*
1. Rheumatic fever	Age-related aortic dilation
2. Infective endocarditis	Annuloaortic ectasia
3. Trauma	Cystic medial necrosis of the aorta (isolated bicuspid valve or Marfan's syndrome)
4. Myxomatous degeneration	Systemic hypertension
5. Congenital AR	Aortitis (syphilis, giant cell arteritis)
6. SLE	Reiter's syndrome
7. RA	Ankylosing spondylitis
8. Ankylosis spondylitis	Behcet's syndrome
9. Takayama's arteritis	Psoriatic arthritis
10. Whipple's disease	Osteogenesis imperfecta
11. Crohn's disease	Relapsing polychondritis
12. Drug induced valvulopathy	Ehlers-Danlos syndrome

173. There are 4 causes of acute aortic regurgitation:

1. Aortic dissection—by disturbing the annulus support for the valve.
2. Bacterial endocarditis—by perforation or paravalvular incompetence or any other inflammation can cause prolapse or eversion of aortic cusp.
3. Prosthetic valve—leakage after surgery.
4. Ruptured sinus of Valsalva—Traumatic causes which are due to non-penetrating cardiac injuries are rare.

174. About 3/4 of the aortic regurgitation patients are males, whereas females predominate with associated mitral valvular disease.

175. About 3/4 of aortic regurgitation patients are of rheumatic origin. Rheumatic etiology is less common in isolated aortic regurgitation.

176. The following 4 pathophysiological changes occur in aortic regurgitation:

1. Regurgitation of diastolic flow increases the volume load. The amount of volume load is influenced by:
   - i. Size of incompetence.
   - ii. Diastolic pressure gradient across the valve.
   - iii. Duration of systole.
   - iv. Chronicity and severity of incompetence.
2. Left ventricular end-diastolic volume gradually increases since it receives blood from left atrium and the systemic circulation.
3. Compensatory dilatation of the left ventricle allows minimal elevation of left ventricular end-diastolic pressure. Compensatory left ventricular hypertrophy normalizes systolic wall stress or afterload.
4. Total left ventricular stroke volume is appropriately increased to maintain effective systemic circulation. Chronic aortic regurgitation with severe left ventricular enlargement can produce the largest left ventricular stroke volume of any disease affecting the left ventricle. Increased left ventricular stroke volume greatly increases the mechanical pressure, volume work, compensatory hypertrophy and myocardial oxygen consumption.
5. Because of the backward flow of blood the forward flow is impaired. This is compensated by peripheral vasodilatation and as well as increased ejection from the left ventricle during the early part of systole. The peripheral pulse pressure is wide because of increased systolic and lowered diastolic pressure. Signs of wide pulse pressure in the form of exaggerated arterial and arteriolar pulsations (water-hammer pulse) are present unless the aortic regurgitation is minor.

6. Slowing of the heart rate increases the diastolic period and increases the regurgitent volume of blood in aortic regurgitation . With good left ventricular function even moderate aortic regurgitation is tolerated well for long periods.
7. If the left ventricular myocardium is failing, the left ventricular diastolic pressure goes up and results in an increase in left atrial pressure and pulmonary congestion.
8. Dilatation of the left ventricle is accompanied with abnormal stress on the papillary muscle complex of the mitral valve. This may result in inadequate apposition of the mitral leaflets and appearance of mitral regurgitation.
   Heart rate exerts minimal influence on the severity of aortic regurgitation.

Following are the clinical manifestations.
Physical findings are caused by large left ventricular stroke volume and rapid diastolic run off.

177. The 4 common symptoms include:

1. Palpitation due to large left ventricular stroke volume and awareness of the heart beat in the left lateral position. Thus, the main symptom is palpitation.
2. Breathlessness: With mild to moderate aortic regurgitation the forward flow can be increased on exercise. Thus breathlessness is not an early symptom.
3. Exertional chest pain: Atypical angina pectoris which lasts for longer duration and can occur at rest. Flushing, palpitation sweating may accompany chest pain.
4. Symptoms of left ventricular failure: Abdominal discomfort, edema of feet, etc.

Patient may remain asymptomatic for many years with aortic regurgitation because of the compensatory mechanism of the left ventricular volume overload.

178. The 4 other unusual symptoms that can occur in severe aortic regurgitation include:

1. Neck pain.
2. Abdominal pain.
3. Postural dizziness.
4. Excessive sweating on the trunk.

Stretching of the carotid sheath by large left ventricular systolic volume causes neck pain and a similar mechanism plays in the abdominal pain. Disturbance in the cerebral circulation with marked pressure changes during the rapid diastolic run off causes the postural dizziness.

179. Inspection: The 4 points—

1. Sudden distension and collapse of larger arteries are visible. Prominent carotid pulsations (Corrigan's sign), visible arterial pulsations over the extremity vessels (dancing peripheral arteries) or visible pulsations of the abdominal aorta are indicative of wide pulse pressure of any cause.
   (Corrigan's pulse: Large volume carotid pulsations seen in patients with severe aortic regurgitation. It refers to what is seen, not what is felt).
2. Head-bobbing motion with each systole (de Musset's sign) due to sudden filling of the carotid vessels in severe aortic regurgitation. Arteriolar pulsations may be seen over the nail bed, uvula, lips, ear lobes and in the eye grounds.
3. Apex beat is displaced inferiorly and laterally.
4. Physical abnormalities of associated disease may be seen, such as asthenic body, long extremities, arachnodactaly of Marfan's syndrome. Bluish discoloration of sclera in osteogenesis imperfecta and subluxation of lens in Marfan's syndrome.

180. On palpation:

1. A rapidly rising 'Water-hammer pulse' which falls suddenly during late systole and diastole.
2. Quincke's pulse—alternate flushing and paling of the skin at the root of the nail is visible when pressure is applied to the tip of the nail.
3. Apex beat has systolic expansion and subsequent retraction in contrast to sustained systolic thrust characteristic of severe aortic stenosis.
4. Carotid pulse may be bisferiens with the systolic waves separated by a through in pure aortic regurgitation or combined with aortic stenosis.
5. Blood pressure recording shows very high pulse pressure. The wider the pulse pressure, the more severe the aortic regurgitation. Sometimes, the systolic blood pressure may be as high as 300 mm Hg. The diastolic pressure may be recorded as zero with severe aortic regurgitation. Sometimes, the severity of aortic regurgitation may not always correlate with the degree of pulse pressure. If the pulse pressure is less than 50% of the peak systolic pressure or if diastolic blood pressure is above 70 mm Hg. Aortic regurgitation may not be hemodynamically severe unless left ventricular failure exists.
   There is exaggeration of systolic pressure difference between the brachial and femoral arteries.
   A disproportionate raise in femoral artery systolic pressure has been designated as Hill's sign. Normal difference between the brachial artery and femoral artery is less the 20 mm Hg, the femoral systolic pressure being higher. Systolic pressure difference between 20–40 mm Hg suggests mild aortic regurgitation. Between 40–60 mm Hg suggests moderate AR and more than 60 mm Hg suggests severe AR.

6. A diastolic thrill is often palpable along the left sternal border.
7. Prominent systolic thrill may be palpable along the carotids. This thrill and accompanying systolic murmur are due to markedly increased left ventricular output and do not necessarily signify coexistence of aortic stenosis.
8. Sometimes a systolic thrill may be palpated with the ejection murmur in acute aortic regurgitation.

181. Physical findings with hyperdynamic pulse in chronic aortic regurgitation named after persons:

Table I-11

1. Corrigan's pulse or water-hammer pulse	Rapid upstroke followed by quick collapse
2. de Musset's sign	Head bobbing with each heartbeat
3. Traube's sign	Pistol-shot sounds heart over the femoral arteries in both systole and diastole
4. Muller's sign	Systolic pulsations of the uvula
5. Duroziez's sign	Systolic murmur over the femoral artery when compressed proximally and a diastolic murmur when compressed distally or systolic-diastolic murmur with increasing compression over the femoral arteries
6. Quincke's sign	Capillary pulsations visible in the nail bed
7. Hill's sign	Popliteal cuff systolic pressure exceeding brachial cuff systolic pressure by > 60 mm Hg
8. Becker's sign	Arterial pulsations visible in the retinal arteries

182. On auscultation:

1. A booming pistol-shot sound can be heard over the femorals.
   A systolic murmur may be heard if pressure is applied to partially occlude the artery proximal to the chest piece and a diastolic murmur if pressure is applied distally.
   This combination of systolic and diastolic murmur is known as Duroziez's sign.
2. Aortic second sound is diminished or absent—scarring of the aortic leaflet margins diminish the aortic second sound.
3. Third heart sound is common—the ventricular gallop reflects the exaggerated diastolic filling, an increase in end-diastolic volume or a decrease in contractile state as evidenced by the left ventricular dysfunction. Fourth heart sound may be heard occasionally.
4. A loud systolic ejection click is sometimes heard along the left sternal border and is produced by aortic distension with greatly increased stroke volume.
5. High pitched blowing decrescendo-diastolic murmur best heard along the left sternal border in the third left intercostal space. The duration of the murmur is correlated with the hemodynamic abnormality. It is holodiastolic in severe regurgitation. When the murmur is soft it is best heard with the diaphragm in the sitting posture, bending forward and breath held in expiration.
6. 'Cooing' or musical blowing of the murmur suggests eversion of the aortic cusp.
7. A systolic ejection murmur that is best heard at the base of the heart is transmitted to the carotids. Sometimes, it may be as loud as grade V or VI without any organic obstruction.
8. Austin-Flint murmur is a soft, low pitched rumbling mid-diastolic or presystolic bruit. It is caused by the displacement of anterior leaflets of mitral valve by the aortic regurgitant stream which produces functional mitral stenosis. It signifies severe aortic regurgitation. It may be difficult to differentiate from diastolic murmur of mitral stenosis, which is associated with loud first sound and opening snap.
   Auscultatory findings are intensified by isometric exercise, such as handgrip exercise which increases systemic resistance. Inhalation of amylnitrate has the opposite effect.

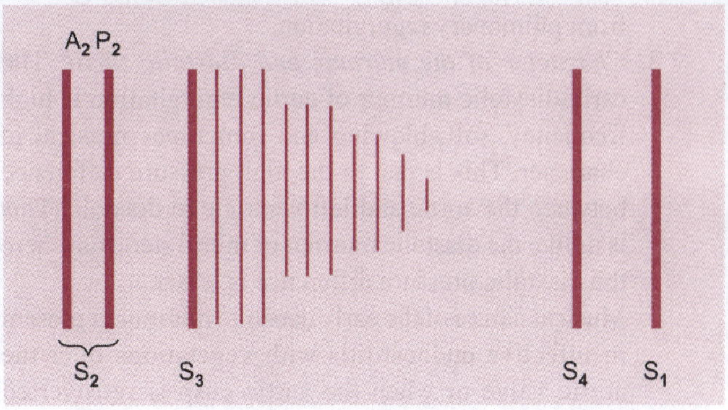

Fig. I-13: Auscultatory findines in aortic regurgitation

- S_1—intensity decreases as LV function worsens
- S_2—may be narrowly split or paradoxically split due to prolonged systolic ejection time
- A_2—may be soft due to poor coaptation
- P_2—may be obscured by the murmur
- S_3—may be present late in the course
- S_4—frequently seen due to LVH and poor LV compliance.

Murmur: Murmur is diastolic, soft and blowing, decrescendo. Heard best at left sternal border. Severity correlates more with duration than intensity. Diagrammatic representation of auscultatory findings in chronic AR.

183. Summary of features of aortic regurgitation murmur:

Table I-12

Features	Description
1. Timing	Early diastolic
2. Site of best audibility	Right 2nd ICS/LSB/Apex/ right sternal border
3. Character	High frequency/soft/blowing/musical
4. Length/grading	< grade 3/6, thrill is rare

1. *Timing*: Many a times, it is not certain between the early diastolic and mid-diastolic timing of the murmur. The bell and diaphragm help to differentiate it. A diastolic murmur best heard with the bell is the mid-diastolic murmur of mitral valve and the one best herd with diaphragm is the early diastolic murmur of aortic regurgitation.
2. *Site of best audibility*: The most common form of aortic regurgitation murmur of rheumatic origin is best heard along the left sternal border but is also well-heard at the right 2nd intercostal space and apex.
   In rare causes of aortic regurgitation, such as syphilis, due to aortic root disease the murmur is best heard along the right sternal border but also along left sternal border and apex.
   The audibility of early diastolic murmur at the right 2nd ICS and apex distinguishes acute aortic regurgitation from pulmonary regurgitation.
3. *Character of the murmur and diastolic thrill*: The early diastolic murmur of aortic regurgitation is high frequency, soft, blowing and sometimes musical in character. This is due to the high pressure difference between the aortic and left ventricle in diastole. This is unlike the diastolic murmur of mitral stenosis where the diastolic pressure difference is lesser.
   Musical nature of the early diastolic murmur is present in infective endocarditis with vegetations over the aortic valve or when the aortic cusp is retroverted as in syphilis. Rough character of the murmur as in aortic stenosis with a thrill suggests a retroverted aortic cusp as in syphilis. This unexpected thrill of aortic regurgitation is often mistaken for systolic thrill.
4. *Length of the murmur*: It is the reflection of the duration of pressure gradient across the aortic and left ventricle in diastole. In the absence of heart failure in chronic aortic regurgitation, a short murmur generally means mild aortic regurgitation and long murmur is associated with moderate to sever aortic regurgitation.

184. The length of early diastolic murmur in aortic regurgitation depends on:

1. Aortic pressure (systemic vascular resistance).
2. Degree of abnormality of the aortic valve.
3. Left ventricular end-diastolic pressure.
4. Probably the direction of the jet of aortic regurgitation.

185. Relation of diastolic murmur to physiological act/maneuver:

Table I-13

1. Respiration	Best heard in expiration in sitting (or standing), leaning forward
2. Isometric hand grip/ vasopressor (phenylephrine)	Increases
3. Amylnitrate inhalation/or sublingual nitrate	Decreases
4. Prompt squatting	Increases

186. The features of the 4 sounds in aortic regurgitation:

Table I-14

1. First sound	Normal with mild AR. Diminished or absent in severe AR
2. Second sound	Normal split with mild AR/ reversed split with severe AR or LV dysfunction. A_2 is diminished or absent in rheumatic valve disease. Accentuated with aortic root disease as in syphilis
3. Third sound	Suggests heart failure or associated mitral regurgitation
4. Fourth sound	Acute AR/aortic dissection with past hypertension and left ventricular hypertrophy

187. Auscultatory features that simulate AV valve diastolic murmurs:

1. Third heart sound as mid-diastolic murmur.
2. Fourth heart sound as presystolic murmur.
3. Third and fourth heart sounds together as mid-diastolic murmur.
4. Early diastolic murmur of aortic regurgitation at apex.

188. The features of Austin-Flint murmur are:

1. It is due to heavy jet of AR falling on anterior mitral leaflet preventing adequate opening.
2. Does not occur with mild AR.
3. Requires at least a moderate AR.
4. Can be mid-diastolic and/presystolic.
5. With premature closure of mitral valve in a severe AR or in acute AR, the presystolic murmur does not occur.
6. Increases with isometric hand grip or vasopressors.
7. Decreases with amylnitrate inhalation or vasodilators.
8. Low pitched, best heard with the bell, unlike the murmurs of AR, which is high pitched and best heard with the diaphragm.

189. Right sided murmurs of aortic regurgitation:

Diastolic murmurs of aortic regurgitation are mostly louder on the left sternal border than on right sternal border. However, some aortic diastolic murmurs are best heard along the right sternal border—in third and fourth intercostal spaces. The third space is most likely to show the difference. Whenever an aortic diastolic murmur is heard louder or equal on the right side as compared with left sternal border, it is usually associated with dilatation and right sided displacement of aortic root. This aortic diastolic murmur has been associated with following conditions:

1. Aortic aneurysm
2. Aortic dissection
3. Hypertension
4. Arteriosclerosis
5. Ventricular septal defect with aortic regurgitation.

Collagen diseases, such as:

6. Rheumatoid spondylitis
7. Marfan's syndrome (a variant of Marfan's syndrome).
8. Osteogenesis imperfecta.

Whenever there is diastolic hypertension, aortic regurgitation, right sided aortic diastolic murmur—it is usually suggestive of aneurysm and/or dissection of first part of ascending aorta—search for other clinical features.

190. Table of causes of right sternal and left sternal border diastolic murmur of AR:

Table I-15

Right sternal border murmur of AR: causes	*Left sternal border murmur of AR: causes*
1. Syphilis	Rheumatic heart disease
2. Marfan's syndrome	Congenital bicuspid valve
3.Ankylosing spondylitis	Infective endocarditis
4. Rheumatoid arthritis	AR with valvular AS
5.Annuloectasis of aortic root	AR with subvalvular fixed AS
6. Reiter's syndrome	Prosthetic AR
7. AR with tetralogy of Fallot	
8. AR with VSD	

The murmur is conducted to the right sternal border with dilated aortic root. In aortic regurgitation of tetralogy of fallot, the jet of aortic regurgitation is directed selectively into right ventricle due to dextroposition of aorta and the murmur may better audible along the right sternal border. Similarly, in aortic regurgitation of ventricular septal defect, the right coronary artery cusp prolapses in to right ventricle due to lack of support. The left sternal border murmur is suggestive of valvular origin for the murmur.

191. Differential diagnosis of AR with conditions associated with wide pulse pressure:

1. Patent ductus arteriosus
2. Arteriovenous fistulae
3. VSD with AR
4. Ruptured sinus of Valsalva
5. Anemia
6. Thyrotoxicosis
7. Pregnancy
8. Anxiety, fever marked bradycardia.

5, 6, 7, 8 are hyperdynamic states.

192. Differential diagnosis of AR with conditions associated with non-rheumatic regurgitant diastolic murmur.

1. Pulmonary regurgitation
2. AR with VSD
3. Ruptured sinus of Valsalva
4. Congenital aorticvalve disease (leaking bicuspid aortic valve or aortic stenosis). Pure congenital AR is extremely rare. Others include Marfan's syndrome, Hurler syndrome.

193. Causes of acute aortic regurgitation and clinical settings.

Table I-16

Causes of acute aortic regurgitation	*Clinical features*
1. Infective endocarditis	Fever Acute pulmonary edema, heart failure Rheumatic heart disease Bicuspid aortic valve
2. Acute aortic dissection	Acute chest pain/back pain Absent or asymmetry of peripheral pulse
3. Trauma a. Blunt injury chest b. Surgical or balloon dilatation	Deterioration postprocedure
4. PTCA guiding catheter interfering with aortic valve closure mechanism	Unexplained hypotension or elevation of pulmonary artery diastolic pressure during PTCA

194. Chest roentgenogram the following 4 points:

1. Varying degree of left ventricular enlargement depending on the degree of aortic regurgitation. Apex is displaced downward, posteriorly and to the left and cardiac shadow may extend below the left dome of diaphragm in frontal plane. Anterior oblique and lateral view show posterior displacement of left ventricle and encroachment on the spine.
   Heart size may be normal in acute aortic regurgitation despite marked venous congestion and pulmonary edema.
2. Ascending aorta and aortic knob may be moderately dilated and extend on the right than the right atrial shadow in frontal plane in primary valvular disease. Prominent dilatation of ascending aorta is a feature of Marfan's syndrome.

3. Aneurysmal dilatation of the aorta may be seen in primary valvular disease in frontal plane and may occupy retrosternal space in lateral view.
4. Syphilitic aortitis is suspected with calcification of the dilated ascending aorta. Calcification of the valve is usually not seen and should suspect the possibility of associated aortic stenosis.

   Fluroscopy reveals vigorous aortic and left ventricular pulsations in opposite directions during systole.

195. Electrocardiogram the 4 points:

There may be no changes in the early stage. The following changes may be seen in severe aortic regurgitation.

1. Left ventricular hypertrophy, left axis deviation and left atrial abnormalities are seen after development of LV dysfunction (Tall R in V5, and deep S in V1). There are also deep 'Q' waves in left chest leads accompanied with tall T waves. The pattern of deep 'Q' and tall T waves has been called the diastolic over loading pattern of the left ventricle.
2. Conduction abnormalities are unusual but can occur after LV dysfunction. Atrial premature beats, ventricular premature beats are common. Sustained supraventricular or ventricular tachyarrhythmias are uncommon in the absence of LV dysfunction or concomittent mitral valve disease.
3. Signs of old myocardial infarction indicates associated coronary artery disease. QRS prolongation indicates diffuse myocardial disease generally associated with patchy fibrosis. These indicate poor prognosis.
4. ST-T wave depression in L!, aVL, V5 and V6 are frequently seen.

In acute aortic regurgitation there may be no evidence of left ventricular hypertrophy and ST-T changes suggest myocardial ischemia.

196. Echocardiography:

It provides information on aortic valve apparatus, aortic root, etiology, severity of aortic regurgitation and measurements of ventricular function.

1. Dilatation of aortic root suggest chronic basis for the aortic regurgitation.

   Diastolic oscillations in the aortic root or ventricular outflow track can be observed with a flail leaflet. Aortic dissection can be seen as a double lumen in the ascending aorta.
2. Dilatation of the left ventricle and left atrium. Left ventricular chamber dimensions and wall thickness gives calculation of chamber volume, stroke volume, shortening fraction, left ventricular mass, end-diastolic and end-systolic wall stress, preload and afterload respectively.

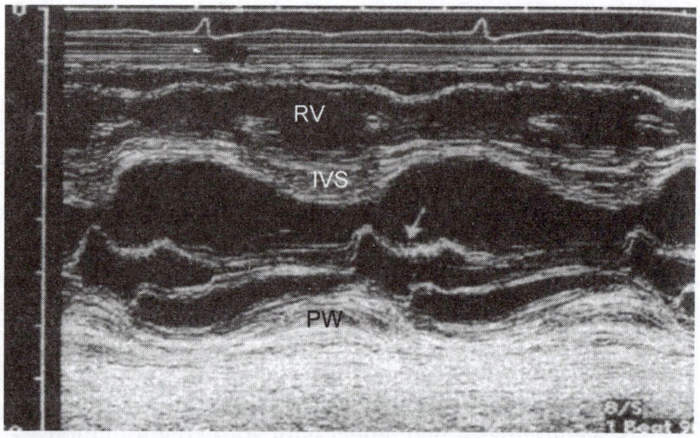

Fig. I-14: M-mode echocardiogram of a patient with aortic regurgitation. Shows mitral valve fluttering during diastole. This is because, the leaflet is caught between the antegrade flow from left atrium and the retrograde diastolic flow of aortic regurgitation stream which is directed toward the mitral valve

Left ventricular end-diastolic pressure may be normal in chronic aortic regurgitation due to increased compliance of volume overload left ventricle. As left ventricular end-diastolic pressure increases, compensatory increase in wall thickness will maintain a near normal end-diastolic wall, stress or preload. Ejection fraction is an index of mechanical performance but it is spuriously preserved since systolic ejection is initiated at a lower left ventricular pressure than normal. End-diastolic pressure-volume wall stress indicates the contractile state and may become depressed before the clinical symptoms of congestive heart failure appear.

3. Mitral valve abnormalities include characteristic diastolic fluttering of the anterior leaflet, premature closure of valve before the onset of QRS complex and thickening of leaflets.
4. Vegetations of endocarditis can sometimes be found on aortic valves.

   Echocardiography is useful before and after surgery. Patients with left ventricular end-diastolic dimension more than 55 mm or heart failure, or failure of significant reduction in heart size are of high-risk group. Doppler, TEE, stress ECHO are also done for some more information.

197. Cardiac catheterization: It helps in 4 ways:

1. Document aortic incompetence and estimate its severity.
2. Evaluate left ventricular function.
3. Identify other abnormalities in the aorta, mitral valve, etc.
4. Detect any defect in coronary anatomy.

Coronary arteriography is indicated in adults over 40 years of age whether the history of chest pain is present or not.

198. Four grades of aortic regurgitation by angiography.

Table I-17

Degree of AR	*LV opacification*	*Rate of clearing*
1. Mild 1+	Fair, incomplete	Rapid
2. Moderate 2+	Faint, complete	Rapid
3. Moderate to severe Intermediate 3+	Equal to aortic opacification	Intermediate
4. Severe 4+	Greater than aortic opacification	Slow

199. The degree of abnormality or positivity of Hill's sign correlates with the angiographic severity of aortic regurgitation.

Table I-18

Hill's sign in aortic regurgitation	*Angiographic correlation*
Lower limb systolic blood pressure	Evaluation of aortic regurgitation
1. < 20 mm Hg	Normal or trivial or mild AR Angiographic 1+ AR Associated coarctation
2. 20–40 mm Hg	Angiographic 2+ AR
3. 40–60 mm Hg	Angiographic 3+ AR
4. > 60 mm Hg	Angiographic 4+ AR

The blood pressure should be measured in all the limbs in all the patients with aortic regurgitation because the Hill's sign aids in the estimation of severity but any asymmetry of pressure gives a clue to the underlying coarctation of aorta or aortic dissection.

200. Medical treatment: The 4 points in management are:

1. *Heart failure:* It can be treated with salt restriction, digitalis, diuretics, vasodilators, such as hydralazine, ACEI and calcium channel blockers have been used in chronic AR to reduce the severity of regurgitant, and to stabilize or delay before the surgical intervention. Long-term vasodilator therapy is not recommended for asymptomatic patients with mild to moderate AR with normal systolic function.
   i. Hydralazine was found to improve LV systolic function and to reduce LV chamber dimensions in some studies.
   ii. Nifedipine was found useful to reduce LV volume and increase in LVEF.
   iii. ACEI was found to decrease in LV volume in some studies. However, ACEI action was seen well when blood pressure was effectively lowered.
   iv. In patient with significant root dilation as in cystic medial necrosis or related conditions (as in Marfan's syndrome). β-blockers are advised to slow the rate at which the aortic root enlarges.

   Medical therapy in acute AR is hemodynamic stabilization before doing surgical intervention. For patients with cardiogenic shock, IV vasodilators are used to reduce the after-load stress on LV, to lower LVEDP and to increase the cardiac output. In severe cases, IV inotropic agents may be needed temporarily. β-blockers may be used with caution when acute AR is caused by aortic dissection.
2. *Infection:* Prophylactic coverage against bacterial endocarditis is indicated during dental procedures, surgical instrumentation of gastrointestinal or genito-urinary tract. Endocarditis should be vigorously treated with suitable antibiotics. Syphilitic aortitis should be treated with full course of penicillin.
3. *Arrhythmias:* These are treated with antiarrhythmic drugs.
4. *Angina:* It is managed with antianginal drugs. They are not very helpful in angina of coronary artery disease or aortic stenosis.

However, one should keep in mind that the primary defect is a mechanical one and medical treatment alone cannot rectify the impaired or defective valve.

201. Surgical treatment.

More risky. Aortic regurgitation patients usually do not become symptomatic until they develop myocardial dysfunction. Timing of surgery is very important. It often does not restore normal left ventricular function. Various methods are indicated depending on the chronicity and other associated lesions. The 4 important methods are:

1. Replacement of aortic valve with a suitable prosthesis or heterograft.
2. Narrowing of the annulus may be possible in cases of aortic regurgitation due to aneurysmal dilatation of the annulus of the ascending aorta or by excising the aneurysm.
3. Excision of aneurysm and replacement of aortic valve with a graft are frequently necessary. This has high risk than simple aortic valve replacement alone.
4. Rarely urgent surgery is needed when a leaflet has been perforated in bacterial endocarditis or acute dissection of the ascending aorta.

Since it is a high-risk operation, surgery should be considered in patients who have free aortic regurgitation with cardiomegaly who have symptoms not responding to medical treatment.

TRICUSPID STENOSIS (TS)

Tricuspid stenosis is most often rheumatic and is associated with mitral stenosis.

Tricuspid stenosis causes obstruction to right atrial emptying.

202. Prevalence, etiology and pathology:

1. Relatively uncommon
2. More common in women than in men
3. More common in India than in USA or Western Europe
4. Does not usually occur as an isolated lesion
5. Almost of rheumatic origin > 90%
6. Most commonly observed in association with mitral stenosis and sometimes with mitral and aortic stenosis. (trivalvular stenosis)
7. In 5–10% of patients it occurs with severe mitral valvular disease
8. Rheumatic tricuspid stenosis is commonly associated with some degree of tricuspid regurgitation.

203. Causes of TS: Tricuspid stenosis is rare as an isolated lesion and is most commonly as part of multi valvular processes:

1. Congenital
2. Rheumatic
3. Infective endocarditis
4. Carcinoid syndrome
5. Malignancy (e.g. myxoma, metastasis)
6. Whipple's disease
7. Fabry's disease
8. Iatrogenic: Methysergide, ergot derivatives anorexigenic agents, prosthetic valve failure.

204. Pathophysiology:

1. A diastolic pressure gradient between the right atrium and ventricle is the characteristic hemodynamic expression of tricuspid stenosis. It increases during exercise and inspiration but reduces during expiration. A mean diastolic pressure gradient of more than 5 mm Hg is sufficient to elevate right atrial pressure to result in systemic venous congestion associated with jugular distension, ascites and edema unless sodium is restricted or diuretics are given.
2. In patients with sinus rhythm right atrial 'A' wave is extremely tall and may even approach the levels of right ventricular systolic pressure.
3. Resting cardiac output is quiet low and fails to rise during exercise. Low cardiac output is responsible for the normal or slightly elevated left atrial, pulmonary arterial and right ventricular systolic pressures despite the presence of even moderately severe mitral stenosis.
4. A mean diastolic pressure gradient across the tricuspid valve as low as 2 mm Hg is sufficient to establish the diagnosis. Right atrial and right ventricular systolic pressures should be noted simultaneously using two catheters or a single catheter with double lumen with proximal opening into the right atrium and distal opening into the right ventricle.

205. Symptoms:

1. Weakness, fatigue are secondary to low cardiac output and discomfort is due to refractory edema and ascites; marked hepatomegaly is common. These symptoms of systemic venous congestion are out of proportion to dyspnea.
2. Some patients complain of a fluttering discomfort in the neck due to giant 'A' waves in the jugular venous pulse.
3. Since it is generally preceded by mitral stenosis, many patients initially have symptoms of pulmonary congestion (paroxysmal nocturnal dyspnea, hemoptysis, acute pulmonary edema). Amelioration of symptoms of pulmonary congestion in a patient with mitral stenosis should rise the suspicion of tricuspid stenosis. Characteristically, the patient of tricuspid stenosis complain of relatively little dyspnea for the degree of hepatomegaly, swelling of the abdomen and anasarca.
4. It is suspected that when the right ventricular failure symptoms persist after adequate mitral valvulotomy. Progressive fatigue, edema, anorexia are common. Orthopnea, paroxysmal nocturnal dyspnea are minimal. Pulmonary edema and hemoptysis are rare.

206. Physical findings:

1. JVP is raised and in patients with sinus rhythm giant 'A' waves are seen. The 'V' waves are less conspicuous since tricuspid stenosis impedes right atrial emptying during diastole. The 'Y' descent is slow and barely seen indicating the absence of normal rapid early right ventricular filling.
2. Signs of congestion: Marked hepatic congestion is seen often resulting in cirrhosis, portal hypertension, splenomegaly, ascites, edema, jaundice and serious malnutrition. There may be prominent presystolic pulsations of the liver.
3. Opening snap of tricuspid stenosis may be heard or recorded phonocardiographically approximately 0.06 second after pulmonary valve closure. It is often difficult to distinguish from opening snap of mitral valve.
4. Diastolic rumbling murmur similar to the quality of murmur of mitral stenosis is heard at the left lower sternal margin and over the xiphoid process. The diastolic murmur and opening snap both are accentuated during inspiration and reduced during expiration.

Since the tricuspid stenosis occurs almost always in association with mitral stenosis, the less common valvular lesion may be missed.

A giant 'A' wave in the jugular venous pulse in the absence of palpable pulmonary valve closure and right ventricular lift of pulmonary hypertension suggest the possibility of tricuspid stenosis.

Signs of multivalvular involvement should be searched. Associated murmurs of mitral and aortic valve disease may be present.

207. Murmur of tricuspid stenosis:

1. It is audible in tricuspid area (4th space, left sternal border), localized to tricuspid area.
2. It is presystolic with or without mid-diastolic component.
3. Rough and rumbling in character.
4. It is increased:
   a. During inspiration
   b. Supine position
   c. Passive leg rising
   d. Rapid deep breathing.

Diastolic murmur of tricuspid stenosis is similar to mitral stenosis. However, the most important difference is the remarkable increase in intensity of murmur with inspiration in tricuspid stensosis. The inspiratory increase is often so explosive that it is often mistaken for a pericardial rub. Absence of this feature should rise doubt about the diagnosis of tricuspid stenosis.

If ordinary inspiration fails to bring in the murmur, passive leg rising in supine position during inspiration generally brings in the murmur. Another way is to ask the patient to breath in and out rapidly 5–6 times and then listening for the murmur during inspiration. The few rapid breaths increase the venous return, which accumulated in the right atrium enhancing the gradient and thereby the murmur. The inspiratory increase is so constant in tricuspid stenosis, that the absence of this feature should rise the doubt about the diagnosis of tricuspid stenosis.

The murmur is best heard at tricuspid area. But occasionally heard at left 3rd space, which can be mistaken for early diastolic murmur of aortic regurgitation or pericardial rub. The murmur may occasionally be heard at the apex in rheumatic tricuspid stenosis. In Ebsteins's anomaly, the displaced tricuspid valve toward the right ventricle and dilated right atrium together can cause murmur being best heard at apex.

The timing of tricuspid stenosis murmur is presystolic with or without mid-diastolic component. The length of the murmur is directly related to the severity of stenosis. The tricuspid diastolic murmurs are earlier in diastole. Because of this, often mistaken for early diastolic murmur of aortic or pulmonary incompetence. But their remarkable increase with inspiration and decrease or disappearance withstanding or expiration differentiate tricuspid stenosis from aortic regurgitation or pulmonary regurgitation.

The murmur of tricuspid stenosis is low frequency and rough and rumbling in character. This is due to low pressure difference between the right atrium and right ventricle in diastole. The murmur is often mistaken for a pericardial rub due to the rough character.

208. Though the length of the murmur is directly related to the severity of tricuspid stenosis in certain conditions the murmur may be shorter for the degree of stenosis.

The conditions where significant tricuspid stenosis is with shorter or no murmur:

1. Ebstein's anomaly of tricuspid valve.
2. Rheumatic tricuspid stenosis with accompanying mitral stenosis, severe pulmonary hypertension, elevated right ventricular end diastolic pressure.
3. Diuretic therapy in tricuspid stenosis.
4. Atrial fibrillation (absent presystolic murmur).

209. Following accompanying features are helpful as they are often indicate to look for the murmur of tricuspid stenosis.

Associated features:

Table I-19

Positive	Negative
1. Puffiness of face, edema feet	Absence of paroxysmal nocturnal dyspnea
2. Prominent 'A' and slow 'Y' in JVP	Absence of right ventricular hypertrophy
3. Tricuspid opening snap	No pulmonary hypertension
4. Associated mitral stenosis	No right ventricular 3rd or 4th sound

1. The exception to the above features are frequent.
2. Many patients with milder degree of tricuspid stenosis do not show puffiness of face or edema feet particularly so when they are receiving diuretics.
3. Paroxysmal nocturnal dyspnea though rare, can occur if the accompanying mitral stenosis is tight or tricuspid stenosis is mild.
4. Significant pulmonary hypertension can occur in spite of tricuspid stenosis.
5. The 'A' wave in JVP is absent in atrial fibrillation and the slow 'Y' descent is an unreliable sign.

210. Roentgenography: There are 4 points to be seen in the chest X-ray of combined tricuspid and mitral stenosis:

1. Marked cardiomegaly with conspicuous enlargement of right atrium giving prominent right border
2. Dilated superior vena cava and azygos vein
3. Less marked dilatation of pulmonary artery
4. Less marked pulmonary congestion than with pure mitral stenosis.

211. ECG—the 4 points to be checked in tricuspid stenosis:

1. In a patient with valvular disease with right-sided heart failure without artrial fibrillation, presence of tall, peaked P waves of right atrial dilatation in LII as well as prominent upright P waves in V1 should suggest the possibility of tricuspid stenosis.
2. There may be depression of PR segment resulting from increased magnitude of the atrial T waves.
3. There are signs of biatrial enlargement with abnormally tall, broad 'P' waves in LII, LIII and aVF since tricuspid stenosis is usually associated with mitral valvular disease,
4. Right atrial dilatation may rotate ventricular septum and affect QRS morphology. It may cause reduction in QRS amplitude in V1 whereas QRS complex may be taller in V2.

212. Echocardiogram: It is most useful investigation. It is more difficult to image.

The changes are similar to those of mitral stenosis:

1. Reduction in the TV orifice is noted in TS.
2. Increased transvalvular velocity.
3. A mean pressure gradient more than 5 mm Hg using continuous wave Doppler is diagnostic.
   TS is more commonly described by the tricuspid diastolic pressure gradient .
4. Calcification and thickening of tricuspid valve often results in multiple or disorganized echos.
5. Reduction in E-F slope of the anterior leaflet.
6. Paradoxical motion of the septal leaflet in diastole.
7. 2D Echo shows diastolic doming of the leaflets, thickening and reduced separation of the tips of the leaflets.
8. 3D Echo shows all TV leaflets, potentially helping for more accurate calculation of TV area.

213. Angiography: Injection of contrast material into right atrium and filming in 30° right anterior oblique demonstrate the tricuspid valve. It shows the following 4 changes:

1. Thickening of tricuspid leaflets.
2. Decreased motility of leaflets.
3. Jet through the narrowed tricuspid orifice.
4. Thickening of right atrial wall.

214. Management: Medical management is similar to those of any other valvular diseases. The 4 points in medical management are:

1. Digitalis.
2. Diuretics.
3. Salt restriction.
   Intensive salt restriction and prolonged diuretic therapy decreases hepatic congestion and improves hepatic function to reduce the risks of subsequent operation.
4. Surgical treatment: Surgery is usually carried out at the time of mitral valve surgery. Tricuspid stenosis is always accompanied by some regurgitation. Simple finger fracture commissurotomy often does not improve and may even cause severe regurgitation for stenosis. Valve replacement is indicated in whom diastolic gradient across the tricuspid valve exceeds 5 mm Hg and tricuspid orifice less than 1.5–2.0 cm^2. Tricuspid valve is replaced under cardiopulmonary bypass. A tissue valve is preferred to a mechanical prosthesis in tricuspid position since the risk of thrombosis is high in the latter.

TRICUSPID REGURGITATION

215. Etiology and pathology:

1. *Functional:* Most common cause of tricuspid regurgitation is functional secondary to marked dilatation of the right ventricle and the tricuspid annulus. Right ventricular hypertension secondary to any form of cardiopulmonary disease can cause tricuspid regurgitation, the most commonly mitral valvular disease, right ventricular infarction, congenital pulmonary stenosis, pulmonary hypertension secondary to Eisenmenger's syndrome and primary pulmonary hypertension, etc.
   It can occur as a complication of right ventricular failure of any other cause, e.g. infarction of inferior wall of right ventricle. Later stages of heart failure due to rheumatic or congenital heart disease with severe pulmonary hypertension, i.e. when the systolic pressure exceeding 60 mm Hg.
   Functional tricuspid regurgitation diminishes or disappears as the right ventricle decreases in size.
2. *Congenital:* Congenitally deformed tricuspid valve in association with endocardial cushion defects like Ebstein anomaly, Marfan's syndrome, etc. In Marfan's syndrome, tricuspid regurgitation occurs as a consequence of dilatation of the annulus of tricuspid valve without dilatation of right ventricle. In infants, tricuspid regurgitation may complicate right ventricular failure secondary to neonatal pulmonary disease with persistence of fetal pulmonary circulation.
3. *Rheumatic:* Organic tricuspid regurgitation of rheumatic origin is often associated with tricuspid stenosis.
4. *Infective:* Infective endocarditis particularly staphylococcal endocarditis in drug addicts.
5. *Ischemic:* Infarction of right ventricular papillary muscle, rupture of chordae tendineae in coronary artery disease and in perinatal asphyxia.
6. *Connective tissue disorders:* Rheumatoid arthritis, systemic lupus erythematosus, etc.

7. *Degenerative:* Myxomatous degeneration of chordae tendineae causing tricuspid valve prolapse usually but not always accompanies mitral valve prolapse.
8. *Miscellaneous causes:* Right atrial myxoma, carcinoid syndrome, thyrotoxicosis, postsurgical, methysergide induced valvular disease, trauma, radiation, etc.

216. Clinical features:

1. Evidence of weight loss, cachexia, cyanosis, mild jaundice, edema and ascites are often present. Fatigue is due to low systemic output. It is possible that with the onset of tricuspid regurgitation, the dyspnea may be relieved to some extent in patients of mitral stenosis.
2. Jugular venous pulse is raised with prominent 'V' waves. The 'V' wave and 'Y' descent become prominent during inspiration. The systolic back flow under pressure results in prominent systolic wave the 'V' wave.
3. A venous systolic thrill and a murmur in the neck may be present in severe tricuspid regurgitation.
4. Pulse is irregular with pulse deficit in atrial fibrillation, which is common in tricuspid regurgitation.
5. Marked hepatomegaly with systolic pulsations is commonly present initially, but in chronic tricuspid regurgitation with congestive cirrhosis, the liver may become firm and non-tender with ascites, pleural effusion and edema. There may be pain in right hypochondrium due to congested liver.
6. A prominent right ventricular parasternal lift; it is hyperdynamic and thrusting in quality.
7. S_3 originating from right ventricle is usually present. It is accentuated during inspiration. P_2 is accentuated when tricuspid regurgitation is associated with pulmonary hypertension.
8. A high-pitched blowing holosystolic murmur of grade 3/6 along the lower left sternal border is present. It can be associated with a thrill. The murmur is intensified during inspiration (Rivero-Carvello's sign), with supine passive leg rising and reduced during expiration, with standing and the Valsalva maneuver. However, when the failing ventricle can no longer increase its stroke volume, the inspiratory augmentation is lost.

217. Summary of systolic murmur in tricuspid regurgitation:

Table I-20

1. Timing	Pansystolic
2. Site of best audibility and conduction	Tricuspid area (left 4th space), no selective conductivity but is often heard to the right of sternum
3. Grading	< 3/6
4. Character	Soft and blowing

The typical murmur of tricuspid regurgitation is pansystolic and is indicative of high right ventricular pressures. The duration of the murmur is indicative of the duration of pressure difference between the right ventricle and right atrium in systole. Non-pansystolic murmur occur with organic tricuspid valve disease and normal right ventricular pressures. The high frequency murmur is suggestive of high pressures in right ventricle. With normal ventricular pressures, the murmur is lower in frequency.

The murmur of tricuspid regurgitation is best audible in tricuspid area and is generally not selectively conducted. It may be heard over the right of the sternum or over the liver. In Ebstein's anomaly the murmur may be best heard laterally at the apex due to displacement of the tricuspid valve. In severe tricuspid regurgitation with enlarged right ventricle forming the apex, the murmur may be audible at apex and even in the axilla and may be mistaken for mitral regurgitation.

218. Associated features with systolic murmur in tricuspid regurgitation:

1. Signs of pulmonary hypertension
2. Hyperkinetic right ventricular impulse
3. Prominent 'V' wave and rapid 'Y' descent in jugular venous pulse
4. Right ventricular S_3

219. Roentgenography: The following 4 signs may be seen:

1. Marked cardiomegaly secondary to the condition responsible for the dilatation of right ventricle.
2. Right atrium is prominent. Fluoroscopy may show systolic pulsation of right atrium.
3. Rarely calcification of tricuspid ring.
4. Evidence of pulmonary arterial and venous hypertension are common.

   Elevation of right atrial pressure, such as distension of azygos vein and the presence of pleural effusion may be seen.

220. Electrocardiogram usually shows nonspecific and characteristic of the lesion responsible for tricuspid regurgitation. The following 4 signs may be present:

1. Right ventricular hypertrophy severe tricuspid regurgitation always show right ventricular hypertrophy.
2. Right atrial hypertrophy.
3. Atrial fibrillation.
4. In rare instances of isolated tricuspid regurgitation—it may show incomplete bundle branch block.

221. Echocardiogram: The following signs may be seen:

1. In tricuspid regurgitation secondary to the dilatation of tricuspid annulus, the right atrium, right ventricle and tricuspid annulus are usually dilated.

2. Right ventricular diastolic overload is evident with paradoxical motion of ventricular septum similar to that of atrial septal defect.
3. Exaggerated motion and delayed closure of tricuspid valve is seen in Ebstein's anomaly.
4. In tricuspid regurgitation secondary to right ventricular dilatation and pulmonary hypertension, the pulmonary valve shows diminished or absent 'A' deflection.
5. Prolapse of the tricuspid valve may be evident in M-mode or 2D echocardiography.
6. Endocarditis may reveal vegetations on the valve or flail leaflets.
7. In tricuspid regurgitation secondary to carcinoid syndrome, the valve leaflets are thickened and retracted, fixed in semi open position throughout the cardiac cycle.
8. Contrast echocardiography: Two-dimensional echocardiogram is recorded while injecting saline or indocyamine green dye into antecubital vein. It is sensitive and specific for tricuspid regurgitation. The microcavities that are produced by the injection are readily visible on echocardiography and normally travel as a bolus through the circulation. In tricuspid regurgitation, these microcavities are seen travelling back and forth across the tricuspid valve and pass into the inferior vena cava and hepatic vein during systole.

Simultaneous echocardiography and phonocardiography studies of tricuspid valve may reveal non-ejection systolic click that occurs at the onset of prolapse originating from the right side of the heart.

222. Cardiac catheterization and angiography:

1. The right atrial and right ventricular end-diastolic pressures are characteristically elevated in tricuspid regurgitation whether it is due to organic disease or secondary to right ventricular systolic overload, e.g. pulmonary hypertension and pulmonary stenosis.
2. The right atrial pressure tracing shows absence of the X descent, prominent V or C-V wave ('ventricularization' of atrial pressure). Increasing resemblance of right atrial pressure pulse to right ventricular pressure pulse indicates the severity of tricuspid regurgitation. A rise or no change in right atrial pressure during inspiration is characteristic. (Normally there is fall in inspiration).
3. Pulmonary artery or right ventricular systolic pressure gives an idea whether the tricuspid regurgitation is primary (disease of the valve or its supporting structure) or secondary to right ventricular dilatation, i.e. functional. A pulmonary artery or right ventricular systolic pressure of less than 40 mm Hg is suggestive of primary etiology whereas a pressure greater than 60 mm Hg favors secondary cause.
4. Right ventriculography helps in the diagnosis and quantitative assessment of tricuspid regurgitation.

223. Management:

Isolated tricuspid regurgitation in the absence of pulmonary hypertension, such as that occurring in infective endocarditis or trauma is usually well-tolerated and does not require surgery. Indeed excision of infective tricuspid valve in narcotic drug addicts is often well-tolerated.

1. Annuloplasty is indicated in tricuspid regurgitation where it is secondary to annular dilatation.
2. In tricuspid regurgitation associated with mitral valve disease, pulmonary hypertension and right ventricular dilatation, the severity of regurgitation should be assessed. Effective surgical correction of mitral valve often results in lowering of pulmonary hypertension and gradual reduction or disappearance of tricuspid regurgitation.
   Mild tricuspid regurgitation disappears after mitral valve surgery. Moderate tricuspid regurgitation may require tricuspid annuloplasty while doing the mitral valve surgery.
   Severe tricuspid regurgitation needs valve replacement.
3. In tricuspid regurgitation due to organic disease, such as in Ebstein's anomaly or carcinoid heart disease, needs valve replacement. The risk of thrombosis in valvular prosthesis is greater in the tricuspid position than in mitral position because of lower pressure and flow rates in the right side of the heart. So, porcine heterograft is preferred to valvular prosthesis. The durability of biological prosthesis up to 10 years has been established.
4. In problematic cases of tricuspid endocarditis in drug addicts, total excision of tricuspid valve without replacement can be tolerated. Valvular replacement frequently results in reinfection in drug addicts when the antibiotic therapy becomes unsuccessful. A diseased valvular tissue should be excised in order to eradicate endocarditis and antibiotics are continued. Most of them tolerate loss of tricuspid valve without great difficulty. However, if the medical management does not control tricuspid regurgitation and if the infection is controlled valve replacement can be done.

PULMONARY VALVE DISEASE

Congenital pulmonary stenosis is described in chapter on congenital heart disease (See Chapter L-59–76).

The pulmonary valve is a trileaflet valve that separates the right ventricle from pulmonary vasculature. So, any abnormality of the valve can produce effects on RV by pressure and/or volume overload .

The most common cause of pulmonic stenosis is congenital. Acquired right ventricular outflow obstruction is extremely rare.

224. Causes of PS:

1. Congenital: The most common. Occurs approximately 10–12% of all adult patients with congenital heart disease.
2. Rheumatic: Uncommon. Usually occurs in multi valvular involvement.
3. Carcinoid heart disease: Caused by typical 'carcinoid plaque'.
4. Rarely, pseudopulmonary valve stenosis occur as a result of right ventricular outflow obstruction from cardiac tumors or from an aneurysm of the sinus of Valsalva.

225. The 4 most common symptoms are:

1. Dyspnea on exertion
2. Angina
3. Palpitation
4. Features of right heart failure

Cyanosis is rare unless there is patent foramen ovale or ASD.

226. The 4 features of general appearance with pulmonary stenosis:

1. Moon face
2. Noonan's syndrome
3. Hypertelorism
4. Angiomatous malformations over the skin.

227. The murmur of pulmonic stenosis.

Table I-21

Features	Description
1. Site of best audibility/ selective conduction	Pulmonary area (Left 2nd and 3rd spaces), conducted to supraclavicular, left side of the neck
2. Timing	Ejection systolic
3. Grade	4/6
4. Length, peaking	Short, moderate, long covering A_2 Peaks in midsystole, late systole

The murmur of pulmonic stenosis is as a rule ejection systolic in timing. A pansystolic murmur is suggestive of either a ventricular septal defect or tricuspid regurgitation. The prominent 'A' wave in JVP, the sustained right parasternal heave, audible S_4, wide split S_2 and the ejection click help to distinguish it from VSD.

The murmur of valvular pulmonary stenosis is generally best heard at the left 2nd or 3rd space but it also audible at 4th space along the left sternal border. It is selectively conducted to the supraclavicular area and left side of the neck. The murmur of ventricular septal defect is generally not conducted to the neck.

The murmur of pure pulmonary stenosis is usually at least grade 4/6 (murmur with thrill). The louder and longer the more severe the stenosis. In tetralogy of Fallot the features are inversely related to the severity of pulmonic stenosis. This is because, in pure pulmonic stenosis, the right ventricle has the obligation to empty only into the pulmonary circulation, as the severity of pulmonic stenosis increases the loudness of the murmur also increases. In TOF, the right ventricle has no obligation to empty into the pulmonary circulation, in view of the associated ventricular septal defect, which allows the right ventricle to decompress into the left ventricle and aorta. The length and loudness of the murmur inversely related to the severity of tetralogy of Fallot.

228. Relation of murmur to physiological act/maneuver:

Table I-22

1. Respiration	Increases with inspiration
2. Posture	Decreases on standing
3. Valsalva maneuver	Decreases or disappears
4. Isometric hand grip	Decreases

229. Accompanying features of pulmonic stenosis murmur:

1. Prominent 'A' wave in JVP
2. Systolic thrill at pulmonary area
3. Sustained parasternal heave of RVH
4. Diminished pulmonic sound
5. Wide split S_2
6. Right ventricular S_4
7. Ejection click
8. The murmur of pulmonary incompetence.

The prominent 'A' wave in JVP has the same significance as the fourth heart sound but is more easily appreciable than fourth heart sound.

A sustained parasternal heave is consistent with pulmonic stenosis but a hyperkinetic impulse suggests ASD. Isolated parasternal impulse without left ventricular impulse rules out ventricular septal defect as the cause of long systolic murmur.

The wide and variable split of S_2 with diminished P_2 distinguishes pulmonic stenosis from VSD. A fixed split occurs with associated ASD or right heart failure.

Presence of S_4 makes TOF unlikely and pure pulmonic stenosis likely. The gradient across the outflow is usually more than 70 mm Hg when S_4 is present.

The murmur of pulmonary incompetence is of low frequency murmur of low pressure localizes the lesion to the valve. A dysplastic valve is not easily amenable for balloon valvuloplasty.

The ejection click not only distinguishes pulmonic stenosis from VSD but also localizes the obstruction of the valve.

230. The murmur of pulmonic stenosis should be differentiated from the conditions which simulate it:

1. Innocent systolic murmur
2. Atrial septal defect
3. Ventricular septal defect
4. Tetralogy of Fallot.

231. Pulmonary stenosis is associated with pulmonary incompetence in the following 4 conditions:

1. Dysplastic valve as in Noonan's syndrome.
2. Infective endocarditis in PS.
3. Postsurgical valvotomy.
4. Postballoon valvotomy.

232. Ejection systolic murmur of grade 3/6 at pulmonary area is one the most common murmurs with otherwise normal cardiovascular system. This physical sign often helps in the diagnosis of following conditions of non-cardiovascular origin:

1. Innocent systolic murmur-functional murmur.
2. Pectus excavataum-functional murmur.
3. Straight back syndrome-functional murmur.
4. Kyphoscoliosis-functional murmur.
5. Anemia-functional murmur.
6. Pregnancy-functional murmur.
7. Thyrotoxicosis-functional murmur.
8. ASD.
9. Mild pulmonic stenosis.
10. Idiopathic pulmonary artery dilatation.
11. Pulmonary arterial hypertension.
12. Hypertrophic obstructive cardiomyopathy.

233. Abnormal split of second heart sound with additional sounds distinguishes the following 4 conditions:

Table I-23

1. Wide 'fixed ' split of S_2, P_2 normal or louder, tricuspid MDM	ASD
2. Wide, variable split, decreased P_2, EC	Mild pulmonic stenosis
3. Close split or single S_2, decreased P_2	Pulmonic arterial hypertension
4. Reversed split, LV S_4, LVH	Hypertrophic obstructive cardiomyopathy

EC: Ejection click; MDM: Mid-diastolic murmur

(See Chapter on Congenital Heart Diseases for Investigations, Management L-69–76)

PULMONARY REGURGITATION

234. Etiology: The following are the common causes:

1. Most common cause is dilatation of the pulmonary ring secondary to pulmonary hypertension of any etiology.
2. Dilatation of pulmonary artery: Idiopathic or secondary to connective tissue disorder, such as Marfan's syndrome.
3. Infective endocarditis.
4. Iatrogenic: Caused during the surgical correction of pulmonary stenosis or tetralogy of Fallot or injury produced by a pulmonary artery flow catheter.
5. Congenital malformations such as absent, malformed, fenestrated or supernumerary leaflets. These are often associated with other congenital anomalies such as tetralogy of Fallot, ventricular septal defect, pulmonary stenosis.

Less common causes:

6. Carcinoid syndrome.
7. Rheumatic involvement: Pulmonary valve is affected by rheumatic fever far less frequently than the other valves.
8. Syphilis.

235. Clinical manifestations:

Isolated pulmonary regurgitation like tricuspid regurgitation causes right ventricular volume overload and tolerated for many years unless it is complicated by pulmonary hypertension, which aggravates right ventricular failure. Pulmonary regurgitation caused by infective endocarditis develops septic pulmonary emobli and severe right ventricular failure.

Physical examination: The following 4 observations are:

1. Palpable left parasternal shift of hyperdynamic right ventricle.
2. Palpable systolic pulsations in the second left intercostal space of enlarged pulmonary artery.
3. P_2 is accentuated in patients with pulmonary regurgitation secondary to pulmonary hypertension. There is wide splitting of S_2 due to prolongation of right ventricular stroke volume. S_3 and S_4 may be heard in the 4th intercostal space of left parasternal area.
4. In the absence of pulmonary hypertension, the diastolic murmur of pulmonary regurgitation is low pitched and is heard in left third and fourth intercostal spaces in the parasternal area. With the development of pulmonary systolic pressure exceeding 70 mm Hg, dilatation of pulmonary annulus results in a regurgitant jet of high velocity. This gives rise to high pitched, blowing decrescendo murmur in early diastole at the left sternal edge, the so called Graham Steell murmur.

It is distinguished from aortic regurgitation from other evidence.

236. Summary of murmur of pulmonary regurgitation in pulmonary hypertension.

Table I-24

Features	Description
1. Timing	Early diastolic
2. Length	Very short to pandiastolic
3. Site of best audibility and conduction	Pulmonary area (left 2nd or 3rd ICS Left sternal border 3rd and 4th ICS Apex if formed by right ventricle
4. Character	High pitched

237. Pulmonary regurgitation murmur relation to physiological act/maneuver.

Table I-25

Features	Description
1. Respiration	May increase with inspiration but often do not increase
2. Posture	Better heard in supine position, passive leg rising
3. Isometric hand grip/vasopressor	No change
4. Amylnitrate inhalation	No change/may decrease

238. Associated signs of severe pulmonary hyptertension with pulmonary incompetence.

1. Loud pulmonary sound
2. Palpable pulsations in left 2nd intercostal space
3. Right ventricular impulse
4. Prominent 'A' wave in JVP
5. Tricuspid regurgitation
6. Right ventricular 3rd or 4th heart sound
7. Right sided Austin-Flint murmur
8. Evidence of mitral stenosis.
   Pre-existing left to right shunt or Eisenmenger syndrome.
   Primary pulmonary hypertension, etc.

239. The significance of Graham Steell murmur.

The presence of Graham Steell murmur in a patient with pulmonary hypertension suggests that the pulmonary artery pressures are in the systemic or suprasystemic range often mean inoperability. In valvular disease, this murmur as a rule indicated underlying severe mitral stenosis or combined mitral stenosis and regurgitation with dominant mitral stenosis. It rarely occurs with mitral regurgitation and never occurs with aortic valve disease.

Table of significance of Graham Steell murmur.

Table I-26

Clinical setting	Significance
1. Pulmonary artery pressure	Near systemic/ systemic or suprasystemic
2. Valvular heart disease	Almost always suggests MS or MS+MR with dominant MS. Rheumatic heart disease is a most likely
3. Left to right shunts	Severe PAH-fixed or hyperkinetic No PAH but dilated PA as in ASD
4. Cyanosis	Eisenmenger syndrome, cyanotic heart disease with pulmonary arterial hypertension as in transposition of Great arteries, double outlet right ventricle, single ventricle, total anomalous pulmonary venous connections

240. Electrocardiogram and roentgenogram shows the following 4 changes:

1. In the absence of pulmonary hypertension, pulmonary regurgitation often shows right ventricular diastolic overload, i.e. rSR' or rsR' pattern in right precordial leads.
2. In pulmonary regurgitation secondary to pulmonary hypertension, there is evidence of right ventricular hypertrophy.

X-ray shows :

3. Enlargement of pulmonary artery and right ventricle.
4. Fluoroscopy shows marked pulsations of the main pulmonary artery.

241. Echocardiogram shows the following 4 changes:

1. Right ventricular dilatation and in patients with pulmonary hypertension, right ventricular hypertrophy as well.
2. Diastolic fluttering of tricuspid valve leaflets similar to mitral valve leaflets in aortic regurgitation.
3. Abnormal septal motion characteristic of volume overload of right ventricle in diastole and /or septal flutter may be seen.
4. The pulmonary valve motion helps to determine the cause of pulmonary regurgitation.
   - Absence of 'A' wave and systolic notching of the posterior leaflets suggest pulmonary hypertension.
   - A large 'A' wave indicates pulmonary stenosis
   - Contrast echo and pulsed Doppler technique are useful in detecting pulmonary regurgitation.

242. Management consists of:

1. Management of right ventricular dilatation or failure.
2. Management of primary condition, such as infective endocarditis.
3. Management of lesion that is responsible for pulmonary hypertension, such as surgical treatment of mitral valvular disease.
4. Replacement of pulmonary valve is rarely necessary in conditions like intractable right heart failure.

243. Drug-induced valve disease:

Drug-induced valvulopathy have been noticed over the last two decades which mimic other causes of valvular disease. Following drugs are noticed to cause the valvular disease:

1. Ergot: Methysergide, ergotamine were reported to cause valve disease in the early 1908.
2. Diet pills: In 1997, Connolly et al. reported that fenfluramine and dexfenfluramine were associated with valve disease with typical histological findings.
3. Recently, valvular disease was reported in 24–28% of patients who are undergoing treatment for Parkinsonism. Ergot derived dopamine agonist (e.g. pergolide, cabergoline have caused the disease).
4. Use of serotonin drugs, e.g. selective serotonin reuptake inhibitors (SSRIs) may give rise to valvular disease but it is not yet fully convincing .

Once the drug induced valve disease is suspected, the drug should be discontinued immediately. Left sided lesions are more. Some improvement in the valve regurgitation has been noticed at follow up intervals of one year.

VALVULAR SURGERY

244. Some historical landmarks in valve surgery:

1. First mitral valvotomy was attempted by Cutler and Levine on May, 20th, 1923 on a 11-year-old girl.
2. Prosthetic aortic valve replacement was done in 1960 by Harkin and in 1961 by Lillihi and Muller.
3. Mitral valve replacement with the ball valve type of prosthesis was done in 1961 by Albert Starr. (Starr-Edward ball valve prosthesis).
4. Tricuspid valve replacement by prosthetic valve was done in 1963 by Starr and his colleagues.

245. The 4 types of operations that can be performed on mitral valve are:

1. Closed mitral valvotomy
2. Open mitral valvotomy
3. Mitral valve repair
4. Mitral valve replacement.

246. The 4 situations where closed mitral valvotomy can be attempted are:

1. Patients with pure mitral stenosis. Mitral valve area below 1.0 cm^2 particularly with normal sinus rhythm.
2. Class II and III heart failure of NYHA.
3. Absence of perivalvular or valvular calcification.
4. Absence of mitral regurgitation.

Patients with atrial fibrillation pose specific problems and need individual assessment of closed or open mitral valvotomy. Pregnancy associated with mitral stenosis pose a specific problem and they frequently abort during first trimester of pregnancy. Mitral valvotomy can also be done safely in second and also in third trimester with safety to the mother as well as the fetus.

247. There are 4 conditions where open mitral valvotomy can be attempted.

1. History of embolic episodes: Clots in the left atrium demonstrated by Echo/angiography.
2. Patients with atrial fibrillation.
3. Patients with restenosis.
4. Patients with extensive damage of mitral valve apparatus like fusion of the subvalvular apparatus, etc.

248. There are 4 conditions where mitral valve repair can be attempted.

1. Patients with acute incompetence caused by rupture of chordae tendineae.
2. Rupture of papillary muscle due to endocarditis, trauma or ischemia.
3. Patients who have annular dilatation, chordal lengthening and mitral valve prolapse.
4. Localized loss of cuspal tissue due to infection, trauma, etc.

There should be little or no calcification and mitral valve should be suitable for repair. This procedure is not usually performed in India due to severe deformity of mitral valve apparatus and the aggressive nature of mitral valve disease.

249. The 4 conditions where mitral valve replacement can be attempted are:

When the valve shows gross distortion by:

1. Extensive fusion of subvalvular apparatus.
2. Extensive calcification of the valve.
3. Extensive vegetation and damage due to endocarditis.
4. Finally when the earlier operation has failed.

250. Prosthesis: The ideal valve prosthesis should have the following characteristics.

1. *Adequate hemodynamic performance:* It should allow free flow of blood across the orifice without causing any mechanical obstruction to the blood flow.
2. *Durability:* The valve should not wear off or deteriorate or vary in size during the life time.

3. *Resistance to infection:* It should avoid bacterial or fungal vegetations over the valve.
4. *Resistance to thrombosis:* It should avoid thrombotic deposition on the valve and prevent consequent thromboembolism.
5. *Ease of insertion:* Insertion should be easy so that average surgeon can perform the valve replacement securely.
6. *Bioincompatability:* The valve should not be rejected by the host. It should not damage the blood elements nor it should excite the immune system to reject.
7. *Silence:* The sound produced by the valve should not be disturbing to the patient. It should be preferably silent.
8. *Economy:* It should be less expensive.

Starr-Edwards ball valve prosthesis, which was introduced in 1961 has undergone lot of modifications in its design. The valve has survived the test of time and is still one of the most popular and durable prosthetic valves in use. Hemodynamic performance is adequate with ball valve prosthesis and excellent with tilting disk and bileaflet valve prosthesis.

251. The following 4 mechanical valves are commonly used:

1. Starr-Edwards: It is a ball valve prosthesis with barium impregnated ball residing inside a stellate cage. Though this valve has been extensively used since 1961. It is not useful in small mitral orifice and of limited use in small ventricle because of its bulky cage design.
2. Bjork-Shiley. It is a tilting disk valve. These are the most common artificial valves used in.
3. Medtronic Hall — India.
4. St Jude valve: It is a bileaflet valve. It is the newest mechanical valve giving good results.

The mechanical valves are generally very durable and carry an operative mortality of an average of 4%. However, the need for anticoagulation and predisposition to thrombotic manifestations makes their use slightly restricted.

252. Biological (or tissue valves):

Homografts: Fresh homografts (Allograft-valves from cadavers) were used in aortic position and proved virtually free from thrombotic complications.

The pioneering work of Sir Brian Barratt Boyce in New Zealand, Sir Donald Ross in United Kingdom and Stanford group in United States of America have contributed a lot. They improved the results and used both free grafts and also stent mounted valves. Successful implantation of aortic valves (Homografts) showed satisfactory functioning for 9–12 years but in mitral position showed malfunctioning after 5 years in 60% of cases.

Advantages of homografts are:

1. Free from thromboembolism
2. No anticoagulants are necessary
3. No hemolysis
4. Low incidence of endocarditis
5. Inaudible
6. Can be used in children; choose your own size
7. Deteriorate slowly—no sudden death
8. Quality of life is excellent. Survival is better than many. Life span is approximately 15 years.

The presence of diastolic murmur appearing after about 10 years indicates deterioration of the valve and it may have to be replaced after 3–5 years as an elective procedure.

253. The 4 advantages of cryo preservation of homografts are:

1. Preserves valve structure intact
2. Prevents degeneration
3. Facilities of stock filling
4. Viability.

254. The 4 advantages of homografts are:

1. Invariably competent.
2. Choose your own size.
3. No distortion.
4. No turbulence.

They give excellent hemodynamic performance.

255. Heterografts: Gluteraldehyde preserved heterografts of bovine or porcine origin have been used extensively. They have low incidence of thromboembolism and no need of anticoagulation. They are contraindicated in 4 situations:

1. Children
2. Chronic renal failure
3. High calcium turnover states
4. Tissue incompatibility.

256. Biological valves are most suited in the following 4 conditions:

1. In patients where anticoagulants are contraindicated like severe bleeding disorders, angiomatous malformations in brain, stomach, etc. and in patients whose occupation makes anticoagulants hazardous.
2. In patients whose social and mental status make them unable to maintain proper anticoagulation regimes.
3. In young women of childbearing age because the anticoagulants (coumadine) cross the placenta and causes fetal malformations. This is a relative indication and should be prepared for second replacement procedure in 10–15 years time.
4. In very elderly over 65 years who can do well for 10–15 years with a tissue valve without the use of anticoagulants.

257. Comparison of mechanical and biological valves:

Table I-27

	Mechanical Valve	vs	Biological Valve
1. Thromboembolism/ Thrombosis	10–14%		0%
2. Anticoagulants	Necessary		Not necessary
3. Hemolysis	Present		Not present
4. Hemodynamics	Good in all positions		Good in aortic position than mitral.
5. Infection	More		Less
6. Durability	More durable		Less durable
7. Young women of child bearing age	Not desirable		Preferable
8. Sound	Audible		Inaudible

258. Postoperative follow-up.

1. *Anticoagulation:* All mechanical valves need anticoagulation. The most common anticoagulant used is heparin sodium. The dose is titrated to prothrombin ratio (PTR) of around 2.5:1. Prothrombin time should be done frequently at least once a month and anticoagulants continued lifelong. Anticoagulation poses the problem of suboptimal or excess dosage leading to thrombosis or bleeding. One is not clear, oral anticoagulants like coumadin group of drugs should be given alone or should be supplemented with antiplatelet drugs. The problem is not mere thrombosis. Excessive tissue response at the valve-heart interface can interfere with the functioning of the prosthesis. Many patients who religiously follow the anticoagulation regime do report unpredictably with embolic problems.
   Avoid green leafy vegetables like spinach and cabbage as they interfere with anticoagulation. Aspirin alone is used recently as an anticoagulant especially in children but its use alone is not universally accepted.
2. *Infective endocarditis prophylaxis:* All the artificial valves are prone to seeding of bacteria. Therefore, antibiotic coverage is given before any dental, genitourinary and rectal procedures. A number of regimes have been used but a single dose of amoxycillin 3 gm IV just before the procedure or combination of gentamicin and cloxacillin 2 hours before and 6 hours after the procedure is satisfactory.
3. *Management of pregnancy:* Warfarin sodium crosses placental barrier and may cause fetal abnormalities. Therefore, in patients with mechanical valves the pregnancy should be planned after consultation with cardiologist. Ideally anticoagulants should be stopped before conception or within a week and patient should be started on injection Heparin 500 IU every 6–8 hours . This should be continued during first trimester. Warfarin can be given in second trimester but should be stopped around 36 weeks. Patient should be hospitalized and heparin is started.
4. *Regular follow-up:* All patients should undergo thorough check up at least once a year by a cardiologist and that should include echocardiogram and Doppler study.

259. There are 4 causes of redo valve surgery:

1. Bioprosthetic valve.
2. Perivalvular leak—suture leak.
3. Valve endocarditis.
4. Valve patient mismatch.
   No tissue valve under seven years of age.

Paper gowns and paper pads are used to prevent infection during surgery. Infection is costlier than paper gowns. No cure of fungal infection of prosthetic valve except replacement. Large perivalvular leak needs valve replacement.

260. Redo surgery after valve repair.

1. Endocarditis
2. Restenosis
3. Stuck valve
4. Paravalvular leak

25–30% of mitral stenosis surgery come for redo surgery.

***261. The following instructions are given to out patients with valvular heart diseases (waiting for CMV/OMV/MV repair/TV repair/AVR/OMV+AVR/PBPV/PBAV/PBMV, etc.**

1. Take injection penicillin (Penidure 12 lakhs) as advised once in 21 days. It is very important as it prevents your heart from getting further damaged. Do not expect it to improve your chest pain/palpitations/breathlessness. For these there are other medicines. But if you stop penidure, there is great risk of your heart valves getting further damaged. It is an armour to protect your heart from further damage. Continue injection penidure up to 60 years of age. Even after operation, it must be continued. Ask doctor for further clarification. Never stop without doctor's permission.
2. Some people are allergic to injection penicillin. For them, there are oral drugs like, pentids, sulfadiazine or erythromycin. If any doctor asks you to stop penicillin injection ask him the dose and name of alternative oral medicine.
3. Avoid pregnancy as a general rule. If pregnancy is necessary, ask doctor's permission. If doctor advises against pregnancy then avoid it otherwise there is danger to the life of both child and mother.

* (From Sri Satya Sai Institute of Higher Medical Sciences, Puttaparti- 515 134 (India)).

4. Avoid heavy work or strain.
5. Take diet with less salt. What is less salt? Do not add salt in your plate. Put minimum salt while cooking food. If any doubt ask doctor for specifying the exact amount by weight (grams per day).
6. If you are taking potklor tonic (red colored tonic), take exact dose. Do not stop it or change dose without consulting doctor as it's dose is related with the urine passing tablet which you are taking.
7. If you get vomiting, go to the doctor, some medicine you are getting may cause vomiting.
8. IE prophylaxis (See the other instructions in IE).

ANTICOAGULATION

262. Indications and precautions.

1. After mechanical valve replacement → Lifelong.
2. After valve repair/bioprosthetic valve→ 3 months.
3. S/p (Percutaneous transluminal mitral commissurotomy (PTMC) for mitral stenosis with atrial fibrillation.
4. Acitron or warfarin must be taken everyday.
5. Prothrombin time test (PTT) once in a month.
6. Keep INR → 2–3 for SVR, MS+AF
7. Keep INR → 2.5–3.5 for MVR, MV repair.
8. Over dosage is dangerous
   Under dosage is equally dangerous.
   What is INR?
   International Normalized Ratio
   Formula PT patient/ISI
   PT reference
   PT—Prothrombin time
   ISI—International sensitivity index

263. Target INR.

1. Mitral valve repair—2.5–3.5
2. Mitral valve replacement—2.5–3.5
3. Aortic valve replacement—2–3
4. Atrial fibrillation—2–3

264. Management of INR.

1. What to do if INR is low?
   Cautious increase of oral anticoagulant.
2. What to do if INR is high?
   Cautious decrease of oral anticoagulant.
3. INR up to 8—stop warfarin.
   Start when INR is < 5.
4. INR > 8—stop warfarin.
   Vitamin K 0.5 mg IV or 5 mg oral.

265. What to do if there is major bleeding?

1. Hospitalization
2. Stop warfarin
3. Vitamin K 5 mg IV
4. FFP 15 mL/kg

266. Warfarin drug interactions.

1. Ibuprofen
2. Diclofenac
3. Celecoxib
4. Rofecoxib
5. Mefenamic acid
6. Piroxicam
7. Ketorolac
8. Dextropropoxyphene
9. Amiodarone
10. Norfloxacin
11. Oflaxacin
12. Cotrimoxazole
13. Clarithromycin
14. Erythromycin
15. Metronidazole
16. Tetracycline
17. Trimethoprim
18. Prolugel course of ampicillin/paracetamol
19. Sodium valproate
20. Statin
21. Omeprazole
22. Esomeprazole

Anticoagulant effect is decreased by:

23. Rifamycin
24. Phenobarbital
25. Carbamazepine
26. Grisofulvine
27. Oral contraceptives
28. Vegetable salads!

Oral anticoagulants are contraindicated in 1st and 3rd trimester of pregnancy.

J Infective Endocarditis

Infective endocarditis is defined as a disease caused by dissemination of an infective agent from a focus of infection on a valve or other part of the endocardium of the heart.

Infective valvular vegetation is the central element of infective endocarditis from pathogenic and clinical point of view.

Incidence of IE is one per 1000 hospital administered patients. An estimated 10,000 to 15,000 new cases of infective endocarditis (IE) are diagnosed each year in united states.

1. There are 4 types of manifestations of infective endocarditis.

1. Subacute bacterial endocarditis (SBE):

   Sir William Osler gave comprehensive description of this condition in 1885.

   It slowly evolves over several weeks. It is caused by organisms of low virulence such as *Streptococcus viridans*, which has limited ability to infect other tissues.
2. Acute bacterial endocarditis (ABE):

   It is often caused by primary pathogens, such as *Staphylococcus aureus*, *Neisseria gonorrhoeae* or *Streptococcus pneumoniae* which can infect other tissues also. It develops in few days or weeks with severe complications. This form of the disease is associated with rapid destruction of endocardial tissue. In practice, the subacute and acute forms however, represents the ends of a continuous spectrum.
3. Native valve endocarditis (NVE) or right sided endocarditis:

   It occurs on normal valves common in parenteral drug addicts with skin cellulitis or septic phlebitis.

   It is also caused by infected peripheral or central venous catheters, transvenous pacing, etc.

   Infecting organisms originate from skin (*Staphylococcus aureus*, *C. albicans*) or infected materials (*Pseudomonas aeruginosa*, *Serratia marcescens*).

   Staphylococcus aureus is the frequent organism.

   Tricuspid valve is the most common site in parenteral drug addicts.
4. Prosthetic valve endocarditis (PVE):

   As the name implies it is the infection of artificial valve.

Common organisms are *Staphylococcus aureus* and *Aspergillus*.

Mortality is as high as 20% for both native and prosthetic valve endocarditis.

2. The following striking changes are found in the epidemiology, clinical features and the underlying heart disease of modern infective endocarditis.

1. The median age of patients has increased from about 30 to 50 years steadily in three decades. It may be partly due to decrease in incidence of rheumatic fever.
2. Male to female ratio has risen

   Approximately 2:1 overall; 5:1 over 60 years of age due to parenteral drug addiction.
3. The proportion of acute cases has increased.
4. An increase of 40% in the proportion without any recognizable heart disease common with acute bacterial endocarditis in children below 2 years and in drug addicts.
5. An increase in the incidence of degenerative diseases as the predisposing factor.
6. An increase in the recognition of previously undiagnosed or nonexistent underlying causes, such as mitral valve prolapse (MVP) or prosthetic valves.
7. Decrease in the proportion with rheumatic heart disease.
8. Change in the microorganism pattern:

Decrease in the proportion of cases due to streptococci and an increase in the proportion of gram-negative bacilli, rickettsial, chlamydial, fungi, and miscellaneous unusual microorganisms.

Previously described classical signs of advanced subacute bacterial endocarditis such as Osler's nodes, clubbing of fingers or Roth's spots are rarely seen now.

The changes may be due to changes in the susceptible population or earlier treatment with antibiotics before advanced manifestations.

Mitral valve prolapse is frequently recognized after the echocardiography which was previously wrongly diagnosed as mild rheumatic valve damage. Though the risk of infective endocarditis is low, it occupies 15–30% of subacute endocarditis.

3. Risk factors associated with infection are:

1. Existing cardiac structural abnormalities 70–75% show MVP with regurgitation is the leading condition. Congenital heart disease 10–20%
2. Immunosuppressed status
3. Pacemaker related infections
4. Prolonged surgery/reoperation
5. Catheter related bacteremia
6. Sternal wound infections
7. Prosthetic valves
8. Drug addicts.

4. The 4 special features of infective endocarditis in parental drug abusers are:

1. Bacteremia—either from direct intravenous injection or secondarily from injection sites—cellulitis, abscess, septic thrombophlebitis. Narcotic addicts rarely use sterile syringes. Endocarditis occurs on normal valves.
2. *Staphylococcus aureus* is the common organism found in about 50% of cases but gram-negative bacilli especially *Pseudomonas* is found in 15% and fungi (*Candida parapsilosis*) in 5%.
3. Acute infective endocarditis with high frequency of *Staphylococcus aureus* is common. This is one of the causes of overall increase in acute cases than subacute cases in the last three decades.
4. The incidence of right sided infective endocarditis or native valve endocarditis (NVE) is higher in parenteral drug addicts.

Tricuspid valve is the most likely site of infection in a drug addict because it faces the incoming infected blood and is sited before the lungs. Tricuspid valve involves in 40–70%. Tricuspid vegetations embolize to the lungs resulting in multiple small radiological opacities due to septic pulmonary infarcts.

Left sided valves are also involved in 50%. More than one valve may be involved on either side. Aortic and/or mitral valve involves in about 30–48%.

Pulmonary valve is affected only in 2% of cases.

Increase in the incidence of infective endocarditis without any previously recognizable heart disease is partly due to increased incidence in parenteral drug addicts and more use of infected peripheral or central venous catheters, or transvenous pacing catheters; increase in procedures like cardiac catheterization, AV shunts for hemodialysis.

5. The bacteria causing infective endocarditis can be described under 4 groups.

1. Organisms causing infective endocarditis tend to be normal commensals from various parts of the body. Overall 80% of cases are due to infection with streptococci or staphylococci.
   About 60% of cases are due to *Streptococcus viridans*, a normal commensal of the oropharynx and are highly susceptible to penicillin.
   The next most common organisms are the group D streptococci, such as *Streptococcus faecalis*, a commensal from the gut or an infecting organism in the urinary tract. Patients are usually of the average age group of 60 years in males and 40 years in females. Many patients give a recent history of urethral catheterization, cystoscopy, prostatectomy, abortion, cesarean section, etc.
2. In drug addicts: Sixty percent of infections are due to *Staphylococcus aureus,* which may arise from a boil or infected spot on the skin.
   - About 50–60% *Staphylococcus aureus*
   - 10–15% streptococci
   - 10–15% gram-negative bacilli
   - Others may be fungal
   - Multiple organisms can be involved.
3. In prosthetic valve endocarditis (PVE) accounts for about 5–15% of all cases of endocarditis. About 1–4% of prosthetic valves may develop infective endocarditis. They are likely to be infected by *Staphylococcus epidermidis* or gram-negative organisms such as bacteroides, *Escherichia coli* or *Haemophilus influenzae*. If PVE occurs within 60 days of operation, it is termed as early. If it occurs after that it is termed as late. Early PVE reflects contamination arising in the perioperative period, mostly during operation. Early PVE is caused by staphylococcal organisms in 45–50% of cases. *S. epidermidis* in about 25–30% of cases and *S. aureus* in 20–25%. Late PVE occurs due to transient bacteriemia arising from dental, genitourinary or gastrointestinal procedures. *Staphylococcus viridans* is responsible

for 25–30% of cases, *Staphylococcus epidermidis* in 21–28%, *Staphylococcus aureus* in 9–12% and fungi in 5–8% and diphteroids. Higher incidence is noticed with black race and longer cardiopulmonary bypass surgery. At present, there is no much differences in PVE at 5 years between mechanical and homografts. However, mechanical valves have a higher risk of PVE in the first 3 months of surgery. The PVE risk is higher after 12 months in porcine valves.

4. In the culture negative cases: In most culture negative cases infective endocarditis (IE) is due to penicillin sensitive streptococci. Rarely a culture negative case may be due to Q fever caused by *Coxiella burnetii* or a fungus such as *Monilia*.

6. There are 4 stages in the pathogenesis of infective endocarditis.

1. Usually there is initial underlying heart disease (congenital or acquired).
2. Endothelial trauma: It is the cause of turbulence of blood flow. This process is exaggerated in abnormal valves or an abnormal jet flow that impinges on endocardium.
3. Nonbacterial thrombotic vegetations—Occurs by deposition of platelets, fibrin, etc., which acts as a nidus for bacterial colonization.
4. Infective endocarditis: Colonization of blood borne bacteria, attached firmly to the vegetations on structures of valve cusps. Fibrin serves to protect the bacteria which are attached firmly in the crypts of vegetations hiding from the usual defence mechanism of the host.

   If the process is seen at stage 3 before superimposed infection, it is termed as nonbacterial thrombotic endocarditis (NBTE) in which blood cultures, etc. are negative.

New mechanism of endothelial damage on previously normal valves is by chronic traumatization by intravenous injection of foreign substances as in parenteral drug addicts. These conditions cause acute bacterial endocarditis.

The vegetations of infective endocarditis vary in size from peanut to large cauliflower like polypoidal masses.

Less pathogenic organisms cause less destruction or ulceration but lead to large polypoidal vegetations.

7. Anatomical location of vegetation where it is predisposed the 4 sites are:

1. In ventricular septal defect—involves the endocardium opposite to the direction of the shunt.
2. In patent ductus arteriosus—involves the pulmonary side of the ductus.
3. In rheumatic valvular lesion—usually on the valve edge along the line of closure.
4. In drug addicts—frequently right sided endocarditis involves tricuspid valve.

Bacterias are deposited on the endothelium in areas of high flow with decreased lateral pressure.

Thrombi develop with endocardial abnormalities, which act as foci for bacterial implantation.

8. Infective endocarditis invades locally from the valves to the following 4 structures.

1. The surrounding mural endocardium causing mycotic aneurysms or abscess.
2. Penetrate valve ring causing conduction defects.
3. Chordae tendinae causing rupture and valvular incompetence.
4. Valve roots—causing para-aortic or paravalvular abscess.

9. After the formation of thrombotic vegetations, several predisposing factors promote bacterial adherence and bacteremia in conditions such as the following 4.

1. Increasing prevalence of drug abuse.
2. Dental causes—dental extraction, etc.
3. Urogenital or gastrointestinal procedures—prostatectomy, rectal or colon surgery, septic abortion, etc.
4. Iotrogenic bacteremia:
   - Procedures like indwelling catheters
   - AV shunts for hemodialysis
   - Cardiac catheterization
   - Pacemakers, cardiac surgery, etc.

10. 4 abnormal valves that are commonly affected are:

1. Bicuspid aortic valve and proposing mitral valves, neither of which may have been recognized previously.
2. Rheumatic valves—That is valves previously damaged by rheumatic fever.
3. Prosthetic valves.
4. Regurgitant mitral or aortic valves are most common to be affected.

In about 30% of cases the condition is thought to occur on a previously normal valve. Partly because the rheumatic fever is becoming less common or unrecognized.

11. The 4 leading underlying congenital heart diseases that are affected are:

1. Bicuspid aortic valve
2. Patent ductus arteriosus
3. Ventricular septal defect
4. Tetralogy of Fallot and other cyanotic congenital heart diseases.

   Atrial septal defect is rarely involved.

12. Order of frequency of valves, involved in infective endocarditis, is

1. Mitral 2. Aortic
3. Tricuspid 4. Pulmonary valve.

Left sided heart valves damaged by rheumatic fever are most commonly involved. Valves damaged by syphilis or arteriosclerosis are also susceptible.

13. In infective endocarditis particularly in drug addicts the order of frequency of valves involved differs as follows:

1. Tricuspid valve in about	54%
2. Aortic valve in about	25%
3. Mitral valve in about	20%
4. Mixed right and left side valve	6%

Pulmonary valve may also be infected. In cases of *Staphylococcus aureus* infection, 75% of times, tricuspid valve is infected. In tricuspid valve endocarditis, though murmurs are frequently absent, pulmonary emboli and pneumonia are common.

14. Host defence is diminished in conditions such as the following 4.

1. Intravenous drug abuse
2. Alcoholic cirrhosis of liver
3. Diabetes
4. Immune deficiency states such as renal failure, immunosuppressive therapy, etc.

So far no case is detected in AIDS autopsies. From recent studies one should conclude that if infective endocarditis develops in AIDS, it is an end stage complication and may present as a nonbacterial thrombotic endocarditis (NBTE).

15. The clinical features of infective endocarditis (IE) result from the following 4 ways.

1. The local intracardiac infectious process and its complications.
2. Constant bacteremia with seeding of distant foci
3. Bland or septic embolization of segments of vegetations to virtually any organ.
4. The development of immune complex associated disease.

16. Intracardiac infection can lead to:

1. Rupture of the:
   i. Valve
   ii. Chordae tendinae
   iii. Interventricular septum
   iv. Papillary muscle.
2. Valve ring abscess particularly with *Staphylococcus aureus*
3. Purulent pericardial effusion
4. Aneurysm of sinus of Valsalva
5. Fistulae between the chambers of heart and pericardium or major vessels
6. Occlusion of the valve orifice by large vegetations such as those caused by fungi or *Haemophilus* species
7. Healing by scar formation may cause valvular stenosis or regurgitation
8. Conduction abnormalities and heart failure.

Cardiac murmurs occur in 90% of cases either due to pre-existing disease or to aortic or mitral regurgitation occurring as a result of destruction of a valve. It is the most common complication of IE. Congestive heart failure occurs in about one-third to half of the cases.

Heart murmurs are almost always present except in acute infections or with right sided infections. The appearance of a new regurgitant murmur or true changes in a pre-existing murmur are uncommon but when present, they suggest acute staphylococcal disease and correlate with development of congestive heart failure.

Contributing factors include valve destruction, myocarditis, coronary artery emboli with myocardial infarction and myocardial abscesses. Rupture of a valve result in acute heart failure.

17. Symptoms of IE usually start within 9 weeks of the precipitating bacteremia. Mean incubation period is about one week for streptococcal endocarditis.

Clinical features of bacteremia are 4.

1. Fever: It is present in almost all cases, although in about 10% of cases there is no fever at the time of presentation. It is usually low grade except with acute disease and is often remittent.
2. Nonspecific symptoms, such as malaise, fatigue, night sweats, anorexia and loss of weight are common particularly with organisms of low pathogenicity, e.g. *Streptococcus viridans*. The infection with organisms of high pathogenicity is usually explosive, e.g. *Staphylococcus aureus*.
3. Splenomegaly occurs in about half the cases as a response to bacteremia.
4. Nonspecific signs like petechiae and clubbing of fingers tend to occur in long duration. Splinter hemorrhages of the finger nails are nonspecific that are found frequently in healthy people as a result of trauma and also in patients with arteritis. Lesions located proximally in the nail bed are more suggestive of IE than the distal lesions. Conjunctival splinters are more specific. Petechial hemorrhages on the neck and chest occur occasionally. They may be due to emboli or vasculitis.

18. Fever is absent in 4 conditions of infective endocarditis.

1. The elderly or those with severe debility.
2. Renal failure
3. Congestive heart failure
4. Those treated with antibiotics.

19. Clinical features due to infected emboli depend on the site of lodgment. Infected arterial emboli break off from the site of infection in almost a third of cases.

1. Emboli originating from the left side of the heart are randomly distributed throughout the circulation causing strokes and ischemia or infarction of the gut, kidney, spleen or limb. Systemic emboli may occur during or after therapy and are recognized in about a third of patients.
2. Emboli in congenital lesions with left to right shunt tend to be swept into the pulmonary circulation causing pleurisy and patchy pneumonia.
3. Very large emboli particularly to extremities suggest fungal infection.
4. Pulmonary emboli may occur in right sided endocarditis—tricuspid valve endocarditis can be seen in left sided endocarditis with left to right cardiac shunts.

Neurological manifestations are common in about one-third of patients with endocarditis. There may be major cerebral embolism, brain abscess, purulent meningitis, cerebral arteritis, cranial nerve palsy.

20. Circulating immune complexes are found in all patients with IE. The development of immune complex associated disease shows the following 4 clinical features.

1. Arthritis: Musculoskeletal complaints may mimic rheumatological disorders. Rheumatoid factor (IgM antibody directed against IgE) develops in about 50% of patients with subacute IE.
2. Glomerulonephritis: Immune complex deposition along the glomerular basement membrane results in the development of glomerulonephritis. Renal disease is present in most patients with IE and is due to glomerulonephritis, infarction or abscesses. Renal insufficiency may result in persistence of fever. Patients with metastatic infection are at high risk of relapse of IE.
3. Osler's nodes: They may occur in about 10–25% of the cases. They are tender, red indurated lesions in the pulps of the fingers and toes, lasting a day or so. They have been attributed to deposition of immune complexes in mucocutaneous vessels. They may also occur in other diseases. They also may be present on the dorsal surfaces, toes, soles, forearm and ears.
4. Other peripheral manifestations: They include Janeway lesions which are transient non-tender macular patches on the palms and soles. They are most commonly seen in acute endocarditis. Roth spots occur in less than 5% of patients with endocarditis. They are hemorrhages with a pale center in the fundus. They are also found in connective tissue disease and hematological disorders.

Although the lesions such as Janeway lesions, Roth spots, Osler's nodes and the petechial hemorrhages are due to microemboli, it is possible that they are due to a form of vasculitis caused by bacterial antigens forming antigen/antibody complexes with the deposition of complement. In support of this, the infective process leads to an intense immune response with elevated levels of immunoglobulin and that as well as being affected by septic emboli. The kidney may be affected by immune complexes causing focal and diffuse proliferative glomerulonephritis. Serial quantitative determination of immune complexes concentration can be used to monitor response to therapy.

21. Clinical picture is caused by 4 factors, which resembles several diseases. The whole field of internal medicine is reflected in a highly interdisciplinary way.

I. Features caused by local invasion of valves:

Valve rupture
Chordae rupture
Valve ring abscess
Aortic root abscess, etc.

This gives rise to breathlessness, chest pain with features of murmur and cardiac failure.

A narrow murmur remains an important finding.

These are misdiagnosed as—

Pulmonary edema
Chronic cardiac failure
Myocardial infarction
Aortic aneurysm
Aortic stenosis
Atrial myxoma, etc.

II. Features caused by systemic infection:

Fever
Anemia
Splenomagaly
Malaise, etc.

The symptoms of fever, chills, rigors, sweat, malaise, lethargy, anorexia, headache, weight loss, backache, arthralgia, myalgia may be present for a long time.

These are often mimicked as—

Occult carcinoma
Lymphoma
Tuberculosis
Arthritis
Osteomyelitis, etc.

PYREXIA OF UNKNOWN ORIGIN (PUO)

III. Features caused by septic embolism
Cerebral embolism
Coronary embolism
Renal embolism
Mesenteric embolism
Retinal embolism
Peripheral embolism
Mycotic aneurysms, etc.
This can cause signs and symptoms of focal weakness, giddiness, hemiplegia, chest pain, acute abdominal pain, loss of vision, cold and painful extremities, etc.
These can cause diagnostic errors.
Most frequent errors caused by septic embolism are:
Stroke
Brain abscess
Meningitis
Pneumonia
Pleuritis
Acute abdomen
Abdominal infections, etc.
Petechiae in the skin, eye, mucosa, Osler's nodes are caused by microembolism of small vessels.
Loss of vision is either by embolisation in the brain or retinal artery or from optic neuritis.

IV. Features caused by immune reactions
Arthritis
Glomerulonephritis
Vasculitis
Disseminated intravascular coagulation
These can give rise to signs of arthritis, uremia, vascular phenomena, clubbing of fingers, etc.
These are misdiagnosed as
Rheumatic endocarditis
Connective tissue diseases
Glomerulonephritis and
Other forms of vasculitis.
Since these features mimic many conditions, it results in late diagnosis. Average duration of symptoms before diagnosis is about 10 weeks!

22. Infective endocarditis is suspected in a known patient of congenital or valvular disease with the following 4 features.

1. Persistent fever with sweating at nights should think in every case of pyrexia of unknown origin (PUO)
2. Unexplained arterial occlusion
3. Anemia
4. Splenomegaly.

Remember absence of fever is a diagnostic pitfall.

Fundoscopic examination should be routine in all patients suspected IE it may reveal chroinic retinitis or/and ophthalmitis.

23. Delay in diagnosis leads to any of the following 4.

1. Embolic stroke
2. Progressive valve damage
3. Heart failure
4. Death.

24. The 4 late features due to delayed diagnosis are:

1. Purpurae
2. Petechial hemorrhages under the finger nails
3. Osler's nodes—painful tender swellings at the finger tips, results probably due to vasculitis than embolism
4. Clubbing is a late sign.

25. Changing pattern of clinical features compared to three to four decades are 4.

1. Gradual increase in number of patients.
2. Afebrility—even during hospital stay.
   Fever is not an invariable accompaniment of endocarditis. It is a diagnostic pitfall.
3. Gradual increase in absence of murmur.
4. Gradual increase in embolic events.
   Splenomegaly has become a rare finding.
   Afebrility can be due to antibiotics given by practitioners before hospital admission.

Higher incidence of embolic complications and of local invasive complications are mainly due to increasing incidence of more virulent microorganisms, such as staphylococci—mostly in drug addicts. There is decrease in number of nonenterococcal streptococci, change in clinical features such as absence of a murmur, fever, signs of fever such as anemia, splenomegaly and increasing incidence of emboli and immunological complications make the diagnostic delay resulting in higher incidence of morbidity and mortality.

The late diagnosis is due to pitfalls in the presentation of present day infective endocarditis, which mimics several conditions as if the whole field of internal medicine is covered in a highly interdisciplinary manner and lack of suspicion and reliance on older and no longer tenable textbook description.

The remarkable regression of heart failure as the leading cause of death from 70% in sixties to 41% in the last decade is mainly due to surgical progress.

26. Investigations.

Routine laboratory tests are 4.

1. Blood counts and urine analysis
   - May reveal raised ESR.
   - Normocytic, normochromic anemia, leukocytosis.

   Urine may show microscopic hematuria, slight proteinuria.

About 50% of patients with IE have a positive serum tests for rheumatoid factor for at least 6 weeks and virtually all patients have circulating immune complexes. These tend to disappear with cure.

2. Blood cultures:
Isolation of an organism is the most important step in the diagnosis of infective endocarditis. Blood cultures should be taken from all patients with fever and heart murmur, unless the disease is clearly due to other cause or the fever within a few days without treatment. Bacteremia is usually continuous 10 to 20 cc of blood is taken, 3 to 5 samples in 24 hours. There is no advantage in taking cultures at any particular time of body temperature. The critical diagnostic finding in IE is bacteremia or fungemia. Blood cultures may be negative in infections with fastidious organisms such as *Haemophilia* or *parainfluenzae*. Fifty percent of patients with candida endocarditis and almost all with *Aspergillus*, *Histoplasma*, *Coxiella burnetii* endocarditis may have negative blood cultures.
3. Roentgenography
4. Electrocardiography:
ECG is taken at the time of admission and repeated at intervals. May reveal otherwise silent myocardial infarction due to coronary embolization. Conduction disturbances develop during endocarditis suggests extension of infection into the myocardium. This may be due to myocarditis or to an abscess located close to the conduction system.

Special investigation is echocardiography—given below in detail.

27. Roentgenography may show 4 important changes.

Most important contribution of chest X-ray in the evidence of early congestive heart failure.

1. Assessment of heart failure helps in management and prognosis.
2. Presence of multiple small patchy infiltrations in the lungs of parenteral drug abuser with fever strongly favors the diagnosis of septic embolic from right sided infective endocarditis.
3. Valvular calcification in a previously abnormal valve.
4. Aorta may show mycotic aneurysm.
Fluoroscopy may reveal abnormal motion of prosthetic valve indicating presence of vegetations or partial dehiscence of the valve from aortic root. This helps to decide whether valve replacement is needed during management of prosthetic valve endocarditis.

28. All patients suspected IE should have baseline and follow-up ECGS:

1. It may show conduction disturbances ranging from 1° to 3° heart blocks due to intramyocardial extensions of infection (especially with PVE).
2. A new AV block suggestive of abscess formation
3. Rarely MI may occur due to embolization and vegetations
4. Nonspecific changes may be seen including arrhythmias.

29. There are 4 major aspects of diagnostic progress.

1. M - Mode and 2D echocardiography
2. Doppler echocardiography
3. Circulating immune complexes
4. Leukocyte scanning.

30. Echo is helpful for both diagnosis and management of IE echocardiogram can detect 75–80% of valve vegetations. It is beneficial in 4 conditions.

1. Identifying high-risk patients with large vegetations—to advise patients for early operation.
2. Identifying unsuspected pre-existing valve lesions
3. Identifying early aortic incompetence—
Premature mitral valve closure due to raised end-diastolic pressure is a useful echo sign of aortic regurgitation which usually requires valve replacement.
4. Identifying severe volume overload left ventricular failure.

Sequential echocardiograms can help in documentation of the response to medical treatment as well as timing for surgery by providing objective assessment of cardiac function. Large mobile vegetations of aortic valve caused by fungi or staphylococci are of high risk.

Color Doppler helps in detecting abnormal turbulence especially due to valvular incompetence.

TTE is also very useful in detecting prosthetic valve endocarditis or pacemaker endocarditis.

31. Echocardiography is of vital importance in the detection of local invasive complication of valvular vegetations such as the following 4.

1. Valve rupture
2. Chordae tendinae rupture
3. Aortic root abscess or paravalvular abscess
4. Myocardial abscess.

32. False positive results with Echo can occur occasionally in 4 conditions which mimic vegetations of endocarditis.

1. Myxomatous degeneration of mitral valve
2. Fibrosis and calcification of valve leaflets
3. Chordal rupture
4. Degenerative thickening of bioprosthesis.

33. The disadvantages of echocardiogram in infective endocarditis are 4.

1. It cannot detect vegetations less than 3 to 4 mm size.

2. It cannot visualize all the leaflets in every patient—all the leaflets of tricuspid, pulmonary, and aortic valves cannot be visualized.
3. Vegetations on prosthetic valves are difficult to demonstrate.
4. It does not differentiate active lesions from healed lesions or acute from subacute form of endocarditis.

So, a negative study by echocardiogram does not rule out infective endocarditis.

Serial phonocardiography and cineradiography are useful in evaluating infection on prosthetic valve. Cinefluoroscopy of the prosthetic valve may show abnormal socking motion of the ring.

34. There are 4 controversial opinions on the prognostic values of echocardiographic information. However, we can conclude that patients without detectable vegetations have:

1. Lower mortality
2. Lesser embolic complications
3. Less congestive cardiac failure
4. Requires less frequent surgery.

35. Effectiveness of the antibiotic therapy is monitored by 4 methods.

1. Minimal inhibitory concentration test (MIC)
2. Minimal bactericidal concentration (MBC)
   Constant bacteremia is a predominant feature of infective endocarditis. 3 to 5 blood samples (average 4) of 20 cc each should be taken at 2–3 hours intervals in 24 hours for culture depending on the condition of the patient to determine bacteremia.
3. Serum bactericidal activity (SBA): to know the adequacy of antibiotic treatment.
4. Last but not the least is the clinical response of the patient to the antibiotic therapy.

36. There are 4 principles to be followed while treating IE with antibiotics.

1. Cure of IE requires sterilization of the vegetations.
2. Isolation of infecting organism is important so as to select an appropriate antibiotic regime.
3. Bactericidal agents are required in high concentration for a long enough time to sterilize the vegetations. If any microorganisms are viable after the antibiotic treatment is discontinued, multiplication and relapse will probably occur. Therefore, the drugs are given for at least 2 weeks after the febrile period. In general, the length of the course is determined by the sensitivity of the organisms.
4. Drugs are given by intravenous bolus and not by continuous infusion.

37. ANTIBIOTIC TREATMENT OF ENDOCARDITIS

There are 4 groups of antibiotic of choice.

1. Penicillins
2. Cephalosporins
3. Aminoglycosides
4. Vancomycin.

Large parenteral doses of antibiotics are necessary to penetrate into the jungle-like meshwork of vegetations in which microorganisms are deeply embedded and highly protected.

38. The 4 commonly recommended drugs and their dosages.

1. Benzyl penicillin 1.2 g (2 mega units) every 4 hours.
2. Gentamicin 1 mg per kg body weight every 8 hours, adjusted to give a peak value of 5-10 mg per liter. Because of its ototoxicity and nephrotoxicity, blood levels should be measured twice per week.
3. Flucloxacillin 2 g every 4 hours.
4. Vancomycin: It is given in patients who are allergic to penicillin. 750 mg every 12 hours together with gentamicin. Blood levels of both drugs should be monitored as the combination is potentially ototoxic.

39. Antibiotic treatment: The 4 stages are—

(80% are gram-positive bacteria)

1. Initial therapy in clinically apparent subacute bacterial endocarditis with penicillin sensitive *Streptococcus* should begin with
   Benzyl penicillin IV + gentamicin to cover *Enterococcus* and other *Streptococcus* for 2 weeks followed by amoxycillin for 2 weeks.
   For less sensitive streptococci—
   —continue gentamicin for 4 weeks.
2. In severely ill patients or with other risk factors such as acute aortic incompetence, prosthetic valve, drug addicts—add oxacillin to cover *Staphylococcus aureus*.
3. In elderly patients with impaired renal function
   —Netilmicin is an alternate to gentamicin.
4. In patients allergic to penicillin—
   —give vancomycin.

If blood cultures are negative after one week, serological tests for *Candida*, *Aspergillum*, *Brucella*, *Coxiella*, *Histoplasmosis*, *Chlamydia*, techoic acid antibody titer for *Staphylococcus aureus* should be performed. Blood cultures should be monitored for another 2 weeks in order to detect rare fastidious organisms.

Staphylococcus aureus or *epidermidis* infective endocarditis should be treated for 6 weeks with pencillinase-resistant penicillin such as oxacillin or every cephalosporin or flucloxacillin 2 g every 4 hours and gentamicin every 8 hours for 2 weeks, followed by flucloxacillin for a further 2 to 4 weeks.

Any *Streptococcus* that is resistant to any β-lactam antibiotic is usually resistant to all β-lactum antibiotics and therefore vancomycin is indicated.

In *Staphylococcus epidermidis,* which is prevalent in prosthetic valve endocarditis is often resistant to methicillin and therefore assumed to be resistant to all β-lactum antibiotics. The combination of vancomycin + rifampicin + gentamicin is a successful regimen in this multiresistant microorganism.

Metronidazole is valuable in endocarditis caused by anaerobes.

Tetracycline combined with clindamycin are useful in *Coxiella* endocarditis.

Any source of infection should be treated if possible, for example, tooth with an apical abscess should be extracted, urinary catheters, etc.

SURGICAL MANAGEMENT OF INFECTIVE ENDOCARDITIS

Surgical progress in infective endocarditis is satisfactory as the morbidity is not greater than mortality by medical treatment and the risk of prosthetic valve is lower after the replacement of the infected native valve.

40. There are 4 absolute indications for surgery.

1. Intracardiac extension of infective vegetations
   - Arteriovenous fistulas
   - Suppurative pericarditis
2. Severe heart failure due to
   - Rupture of valve
   - Rupture of chordae
   - Rupture of sinus valsalva
   - Rupture of septum
3. Failure of medical therapy with persistent bacteremia due to resistant organisms
4. Fungus infections—debridement and valve replacement combined with amphotericin B therapy.

41. There are 4 relative indications for surgery.

1. Early mitral valve closure or sign of acute aortic incompetence
2. Moderate heart failure
3. Recurrent embolization
4. Infections such as
   - *Coxeilla*
   - Gram-negative bacteria
   - *Staphylococcus aureus*

Replacement after antibiotic treatment of these organisms which had been presumed effective. Endocarditis due to *Staphylococcus aureus* is a rapidly progressive destructive process which demands urgent valve replacement if there are early signs of incompetence.

42. There are 4 controversial indications for surgery:

1. Large mobile or even just visible vegetations
2. First major embolus
3. Mild heart failure
4. Relapse.

43. There are 4 absolute indications for surgery with prosthetic valve.

Local and paravalvular invasion causes moderate to severe hemodynamic disturbance due to

1. Unstable prosthesis
2. Valvular obstruction
3. Intramyocardial extension
4. New periprosthetic leak

Early prosthetic valve infective endocarditis due to *Staphylococcus epidermis* and gram-negative bacteria is a relative indication for surgery but in the presence of fungitis an absolute indication.

44. Prophylaxis of infective endocarditis.

Currently, 40–50% of infective endocarditis cases occur in patients without previously known heart disease and only 20% occur after procedures for which prophylaxis is needed.

Higher risk of developing infective endocarditis is with heart disease in any of the 4 conditions.

1. Prosthetic valve
2. Surgically constructed systemic pulmonary shunts
3. Acquired valve disease
4. Most congenital malformations.

45. Lower risk of developing endocarditis with heart disease which should also receive prophylaxis. The 4 conditions are:

1. Mitral valve prolapse
2. Asymmetrical septal hypertrophy
3. Tricuspid valve disease
4. Pulmonary valve lesion.

Prophylaxis in all patients with mitral valve prolapse to all procedures which cause bacteremia is controversial. It is a frequent condition occurring in 6–10% of population. Endocarditis is five times greater in patients with mitral valve prolapse. Prophylaxis of antibiotics in patients with auscultatory sign of pansystolic murmur indicating mitral incompetence is reasonable.

46. Prophylaxis is not usually required in heart diseases such as the following 4 conditions.

1. Atherosclerotic arterial plaques
2. Coronary artery bypass graft

3. Isolated atrial septal defect
4. Transvenous pacemaker.

***47. Antibiotic prophylaxis cover should be given to all patients for the following 4 procedures.**

1. *Oral surgery:* 'Degerming' of mouth with antiseptic before dental procedures decreases frequency and intensity of bacteremias.
   —Dental extraction, tonsillectomy, adenoidectomy, etc.
2. *Gastrointenstinal procedures:* Esophageal dilation sclerotherapy for esophageal varices, colon or rectal surgery.
3. *Genitourinary procedures:* Prostatic surgery, septic abortion, etc.
4. *Iatrogenic:*
   Procedures like urinary catheterization
   Indwelling catheters
   Cystoscopy
   AV shunts for hemodialysis
   Pacemakers
   Cardiac catheterization
   Amoxyllin is the standard prophylaxis
   Single dose of 3 g one hour before dental procedures.
   Erythromycin or clindamycin is given for patients with penicillin allergy.
   Vancomycin is given to prevent bacteremia as well as multiplication and adherence.
   – Given in patients with prosthetic valve.

***48. The following instructions are given to outpatients waiting for surgery.**

IE prophylaxis means that you have to take certain precautions in your lifestyle. It is not a medicine. It is a set of very important precautions which must be maintained. They are:

1. Whenever you get any fever or cough and cold, go to local doctor and get appropriate antibiotic treatment.
2. If you get any injury like cuts or bruises, immediately go to the doctor, get dressed and antibiotic treatment.
3. If any other minor surgical procedures like catheterization, removal of tooth, hemarrhoidectomy, etc. is done, tell the doctor that you are under IE prophylaxis. He will give you adequate antibiotic treatment.
4. Regularly brush you teeth and keep good dental hygiene.

49. The following schedule for antibiotic administration may be followed:

A. For dental procedures and surgery in upper respiratory tract (Prophylaxis directed against *S. viridans*):
   Use oral amoxycillin:
   Dose: Adults (wt > 25 kg)—3 g amoxycillin po 1 hour prior to procedure and 1.5 g 6 hours after the initial dose.
   Children (wt < 25 kg)—1 g amoxycillin po 1 hour prior to procedure and 500 mg 6 hours after the initial dose.
   For Patients Allergic to Penicillin
   Use erythromycin (Stearate):
   Dose: Adults 1 gram orally 2 hours prior to procedure and 500 mg 6 hours after initial dose.
   Children 20 mg/kg. Orally one hour prior to procedure 10 mg. 6 hours after procedure.
B. For gastrointestinal and genitourinary surgery (Prophylaxis directed against enterococci):
   Use Ampicillin + Gentamicin:
   Dose: Adults 2 g Ampicillin 7 1.5 mg/kg Gentamicin IM/IV 30 minutes before the procedure and 1.5 g Amoxicillin, 6 hours after the initial dose.
   Children ampicillin 50 mg/kg IM/IV and Gentamicin 2 mg/kg IM/IV 30 minutes before the procedure, and 500 mg. Amoxicillin 6 hours after initial dose.
   For Patients Allergic to Penicillin or Ampicillin
   use Vancomycin + Gentamicin
   Dose; Adults 1 g Vancomycin, given IV over 60 minutes and 1.5 mg/kg Gentamicin IM/IV, given 60 minutes before the procedure. Doses may be repeated 8–12 hours later.
   Children: Vancomycin 20 mg/kg and Gentamicin 2 mg/kg. Timing as above.
C. For dental procedures and surgery in the upper respiratory tract in the patients at high risk for endocarditis (e.g. patients with prosthetic valves)
   Use Ampicillin + Gentamicin
   Dose: As outlined above
D. *For Patients Allergic to Penicillin*
   Use Vancomycin
   Dose: As outlined above: (Gentamicin is not necessary)
   Please note that the possibility of endocarditis should be suspected in those patients whenever he/she is febrile and it may then, be necessary to collect blood for culture.

*(From Sri Satya Sai Institute of Higher Medical Sciences, Prasantigram, Puttaparti–515 134 (India))

K Cardiomyopathies and Myocarditis

The term cardiomyopathy is defined as an intrinsic disease of the myocardium itself leading to myocardial dysfunction in which there is no structural deformity of the heart.

1. **Cardiomyopathy is a progressive heart muscle disease and should be considered when there is unexplained cardiomegaly or cardiac failure after the following 4 major causes are excluded.**

   1. Congenital 2. Rheumatic (valvular)
   3. Hypertensive 4. Ischemic.

   There are disagreements in the definition and inclusions of specific causes.

2. **Cardiomyopathies can be clinically described into 4 types—(This is done to fit into 4) based on pathological and hemodynamic features. This classification indicates whether the management should be medical or surgical. Clinical classification is more useful for the practitioners. (Recent literature is extensive and has concentrated on molecular biology and pathogenesis rather than its clinical management).**

   1. *Dilated (Congestive) cardiomyopathy (DCM):*
      It comprises the largest group.
      Cardiomegaly with impairment of systolic pump function resulting in left sided heart failure and later right sided heart failure are seen.
      Symptoms of AV valve regurgitation are seen.
      Dilatation is early—so, dilated cardiomyopathy (DCM) is preferred. Congestion is a late manifestation.
   2. *Restrictive cardiomyopathy (RCM):* Ventricular walls become rigid and impede ventricular filling and presence of clots are common. Impairment of diastolic function is the hallmark. It may simulate chronic constrictive pericarditis.
   3. *Hypertrophic cardiomyopathy (HCM):* It is also known as idiopathic hypertrophic subaortic stenosis (IHSS), hypertrophic obstructive cardiomyopathy and muscular subaortic stenosis. It is mainly the systolic dysfunction characterized by the dynamic left ventricular outflow obstruction due to mid-systolic opposition of the anterior mitral valve leaflet against asymmetrical hypertrophied septum resulting in narrowing of subaortic area. The ventricular septum bulges into the left ventricle, the malaligned mitral valve causes obstruction in the left ventricular outflow during systole. It may stimulate aortic stenosis.
      It can be subdivided into 4 types:

      Familial

      Idiopathic hypertrophic subaortic stenosis (IHSS)
      i. With ventricular outflow obstruction
      ii. Without ventricular outflow obstruction

      Nonfamilial

      i. With ventricular outflow tract obstruction
      ii. Without ventricular outflow tract obstruction.
   4. *Obliterative cardiomyopathy (OCM) (Endomyocardial fibrosis- EMF):*
      Most commonly seen in children and young adults in tropical and subtropical Africa particularly Uganda and Nigeria. It is the frequent cause of heart failure in Africa accounting for 1/4th of deaths due to heart disease. It is particularly common in Kerala in India. It is characterized by endomyocardial fibrosis of right and left inflow tracts. It may be dominant left ventricular endomyocardial fibrosis (LVEMF) or right ventricular endomyocardial fibrosis (RVEMF).
      Proliferation of elastic tissue of endocardium is seen.

3. Familial hypertrophic cardiomyopathy gene test.

Gene	Name	Locus
MHY7	Myosin heavy chain 7	14q12
MVBPC3	Myosin-binding protein C	11p11.2
TNNT2	Troponin T2	1q32
TNNI3	Troponin 1	19q13.4
TPM1	Tropomyosin 1	15q22.1
ACTC	Actin, α	15q14
MYL2	Myosin regulator light chain	12q23-q24.3
MYL3	Myosin essential light chain	3p

Gene test is available through laboratory for Molecular Medicine, Harvard Medical School.

Eight genes included in panel of only commercial available. Detection rate in patients with clinical symptoms HOCM—55–70%.

A poor prognosis and higher risk of sudden death are associated with certain mutations – in the β-myosin heavy chain.

Troponin: T mutations are associated with higher mortality even in the absence of hypotrophy.

4. Primary cardiomyopathies are of 4 types: (etiology is not known).

1. Idiopathic (D/R/H)
2. Familial (D/H)
3. Endomyocardial fibrosis (R/O)
4. Eosinophilic endomyocardial disease (O). (also called Loeffler's endocarditis and Fibroplastic endocarditis)

If the myocardial disease is secondary to a systemic disease, it is termed as secondary cardiomyopathy.

5. Cardiomyopathies which are reversible can be described into 4 groups by its etiology (D).

1. *Physiological peripartum cardiomyopathy (D)*
   Unexpected and unexplained heart failure in late pregnancy or purperium is seen in multiparous black women above 30 years age. Further pregnancies should be avoided particularly if cardiomegaly persists.
2. *Deficiency and drugs (D)*
   Nutritional: Alcoholic abuse—Alcoholic cardiomyopathy is the major form of secondary DCM in Western countries.
   Thiamine deficiency
   Protein deficiency
   Selenium deficiency
   Electrolytes: Phosphate deficiency (Hypophosphatemia)
   Drugs: Emetine, arsenic, isoproterenol, chloroquine, phenothiazines, etc.
   Cytotoxic drugs, e.g. adriamycin, bleomycin, cyclophosphamide anesthetic gases, poisons
   Heavy metals—Cobalt, cadmium, lead, etc.
   Radiation.
3. *Infective (D)*
   Viral myocarditis
   Bacterial myocarditis
   Fungal myocarditis
   Rickettsial
   Protozoal myocarditis
   Metazoal myocarditis
   Serum antibody titers for enteroviruses, toxoplasma, cold agglutinin, ASO (infective and toxic) may be needed to detect.
4. *Metabolic (D)*
   Diabetes mellitus
   Hyperthyroidism
   Hypothyroidism
   Hyperkalemia
   Hypokalemia
   Hypophosphatemia
   Hypocalcemia
   Pheochromocytoma
   Uremia.

6. Cardiomyopathies which are difficult to reverse the pathogenesis can be described into 4 groups by their etiology. (Irreversible or difficult to reverse)

1. *Familial storage disease (D/R)*
   i. Glycogen storage disease
   ii. Mucopolysaccharidosis
   iii. Lipidosis
2. *(R/D Connective tissue disorders)*
   i. Rheumatoid arthritis
   ii. Polyarteritis nodosa
   iii. Systemic lupus erythematosus
   iv. Scleroderma
   v. Dermatomyositis
3. *Infiltrations and granulomas*
   i. Amyloidosis (R/O)
   ii. Sarcoidosis (D/R/O)
   iii. Malignancy (O)
   iv. Hemochromatosis (O)
4. *Neuromuscular (D)*
   i. Muscular dystrophy
   ii. Myotonic dystrophy
   iii. Friedreich's ataxia (D/H)
   iv. Refsum's disease

7. The 4 types of diseases that affect the heart.

1. Diseases that affect the endocardium, e.g. rheumatic valvular disease.
2. Diseases that affect the myocardium, e.g. IHD, cardiomyopathies.
3. Diseases that affect the pericardium, e.g. pericarditis
4. Diseases that affect the heart from outside.
   For example, thyrotoxicosis, glycogen storage diseases, rheumatoid arthritis, diabetes mellitus.
   A detailed study of dilated cardiomyopathy is necessary since it comprises the largest group.

8. The 4 important points to know in DCM.

1. Dilatation of LV, LV + RV, RV
2. Hypertrophy is little or no hypertrophy
3. Poor systolic function
4. It is primarily a myocardial disease.

9. The symptoms are mainly due to contractile dysfunction caused by the following 4 manifestations.

1. Congestive heart failure } Common
2. Arrhythmias } Common
3. Transient systemic emboli
4. Pulmonary embolism.

10. The 4 points which go in favor of DCM:

1. Q waves below 16 years of age
2. Poor systolic function with global hypokinesia
3. Systolic murmurs of MR and/or TR
4. Transient hypertension with heart failure, which responds to treatment of congestive heart failure without antihypertensive drugs.

11. The 4 points which go against the diagnosis of DCM:

1. Typical history of ischemic heart disease with Q waves in those above 30 years of age. Regional thinning of myocardium is seen in echocardiogram.
2. Diastolic murmurs
3. Hypertension that requires treatment
4. Congenital or pulmonary heart diseases.

12. The 4 important signs to look in the X-ray chest for DCM:

1. LV dilatation—Moderate to marked generalized cardiac enlargement; enlargement may be often due to associated pericardial effusion
2. Left atrial enlargement
3. Pulmonary venous congestion
4. Interstitial or alveolar congestion.
   (Note: No valvular calcification)

13. The 4 important points to be observed in ECG of DCM.

1. Chamber hypertrophy
   Ventricular enlargement with or without strain
   LVH or LVH + RVH or RVH
   Left atrial enlargement
2. Nonspecific ST-T changes are almost universal
3. LBBB or RBBB without specific pattern. Sometimes, the symptomatic LBBB may suggest a presymptomatic QRS widening with LBBB stage of DCM
4. Arrhythmias: Sinus tachycardia, AF, ventricular tachycardia, ventricular arrhythmias
   AV blocks are rare.

14. The 4 points to be observed in echocardiogram.

1. Dilatation of the ventricles without hypertrophy
2. Systolic dysfunction—global hypokinesia—dyskinesia
3. Pericardial effusion is often present
4. Mural thrombi (Mural thrombi are more in Western series than in Indian series).

15. The following 4 points are to be observed which may determine the prognosis of DCM.

1. Symptoms of congestive heart failure } Good prognosis
2. Symptoms of myocarditis } Good prognosis
3. Angina } Bad prognosis
4. Tachycardia } Bad prognosis

16. Poor prognosis is expected in a patient with any of the 4 situations.

1. More than 55 years age
2. Low ejection fraction
3. Large end systolic volume
4. Increase in LVEDP of more than 20 mm Hg.

17. The 4 important conditions, which are sometimes difficult to differentiate from DCM.

Following points help to differentiate from these conditions.

1. Myocardial infarction with Q waves (typical transmural infarction): Regional thinning of the ventricular wall and regional wall motion abnormality in echocardiogram is the hallmark of MI.
2. Coronary artery embolism: DCM and coronary artery embolism may coexist.
   Small coronary arteries may be involved when other coronary arteries are normal. Ventricles are dilated and selective arteriograms are normal in DCM. These patients are sometimes wrongly diagnosed as coronary heart disease and since they are in the younger age group, many are included under precocious ischemic heart disease.

3. Hypertension with congestive heart failure.
   They have hypertrophied ventricles, LV wall is thicker than normal, whereas LV is dilated and the wall is thinner in DCM.
4. Viral myocarditis with congestive heart failure.
   Natural history of the patient is different. Some may die during an acute fulminant attack, others may have excellent prognosis and may return to 'normal', whereas in DCM even after initial improvement there is a gradual progression of the disease either slow or rapid. Isolation of the virus from the throat, stool, blood and presence of high antibody titers would help in the diagnosis of viral myocarditis.

18. It is worth to mention here about anomalous left coronary artery from pulmonary artery (ALCAPA) as a cause of congestive cardiomyopathy since the diagnosis can be made by electrocardiogram and the treatment is specific.

There are 4 points in the diagnosis and treatment of DCM due to ALCAPA.

1. It is suspected when the patient presents with congestive cardiomyopathy with or without a mitral regurgitation murmur.
2. Diagnosis is made from the electrocardiogram, which shows anterolateral myocardial infarction pattern.
3. Diagnosis is confirmed by aortic root angiogram which shows a large right coronary artery and absence of the origin of left coronary artery from the aorta.
4. Treatment is surgical: Transplantation of left coronary artery origin from the pulmonary artery to aorta through a graft.

19. Clinical manifestations in cardiomyopathies help to differentiate the 4 types.

1. *Dilated Cardiomyopathy (DCM):*
   Chambers dilated, muscle weakness present.
   Signs and symptoms are due to left sided heart failure and later right sided heart failure.
   Arrhythmias, AV valve regurgitation are seen.
2. *Restrictive cardiomyopathy (RCM):* Walls are rigid causing resistance to ventricular filling.
   Signs and symptoms are like those in constrictive pericarditis such as edema, ascites, enlarged and tender liver.
   Diastolic function is mainly impaired.
   Physical examination may reveal signs of systemic diseases like amyloidosis and iron-storage disease.
3. *Hypertrophic obstructive cardiomyopathy (HOCM):*
   Left ventricular hypertrophy of a non-dilated chamber without any obvious cause like hypertension or valvular disease is seen.
   Preload and after load are decreased.
   Dynamic LV outflow obstruction occurs due to mid systolic opposition of anterior mitral valve leaflet against asymmetrical hypertrophied septum.
   Symptoms are like those of aortic stenosis.
   Patients may not have symptoms or may have:
   i. Breathlessness
   ii. Chest pain
   iii. Syncope
   iv. Sudden death
   The shortness of breath is caused by diastolic dysfunction, low cardiac output and hyperventilation. The angina is caused by relative ischemia resulting from hypertrophy, microvascular changes and/or coronary artery disease. The syncope is caused by arrhythmia, low left ventricular volume or inappropriate vasodilatation. Sudden death is most common in adolescence and early adulthood. Patients who fear of sudden death may manifest itself as avoidance of physical activity, a tendency to hyperventilation and disability that is not strictly attributable to the disorder.
   Conditions, which increase myocardial contractility such as exercise, digitalis, isoproterenol and those that reduces ventricular volume, such as sudden standing, nitroglycerin, amylnitrate, Valsalva maneuver cause increase in left ventricular obstruction. On the other hand, increase in arterial pressure by squatting, phenylephrine, increase in venous return by raising the legs, increase in blood volume reduces the left ventricular obstruction.
   Angina pectoris symptoms are the result of obstruction to the coronary vessels. There can be syncope or may be sudden death in children and young adults during or after physical exertion.
4. *Obliterative cardiomyopathy (OCM):*
   Common in children and young adults in tropical and subtropical Africa. Signs and symptoms depend on which ventricle and AV valve is predominantly involved.
   Left sided involvement results in pulmonary congestion while right sided involvement shows similar to constrictive pericarditis.

20. Jugular venous pulse and carotid pulse in cardiomyopathies help to differentiate 4 types.

1. **DCM**: JVP raised. Pulse pressure is small.
2. **RCM**: JVP raised but does not fall normally or it may raise with inspiration (Kussmaul's sign).
3. **HOCM**: Rapidly raising carotid pulse.
   (Spike-and dome-shaped carotid artery pulse tracing).
4. **OCM**: Earlier dominant 'a' wave in JVP is replaced by dominant 'V' wave with the progression of the disease.

21. Apical impulse in cardiomyopathy helps to differentiate the 4 types.

1. **DCM:** Not often felt because of feeble heart.
2. **RCM:** Apex is usually easily palpable (In contrast to constrictive pericarditis).
3. **HOCM:** Double or triple apex beat apex is forcible or heaving. Fourth heart sound may be palpable resulting in double apical impulse.
4. **OCM:** Apical impulse is not often felt.
   (Apex may be obliterated by thrombus and fibrous tissue).

22. Auscultation helps to differentiate the 4 types of cardiomyopathies.

1. **DCM**: S3, S4 common, gallop rhythm.
   Murmurs of atrioventricular valve regurgitation (MR and/or TR regurgitation murmurs)
   Mitral regurgitation murmur is not pansystolic.
2. **RCM:** Sounds may be distant (in contrast to constrictive pericarditis) S3, S4 common.
3. **HOCM:** S4 heard. S2 may be normally split, single or paradoxically split depending on the severity of the left ventricular outflow obstruction.
   Harsh crescendo-decrescendo (diamond shaped) systolic murmur best heard at the lower left sternal border and at apex where it is holosystolic and blowing due to mitral regurgitation.
   The systolic murmur is caused by narrow left ventricular outflow tract and often some mitral regurgitation. The murmur is augmented by reduction in left ventricular size as occurs on standing up from sitting and transiently abolished by squatting. Patients with apical or concentric hypertrophy usually do not have murmurs.
   It simulates aortic stenosis. Carotid up stroke and systolic murmur increases with Valsalva maneuver.
4. **OCM:** Mitral regurgitation murmur is not pansystolic.

23. X-ray chest in cardiomyopathy helps to differentiate the 4 types.

1. **DCM:** Moderate to marked generalized cardiomegaly.
   Enlargement may be often due to pericardial effusion.
   Left atrial enlargement.
   Pulmonary venous hypertension.
   Interstitial or alveolar congestion.
   (No AV valvular calcification as in rheumatic valvular disease).
2. **RCM:** Mild cardiac enlargement and pulmonary venous hypertension.
   (No pericardial calcification as in constrictive pericarditis).
3. **HOCM:** Mild-to-moderate cardiac enlargement (Lack of calcification helps to differentiate from rheumatic aortic stenosis).
4. **OCM (EMF):** Small areas of outpouching like small ventricular aneurysms may be seen.
   Normal or mild cardiac enlargement.

24. ECG in cardiomyopathies helps to differentiate 4 types.

No one with cardiomyopathy has normal ECG

1. **DCM**: LVH or LVH + RVH or RVH
   Left atrial enlargement.
   Nonspecific ST-T changes are almost universal
   LBBB or RBBB without specific pattern.
   Arrhythmias—especially atrial fibrillation.
   APCs, PVCs, VT, ventricular arrhythmia's.
   AV blocks are rare.
2. **RCM**: Low voltage QRS or loss of R wave progression in chest leads.
   Nonspecific ST-T changes
   Various conduction defects.
3. **HOCM**: There is no typical pattern. A pattern of LVH with strain or no typical pattern.
   Deep, broad Q's in LI, aVL, V5, V6 are present. They are not due to old MI but abnormal depolarization of asymmetrical septal hypertrophy.
   LAD; evidence of left and right atrial enlargement, short PR with slurring of upstroke.
   Deep S wave, poor R wave progression.
   Tall initial R in V1, LBBB
   AF, AT, VT,
   Giant T wave inversion in the left ventricular leads is a rare form of apical hypertrophy.
   WPW type may be present.
4. Characteristic ECG in DCM of neuromuscular disorders
   In Ducchenne's progressive muscular dystrophy—Prominent R in right precordial leads and R ; S > 1:1 with deep Q wave in limb and precordial leads.
   Myotonic dystrophy is characterized by disorders of impulse formation and conduction.

25. Echocardiogram in cardiomyopathy helps to differentiate the 4 types:

1. **DCM:** LV dilatation with normal or minimal thickening of the walls (No hypertrophy)
   Systolic dysfunction with global hypokinesia or dyskinesia.
   Pericardial effusion is often seen.
   Mural thrombi may be seen.
2. **RCM**: Symmetrically thickened LV wall with normal systolic function.
   Diastolic function is impaired.

'Speckled' appearance of thickened myocardium is seen in RCM of amyloidosis.

CT, MRI and endomyocardial biopsy may be required to establish the diagnosis.

3. **HOCM**: LVH with asymmetrical septal hypertrophy (ASH) 1.3 times of LV free wall (> 13 mm).
   Premature closure of the aortic valve
   Resting gradients >30 mm Hg
   Provocable gradients >50 mm Hg
   Normal or increased motion of the posterior wall
   Reduced rate of closure of the mitral valve in mid-diastole
   Mitral valve prolapse with regurgitation
   Maximal left ventricular diastolic wall thickness >15 mm
   The diagnosis of HOCM is based on resting gradient >30 mm Hg or provocable gradient >50 mm Hg.
   Induction of obstruction and therefore gradients can be accomplished with substance like amyl nitrate, isoproterenol, dobutamine or maneuvers like Valsalva maneuver, exercise that decrease LV preload or increase in contractility. Recognition of MR or mitral valve anomalies have effect on medical or surgical strategies
   Left ventricular cavity is decreased with increased posterior wall activity.
   Systolic anterior motion (SAM) of mitral valve against hypertrophied septum and mid-systolic closure of the aortic valve is seen thus narrowing the outflow tract.
   Unusual 'ground-glass' appearance of hypertrophied septum due to changes in cellular architecture and fibrosis.
4. **OCM:** Both ventricles are markedly thickened.
   Size of the ventricular cavity is compromised due to large mural thrombi.

26. Uses of MRI.

1. It can detect LV hypertrophy missed by echocardiography, specially in the anterolateral and basal left ventricular free walls.
2. Myocardial scar often detected as delayed hyper-enhancement with gadolinium—contrast MRI.
   It may be a predictor of sudden cardiac death (SCD) in the HCM patients.
3. Evaluation of regional myocardial function with use of Cine-MRI.
4. Improved detection of MR, SAM, abnormal papillary muscle and diastolic dysfunction.

27. Cardiac catheterization in cardiomyopathy helps to differentiate the 4 types.

1. **DCM:** Dysfunction and dilatation of left ventricle with diminished cardiac output. LVED, left atrial and pulmonary wedge pressures are usually elevated. RVED, right atrial and central venous pressures are elevated when right sided heart failure supervens.
2. **RCM:** Normal systolic function.
   Ventricular diastolic pressure pulse shows a dip and plateau configuration resembling that of constrictive pericarditis. It may show elevated filling pressure and square root sign in ventricular pressure tracing.
3. **HOCM:** Systolic function is vigorous.
   Obstruction of dynamic LV outflow tract.
   Filling pressures are elevated on both sides.
   Subaortic or midventricular outflow gradient on catheter pull back.
   Spike- and dome-pattern of aortic pressure tracing—a consequence of outlet obstruction.
   Increased RVEDP and LVEDPs.
   Increased pulmonary capillary wedge pressure.
   Increased V wave on wedge tracing—it may result from MR or elevated LA pressure.
   Increased pulmonary arterial pressure.
4. **OCM:** Changes are different in OCM of isolated right ventricular endomyocardial fibrosis (RVEMF) from that of biventricular EMF. In isolated RVEMF, pulmonary wedge pressure and pulmonary artery pressure are normal. When the ventricular diastolic pressure is higher than the pulmonary diastolic pressure, it suggests a passive diastolic flow across the pulmonary valve.
   It may be necessary to increase the left ventricular contractility by utilizing isoprenaline to document the obstruction or increase the magnitude of obstruction during cardiac catheterization.

28. Angiocardiography in cardiomyopathies helps to differentiate the 4 types.

1. **DCM:** Ventricular chambers are dilated.
   Diffusely hypokinetic left ventricle with some degree of mitral regurgitation.
   Selective arteriograms are normal thereby excluding the ischemic cardiomyopathy. It can distinguish the cause of poor left ventricular function as a result of coronary artery disease.
2. **RCM:** Normal to mild cardiac enlargement.
3. **HOCM:** Selective angiocardiography shows obstruction by hypertrophied muscle, degree of mitral regurgitation and outlines the size of the ventricular cavity.
4. **OCM (EMF):** Shows irregular ventricular cavity with mild-to-moderate regurgitation, residual end systolic volume and small areas of outpouching like small ventricular aneurysms.

29. Endomyocardial biopsy sometimes reveals specific etiologies like the following 4 conditions.

1. Myocarditis

2. Amyloidosis, sarcoidosis
3. Adriamycin toxicity
4. Endomyacordial fibrosis.

Which patient should be subjected to endomyocardial biopsy remains controversial.

30. Alcoholic cardiomyopathy is the major reversible form of secondary dilated cardiomyopathy (DCM). It is common in the West. Thiamine enriched flour is used in the Western diet. It should be differentiated from cardiomegaly due to thiamine deficiency (Beriberi) which is common in Far East where polished rice is the major diet.

Table K-1

Alcoholic cardiomyopathy	*Thiamine deficiency (Beriberi)*
1. **History** Usually associated with alcoholic consumption in large quantities for many years, not associated with other effects of alcohol like cirrhosis liver, etc. may be associated with thiamine deficiency	Usually associated with generalized malnutrition, peripheral neuropathy, glossitis, anemia. Thiamine deficiency per se may not be the cause of cardiomyopathy
2. **Clinical manifestations of CVS** Symptoms of low output failure and systemic vasoconstriction.	Symptoms of high output failure with tachycardia, increased cardiac output and often with increase in left and right ventricular filling pressures. Systemic vascular resistance is decreased due to vasomotor depression Biventricular failure Retention of sodium and water leads to edema
3. **CVS examination** Narrow pulse pressure S3, S4 common MR and/or TR murmurs are common	Wide pulse pressure with tachycardia. Frequent systolic murmur at the apex
4. **ECG** Diffuse non-specific ST-T changes	Decreased voltage, Prolonged Q-T interval, T wave abnormalities

31. Thiamine (Vitamin B_1) deficiency causes total body capillary dilatation. In order to fill the dilated vascular bed, a marked hyperkinetic state is produced with the signs of

1. Tachycardia
2. High venous pressure
3. Cardiomegaly
4. Peripheral edema

It is seen in alcoholic patients who resort to an enormous intake of beer. The cardiomyopathy that occurs due to alcohol, thiamine deficiency or both combindly should be differentiated. An acute, fulminent, nonedematous form characterized by cardiovascular collapse and death within hours or days is known as shoeshine beriberi (*shoo* damage: *shin* = heart—Japanese).

32. Restrictive cardiomyopathy (RCM) is difficult to distinguish from constrictive pericarditis. The differentiation is important because the constrictive pericarditis is curable by operation. The following points help to differentiate the two conditions.

Table K-2

	Restrictive cardiomyopathy (RCM)	*Constrictive pericarditis*
1. History	Chronic inflammatory disease Tuberculosis Multisystem involvement Renal disease (amyloid)	Open heart surgery Tuberculosis Radiotherapy
2. Physical examination	MR,TR murmurs common Kussmaul's sign rare Apical pulse prominent, usually palpable Sounds are distinctly heard S3, S4 common	Chest scars Tattoos (previous radiotherapy) Kussmaul's sign Apex impalpable Pericardial knock *Friedreich's sign
3. ECG	Low voltage (clinically in amyloidosis) LAD, pseudo-infarction changes, nonspecific ST-T AF Conduction disturbances or delay	Low voltage (< 50%) ST↑ with concavity upwards in most leads Reciprocal ST changes absent No Qs
4. Echocardiogram Doppler Echo Tissues Doppler imaging E Color M-mode flow propagation velocity (VP)	Increase wall thickness 'Speckling' of intraventricular septum Thickened valves Giant atrial enlargement Diastolic function impaired Mitral and tricuspid valvular regurgitation < 8 (cm/s) < 45 (cm/s)	Pericardial thickening Normal chamber wall thickness 'Septal bounce' due to rapid early diastolic filling with abrupt displacement IVS >25% reduction in mitral inflow E wave velocity with inspiration Increased flow across tricuspid valve with inspiration >8 (cm/s) >100 (cm/s)
5. Cardiac catheterization	VEDP often > 5 mm Hg greater than RVEDP, but RVEDP may equal LVEDP	RVEDP = LVEDP (< 5 mm Hg difference) RVSP < 50 mm Hg RAP > 15 mm Hg RVEDP < 1/3 RVSP Significant changes with respiration

Contd...

Contd...

	Restrictive cardiomyopathy (RCM)	*Constrictive pericarditis*
6. MRI/CT chest	Pericardium usually normal	Pericardium thickened
7. Endomyocardial biopsy	May revel specific histology clinches diagnosis (e.g. amyloidosis, sarcoidosis, hemochromatosis)	Usually normal
8. Management	Management of HF itself, AV block and symptomatic bradycardia commonly co-exit requiring pacemaker Surgical treatment—heart transplantation	Medical—nonspecific for viral or idiopathic pericarditis Specific tuberculosis, amebiasis, hydatid cyst, collagen disease Surgical—pericardiectomy for chronic constrictive pericarditis

33. Involvement of the heart in primary amyloidosis is the frequent cause of death. There are 4 clinical modes of presentations of CVS in amyloidosis either alone or in combination.

1. Systolic dysfunction
2. Diastolic dysfunction
3. Arrhythmias
4. Orthostatic hypotension.

34. Cardiac hypertrophy is of 4 types.

1. Concentric hypertrophy: Left ventricular wall is thick but cavity is small.
2. Eccentric hypertrophy: Dilatation of the ventricle without thickening of the ventricular walls.
3. Asymmetrical hypertrophy.
4. Apical hypertrophy: Hypertrophy confined to apical area only.

35. Management of cardiomyopathies consists of 4 steps.

1. **General measures:**
   Prolonged bed rest
   Avoidance of alcohol
   Avoidance of toxins
   Avoidance of drugs that may cause cardiomyopathy
   Correction of nutritional deficiencies, e.g. thiamine, protein, etc.
   Weight reduction in obese patients.
2. **Treatment of heart failure itself:**
   Conventional treatment of heart failure and maintenance of sinus rhythm is important.

Restriction of salt

a. Eliminate salt shakar at table sodium will be restricted to 1.6 to 2.8 g/daily.
b. Eliminate salt in cooking and at table sodium will be restricted to 1.2 to 1.8 g/daily.
c. Institute A and B + low sodium diet sodium will be restricted to 0.2 to 1 g/daily.

Diuretics

a. Moderately effective (thiazide).
b. Loop diuretic (Frusemide, ethacrynic acid, bumetanide).
c. Loop diuretic + distal tubular (potassium-sparing) diuretic.
d. a + b + c.

Digoxin

Digitalis toxicity is not a problem in DCM. Avoid rapid digitalization, 0.25 mg od is usually sufficient. Adjust the dose according to the age. For example, above 65 years. 0.125 mg od increased dose may be necessary in atrial fibrillation.

Digitalis 0.25 mg tds is dangerous.

Digitalis, diuretics, nitrates, β-stimulators are best avoided in LV outflow tract obstruction, e.g. HOCM.

3. **Specific treatment depends on the type of cardiomyopathy.**

Vasodilators—like hydralazine or sorbitrate in a single dose per day is added to the digitalis, diuretic treatment in DCM. Even both may be added.

Enzyme inhibitors, e.g. captopril, enalapril are reserved in advanced cases of DCM.

Newer cardiotonic drugs like amrinone or milrinone may be tried in DCM.

Anticoagulants—given in all cases of cardiomyopathies who do not have any contraindication to prevent pulmonary or systemic embolism.

β-*blockers*—help in relieving angina dyspnea and syncope to some extent in hypertrophic obstructive cardiomyopathy (HOCM). In HOCM in whom the gradient is not present at rest across LV or RV outflow tract and is present only on inotropic provocation (use of isoproterenol) and in whom the gradient can be completely abolished react better with initial trial with oral β-blockers. Useful in infants and young children with mild or no symptoms. There is no evidence that β-blockers protect against sudden death in HOCM, which is mostly due to dysarrhythmias.

They act by inhibition of sympathetic stimulation brought by the negative inotropic and chromotropic properties of the drugs. β-blockers diminish myocardial oxygen requirement and augment diastolic filling which alleviate angina and the detrimental effect of LV outflow obstruction, respectively.

β-blockers and α-blockers combindly (carvedilol, labetalol) should probably not to be used as the first line drug because of their additional vasodilating properties.

C/I to the β-blockers are bronchial asthma, lung disease, a high degree of heart block in the absence of pacemaker and decompensated LV systolic dysfunction.

Calcium channel blockers like verapamil, nifedipine, diltiazam may reduce the ventricular rigidity and reduce the increased diastolic pressure in HOCM. These drugs may be promising in the near future.

They are considered to be second-line agents when β-blockers are not successful or contraindicated in HCM. They have a negative inotropic effect and reduce the heart rate and blood pressure. They may also have beneficial effects on diastolic function by improving rapid diastolic filling although at the expense of higher LV end-diastolic pressures.

C/I to the use of calcium blockers include the presence of conduction system disturbances in the absences of pacer or in the presence of systolic dysfunction.

Cortisones and immunosuppresive agents are useful in cardiomyopathies associated with connective tissue disorders, granulomas, eosinophilic endomyocardial disease (EMF also called Loeffler's endocarditis or Fibroplastic endocarditis).

Steroids are not much useful in DCM; on the other hand, they may be dangerous in myocarditis.

Antiarrhythmic agents to maintain sinus rhythm is of paramount importance. Sometimes digitalis alone controls the arrhythmias of APCs, PVCs in DCM.

Atrial fibrillation.

Direct current cardioversion (DCC) for unstable symptoms.

β-blockers and/or verapamil for rate control.

Disopyramide or sotalol for maintaining normal sinus rhythm.

Amiodarone for refractory cases.

DDD pacing with nodal ablation in patient with (dual chamber) persistent symptoms who fail medical therapy.

Anticoagulants for recurrent or chronic AF.

Ventricular tachycardia (VT): Amiodarone or AICD (Automatic implantable cardioverter defibrillator) for NSVT (Non-sustain ventricular tachycardia) in high-risk patients.

AICD with pacing for cardiac arrest survivors.

Transplantation for refractory VT.

Beneficial effects of antiarrhythmic drugs in HOCM is not yet established.

Drugs are used to treat the associated conditions like diabetes mellitus, hypo- or hyper-thyroidism, etc.

Antibiotics are used as prophylaxis for endocarditis.

Phlebotomy is indicated in early stages when associated with hemochromatosis. Subcutaneous desferrioxamine is given to reduce the body iron stores but whether it produces improvement is doubtful.

Dialysis

4. **Surgical management**:

   Myotomy/myectomy: Resection of some of the hypertrophied septum is indicated in HOCM particularly in those with dyspnea or paroxysmal nocturnal dyspnea and those with more fixed gradients across the outflow tract. A new approach is to perform the myotomy/myectomy with laser with similar results as are obtained with the conventional blade approach.

   Superior vena cava to pulmonary artery shunt is adviced in dominant RVEMF to reduce venous return to right side thereby helping to decrease the size of right atrium and to postpone the development of atrial arrhythmia's.

Radical stripping of fibrous endocardium with mitral and/or tricuspid valve replacement is done in endomyocardial fibrosis (EMF). In isolated RVEMF, a modified Glenn's operation may prolong the life.

Permanent pacemaking may be very useful in cardiomyopathy associated with myotonic dystrophy, which is characterized by disorders of impulse formation and conduction, which can cause syncope and sudden death.

Implantation of automatic internal defibrillator should be considered in appropriate patients.

Assisted circulation by intra-aortic balloon, left ventricular assist device, artificial heart. The cardiac assist devices are used as a bridge to cardiac transplantation.

Dynamic cardiomyopathy: In this procedure skeletal muscle like latissimus dorsi, which has a high proportion of fast twitch type 'A' fibers are electrically stimulated and converted to type 'C' slow twitch fibers. This conditioned latissimus dorsi is then wrapped around the heart and electrically stimulated in synchrony with ventricular systole of the heart using an implant pacemaker. It improves around 30% of cardiac output. It should be preferably done when the patients are in NYHA class II or III and should not be delayed till NYHA class IV.

Heart transplantation is the last trial in DCM in suitable patients.

MYOCARDITIS

Myocarditis is a generalized inflammation of the heart muscle, which is most often caused by viral infection (viral myocarditis). Myocarditis is potentially very dangerous, even fatal. The heart muscle may be weakened to the point of heart failure, or the heart muscle may be prone to abnormal electrical discharges and rhythm disturbances resulting in potentially fatal arrhythmias. Though most cases are not fatal and can be treated, a severe case of myocarditis can cause dilated cardiomyopathy (DCM) which is much more serious condition. Many idiopathic dilated cardiomyopathies arise from mild or subclinical episodes of myocarditis with associated necrosis or degeneration or both. This disease is also known as inflammatory cardiomyopathy.

The inflammatory process of cardiac muscle results from infections. The commonest is the group B Coxsackie viruses or CVB which were identified in the early 1950s as agents of human heart disease.

Myocarditis is also present in hypersensitivity states such as acute rheumatic fever.

Average age of a patient having myocarditis is 42 years old. Males get it more often than females.

Usually, myocarditis clears up by itself without sequelae.

Myocarditis is known to cause sudden cardiac death.

36. Myocarditis is classified into 4 clinicopathological conditions.

1. *Fulminant myocarditis (13%):* Usually, has a clear onset it can result in either complete spontaneous recovery or rapidly progressive detrition and death; histologically multiple active foci of inflammation infiltrates with complete resolution.
2. *Acute myocarditis (65%):* It has an indistinct onset often incomplete recovery and subsequent dearth histologically active or fordessive inflammatory infiltrate that resolve.
3. *Chronic active myocarditis (11%):* Clinically presents as acute myocarditis but usually progress to mild or moderate cardiac dysfunction. Histologically shows ongoing fibrosis suggesting chronic inflammatory changes.
4. *Chronic persistent myocarditis (7%):* It has distinct onset histologically shows active borderline inflammatory infiltrates usually there is no cardiac compromise.
   Histological classification of myocarditis also called Dallas classification (1986) is also present.

37. The causes of myocarditis are:

I. *Infectious causes*
1. Viruses: Group B Coxsackie viruses are the commonest causes. Other viruses are coxsackie a, poliomyelitis, influenza, adeno, echovirus, rubella, herpes viruses, mumps, rubrota, hepatitis B or C, HIV virus, Epstein-Barr virus, cytomegalovirus, parvovirus B19.
2. Bacterial diphtheria (acute), tuberculosis (chronic), legionella, clostridium, streptococci, staphylococci, salmonella, shigella.
3. Protozoal—treponema cruzi (chagas disease), toxoplasmosis gondii, trichinosis, schistosomiasis.
4. Fungal actinomycetes, histoplasmosis, cryptococcosis, aspergillosis, coccidiomycosis.
5. Helminths—trichinosis, schistosomiasis.
6. Spirochetes—borrelia burgdorferi (Lyme diseases).

II. *Noninfectious causes*
1. Hypersensitivity states.
2. Acute rheumatic fever, giant cell myocarditis, Lyme myocarditis, eosinophilic myocarditis.
3. Physical agents heart stroke, hypothermia.
4. Chemical agents hydrocarbons, carbon monoxide, thallium, lead, arsenic, cobalt.
5. Radiation agents—irradiation
6. Cardiotoxic drugs—catecholamines, amphetamine, cocaine, chemotherapeutic drugs, e.g. anthracyclines, fluorouracil, streptomycin, cyclophosphamide, interleukins-2, trastuzumab (Herceptin), small pox vaccine.
7. Collagen vascular diseases—systemic lupus erythematsus (i.e. lupus carditis, Wagner's granulations or Churg-Straus syndrome, polymyositis or dematotomyosites, scleroderma.
8. Systemic diseases—sarcoidosis, gaint cell myocarditis, Kawasaki's disease, large vessel vasculitis, e.g. polyarthritis nodosa, Takayasu's arteritis, inflammatory bowel diseases (e.g. ulcerative colitis, Crohn's disease).
9. Bites and stings; venous snake, scorpions, wasps and beak wider spiders.
10. Child bish—peripartum cardiomyopathy.
11. Alloantigens; post-transplantation, cellular rejection.

38. Symptoms

1. The hallmark symptom of those found are fatigue, dyspnea, edema
2. Fever flu like symptoms—arthralgia, malaise, sweats or chills, h/o pharyngitis, tonsillitis, URTI, 1 or more weeks before
3. May be asymptomatic or common manifestation with chest pain, which may mimic acute myocardial infarction or symptoms of lung congestion. Chest pain is frequently associated with acute pericarditis, known to cause sudden death, when it is caused by Coxsackie B strain or echovirus

4. Palpitation caused by arrhythmia—infective illness with regular heartbeaor chest pain—suspect myocarditis, arrhythmias or heart block/Stokes-Adams syndrome attack ventricular tachyarrhythmias or even sudden cardiac death.

Myocarditis may not be detected because it may not cause any problem or symptoms that patient can feel and go to the doctor.

39. Physical examination:

1. May be normal in patients who have ECG abnormalities In more severe cases
2. S1 may be muffled and S3 may be present
3. Murmur of mitral regurgitation
4. Pericardial friction rub when associated with pericarditis.

Clinical diagnosis is difficult and many times it arrived at only after more common pediatric problems including asthma, recurrent vomiting and chronic viral illness such as mononucleosis are excluded. Viral myocarditis is preceded many times by a flu-like illness or gastroenteritis. When patients present with classical findings of congestive heart failure, tachypnea, tachycardia and hepatomegaly, the diagnosis is more apparent. Occasionally, the patients present with respiratory distress or shock. Acute myocarditis usually presents with symptoms of mild to moderate congestive heart failure from left ventricular dysfunction.

40. Specific findings in special situations are as follows:

1. Sarcoid myocarditis—lymphadenopathy also with arrhythmias, and sarcoid involvement in other organs (up to 70%)
2. Acute rheumatic fever (effects heart in 50–90%) associated symptoms of polyarthralgia, subcutaneous nodules, erythema marginatum, i.e. Jones Criteria
3. Allergic—hypersensitivity or allergic myocarditis, purities maculopapular rash or any drug allergy
4. Giant cell myocarditis—there can be sustained ventricular tachycardia rapidly progressive heart failure.

41. Investigations.

1. Complete blood count—leukocytosis (often lymphocytosis), increase in eosinophilia may suggest hypersensitivity esinophilic (myocarditis).
2. Elevated acute phase reactants—rise in ESR, C-reactive protein, help to moniter progress, also through they have low specificity tumor necrosing factor (TNF), interleukins, interferons-α, serum soluble FAS and soluble FAS ligand levels rise of these markers indicates more prognosis.
3. ECG.
4. Serial ECG 24 hours.
5. Chest X-ray.
6. Echo.
7. Isolation of virus.
8. Serum viral antibody usually increased to fourfold or more.
9. Anticardiac antibodies titers.
10. Rheumatologic screening.
11. Cardiac catheterization.
12. Endomyocardial biopsy.

Disease specific test are indicated

1. SLE—anti ds DNA.
2. Polymyositis—anti jo.
3. Wasner's granulomatosus—ANCA (antineutrophil cytoplasmic antibody).
4. Scleredema—antisclerosis.

42. Treatment:

1. General measures: Strenuous activity should be avoided. Prolonged bed rest for more severe cases.
2. Analgesics or anti-inflammatory drugs to relieve pain
3. Antibiotics when myocarditis is due to bacterial infection
4. Congestive heart failure: Most patients respond to
   i. Bed rest
   ii. Salt restriction
   iii. Digitalis—some patients appear to be sensitive to digoxin
   iv. Diuretics

   Afterload reduction with ACE inhibitors, such as captopril or enalapril.

   Congestive heart failure and inflammatory myocarditis appear to respond to immunosuppression with prednisone and azathioprine in some cases.
5. Arrhythmias are to be treated by antiarrhythmic group of drugs—Difficult to control arrhythmias
6. Occasionally, patients experience profound cardiovascular collapse which requires high dose ionotropic support and mechanical ventilation
7. Anticoagulant therapy to prevent blood clots is used in some patients with severe myocarditis
8. Cardiac transplantation may be done when it is very severe.

   Death is due to heart failure, arrhythmias or heart block.

   Most often self-limited without sequelae.

   Recur and acute myocarditis may progress to chronic.

43. Some specific types of myocarditis. Four types are well known.

1. Chagas' disease
2. Giant cell myocarditis
3. Lyme carditis
4. Radiation myocarditis.

44. Some rare causes are:

1. Toxoplasmosis
2. Cytomegalovirus
3. Esinophilic myocarditis
4. Myocarditis and SIDS (sudden infant death).

Chagas' disease: It is caused by the protozoan *Trypnosoma cruzi,* carried by the cone nosed bug. It is one of the most common cause of heart disease found in Central and South America. 20% of population may be affected in rural areas. It produces extensive myocarditis which typically becomes evident after the initial infection. May develop into chronic myocardial damage typically appearing 20 years after the initial infection.

45. It is characterized by—:

1. Dilatation of several cardiac chambers
2. Fibrosis and thinning of ventricular walls
3. Aneurysm formation in areas of thinning (especially at the apex)
4. Mural thrombi.

Characteristics of the disease are congestive heart failure, heart block or arrhythmias. Chronic and progressive to heart failure often predominantly right sided failure is the rule.

ECG typically shows RBBB. LAHB pattern which may progress to complete heart block. Echocardiogram shows unique pattern of hypokinesia of posterior of left ventricular wall and relatively preserved septal motion. Ventricular arrhythmias are common and are particularly seen during and after exertion. Cause of death is either heart failure or arrhythmia.

46. Treatment is directed toward heart failure and arrhythmias. It consists of:

1. Standard therapy for heart failure
2. Antiarrhythmic drugs
3. Pace maker for complete heart block
4. Antiprotozoal therapy against Trypnosoma cruzi.

Giant-cell myocarditis: It is a rare form of myocarditis of unknown etiology although it occurs in association with thymoma, systemic lupus erythematosus and thyrotoxicosis. It is characterized by the presence of multinucleated giant cells in the myocardium. It is rapidly fatal disorder that usually affects otherwise healthy individuals of young and middle age of either sex. The median survival is 5.5 months from onset of symptoms with an overall mortality of 90%.

The best treatment is heart transplantation, however patients often die before a donor heart can be obtained.

It is observed that immunosuppression including cyclosporine and steroid may increase survival four-fold.

Lyme carditis: It is caused by the hypersensitivity to circulating immune complexes in response to a bite of tick-borne agent.

Patient may present with headaches, fever, fatigue and syncope.

Conduction abnormalities are the more common manifestations. which results in complete heart block and syncope.

Concomitant myopericarditis is not uncommon and mild left ventricular dysfunction may occur.

Prednisone may be efficacious in ameliorating heart block.

Penicillin or tetracycline is used to treat accompanying skin rash.

Radiation myocarditis: Acute and chronic cardiac complications may result from the use of ionizing radiation in the treatment of carcinoma of the lung or breast, lymphoma or Hodgkin's disease.

Occasionally, patient have acute pericarditis. The most common presentation is that of chronic pericardial effusion or constriction occurring months or years after exposure (in rare cases up to 10 years).

Myocarditis and SIDS (Sudden Infant Death)

47. Myocarditis can cause sudden death or heart failure. The infants with heart failure will present as:

1. Fatigue
2. Difficulty in drinking the whole bottle—sweating with exertion during feeding
3. Tachypnea
4. Tachycardia.

   Sudden infant death (SIDS) can be hereditary when not caused by a virus, as in muscular dystrophy or Pompe's disease.

L Congenital Heart Diseases

Congenital means inborn or existing at birth. Congenital heart disease (CHD) is a structural abnormality of the heart present from birth. The terms such as congenital heart defect, congenital heart disease and congenital cardiovascular diseases are used. The word 'defect' is more accurate than 'disease'. Congenital heart diseases are really anomalies, not diseases. The anomalies are followed animal models during evolution like two chamber heart, three chamber heart, etc. So why not the term congenital 'anomalies' which is more appropriate.

In India, an estimated 2,50,000 children are born with congenital heart disease each year and of these approximately 80,000 newborns would require medical intervention in the neonatal period. The disheartening situation is that only 3% of the affected infants seem to get timely intervention. The remaining 97% of infants with serious heart problems do not survive. Ignorance and poverty are obstacles to approach the pediatric cardiology facilities and account for high mortality.

1. Congenital heart diseases can be classified into 4 groups.

1. Acyanotic heart diseases with normal pulmonary flow, i.e. without shunt.
   - Malposition of the cardia
   - Coarctation of the aorta
   - Aortic stenosis (AS)
   - Pulmonary stenosis (PS)
   - Endomyocardial disease
   - Malformation of aortic arch
   - Cor triatriatum.
2. Acyanotic heart diseases with increased pulmonary blood flow, i.e. with shunt.
   - Atrial septal defect (ASD)
   - Ventrticular septal defect (VSD)
   - Patent ductus arteriosus (PDA)
   - Aortopulmonary septal defect
   - Endocardial cushion defects
   - Partial anomalous pulmonary venous connections (PAPVC).
3. Cyanotic heart diseases with normal or decreased pulmonary flow.
   - Tetralogy of Fallot (TOF)
   - Tricuspid atresia (TA)
   - Pulmonary atresia (PA)
   - Severe pulmonary stenosis
   - Double outlet right ventricle with PS.
4. Cyanotic heart diseases with increased pulmonary blood flow.
   - Transposition of great arteries (TGA)
   - Hypoplastic left heart syndrome
   - Preductal coarctation
   - Total anomalous pulmonary venous connection (TAPVC)
   - Truncus arteriosus
   - Double outlet right ventricle (DORV)
   - Ebstein anomaly of tricuspid valve
   - Eisenmenger's syndrome (Reversed shunt)
   - Cyanotic patients have either pulmonic stenosis or pulmonary arterial hypertension.

2. Congenital heart diseases can also be classified in other way into 4 groups depending on hemodynamic, anatomic and radiographic factors.

1. Systemic and pulmonary circulation communication without cyanosis (left-to-right shunts):
   - Atrial septal defect (ASD)
   - Ventricular septal defect (VSD)
   - Patent ductus arteriosus (PDA)
   - Aortopulmonary septal defect (AP window)

- Aortic sinus aneurysm and fistula
- Coronary arteriovenous fistula
- Anomalous pulmonary origin of coronary artery
- Persistent truncus arteriosus.

2. Obstructive valvular and vascular lesions with or without right and left shunt:
   - Pulmonary stenosis with intact ventricular septum
   - Fallot's tetralogy
   - Ebstein's anomaly
   - Tricuspid atresia
   - Coarctation of aorta.
3. Abnormalities in the origin of the great arteries and veins, the transpositions:
   - Aortic stenosis
   - Pulmonary stenosis
   - Transposition of the great arteries (TGA)
   - Transposition of the pulmonary veins.
4. Malposition of the heart—Dextrocardia.

   About 1% of live births are complicated by cardiovascular malformation with overall male preponderance.

3. The prevalence of congenital heart diseases in India is not known. There is no known etiology of congenital heart diseases, but a few associations with some conditions reveal that a combination of genetic and environmental interactions probably play a major role. The 4 major associated factors are:

1. Environmental factors: Association of patent ductus arteriosus (PDA) in children born at high altitudes.

   Infections: Association of PDA and VSD with rubella infection during pregnancy.

   Chickenpox during first trimester of pregnancy is commonly associated with congenital heart disease.

   Viral illness in the last trimester may produce myocarditis in the newborn.
2. Hereditary factors: Incidence of congenital heart disease in siblings is significantly higher than in the general population.

   Diabetes mellitus in parents, grandparents may be recorded in cases of transposition of great arteries and hypoplastic left heart syndrome. Children of patients surgically treated for congenital heart disease have ten times more chance of having congenital heart disease. The strongest familial tendency is known in ASD associated with bony abnormalities (Holt-Oram syndrome).
3. Association with other congenital malformations caused by genetic and chromosomal aberrations.

   Association of AV canal defects with Down's syndrome. Marfan's syndrome, Ellis-van Creveld syndrome are known genetic disorders associated with congenital heart disease.

   Chromosomal aberrations as seen in Mongolism, Turner's syndrome and trisomy syndromes are associated with congenital heart disease.
4. Association of drugs like lithium during pregnancy with Ebstein anomaly.

   Thalidomide which is banned now was responsible for TOF.

   Dextroamphetamines can be the cause of transposition of great arteries.

   Oral antidiabetic drugs like to tolbutamide, chlorpropamide may cause congenital heart disease (CHD).

   Use of anticonvulsants like phenytoin, and paramethadione, trimethadione in the first trimester is associated with various CHD.

   Stilbesterol may cause transposition of great vessels ingestion of nicotine and smoking may cause PDA, TOF.

   Exposure to radiation in the first trimester is associated with various CHD.

   Some prescription drugs and over the counter medicines, as well as alcohol and "street" drugs, may increase the risk of having a baby with congenital heart disease.

   Other factors that affect the heart's development are under study. The fact is that we do not know what causes most congenital cardiovascular defects.

4. Heart starts beating from the 4th week of intrauterine life.

5. There are 4 congenital anomalies where male sex is predominant.

1. Aortic stenosis (AS)
2. Coarctation of the aorta
3. Tetralogy of Fallot (TOF)
4. Transposition of great Arteries (TOGA)

   PDA and ASD are more common in females.

6. The incidence of male to female ratio of coarctation of aorta is 4:1.

7. Commonest congenital heart diseases.

1. Commonest congenital cardiac anomaly—bicuspid aortic valve.
2. Commonest congenital cardiac anomaly encountered as one of the many congenital anomalies—ventricular septal defect (VSD).
3. Commonest congenital anomaly with cyanosis at birth—transposition of great vessels.
4. Commonest congenital cyanotic heart disease above the age of 2 years is tetralogy of Fallot (TOF). It constitutes about 3/4th of all blue patients.

8. The 4 commonest congenital heart diseases surviving into late adulthood without treatment (uncorrected).

1. Bicuspid aortic valve—commonest congenital malformation without manifestations.
2. ASD—Predominant in females.
3. PDA—Predominant in females.
4. Mild pulmonary stenosis.

9. The 4 congenital anomalies that produce cyanosis at birth—Blue baby.

1. Transposition of great arteries.
2. Pulmonary atresia
3. Tricuspid atresia
4. Total anomalous pulmonary venous connection (TAPVC).
   (Cyanosis appears beyond one month in 'tetralogy of Fallot').

10. When cyanosis is delayed, the following are considered.

1. When occurs after a month with crying, feeding or warm bath or only with syncope—suggests tetralogy of Fallot.
2. When delayed for years and associated with palpitation with little dyspnea on exertion–suggests Ebstein's anomaly.
3. When delayed until adolescence or middle age suggests atrial septal defect with Eisenmenger's syndrome.
4. When delayed for years with differential cyanosis and clubbing suggests patent ductus arteriosus with Eisenmenger's syndrome.

11. The common causes of congestive heart failure (CHF) depending on the age are:

1. In the first 24 hours after birth
   - Pulmonary atresia
   - Mitral or aortic atresia
   - Hypoplastic left heart syndrome
2. In infancy and childhood
   - Congenital heart disease
3. In adolescence
   - Rheumatic heart disease
4. In adults
   - HT, IHD, valvular disease.

12. Some syndromes associated with congenital heart diseases are:

1. Marfan's syndrome – Aortic and mitral regurgitation.
2. Turner's syndrome – Coarctation of aorta.
3. Down's syndrome (Mongolism) – Endocardial cushion defect, osteum primum type ASD.
4. Holt-Oram syndrome – ASD with MS.

13. The 4 common types of defects which are encountered in some congenital heart diseases.

1. Commonest type of ASD—Osteum secondum type.
2. Commonest type of VSD—Membranous type.
3. Commonest site of coarctation of the aorta—Descending aorta.
4. Commonest site of pulmonary artery stenosis—Valvular (infundibular in TOF).

14. A good number of congenital heart diseases are associated with characteristic changes in the extremities.

The following are few examples:

1. Short stature, cubitus valgus, medial deviation of the extended forearm are characteristic of Turner syndrome—associated with coarctation of aorta as a common abnormality.
2. Short stature, web neck, cubitus valgus and hypogonadism found in males occur in Ullrich-Noonan syndrome – associated with pulmonary stenosis as a common abnormality.
3. Thumb with an extraphalanx ("fingerized thumb"):
   a. It may lie in the same plane as the fingers making it difficult to oppose the thumb and fingers—associated with atrial septal defect.
   b. There may be distal radial and ulnar deformities causing difficulty in supination and pronation—when both are present—called Holt-Oram syndrome—associated with atrial septal defect of secundum type, pectus deformities of the sternum may also occur.
4. Arachnodactyly:
   a. Fingers are slender and long ("Spider fingers"): It is characteristic of Marfan's syndrome—associated with aortic regurgitation or mitral valve prolapse.
   b. Thumb sign: when a fist is made over the clenched thumb, the thumb should not extend beyond the ulnar side of the hand, but it usually does so in Marfan's syndrome.
   b. Wrist sign: When the wrist is encircled by the thumb and little finger, the little finger will overlap at least 1 cm in 80% of patients with Marfan's syndrome.
   c. An incomplete form of Marfan's syndrome with kyphoscoliosis, pectus carinatum (pigeon breast) and long extremities may occur in homocystinuria in which thrombosis of intermediate-sized arteries cause myocardial infarction.

15. Bradydectyly: Short fingers are associated with 4 congenital cardiac anomalies.

1. Turner's syndrome
2. Down's syndrome
3. Ellis-van Creveld syndrome
4. Mucopolysaccharidosis.

16. The cardiac lesions that are expected with Ellis-van Creveld syndrome are (chondroectodermal dysplasia, an extra finger and often an extra toe, hypoplastic finger nails, and dwarfism):

1. About two-thirds of patients have an atrial septal defect of ostium primum type
2. Ventricular septal defect
3. Single ventricle
4. Patent ductus arteriosus.

Upper lip of these patients is 'tied' down to the alveolar ridge by multiple frenula. Trisomy 13–15 syndrome also involves polydactyly. These patients tend to have a ventricular septal defect, patent ductus arteriosus and dextrocardia with mental retardation and cleft palate.

17. There are 4 cardiac anomalies that are associated with hypertelorism (widely set eyes).

1. Pulmonary stenosis especially when associated with atrial septal defect.
2. Noonan's syndrome.
3. Hurler's disease or gargoylism with mitral regurgitation.
4. Supravalvular aortic stenosis.

18. There are 4 main circulatory changes at birth which have diagnostic importance.

1. The oxygen and nutritional requirements of the fetus are derived from the mother through the placenta. The lungs are sparingly perfused. Immediately after birth, the lungs expand and provide oxygenation of blood. The increased flow of blood to the pulmonary artery, passing through the lungs, reaches left atrium by pulmonary veins and increases the left atrial pressure. The effect of increased left atrial pressure causes septum primum to approximate with septum secundum resulting in functional closure of the foramen ovale.
2. Blood flows from the pulmonary artery to the aorta by ductus arteriosus in the fetus.
   Clamping of the umbilical cord immediately after birth increases the systemic vascular resistance. Thus the systemic pressure increases, while the pulmonary artery pressure falls due to lowering of the pulmonary vascular resistance. This results in reversal of flow of blood through the ductus arteriosus. The blood flows from the aorta to the pulmonary artery. The ductus arteriosus constricts and closes off. Thus, the pulmonary and systemic circulations are separated from each other immediately after birth.
3. At the time of birth, the pulmonary pressure and resistance are equal or only slightly lower than systemic pressure. Therefore, even when there is an abnormal communication like ASD,VSD or PDA, there is very little flow from left-to-right side. The pulmonary vascular resistance falls fairly rapidly to reach normal adult levels by 2 to 3 weeks in normal children. In the presence of VSD or PDA, however, the fall in pulmonary vascular resistance and pressure is slower and reaches adult levels around 6 to 10 weeks.
   Since there is very little flow across the abnormal communication like ASD, VSD or PDA, they do not manifest in the first few days of life. The VSD or PDA murmur tends to appear at the end of first week of life. It gradually increases in intensity as the pulmonary pressure and resistance falls and maximum shunt would become apparent only 6 to 10 weeks or more when the pulmonary resistance reaches its lowest value.
   In ASD, the right ventricular hypertrophy present at birth, prevents a large shunt. Thick right ventricle cannot expand well in diastole to accommodate large volume of blood. The right ventricle takes 6 months or more to regress. Thus the appearance of murmur in ASD takes even 6 months or longer, before the patients are usually identified.
4. Obstructive lesions like aortic stenosis or pulmonary stenosis and valvular leaks like mitral or tricuspid regurgitation are operative from birth. As such, the murmur of obstructive lesion as well as valvular leaks would be audible soon after birth.

19. Comparison of pressures and resistance in right and left sided chambers and vessels at birth to adults.

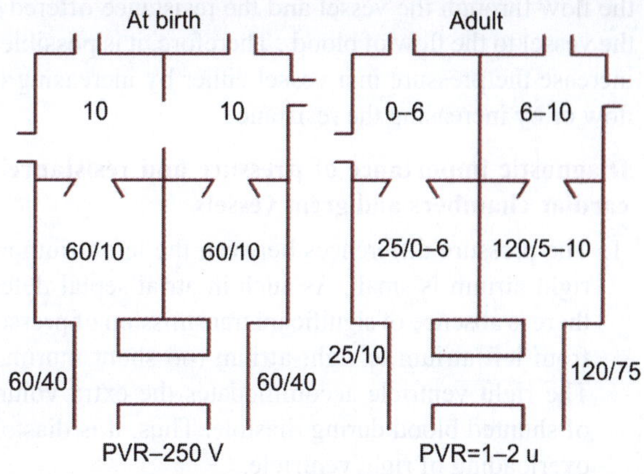

Fig. L-1: Pressure and resistance in the right and left-sided chambers and vessels at birth compared to adults

Table L-1: Pressure and resistance in the pulmonary and systemic circulation

Pressures in mm Hg			
1. SVC	0–6	P W P	6–10
2. RA	0–6	L A	6–10
3. RV	25/0–6	L V	80–120/5–10
4. PA	25/10 (mean 15)	Aorta	80–120/60–85
Resistance (dynes/sec/cm² or units)			
Pulmonary	80–240 or 1–3 units	Systemic	800–1600 or 10–20 units

SVC = Superior vena cava; RA = Right atrium; RV = Right ventricle; PA = Pulmonary artery;
PWP = Pulmonary wedge pressure; LA = Left atrium; LV = Left ventricle

The Fig. L-1 and Table L-1 show that the pressures in the right sided chambers and pulmonary artery are lower than the left side. Therefore, whenever there is a communication between the two sides the flow will be from left-to-right side. The pressure is measured in mm of mercury, flow in liters/min and resistance in dynes/sec/cm^5 or units (80 dynes sec/cm^5 = 1 unit).

According to Poiseuille's equation, modified for application to blood flow through vessels.

Pressure = Flow × Resistance

It serves a useful purpose in understanding the hemodynamics in pulmonary and systemic circulation though it is not strictly accurate.

When this equation is applied to systemic circulation—

Systemic pressure = Systemic flow × Peripheral vascular resistance.

Similarly for pulmonary circulation.

Pulmonary arterial pressure = Pulmonary flow × Pulmonary vascular resistance

It is obvious that the pressure in a vessel is dependent on the flow through the vessel and the resistance offered by the vessel to the flow of blood . Therefore, it is possible to increase the pressure in a vessel either by increasing the flow or by increasing the resistance.

20. Diagnostic importance of pressure and resistance in cardiac chambers and great vessels.

1. The pressure differences between the left atrium and right atrium is small. As such in atrial septal defect, there is absence of significant transmission of pressure from left atrium to right atrium (no shunt murmur). The right ventricle accommodates the extra volume of shunted blood during diastole. Thus, it is diastolic overloading of right ventricle.
2. In ventricular septal defect, the systolic pressures of left ventricle and the right ventricle is at a considerable difference whereas difference in diastolic pressure is not much. Therefore, the blood from the left ventricle to right ventricle occurs during systole (so, the shunt murmur is pansystolic). The flow depends on the size of the defect. The smaller the defect, the less the transmission of left ventricular pressure to the right ventricle. In larger defects, the pressures in the two ventricles may be identical. Then, the flow of blood from left-to-right will depend on the pulmonary vascular resistance.
   In ventricular septal defect, the shunt from left ventricle to right ventricle is during systole. When the shunted blood is reaching the right ventricle, the right ventricle is also actively contracting and becoming smaller. This results in the flow from the left ventricle directly going to pulmonary artery more or less directly. The right ventricle acts simply as a conduit and shunt is not a volume load for the right ventricle. The shunted blood passes through the lungs and finally gives rise to diastolic volume over load of left ventricle.
3. In patent ductus arteriosus, there is considerable difference in pressure between the aorta and pulmonary artery, both in systole and diastole. This results in blood flow from aorta to pulmonary artery in both phases of cardiac cycle (so, the shunt murmur is in systole and diastole, i.e. continuous murmur). The pressure transmission from aorta to pulmonary artery is determined by the size of the ductus. With a large PDA, the pressures in the aorta and pulmonary artery become identical. The flow into the pulmonary artery then depends on the pulmonary vascular resistance. If the pulmonary vascular resistance is low, there will be flow of blood from the aorta to the pulmonary artery. In PDA, the flow from the aorta to pulmonary artery is both systolic and diastolic. Thus, it results in a systolic as well as diastolic volume load of the pulmonary artery. For the left ventricle, the PDA results in a diastolic volume overload.
4. Pressure in a vessel is dependent on the flow through the vessel and resistance offered by the vessel.

Increase in flow through the pulmonary artery means a left-to-right shunt as seen in ASD, VSD or PDA. Generally, the increase in flow is not associated with significant increase in pressure as the resistant falls or remains the same. The distensible character of pulmonary artery is so much that it accommodates almost three times its normal flow without increase in pressure. Hence, large left-to-right shunts can be present without an increase in pulmonary artery pressure. Increase in pulmonary vascular resistance means obstructive disease in the pulmonary circulation. The pulmonary vessels develop medial hypertrophy in the beginning and later intimal changes are added to increase further obstruction. After a certain stage, it is an irreversible process. The increase in resistance to flow in the pulmonary circuit causes reduction in flow. The increase in pulmonary artery pressure is associated within normal resistance is called hyperkinetic pulmonary arterial hypertension. Whereas when the pressure is increased due to increase in pulmonary vascular resistance is called obstructive pulmonary arterial hypertension. Clinically, both situations can be identified separately from each other.

(Diagnostic importance of second heart sound—See Chapter A 158–167)

21. Various congenital heart diseases produce one or more of the following 4 consequences.

1. Arterial unsaturation, i.e. mixing of unsaturated blood with saturated blood.
2. Ventricular overload: Over work of either or both ventricles due to systolic or diastolic overloading.
3. Reduced systemic output.
4. Pulmonary arterial hypertension.

These can lead to retardation of growth and development.

22. Arterial unsaturation causes 4 common clinical manifestations (Caused by R to L shunt).

1. *Cyanosis:* It is the bluish or purplish discoloration imparted to the skin and mucous membranes. Cyanosis with a murmur near the base than the apex and its usual harsh character in general distinguishes congenital from acquired lesion.

   Unoxygenated blood is entering the systemic circulation through a right-to-left shunt or the blood passing through the lungs is not getting fully oxygenated. In the lungs, it is called pulmonary venous unsaturation and indicates severe lung disease. Presence of central cyanosis always indicates presence of heart disease if lung disease has been excluded.

   Cyanosis is clinically visible when the arterial oxygen saturation falls to 60–65% and primarily it depends on reduced hemoglobin of at least 5.0 g in the capillaries which is about 1/3rd of the average (13.5–14 g) hemoglobin content. Cyanosis is occasionally due to an abnormal hemoglobin such as sulfmethemoglobin or methemoglobin. Higher the absolute concentration of circulatory hemoglobin, the more easily will cyanosis be seen. For example, an 80% saturation with 10 g of hemoglobin would produce 2 g of reduced hemoglobin whereas the same percentage of saturation in a person with 15 g hemoglobin would produce 3 g of reduced hemoglobin.

   Cyanosis may be masked or reduced in the presence of significant anemia or polycythemia.

   Cyanosis is of 4 types.
   i. Central (with arterial unsaturation)
   ii. Peripheral (without arterial unsaturation)
   iii. Differential
   iv. Reversed differential cyanosis.

   Central cyanosis: A condition in which the arterial blood has a reduced saturation with oxygen. When it is severe and chronic, polycythemia and clubbing accompany. It is more generalized, severe and likely to occur with right-to-left shunts as also with pulmonary disease and is present on buccal mucosa and nails as well. The importance of knowing central cyanosis need not be elaborated. The following is an example.

   An acyanosed patient with biventricular enlargement, a small aorta and plemorphic lung fields usually indicates VSD. In a deeply cyanosed patient however, such a combination would suggest the transposition of great vessels.

   Peripheral cyanosis: It does not necessarily mean presence of heart disease. Peripheral cyanosis is the result of increased oxygen extraction from the blood by the tissues. Peripheral cyanosis in milder form occurs with low cardiac output states, which affects the nails, tip of the nose, and the ear lobes, etc. but the mucous membrane of the mouth and tongue do not show cyanosis. Extremities are cold and clammy and the pulses are weak. Arterial desaturation is usually absent. There is wide AV oxygen difference.

   Differential cyanosis: There is a difference in the degree of cyanosis between various parts of the body.
   a. The toe nails are more blue in pulmonary hypertension with right-to-left shunt and preductal coarctation with systemic right ventricle.
   b. Hand nails are relatively more blue as compared to toe nails in simple transposition of great arteries.
   c. In hypoplastic left heart syndrome with a small aortic opening and the VSD, right side of the head and neck are somewhat pinker as compared to the rest of the body.

   Reversed differential cyanosis: When the cyanosis and clubbing of fingers are greater than those of toes—suggests complete transposition of great vessels with either a preductal coarctation or complete interruption of the aortic arch. Slightly less cyanosis of the left arm compared to the right arm favors coarctation rather than complete aortic interruption (see A.39-4)
2. *Clubbing:* In severe cases clubbed fingers and toes are blue and have wide thick ends with convex finger nails, generally late in appearance after second year. Clubbing in children always indicate cyanotic CHD. However, cirrhosis liver, lung abscess, bacterial endocarditis may occasionally be responsible.

3. *Polycythemia:* Occurs as a compensatory mechanism to increase the oxygen carrying capacity. < 75% high level of hematocrit values have the disadvantages secondary to the high blood viscosity, which outweigh the advantage of increase in oxygen availability.
4. Dyspnea, hypoxic or cyanotic spells occur because of increased oxygen demand during work and exercise. Arterial unsaturation increases further during exercise adding to the patient's problem.

23. The following 4 conditions are examples of differential cyanosis:

1. Preductal coarctation with systemic right ventricle—toe nails are more blue.
2. Transposition of great arteries—hand nails are relatively more blue compared to toe nails.
3. Patent ductus arteriosus with reversal of shunt—toe nails are more blue.
4. Hypoplastic left heart syndrome with a small aortic opening and ventricular septal defect—right side of the head and neck are somewhat pink as compared body.

24. Peripheral cyanosis occurs in:

1. Cold temperature
2. Shock
2. Cardiac failure
3. Peripheral vascular disease.

25. Ventricular overload has the following 4 affects.

1. Systolic overload occurs when there is increased resistance to ventricular outflow. For example, pulmonary stenosis (PS) on the right side, aortic stenosis (AS) on the left side.
2. Diastolic overload results from increased blood volume during diastole.
   Left ventricular diastolic overload, e.g. PDA, AR.
   Right ventricular diastolic overload, e.g. ASD.
3. Concerned ventricle dilates and undergoes some hypertrophy to increase it's stroke output.
4. Signs and symptoms of left or right sided congestive heart failure appear much earlier in diastolic overload patients than those with systolic overload.

26. Reduced systemic output may be the result of following 4 situations:

1. Lesser degree of inadequate cardiac output is common with congenital heart disease, which results in physical under development with little or no effect on mental development.
2. The inadequate output commonly results from lesions that cause congestive heart failure.
3. Anomalies that do not allow adequate left ventricular output under adequate pressure.
   For example, complete interruption of the circulation at the aortic, mitral or at the level of aortic arch.
4. Anomalies that do not allow left ventricular output with adequate oxygen content to maintain life.
   For example, complete transposition of great arteries or pulmonary veins.

Death occurs within few weeks of life in these conditions.

27. Pulmonary arterial hypertension (PAH) in congenital heart diseases has the following 4 characters:

1. It is frequently seen in lesions with systemic and pulmonary circuit communications.
2. Transmission of blood flow from high pressure to low pressure is most likely cause.
   - From left atrium to right atrium—ASD
   - From left ventricle to right ventricle—VSD
   - From aorta to pulmonary artery—PDA.
3. Incidence varies with different lesions being least in atrial septal defect (ASD) and commonest in ventricular septal defect (VSD). It is not known why patients with similar size defects behave differently as far as development of pulmonary arterial hypertension is concerned.
4. Susceptibility: Individual susceptibility to pulmonary vascular bed may be an important factor in the incidence.
   Severe pulmonary arterial hypertension (PAH) is associated with large left-to-right shunts which is said to be hyperkinetic. On the other hand, left-to-right shunt may be small or absent but the pulmonary vascular resistance may be very high which is said to be obstructive pulmonary arterial hypertension or pulmonary vascular disease.
   From the practical point, the hyperkinetic pulmonary arterial hypertension can be surgically corrected with long-term excellent results. On the other hand, severe obstructive pulmonary vascular disease is currently incurable except by heart-lung transplantation.

28. When a family physician or pediatrician comes across a child with a heart murmur, one has to answer the following 4 questions for evaluation:

1. Does the child have heart disease?
2. Is it a congenital heart disease?
3. If it is congenital heart disease, what is the lesion?
4. What is the severity of the lesion?

First, one has to decide whether the murmur is due to heart disease or is it the so called 'functional' murmur. If it is heart disease, we have to separate congenital from acquired heart disease.

Then specific diagnosis is based on classical features of the individual lesion. X-ray, ECG and echocardiogram help in the diagnosis. Once the specific diagnosis is made, the decision to be made as to what is to be done for the patient depends on the severity of the lesion. One should always remember, that palliative or curative treatment is entirely surgical. Diagnosis should be accurate. Wrong diagnosis results in loss of patient during surgery. The surgical decision depends on the type and severity of the condition.

29. Assessment of a child for the presence of heart disease.

The child is assessed for the presence or absence of heart disease with the guidelines suggested by Nadas' criteria. The criteria are divided into major and minor criteria. Presence of one major or two minor criteria are essential for indicating the presence of heart disease.

There are 4 major criteria:

1. Systolic murmur of grade III or more in intensity
2. Diastolic murmur
3. Cyanosis
4. Congestive cardiac failure.

The systolic murmurs are classified into ejection systolic murmurs and pansystolic murmurs. A pansystolic murmur is always abnormal, no matter what its intensity is. There are only 4 lesions, which produce pansystolic murmur and these are ventricular septal defect, mitral regurgitation and tricuspid regurgitation and aortic stenosis (See Chapter I point I-97).

An ejection systolic murmur can be due to an organic cause or functional murmur. An ejection systolic murmur associated with a thrill is always an organic murmur. Grade III ejection systolic murmur of a functional type may be heard in anemia or high fever specially in smaller children. Almost 50% of children around the age of 5 years may have a soft ejection systolic murmur.

When a murmur is accompanied by a normal second sound, then it is unlikely to be significant.

X-ray, ECG and Echo help and if they are normal one can probably exclude heart disease.

Presence of diastolic murmur always indicates an organic heart disease. The only two exceptions are severe hypertension and severe anemia. In severe systemic hypertension, reduction of blood pressure may cause an aortic regurgitation murmur to disappear. Anemia may result in delayed diastolic murmur across the mitral and tricuspid valves.

Cyanosis (See point 22).

Congestive Cardiac Failure (See point 220-243).

Minor criteria includes:

a. Systolic murmur less than Grade III in intensity
b. Abnormal second sound
c. Abnormal chest roentgenogram
d. ECG
e. Abnormal blood pressure.

Abnormal second sound always indicates the presence of heart disease. It is included in minor criteria only because the auscultation is an individual and subjective finding and no one is perfect in auscultation and anyone can be wrong. If the auscultatory finding is supported by the phonocardiogram it becomes an objective evidence and indicates the presence of heart disease.

The reason to include anormal X-ray in minor criteria is twofold. In infants and smaller children, the heart size varies considerably in expiration and inspiration. If there is a cardiomegaly in a good inspiratory film, it is highly suggestive for the presence of heart disease. It is difficult to assess the heart size in the presence of thymus in children below the age of two years. A relatively large thymic shadow may suggest cardiomegaly. Fluoroscopy is helpful in differentiating the thymus shadow from the heart.

Abnormal ECG

Abnormal blood pressure: It is difficult to obtain blood pressure in smaller children. If the cuff is small, it would falsely give high reading whereas if it is too large, it gives low readings. The blood pressure cuff should cover at least two-thirds of the length of the arm and most of the circumference.

On the basis of the presence of one major or two minor criteria a decision is taken whether the child has heart disease. The advent of two-dimensional echocardiogram with color Doppler has replaced the other criteria.

Most of the congenital heart diseases can be diagnosed accurately by the two dimensional echocardiogram with Doppler. The importance of other investigations are becoming less.

30. The main value of ECG in pediatric use is in finding the mean QRS axis, right or left atrial hypertrophy, right or left ventricular hypertrophy. Based on voltage criteria of ventricular hypertrophy are not diagnostic as the voltage can be affected by other changes such as:

1. Blood viscosity
2. Electrolyte imbalance
3. Position of the electrode on the chest wall
4. Thickness of the chest wall.

If the patient is asymptomatic, physical examination and X-ray are normal but the ECG is abnormal the presence of heart disease is unlikely.

SPECIFIC CARDIAC DEFECTS

MALPOSITION OF CARDIA

31. There are 4 types of cardiac malpositions.

1. Dextrocardia with situs inversus (abdominal viscera)
   - Mirror image dextrocardia—situs inversus totalis
   - Dextrocardia—apex on right side
   - Situs inversus—stomach on right side.

   There is a tendency for these patients to develop non-cardiac lesions like Kartagener's triad—dextrocardia, sinusitis and bronchiectasis (Dextroversion).

2. Dextrocardia with situs solitus
   - Dextrocardia—apex on right side
   - Situs solitus—stomach on left side
   - Aortic knob also on left side.
3. Levocardia with situs inversus (Levoversion)
   - Levocardia—apex on left side
   - Situs inversus—stomach on right side.

   This is associated with incidence of cyanotic congenital heart diseases.
4. Cardiac malpositions with indeterminate situs: Heart may be either left sided or right sided. The situs is ambiguous showing aorticogastric bubble indifference, i.e. aortic knob and the stomach are not on the same side and therefore situs is unpredictable. Left atrium tends to be on the left side of the aorta. In these conditions, interruption of inferior vena cava with azygos continuation is almost present.
   - Levocardia with situs solitus—normal
   - Levocardia—apex on left side
   - Situs solitus—stomach on left side.

   Dextrocardia is associated with least number of other abnormalities of the heart than dextroversion and levoversion.

32. Some observations are made on the severity of the cardiac defects in association with malposition of the heart.

1. Mirror image dextrocardia occurs more frequently in an otherwise normal person.
2. Dextrocardia without situs inversus shows cardiac malformations as a rule.
3. In normal position of the heart with situs inversus, the heart is always seriously malformed.
4. In cardiac malposition with indeterminate visceral situs, there is a striking association of complex multiple cardiac anomalies which usually include systemic and pulmonary venous abnormalities, ASD,VSD and endocardial cushion defects along with asplenia or polysplenia.

Transposition of great arteries occur frequently in cardiac malposition and double outlet right ventricle is common in asplenia.

(For ECG findings in dextrocardia – See Chapter Q point 205)

33. The Kartagener syndrome is associated with the following 4 features:

1. Dextrocardia (Situs inversus)
2. Bronchiectasis
3. Sinusitis
4. Sterility.

Coarctation of Aorta

Coarctation of the aorta is a condition in which the aorta is narrowed just distal to the origin of left subclavian artery, the site corresponding to the insertion of ligamentum arteriosm, (or ductus arteriosus). This condition is due to the defect in development of the tunica media of the aorta.

34. The incidence of coarctation of aorta has the following 4 features:

1. The incidence is approximately 8% of congenital heart diseases next in frequency to VSD and PDA.
2. Greater preponderance of its incidence in males. Twice as common in males as in females.
3. Frequent in patients with Turner's syndrome
4. Common association with other anomalies like bicuspid aortic valve, PDA, VSD, ASD, AS, MR, berry aneurysms of 'circle of Willis'. 40–80% may have a bicuspid aortic valve.

35. Clinical manifestations.

Clinical features depend on the site and extent of obstruction and presence of associated cardiac anomalies which occur frequently. Majority of children and young adults with postductal coarctation are asymptomatic.

1. *History:* Headache, epistaxis, cardiac symptoms may be present from hypertension in the upper part of the body. Weakness or cramps in the legs, cold extremities, claudication with exercise may result from decreased circulation in the lower limbs.

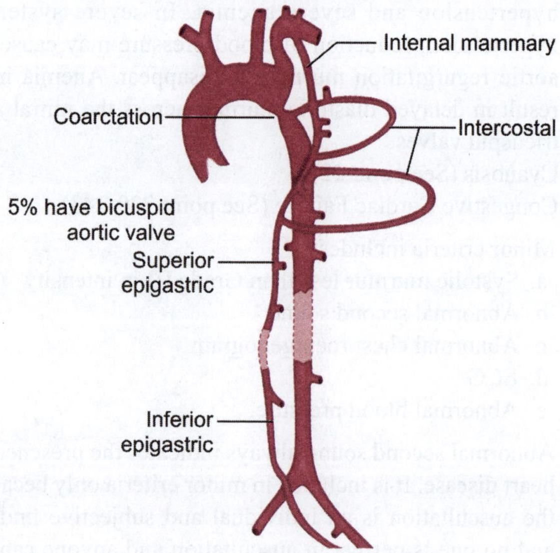

Fig. L-2: Coarctation of aorta

2. *Inspection:* Some individuals may show overgrowth of upper extremities and chest in isolated postductal coarctation. This is characteristically associated with diminished or delayed or even absent femoral pulse.
   Differential cyanosis may be seen. It occurs from preferential shunting of unsaturated pulmonary arterial blood through a patent ductus to the lower parts of the body in preductal coarctation. The toe nails are more blue in preductal coarctation.
   Presence of dilated and tortuous collaterals may be present in the arms around and in between the scapula when the patient bends forward with the arms hanging.
3. *Palpation:* Pulse and BP are markedly diminished or delayed in femoral pulse and a low or unobtainable blood pressure in the lower limbs with hypertension in the upper limbs are the basic clues to the diagnosis. As a rule if the femorals are well felt in an infant, the diagnosis can be excluded. Rarely there can be difference in systolic pressure between two arms when the subclavian artery is at or below the obstruction.
   In the very young infants, it is important to feel both the brachial and carotids. Weak or absent pulse in all sites is characteristic of aortic stenosis or aortic atresia.
   Enlarged and tortuous pulsatile collaterals (Sussman's sign) may be palpated in intercostal spaces, interiorly in the axilla or interscapular area posteriorly. Systolic thrill may be palpable in the suprasternal notch and carotid vessels.
   Heaving apex is felt.
4. *Auscultation:*
   First sound is accentuated followed by a constant ejection click. Second sound is normal splitting with loud A_2
   - S_3 with left ventricular failure
   - S_4 with severe hypertension
   - Moderately loud systolic murmur at the base of the heart
   - Soft systolic bruit may be heard in the interscapular area due to collateral circulation
   - Murmurs over the heart from coexistent conditions like VSD, PDA, AS may be heard.
   - Continuous murmur may be audible over the collaterals but are uncommon.

36. When coarctation occurs proximal to the ductus arteriosus, i.e. preductal coarctation—the following clinical features are present in early life.

1. Differential cyanosis due to shunting of unsaturated pulmonary arterial blood through patent ductus arteriosus to the lower parts of the body.
2. Right ventricular hypertrophy (develops in utero).
3. Pulmonary hypertension.
4. Congestive heart failure.

37. Roentgenogram—may be normal in early childhood. It may show:

1. Dilated left subclavian artery, high on the left mediastinal border.
2. Dilated ascending aorta. Pre- and post-stenotic dilatation above and below it giving a configuration of '3' sign.
3. Barium swallow shows characteristic 'E' sign.
4. Notching of ribs due to erosion of dilated and tortuous collaterals which increases with age. Usually seen between 6–12 years of age.

38. ECG, echocardiogram, cardiac catheterization and digital subtraction aortogram (DSA) are indicated to:

1. Reveal left ventricular hypertrophy of varying degree.
2. Identify associated malformations.
3. Determine the length and size of coarctation.
4. Localise the accurate site of obstruction.

39. Echocardiography: most useful in infants and children. Suprasternal notch view is most useful in adults help to determine.

1. LV size, ascending aorta size.
2. Aortic valve anatomy and function (bicuspid aortic valve is a common association).
3. Color Doppler to localize the site of turbulence.
4. Continuous wave Doppler to assess the pressure gradient. Persistence of flow in diastole (widening of the flow profile from systole into diastole) is seen in severe narrowing.

40. Magnetic resonance imaging (MRI): It is used as a first line of investigation before cardiac catheterization.

1. It clearly demonstrates the precise anatomy.
2. Helps in decision making regarding surgery.
3. Serial MRIs may be used to follow results of therapeutic procedures.
4. It is also useful to identify the intracranial vessels for associated berry-aneurysm.

41. In untreated cases of coarctation of the aorta death occurs due to any of the following 4 causes:

1. Left ventricular failure.
2. Rupture of the aorta in dissection of the aorta.
3. Cerebral hemorrhage from severe hypertension.
4. Infective endocarditis—infection of the bicuspid aortic valve which is present in about 50% of the patients.

42. The treatment of uncomplicated coarctation of aorta is mainly surgical. It should be surgically corrected in all symptomatic and in asymptomatic children around the age of 4 years. The risk is more beyond the age of 15 years because the tissues become more friable.

There are 4 methods of correction.

1. Resection and direct end-to-end anastomosis.
2. Prosthetic tubular Dacron graft may be necessary if the resected segment is long.
3. Subclavian flap aortoplasty or Dacron patch aortoplasty.
4. Recent introduction of percutaneous balloon dilatation (angioplasty) of the coarctation of the Aorta is encouraging. It helps in relief of recoarctation after surgery with successful results. It could be done in very small infants also.

Surgery by resection of coarctation does not guarantee freedom from complications like dissection of aorta. Systemic hypertension can persists following operation and recoarctation can also occur. This has been explained that coarctation of aorta is not a localized disease alone at the junction of arch and descending aorta alone but it is a generalized weakness of the arterial media. There can be failure of expansion of the surgically anastomosed site.

43. There are 4 postoperative complications which are not uncommon in coarctation of the aorta.

1. Sudden hypertension during postoperative period. Abdominal pain, abdominal distension are associated with mesenteric arteritis.
2. Residual hypertension especially in patients who have undergone repair at an older age.
3. Restenosis.
4. Aneurysmal dilatation after balloon angioplasty.

Congenital Aortic Stenosis

(See Chapter I Valvular Heart Diseases 129–170)

Aortic stenosis is defined as subtotal obstruction of varying degrees to the left ventricular outflow.

44. The 4 abnormalities that cause obstruction in order of decreasing frequency are

1. Congenital valvular stenosis (Obstruction at valve level—commonest).
2. Congenital subvalvular stenosis (Obstruction below the valve).
   It is caused by a thin fibrous membranous diaphragm immediately below the aortic valve or from a thick fibrous ring encircling the left ventricular outflow tract.
3. Congenital supravalvular stenosis (Obstruction above the valve).
   It is a localized or diffuse narrowing of the ascending aorta above the level of the coronary arteries.
   Rarely the valvular and subvalvular stenosis may co-exist producing tunnel-like tract narrowing the left ventricular outflow tract.
4. Congenital aortic stenosis associated with other congenital anomalies such as patent ductus arteriosus, coarctation of aorta. Coarctation of the aorta is the most common associated anomaly. Hemodynamics of congenital aortic stenosis are same as acquired aortic stenosis except that a persistent patent ductus arteriosus or stretched foramen ovale in the immediate postnatal period decreases left atrial pressure and lessen the severity of pulmonary edema.

Note: Congenital bicuspid aortic valve, which may not be stenotic is the most common congenital anomaly.

45. Subvalvular aortic stenosis can be described in 4 varieties:

1. Discrete membranous subvalvular stenosis: The membrane is with a central or eccentric hole at left ventricular outflow tract.
2. Fibromuscular subvalvular stenosis: Fibromuscular tissue extends from septal wall of the left ventricle to the anterior leaflet (aortic) of the mitral valve.
3. Idiopathic hypertrophic subaortic stenosis (IHSS) also called as asymmetrical septal hypertrophy (ASH) or hypertrophic obstructive cardiomyopathy (HOCM), asymmetrical septal hypertrophy with ventricular outflow obstruction.
4. Asymmetrical septal hypertrophy without ventricular outflow obstruction.

46. There are 4 characters of supravalvular aortic stenosis.

1. It is rare. It is associated with characteristic 'elfin' facies, mental retardation, dental abnormalities, strabismus; and peripheral arterial stenosis.
2. It is closely related to idiopathic hypercalcemia or may be due to hypervitaminosis D.
3. Since the obstruction is above the aortic valve, the pressure in the segment of the aorta below the obstruction is also elevated resulting in loud A2.
4. The jet through the supravalvular narrowing may be directed toward the innominate artery resulting in a slightly higher systolic pressure in the right arm compared to the left arm.

47. Valvular aortic stenosis occurs in about 4% of patients with congenital heart disease.

48. Aortic stenosis is 4 times more common in males than in females.

49. The rigid aortic stenotic valve causes obstruction to the left ventricular outflow. The severity of the aortic stenosis is judged:

1. Mainly by the peak systolic pressure gradient across the aortic valve and size of the aortic orifice.

In the presence of normal cardiac output:
- A pressure gradient of 75 mm Hg or more and aortic orifice less than 0.5 cm^2 per square meter of body surface is considered severe.
- A gradient between 50 and 75 mm Hg and aortic orifice 0.5 and 0.8 cm^2 is considered moderate.
A gradient of less than 50 mm Hg or orifice greater than 0.9 cm^2 per square meter of body surface is considered mild.

2. By thickening and calcification of the valve with age.
3. By poststenotic dilatation of ascending aorta.
4. By concentric hypertrophy of left ventricle.

50. Symptomatology: May be asymptomatic in most children with normal growth and development. Sudden death is common with severe obstruction. The 4 symptoms of severe obstruction are:

1. Easy fatigue with feeding infants.
2. Breathlessness—and 2 are suggestive of left ventricular failure.
3. Chest pain—suggestive of inadequate coronary blood flow.
4. Exertional syncope—suggestive of inadequate cerebral blood flow during exercise.

PHYSICAL EXAMINATION

51. The 4 important palpatory findings are:

1. Pulse is of low volume (Pulsus parvus). Slow rising carotid pulse distinguishes stenosis from aortic sclerosis.
2. Narrowed pulse pressure: Less than 20 mm Hg suggests severe stenosis.
3. Apex is heaving and sustained though heart is not usually detectably enlarged for palpation or percussion.
4. Systolic thrill along the right upper sternal border, aortic area conducted along the carotids.

52. The 4 important auscultatory findings are:

1. Second sound may be closely split due to delay in closure of the stenotic valve 'paradoxical splitting'. Aortic valve closure sound is delayed to occur after the pulmonic valve closure.
Third heart sound may be heard. A fourth heart sound heard in patients between 12 and 40 years of age is usually suggestive of severe obstruction.
2. A systolic ejection click immediately preceding the murmur can be heard only if the valve is pliable.
3. A systolic murmur may be detected within the first 24 to 48 hours after birth which leads to the discovery of this anomaly. The murmur may be detected in the first year of life in less than half of the patients.
Increased stenosis gives rise to a harsh systolic spindle-shaped murmur loudest over the aortic area with radiation into the carotids and down the left sternal border.
4. An early diastolic blowing murmur may be heard in associated aortic regurgitation. This is common with congenital bicuspid valve or with infective endocarditis.

53. X-ray chest: It may be normal in the early stage. In severe obstruction, it shows:

1. Left ventricle may be enlarged. Cardiac enlargement indicates severity of the disease in most of the cases.
2. Poststenotic dilatation is characteristic.
3. Calcification can be seen with increasing age.
4. Children with left ventricular failure may show left atrial enlargement and pulmonary edema.

54. Electrocardiogram: It may be normal in early stage. In severe obstruction, it may show:

1. Small anterior QRS forces, abnormally large posterior forces as SV1 of 30 mm or more. LVH with strain pattern in severe obstruction.
2. Absent Q waves in leads V_5 and V_6.
3. Abnormal T waves. A superior T wave vector in the frontal plane suggests severe obstruction.
4. Abnormal ST segment. Watch the ST segment during exercise in lead V_5 through V_7 to detect the development of significant pressure gradient, which is a threat leading to sudden death.

55. Echocardiography: The 4 distinctive findings of echocardiography are:

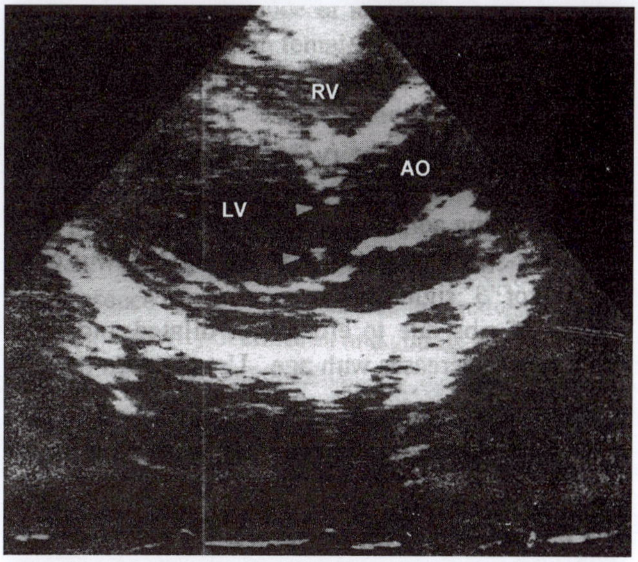

Fig. L-3: Two-dimensional echocardiogram: Parasternal long axis view of a patient with a membranous discrete subaortic stenosis. The arrow heads indicate the echoes from the sub-valvular membrane between the left ventricle (LV) and aorta (AO). RV = Right ventricle

1. Congenital bicuspid valve can be seen. It can distinguish valvular from supravalvular and subvalvular obstruction.
2. Abnormal eccentric closure of the aortic cusps, vegetation and calcification of leaflets can be seen.
3. It can estimate the thickness of posterior wall of left ventricle and septum and can predict the systolic pressure gradient across the left ventricular outflow obstruction. It can estimate the size of left ventricle, mitral valve annulus and aortic root.
4. Poststenotic dilatation of aorta can be seen.

56. The following 4 observations are made in cardiac catheterization and left ventriculography:

1. Systolic pressure gradient between the left ventricle and central aorta can be documented. The gradient may be relatively less if the left ventricular output is markedly diminished even in the presence of severe obstruction. Left ventricular end-diastolic pressure is usually markedly increased.
2. In infants with severe obstruction but who are asymptomatic, there often exists a left-to-right shunt through a stretched foramen ovale. Pulmonary arterial hypertension and right ventricular hypertrophy are the rule. There may be also a right-to-left shunt through a patent ductus arteriosus, which temporarily reduces the congestion of the pulmonary venous bed and provides systemic arterial perfusion.
3. Left ventricular angiography will confirm the site of obstruction and size of the ventricular cavity.
4. Thickened aortic leaflets with a central or eccentric jet of contrast material entering the ascending aorta can be noted. Poststenotic dilatation is characteristic.

57. Medical treatment consists of the following 4 steps.

1. Avoiding strenuous work, isometric exercise. Careful follow-up of infant or child is necessary.
2. Management of cardiac failure.
3. Management of angina.
4. Prophylaxis against bacterial endocarditis.

58. Surgery is recommended.

1. If the child is symptomatic, shows enlargement of the heart or heart failure even if the pressure gradient is 40 mm or less.
2. If the peak systolic pressure gradient is 75 mm Hg or more.
3. If the calculated aortic valve area is 0.5 cm^2/m^2 or less.
4. If the ECG shows clear ST changes at rest or exercise.

59. Percutaneous balloon dilatation of aortic stenosis is tried in some centers. It is a nonsurgical palliative procedure. No patient is excluded for balloon aortic valvuloplasty on the basis of:

1. Age
2. Clinical condition
3. Valve morphology
4. Valve calcification.

60. Surgery is done under cardiopulmonary bypass, hypothermia and cardioplegia.

It consists of:

1. Relief of valvular stenosis by careful incision in the middle of each fused but well supported commissure. Mild aortic regurgitation is common after surgery. Conservative attitude is necessary during surgery. Moderate residual stenosis is preferred to aortic incompetence.
2. Secondary valvotomy for recurrent or residual stenosis.
3. Aortic valve replacement in cases of calcification and restenosis of the valve. Preference is given to salvage the child's own valve as long as possible because an ideal valve substitute for pediatric surgical use does not exist.
4. Repair of associated anomalies.

Pulmonary Stenosis

61. The parts of pulmonary artery in order from below upwards are:

1. Infundibular portion
2. Valve portion
3. Supravalvular portion
4. Peripheral pulmonary portion.

62. Pulmonary stenosis can be classified into 4 types depending on the site.

1. *Valvular stenosis:* It is the most common among these defects and accounts for about 10% of the congenital heart diseases.

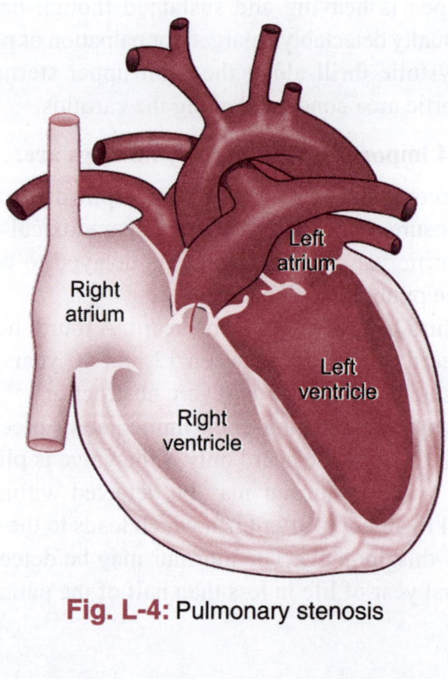

Fig. L-4: Pulmonary stenosis

a. With intact ventricular septum: It is the most common form of isolated right ventricular outflow obstruction.
b. The valve cusps are fused to form a cone or dome-shaped structure with reduction of the diameter, a few millimeters in severe cases.
2. *Infundibular stenosis:* It is at subvalvular level and is commonly seen with other associated cardiac anomalies.
3. *Supravalvular stenosis:* Rare. There may be a history of maternal rubella.
4. *Peripheral pulmonary stenosis:* The narrowing can be at multiple sites, may be associated with supravalvular stenosis. There is often a history maternal rubella. Valvular and infundibular stenosis are important, the others being rare.

63. 1/4th of the patients with pulmonary stenosis may have atrial shunt.

64. Supravalvular stenosis is rare and it may be associated with:

1. Nerve deafness
2. Cataract
3. Microcephaly
4. Other congenital cardiac anomalies.

65. Pulmonary stenosis may occur as an isolated lesion—but it is also a common accompaniment of other congenital heart diseases. It is associated with the following varieties of congenital heart diseases.

1. Stenosis of pulmonary valve or infundibular stenosis with a normal aortic root.
2. Pulmonary atresia.
3. Tricuspid atresia.
4. Fallot's tetralogy.
5. Pulmonary stenosis in double outflow tract right ventricle—in which the stenosed pulmonary artery and aorta arise from the right ventricle, where there is VSD.
6. Transposition of the great vessels with pulmonary stenosis.
7. Common ventricle with pulmonary stenosis.
8. Anomalous muscle bundle of the right ventricle.
As the right ventricle hypertrophies to overcome the obstruction at valve level, the infundibular walls are so thickened that with each ventricular systole they approximate to each other to cause obstruction.

66. Hemodynamics of pulmonary stenosis.

1. Flow across the narrow pulmonary valve results in pulmonary ejection stystolic murmur.
2. To keep the flow normal right ventricle increases its systolic pressure and develops concentric right ventricular hypertrophy.
The degree of obstruction is assessed by mean systolic pressure gradient and the amount of blood flow across the valve. The stenosis is said to be mild when the pressure gradient is below 50, moderate between 50 to 80, severe above 80 mm Hg. The systolic pressure in the right ventricle may exceed left ventricular systolic pressure since the septum is intact.
3. The right ventricular systole is prolonged because of the obstruction resulting in delayed closure of the pulmonic component (P_2) of the second sound.
4. The delay in P_2 results in a widely split second sound. The split is variable becoming wider in inspiration. The width of the split is directly proportional to the severity of obstruction. Thus, the more severe the pulmonary stenosis, the longer the systolic murmur and wider the splitting of second sound.
5. In valvar pulmonic stenosis a pulmonary ejection click is audible during expiration but tends to disappear during inspiration. It precedes the start of the murmur. The more severe the pulmonary stenosis the closer the click to the first sound.
In severe pulmonic stenosis the click almost merges with the first sound which then appears to be louder in expiration compared to inspiration.
6. In severe cases with marked right ventricular hypertrophy, the right ventricular diastolic pressure also increases and failure develops.
7. Right atrial pressure also increases as a result of right ventricular failure to be able to fill the right ventricle and results in a right atrial fourth sound (S_4) as well as prominent 'A' wave in the jugular venous pulse.
8. There can be right-to-left shunt across the patent foramen ovale leading to arterial unsaturation and central cyanosis.
Atresia of the pulmonary valve is usually associated with hypoplastic right ventricle and interatrial communication. Infants with pulmonary artery stenosis often die from hypoxia.

67. Symptoms: Most of the infants are asymptomatic; but symptoms are common with severe obstruction.

The 4 most common symptoms are:

1. Dyspnea on exertion
2. Fatigue
3. Palpitation
4. Chest pain.

They may present with symptoms of heart failure in severe obstruction. Cyanosis is rare unless there is patent foramen ovale or atrial septal defect. Syncope is rare. Growth and development are normal. May present with round facies.

68. Patients with dysplastic valve usually will have non-cardiac abnormalities such as:

1. Short stature
2. Hypertelorism
3. Ptosis
4. Mental retardation.

69. Patients of pulmonary stenosis may have characteristically associated with the following signs:

1. Round face
2. Hyperteleorism
3. Portwine angiomatous malformation over the skin
4. Turner phenotype without chromosomal abnormalities (Noonan's syndrome).

70. The 4 important signs of pulmonary stenosis are:

1. Jugular venous pulse shows a prominent 'A' wave.
2. Hepatomegaly and even pulsatile liver.
   A prominent 'A' wave in the jugular venous pulse, presystolic pulsations in the liver and a fourth heart sound are indicative of severe atrial contraction.
3. Prominent sustained right ventricular parasternal lift, increasingly forceful with severe obstruction.
   Systolic thrill in the suprasternal notch and left upper sternal border.
4. First sound is normal.
   Second sound is wide and fixed split with a late soft pulmonary component due to prolonged left ventricular ejection.

With mild pulmonary stenosis, the split is normal and the intensity of second sound is also normal.

With moderate pulmonary stenosis the split is wide and variable.

With severe pulmonary stenosis the split further widens. In critical pulmonary stenosis, the P_2 is also diminished in intensity and may be so widely split in expiration that further widening during inspiration may not be appreciated on auscultation suggesting fixed split second sound.

A pulmonary ejection click varying with respiration follows the first sound.

Fourth sound is heard if the obstruction is severe.

A harsh systolic murmur, crescendo-decrescendo in shape best heard in the left upper sternal space with radiation toward the left clavicle is characteristic. The duration and intensity of the murmur correlates with the severity of obstruction. In severe pulmonary stenosis, the peak intensity of the murmur as well as the duration of the systolic murmur gets delayed. With moderately severe pulmonary stances the peak intensity of the murmur as well as the duration of the systolic murmur get delayed.

In patients with congestive heart failure, a systolic murmur due to tricuspid regurgitation may be heard at the lower sternal border.

A harsh systolic murmur often with a thrill in the second left intercostal space with faint or absent pulmonary second sound indicates pulmonary stenosis.

71. Chest roentgenogram.

1. Heart size may be normal or slightly increased. Significant enlargement in severe obstruction is an ominous sign.
2. Main pulmonary artery and proximal left pulmonary artery are prominent as a result of poststenotic dilatation. It is not a feature of supra or subvalvular stenosis.
3. Pulmonary oligemia.
4. Calcification of the valve may be seen in adult patients.

72. Electrocardiogram.

1. Right ventricular hypertrophy. The degree of right ventricular hypertrophy is a useful index of severity of pulmonary stenosis.
2. Right ventricular strain pattern. The systolic overloading pattern in the ECG is suggested by a pure 'R' or 'qR' type of complex in V4R and V1 leads. This is not very specific and the rSR complex type can be present.
3. Right axis deviation.
4. Tall 'P' wave of right atrial hypertrophy.

73. Echocardiogram.

1. Exaggeration of the maximal 'A' wave depth of the pulmonary valve is demonstrated with inspiration.
2. Right ventricular hypertrophy.
3. Doppler studies show the severity of obstruction.
4. Demonstrates associated anomalies.

74. Cardiac catheterization and angiocardiography show the following 4 observations:

1. It demonstrates systolic pressure gradient between the right ventricle and pulmonary artery, raised right ventricular pressure and a normal or decreased pulmonary artery pressure. A gradient exceeding 50 mm Hg suggests significant severe stenosis.
2. Right ventricular end-diastolic pressure and right atrial 'A' wave may be elevated. Systemic oxygen unsaturation is present in severe obstruction and patent foramen ovale or atrial septal defect.
3. Right ventricular angiography demonstrates dome shaped valve leaflet with a jet of contrast material entering the distal dilated pulmonary artery.
   Doming is not a feature of dysplastic valve.
4. Infundibular subvalvular narrowing secondary to muscular hypertrophy may be seen.

75. Assessment of severity of pulmonary stenosis.

1. Symptomatic patients (patients with mild to moderate pulmonary stenosis are asymptomatic).
2. Cardiac enlargement.

3. Cyanosis.
4. Closer the pulmonic ejection click to the first sound.
5. Wider the splitting of the second sound.
6. Longer the systolic murmur.
7. Taller the 'R' wave in V1 in ECG.
8. Pulmonary oligemia.

Murmur ending before, at or beyond the aortic component of the second sound indicate moderately severe, severe and critical pulmonary stenosis respectively.

A pure 'R' in V1 of 20 mm suggests systemic pressure in the right ventricle. If the appearance of the 'S' wave in precordial leads is shifted to the left it suggests severe pulmonic stenosis.

76. Management: It depends on the severity of obstruction.

Medical management

1. Unlike valvar aortic stenosis, the valvar pulmonic stenosis generally does not increase in severity with time. Therefore, the patient of mild pulmonary stenosis should be left as such.
2. Treatment of heart failure.
3. Treatment of arrhythmias.
4. Prevention of infective endocarditis.

77. The indications for surgery is assessed during cardiac catheterization in the following way:

1. If the right ventricular pressure is 75 mm Hg or more send for surgery.
2. If the right ventricular pressure is below 50 mm Hg patient should be followed without operation.
3. If the right ventricular pressure is between 50 and 75 mm Hg should be exercised.
4. If the exercise right ventricular pressure reaches the systemic pressure level, sent up for surgery.

The surgery is done under cardiopulmonary by pass with a low-risk of around 1% in valvar pulmonary stenosis. The risk is higher for infundibular pulmonary stenosis since right ventriculotomy has to be done.

78. Prior to mid-1980s, the only treatment for PS was an open surgical procedure. In the early 1980s, the first case reports of nonsurgical treatment of valvar PS were reported. Nonsurgical opening of the pulmonic valve by balloon pulmonary valvuloplasty, or BPV is now the procedure of choice for relief of nearly all cases of valvar PS. The 4 steps in BPV are:

1. Cardiac catheterization procedure is done as usual.
2. The balloon valvuloplasty catheter is threaded over the guidewire and the balloon is positioned such that its center is in the annulus.
3. The dilatation is performed by inflating the balloon with dilute contrast under fluoroscopy and observing

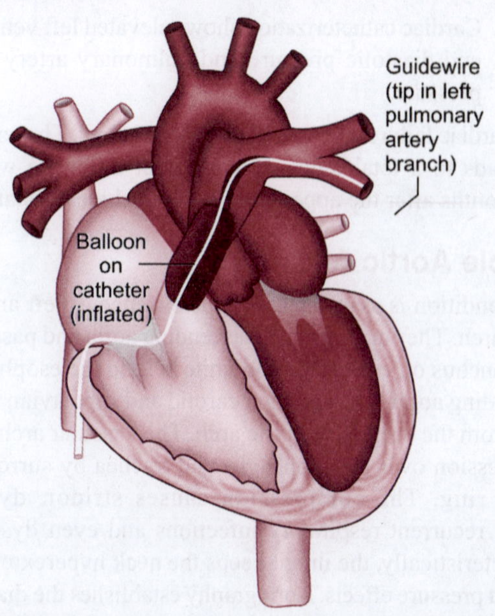

Fig. L-5: Balloon dilatation of pulmonary stenosis

that the balloon remains centered and for inflation of the balloon to its full diameter.
4. Usually, this is repeated two or three times to ensure that maximal effect has been achieved.

ENDOCARDIAL FIBROELASTOSIS

A rare anomaly, noted in infancy, is characterized by proliferation of elastic and collagenous fibers within the endocardium. Endocardium becomes thick and exhibits a smooth, glistening, milky white appearance.

It affects the left ventricle extensively, occasionally left atrium, less commonly right side.

It causes restrictive type of cardiomyopathy with left ventricular hypertrophy and left ventricular dilatation. The condition may be primary or secondary. Secondary forms are noted in association with congenital anomalies like coarctation of Aorta, aortic stenosis, aortic atresia, ventricular septal defect, patent ductus arteriosus, mitral atresia, pulmonary stenosis and glycogen storage disease of the heart. In some cases, there is previous history of viral infection (Coxsackie B or mumps).

The condition presents with congestive cardiac failure in infancy. A systolic murmur of mitral incompetence may present.

79. Investigations.

1. Chest roentgenogram shows marked cardiomegaly and there may be left lower lobe collapse due to pressure on the left lower lobe bronchus.
2. ECG shows left ventricular hypertrophy.
3. Echocardiogram shows left ventricular dilatation with decreased wall motion.

4. Cardiac catheterization shows elevated left ventricular end-diastolic pressure and pulmonary artery wedge pressure.

Cardiac failure responds poorly to treatment. The condition leads to a fatal outcome and infant often die within 6 months after the appearance of clinical manifestation.

Double Aortic Arch

This condition is associated with persistence of left and right aortic arch. They arise from the ascending aorta and pass above the bronchus on either side and unite behind the esophagus to descending aorta. The common carotid and subclavian arteries arise from the respective aortic arch. The vascular arch causes compression over the esophagus and trachea by surrounding like a ring. The compression causes stridor, dyspnea, cough, recurrent respiratory infections and even dysphagia. Characteristically, the infant keeps the neck hyperextended to prevent pressure effects. Aortography establishes the diagnosis.

Surgical correction is made by the division and ligation of the smaller aortic arch. Fortunately, the condition may remain asymptomatic in many cases and the patient leads a normal life.

Right Sided Aortic Arch

The disappearance of the left fourth aortic arch instead of the right during 5th and 6th weeks of embryonic life resulting in occurrence of right aortic arch. The left subclavian artery has an aberrant origin. Majority of patients remain asymptomatic.

Bicuspid Aortic Valve

Bicuspid aortic valve forms the most common congenital anomaly of the cardiovascular system and is seen frequently with congenital aortic stenosis, and in some patients with aortic incompetence and coarctation of aorta. It can become the seat of infective endocarditis.

Coronary Arteriovenous Fistula

It is an uncommon anomaly consisting of an abnormal communication between the right coronary artery and right atrium or right ventricle. It causes progressive right-to-left shunt. The volume of the shunt is generally low. It causes a loud superficial continuous murmur at the lower midsternal area. Coronary arteriography helps in diagnosing the shunt.

Abnormal Origin of the Left Coronary Artery

Rarely the left coronary artery may take origin from the pulmonary artery. This causes relative ischemia of the region supplied by the left coronary artery and there are progressive signs of cardiac failure, developing in infancy. Those who survive the condition, develop collateral circulation from the right coronary artery.

It may present with evidence of:

- Myocardial ischemia of the papillary muscle
- Electrocardiogram shows evidence of anterolateral myocardial infarction.
- The treatment consists of ligation of left coronary artery at its origin or its anastomosis to the aorta through a graft.

Aortic Sinus Aneurysm

It is a congenital weakness in the wall of aorta just above the aortic valves near the origin of the coronary arteries. It causes progressive aneurysmal dilatation of aortic sinus of Valsalva, especially right coronary sinus. This is recognized in adult life when it ruptures into the right ventricle or rarely into the right atrium. Rupture is associated with sudden onset of excruciating pain in the middle of the chest, dyspnea and features of cardiac failure. There is volume overload of ventricles. Pulse is collapsing and there is loud superficial continuous murmur over the sternal area. The condition may be associated with conducton disturbance. Surgical correction is done by excision of the aueurysm and repair of the defect.

Mitral Stenosis (see Chapter I 1–63)

It is an uncommon congenital anomaly and may be associated with aortic atresia and other cardiac anomalies. Very rarely, it can be an isolated disorder. The valve is narrowed by fused commissures or the leaflets may be thickened and tethered. Sometimes, the thickened short chordae tendinae may converge on a single hypertrophied papillary muscle like a 'parachute'.

Mitral Regurgitation (see Chapter I 64–108)

Mitral regurgitation may occur with other cardiac anomalies. It may result from the papillary muscle ischemia or cleft deformity of the mitral valve The pansystolic murmur radiates more posteriorly unlike that encountered in rheumatic mitral regurgitation.

COR TRIATRIATUM

It is a rare congenital anomaly in which all the pulmonary veins join together to form a common chamber and empty into the left atrium through a small opening. It is a kind of supravalvular mitral stenosis. This common chamber is usually situated inside the left atrium. Its major complication is secondary pulmonary hypertension.

80. The 4 common left-to-right shunts with increased pulmonary blood flow are:

1. ASD of the osteum secundum
2. VSD
3. PDA
4. Endocardial cushion defect (ASD of the ostium primum type).

ATRIAL SEPTAL DEFECT (ASD)

It is defined as interatrial communication due to true deficiency in the atrial septum. It should be distinguished from valvular patent foramen ovale, which may persist into adulthood.

81. Characteristics of ASD.

1. ASD is the most common congenital heart defect next to bicuspid aortic valve and mitral valve prolapse.
2. It occurs approximately 5–10% of congenital heart disease.
3. It is the most common acyanotic stent lesion in adults.
4. It may go unrecognized into the adulthood as the clinical features can be subtle.

82. Atrial septal defect is classified into 4 types according to its site and origin.

1. *Osteum secundum type:* It is the most common variety. It occurs in the region of fossa ovalis near the middle of the septum. It does not involve the atrioventricular valves.
2. *Osteum primum type:* It occurs in the lower part of the septum continuous with atrioventricular valves. It is associated with a cleft in the anterior leaflet of the mitral valve with or without cleft in the septal tricuspid leaflet considered as endocardial cushion defect.
3. *Sinus venosus type:* It occurs high in the septum near the entry of superior vena cava as a sinus venosus defect often associated with anomalous termination of right pulmonary veins into the superior vena cava.
4. Defect near the inferior vena cava or coronary sinus. It occurs near the opening of inferior vena cava. Rarely the septum may be totally absent resulting in single atrium.

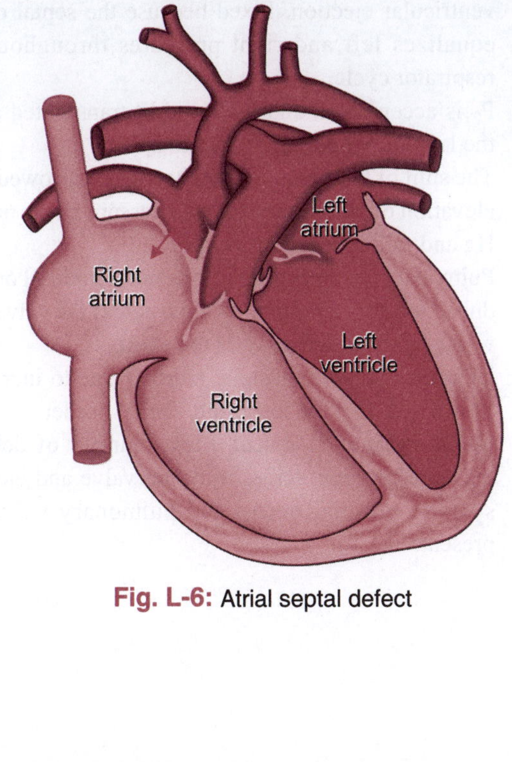

Fig. L-6: Atrial septal defect

83. 3/4th of the defects (75–80%) are considered to be secundum type.

84. 1/4th of the defects (20–25%) are considered to be primum type with associated atrioventricular canal defects.

85. Incidence and morbidity.

1. It is relatively common and is found in about 10% of children surviving beyond first year of life with congenital heart diseases.
2. It is most frequently encountered congenital heart disease in adults next to bicuspid aortic valve.
3. It is common in females with a male/female ratio of approximately 1:2.
4. Patients with atrial septal defect of secundum and sinus venosus type rarely die before the fifth decade whereas osteum primum defect is often associated with high morbidity and mortality rate in infancy and childhood.

86. There are 4 major noncardiac congenital anomalies (mostly skeletal deformities) that are associated with atrial septal defect.

1. Ellis-van Creveld syndrome: Chondrodystrophic dwarfism, nail dysplasia and polydactyly.
   (Example of Mendelian autosomal recessive transmission)–ASD or single atrium
2. Holt-Oram syndrome: Skeletal deformities of upper limb and hypoplasia of the clavicles.
   (Example of autosomal dominance)
3. TAR: Thrombocytopenia—absent radius syndrome.
4. Trisomy-21 (Down's syndrome/Mongolism): Hypotonia, hyperextensible joints, mongoloid facies, mental retardation—endocardial cushion defect, ASD or VSD or TOF.
   (Lutembacher's syndrome—associated with mitral stenosis)

87. Hemodynamics—It can be described in 4 stages:

The hemodynamics of atrial septal defect mainly depends on the size of the defect, compliance of the ventricle, relative resistance in the pulmonary and systemic circulation. A defect of 1 cm or more in diameter is responsible for clinical manifestations.

1. In smaller defect, the left atrial pressure is greater than right atrial pressure and the flow is from left-to-right. The left-to-right shunt is thus silent on auscultation.
2. In larger defect the pressure becomes equal leading to a bidirectional shunt with predominant left-to-right shunt. The right atrium receives blood not only through the superior and inferior vena cava but also the oxygenated blood shunted from the left atrium. The right atrium enlarges in size to accommodate the extra volume of blood. The large volume of blood received by the right atrium passes through a normal sized tricuspid valve, producing a delayed diastolic murmur heard at the lower left sternal border.
   Shunt is only from left-to-right in the presence of normal vascular resistance and normal compliant right ventricle.
3. The left-to-right shunt causes diastolic overloading of right ventricle and increased pulmonary blood flow. Right ventricle enlarges to accommodate the large volume of blood reaching it. Large volume of blood from the right ventricle passing across the normal pulmonary valve produces a pulmonary ejection murmur. Later, there may be marked right ventricular hypertrophy and marked elevation of pulmonary arterial pressure. The large volume also results in prolonged ejection phase of the right ventricle. The pulmonary valve closes late and the pulmonary second sound, P_2 is delayed. Since the right ventricle is fully loaded, further increase in the right ventricular volume during inspiration cannot occur. The second sound is widely split and fixed. The P_2 is also accentuated. The cardiac apex is formed by the elnarged right ventricle and the accentuated P_2 is well-audible at the apex as well. Hence, the audible P_2 at the apex in ASD does not mean pulmonary arterial hypertension. The pulmonary blood flow may be 3 to 6 times greater than systemic blood flow. The pulmonary artery and its branches enlarge to accommodate the left-to-right shunt and the lung fields appear plethoric.
4. Reversal of shunt occurs when the pulmonary vascular resistance exceeds that of systemic vascular resistance (Eisenmenger's syndrome).
   Pulmonary vascular changes occur more slowly in atrial septal defect compared to ventricular septal defect and patent ductus arteriosus with similar sized communication. Generally, it will be tolerated as the pulmonary vascular resistance is low in children and young adults.

88. Symptomatology.

Atrial septal defect can exist without any symptoms until the adult life. Patients with secundum type may begin to present symptoms in the fourth or fifth decade. Osteum primum defect children develop the symptoms at a very early age.

1. Some children show under development.
2. Some children have recurrent respiratory infection.
3. After fourth decade, good number of patients develop symptoms of palpitation and breathlessness due to atrial arrhythmia, pulmonary arterial hypertension.
4. Severe breathlessness develop with reversal of shunt and congestive heart failure.

89. The important clinical signs are:

1. Right ventricular systolic lift along the left sternal border—parasternal impulse.
2. A systolic thrill may be palpable at left 2nd intercostal space in 10% of patients.
3. Cardiac enlargement is usually mild to moderate. Marked cardiomegaly suggests additional lesions like mitral stenosis in Lutembacher's syndrome or mitral regurgitation.
4. First sound is normal or may be accentuated due to loud tricuspid component of the first sound.
5. Second sound is widely split and fixed. Second sound is wide because of delay in hypertrophied right ventricular ejection. Fixed because the septal defect equalizes left and right pressures throughout the respirator cycle.
6. P_2 is accentuated and widely split transmitted along the left sternal border and up to apex.
   The split of the second sound becomes narrowed with elevation of pulmonary arterial pressure above 60 mm Hg and fall in the shunt volume.
7. Pulmonary ejection systolic murmur (Grade III or less) due to increased pulmonary flow across the valve. It is widely transmitted all over the chest.
8. Delayed tricuspid diastolic murmur due to increased flow is heard at the lower left sternal border.
   Shunt murmur is absent. Flow murmur of delayed diastolic murmur across tricuspid valve and ejection systolic murmur across the pulmonary valve are present.

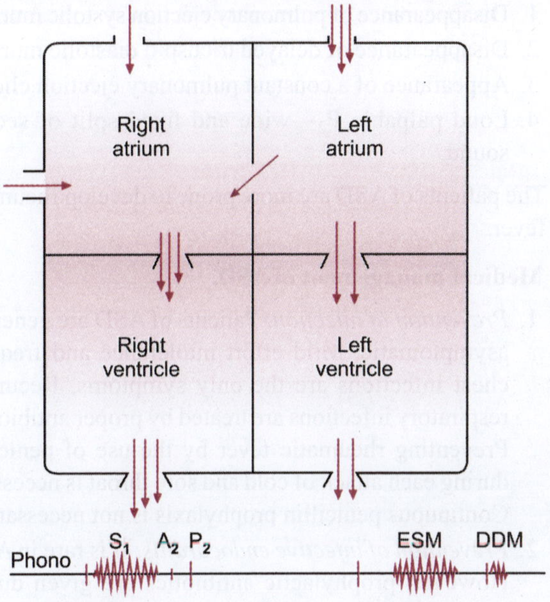

Sounds:
- S_1 Accentuated—Loud
- S_2 Wide-fixed split, P_2^{++}
- X Inconstant (infrequent).

Murmurs:
- Shunt murmur—absent
- Flow murmur—delayed diastolic
- Pulmonary—ejection systolic.

Fig. L-7: Auscultatory findings in ASD

90. A pansystolic murmur of mitral regurgitation at the apex in a patient with other findings of atrial septal defect suggest the following 4 possibilities:

1. Ostium primum defect in which ECG shows left axis deviation of more than –30° (ostium primum type ASD).
2. Floppy posterior leaflet of the mitral valve with a midsystolic click or even a pansystolic murmur.
3. Ostium secundum defect may be associated with rheumatic mitral regurgitation, which is not an uncommon association in India.
4. ASD secundum defect may very rarely be associated with cleft mitral valve resulting in mitral regurgitation.

The last three conditions have right axis deviation in ECG.

91. There are 4 signs to be looked in X-ray chest in ASD.

1. Right atrial dilatation.
2. Right ventricular dilatation.
3. Dilatation of pulmonary artery and its branches. (Dynamic pulsations 'Hilar dance' is seen on screening).
4. Increased pulmonary vascular markings—pulmonary plethora.

Ascending aorta is not conspicuous. There is no left atrial enlargement unlike patent ductus arteriosus or ventricular septal defect. The barium filled esophagus in anterior oblique view shows definite absence of left atrial enlargement.

92. There are 4 ECG changes to be looked in ASD.

1. Right axis deviation.
2. Right atrial hypertrophy and right ventricular hypertrophy. Degree of right atrial and right ventricular hypertrophy varies with each type of defect depending on the height of pulmonary arterial pressure.
3. The characteristic configuration of the precordial leads in V1 is rSR' pattern indicating incomplete right bundle branch block (complete right bundle branch block in 10%) in secundum type.
4. Right bundle branch block with left axis deviation beyond – 30° and prolongation of PR interval occurs in ostium primum defect.

First degree AV block in sinus venosus type ASD.

93. There are 4 echocardiography findings in ASD.

1. Evidence of volume overload on the right side of the heart is identified as right atrial, right ventricular and pulmonary dilatations.
2. Anterior systolic (Paradoxical ventricular septal motion) or flat interventricular motion.
3. 2D Echo visualizes the atrial septal defect of secundum type preferably from the subcostal approach with 90%

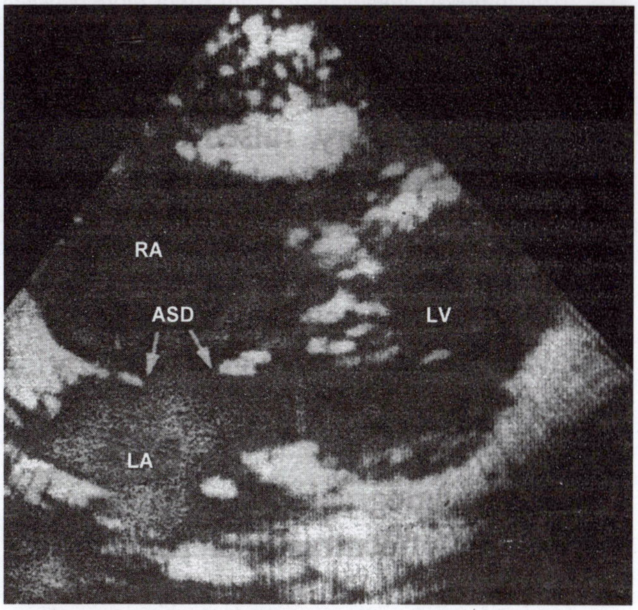

Fig. L-8: Two-dimenstional echocardiogram: Subcoastal view from a patient with atrial septal defect (ASD) secondum type; RA = Right atrium; LA = Left atrium; LV = Left ventricle sensitivity. Sinus venosus defects are more difficult to identify, the success rate being about 50%.

4. Associated abnormalities such as endocardial cushion defects with osteum primum defect, mitral valve prolapse, etc.
   Transesophageal Echo is helpful in identifying the difficult types of ASD.

94. Cardiac catheterization and angiography.

1. Passage of the catheter across the atrial septal defect confirms the diagnosis. The catheter, if passed from the inferior vena cava usually passes central atrial opening easily.
2. Catheter may enter high into the right pulmonary vein from right atrium in sinus venosus defect.
3. Catheter passes low in osteum primum defect.
4. Serial estimation of oxygen saturation or indicator dilution curve techniques may indicate magnitude of the shunt. Increased oxygen saturation is found in right atrium, right ventricle and pulmonary artery —compared with superior and inferior vena cava. Increased oxygen saturation in superior vena cava is found in sinus venosus defect.
5. Pulmonary arterial and right ventricular pressures are usually normal or slightly elevated in young patients in spite of large shunts. Pulmonary arterial hypertension is frequent in older patients. A systolic pressure gradient up to 20 mm Hg of right ventricular outflow is accepted. Right atrial and left atrial pressures are identical. A mean pressure gradient of 3 mm Hg or more between the two atria should raise the suspicion of atrial septal defect associated with left atrial hypertension, or partial anomalous pulmonary venous connections or left ventricular-right atrial communication.
6. Left ventricular angiogram is helpful in endocardial cushion defects. It frequently demonstrates 'goose neck' deformity of the left ventricular outflow tract caused by abnormal anterior mitral valve leaflet. It may also demonstrate mitral regurgitation.
7. Indicator-dilution curves and selective angiography will help in demonstrating the number and location of the anomalous veins.
8. Partial anomalous pulmonary venous connections (PAPVC) can be demonstrated. They are generally associated with sinus venous defect or occasionally with primum or secundum type defects or they may not be associated with any interatrial septal defect.

95. Complications: Pulmonary arterial hypertension due to pulmonary vascular obstructive disease is rare in ASD patients before the age of 20 years. It is recognized by the:

1. Disappearance of pulmonary ejection systolic murmur.
2. Disappearance of delayed tricuspid diastolic murmur.
3. Appearance of a constant pulmonary ejection click.
4. Loud palpable P_2—wide and fixed split of second sound.

The patients of ASD are more prone to develop rheumatic fever.

96. Medical management of ASD.

1. *Prevention of infection:* Patients of ASD are generally asymptomatic. Mild effort intolerance and frequent chest infections are the only symptoms. Recurrent respiratory infections are treated by proper antibiotics. Preventing rheumatic fever by the use of penicillin during each attack of cold and sore throat is necessary. Continuous penicillin prophylaxis is not necessary.
2. *Prevention of infective endocarditis:* It is rare in ASD. However, prophylactic antibiotics are given during dental procedures, instrumentation of GU or GI systems, etc.
3. *Management of arrhythmias:* Atrial fibrillation, supraventricular tachycardias.
4. *Management of cardiac failure:* Congestive cardiac failure is rare.
   Infants and children are followed at yearly intervals.

97. Surgical management of ASD.

Closure of atrial septal defect is done between 3–6 years age in uncomplicated cases under cardiopulmonary bypass where there is a significant left-to-right shunt. (Pulmonary-to-systemic flow ratios exceeding approximately 1.5–1.0)

1. By direct suture in secundum type.
2. By pericardial or Dacron graft in secundum type.
3. In sinus venosus type: The repair is done with a pericardial or tubular Dacron patch from above into the abnormally draining vein/veins down to and around atrial septal defect. It is placed in such a way so as to divert pulmonary venous blood across the defect into the left atrium and to divert superior vena cava blood into right atrium.
4. Repair of associated endocardial cushion defects as in osteum primum defect.
   Osteum secundum defects are easy to correct whereas osteum primum defects are more complex.

Recent advancement by nonsurgical method is by closure of the atrial septal defect by catheter method. The closure is made by passing the catheter with a device at its tip to close the defect. Rashkind et al have used umbrella type device to close the ASD by transcatheter method.

98. Contraindications for surgery.

1. Small defects.
2. Trivial left-to-right shunts.
3. Severe pulmonary vascular diseases without significant left-to-right shunt.
4. Severe pulmonary hypertension with reversal of shunt —Eisenmenger's syndrome.

SINGLE ATRIUM

99. The 4 anatomical features are:

1. Common atrial chamber due to failure of development of interatrial septum.
2. The vena cavae and pulmonary veins drain directly into the large single chamber.
3. Persistence of the left superior vena cava.
4. Commonly associated with cleft mitral valve.

The functional abnormality is similar to ASD. The symptoms develop early. Pulmonary hypertension is not a feature. The main axis in the electrocardiogram is superiorly oriented.

VENTRICULAR SEPTAL DEFECT (VSD)

Ventricular septal defect is the opening in that part of the ventricular septum that separates the two ventricles. (Left ventricular and right atrial communication is a special type) The systolic pressure in the left ventricle is normally about six times than that of right ventricle so the blood flows from the left-to-right ventricle in ventricular septal defect.

Isolated ventricular septal defect is the most common congenital heart disease second only to bicuspid aortic valve.

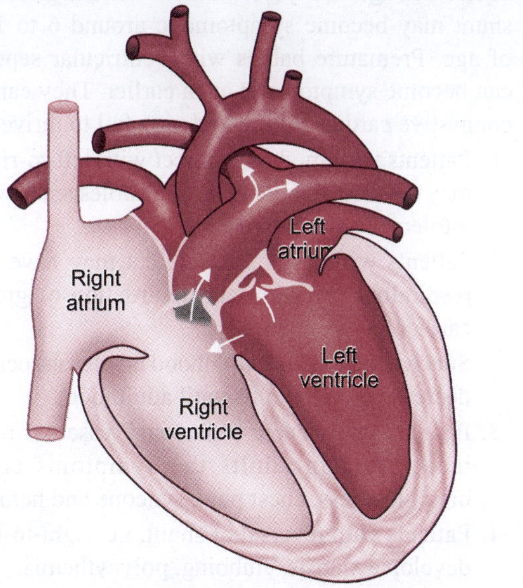

Fig. L-9: Ventricular septal defect

100. It is one of the most common congenital defects. True incidence is difficult to estimate due to spontaneous closure by 6 months.

1. 15–20% spontaneously close by 6 months.
2. About 2 per 1000 live births.
3. Isolated VSDs account for about 25% of all congenital heart diseases.
4. Males and females are affected equally.

Isolated VSD account for about 10% of adult patients with congenital heart defects. This indicates that the natural closure of the defects, improved diagnosis and subsequent surgical closure.

In general, nearly 30% of perimembranous defects close spontaneously, and about 75–80% of all small VSDs spontaneously close by 10 years age.

101. The clinical manifestations depend on 4 factors. Its site, number, size and associated other congenital anomalies.

1. *Site:* Membranous, muscular and bulbar part of the septum. Membranous septum is the most commonly affected part. Defect can exist in the muscular septum towards the apex of right ventricle (Roger's disease) 90% are located at the membranous part with a variable extension into the muscular part.
2. *Number:* May be single or multiple defects.
3. *Size:* Variable in size from small to very large size.
4. *Association with other anomalies:* Can exist as an isolated defect or it can exist with other anomalies like TOF, PS, PDA, coarctation of aorta, transposition of great arteries, truncus arteriosus and tricuspid atresia. It is the most common congenital anomaly encountered as one of the many congenital anomalies.

102. 3/4th of the ventricular septal defects are:

1. Paramembranous—most common type—have higher rate of spontaneous closure.
2. Occur at the outflow portion of the right ventricle.
3. Immediately below the crista supraventricularis or subaortic.
4. Posterior to the papillary muscle of the conus.

103. The 4 most common congenital anomalies that are associated with ventricular septal defect in order of decreasing frequency are:

1. Obstructive anomalies of the Aorta.
   Most commonly coarctation of aorta, bicuspid aortic valve.
2. Additional shunts.
   Most commonly ASD and PDA.
3. Intracardiac obstructions
   PS, TOF, subaortic stenosis, mitral stenosis, anomalies of bundle of right ventricle.
4. Incompetent valves.

104. Ventricular septal defect (VSD) can be distinguished into 4 grades.

1. Small defect less than 0.5 cm^2 diameter—L to R shunt. No elevation of right ventricle or pulmonary artery pressure. Defect may sometimes close spontaneously.
2. Defect is 0.5–1.0 cm^2 diameter—resistance to L to R shunt, progressive volume over load of both ventricles. Development of mild to moderate pulmonary hypertension
3. Defect greater than 1.0 cm^2 diameter—Right and left ventricles exhibit free communication and their pressure is same.
4. Pulmonary resistance greater than systemic resistance—shunt gets reversed, R to L shunt—Eisenmenger's syndrome. This is noted in young adults. The magnitude of left-to-right shunt is determined by the pulmonary vascular resistance. There is volume overload of the left ventricle which may lead to its failure.

105. Hemodynamics.

1. A ventricular septal defect results in shunting of oxygenated blood from the left ventricle to right ventricle. The left ventricle starts contracting earlier than right ventricle. As there is high pressure in the left ventricle, the flow of blood from left ventricle to right ventricle starts very early in systole and a high pressure gradient is maintained between the two ventricles throughout the systole. Therefore, the murmur resulting from left-to-right shunt starts early masking the first sound and continuous throughout the systole with almost the same intensity appearing as a pansystolic murmur on auscultation and palpable as a thrill.
2. At the end of systole, the decreasing left ventricular pressure becomes lower than the aortic pressure. This results in closure of aortic valve and occurrence of A_2. However, even at this time, the LV pressure is higher than RV pressure and left-to-right shunt continues. Therefore, the pansystolic murmur of the shunt continues to end beyond A_2, completely masking it.
3. The left-to-right shunt occurs during systole at a time when the right ventricle is also contracting and its volume is decreasing. The bloodstream of left-to-right shunt, therefore is directed toward the pulmonary artery. This flow of blood across the normal pulmonary valve results in an ejection systolic murmur at the pulmonary valve. However, this ejection systolic murmur cannot be separated from the pansystolic murmur. The ejection systolic murmur has a selective transmission of the pansystolic murmur to the upper left sternal border where its ejection character can be recognized since it does not mask the A_2.
4. The increased volume of blood passing through the pulmonary circulation results in pulmonary plethora recognized in the X-ray chest.
5. The large volume of blood finally reaches the left atrium resulting in left atrial enlargement.
6. The large volume of blood, while passing through a normal mitral valve results in delayed diastolic murmur at the apex and is directly related to the size of the shunt. The large flow across the normal mitral valve also results in accentuated first sound not appreciated at the bed side as it is drowned by the pansystolic murmur.
7. Since the left ventricle has two outlets, the aortic valve allowing forward flow and the ventricular septal defect resulting in a backward leak, it empties relatively early. This results in an early aortic valve closure sound (A_2)
8. Since the ejection into the right ventricle and pulmonary artery is increased because of the left-to-right shunt the pulmonary component is delayed. Therefore, the second sound is widely split but varies with respiration in patients of VSD with a large left-to-right shunt. There is also an increase in the intensity of P_2.

106. Symptomatology.

It varies greatly with patient's age, size of the defect and level of pulmonary vascular resistance.

Many infants and children remain asymptomatic when the defect is isolated and small. In half the number of infants the defect may close spontaneously during childhood before the age of 3 years. Babies with large left-to-right shunt may become symptomatic around 6 to 10 weeks of age. Premature babies with ventricular septal defect can become symptomatic even earlier. They can develop congestive cardiac failure and may fail to thrive.

1. Patients with moderate defect with left-to-right shunt may develop symptoms in late adolescence with effort intolerance and fatigue.
2. Patients with large sized defect may have recurrent respiratory infection and retardation of growth and cardiac failure in infancy.

   Survival beyond the childhood is often associated with decrease of symptoms until adulthood.
3. Patients with severe pulmonary vascular resistance, most often in adults the symptoms consist of breathlessness, chest pain, syncope and hemoptysis.
4. Patients with reversal of shunt, i.e. right-to-left shunt develop cyanosis, clubbing, polycythemia.

107. The 4 clinical signs in moderate to large sized VSD.

1. Cardiomegaly: Pericardium is hyperkinetic. Heart size is moderately enlarged with left ventricular type of apex. Left ventricular or biventricular pulsations are generally well-palpable. Only right ventricular pulsations are present in presence of severe pulmonary arterial hypertension.

   Left atrium enlarges in size by receiving large volume of blood.

   Pulse pressure is relatively wide.
2. Prominent parasternal systolic thrill in the 3rd and 4th left intercostal space. It disappears with development of pulmonary arterial hypertension and reduction of left-to-right shunt.
3. The first and second sounds are masked by a pansystolic murmur at the left sternal border.

   The second sound can however be made out at the second intercostal space or higher. Second sound is normal or closely split and varies with respiration, widely split when there is disparity in size of hypertrophied ventricles.

   Third sound is heard at the apex due to increased volume of blood entering the ventricle.
4. A loud pansystolic murmur that results from flow across the defect is harsh, generally loud at the lower 3rd and 4th intercostal space to the left of sternal border with no specific radiation or change with respiration.

   A mid or delayed diastolic rumbling murmur starting with third heart sound due to increased flow across the mitral valve is present at the apex in large shunts. The intensity and duration of delayed diastolic murmur at the apex is directly related to the size of the shunt.

   A basal midsystolic ejection murmur may be present because of increased pulmonary blood flow. The thrill and murmur diminish in their intensity with increasing pulmonary arterial dilatation and reduction of left-to-right shunt. In patients with severe pulmonary arterial hypertension with almost no left-to-right shunt or reversed shunt, the systolic murmur may be very short or absent and an early diastolic murmur of pulmonary regurgitation may be heard at the left upper sternal edge.

   Sounds:
   - S_1 masked by murmur
   - S_2 masked by murmur at left lateral sternal border widely split at 2nd LICS but mobile
   - S_3 with small left-to-right shunts.

   Murmurs:
   - Shunt murmur: Pansystolic
   - Flow murmurs: Pulmonary ejection systolic murmur
   - Mitral delayed diastolic murmur.

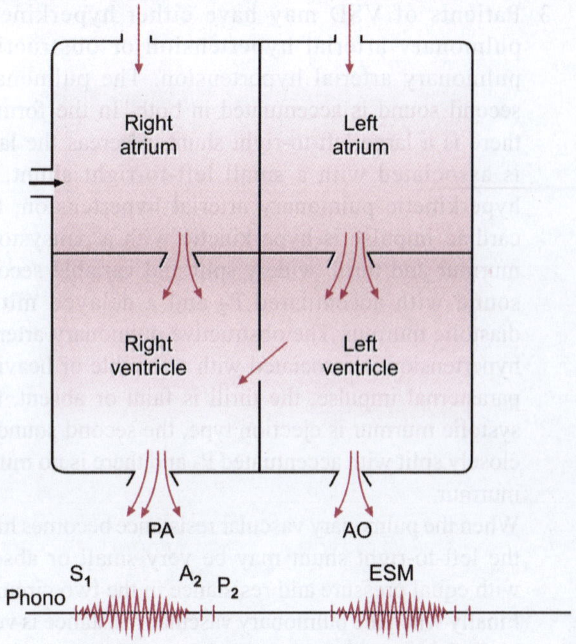

Fig. L-10: Auscultatory findings in VSD

108. Functional disturbance and assessment of severity of ventricular septal defect depend on 4 factors. Mainly on its size and status of the pulmonary vascular bed than on its site.

1. Size of the defect: In small defects, the left-to-right shunt murmur continues to be pansystolic but the shunt is small, the second sound is normally split and the intensity of the pulmonary second sound is normal. There is also absence of the delayed diastolic murmur.

   If the VSD is very small, it acts as a stenotic area resulting in an ejection systolic murmur. This is the most common cause of the functional systolic murmur in children, which disappear as they grow older because of the spontaneous closure of small ventricular septal defects.

   In small defects, the high velocity jet from high pressure left ventricle to low pressure right ventricle has no significant hemodynamic effect. The effects are seen with moderate to large size defect.
2. In a large ventricular septal defect with low pulmonary vascular resistance, a large left-to-right shunt increases pulmonary blood flow, being twice or more than the systemic blood flow.

   The right ventricular pressure increases and the difference in the systolic pressure between the two ventricles decreases, the left-to-right shunt murmur becomes shorter and softer and appears as an ejection systolic murmur. The pulmonary artery pressure is increased resulting in an accentuated pulmonary second sound.

3. Patients of VSD may have either hyperkinetic pulmonary arterial hypertension or obstructive pulmonary arterial hypertension. The pulmonary second sound is accentuated in both. In the former, there is a large left-to-right shunt, whereas the later is associated with a small left-to-right shunt. In hyperkinetic pulmonary arterial hypertension, the cardiac impulse is hyperkinetic with a pansystolic murmur and thrill, widely split and variable second sound with accentuated P_2 and a delayed mitral diastolic murmur. The obstructive pulmonary arterial hypertension is associated with a forcible or heaving parasternal impulse, the thrill is faint or absent, the systolic murmur is ejection type, the second sound is closely split with accentuated P_2 and there is no mitral murmur.
   When the pulmonary vascular resistance becomes high the left-to-right shunt may be very small or absent with equal pressure and resistance in the two circuits. Finally when the pulmonary vascular resistance is very high, there may be reversal of shunt with unsaturated blood being directed to left ventricle into the systemic circulation (Eisenmenger's syndrome).
4. Presence or absence of associated pulmonary stenosis affects the function very much.
   In the presence of infundibular pulmonic stenosis, the right ventricular pressure increases and the VSD murmur becomes an ejection systolic murmur. The pulmonary arterial pressure is normal or decreased and the P_2 is diminished in intensity and as well as delayed in timing resulting a widely split, variable second sound with soft P_2.

109. On the basis of assessment of clinical findings, it is possible to differentiate the size of the VSD.

1. Very small VSD
2. Small VSD
3. Medium sized VSD
4. Large VSD.

It is also possible to differentiate whether there is associated pulmonary stenosis or pulmonary arterial hypertension of the hyperkinetic or obstructive type.

110. Systolic murmur of VSD is differentiated from systolic murmur of mitral regurgitation.

Table L-2

VSD	MR
1. Murmur is compared to a leaf in a pot—moves from place to place	Localized to apex
2. Diffusely heard in left and right side	Radiates to axilla
3. Not influenced by respiration	Decreases in intensity with inspiration, increases on expiration Hand grip increases the intensity
4. Never have associated ejection systolic murmur	Have associated ejection systolic murmur

111. There are 4 X-ray findings in large sized VSD. It is often helpful in distinguishing the degree of left-to-right shunt.

1. Left atrial dilatation in large size defect.
2. Cardiac silhouette is of left ventricular type with heart size depending on the size of the left-to-right shunt. The bigger the left-to-right shunt, the larger the heart. Biventricular hypertrophy.
   Patients with small size VSD or associated pulmonary stenosis or pulmonary arterial hypertension have a normal sized heart.
3. Prominent pulmonary artery segment (The aorta appears normal or smaller than normal in size).
4. Increased pulmonary vascular markings—Pulmonary plethora.

Pulmonary vasculature is normal with small defects if there is associated pulmonary stenosis. A small or normal sized heart with normal pulmonary vascular markings suggest hemodynamically insignificant lesion, whereas cardiomegaly, left atrial and left ventricular enlargement suggest large left-to-right shunt. A large defect with small heart and oligemic lungs suggest the pulmonary vascular disease.

112. ECG changes are variable. All children are born with right ventricular hypertrophy. Therefore, initially all patients of VSD have right ventricular hypertrophy. Right ventricular hypertrophy regresses more slowly because of the fall of pulmonary vascular resistance due to ventricular septal defect and slow regression of pulmonary arterial hypertension.

1. No change is seen in smaller defects.
2. In large left-to-right shunts without pulmonary arterial hypertension shows left ventricular hypertrophy by the time they are 6 months to 1 year old. The mean QRS axis in the frontal plane generally lies between –30° to + 90°. Right axis deviation suggest elevated right ventricular and pulmonary artery pressure.
3. Biventricular hypertrophy is seen with large left-to-right shunt. There are, however, no ST and T changes suggestive of left ventricular strain pattern.
4. Isolated right ventricular hypertrophy is seen with severe pulmonary arterial hypertension.
   RBBB may occur after surgical correction.

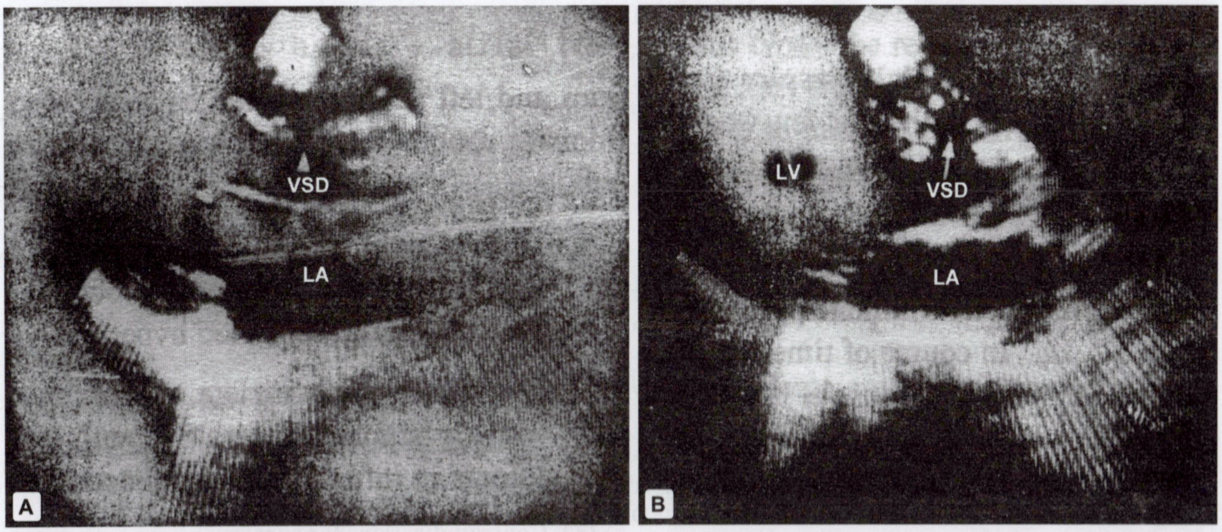

Fig. L-11: Two-dimensional echocardiogram: Long axis view of a patient with a membranous ventricular septal defect. A. Discontinuity of echoes from the ventricular septal defect (VSD) can be seen; B. Contrast Echo: Contrast injection fills the right ventricle. LA = left atrium; LV = left ventricle; VSD = Ventricular septal defect

113. Echocardiography specially two-dimensional echocardiogram demonstrates the following with moderate to large sized VSD.

1. Ventricular septal defect is identified specially in apical four chamber view.
2. Biventricular enlargement.
3. Pulmonary artery dilatation.
4. It differentiates a large ventricular septal defect from a single ventricle. It is important because surgical correction of single ventricle is met with little success.

114. Cardiac catheterization and angiogram in ventricular septal defect.

1. Increased right ventricular oxygen saturation reflects left-to-right shunt in ventricular septal defect. No change is seen with small defects.
2. Routine right heart pulmonary and systemic arterial pressures are noted and blood samples are taken. Right ventricular and pulmonary arterial systolic pressures are normal with small defects. These pressures are at the systemic levels in large defects and the mean left atrial pressure may be elevated to 10–15 mm Hg. Assessment of left atrial or pulmonary artery wedge pressure and left ventricular-end-diastolic pressure may help in the possible assessment of left ventricular obstruction.
3. Selective left ventricular angiography in the antero-posterior, lateral and oblique views demonstrate the spatial relationship of the great arteries to each other and to the ventricles. It demonstrates the exact site, size and number of ventricular septal defects.
4. Ascending aortic angiogram is necessary to rule out the associated conditions like patent ductus arteriosus, aortic regurgitation, coarctation of aorta, etc.

115. Increased oxygen saturation at the level of the right ventricle differentiates ventricular septal defect from:

1. Truncus arteriosus
2. Aorto-pulmonary septal defect (Aorto-pulmonary window)
3. Single ventricle
4. Isolated large patent ductus arteriosus.

116. Course of VSD.

1. Spontaneous closure can occur in small ventricular defects. In about 90% of patients who have spontaneous closure, it occurs by the age of three years, though it may occur as late as 25 years or more.
2. Patients with uncomplicated VSD may develop pulmonic stenosis due to hypertrophy of the right ventricular infundibulum.
3. May develop hyperkinetic pulmonary arterial hypertension or obstructive pulmonary arterial hypertension.
4. Rarely develop arterial hypertension due to prolapse of the right coronary or the non-coronary cusp of the aortic valve.
   Development of the pulmonary arterial hypertension is a dreaded complication since it is of the obstructive type, which makes the shunt reversible, from right-to-left and make the patient inoperable.

117. Complications of VSD.

1. May develop congestive cardiac failure in infancy which is associated with high mortality. May develop congestive cardiac failure in adults life around the age of 30 to 40 years.
2. VSD is the most common congenital anomaly

complicated by infective endocarditis. The incidence of infective endocarditis is small enough, that cannot be considered as an indication for surgery in small defects.
3. Recurrent chest infections.
4. Anemia and others.

MANAGEMENT

118. Medical management.

1. Control of congestive cardiac failure. Management of congestive cardiac failure is common in infants with large left-to-right shunt.
2. Prevention and treatment of recurrent respiratory infections.
3. Prevention and treatment of infective endocarditis. Risk of bacterial endocarditis is higher in patients with small or moderate sized defects than those with larger ones. VSD is the most common congenital anomaly complicated by infective endocarditis. Proper prophylaxis before any minor surgical procedure is essential.
   In a patient with culture proven endocarditis, 4 to 6 weeks of antibiotics should be given parenterally before consideration for intervention.
4. Recent data suggests that selective pulmonary vasodilators including:
   i. Nitric oxide
   ii. Prostacyclin analog
   iii. Endothelium receptor antagonists
   iv. Phosphodiesterase-5 inhibitors may be beneficial in these patients.

The patient of VSD should be watched carefully to assess the development of either pulmonary stenosis, pulmonary arterial hypertension or aortic regurgitation.

119. Surgery is indicated in:

1. Congestive cardiac failure occurring in infancy and is not responding to medical management.
2. Large left-to-right shunt with pulmonary to systemic ratio exceeding 1.5:1.0 or 2.0:1.0 regardless of level of pulmonary arterial pressure (pulmonary flow more then twice the systemic flow).
3. Associated with pulmonary stenosis or pulmonary arterial hypertension.
4. Associated with aortic regurgitation.

120. Surgical management.

1. Palliative surgery is indicated in infants with large left-to-right shunts where definitive closure is risky. Pulmonary artery banding is done to protect pulmonary vasculature followed sometime later by corrective surgery.
2. Transcatheter closure with the RVD can be attempted. Definitive surgery:
3. Primary patch closure of the defect by Dacron is done before the age of two years by utilizing the technique of hypothermia
4. In older children, definitive surgery is done by the use of cardiopulmonary bypass.
   The operation can be done through the right atrium which is preferred approach or through a right ventriculotomy which leaves majority of patients with a right bundle branch block.

121. Complications of surgery are:

1. Complete heart block
2. Bifascicular block
3. Right bundle branch block
4. Reopened or residual ventricular septal defect.

122. Contraindications for surgery.

1. Small defect: Spontaneous closure occurs in significant number of patients.
2. Elevated pulmonary vascular resistance to a level, which eliminates left-to-right shunt and carries increased risk.
3. Significant elevation of pulmonary vascular resistance.
4. Eisenmenger's syndrome.

SINGLE VENTRICLE

A single ventricle occurs from the absence of interventricular septum. It maintains both systemic and pulmonary circulations. Often there is transposition of great vessels and the clinical picture simulates that of VSD.

PATENT DUCTUS ARTERIOSUS (PDA)

Patent ductus arteriosus is the persistence of normal fetal vascular channel communicating pulmonary artery to the aorta.

It occurs in approximately 1 in 2000 live births. In infants, the incidence is 10–20%, 12% of all congenital defects.

123. There are 4 anatomical points to know about PDA.

1. The opening is situated just distal to the origin of the left pulmonary artery below and just distal to the origin of the left subclavian artery above.
2. Aortic side opening is larger than the pulmonary side opening.
3. The channel undergoes functional closure after birth and complete closure within 2 to 3 weeks, and becomes ligamentum arteriosum. It may remain patent as long as 8 weeks.
4. The recurrent laryngeal branch of left vagus nerve hooks around its lateral and inferior aspects.

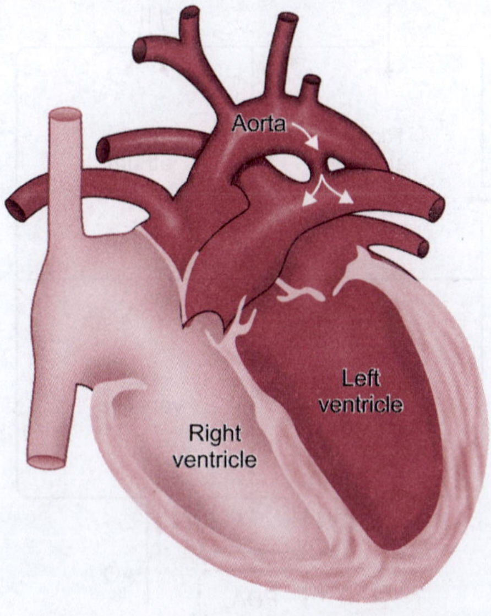

Fig. L-12: Patent ductus arteriosus

124. PDA may exist in an isolated form or may coexist with other anomalies. The 4 common coexisting conditions are:

1. Coarctation of aorta
2. Ventricular septal defect
3. Pulmonary stenosis
4. Aortic stenosis.

In certain anomalies, so-called ductus dependent conditions such as pulmonary atresia, aortic arch interruption anomalies, persistent patency of the ductus is desirable since it plays a vital role in the maintenance of pulmonary and systemic blood flow.

125. Patent ductus arteriosus is the most common type of extracardiac shunt occurring more frequently in:

1. 3 to 4 times more common in females
2. Premature infants especially those with asphyxia or respiratory distress syndrome
3. Children born at high altitudes
4. Children born to those mothers who are affected by rubella in the first trimester of pregnancy.

126. The hemodynamic effects of PDA depends on its size—not only its cross-sectional area but also to its length of the channel and pulmonary vascular response.

1. Small PDA is associated with a normal pulmonary arterial pressure and left-to-right shunt and may be asymptomatic.
2. When the patency of the ductus is moderate or large, the aortic pressure is directly transmitted into pulmonary vasculature and leads to pulmonary hypertension. In majority of cases the flow is from left-to-right, occurs both during systole and diastole, as a pressure gradient is present throughout the cardiac cycle between the two great arteries, if the pulmonary artery pressure is normal. The flow of blood results in a murmur which starts in systole, after the first sound and reaches a peak at the second sound. The murmur then diminishes in intensity and is audible during diastole. Thus, it is a continuous or machinery murmur.
3. The PDA results in systolic as well as diastolic overloading of the pulmonary artery. There is an increased flow of blood through the lungs to the left atrium. The left atrium enlarges in size to accommodate the increased blood flow.
4. The increased blood flow across the normal mitral valve results in accentuated first sound and a delayed mitral diastolic murmur. The intensity of the delayed diastolic murmur is directly related to the size of the left-to-right shunt. There is no delayed diastolic murmur with small shunts.
5. Third sound is heard in moderate sized shunts due to rapid early filling of the left ventricle. Large shunts give rise to delayed mitral diastolic murmur.
6. Left ventricle enlarges in size to accommodate large volume of blood that reaches it during diastole as in VSD. This results in prolongation of the left ventricular systole and increase in left ventricular size.
7. The prolongation of the left ventricular systole causes delayed closure of the aortic valve and a late aortic second sound, A_2. With large left-to-right shunt second sound S_2, may be paradoxically split.
8. The large left ventricular volume is ejected into the aorta during systole results in dilatation of the ascending aorta. A dilated ascending aorta results in an aortic ejection click, which is heard all over the precordium and precedes the start of continuous murmur. The increased volume of blood passing through a normal aortic valve results in an aortic ejection systolic murmur, but it is drowned by the loud continuous murmur and is not usually made out.

127. Clinical features: They vary with age, size of the shunt and the pulmonary vascular status. Generally small PDA exists without any symptoms in infancy and childhood and the condition may be recognized by its characteristic murmur during routine examination.

1. A large left-to-right shunt at high pressure especially in infants may cause heart failure in the first few weeks or months of life. If it does not occur during infancy, it is most unlikely to occur before the third decade.
2. Respiratory distress symptoms are more frequent in premature infants than with full-term infants particularly with birth weight less than 1.5 kg.

In course of time the respiratory distress symptoms often blend with those of heart failure.

Increase in carbon dioxide retention causes increase in ventilatory or oxygen requirements, presents with episodic apnea and bradycardia. Repeated respiratory infections, palpitation, breathlessness are the common presenting symptoms. Growth may be affected with heart failure.

3. With the reversal of shunt, the unsaturated blood from the pulmonary artery reaches the descending aorta and produces characteristic differential cyanosis. The toes exhibit cyanosis and clubbing whereas the fingers remain acyanotic. Diffuse cyanosis may be present if there is pulmonary edema.
4. The flow from the aorta to the pulmonary artery is a leak from the systemic flow. This results in bounding pulse with wide pulse pressure known as Corrigan or water hammer pulse.

   Presence of prominent carotid pulsations in a patient with left-to-right shunt is a strong indication of PDA. Apex is hyperdynamic when there is left ventricular hypertrophy.
5. Systolic or continuous thrill in the left second intercostal space in the parasternal region.
6. First sound is accentuated and second sound is narrowly or paradoxically split with large left-to-right shunt. The pulmonary second sound is louder than normal. It is difficult to hear the second sound in PDA since the maximum intensity of the continuous murmur occurs at the second sound and thereby masking the second sound. Clinically, there is no point in evaluating second sound in the presence of continuous murmur.
7. A harsh continuous 'machinery murmur' in the left second intercostal space radiating to the left clavicle and along the left sternal border. The murmur starts after the first sound and accentuates in the late systole and continues into diastole through the second sound. The murmur diminishes in intensity and is heard only during a part of the diastole. The peak at the second sound differentiates the PDA murmur from other causes of continuous murmur. The systolic portion of the murmur is very grating and rough. It appears to be broken into multiple sysolic sounds—the multiple clicks. The continuous murmur indicates the presence of both systolic as well as a diastolic difference in pressure between the aorta and pulmonary artery, thus excluding significant pulmonary arterial hypertension. There is a third sound at the apex followed by a delayed diastolic murmur in large shunts.

   When the pressure difference between the aorta and pulmonary artery is low, only systolic murmur is audible instead of continuous murmur.

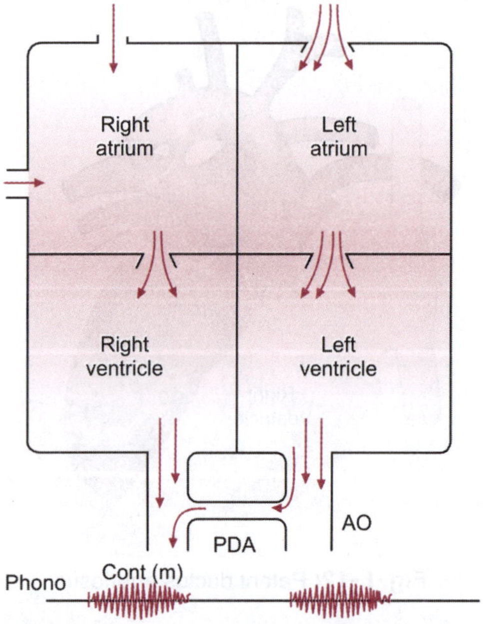

Fig. L-13: Auscultatory findings in PDA

8. Pulmonary hypertension gives rise to early diastolic blowing murmur of pulmonary incompetence (Graham-Steell) or no murmur is audible at all. Second sound is normally split with normal or accentuated pulmonary component.

   Sounds:
   - S_1—accentuated—loud M_1
   - S_2—normal splitting and movement
   - Single or paradoxical P_2
   - S_3—with small left-to-right shunt

   X—Constant.

   Murmurs:
   - Shunt murmur: Continuous (machinery) murmur
   - Flow murmurs: Mitral delayed diastolic
     Aortic ejection systolic (drowned).

128. The PDA should be distinguished from the following 4 important conditions where continuous murmur is present.

(See the causes of continuous murmur 250)

1. A continuous murmur is heard in truncus arteriosus at the interscapular area.
2. A venous hum heard over the base of the neck on the right side—disappears in supine position and increases in inspiration.
3. Sudden onset of continuous murmur at lower level of the precordium is associated with rupture of sinus of Valsalva.
4. Peripheral murmur with cyanosis is associated with pulmonary arteriovenous fistula.

PDA is difficult to differentiate from aortopulmonary window and VSD with prolapse of aortic valve cusp into the septal deficiency.

129. Following are chest roentgenogram findings but they depend on the magnitude of the shunt.

1. Prominent aortic arch is seen in PDA unlike ASD or VSD.
2. Prominent pulmonary artery and its branches.
3. In large shunts, left atrium is enlarged as evidenced by indentation on a barium filled esophagus or elevation of left main stem bronchus.
4. Left ventricular hypertrophy.
5. Increased pulmonary flow—pulmonary plethora.
6. Signs of pulmonary edema when there is heart failure.
7. In older patients with Eisenmenger's complex central pulmonary arteries are prominent with rapid tapering to the periphery of the lung fields.
8. Fluoroscopy may reveal pulsating aortic knob.

130. Electrocardiogram may show the following 4 changes:

It is normal with a small shunt.

1. Axis may be normal with left ventricular dominance or hypertrophy or there may be left axis deviation.
2. Left atrial hypertrophy is probably the most common abnormality—P is notched and wide.
3. Left ventricular hypertrophy with volume overload type—seen in the left precordial leads.
   It never shows ST and T changes suggestive of left ventricular strain pattern in uncomplicated PDA below the age of 15 years. Presence of ST and T changes suggest the presence of additional aortic stenosis or left ventricular fibroelastosis.

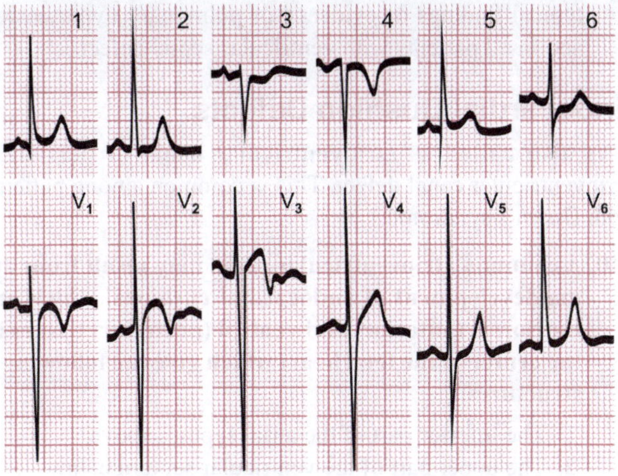

Fig. L-14: ECG from a patient with PDA. Note LV diastolic overload; high voltage QRS complexes

4. Right ventricular hypertrophy is seen with pulmonary hypertension.

131. Assessment of severity.

1. Larger the heart size, the larger the left-to-right shunt.
2. Absence of third heart sound and delayed diastolic murmur indicates a small left-to-right shunt.
3. Presence of third sound indicates moderate left-to-right shunt whereas audible delayed diastolic murmur suggests a large left-to-right shunt.
4. The wider the pulse pressure, larger the shunt.

132. Echocardiogram shows:

1. Dilated pulmonary artery and large aorta
2. Left atrial enlargement
3. Left ventricular enlargement. Left ventricular end-diastolic volume is increased and circumferential fiber shortening is significantly increased
4. Doppler and 2D Echo detects the patent ductus arteriosus and quantitation of flow.
   TEE is more useful.

133. There are 4 points to demonstrate in the cardiac catheterization and angiography.

1. The catheter enters patent ductus arteriosus easily from the pulmonary artery and thereafter enters the descending aorta easily except when the ductus is too small.
2. The oxygen saturation is increased in pulmonary artery to a degree relative to the size of the shunt.
3. Pulmonary arterial and right ventricular pressures are elevated in large shunt.
4. Ascending aortic cineangiography delineates the ductus arteriosus and shows early opacification of pulmonary arteries.

134. There are 4 important complications of patent ductus arteriosus.

1. Congestive heart failure
2. Bacterial endocarditis
3. Pulmonary hypertension with reversal of shunt—Eisenmenger's complex
4. Rarely aneurysm and dilatation with compression of recurrent laryngeal nerve and rupture of the ductus.

135. Management.

1. Treatment of heart failure and respiratory infection. Improvement of oxygenation in premature infant promotes spontaneous closure of the ductus. Relation of intravenous fluids to the incidence of ductus in the premature infants has been documented. So, it can be iatrogenic.

2. Pharmacological closure of the ductus in premature infants by prostaglandin inhibitors, aspirin, indomethacin has been tried. Prostaglandin inhibitors are not effective in full-term children because patent ductus arteriosus in them is a true mechanism.
3. Catheter closure—transfemoral catheter closure using a prosthesis—Rushkind umbrella device (RUD).
4. Direct surgical closure.
   Primary prevention is by decreasing the incidence of prematurity. Immunization of children in those born with rubella syndrome.

136. There are 4 ductus dependent congenital anomalies where the closure of ductus after delivery produces deterioration of the clinical condition.

1. Pulmonary atresia
2. Tricuspid atresia
3. Transposition of great arteries with restricted ASD
4. Aortic arch interruption anomalies.

137. Maintenance of patency is attempted in ductus dependent conditions since it plays a vital role in the maintenance of pulmonary and systemic flow. There are 4 steps of treatment for the maintenance of patency.

1. Prostaglandin EI intravenously or through umbilical artery—0.1 μg/kg/min.
   If there is improvement in arterial oxygen saturation or pH.
2. Maintenance of dose of 0.01–0.075 μg/kg/min is continued.
   If no initial improvement.
3. Dose is increased to 0.4 μg/kg/min.
4. Metabolic acidosis is corrected by IV sodabicarbonate 0.5 μg/kg.

Aortopulmonary Septal Defect

It is a very rare anomalous communication between the left side of the ascending aorta and the right side of the main pulmonary trunk just above the semilunar valves. It is usually wide. Unusually, it is narrow.

138. 4 names (synonyms) are given to this deficiency of septum that divides primitive truncus arteriosus.

1. Aortopulmonary septal defect
2. Aortopulmonary window
3. Aortic septal defect
4. Partial truncus arteriosus.

139. Clinical features of aortopulmonary septal defect are similar to PDA. Those with small defects are similar to those with small PDA and those with large defects are similar to those with large PDA.

The following are the 4 distinguishing points of these two conditions.

Table L-3

Aortopulmonary septal defect	*Patent ductus arteriosus*
1. *Clinical features*	
A harsh systolic murmur is heard at the lower sternal border	A harsh continuous machinery murmur is heard in left 2nd ICS radiating to the left clavicle and along the left sternal border
2. *X-ray chest*	
Biventricular hypertrophy similar to that of large VSD is seen. Isolated right ventricular dilatation in young infants and old patients with pulmonary vascular disease Aortic knob not enlarged	Left atrium and left ventricular enlargement is seen Right ventricular enlargement depends on the status of the ductus—enlarges in wide opening Aortic knob is enlarged Fluoroscopy may reveal pulsating aortic knob
3. *Cardiac catheterization and aortogram*	
Venous catheter may cross defect and enter the ascending aorta Aortography demonstrates defect and associated anomalies	Catheter enters easily from the pulmonary artery thereafter descending aorta easily. Aortography delineates the ductus arteriosum
4. *Surgical management*	
Surgical risk is very high transaortic obliteration of septal defect by Dacron patch under cardiopulmonary bypass. Aortic valve leaflets, coronary arterial ostia, orifice of the pulmonary artery should be identified and protected	Surgical risk is very low with very good result. Closure of the ductus by transcatheter closure using prosthesis or by direct surgical closure

Catheterization and aortography is recommended in patients suspected of patent ductus arteriosus with any typical findings or evidence of pulmonary hypertension and in all patients with ventricular septal defect.

Endocardial Cushion Defects

It is also called as atrioventricular canal or persistent atrioventricular canal defect. This is common among patients with Down's syndrome.

140. A common atrioventricular canal may result from the maldevelopment of endocardial cushions, which are the dorsal (anterior) and ventral (posterior) tissues in the center of the fetal heart which give the following 4 structures:

1. The inferior part of the atrial septum above.
2. The upper part of the ventricular septum below.
3. The medial (anterior) leaflet of the mitral valve to the left side.
4. The septal leaflet of the tricuspid valve to the right side.

141. Any type of combination of endocardial cushion defect can occur. When there is defect of all 4 of the above structures, a complete AV canal results.

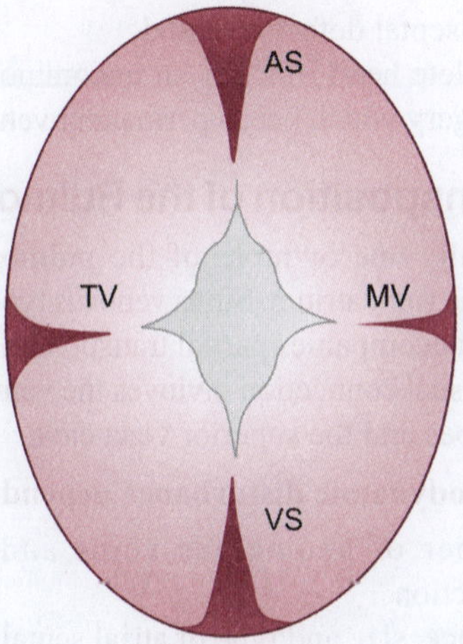

Fig. L-15

1. If the lower part of the atrial septum (AS) does not develop, an ostium primum ASD results.
2. If the upper part of ventricular septum (VS) does not develop, a VSD results.
3. If the medial cushion part of the mitral valve does not develop, a cleft mitral leaflet results.
4. If the medial part of the tricuspid valve does not develop, cleft tricuspid leaflet results.

142. There are 4 characteristic anatomical features of this defect.

1. Ostium primum type of atrial septal defect; the defect is situated at the lower end of the interatrial septum and is large. Upper margin is crescent shaped and there is no septum in the lower margin and is bounded by mitral and tricuspid valve—incomplete type.
2. Ventricular septal defect is present below the mitral and tricuspid valve in addition to atrial septal defect—complete type.
3. Anterior leaflet of mitral valve has a cleft and there is an abnormal attachment of the chordae tendineae to result in mitral incompetence in both types.
4. Septal leaflet of tricuspid valve may show similar deformity but less frequently.

143. Hemodynamics.

1. Left-to-right shunt in incomplete type is at the atrial level and shows features of atrial septal defect and mitral incompetence unlike secundum type.
2. Complete type shows left-to-right shunt at atrial and ventricular level.
3. If the ventricular septal defect is large the right ventricle and pulmonary arterial pressures rise similar to large ventricular septal defect.
4. Coexistence of mitral regurgitation causes shunting of blood from left ventricle to right atrium.

144. Clinical features.

1. Mild mitral regurgitation is tolerated quite well. Moderate to severe mitral regurgitation is associated with easy fatiguability, frequent respiratory infections, underdevelopment and cardiac failure. Patients with complete atrioventricular canal defect are very sick.
2. In incomplete type, the findings are those of atrial septal defect unless the mitral valve is incompetent. In mitral regurgitation, the findings are of the mitral regurgitation.
3. In complete type the findings are that of ventricular septal defect and mitral regurgitation.
   Pulmonary second sound split suggests an associated atrial septal defect.
4. In some, murmurs of mitral and tricuspid regurgitation are found.

145. Chest roentgenogram.

1. Marked cardiac enlargement
2. Pulmonary hyperemia

} Features of complete atrioventricular canal defect

3. Combined ventricular dilatation distinguishes primum defect with mitral regurgitation from secundum type of atrial septal defect.
4. Absence of left atrial dilatation with clinical and radiological findings of large left-to-right shunt would suggest complete atrioventricular canal defect.

146. Electrocardiogram: This is helpful in distinguishing atrioventricular canal defects from those with isolated atrial septal defect or ventricular septal defect.

1. Characteristic superior orientation of mean QRS axis in the frontal plane lying between 0–150° in 90–95% of cases. 70% with partial canal will have axis between 0–90° and 20% will have an axis between –91° to –150°.
2. PQ interval is prolonged in both partial and complete type.
3. Biatrial hypertrophy.
4. Biventricular hypertrophy.

A left axis deviation is so common with endocardial cushion defect and so rare with atrial septal defect, at higher levels, that differentiation of the ASD primum from the secondum and sinus venosus defects is quiet possible.

147. Echocardiogram: 2D echocardiogram visualizes

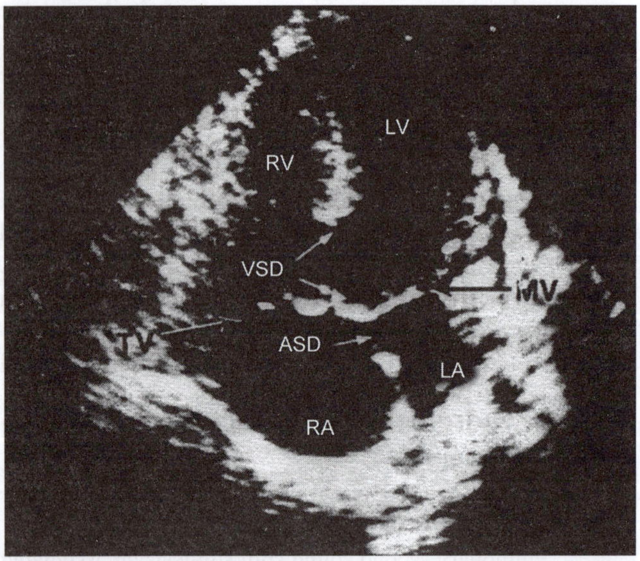

Fig. L-16: Two-dimensional echocardiogram: Apical four chamber view of a patient with endocardial cushion defect. Shows perimembranous ventricular septal defect (VSD) and atrial septal defect (ASD) of primum type. LA = left atrium; LV = left ventricle; RA = right atrium; RV = right ventricle; MV = mitral valve; TV = tricuspid valve

1. Atrial septal defect.
2. Mitral valve attachment to the ventricular septum in incomplete type.
3. Atrial and ventricular components of complete canal.
4. Displaced and cleft anterior leaflet of mitral valve with or without associated atrial or ventricular septal defect.

Echo with transesophageal probe is very helpful in detecting the difficult cases.

148. Cardiac catheterization and angiography.

1. Catheter passes across ventricles easily.
2. Increased oxygen saturation between superior vena cava and right atrium is present in both incomplete and complete type.
3. Right ventricular and pulmonary arterial systolic pressure in excess of 60% of systemic systolic pressure favors the presence of complete canal.
4. Left ventricular angiography demonstrates characteristic goose-neck (swan) deformity of the left ventricular outflow tract.

149. Surgical management.

1. Palliative surgery: Pulmonary banding deserves consideration in a very sick, small infant with large ventricular septal defect and a markedly increased pulmonary blood flow.
2. The atrioventricular canal defect is corrected by pericardial patch.
3. Cleft in the mitral valve is closed.
   Valve may require replacement.
   Atrial septal defect is closed.
4. Complete heart block is an uncommon complication of surgery which needs permanent ventricular pacing.

Partial Transposition of the Pulmonary Veins

In this anomaly, one or more of the pulmonary veins are connected to the right atrium. Sinus venosus type of atrial septal defect usually accompanies partial transposition of pulmonary veins and the usual connection invloves the veins of right upper and middle lobes and the superior vena cava.

150. The hemodynamic disturbance depends on 4 factors.

1. Number of anomalous veins and their site of connection.
2. Presence, size and type of atrial septal defect.
3. State of the pulmonary vascular bed.
4. Other associated defects.

Physical findings are similar to that of atrial septal defect in isolated partial transposition of pulmonary veins.

151. 'Scimitar syndrome' is a characteristic roentgenographic finding which consists of:

1. Partial transposition of pulmonary veins associated with.
2. Pulmonary parenchymal abnormalities.
3. Hypoplasia of right pulmonary artery and lung.
4. Dextroposition of the heart.

A crescent-like shadow is seen in right lower lung field which is produced by the anomalous venous channel.

TETRALOGY OF FALLOT

It is the most common cyanotic congenital heart disease above the age of 2 years comprising 10% of all congenital heart diseases. It occurs in approximately 1 in 3000 live births.

152. The 4 components of tetralogy of Fallot are:

1. Pulmonary stenosis giving rise to right ventricular outflow obstruction.
2. Ventricular septal defect.
3. Dextroposition of aorta overriding the ventricular septal defect.
4. Right ventricular hypertrophy.

The term pseudotruncus arteriosus is applied when the obstruction is complete.

153. The 4 anatomical features of tetralogy of Fallot are:

1. Ventricular septal defect: It is located at the upper part of the septum just below the aortic valve and is approximately the size of the aortic orifice.

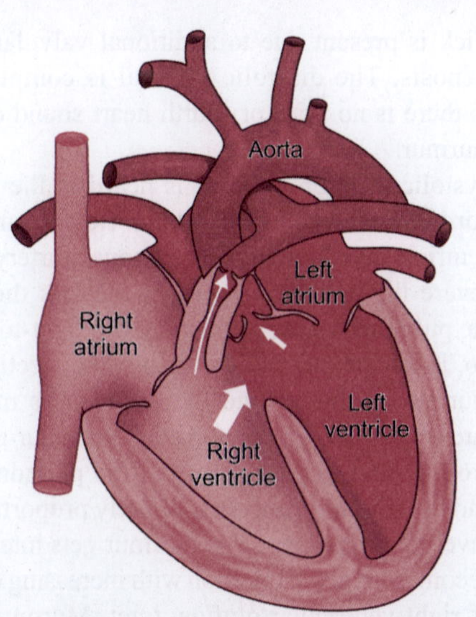

Fig. L-17: Tetralogy of Fallot: The stenosis is in the infundibulum of right ventricle

2. Pulmonary valve is bicuspid or unicuspid. Pulmonary stenosis is generally infundibular but may be both infundibular and valvular. Right ventricular outflow tract obstruction is the cause of right-to-left shunt.
3. Aorta has biventricular origin and its root is displaced anteriorly overriding the septal defect. Aorta is wider than normal. Sometimes, the aortic arch is right sided.
4. Right ventricular hypertrophy is the normal consequence of various abnormalities.

Rarely, it is associated with atrial septal defect when it is referred as pentalogy of Fallot.

154. There are 4 hemodynamic consequences of tetralogy of Fallot.

1. Ventricular septal defect is as large as the aortic orifice, so both ventricles and aorta essentially have the same systolic pressures. Since the pressure in right ventricle cannot exceed the left ventricular pressure due to large ventricular septal defect the right ventricle is otherwise 'protected' from excessive work. Since the right ventricle is effectively decompressed by the VSD, congestive cardiac failure never occurs in TOF.
   When the right ventricular pressure is high as the left ventricular or the aortic pressure, a right-to-left shunt appears to decompress the right ventricle. When the right and left ventricular pressures have become identical, increasing severity of pulmonary stenosis, reduces the flow of blood into the pulmonary artery and increases right-to-left shunt. As the systolic pressures between the two ventricles are identical, there is little or no left-to-right shunt and the VSD is silent. The right-to-left shunt is also silent since it occurs at insignificant difference in pressures between the right ventricle and the aorta. So, there is no shunt murmur.
2. Since there is severe pulmonary stenosis with large ventricular septal defect, a right-to-left shunt is present. The clinical features depend on the ratio between the resistance to the flow into the pulmonary artery and resistance to flow into the aorta. When the resistance to the right ventricular flow is low, the pulmonary flow may be twice the systemic flow and the arterial oxygen saturation may be within normal limits and there may be no cyanosis—referred to as acyanotic tetralogy of Fallot. Whereas, when the resistance to the pulmonary flow is great, sometimes even three to four times the systemic resistance with right-to-left shunt, arterial oxygen unsaturation and subsequent cyanosis, polycythemia, etc. are present.
   Physiologically, the pulmonary stenosis causes concentric hypertrophy of right ventricle without cardiac enlargement and an increase in right ventricular pressure. Concentric right ventricular hypertrophy reduces the distensibility of the right ventricle during diastole. The right atrial contraction at the end of diastole causes relatively large 'A' wave in jugular venous pulse. They may become too tall when right ventricular dysfunction is present.
   The flow from the right ventricle into the stenosed pulmonary artery produces an ejection systolic murmur. The more severe the pulmonic stenosis, the less the flow into the pulmonary artery and bigger the right-to-left shunt. Thus, the more severe the pulmonary stenosis, the shorter the ejection systolic murmur and the more cyanosis. The right ventricular outflow obstruction results in a delay of the P_2, i.e. the pulmonary artery pressure is reduced, P_2 is also reduced in intensity. The late and soft P_2 is generally inaudible in TOF.
3. Squatting relieves breathlessness and faintness after exercise in tetralogy of Fallot. The exact cause is not known.
   The arterial oxygen saturation returns to its resting value more rapidly after squatting. The pressure on the abdomen with folded legs causes compression of abdominal aorta and femorals which increases the peripheral vascular resistance and decreases the flow from the aorta. Squatting usually increases venous return resulting in increased right ventricular stroke volume pressure and pulmonary blood flow.
4. Severity of the cyanosis is directly proportional to the severity of pulmonary stenosis whereas the intensity of the systolic murmur is inversely proportional to the severity of pulmonary stenosis. Cyanotic spells may result from decrease in peripheral resistance and systemic arterial pressure resulting in decrease of right ventricular pressure and pulmonary blood flow. Worsening of cyanosis during crying, feeding,

breath holding, etc. are presumably due to decrease in pulmonary blood flow.

155. Clinical features of tetralogy of Fallot.

Symptoms may start in infancy but generally little later and progressive. The majority of children are first brought around 6 months of age for cyanosis.

1. The most common symptoms are dyspnea on exertion and exercise intolerance. Children assume squatting position as soon as they become dyspnic while resting after exercise. Squatting after exertion is common in children between 2–10 years and is pathognomonic of tetralogy of Fallot. Although squatting is not specific for TOF, it is the most common congenital lesion in which squatting is noted.
   Anoxic spells occur more commonly after waking up or following exertion. The child starts crying, becomes dyspnic, bluer than before and may loose consciousness. Convulsions occur frequently from once in a few days to numerous attacks every day.
2. Cyanosis at birth or develops before one year.
   If the right ventricular outflow tract obstruction is severe, marked cyanosis is seen from birth or when the ductus closes. Sudden increase in cyanosis, associated with hypoxic spells are common between 2 months and 2 years. Infection and exertion aggravate the cyanosis. Prolonged severe cyanotic episodes can lead to syncope, convulsions and even death. Central cyanosis is increased by exertion or emotional stress.
3. General growth is retarded, underdeveloped and undernourished. Growth is generally normal unless there is severe cyanosis.
4. Severe clubbing of fingers and toes. Clubbing occurs after 3 months of age and is proportional to the severity of cyanosis.
5. Slightly prominent 'A' wave in jugular venous pulse. Concentric hypertrophy of right ventricle reduces the diastolic filling. The right atrial contraction at the end of diastole causes a relatively large 'A' wave, but they are not too tall unless the right ventricular dysfunction is present. Heart size is normal with a mild right ventricular parasternal heave. Apex is difficult to palpate. Systolic thrill may be felt in the 3rd intercostal space along the left sternal border.
6. First sound is normal. Second sound is single and the pulmonary component is not heard. Since the pulmonary artery pressure is reduced, the P_2 intensity is reduced. The right ventricular outflow obstruction causes delay of the P_2. The soft and delayed P_2 is generally inaudible in TOF. Thus, the audible S_2 is single and is A_2. Since the aorta is somewhat displaced anteriorly, the audible A_2 is quiet loud. Ejection click is more frequent due to a large aorta or inconstant ejection click is present due to additional valvular pulmonic stenosis. The diastolic interval is completely clear as there is no third or fourth heart sound or diastolic murmur.
7. Systolic ejection murmur is heard in the left sternal border. It is produced by the flow from the right ventricle into the stenosed pulmonary artery. The more severe the pulmonic stenosis, the less the flow into the pulmonary artery and more the right-to-left shunt. So, in severe pulmonic stenosis, the ejection systolic murmur is shorter and the cyanosis is more. Thus, intensity of the ejection systolic murmur is inversely proportional to the severity of the pulmonic stenosis and severity of cyanosis is directly proportional to the severity of istenosis. The murmur gets intensified and becomes longer in duration with increasing obstruction of right ventricular outflow tract. Murmur decreases in intensity during hypoxic spells, polycythemia, decreased systemic vascular resistance.
8. A continuous murmur over the paravertebral area may indicate collateral circulation to the lungs through bronchial arteries.
   Sounds:
   - S_1—Normal
   - S_2—Single—only A_2 heard
   - P_2—Soft and delayed, inaudible
   - X—Constant, more frequent

   Inconstant: If valvular PS
   Murmur: Shunt murmur absent
   Flow murmur: Pulmonary ejection systolic murmur
   The smaller the flow, the shorter the murmur.

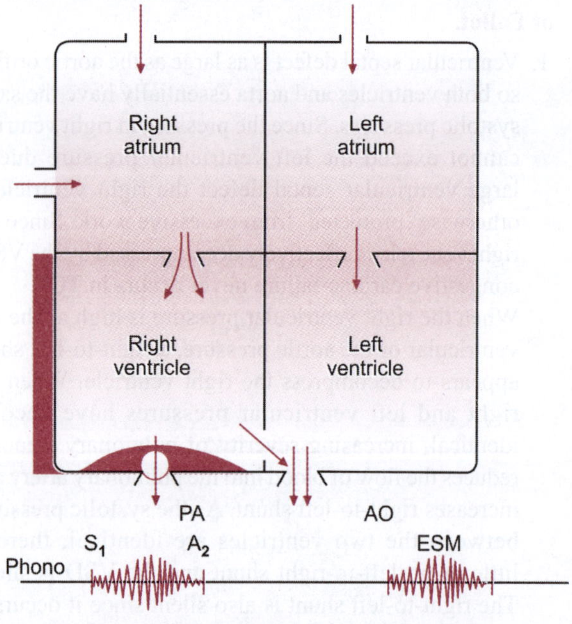

Fig. L-18: Auscultatory findings in TOF

156. Congestive cardiac failure is rare in TOF because ventricular septal defect is always large enough to allow free flow to the right-to-left shunt. Since the right ventricle is protected by the effective decompression by the ventricular septal defect, congestive failure never occurs in TOF. The 4 exceptions are the presence of:

1. Anemia
2. Infective endocarditis
3. Systemic hypertension
4. Unrelated myocarditis.

It is the prime duty of the physician to prevent or treat these complications before palliative or corrective surgery.

157. The 4 important findings in chest roentgenogram are:

1. Normal sized boot-shaped heart with elevated apex. Right ventricular enlargement is seen in lateral view.
2. The pulmonary segment is concave in the region of the pulmonary conus. The concavity of the pulmonary conus and elevated apex gives boot-shaped contour. The absence of pulmonary artery segment gives it the shape described as "Corur en Sabot".
3. Pulmonary vascularity is reduced—pulmonary oligemia.
4. Aortic shadow is prominent. Aortic knuckle may be right sided in some cases.

158. Check the following 4 findings in electrocardiogram.

1. Right ventricular hypertrophy
2. Right axis deviation between +90° and +210°.
3. Right atrial hypertrophy—P 'Pulmonale' may present in some patients.
4. If the axis is superior, suspect single ventricle, double outlet right ventricle with pulmonary stenosis, endocardial cushion defect.

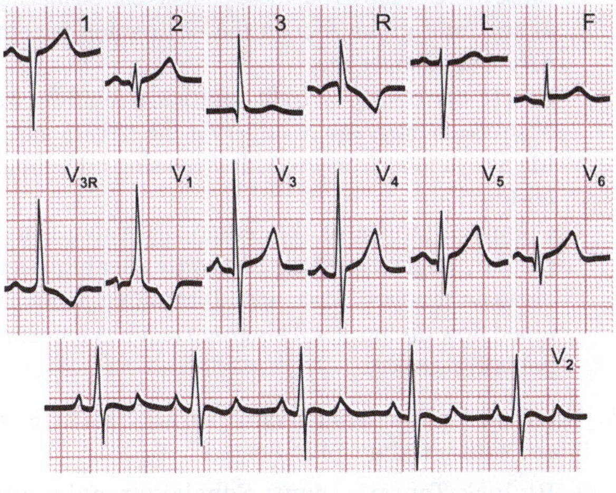

Fig. L-19: ECG of tetralogy of Fallot: Note marked RAD (+150°) with RVH. T waves become upright in V_2

159. Echocardiogram is a very useful tool in TOF. It helps in finding out some of the associated anomalies.

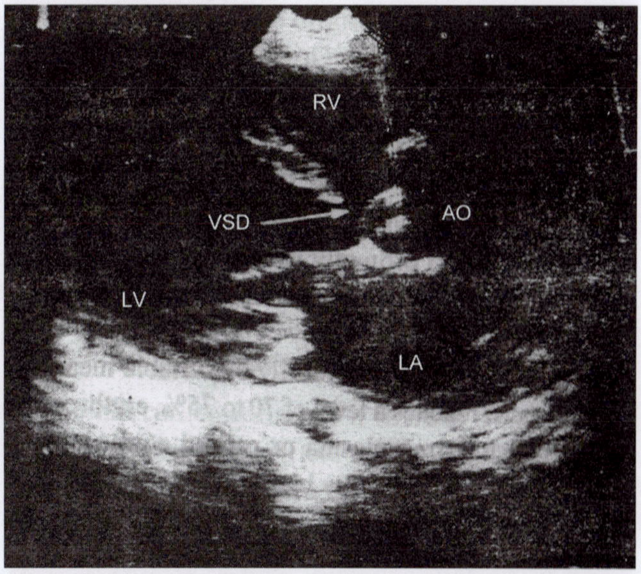

Fig. L-20: Two-dimensional echocardiogram: Parasternal long axis of a patient with Fallot's tetralogy. Aorta (AO) is overriding the ventricular septal defect (VSD). LA = left atrium; LV = left ventricle; RV = right ventricle

1. It demonstrates the discontinuity of the ventricular septum with aortic wall by lack of echoes.
2. Right ventricular hypertrophy.
3. Narrowing of the outflow tract.
4. Anteriorly displaced dilated aorta.
5. Small pulmonary artery.
   Pulmonary valve may be difficult to identify. If this could not be recorded, truncus arteriosus and ventricular septal defect with pulmonary atresia could not be excluded.
6. Left atrium is small in tetralogy of Fallot whereas normal or enlarged in truncus arteriosus.
7. Anterior mitral valve continuation with posterior aortic wall excludes double outlet of the right ventricle with pulmonary stenosis.
8. Associated endocardial cushion defects can be recorded.

160. Cardiac catheterization in tetralogy of Fallot.

1. Right ventricular, left ventricular and aortic systolic pressures are equal.
   - Right atrial pressure is almost normal.
   - Systemic pressure gradient across the right ventricular outflow tract can be recorded if the valve is crossed. If the pulmonary artery is entered, pressure is normal or low.

2. Catheter easily passes from right ventricle into the aorta
3. Aortic and left ventricular oxygen saturations are reduced
4. If there is associated atrial septal defect, there will be an additional right-to-left or bidirectional shunt at atrial level.

161. Cineangiography demonstrates.

1. Site and severity of obstruction
2. Site and size of the ventricular septal defect
3. Position and size of the pulmonary arteries
4. Position and size of aorta and coronary anomalies if any.

162. Complications of tetralogy of Fallot are:

1. Iron deficiency anemia
2. Infective endocarditis
3. Hypoxic spells
4. Paradoxic embolism
5. Polycythemia
6. Coagulation defects
7. Cerebral infarction
8. Cerebral abscess.

163. TOF patients die in infancy or childhood if not managed properly. Patients rarely reach middle age. Death usually results from 4 causes.

1. Hypoxic episodes
2. Infective endocarditis
3. Cerebral abscess
4. Cerebrovascular accidents.

164. Medical management: It is primarily directed toward the prevention and treatment of complications.

1. Iron deficiency anemia is treated with iron supplementation
2. Infections are treated promptly with suitable antibiotics. Prophylactic antibiotics are recommended for prevention of infective endocarditis.
3. Hypoxic spells are treated carefully by suitable measures.
4. If the hematocrit reaches a level of 70–75%, erythropheresis is done using fresh frozen plasma or colloid equivalent. This will temporarily relieve viscosity but definitive surgery is indicated.

165. There are 4 important steps in the treatment of paroxysmal cyanotic spells of tetralogy of Fallot. (see 276)

1. Oxygen in high concentration—Place the child in knee-chest position.
2. Injection morphine 0.1–0.2 mg/kg.
3. Correction of dehydration with intravenous fluids and metabolic acidosis with IV sodium bicarbonate.
4. Vasopressors, β-adrenergic blockers or general anesthesia in severe attacks with prolonged hypoxic spells.

Propranolol should be given orally for prevention and intravenously for severe hypoxic spells.

166. There are 4 ways of management of children with TOF who are symptomatic and progressive.

1. In a severely cyanotic newborn, prostaglandin is administered to open the ductus until the surgery is done—as with pulmonary atresia.
2. Palliation with propranolol followed by delayed correction.
3. Palliative surgery with a shunt from systemic artery to the pulmonary artery and delayed correction.
4. Early corrective surgery.

167. The aim of the surgery is:

1. Complete closure of the ventricular septal defect with a Dacron patch to the right of the aorta accommodating its dextroposition.
2. Relief of right ventricular outflow obstruction.
3. Preservation of sinus rhythm.
4. Preservation of competent pulmonary valves.

168. The severity of the clinical features is directly related to the degree of right ventricular outflow obstruction/ hypoplasia. The presence of small pulmonary arteries or pulmonary atresia needs two stage operation. There are 4 guidelines to observe while deciding surgery with reference to the right ventricular outflow obstruction.

1. Patients with only pulmonary valve stenosis and mild infundibular hypertrophy are the least cyanotic and they can be managed easily. Adequate pulmonary valvotomy preserves the valve. Infundibulectomy with or without a patch relieves right ventricular infundibular obstruction.
2. Moderate right ventricular outflow obstruction may cause more cyanosis but these patients can be managed as the mild group though the obstruction becomes severe at younger age.
3. Severe narrowing of right ventricular outflow tract obstruction may require surgery in the early months of life as cyanosis worsens with increasing infundibular obstruction.
4. Complete atresia of the pulmonary valve usually requires surgical intervention shortly after birth as the ductus arteriosus closes and all effective pulmonary blood flow disappears. This group requires immediate palliative surgery.

169. There are 4 methods of palliative surgery in a high-risk infant with tetralogy of Fallot.

1. Blalock-Taussig shunt: Subclavian-pulmonary anastomosis. The divided end of the right subclavian artery (usually on the opposite side of the aortic arch)

is anastomosed to the cephelad side of the pulmonary artery of the same side. This was the first palliative surgery done for TOF and is still preferred method to increase the pulmonary blood flow with less complications.
2. Pott's shunt: The descending aorta is anastomosed to the pulmonary artery.
3. Waterson's shunt: The ascending aorta is anastomosed to the right pulmonary artery.
4. Valvulotomy/transventricular infundibulectomy.

The definitive surgery is done at a later date when the risk is less. Potts shunt and Watterson shunt were abandoned owing to associated uncontrolled pulmonary blood flow progressing to pulmonary hypertension.

170. Incredible risk factors of corrective surgery are:

1. Pulmonary arterial problem
2. Previous palliative procedure
3. Size of the patient
4. Hematocrit
5. Transluminar patch
6. Early operation
7. Absent pulmonary valve
8. Major associated anomaly.

171. There are 4 points to observe in definitive corrective surgery of tetralogy of Fallot. It is done under cardiopulmonary bypass.

1. Closure of the ventricular septal defect with a Dacron graft patch to the right of aorta accommodating into dextroposition. Careful suturing of the Dacron graft is made with a continuous suture with stitches placed so as to avoid the area occupied by the bundle of His.
2. Release of right ventricular outflow tract obstruction across the pulmonary annulus extending to pulmonary artery and patching with pericardium or prosthetic material. Obviously the valve function is destroyed by this procedure but usually valvular incompetence is better tolerated than obstruction. Need of transannular patch at the time of repair is based on pulmonary annular diameter and the ratio of right ventricular to left ventricular systolic pressure. These can be predicted with reasonable accuracy by preoperative angiography and annular measurements during surgery. Relief of right ventricular outflow tract obstruction without right ventriculotomy is preferred to preserve right ventricular function. Precise calculation and operative judgment of enlarging the outflow tract region gives good results.
3. In the absence of continuity of right ventricle and pulmonary artery, a prosthetic conduit is used to connect these structures. In infants and children, conduit may not contain valve but in older patients, a valvular conduit gives good results.
4. Correction of associated anomalies, if any.

172. Complications after repair of TOF.

1. Residual ventricular septal defect
2. Residual pulmonary stenosis
3. Right ventricular aneurysm
4. Right ventricular dysfunction
5. Pulmonary regurgitation
6. Tricuspid regurgitation
7. Complete heart block
8. RBBB with or without left anterior hemiblock.

Prognosis of corrective surgery is usually good. Early primary closure in infancy gives better results and improved long-term left ventricular function. Surgery carries more risk in adults than in children.

173. Prognosis after surgery is predicted by the following 4 factors:

1. Residual ventricular septal defect
2. Distal pulmonary stenosis
3. Pulmonary regurgitation
4. Impaired right ventricular function.

Tricuspid Atresia

Tricuspid atresia is a condition where the tricuspid valve is absent or imperforate. There are many ways the valve can be imperforate—the leaflets of the valve may be formed but tightly stuck to each other, or may not be formed at all, with muscle tissue of the heart forming a wall where the valve should have been.

The right ventricle is hypoplastic.

174. The hemodynamic consequences depend on the presence of other defects.

1. Cyanosis: As the blood cannot pass to the right ventricle and pulmonary artery and the lungs for oxygenation.
2. Risk of paradoxical embolism.
3. In the absence of tricuspid valve, blood cannot flow across the valve from right atrium to right ventricle. And if there is no alternate route, circulation of blood is not possible. But mother nature always has the solution to such problems ready.
These children usually have associated atrial septal defect (ASD) blood flows from right atrium to left atrium. It then flows into the left ventricle from where it may take a variable path.
4. Further course depends on the presence of other defects, such as pulmonary stenosis (PS) and transposition of great arteries (TGA). In the presence of pulmonary stenosis, deep cyanosis will be present necessitating

early repair. If there is transposition of great arteries, blood flow into the aorta may be reduced. Left ventricle, therefore, maintains both the systemic as well as the pulmonary circulation. The oxygen saturation in the pulmonary artery and the aorta is identical. The saturation of blood in the aorta depends on the size of pulmonary blood flow. The larger the pulmonary blood flow, the more the oxygenated blood coming back to the left atrium to mix with the unoxygenated blood coming from the right atrium and the higher the final mixed sample saturation.

A small ventricular septal defect (VSD) is always present.

175. Clinical features: It depends on the state of pulmonary blood flow which may be diminished or increased. 90% of patients have diminished pulmonary blood flow. Symptoms and physical signs are more or less similar to TOF. They are cyanotic from birth. Anoxic spells and squatting may be present. The patients are relatively sicker than patients of TOF. Features suggesting tricuspid atresia are:

1. Left ventricular type of apical impulse
2. Prominent large 'A' wave in JVP
3. Enlarged liver with presystolic pulsations
4. First sound is of mitral component.

Patients of tricuspid atresia with increased pulmonary blood flow cannot be generally diagnosed accurately clinically.

176. The 4 findings in chest roentgenogram are:

1. Cardiac silhouette is left ventricular type with a broad apex.
2. Right atrium is enlarged.
3. Superior vena cava shadow is prominent.
4. Lungs are oligemic.

177. Check the 4 findings in the electrocardiogram.

1. Left axis deviation
2. Left ventricular hypertrophy
3. Right atrial hypertrophy—P 'Pulmonale'
4. May show left atrial hypertrophy.

Medical management is similar to TOF. Surgery is done to prolong the life of these patients. There is no definitive operation since the absence of right ventricular inflow portion cannot be corrected.

Surgery is mainly palliative Fontana operation. This consists of anastomosing the right atrium to the pulmonary artery, and closing the ASD. Blood entering the right atrium from the veins passes across this surgical connection into the pulmonary artery and to the lungs. It completely bypasses the right ventricle.

Pulmonary Atresia

No pulmonary valve exists.

178. Hemodynamics.

1. As the pulmonary valve does not exist, the blood cannot flow from the right ventricle into the pulmonary artery and on to the lungs. The right ventricle acts as a blind pouch that may stay small and not well developed. Tricuspid valve is often poorly developed, too.
2. ASD is usually present through which blood passes to the left atrium and left ventricle.
3. The left ventricle pumps the unsaturated oxygen blood to the body.
4. The child appears cyanotic.

The only source of lung blood flow is the patent ductus. If the PDA narrows or closes, severe cyanosis develops. Early management includes using a drug to keep the PDA from closing. (L-133)

Surgery is by creating a shunt between aorta and pulmonary artery to help the blood flow to the lungs. If the right ventricle is too small to be a pumping chamber, the right atrium is directly connected to the pulmonary artery (Fontana operation).

COMPLETE TRANSPOSITION OF THE GREAT ARTERIES

This condition is an abnormal origin of the great arteries as aorta arising from the right ventricle and pulmonary trunk from the left ventricle. The incidence is approximately 20–30 in 1 lakh live births: This is also known as dTGA in which 'd' refers to the dextroposition of the bulboventricular loop, which is characterized by right-sided RV. The coronary anatomy was also variable.

179. The 4 anatomical features of transposition of the great arteries are:

1. Aorta arises from right ventricle.
2. Pulmonary artery arises from left ventricle.
3. Aorta is located to the right and anterior to the pulmonary artery.
4. Aortic valve level is higher than usual.

180. Some epidemiological features of transposition of the great arteries.

1. It is an important cyanotic congenital heart disease in infancy barring tetralogy of Fallot and account approximately 10% of all cyanotic heart diseases.
2. It occurs frequently in the offspring of diabetic mothers.
3. More males are affected than females. Male to female ratio is 2:1.
4. It is the common cause of death from congestive cardiac failure in congenital heart disease in the first 2 months of life.

181. Hemodynamics in transposition of great arteries.

1. The systemic venous return is conducted back to the systemic arterial system due to the origin of aorta from right ventricle.
2. Pulmonary venous return back to the pulmonary arterial system due to the origin of pulmonary artery from left ventricle.
3. There is mixing or interchanging of blood. Hemodynamic effects depend on the combination of associated defects particularly which can cause mixing of blood. There must be a communication such as ASD, VSD, PDA or patent foramen ovale for survival.
4. The right ventricle is the systemic ventricle and its systolic pressure is same as systemic arterial pressure.

182. The life can be sustained if there is a communication either in the atrium, ventricle or persistent ductus. Rarely a patient survives into young adult life. Those who live beyond infancy may have any of the following 4 associated anomalies:

1. Large ventricular septal defect
2. Large atrial septal defect
3. Single ventricle
4. Pulmonary stenosis.

183. Clinical features of transposition of the great arteries.

The clinical features depend on the associated anomalies such as ASD, VSD, PDA, patent foramen ovale. Absence of these produce severe hypoxia.

1. Significant cyanosis at birth or few hours or days is the presenting symptom or sign and it is progressive. Infants with large ventricular septal defect and significant pulmonary stenosis may present within the first few days of life with cyanosis if the pulmonary stenosis is severe. They present little late with cyanosis if the pulmonary stenosis is mild or moderate. Infants with large ventricular septal defect present with signs of congestive cardiac failure with mild cyanosis.
2. Tachycardia, breathlessness, and failure to thrive are characteristic.
3. Retardation of growth.
4. Signs of congestive cardiac failure are seen. Congestive heart failure is the common cause of death from congenital heart disease.
5. Forceful or hyperdynamic right ventricular lift.
6. First sound is loud. Second sound is single due to poor pulmonary valve or may be narrowly split confirming the presence of two semilunar valves.
7. Systolic murmur may present or absent. Stenotic murmur of greater intensity and duration may be present than expected in tetralogy of Fallot with similar degree of cyanosis.
8. Gallop rhythm.

184. Chest roentgenogram is highly suggestive. The 4 characteristic findings are:

1. Cardiomegaly after the first few days.
2. Heart may resemble egg-on-side appearance.
3. Supracardiac shadow is narrow.
4. Pulmonary vascular markings increased.

185. Electrocardiogram in cases of intact ventricular septum shows.

1. Peaked 'P' waves by 2nd or 3rd day.
2. Persistent upright T waves in V1, V3R after 4 days. It gives a clue that right ventricular systolic pressure is at systemic level.
3. Right ventricular hypertrophy may appear after 4 days.
4. Right axis deviation with marked right ventricular hypertrophy in older infants.

186. Echocardiogram: Two-dimensional study helps in identifying.

1. Origin of the aorta from the right ventricle.
2. Origin of the pulmonary artery from the left ventricle.
3. Associated other anomalies.
4. Atrial septal opening using subxiphoid approach—which can help in judging the success of balloon septostomy or surgical septectomy.

187. Cardiac catheterization and angiography are performed as an emergency specially in a very sick and severely cyanotic newborn.

1. Pulmonary arterial oxygen saturation is invariably higher than the systemic arterial oxygen saturation.
2. The right ventricular pressure is at systemic level; the left ventricular pressure is lower but it can be at systemic level if there is a large ASD, VSD or PDA with pulmonary stenosis. A wide pressure difference between the two atria or ventricles is suggestive of intact atrial or ventricular septum.
   Selective ventricular angiography demonstrates.
3. Anteriorly placed aorta arising from the right ventricle.
4. Posteriorly placed pulmonary artery arising from the left ventricle.

188. Management: 90% mortality by the first year of life and still worse outcomes without associated lesions for adequate mixing of blood.

At birth, the infants are treated with intravenous prostaglandin E to keep the ductus arteriosus (patent) open and some may undergo Raskind palliative surgery to improve oxygenation until definitive surgery.

It responds poorly to the medical treatment. It consists of management of hypoxia, congestive heart failure, infections, endocarditis, etc. and prevention of hypothermia and hypoglycemia.

Surgical Management

An immediate palliative procedure should be done for the survival of infant. An adequate interatrial opening is necessary whether it is created by balloon-induced septostomy or surgically created. Infants will do better during the first week with intact ventricular septum. This is followed later by corrective surgery—Senning operation or Mustard operation.

1. First step is to do balloon atrial septostomy (Rashkind procedure) without any delay. The benefit of this is determined by increase in systemic arterial oxygen saturation above 60% or PO_2 above 30 mm Hg. The adequacy of the opening can also be noticed by two-dimensional echocardiography.
   If the opening is inadequate.
2. Surgical atrial septectomy (Blalock-Hanlon) is performed without delay or corrective surgery if possible.
   If balloon-septostomy is not satisfactory but the size of the interatrial opening is adequate, judged by echocardiography a trial of intravenous arterial 'switch' operation now appears to be giving encouraging results as a palliative surgery though not superior or alternative to atrial septostomy, etc.
   Prostaglandin EI is recommended.
3. Systemic-to-pulmonary arterial shunt is performed in severe left ventricular outflow obstruction and decreased pulmonary blood flow.
   Pulmonary artery banding within the first 2 or 3 months may help in reducing the pulmonary arterial hypertension as an adjuvant in ventricular septal defect and pulmonary arterial hypertension to prevent severe pulmonary vascular obstructive disease.
   If the response is still not satisfactory.
4. Corrective surgery—Senning operation or Mustard operation is performed.

Repair of the basic defect is performed allowing venous return to flow across mitral valve to the left ventricle and pulmonary artery while the pulmonary venous blood is allowed to reach the right ventricle through the tricuspid valve on to the aorta.

External conduit is created with an aortic homograft between right ventricle and pulmonary artery in those children with ventricular septal defect. Ventricular septal defect repair is done so that the left ventricle ejects into the aorta.

CORRECTED TRANSPOSITION OF THE GREAT ARTERIES

The condition is associated with malformation and transposition of the ascending aorta and right-to-left reversal of the ventricles.

189. The 4 anatomical features are:

1. Aorta arises anteriorly and to the left of the pulmonary artery.
2. Functional right ventricle has the anatomic structure of the left ventricle and the atrioventricular valve resemble the bicuspid mitral valve.
3. The left ventricle has the anatomic structure of right ventricle but functions like the left ventricle and the atrioventricular valve resembles the tricuspid valve.
4. The aorta and pulmonary artery arise from the left-and right-sided ventricles, respectively.

The coexisting cardiac malformations especially VSD determine the symptomatology.

The condition may exhibit frequent arrhythmias and atrio-ventricular conduction disturbances. The abnormality is proved by the angiocardiogram.

When the condition exists as an isolated anomaly, it does not present with any symptoms and is compatible with normal life.

Hypoplastic Left Heart Syndrome

The term refers to the presence of obstructive lesion on the left side of the heart in association with hypoplasia of the left ventricle. The condition is associated with atresia of the aorta and mitral valve and atresia or hypoplasia of the aortic arch. There is right ventricular hypertrophy. The condition presents with sudden onset of cardiac failure in infants and is associated with high mortality.

190. Underdevelopment of the left side of the heart characterized by 4 features:

1. Aortic valve atresia
2. Hypoplastic ascending aorta
3. Hypoplastic/atretic mitral valve
4. Endocardial fibroelastosis.

191. The 4 hemodynamic manifestations are:

1. Pulmonary venous return is diverted from left atrium to right atrium through atrial septal defect.
2. Right ventricle supplies pulmonary artery, ductus arteriosus, descending aorta (antegrade flow), aortic arch, ascending aorta, coronary circulation (retrograde flow).
3. Leads to right ventricular overload.
4. Results in congestive heart failure.

Cause of 25% of cardiac deaths in 1st week of life. Prognosis is 100% fatal by 6 weeks.

Treatment consists of Norwood procedure (palliative)—three stage surgery that results in the right atrium feeding the pulmonary circulation and the right ventricle feeding the systemic circulation.

Heart transplantation is the treatment of choice.

TRANSPOSITION OF PULMONARY VEINS

192. There are 4 pulmonary veins, two from each lung. They are devoid of valves. Unlike other veins, they contain oxygenated blood. They bring oxygenated blood from the lungs to the atrium.

193. Transposition of pulmonary veins is a rare cyanotic heart disease where all the pulmonary veins connect either to the right atrium or to the systemic veins, the condition is called total anomalous pulmonary venous connection (TAPVC).

There are 4 types of transposition of pulmonary veins (total anomalous pulmonary venous connection TAPVC).

Supradiaphragmatic

Type-I: Supracardiac—where pulmonary veins drain into superior vena cava.

Type-II: Cardiac—where pulmonary veins drain into right atrium.

(Sometimes pulmonary veins may drain into coronary sinus or vena azygos).

Subdiaphragmatic

Type-III: Subdiaphragmatic—where pulmonary veins open into inferior vena cava or branches of hepatic venous system.

Type-IV: Where pulmonary veins open into multiple sites: very rare.

194. Characteristic physical findings in TAPVC are presence of multiple heart sounds. They are heard in the following manner.

1. First sound followed by an ejection click.
2. Fixed widely split second sound with an accentuation of pulmonary component.
3. Third heart sound.
4. Fourth heart sound.
   A midsystolic murmur can be heard along the left sternal border.

195. X-ray chest: Specific site of anomalous connection may give rise to a characteristic appearance of cardiac silhouette.

1. Prominent right atrium.
2. Prominent right ventricle.
3. Pulmonary plethora and enlarged pulmonary arterial segments.
4. If the left superior vena cava is persistent, the cardiac contour will show 'figure-of-eight' or 'snow-man' appearance due to large supracardiac shadow.

The management is like that of any cyanotic heart disease and needs lifesaving palliative procedure followed by corrective surgery.

DOUBLE OUTLET RIGHT VENTRICLE

A rare anomaly showing the origin of the aorta and pulmonary artery from the right ventricle. The condition is associated with ventricular septal defect. Sometimes there may be pulmonary stenosis in addition. The aorta is transposed so as to take its origin from right ventricle and the aortic and pulmonary valves remain side by side and the condition may present like ventricular septal defect of tetralogy of Fallot.

TRUNCUS ARTERIOSUS

It is a rare anomaly due to failure of development of septum between the aorta and pulmonary artery.

196. The anatomical features are:

1. Single vessel arises from both ventricles-truncus
2. Single valve
3. Generally truncus overrides a ventricular septal defect
4. Absence of outflow tract of the right ventricle.

197. 4 cusps are present in truncus arteriosus—quadricuspoid single valve.

198. Truncus arteriosus anomaly is classified into 4 types:

Type-I: Ascending aorta and main pulmonary artery arise from the truncus and the pulmonary artery divides into right and left pulmonary artery branches.

Type-II: Absence of the main pulmonary artery and right and left pulmonary arteries may arise independently from the posterior aspect of truncus arterious.

Type-III: Right and left pulmonary arteries arise from the lateral aspect of the truncus arteriosus.

Type-IV: Pulmonary arteries arise from the lateral aspect of descending aorta or there can be complete absence of them.

Type I, II and III may have normal pulmonary vascular resistance and they are like left-to-right shunt with mild cyanosis. Type IV shows increased pulmonary vascular resistance with marked cyanosis as in tetralogy of Fallot or Eisenmenger's syndrome. Surgical repair is possible in Type I, II and III with reconstruction of pulmonary outflow tract from right ventricle and closure of ventricular septal defect.

199. Truncus arteriosus should be distinguished from the following 4 anomalies.

1. Pulmonary atresia—small left ventricle and pulmonary oligemia.
2. Eisenmenger's complex.
3. Transposition of great vessels.
4. Tetralogy of Fallot.

EBSTEIN'S ANOMALY

Incidence is about 0.5% of congenital anomalies. The natural history varies from early death to adult survival depending on the degree of tricuspid valve involvement and types of arrhythmias that occur with increased risk of sudden death. There is an association with maternal lithium use. But most of them are sporadic.

200. It is a relatively infrequent anomaly of tricuspid valve with diminished pulmonary blood flow. There are 4 anatomical features of this anomaly.

1. Posterior leaflet and often medial (septal) leaflet of tricuspid valve are attached to the ventricular wall far below the annulus fibrosis. The leaflets originate from the ventricular wall than from atrioventricular ring. The anterior leaflet is attached normally to the annulus. Papillary muscles of the chordeae are usually malformed. Malformed and fused leaflets causes obstruction to the flow of blood into the right ventricle thereby diminishing the pulmonary blood flow. The tricuspid valve is generally incompetent.
2. Right ventricle is small: A portion of right ventricle proximal to the valve is continuous with right atrium and behaves like right atrium as 'atrialized' portion of right ventricle. However, the contraction of this is poor. Hypoplasia or atrophy of the right ventricular myocardium is common.
3. The right atrium is large.
4. The foramen ovale is usually present.

A right-to-left shunt of blood at the atrial level is present.
A varying of tricuspid incompetence is present.

201. Hemodynamics: The clinical features depend on the following:

1. There is obstruction to the right ventricular filling due to decrease in size of the right ventricle, a part of which is continuous with the large right atrium. The symptoms result from right ventricular dysfunction. The downward displaced septal leaflet can create accessory pathways and clinical Wolf-Parkinson-White syndrome is found in 10–25% of patients. The combination of atrial flutter or fibrillation conducted through the accessory pathway is poorly tolerated.
2. Tricuspid regurgitation.
3. Right atrium dilates to accommodate more blood
4. There is generally right-to-left shunt across foramen ovale resulting in cyanosis.

The more the tricuspid valve malformation, worse the cyanosis.

202. Symptoms.

1. Effort intolerance and fatigue with moderate cyanosis with clubbing is seen in children. Only few children with intact atrial septum do not develop cyanosis.
2. Symptoms of right heart failure develop in early infancy.
3. Palpitation due to supraventricular arrhythmias is a common occurrence.
4. Occasionally, syncope occurs due to arrhythmias or low cardiac output.

203. Signs.

1. Cyanosis and clubbing is present.
   Jugular venous pulse shows prominent 'V' waves but there is no venous engorgement.
   Apical impulse suggestive of left ventricular hypertrophy is unremarkable
2. Systolic thrill at the lower left sternal border.
   Enlarged liver with prominent systolic pulsations.
3. Wide splitting of the first and second sound. The second sound is widely split but variable with a soft pulmonic component. A right ventricular third sound/and or right atrial fourth sound may give rise to a characteristic cadence. Thus, the triple or quadruple sounds are usually heard.
4. The most common auscultatory findings are the regurgitant murmur of tricuspid regurgitation, gallop rhythm, multiple ejection sounds, and a widely split S_2. There may be mild systolic ejection murmur or a loud pansystolic murmur. There is also a short tricuspid delayed diastolic murmur. Both the systolic and diastolic murmurs produced at the tricuspid valve may have a scratchy character not unlike the pericardial friction rub.

Ejection systolic murmur of pulmonary stenosis.
The heart sounds and murmurs are accentuated during inspiration.

204. Chest roentgenogram shows:

1. Right atrial enlargement
2. Small right ventricle
3. Small pulmonary artery
4. Balloon-shaped heart giving a stencilled effect in the background of clear lung fields.

Pulmonary vascularity is reduced if the right-to-left shunt is large.

205. Electrocardiogram shows:

1. Giant peaked 'P' waves (Himalayan P waves).
2. Prolonged PR interval.
3. Incomplete or complete right bundle branch block.
4. Wolf-Parkinson-White syndrome may be noticed frequently in about 10% of cases with short PR and initial slurring of QRS—delta wave.

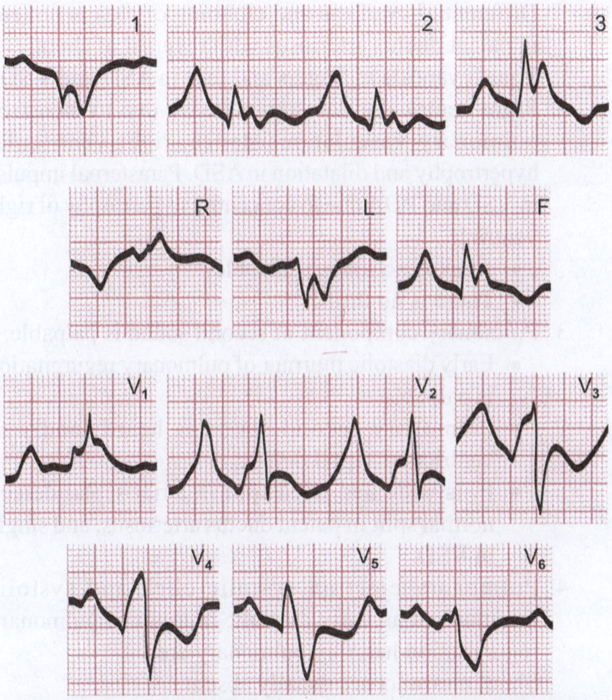

Fig. L-21: Electrocardiogram of a patient with Ebstein's anomaly. Note: giant P waves, low voltage, atypical RBBB

206. Echocardiogram.

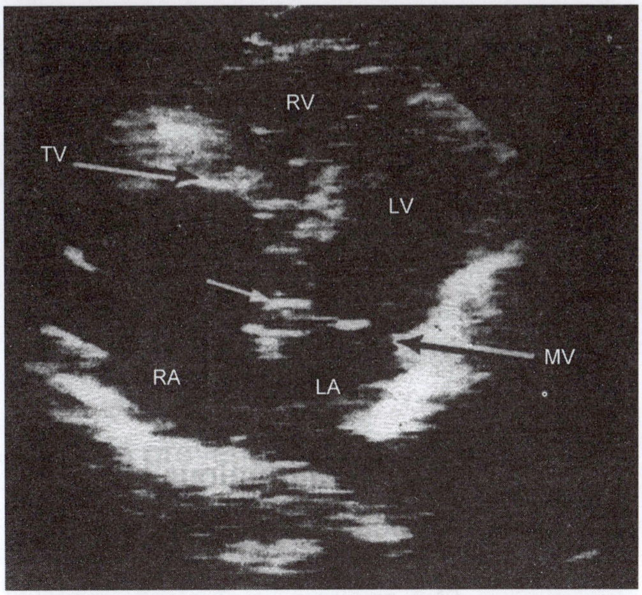

Fig. L-22: Two-dimensional echocardiogram of a patient with Ebstein's anomaly. Apical four chamber view. The tricuspid valve (TV) is displaced from the tricuspid annulus. Right ventricular volume is decreased; right atrial volume is increased. LA = Left atrium; LV = Left ventricle; MV = Mitral valve; RA = Right atrium; RV = Right ventricle

1. A large tricuspid valve with large anterior leaflet.
2. Marked displacement of tricuspid apparatus into right ventricular cavity.
3. Marked delay in closure of the tricuspid valve and it occurs after mitral valve closure.
4. Large right atrium and a small right ventricle.

207. Cardiac catheterization and angiocardiography: There is high-risk of cardiac catheterization due to frequent arrhythmias in this condition. The risk can be minimized by prompt cardioversion.

1. An intracardiac electrocardiogram with electrode proximal to the tricuspid valve during cardiac catheterization reveals.
   Right ventricular complex with the pressure recorded is that of right atrium. This is a good evidence of tricuspid valve displacement with an 'atrialized' portion of right ventricle.
2. It is difficult to enter into pulmonary artery but it is important to exclude associated pulmonary atresia in a cyanotic child.
3. Right ventricular angiography demonstrates abnormal attachment of the displaced tricuspid leaflets as a large sail or notch.
4. Left ventricular angiography should also be considered because of the frequent associated anomalies of left ventricle and mitral valve.

208. Medical management mainly consists of treatment of:

1. Right sided cardiac failure
2. Rhythm disturbance
3. Infective endocarditis
4. Cyanosis.

209. Surgical management consists of:

1. Reconstruction or replacement of displaced tricuspid valve with a porcine heterograft.
2. Plication of atrialized portion of right ventricle is desirable when the chamber contracts poorly or paradoxically.
3. Closure of atrial septal defect.
4. Surgical ablation of abnormal pathway of WPW syndrome during operation. Repair need not necessarily make free from supraventricular arrhythmias.

EISENMENGER'S SYNDROME

This term is used for pulmonary hypertension caused by reversal of shunt, i.e. left-to-right shunt in the beginning reverses to right-to-left shunt later, or bidirectional. This condition refers to the existence of large communication at the level of the atrium (ASD), ventricle (VSD) or aortopulmonary artery (PDA). Eisenmenger's 'complex' consists of pulmonary arterial hypertension with a ventricular septal defect providing the right-to-left shunt.

210. The progression or severity depends on the following 4 factors:

1. Prolonged exposure to large pulmonary blood flow.
2. High pulmonary arterial pressure.
3. Non-regression of fetal type of pulmonary vasculature.
4. Possible genetic predisposition.

Irreversible changes of pulmonary vascular disease may occur very early in life or may be delayed for several years.

211. Hemodynamics:

Pulmonary arterial hypertension is due to pulmonary vascular obstructive disease.

1. If a shunt is present at ventricular level (VSD) or pulmonary arterial level (PDA), the right ventricular pressure cannot go beyond systemic pressure. The right-to-left shunt decompresses the right ventricle. Thus, the right ventricle shows concentric hypertrophy without dilatation. This gives rise to mild parasternal impulse without a significant heave. In right-to-left shunt at atrial level (ASD) indicates right ventricular failure to accommodate the volume and push into the pulmonary artery. It results in parasternal heave and cardiac enlargement. The right ventricular pressure may be higher than systemic pressure.
2. A right-to-left shunt at atrial or ventricular level reaches the ascending aorta and is thus distributed to the whole systemic circulation. This results in equal cyanosis of fingers and toes. A right-to-left shunt of PDA is directed downwards into the descending aorta distal to the left subclavian artery. This results in differential cyanosis—fingers remain pink whereas toes show cyanosis. So, the differential cyanosis is diagnostic of pulmonary arterial hypertension with patent ductus arteriosus.
3. Pulmonary second sound is loud. P_2 is widely split and fixed in ASD, normal split in PDA and single in VSD. Pulmonary artery hypertension gives pulmonary ejection systolic click which unlike in valvular pulmonary stenosis, is well heard in both during inspiration and expiration.
4. A functional pulmonary regurgitation murmur can be present.

212. Signs of Eisenmenger's syndrome.

1. Central cyanosis and clubbing. Prominent 'A' wave in the jugular venous pulse.
   Differential cyanosis and clubbing of toes is noticed in patent ductus arteriosus with reversal of shunt. Equal cyanosis in fingers and toes in ASD and VSD.
2. Right ventricular parasternal heave due to increased pulmonary vascular resistance, right ventricular hypertrophy and dilatation in ASD. Parasternal impulse in VSD and PDA due to concentric hypertrophy of right ventricle.
   - Apex is no longer palpable.
   - There is no thrill.
3. Pulmonary component of second sound is palpable.
   - Early diastolic murmur of pulmonary regurgitation is palpable.
   - Pulmonary second sound is heard loudly in ventricular septal defect.
   - P_2 is wide and fixed split in atrial septal defect; normal split in patent ductus arteriosus, and single in VSD.
4. Pulmonary ejection systolic click and systolic murmur and an early diastolic murmur of pulmonary regurgitation heard in pulmonary area.
   Shunt murmurs are usually absent.

Sounds:

- S_1 Normal
- S_2 wide and fixed split in ASD
  - Normal split in PDA
  - Single in VSD
  - P_2 accentuated
- X inconstant (P constant)
- S_3 RV in ASD
- S_4 RA in ASD.

Murmurs:

- Ejection systolic murmur
- Pulmonary regurgitant murmur (Graham Steell).

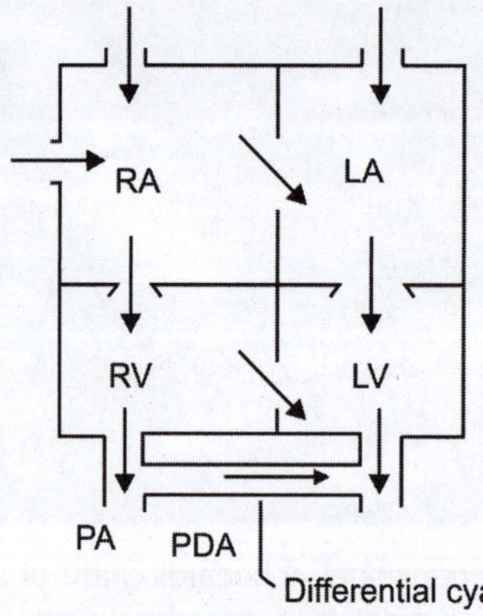

Fig. L-23: Auscultatory findings in Eisenmenger's syndrome

213. Investigations:

1. *X-ray chest:*
   - Enlarged right ventricle
   - Enlarged pulmonary artery and its branches
   - Peripheral lung fields are clear. Thus the hilar areas suggests pulmonary plethora whereas peripheral lung fields show oligemia.
2. *ECG:* Right axis deviation.
   Right ventricular hypertrophy. P 'Pulmonale' may be present.
3. *Echocardiography:* It may show dilated pulmonary artery, dilated right ventricle and right atrium. Pulmonary valve may show absent 'A' wave with midsystolic notch and flutter indicating significant pulmonary hypertension.
4. *Cardiac catheterization:* Pressure in the pulmonary artery, right ventricle and aorta are nearly the same and pulmonary vascular resistance is markedly increased. Pulmonary artery pressure is equal or greater than systemic vascular pressure. There is fall in oxygen saturation beyond the location of the shunt.
   Angiocardiogram—Demonstrates the location of the shunt.

214. Treatment of Eisenmenger's syndrome.

No specific treatment. Therefore, the treatment is directed to management of cardiac failure and prevention of infection.

1. Diuretics
2. Antibiotics
3. Periodic venesection: Phlebotomy.
4. Correction of iron deficiency anemia: Oxygen supplementation is needed in air-travel if the cabin pressure is permitted to decrease below that of sea level.

Transient symptomatic relief from severe polycythemia may be obtained by erythropheresis.

If the time for surgical correction is lost, closure of the defect simply advances to death from right heart failure. Therefore, early detection and early closure of large left-to-right shunt is essential to prevent Eisenmenger's syndrome. Pulmonary arterial hypertension below the age of 2 years is generally reversible.

215. 4 complications to be anticipated are:

1. Syncope
2. Hemoptysis
3. Brain abscess
4. Hyperuricemia.

216. Progress: It is generally progressive downhill resulting in death in the twenties or thirties. Most patients die because of:

1. Pulmonary infarction
2. Congestive heart failure
3. Cardiac arrhythmias
4. Cerebral infarction or abscess.

Pregnancy should be avoided. No successful surgical treatment is presently available. So early detection and correction of the shunt is essential.

MARFAN'S SYNDROME

217. It is an autosomal dominant generalized disorder of due to malformation of chromosome 15, affecting connective tissue mainly of CVS, eyes, skeletal system and others.

1. *Cardiovascular system:* About 90% have CVS abnormalities. Weakness in the media of aorta causes aneurysmal dilatation and dissecting aneurysm of the proximal portion of the ascending aorta. There may be mitral valve prolapse or severe mitral valve regurgitation but less common than severe aortic valve disease.
2. *Eyes:* Weakness of the supporting tissue of the lens causes bilateral subluxation or dislocation of the lens (Ectopia lentis) and myopia.
3. *Skeletal system:* Extremities are long and thin (dolichostenomelia), excessively long finger bones (arachnodactyly). 'Spider fingers' are found in many patients. (see L-14 for "Thumb sign", "Wrist sign")
   Long limbs and fingers includes arm spaces exceeding height. Tall, thin stature.
   Narrow and/or sharp future face—this can include a narrow mouth with high arched palate and consequently crowded teeth.
   Sternal displacement causes pushed-out 'pigeon breast' (Pectus carinatum), or caved-in (Pectus excavatum)
   Scoliosis.
4. *Other manifestations:*
   - Very loose and injury prone joints, laxy joints
   - Muscle hypotonia
   - Sparse subcutaneous fat
   - Striae especially over the skin of the pectoral, deltoid and thigh areas
   - Decreased elasticity of the lung tissue. Lung cysts with spontaneous pneumothorax occasionally may occur. Collapsed lung for no apparent reason may be seen.

Most people of Marfan's syndrome do have floppy mitral valve (MVP), but most people who have MVP do not have Marfan's.

The serious problem of Marfan's syndrome arises from a weak and rupture-prone aorta and suboptimal heart valves. The blood vessels are less flexible than normal. The aorta is subjected to full force of the heart beat. This pounding force can over time, wear down the aorta to widen and dilate resulting so far that it actually rips until it ruptures, which can drop in less than a heart beat permanently.

The survival needs immediate surgical intervention. The treatment consists of replacement of aortic arch with a Dacron—graft and replacement of aortic valve with a mechanical valve. Anticoagulation medication for lifelong is needed to prevent the formation of blood clots.

With the advent of modern medication and surgical techniques, it is also manageable as long as you are aware of the problem and taking corrective action. Often β-blockers are prescribed to lower the blood pressure and lessen the stress on the aorta and valves.

Is there a cure? Unfortunately, no.

Marfan's syndrome as with many other genetic disorders, is not amenable to cure, per se. This is because, every single, copy of chromosome 15, is all over the body, is messed up. The problem with chromosome 15 is that it is in use all over the body, in absolutely in every single system. For the syndrome to be 'cured' every one of those copies would have to be fixed and these are millions. This is beyond the boundaries, of what can be done at the present day knowledge.

As recently as 1970s, the lifespan for anyone affected by Marfan's syndrome was only in the mid-40s, but recent advances in surgery and medication have extended that until half of all of those affected live past the age of 70s—a normal lifespan.

218. Hurler's syndrome (gargoylism).

It is a rare autosomal recessive metabolic disorder in which abnormal glycoproteins are deposited in most of the organs. The 4 characteristic features are:

1. Dwarfism
2. Mental retardation
3. Deafness
4. Cardiomyopathy.

The heart valves may be thickened.

LEFT-TO-RIGHT SHUNTS

219. Causes of L to R shunts.

1. ASD
2. VSD—including left ventricular right atrial shunts
3. PDA or other aortopulmonary communications
4. Anomalous drainage of pulmonary veins to right atrium or superior vena cava.

220. Differences between the L to R shunt and R to L shunt.

Table L-4

In all L to R shunt	*In all R to L shunt*
1. No cyanosis	Cyanosis is present
2. Aortic arch is small	Aortic arch is large
3. Pulmonary artery and its branches are prominent. Pulmonary markings are prominent than normal—'pulmonary plethora' Pulmonary arterial hypertension develops when pulmonary vascular resistance equal to or greater than systemic vascular resistance resulting in bidirectional or R to L shunt, i.e. reversal of shunt —Eisenmenger's syndrome	Pulmonary artery and its branches are less prominent Pulmonary markings are less prominent than normal pulmonary oligemia. Once L to R shunt becomes reversal, R to L shunt occurs Cyanosis appears Eisenmenger's syndrome and the condition becomes inoperable
4. Right ventricular hypertrophy is seen	Left ventricular hypertrophy is seen

221. There are 4 common complications to be looked into the left-to-right shunts.
(The commonest L to R shunts in congenital heart diseases are ASD, VSD and PDA).

1. Congestive cardiac failure: Common in VSD and PDA—because they are high pressure shunts. Uncommon in ASD because of low pressure shunt. Patients with L to R shunt who do not develop congestive heart failure in the first year of life will not generally develop till the age of 10 years unless there are other complications like infections, anemia or other congenital anomaly.
2. Repeated respiratory infections: Repeated attacks of bronchitis, bronchopneumonia, pneumonia may occur about 4 to 6 times in the first year of life, and tend to persist for a longer time. Dilated pulmonary vessels compress the soft thin bronchioles in children causing stasis and infection.
3. Infective endocarditis: Rare below the age of 2 years. Common in VSD, can occur in PDA rare in ASD. VSD is the commonest congenital anomaly complicated by infective endocarditis. Preventive care is important.
4. Pulmonary arterial hypertension.

Develop pulmonary vascular obstructive disease—the Eisenmenger syndrome.

Later, L to R shunt gradually disappears and right-to-left shunt or cyanosis appears and the patient becomes inoperable.

CONGESTIVE CARDIAC FAILURE

(See Chapter C-Heart Failure)

Children with heart failure differ from adults. There are maturational differences in contractile function with improvement from early fetal gestation to the adult. This is likely to have an effect on immature subject. There are congenital, structural, genetic causes of heart failure in the fetus, infant and child that are either modified by adulthood or lead to early death such that the causes of heart failure in infancy are largely due to congenital heart disease, in the old children it is rheumatic fever/rheumatic heart disease whereas this is not the case in adult. The most common cause of heart failure in children is ventricular septal defect in which myocardial function is frequently normal. Therefore, in young patients with heart failure, the systemic output is most often normal, but excessive preload, afterload or pulmonary blood flow leads to pulmonary edema.

The majority of children with heart failure have surgically correctable cause. However, for medical management of heart failure in children, there are no long-term prospective randomized, double blind placebo-controlled data available. Essentially every form of treatment has either been proposed as successful or unsuccessful on the basis of uncontrolled trials. Patients of congenital heart disease have a relatively better myocardium. If a patient of congenital heart disease does not develop heart failure within the first year of life, he is not likely to do so in the next 10 years, unless the case is complicated by anemia, infection or bacterial endocarditis.

222. Causes of congestive cardiac failure:

Infants:
1. Congenital heart disease
2. Myocarditis and primary myocardial disease
3. Paroxysmal tachycardia
4. Anemia.

Miscellaneous causes:
5. Infections
6. Neonatal asphyxia/upper respiratory obstruction
7. Hypoglycemia
8. Hypocalcemia.

Children:
1. Rheumatic fever and rheumatic heart disease.
2. Congenital heart disease complicated by anemia, infection, endocarditis. Hypertension is another cause with glomerulonephritis.
3. Myocarditis and primary myocardial disease.
4. Upper respiratory obstruction.

Uncommon causes of congestive failure in infants and children include upper respiratory infection, hypoglycemia, neonatal asphyxia and hypocalcemia.

223. Any of the following 4 groups of congenital heart disease of patients can develop congestive cardiac failure in early infancy.

1. Left-to-right shunts
2. Right-to-left shunts
3. Obstructive lesions
4. Transpositions.

Patients with left-to-right shunts tend to develop congestive cardiac failure around 6 to 8 weeks of life. Pulmonary vascular resistance is high at birth and the pulmonary artery pressure is more or less equals the systemic pressure. Fall in the pulmonary vascular resistance occurs maximum in the first few weeks of life and then more slowly for a few months. The left-to-right shunt is small, whether the communication is at the atrial (ASD), ventricular (VSD) or pulmonary artery level (PDA). The size of the shunt gradually increases and reaches its maximum around the age of 6 weeks. If the infant is going to develop heart failure on the basis of a large shunt, he will do so at this time. The chances of increase in the shunt after a few months of life are minimal. Therefore, if congestive cardiac failure does not occur at this time, it is not likely to occur unless it is complicated by anemia, infection, endocarditis. Digoxin and diuretics are indicated. Oxygen administration is generally withheld because of properties of pulmonary vasodilatation and systemic vasoconstriction.

Patients with right-to-left shunts at ventricular or pulmonary artery level have either pulmonary stenosis or pulmonary arterial hypertension. Since the right ventricle is decompressed by the right-to-left shunt, congestive failure does not occur. Right-to-left shunt at the atrial level can be secondary to obstruction at the right ventricular outlet or inlet. The ventricular outlet obstruction cause congestive failure in the first few days of life. If the obstruction is severe or there is atresia, heart failure develops late when there is less severe obstruction. Tricuspid atresia is the commonest obstruction at the right ventricular inlet. Tricuspid atresia is a mechanical obstruction and does not represent congestive failure.

Obstructive lesions: (e.g. hypoplastic left heart syndrome, interrupted aortic arch, coarctation of the aorta).

Congestive cardiac failure is relatively a late manifestation of congenital obstructive lesions. However, atresia or severe stenosis of aortic, pulmonary, mitral valves cause congestive failure within few days. They may be asymptomatic for many years if the lesion is mild.

Coarctation of the Aorta can cause congestive failure within the first few months of life. If the symptoms do not manifest in the first year of life, collaterals develop and prevent heart failure. Therefore, the obstructive lesions result in congestive failure either soon after birth or later when the child is older. Prostaglandin EI is given to dilate the ductus arteriosus, and oxygen is withheld because it can constrict the ductus. The infant usually undergoes intubation and hypoventilation to increase pulmonary vascular resistance and force blood into the systemic circulation. Digoxin and diuretic drugs may be given.

Transpositions: Transposition of great arteries (TGA) or of the pulmonary veins manifest congestive failure within the first 2 or 3 months of life, former earlier than the later. Transpositions of pulmonary veins develop congestive failure somewhat later, usually by the age of six to eight weeks, following the fall in pulmonary vascular resistance as in patients with left-to-right shunts.

Any of the 4 groups of patients can develop congestive cardiac failure in the early infancy. They are unlikely to develop it subsequently unless there are complications.

224. The time of onset of congestive cardiac failure is so precise that it can be used as an aid in the differential diagnosis of causative lesions. The following 4 examples:

Table L-5

Age	Lesion
Birth to 1 week	Pulmonary, aortic and mitral atresias within 72 hours Hypoplastic left and right heart syndromes, transpositions and malpositions of great arteries
1 to 4 weeks	Transposition and malposition complexes, endocardial fibroelastosis, coarctation of aorta
1 to 2 months	Transposition and malposition complexes, endocardial cushion defect, VSD, PDA. total anomalous pulmonary venous connection, anomalous left coronary artery from pulmonary artery
2 to 6 months	Transposition and malposition complexes, VSD, PDA, total anomalous pulmonary venous connection, aortic stenosis, coarctation of aorta

225. Myocardial disease: Coxsackie B virus infection is the most common cause of myocarditis which may occur from the age of few hours to 7 weeks. It is relatively less common later.

There are 4 important primary myocardial diseases that cause CCF:

1. Glycogen storage disease
2. Endocardial fibroelastosis
3. Medial necrosis of coronary arteries
4. Anomalous origin of left coronary artery from pulmonary artery (ALCAPA).

Although the last is a congenital anomaly, it is included in the primary myocardial disease group, since its presentation is identical to this group.

226. The 4 features of myocarditis and primary myocardial disease are

1. Cardiac enlargement predominantly involving left ventricle
2. Absence of significant murmurs
3. Congestive failure
4. Gallop rhythm.

227. The 4 ECG changes in myocardial disease and primary myocardial disease are:

1. Conduction disturbances
2. Arrhythmias
3. Left ventricular hypertrophy
4. Nonspecific ST and T changes.

Low voltage may be seen in myocarditis.

Tall voltage is seen in glycogen storage disease and fibroelastosis over the left chest leads.

Anomalous origin of left coronary artery from pulmonary artery patients show anterolateral myocardial infarction pattern.

228. 4 features of CCF caused by paroxysmal supraventricular tachycardia are:

1. 3/4th of patients are below the age of 4 months
2. Males predominate
3. Heart rate above 180/minute
4. Tendency to recurrence if the tachycardia is after 4 months of age.

Usually, there is no failure in the first 24 hours. About 20% develop congestive failure if tachycardia persists for 36 hours and almost 50% will do so in 48 hours.

229. Some features of CCF due to anemia and infection.

1. Hemoglobin levels of 5 g/dL in a normal heart can result in congestive failure. In a heart compromised by disease, congestive failure may be precipitated even with 7 or 8 g/dL. Younger the infant the more susceptible to develop failure.
2. Sever infections of upper and lower respiratory tract may cause CCF. Sometimes, it may be difficult to differentiate pulmonary infection from cardiac failure in infants, as tachycardia, tachypnea and palpable liver may present in both. Differentiation of simple infection is made on the presence or absence of cardiac enlargement. Diagnosis of cardiac failure in the absence of cardiac enlargement is equivocal except in neonates.
3. The three conditions where CCF may result without cardiac enlargement are—congenital mitral stenosis, cor triatriatum, and the obstructive variety of total anomalous pulmonary venous connections, which are all physiologically identical.
4. In older children, congestive failure occur in congenital heart disease complicated by systemic or endocardial infection, anemia unrelated to myocarditis and systemic hypertension.

   Nonspecific obstructive aortitis is a common cause, if complicated congenital heart disease and systemic hypertension from renal parenchymal disease are excluded.

230. The features of CCF due to rheumatic heart disease.

1. Acute rheumatic fever with carditis and rheumatic heart disease is the most comman cause of congestive failure in older children.
2. The manifestations of rheumatic disease are different in India. Symptomatic mitral stenosis occurs at an early age without the latent period of two decades as seen in western countries.
3. A child with rheumatic heart disease with congestive failure may not have active carditis.
4. Patients of gross mitral or aortic regurgitation with congestive failure frequently present without evidence of rheumatic activity.

Clinical Features

The recognition of CCF in older children are same as in adults. The recognition in infants and small children is based on subtle signs and symptoms and is difficult to recognize.

231. Symptoms of congestive heart failure in infants and children are:

1. Poor weight gain or absence of weight gain. It can be due to small feeds because of easy fatiguability or excessive loss of calories from increased work of breathing associated with CCF.
2. Difficulty in feeding.
3. Breaths too fast.
4. Breaths better when held against the shoulder which is equivalent of orthopnea in older children or adults.
5. Persistent cough or wheezing.
6. Irritability or excessive perspiration and restlessness.
7. Puffiness of face.
8. Pedal edema.

7 and 8 may cause weight gain.

232. Signs of congestive cardiac failure in infants and children.

Table L-6

Left sides failure	Right sided failure	Combined failure (Failure of either side)
1. Tachypnea	Hepatomegaly	Cardiac enlargement
2. Tachycardia	Puffiness of face	Gallop rhythm (S_3)
3. Cough	JVP raise	Peripheral cyanosis
4. Ronchi or rales	Edema feet	Small volume pulse

The infant or child with heart failure is generally tachypneic with a respiratory rate (taken while asleep) greater than 60 breaths per minute at < 2 years old and > 40 breaths/min at ~2 years old. The tachycardia needs close inspection because it is generally unlabored and the infant may appear to be comfortable. The presence of intercostal retraction may indicate associated pulmonary infection or impending cardiovascular collapse.

The pulse volume should be obtained in all 4 extremities and both carotid arteries. Blood pressure reading should be obtained in all 4 extremities. Infants with obstruction to systemic ventricular outflow such as that found in critical aortic stenosis may have diffusely reduced pulse volume whereas in coarctation of aorta or interruption of the aortic arch, there may be differential pulse volume between the arms and legs. If the coarctation involves the left subclavian artery, and there is retroesophageal right subclavian artery originating below the coarctation level, the only normal pule may be the carotids.

In a patient with signs and symptoms of heart failure, a diuretic, such as furosemide may be given before diagnostic testing is completed. Oxygen administration is generally withheld until an anatomic diagnosis can be made. In patients with anatomic outflow obstruction such as hypoplastic left heart syndrome in which the entire systemic flow is through the ductus arteriosus, administration of oxygen may constrict the ductus and reduce the systemic flow.

233. Diagnostic evaluation of subacute or chronic heart failure in infants and children.

1. Chest X-ray
2. ECG including Holter's monitor
3. Two-dimensional Echo Doppler
4. Cardiac catheterization/coronary arteriography to determine coronary anatomy if not established by 2D Echo.

In fetus, repeated echocardiogram for paroxysmal arrhythmia if there is evidence of hydrops fetalis.

Blood serum, glucose, calcium, electrolytes, creatinine tests for abnormalities that may accompany or cause heart failure. Carnitine and selenium deficiency if there is family history of early cardiac deaths.

Chest X-ray is helpful to detect plural effusion, pneumonia or anatomical abnormalities such as diaphragmatic hernia. It will also confirm the diagnosis of pulmonary over circulation.

ECG may be helpful in the diagnosis of tachycardia or bradycardia that can cause heart failure. Chronic arrhythmias of any sort can cause cardiomyopathy. Occasionally, wide Q waves of anomalous origin of left coronary artery from the pulmonary artery may be of diagnostic value.

Essential diagnostic test is the transthoracic Doppler two-dimensional echocardiogram. This reveal congenital heart disease of left-to-right shunt, right-to-left shunt, systemic outflow obstruction, pericardial effusion/tamponade. Dilated poorly functioning of the heart where a correctable cause is abnormal origin of left coronary artery from pulmonary artery. Other causes include acute myocarditis, acute presentation of chronic cardiomyopathy.

Normally functioning heart with dilated chambers, especially right ventricle and right atrium may indicate a congenital extracardiac arteriovenous fistula found most commonly in the cerebral or hepatic circulation, chronic severe anemia may also present with this Echo picture.

234. Management of cardiac failure (See Chapter C-Heart Failure).

It consists of correction of inadequate cardiac output for tissue oxygenation at rest or during stress.

There are 4 steps to correct inadequate cardiac output (See Chapter C- Heart Failure point 12)

1. Reducing cardiac work
2. Augmenting myocardial contractility
3. Increasing cardiac performance by reducing the heart size
4. Correcting the underlying cause.

235. Cardiac work is reduced by:

1. Rest—by restricting the patients activities.
2. Sedatives.
3. Correcting precipitating or aggravating causes like anemia, infection specially pulmonary infection, obesity, thyrotoxicosis, etc.
4. Vasodilators.

Neonates with CCF are nursed in an incubator. The baby is kept in an incline position of about 30°. This helps to pool the edema fluid to the dependent parts and reduces lung congestion, thus reducing the work of breathing. Humidified oxygen at 40–50% concentration is given to improve impaired oxygenation secondary to pulmonary congestion, with improved tissue oxygenation. If the cardiac output improves, the heart work is reduced.

236. Sedatives: Injection of morphine sulfate in doses of 0.05 mg/kg SC is given for sedation if the infant or child is irritable, restless or dyspneic. Sedatives help by:

1. Restricting the physical activity, and respiratory effort and keep the child in bed.
2. Reduces anxiety in children thereby reducing catecholamine secretions thus reducing the cardiac work.
3. Diminishes venous return, respiratory rate as well as heart rate.
4. Reduces oxygen requirement for body tissues and thus reduces the cardiac workload.

237. Anemia: causes tachycardia and a hyperkinetic circulatory state. Cardiac work load is reduced by correction of anemia. It is treated by:

1. 3–5 mL of packed cells/kg body weight every 12 hours.
2. Half of the digitalizing dose of digoxin is given before intravenous infusion to prevent worsening of CCF.
3. IV furosemide is given if there is worsening of congestive failure.
4. Supplemented by oral hematinics.

238. Vasodilators (see Chapter C- point 130–141).

Vasodialtors act by reducing the arteriolar and venous vasoconstriction, thus reducing the cardiac work. Vasodilators are indicated only in the presence of severe CCF with significant elevated left ventricular filling pressures. They may be lifesaving in pulmonary edema where IV nitroprusside is indicated.

1. Nitrates are preferential venodilators.
2. Hydrallazine is an arteriolar dilator.
3. Sodium nitroprusside and prazocin has both arteriolar and veno dilatation.
4. ACEI act by combination of arteriolar and veno dilatation combination of isosorbide dinitrate and hydrallazine given orally is very effective. IV vasodilators should not be given in the absence of hemodynamic monitoring as the patient can go into hypotensive shock.

239. Augmenting myocardial contractility (See Chapter C-Point 70–82).

In the infant or child acute heart failure accompanied by decreased ventricular function, principles similar to those described for adults are followed. Diuretics are given cautiously because an acute decrease in preload may lead to hypotension. IV inotropic agents used in children (dopamine, dobutamine, epinephrine, isoproteronol) are generally similar use to those in adults. In equivalent doses, dopamine may be less effective in infants because of maturational differences in norepinephrine stores. IV digoxin may be used. However, in acute setting with changing renal perfusion and function, change in potassium and calcium concentrations, digoxin concentration and effects may be unpredictable. The use of digoxin in these settings may be unpredictable. Amrinone has been used as both a primary ionotropic agent and as a systemic vasodilator. Other systemic vasodilators, such as sodium nitroprusside, hydrallazine, nitroglycerin have also been used. Ventricular assist divices for both right ventricle and left ventricle are being developed for pediatric use.

Digoxin:

1. Increases force of contraction
2. Decreases heart rate

3. Increases ejection fraction
4. Increases cardiac output.

240. Digitalis dosage of infants and children are made in the following way:

Table L-7

	Digitalization in first 24 hours Dose	Daily maintenance
1. Premature	0.04 mg/kg × 8th hrly	1/4
2. Birth to 1 year	0.08 mg/kg × 8th hrly	1/4 to 1/3
3. 1 to 3 years	0.06 mg/kg × 8th hrly	1/4
4. Above 3 years	0.04 mg/kg × 8th hrly	1/4

(Parenteral dose = Oral dose × 0.7)

Digoxin is available in tablet, elixir and parental forms. Lanoxin elixir (1 mL = 0.05 mg) is unstable in summer, loses its potency in 3 to 6 months.

Parenteral digoxin 0.5 mg/2 mL is available. Infants tolerate digoxin well. Unlike adults, children should be digitalized in 24 hours. They are too sick for slow digitalization. Once digitalis is started, it should be continued for a number of years. Early discontinuation may result in reappearance of congestive failure resistant to therapy.

241. Digitalis is used with caution in the following 4 conditions:

1. Premature neonates
2. Very cyanotic patients
3. Congestive failure due to myocarditis
4. Congestive failure associated with very large heart.

Half the calculated dose is used in digitalizing as well as the maintenance dose initially in these situations. The PR interval in ECG is a useful indicator of toxicity in children. If the PR interval widens to one and a half times of the initial PR interval, digitalis toxicity is present. In infants, the upper limit of normal PR interval is 0.14 sec.

242. Improving the cardiac function by reducing the heart size (See Chapter C -Point 92–93).

The drugs useful in reducing the heart size are digitalis and diuretics.

Diuretics: Orally furosemide is commonly used.

1. Diuretics should preferably be started after complete digitalization.
2. The use of diuretics in infants and smaller children are limited to those cases where congestive failure cannot be adequately controlled with digitalis.
3. Oral furosemide is the commonly used drug. Its action starts within 20 minutes.
4. It is necessary to have frequent checks of serum electrolytes to prevent serious electrolyte imbalance.

Restriction of salt intake is not possible to practice in infants, since low sodium milks are not easily available. Salt free diets are unpalatable. The child stops eating and starts loosing weight. Hence, low sodium diets should be used only if the congestive failure cannot be controlled with digitalis and diuretics.

CCF increases caloric requirements. Concentrated milk formulae supplemented by soluble protein preparations provide more calories.

As long as the dose of furosemide is < 2 mg/kg per day orally is given, excess potassium loss generally does not occur. At higher doses, spiranolactone generally is added, potentially obviating the need for potassium supplementation.

243. Correction of underlying causes: Cardiac catheterization with angiocardiography may be necessary for the specific diagnosis of congenital anomaly. Many of these conditions are tackled by curative or palliative surgery. In any patient of rheumatic heart disease, if active carditis has been excluded and an adequate trial has been given to medical management, operation treatment should be considered.

Management of infants and children with heart failure may differ from adults in the following 4 conditions.

1. *Congenital heart disease with left-to-right shunt:* In an infant with large left-to-right shunt, the choice for continued medical management is weighed against the severity of heart failure, natural history of defect, and expected success of operation. For example, in an infant with large ventricular septal defect (VSD), there is approximately 50% probability that the defect will become small enough, not to require surgical intervention. Surgery is postponed as long as the infant is gaining weight and free of lower respiratory tract infection. If the infant has still a large defect after 6 months of age, increasing consideration is given for repair, especially in the presence of elevated pulmonary artery pressure. The greatest controversy has surrounded the use of digoxin in infants with left-to-right shunt. In premature infant with patent ductus arteriosus, the risk of digoxin toxicity and the lack of demonstrated benefit do not justify the use of digoxin. The controversy currently surrounds with VSD in whom, contractility, as measured by load-dependent indexes frequently normal. The results and recommendations are contrary. In the study by Kimbell et al, digoxin did not change symptoms, although combination of digoxin and furosemide did provide an increase in contractility over that at baseline. In the study of Colon and Sanders digoxin was found to be useful. It appears that in certain children with a

large left-to-right shunt and symptomatic heart failure, digoxin may be beneficial.

Finally, controversy surrounds the use of vasodilators. In a large interventricular communication in which right ventricle and left ventricle systolic pressures are equal, the amount of left-to-right shunt is dependent on the balance of pulmonary and systemic vascular resistance. Because there are no specific vasodilators that affect the pulmonary and systemic circulations differentially and in the same direction, it is to be expected that some might improve and others might not. It appears that captopril and enlapril are most beneficial in children with either elevated systemic vascular resistance (> 20 U/m^2) or those without markedly elevated pulmonary arteriolar resistance (< 3.5 U/m^2). These infants must be monitored closely for hypotension or worsening heart failure.

2. *Eisenmenger's syndrome with heart failure (See Point 208–214).*

   The type of heart failure generally found in patients with Eisenmenger's syndrome is right sided heart failure with:

   i. Tricuspid regurgitation
   ii. Hepatomegaly
   iii. Peripheral edema
   iv. Low cardiac output.

   A diuretic may relieve painful hepatic congestion and edema. Digoxin is freqently used although the benefit has not been studied. Phlebotomy is done to reduce the viscosity of blood and high hematocrits to decrease symptoms of headaches, muscle and joint aches but its effect on myocardial function is undemonstrated.

   If patients with Eisenmnger's syndrome are treated with a vasodilator, there is a risk that with relatively fixed pulmonary arteriolar resistance; there will be a greater vasodilating effect on systemic vasculature, in increase in right-to-left shunt and a decrease in systemic arterial saturation. Vasodilators usually are not given due to this reason unless the shunt has been corrected previously.

   Heart/lung transplantation should be considered in those with Eisenmenger's syndrome.

3. *Heart failure due to arrhythmias:* Acute paroxysmal tachyarrhythmias or bradyarrhythmias may cause heart failure and elimination of the arrhythmia is the treatment of choice. Chronic incessant tachyarrhythmias (e.g. atrial ectopic tachycardia, permanent junctional reciprocating tachycardia, atrial flutter or ventricular tachycardia) that are present > 10% of the day may cause chronic heart failure. These arrhythmias may cause a dilated poorly functioning heart or diastolic dysfunction. The identification of the tachyarrhythmias generally is not difficult. However, in some patients, a right atrial ectopic focus tachycardia may masquerade as sinus tachycardia. In these patients, atrial ectopic tachycardia is more likely if the P wave is negative in lead V_2 or if the heart rate is > 150% of the upper limit of normal for age. The causative nature of the tachyarrhythmias has been demonstrated by the eventual normalization of cardiac size and function after definitive treatment of tachyarrhythmias.

   Vagal stimulation, specially eye ball pressure in supraventricular tachycardia is contraindicated in infants for fear of damage to the eye. The treatment of choice lies between digoxin, propranolol and verapamil. Verapamil is safe and rapidly acting drug when given intravenously. The dose is 0.75–1 mg for newborns, 0.75–2 mg for infants and 2–3 mg for children between 1–5 years. Once, tachycardia is controlled, the child should be given digoxin for 2–3 years for prevention of recurrence.

4. *Congestive cardiomyopathy:* Idiopathic dilated cardiomyopathy must be diagnosed by exclusion. Cardiac catheterization is advised if echocardiogram has not demonstrated normal proximal coronary anatomy. If there is no anatomic cause, myocardial biopsy may be performed to diagnose myocarditis. Metabolic and genetic familial causes of congestive cardiomyopathy, such as carnitine and selenium deficiency are more common than in adults. Family history of early deaths from heart disease should be sought. Most recently, ACE inhibitors such as enalapril and captopril showed benefits which are refractory to digoxin and furosemide. Platelet antagonists should be considered as prophylaxis against stroke. At present, no form of therapy in children markedly affects longevity, because the prognosis is so poor in many patients, heart transplantation should be considered.

   There is evidence to suggest that steroids may be hazardous in patients with coxsackie myocarditis. Steroids should be avoided in patients with myocarditis, unless they have serious conduction disturbances or peripheral vascular failure. Patients with endocardial fibroelastosis respond well to digitalis. Once digitalis has been started in these patients it should be continued for years. Early discontinuation may result in reappearance of congestive heart failure resistant to therapy.

   Uncommon causes of congestive heart failure in infants and children include upper respiratory infection, hypoglycemia, neonatal asphyxia and hypercalcemia. Appropriate treatment depends on high index of suspicion.

244. Heart failure in the fetus: It is demonstrated in the fetal echocardiogram by 4 findings:

1. Plural effusion
2. Pericardial effusion
3. Ascites
4. Skin edema.

Fetal heart failure by congenital heart disease is an ominous sign and may be associated with spontaneous abortion. The most common cause for fetal heart failure is sustained supraventricular tachycardia. High-index of suspicion of an arrhythmia is needed if there are signs of heart failure and the heart is anatomically normal. The arrhythmia is treated initially with digoxin given to the mother. There are reports of success with verapamil, flecainide, procainamide and amiodarone. The majority of fetuses with supraventricular tachycardia can be treated successfully, with only a minority requiring early delivery.

245. Summary of heart failure in the fetus, infant and child.

1. Majority of infants with heart failure have a surgically correctable cause.
2. Initial laboratory tests should include CBC, Urine analysis, serum electrolytes, glucose, calcium creatinine, chest X-ray and ECG. The essential diagnostic study is the transthoracic Doppler-2D echocardiogram.
3. In infants with heart failure, oxygen administration generally is withheld until an anatomic diagnosis is made.
4. Heart failure with left-to-right shunt is managed initially with intravenous furosemide. Oxygen is withheld because of its properties of pulmonary vasodilatation and systemic vasoconstriction.
5. Infants with heart failure due to systemic outflow obstruction should receive prostaglandin EI to dilate the ductus arteriosus and oxygen should be withheld.
6. A diagnosis of idiopathic dilated cardiomyopathy is made by exclusion. Cardiac catheterization is performed if two-dimensional echocardiogram has not demonstrated the proximal coronary anatomy. If no anatomic cause is demonstrated, myocardial biopsy is indicated.
7. The management principle and drugs used to treat dilated cardiomyopathy in children are similar to those used in adults.
8. Controversy surrounds the use of dioxin in infants and children, but it may be useful in those with symptomatic heart failure.
9. ACE inhibitors are most beneficial in children with either elevated systemic vascular resistance or those without markedly elevated pulmonary vascular resistance.
10. Vasodilators are generally contraindicated in Eisenmenger's syndrome unless the shunt has been surgically corrected.
11. Chronic incessant tachyarrhythmias that are present > 10% of the day may cause dilated cardiomyopathy and heart failure.
12. The most common cause of fetal heart failure is sustained supraventricular tachycardia, which is treated by administering digoxin to the mother.

CYANOTIC HEART DISEASES

246. Following are some of the cyanotic heart diseases.

1. Tetralogy of Fallot (TOF). It is the commonest of the cyanotic heart diseases.
2. Complete AV canal with severe pulmonary stenosis (PS).
3. TGA with severe PS.
4. Double outlet right ventricle with severe PS.
5. Single ventricle with PS.
6. Tricuspid atresia with PS.
7. Corrected L-TGA with large VSD and severe PS.
8. Pulmonary atresia (PA).

Severe pulmonary stenosis is the common factor among these defects which results in reduction of pulmonary blood flow. Patients who are cyanotic have either pulmonary stenosis or pulmonary arterial hypertension.

247. Major complications in cyanotic heart diseases result from:

1. Severe hypoxia
2. Metabolic acidosis
3. Polycythemia
4. Paradoxical embolization from intracardiac shunt.

248. An alarming complication of cyanotic spells in congenital heart disease is known by various names like:

1. Tet
2. Hypoxic spells
3. Anoxic spells
4. Blue spells.

This is characterized by paroxysmal attacks of dyspnea causing hyperpnea and roller back of eyes. Such attacks may occur as early as one month or delayed to 12 years. Peak frequency is 2–3 months. Such paroxysms may occur at anytime but majority occur in the morning on awakening. Crying, feeding, defecation are frequent precipitating events as they all increase oxygen demand and cause increase of PCO_2 all of which increase the right-to-left shunt thereby increasing hypoxia besides causing increased oxygen consumption due to increased work of breathing. Several causes have been suggested including increase in RVOT obstruction, acute rise of pulmonary vascular resistance and/or sudden decrease of systemic vascular resistance. Regardless of exact cause, the result is reduced pulmonary flow relative to systemic flow.

If convulsions are untreated cerebrovascular accidents and death may occur.

249. Emergencies in congenital cyanotic heart diseases.

Clinical Approach and Symptomatology

1. *Age of onset:* Age of onset of cyanosis is important as conditions like:
   - Transposition of great arteries
   - Pulmonary atresia
   - Tricuspid atresia
   - TAPVC
   - Produces cyanosis at birth—Blue baby.
   - Whereas in tetralogy of Fallot (TOF) the cyanosis appears beyond the first month.
2. *Easy fatigubility:* The child gets tired very easily. The small infant may get tired while feeding and leaves the feed in between. This is an ominous sign of low cardiac reserve.
3. *Squatting:* The child sits down in squatting position after playing for a short while. Infant may roll his legs on his abdomen. Compression of the abdomen in this position compresses the aorta and femoral artery with raised pressure and reduction in right-to-left shunt.
4. *Failure to thrive:* Infants may not gain weight because of increased metabolic activities of heart and poor feeding. In older children puberty may be delayed, probably because of tissue hypoxia.
5. *Recurrent chest infection:* Infants with increased pulmonary blood flow have history of recurrent chest infection.
6. *Chest pain:* Scratch marks on the anterior chest wall are indirect pointer of chest pain in small infants, who cannot complain of chest pain. This may be seen in hypercyanotic spells and anomalous origin of coronary artery.
7. *Hypercyanotic spell:* Characteristically seen in TOF, precipitated in conditions with increased oxygen demand like feeding, defecation, playing. Child may get convulsions, hemiplegia or rarely death may occur.
8. History of exposure to drugs like nitrates, aniline dyes, prilocaine may cause cyanosis due to methemoglobinemia. History of taking drugs during pregnancy should be asked in detail. History of maternal consumption of alcohol, nicotine, smoking, etc. should be asked.

Exposure to radiation in first trimester.

Family history of diabetes in parents, grandparents may be recorded in cases of transposition of great arteries and hypoplastic left heart syndrome.

250. Some of the following general features in congenital cyanotic heart diseases may be recorded.

1. Rounded face in pulmonary stenosis.
2. Child with features of Down's syndrome usually have endocardial cushion defect.
3. Rocker bottom feet, umbilical hernia and double outlet right ventricle are present in 13–1 trisomy while 16–18 trisomy cases usually have VSD and PDA.
4. Congenital rubella syndrome in a mentally retarded child with cataract usually have pulmonary artery stenosis or PDA.

Clubbing is usually seen in older children. Growth and development, nutritional status are assessed. They are usually below normal.

251. CVS examination.

1. Pulse
   - Weaker pulse in the legs than in arms in coarctation of aorta
   - Plateau pulse in aortic stenosis
   - Dominant 'A' wave of jugular venous pulse reflects vigorous right atrial contraction due to diminished compliance of right ventricle. Large systolic CV waves are present in tricuspid regurgitation.
2. Blood pressure
   - Low BP in shock and septicemia, etc.
   - Decreased pulse pressure in pulmonary stenosis, aortic stenosis
   - Wide pulse pressure may occur in truncus arteriosus, PDA, etc.
3. Palpation and percussion
   - Apex on right side in dextrocardia
   - Systolic expansion of pulmonary artery in pulmonary hypertension
   - Systolic thrill in TOF, VSD, AS, PS, PDA, etc.
   - RV systolic lift at left sternal border
   - Cardiomegaly is usually present in big L to R shunts with congestive cardiac failure
   - Congestive cardiac failure in infants may be yet another presentation which is detected only by the presence of hepatomegaly.
4. Auscultation
   - Second sound is loud and single in TOF, TA and pulmonary hypertension, etc. It is of aortic origin in the former and pulmonary origin in the later
   - Systolic murmur is present in TOF, PS, VSD, etc.
   - Continuous murmur is heard in PDA, truncus arteriosus, posteriorly over the chest in prominent bronchial collaterals and others. All cyanotic children ultimately develop bronchopulmonary collaterals as part of natures compensatory mechanism.

These help by relieving few symptoms as the child grows

- Early diastolic murmur is present in pulmonary hypertension (Eisenmenger syndrome)
- Decrescendo diastolic murmur may be heard in pulmonary valvular regurgitation.

252. Continuous murmur is heard in:

1. Patent ductus arteriosus (PDA)
2. Coronary arteriovenous fistula
3. Ruptured sinus of Valsalva—fistula into right side
4. Aortic pulmonary septal defect
5. Systemic arteriovenous fistula over the chest
6. Bronchial collateral murmurs
7. Pulmonary arteriovenous fistula
8. Peripheral pulmonic stenosis—bronchial artery anastomosis in pulmonary atresia
9. Venous hum including the one which is associated with total anamolous pulmonary venous connection (Artificial ductus in Blalock or Waterson shunt)
10. Small atrial septal defect associated with mitral stenosis
11. Truncus arteriosus
12. Blalock-Taussig shunt.

Impression of continuous murmur due to a combination of pansystolic murmur and regurgitant diastolic murmur occurs most commonly with ventricular septal defect associated with aortic regurgitation.

Combination of aortic stenosis and aortic regurgitation never gives an auscultatory impression of a continuous murmur since a gap between the two murmurs can always be appreciated (to and fro murmur).

253. Characterstic murmurs of congenital heart diseases: It is wise to repeat the important murmurs at this juncture.

1. *Ventricular septal defect:* It is the most common congenital lesion encountered as one of the many congenital anomalies. It produces a pansystolic murmur often associated with a thrill. It is widely spread but best heard along the lower left sternal border. It may be soft during early infancy or childhood. In large defects, it may cause early diastolic flow murmur over the mitral area which is low pitched, short and usually weak. In pulmonary hypertension, there is loud single second sound over the pulmonary area in first and second left intercostal spaces parasternally.
2. *Atrial septal defect:* A pulmonary ejection murmur is occasionally associated with a systolic thrill. Wide, fixed split of second sound is the characteristic finding. A low pitched early diastolic murmur over the tip of the sternum is due to increased blood flow through the tricuspid valve.
3. *Aortic stenosis:* It produces a loud and harsh systolic murmur with crescendo-decrescendo type best heard over the aortic area but it is usually transmitted over the pericardium and neck vessels. An aortic thrill is felt at the base of the heart along the carotids and in suprasternal notch.
4. *Pulmonary stenosis:* It produces similar loud and harsh systolic murmur except that it is best heard in the pulmonary area. Second sound in the pulmonary area is either diminished or absent.
5. *Patent ductus arteriosus:* It produces a loud continuous crescendo-decrescendo murmur with its peak intensity in late systole and wanes in mid-diastole or late diastole. It is the best heard over the pulmonary area. The murmur usually cannot be detected in diastole in the first year of life; later typical continuous or machinery murmur appears. A systolic thrill is usually present at the site of maximum intensity.
6. *Tetralogy of Fallot (TOF):* It has a typical murmur of pulmonary stenosis. The single sound in the pulmonary area arises from the anteriorly displaced aortic valve. Cyanosis appearing over the age of 2 years is usually due to TOF, especially if cyanosis and shortness of breath are relieved by squatting. Whenever cyanosis appears after the first weak of life, it usually suggests TOF.
7. *Transposition of great vessels:* It is a common cause of cyanosis at birth that is aggravated by crying. It may produce no murmur at all or it may produce the murmur of pulmonary stenosis or an associated ventricular septal defect.
8. *Coarctation of aorta:* It may not produce characteristic murmur but moderately loud systolic murmur may be heard over the obstruction in the interscapular and left supraclavicular areas. Widespread soft systolic bruit due to collateral circulation may be heard. It is diagnosed by weaker pulse and blood pressure in the lower extremities than in the upper extremities. Hence, checking the pulse and blood pressure in the lower extremities is essential in a child with a murmur.

254. Knowing when a murmur first appeared is often significant in the following way:

1. A harsh murmur present on the day of birth is almost always due to either pulmonary stenosis or aortic stenosis. Any significant obstruction of the pulmonary or aortic valve creates turbulent flow immediately after birth.

2. A murmur that first appears several days after birth suggests either patent ductus arteriosus or ventricular septal defect. This delay is because the pressure in the right ventricle and pulmonary artery, elevated at birth, does not fall immediately to adult levels. The elevation of pressure tends to equalize the pressure between the right and left ventricle and reduces turbulent flow through the defect.
3. A murmur that first appears several months or even years after birth suggests atrial septal defect or acquired heart disease. The murmur of an atrial septal defect is delayed longer because of closer approximation of pressures in the atria and their greater dispensability in early childhood apparently reduces shunting of blood and hence the turbulence.
4. A murmur that first appears several years after birth suggest acquired heart disease.

The significance of soft murmurs that disappear between birth and 2 years of age is also important. These probably represent delayed closure of a patent ductus arteriosus. Most of them close within 3 months but some may take longer time. Hence, all murmurs in the neonatal period need close follow-up since they may become louder, which suggest possibility of an organic lesion.

255. The following 4 innocent systolic murmurs occur frequently in children.

1. *Vibratory murmur:* It is an early to midsystolic murmur over the 3rd and 4th left intercostal space, diminishes or disappears when the patient is upright (not more than Grade III on a scale of VI).
2. *Pulmonary ejection murmur:* It is also early to midsystolic, well-localized over 2nd or 3rd left intercostal spaces parasternally. It rarely exceeds Grade III. This is produced by increased pulmonary blood flow, such as anemia, anxiety or exercise. It can be differentiated from ASD by wide and fixed P_2 split.
3. *Cardiorespiratory murmur:* It occurs in middle or late systole over any part of pericardium or at the heart-lung margins, often called as 'systolic whoop'.
4. *Carotid bruit:* It occurs in early to mid-systole over right neck vessels. It can be differentiated from aortic stenosis by its absence over aortic area.

Innocent murmurs are frequently heard on the back particularly in thin-chested children.

(*Note:* Venous hum is the only innocent murmur heard in diastole over the base of the heart and neck vessels. It disappears when neck veins are occluded or patient is in supine position or when the head is turned to one side.)

256. Investigations.

1. Hematocrit is usually elevated to 55–60%. Hematocrit beyond 65% increases blood viscosity.
2. Hemoglobin of 12% in a cyanosed child is relative anemia which should be treated with iron. Hemoglobin electrophoresis is done in suspected cases of methemoglobinemia.
3. ESR is raised in anemia and infections.
4. Blood culture is useful in septicemia and subacute bacterial endocarditis.
5. PO_2.
6. PCO_2.
7. pH.
8. Oxygen saturation, etc. are estimated.

Routine blood counts, blood sugar, serum electrolytes are useful parameters.

257. Detection of enzyme disorders when inborn errors of metabolism is suspected in cases of:

1. Pompe's disease	– Glycogen storage disease of heart
2. Homocystinuria	– Aortic and pulmonary arterial dilatation, intravascular thrombosis.
3. Mucopolysaccharidosis Hurler, Hunter syndromes	– Multivalvular, coronary and great artery disease and cardiomyopathy.
4. Morquio, Scheie, Morateaux-Lamy	– Aortic incompetence

258. X-ray chest is useful for evaluation of:

1. Heart size
2. Shape
3. Pulmonary vascularity
4. Visceroatrial situs.

259. Some classical diagnostic features in X-ray chest are:

1. Boot-shaped heart in tetralogy of Fallot (TOF).
2. Egg-shaped heart in transposition of great arteries (TGA).
3. Snowman's or 'figure-of-eight' appearance in total anomalous pulmonary venous connection (TAPVC).
4. 'Scimitar' sign in partial anomalous pulmonary veins (PAPV).

Important features in the lung fields are also considered. Pulmonary plethora is seen in L to R shunts, e.g. transpositions with VSD, persistent truncus, single ventricle, whereas oligemia is seen in defects associated with pulmonary stenosis, e.g. TOF, pulmonary atresia, transposition with pulmonary stenosis and double outlet right ventricle with pulmonary stenosis.

260. X-ray chest in pulmonary hypertension reveals:

1. Enlargement of right ventricle
2. Conspicuously enlarged pulmonary artery
3. Prominent hilar pulmonary vascular markings
4. Attenuated peripheral vessels.

261. Some diagnostic features in ECG are:

1. Incomplete RBB in ASD of the secundum type.
2. Left axis deviation in:
   a. Tricuspid atresia
   b. Ostium primum ASD
   c. AV canal defects
   d. Univentricular heart.
3. Sudden transition of R waves from V_1 to V_4 seen in TOF.
4. Himalayan P waves in Ebstein anomaly of tricuspid valve.

262. Echocardiography with Doppler is the single most important noninvasive diagnostic tool in congenital heart diseases since it shows:

1. Structural abnormalities even in the most complex cardiac anomalies and their spatial relationship to each other—ventricular and interatrial defects.
2. The complete intracardiac and great vessel anatomy and concomitant valvular lesions—valve stenosis, endocardial vegetations.
3. Doppler shows the direction of blood flow and helps in calculating pressures and pressure gradients.
4. Contrast Echo may help to know the direction of flow in a shunt.

263. Cardiac catheterization and angiocardiography aim to know the following:

1. To precisely demonstrate the anatomy of the defect. To do differential oximetry and determine the level and direction of shunts.
2. To measure the various pressures and pressure gradients.
3. To calculate flow rates and flows across shunts.
4. To calculate pulmonary vascular resistance (PVR) and cardiac output.

Because of its invasive nature their use is restricted. Nowadays, cardiac catheterization is used as a therapeutic procedure in certain specific indications. Angiography also demonstrates flow of blood and obstructions.
All this information helps in assessing the operability and probable outcome of surgery.

264. Management:

General measures:

1. Maintenance of nutritional status—by proper caloric intake.
2. Maintenance of thermoneutral environment more so in a sick newborn—servo control is very useful for optimum oxygen utilization.
3. Maintenance of fluid and electrolyte balance:
   A constant check is necessary especially in cases if decongestive therapy and diuretics are given. Fluid requirement is curtailed in premature PDA and CHF. Salt restriction is not usually recommended.
4. Correction of metabolic derangement:
   Hypoglycemia, hypocalcemia, hypokalemia, hyponatremia—should be looked for and corrected. Routine immunization should be followed.

265. Approach to a cyanotic new born should be as follows:

1. Differentiate between severe pulmonary disease and congenital heart disease.
2. Correction of metabolic acidosis with sodium bicarbonate (0.5 mg/kg).
3. Effective oxygen delivery—use mechanical ventilator if necessary.
4. In case of PDA dependent cyanotic disease, administration of prostaglandin EI is considered. (L-135)

266. The following are helpful in differentiating pulmonary from cardiac etiology of cyanosis in the new born.

1. History of meconium aspiration favor pulmonary origin.
2. Associated hypoglycemia and hypocalcemia favors pulmonary etiology.
3. Administration of 100% oxygen for 5–10 minutes increases bronchial arterial oxygen saturation in pulmonary diseases.
4. 2D echocardiography differentiates the two forms of cyanosis.

267. Medical management of congenital cardiac emergencies consists of congestive cardiac failure, cyanosis and cyanotic spell.

The mainstay of the treatment is:

1. Oxygen therapy (humidified oxygen)
2. Diuretic and digoxin
3. Morphine
4. β-blockers
5. Correction of acidosis by sodium bicarbonate
6. Ventilatory support
7. Inotropics may be needed
8. Infusion of prostaglandin E_1 or E_2 in ductus dependent patients as a lifesaving measure.

The other general measures include antibiotics for prophylaxis against endocarditis, prevention of dehydration in polycythemia.

268. Treatment of congestive heart failure.

Congestive heart failure in a cyanotic heart disease is mostly seen in defects associated with increased pulmonary blood flow and pulmonary hypertension like TGA, TAPVC and late-onset cyanosis in Eisenmenger's syndrome.

Clinical features are same as in adults except that edema is not usually seen in neonates and infants.

Treatment consists of:

1. Oxygen
2. Digitalis and diuretics
3. Peripheral vasodilators
4. Correction of acidosis.

269. Immediately after birth, there is fall in pulmonary arterial pressure, resistance and vascular tone and a gradual reduction in the thickness of media of the pulmonary arterioles and widening of the lumen.

Thus pulmonary circulation of the normal adult has evolved from:

1. High pressure to low pressure
2. High resistance to low resistance
3. Highly reactive vascular bed to low reactive bed
4. Relatively small cross-sectional area to large cross-sectional area.

Pulmonary hypertension is a frequent complication of congenital heart disease. Status of the pulmonary vascular bed may be the principal factor to determine the clinical features, prognosis and indications for surgery.

The blood flow will be in the direction of least resistance. The basic physical characteristics of any fluid in motion apply to the hemodynamics in cardiac defects.

Thus in ASD or simple VSD the shunt is from left-to-right because the pressure in the left side is more than the right side. Later, during the natural course of the disease when the pulmonary vascular resistance increases there is reversal of the shunt as the right sided pressure increases to a level more than the left side. This results in mixing of desaturated blood in the left side thus causing clinical cyanosis.

Thus, no child should be allowed to end up with Eisenmenger's syndrome with the advent of infant surgery in VSD, ASD, PDA and others.

270. There are 4 important general factors to know in pulmonary hypertension in congenital heart diseases of left-to-right shunts.

1. More frequent in PDA and VSD.
2. Rare in ASD below the age of 20 years.
3. Generally starts from 1 to 10 years of age.
4. Children of VSD with pulmonary hypertension should be operated below 3 years of age because it is not reversible after the age of 3 years.

271. Incidence of brain abscess and embolus are relatively high, about 2–4% in cyanotic and polycythemic children. They often have previous microcirculatory damage of the central nervous system.

272. Treatment of infections: Appropriate antibiotics are given based upon culture and sensitivity in cases of septicemia, bronchopneumonia and bacterial endocarditis.

Prophylaxis of infective endocarditis is considered in the following 4 groups.

For tonsillectomy, adenoidectomy, bronchoscopy, dental procedures, instrumentation, etc.

1. For most patients
   Proc penicillin 600,000 units + Cryst penicillin 200,000 units IM.
   or Penicillin 'U' orally 500 mg or 12,00,000 Cryst penicillin one hour before the procedure.
2. For patients allergic to penicillin
   Erythromycin—500 mg two hours before and 250 mg × 6th hourly for 2 days.
   Children—20 mg/kg, 10 mg/kg × 6th hourly for 2 days.
3. For GI or GU operations, or any operation or infected tissues.
   For most patients:
   Penicillin as above + SM 1 g/day on the day and for 2 days following.
   Children: Streptomycin—40 mg/kg.
   or Ampicillin + Streptomycin—
   Ampicillin 50 mg/kg oral or IM 1st dose and 25 mg/kg subsequently.
4. For patients allergic to penicillin
   Erythromycin as above + Streptomycin as above.

273. Maintenance of some specific complications.

1. Arrhythmias: PAT, AF or heart blocks, etc. are corrected with drugs, DC cardioversion or pacing.
2. Cardiogenic shock:
   Dopamine 2–2.5 μg/kg/min IV infusion or
   Dobutamine 2–15 μg/kg/min IV infusion or
   Isoproteronol 0.1–1 μg/kg/min IV infusion.
3. Maintenance of ductus:
   Patency of ductus is maintained in cases of tricuspid atresia, pulmonary atresia, transposition of great arteries till some intervention is done.
   Prostaglandin E 0.05–0.1 μg/kg/min IV
   Closure of ductus in a premature infant is brought about with indomethacin or prostaglandin synthesis inhibitor in doses of 0.1–0.3 mg/kg every 12–24 hours for 1–3 doses.

4. Maintenance of pulmonary hypertension:
   To reduce pulmonary vascular resistance in a case of persistent fetal circulation.
   Tolazoline 1 mg/kg IV as a bolus followed by 2 mg/kg IV/hour

274. Polycythemia secondary to hypoxia leads to increased viscosity. The treatment consists of:

1. Prevention of dehydration.
2. Relative anemia or a normal hemoglobin with hematocrit level below 65% generally reflects iron deficiency and should be treated with iron. Response to iron therapy is very gratifying. Hemoglobin of 12 g is relative anemia and iron therapy should be given.
3. Severe anemia or hypovolemia may require blood transfusion.
   Anemia in the presence of cyanosis may lead to poor effort tolerance, greater dyspnea and even increased frequency of anoxic spells.
   Exchange transfusion is done in extreme situation of hemoglobin M disease.
4. Phlebotomy is advised if the hematocrit levels are above 65% and/or heart failure is present. It improves hemostasis temporarily in polycythemic patients with hematocrit above 65%. It should not be recommended for simple fear of stroke. Volume replacement is done with frozen plasma.

275. Cyanotic spells—especially in tetralogy of Fallot's (TOF) consists of:

1. Paroxysms of dyspnea
2. Cyanosis
3. Unconsciousness
4. Convulsions even caused by cerebral anoxia.
   The affected child assumes a characteristic squatting posture after walking a variable distance. Walking causes further arterial unsaturation. It is quickly restored to normal by assuming this posture either by increasing systemic venous return or by increasing the peripheral vascular resistance thereby reducing the right-to-left shunt.

276. Treatment of hypoxic spells are aimed at:

1. Improving PO_2.
2. Correcting acidosis.
3. Decreasing right ventricular outflow tract (RVOT) obstruction thereby improving pulmonary blood flow.
4. Reducing PVR:SVR ratio.
   (Pulmonary vascular resistance: Systemic vascular resistance ratio).

277. Occurence of anoxic spells in congenital cyanotic heart disease varies in:

1. *Incidence:* Varies from 20–70%.
2. *Age:* May occur as early as one month or delayed till 12 years.
3. *Time:* Majority occur in the morning on awakening.
4. *Precipitating events:* Crying, feeding, defecation, playing, etc.

These events increase oxygen demand and increase of PCO_2 and fall of blood pH and PO_2 all of which increase right-to-left shunt.

278. Following treatment is useful in anoxic spells.

1. Knee chest or knee elbow position.
2. 100% oxygen administration/40% moist oxygen inhalation.
3. Morphine sulfate 0.1–0.2 mg/kg IV or SC.
4. Correction of acidosis.
   - Empirically: Sodium bicarbonate 0.5–1.0 mg/kg IV may be given before the availability of laboratory data.
   - IV sodium bicarbonate is given when PO_2 is below 40 mm Hg. Acidosis is calculated from the formula.
     Total base deficit = 0.3 × Body weight in kg × Base deficit in mEq.
   - Half the calculated dose should be given over 30 minutes.
   - Next step is to tackle infundibular obstruction and/or systemic vascular resistance.
5. Propranolol 0.05–0.1 mg/kg may be given IV during spell to be followed by oral maintenance therapy with 0.5–1.0 mg/kg 4 to 6 hourly.
6. Vasopressors: Phenylephrine 0.02 mg/kg IV followed by 2–5 mEq/kg continuous drip may reverse a spell. Methoxamine (vasoxyl) 0.1 mg/kg IM or IV drip may also be used instead.
7. Glucose supplement to correct hypoglycemia resulting from increased utilization and depleted stores.
8. Lastly, general anesthesia may be necessary to terminate the attack.

279. Majority of infants with heart failure or cyanosis have a surgically correctable cause and surgical correction is class I indication for treatment of such patients. The major consideration in these patients is the timing of operation, especially for those in whom the defect may become smaller, e.g. VSD.

Surgically correctable cyanotic heart diseases can be prognostically classified into 4 groups in the following way:

I. **Cyanosis associated with decreased pulmonary flow with low risk.**
   1. Tetralogy of Fallot.

2. ASD with pulmonary stenosis and right-to-left shunt.
3. Vena caval anomalies to left atrium.

II. **Cyanosis associated with decreased pulmonary flow with high risk.**
1. Tricuspid atresia
2. Pulmonary atresia
3. Persistent truncus arteriosus with hypoplastic pulmonary arteries.

III. **Cyanosis associated with increased pulmonary flow with low risk.**
1. Total anomalous pulmonary venous return with normal pulmonary vascular resistance.
2. Transposition of great arteries with intact ventricular septum.
3. Congenital pulmonary arteriovenous fistula.

IV. **Cyanosis associated with increased pulmonary flow with high risk.**
1. Transposition of great arteries with VSD or PS
2. Double outlet right ventricle
3. Truncus arteriosus
4. Complete atrioventricular canal defects
5. Single ventricle.

280. The following palliative surgical procedures are described in congenital heart diseases.

1. Septostomy and septectomy in TGA, TA, TAPVC, etc.—to allow mixing of blood. Opening is made in the interatrial septum. It is useful in transposition of great arteries. It helps the child by reducing cyanosis.
2. *Shunt or shunting procedure:* The operation of forming a passage between blood vessels to divert blood from one part of the body to another. It is used to reduce the cyanosis in infants with severe tetralogy of Fallot and those with tricuspid atresia or pulmonary atresia.
   i. Blalock-Taussig shunt (BT and modified BT shunt): It consists of anastomosis of left subclavian artery with left pulmonary artery. It is always done on the side opposite of the aortic arch.
   ii. Bilateral bidirectional Glenn shunt: It consists of anastomosis of superior vena cava and the right pulmonary artery.
   iii. To increase the pulmonary blood flow without being dependent on ductus.
   Pott's shunt: It consists of anastamosis of descending aorta with the pulmonary artery.
   iv Waterson's shunt: It consists of anastamosis of ascending aorta and right pulmonary artery Davidson's shunt.

   Transannular patch: Some prefer to put transannular patch instead of shunt. It gives better palliation and growth of the pulmonary arteries.
3. *Banding of the pulmonary artery:* A procedure in which a band is placed around the pulmonary artery to narrow it and reduce the blood flow and high pressure in the lungs. The band can be removed when the child is older and fix the defect with open heart surgery.

   To decrease the pulmonary blood flow in VSD with coarctation, AV canal defects, etc.
4. *Fontana operation:* A procedure in which the right atrium is connected to the pulmonary artery either by direct anastamosis or by a conduit. This allows blood to bypass an incomplete or underdeveloped right ventricle, as in tricuspid atresia and pulmonary atresia. The atrial defect is also closed to relieve cyanosis.

   A valve is kept between the right atrium and inferior vena cava to prevent the backward flow of blood into the inferior vena cava.
5. *'Arterial Switch' of Jatene is modified by the Le Compte and others:* A surgical procedure in which the major arteries are switched in babies with transposition of the great arteries. The aorta is connected to the left ventricle. The pulmonary artery is connected to the right ventricle. This arterial switch procedure may be done in the first few weeks after birth and in infants as small as 2.5 kg or depending on various factors, slightly later. If there is large ventricular septal defect or other defects related to the transposition, the repair gets more complicated. Then other surgical procedure may be needed.
6. *Balloon valvuloplasty:* A procedure in which a special catheter containing a deflated balloon is inserted into the opening of a narrowed heart valve. When the balloon is inflated, the valve is stretched open and the balloon is removed. The procedure is used with favorable results to improve blood flow in pulmonary stenosis. It is also used in some cases of aortic stenosis, where the long-term results are still being studied.
7. *Ross procedure:* A procedure in which a person's diseased or abnormal aortic valve is replaced with the patient's own pulmonary valve (pulmonary autograft). A homograft valve (valve from a human donor) is then placed where the pulmonary valve was.
8. *Venous switch or intra-atrial baffle:* A procedure that creates a tunnel inside the atria to help correct transposition of the great arteries. It redirects oxygen-rich blood to the right ventricle and aorta, and redirects venous blood to the left ventricle and pulmonary artery. In the Mustard procedure, the intra-atrial baffle is made of tissue from the pericardium. In the Senning procedure, the intra-atrial baffle is made of flaps from the atrial wall.

281. Fontana operation: This procedure is devised for patients of tricuspid atresia. The right atrium is anastomosed to the pulmonary artery by various methods. The main pulmonary artery is ligated off. The results of the procedure are good. Many surgeons modified this procedure for use in various other congenital heart anomalies.

Palliative surgery is done as a life-saving procedure to help the infant to live till the corrective surgery is undertaken when possible.

In experimental studies it was seen that the right ventricle could be bypassed without any hemodynamic derangements. Right atrium was anastomosed with pulmonary artery. Main pulmonary artery was ligated off. Modified procedures are used in other defects. Currently, it can also be used for pulmonary stenosis with intact ventricular septum, DORV with PS and univentricular heart.

It is indicated in:

1. Mainly tricuspid atresia

It can also be used for:

2. Pulmonary atresia with intact ventricular septum
3. Double outlet right ventricle (DORV)
4. Univentricular heart.

With improvements and modifications of the original procedure, the mortality has come down to 5–10%.

282. Therapeutic cardiac catheterization is helpful in the following 4 conditions:

1. Balloon atrial septostomy for TGA, TA, TAPVC. It is a life-saving procedure
2. Balloon valvotomies and volvuloplasties.
3. Button or umbrella devices to close some ASDs and VSDs.
4. Rashkind umbrella device (RUD) to close some ideal PDAs.

Balloon atrial septostomy lowers the left atrial pressure and provides mixing of the systemic and pulmonary venous blood at the atrial level. This results in relieving hypoxia as well as pulmonary congestion.

283. The following 4 conditions can be corrected with the help of balloon-catheter.

Percutaneous balloon-catheter procedures are used to correct some of the defects and is a palliative life-saving procedure in some conditions. Atrial septostomy (Rashkind procedure) is performed with a balloon catheter—to create an atrial septal defect to permit mixing of arterial and venous blood. It is primarily used as a life-saving procedure in transposition of great arteries. Likewise several conditions can be corrected with percutaneous catheter procedure.

1. Aortic valvotomy in aortic stenosis
2. Pulmonary valvotomy in pulmonary stenosis
3. Coarctation of aorta
4. Pulmonary artery branch stenosis.

284. Transcatheter occlusive procedures are used to correct some of the congenital heart diseases. Portman et al in 1971 reported closure of patent ductus arteriosus. Since then many successful cardiac defects were treated. They include:

1. Aortopulmonary collaterals
2. Atrioventricular fistulas
3. AV shunts
4. Septal defects.

Rashkind umbrella device (RUD) has found great use.

285. Arterial 'Switch' operation now appears to be an attractive better palliative surgery if not superior or alternative to palliative atrial septostomy, etc. It should usually be preceded by:

1. Cardiac catheterization
2. Balloon-atrial septostomy
3. Infusion of prostaglandin EI to keep the ductus open
4. Left ventricular systolic pressure at or near systemic levels until the switch can be accomplished.

286. 'Blalock-Taussig shunt'—Left subclavian and left pulmonary artery anastomosis—is performed to increase the pulmonary blood flow. It can be done in the following 4 conditions:

1. Tetralogy of Fallot
2. Double outlet right ventricle with pulmonary stenosis
3. Single ventricle with decreased blood flow to lungs
4. Transposition with pulmonary stenosis.

287. Pulmonary artery banding is usually done within the first 2 or 3 months of life to prevent severe pulmonary vascular obstructive disease. It can be tried in cases of increased pulmonary blood flow with pulmonary arterial hypertension as in:

1. Corrected transposition with ventricular septal defect (VSD)
2. Large ventricular septal defect or difficult multiple ventricular septal defects
3. Atrioventricular canal defects
4. Truncus arteriosus.

288. Pulmonary artery is initially banded in some conditions to:

1. Increase the left ventricular pressure
2. Stimulate left ventricular hypertrophy
3. Achieve good left ventricular function
4. Accomplish normal sinus rhythm.

Pulmonary artery banding is usually avoided because of its inherent complications and mortality.

289. Indications of conduits in surgery for congenital heart disease:

1. Truncus arteriosus
2. Pulmonary atresia with ventricular septal defect
3. Transposition of great arteries with ventricular septal defect
4. Left ventricular outflow obstruction.

Conduits can be homografts (from cadavers), xenografts (from animals), synthetic materials like Dacron. Non-synthetic conduits are prone to degeneration and calcification over a period of time. Dacron conduits require anticoagulation with its inherent risk. The bigger problem is that it does not grow with the child so there is patient-conduit mismatch and thus may require replacement.

290. Definitive surgical treatment—To know when to operate, when not to operate is important.

Only a few important conditions are mentioned here:

1. *PDA:* Simple ligation or division and suturing of PDA. The mortality is nearly zero.
2. *ASD:* Patch closure with pericardial graft or direct suturing of a secundum ASD under cardiopulmonary bypass (CPB).
   ASD is completely curable with very little mortality.
3. *VSD:* Patch repair of VSD.
   Mortality is 1–2%.
4. *TOF:* Total correction is preferred for all children over 1 year of age with suitable anatomy. The procedure aims at closing the VSD, relieving PS and PVOT obstruction. Overall mortality varies from 2–5%.

With great advancements in cardiac surgery, more than 99% of congenital cardiac defects could be corrected by surgery with acceptable mortality. Cardiac surgery does not stop here. Intrauterine diagnosis and correction is now being undertaken at a few advanced centers for a few selected conditions.

Pulmonary hypertension associated with increased blood flow as in left-to-right shunts greatly benefit by surgical correction. When the pulmonary hypertension is due to decreased pulmonary blood flow (as when the pulmonary vascular resistance increases) the patient's signs and symptoms decreases. This is not to be taken as an improvement but this becomes an indication for urgent surgery. If surgery is delayed anymore and there is reversal of the shunt seen by the appearance of cyanosis, then surgery cannot be performed. The quality of such children is poor and their lifespan is diminished. So, no child is allowed to end up with Eisenmenger's syndrome with the advent of infant surgery. The only modality of treatment available for these patients is a complete heart-lung transplant as the pulmonary changes are irreversible.

INDIVIDUAL PREVENTION AND PREVENTIVE PROGRAM

291. Prevention of congenital heart disease starts from 'in utero' and strictly even before pregnancy with marriage counseling. Mother's health plays an important role in the prevention.

1. Marriage counseling: To prevent transmission of genetic disorders. The genetic transmission rate is high if both partners are affected.
2. Correction of severe anemia and other deficiency diseases.
3. Use of drugs by strict supervision by a doctor.
4. Stop smoking or ingestion of alcohol.

292. Preventive program:

Preventive program depends on the cause of the disease. Congenital anomalies appear to result from complex interaction of multifactorial genetic and environmental systems. No cause is yet known in more than 90% of CVS anomalies.

1. Immunization of children against Rubella.
   Rubella vaccine that has been developed may lessen maternal rubella and its cardiac consequences.
2. Strict drug testing in animal models.
   New drugs that may be teratogenic when taken in early pregnancy are abandoned. This reduces the chances of another thalidomide tragedy. No medication is taken during pregnancy without prior consultation with a physician.
3. Appropriate use of radiological equipment and techniques to reduce gonadal and fetal radiation exposure which are potential hazards of birth defects.
4. Detection of abnormal chromosomes in fetal cell obtained from amniotic fluid in occasional pregnancies. The presence of cardiac anomalies may exist as one component of a multiple system involvement in Down's trisomy 13–15 (D) 17–18 (E), Turner's syndromes. Similarly detection of such cells of the enzyme disorders observed in Hurler's syndrome, homocystinuria or Pompe's disease may help to predict some cardiac anomalies.

293. Instructions to patients of children with congenital heart disease.

Do Not Panic: Many heart diseases will not hamper the child's growth and development. He can lead a normal active life, play and go to school.

Inform the teacher about the heart condition so that special care is taken.

1. Let the child avoid any strenuous exercise, let not the child be fatigued by excess travel.
2. Do not subject the child to sudden changes in temperature and altitude.
3. Give all immunizations at the right time.
4. Prevent infective endocarditis.

Diet:

5. Practice hygiene while feeding.
6. Give plenty of fluids to avoid dehydration.
7. Supplement diet with iron rich foods.
8. In case of a 'spell' (recognized by restlessness, deep breathing, blueness, and inconsolable cry). Keep the child in a "knee-chest" position (knees pressed firmly against the abdomen) and consult a doctor.

M Pulmonary Hypertension and Pulmonary Embolism

The pulmonary circulation is a low pressure system within which the normal systolic pressure is 15–30 mm Hg and the normal diastolic pressure is 5–15 mm Hg. Anything that exceeds 30/15 mm Hg is considered as pulmonary hypertension.

1. One should know the following 4 features while describing the pulmonary hypertension .

1. Pulmonary hypertension denotes a deviation of either pulmonary arterial or pulmonary venous pressure.
2. This can be brought about by a number of causes which may produce transient or permanent changes in the lungs and pulmonary vasculature.
3. There are two hemodynamic syndromes to be distinguished.
   i. *Pulmonary arterial hypertension* in which the arterial pressure is raised but the capillary and venous pressure is usually normal.
   ii. *Pulmonary venous hypertension* or congestion in which pulmonary pressure is usually slightly raised.
4. As these two conditions differ entirely in etiology, pathology, and radiological appearances, the conditions should be described with qualifying adjectives of arterial or venous to identify the pulmonary arterial hypertension and pulmonary venous hypertension.

Pulmonary edema is the main feature to distinguish these two syndromes. Since pulmonary venous hypertension occurs very frequently and not pulmonary arterial hypertension.

2. The 4 factors which control the pulmonary arterial pressure are:

1. The output of the right ventricle (blood volume).
2. The resistance of the blood flow offered by the pulmonary vascular bed.
3. Lung elasticity.
4. The degree of lung inflation with air.

3. The 4 factors which influence the pulmonary venous pressure are:

1. The efficiency of the left ventricle—any cause of the left ventricular failure. For example,
   a. Hypertension.
   b. Aortic valve disease.
   c. Ischemic heart disease.
   d. Cardiomyopathy.
2. Obstruction to mitral valve:
   a. Mitral stenosis.
   b. Mitral regurgitation.
   c. Left atrial tumor or myxoma.
   d. Ball valve thrombus.
3. Pulmonary capillary or pulmonary venous disease. For Example,
   a. Veno-occlusive disease
   b. Thrombosis
   c. Mediastinitis
   d. Tumor infiltration.
4. Constrictive pericarditis:
   Pulmonary venous hypertension is present when the venous pressure rises above 20–25 mm Hg.

4. There are 4 conditions where pulmonary arterial hypertension occurs.

One primary cause and three secondary causes. They are:

1. Primary pulmonary hypertension: Cause is not known.
   - No parenchymal pulmonary pathology
   - No primary cardiac disease
     – Irreversible.

   Secondary to:
2. Increased pulmonary capillary pressure, e.g. left ventricular failure, mitral valvular disease - Mitral stenosis is the most common cause. It causes sustained rise in pulmonary venous pressure—reversible if the cause is treated.
3. Increased blood flow as in left to right shunts. For example, ASD, VSD, patent ductus arteriosus.
   - Reversible if the cause is treated.
4. Increased pulmonary vascular resistance.
   - Irreversible in repetitive thromboembolism.

5. There are 4 steps in the mechanism of pulmonary hypertension in left ventricular failure (or mitral stenosis with elevated left atrial pressure).

1. Rise in left atrial pressure: It is reflected in the pulmonary veins.
2. Rise in pulmonary venous pressure: The reserve capacity of pulmonary bed is much less than that of systemic venous bed. The capacity of the pulmonary venous bed is sufficient to accommodate some rise in pulmonary venous pressure without an increase in pulmonary arterial pressure.
3. Rise in pulmonary capillary pressure: As the pulmonary venous pressure rises, the pulmonary capillary pressure also rises. When the pulmonary capillary pressure exceeds the colloid osmotic pressure of the plasma (28 mm Hg) fluid exudates into alveolar air spaces resulting in pulmonary edema.
   Pulmonary edema produces complex effects, including interference with gas exchange, alteration in the ventilation perfusion ratio with 'shunting' of unoxygenated blood through the lungs, and decrease in lung compliance (Stiff lungs) increasing the work of breathing. Edema of the mucosa of smaller air passages may produce airways obstruction, and distended smaller blood vessels may rupture with hemoptysis.

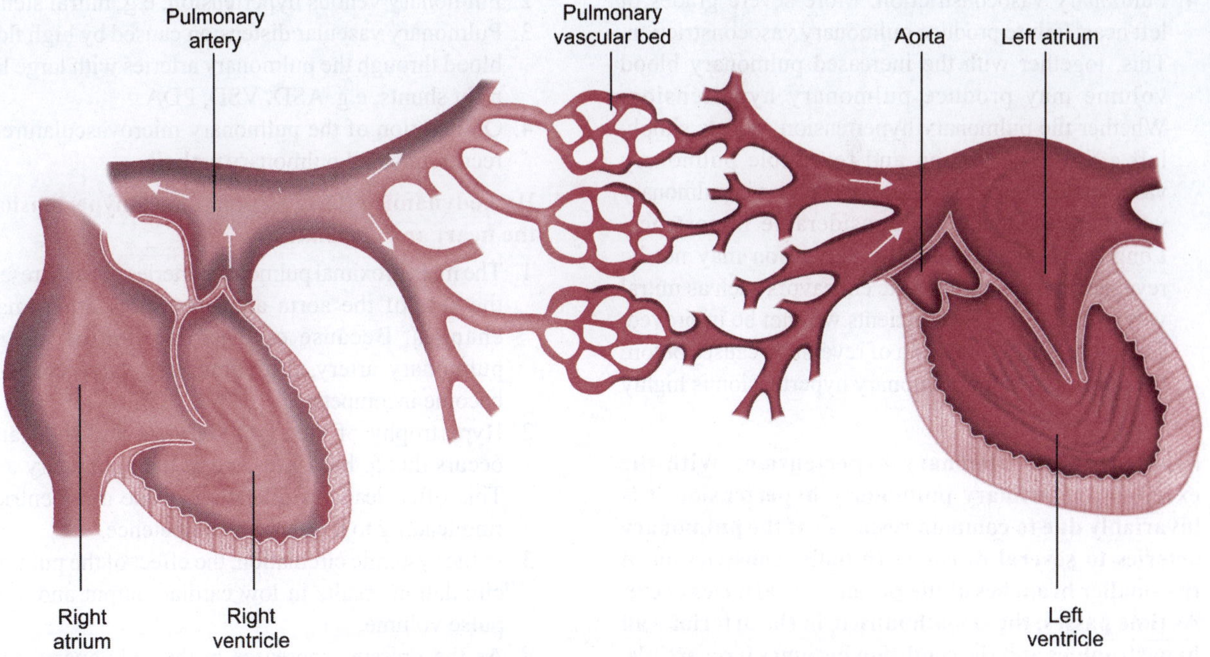

Fig. M-1: Pulmonary circulation (Diagrammatic)

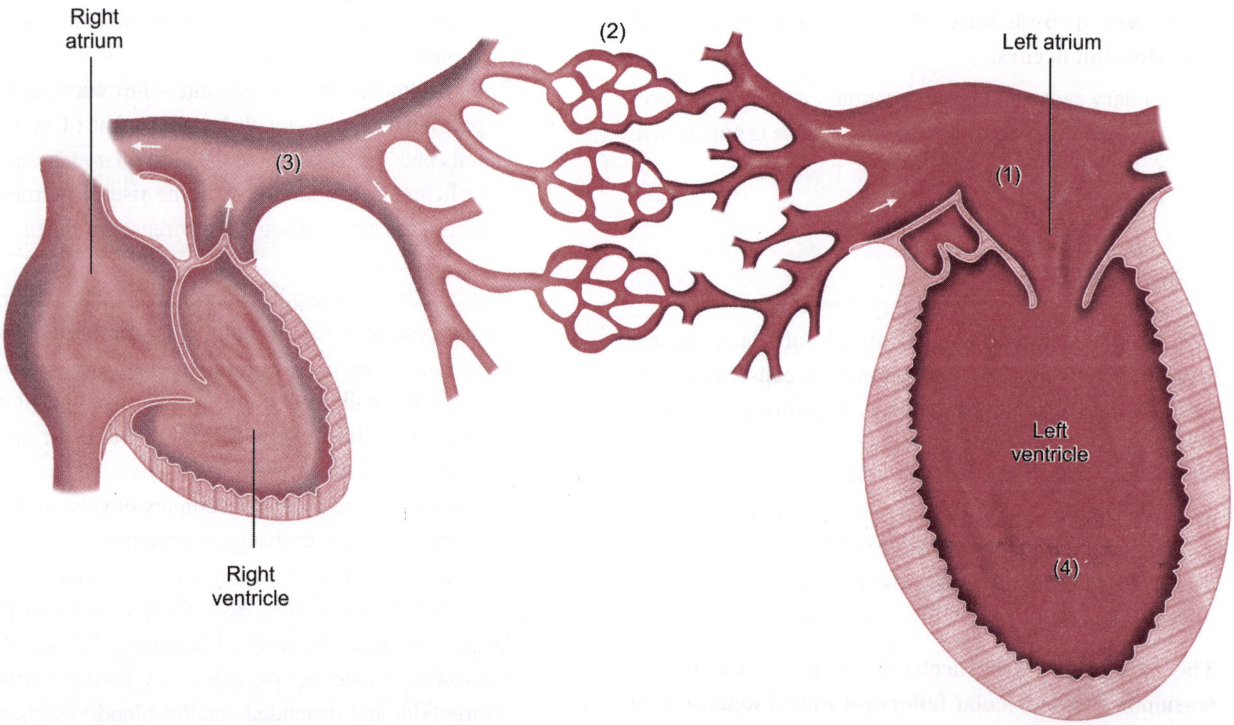

Fig. M-2: 1. Elevation of left atrial pressure, 2. Pulmonary vasoconstriction, 3. Pulmonary hypertension, 4. Left ventricular enlargement

4. Pulmonary vasoconstriction: More severe grades of left heart failure produce pulmonary vasoconstriction. This, together with the increased pulmonary blood volume may produce pulmonary hypertension. Whether the pulmonary hypertension reflects simply left atrial hypertension and reversible pulmonary vasoconstriction or a more permanent rise in pulmonary vascular resistance has considerable importance. Long standing pulmonary hypertension may not be reversed by such therapeutic endeavors such as mitral valve surgery and such patients will not be improved. Therefore, early correction of reversible causes before the development of pulmonary hypertension is highly rewarding.

6. **Mechanism of pulmonary hypertension: With the exception of primary pulmonary hypertension it is invariably due to common response of the pulmonary arteries to several diseases. Initially, constriction of the smaller branches of the pulmonary arteries occur. As time passes, the smooth muscle in the arterial wall hypertrophies and the condition becomes irreversible.**

There are 4 groups of conditions which may result in spasm of the pulmonary vasculature and pulmonary hypertension.

1. Alveolar hypoxia, e.g. severe chronic obstructive airways disease.
2. Pulmonary venous hypertension, e.g. mitral stenosis.
3. Pulmonary vascular distension caused by high flow of blood through the pulmonary arteries with large left to right shunts, e.g. ASD, VSD, PDA.
4. Obliteration of the pulmonary microvasculature, e.g. recurrent small pulmonary emboli.

7. **Hemodynamic effects of pulmonary hypertension on the heart and circulation.**

1. The main proximal pulmonary arteries dilate to resemble the size of the aorta and may show atheromatous changes. Because of the dilatation of the main pulmonary artery, the pulmonary valve cusps may become incompetant.
2. Hypertrophy of the right ventricle and right atrium occurs due to back pressure in the pulmonary artery. This often leads to dilatation of the atrioventricular ring leading to tricuspid incompetence.
3. In the systemic circulation, the effect of the pulmonary circulation results in low cardiac output and a small pulse volume.
4. As the pressure increases in the pulmonary system, it becomes equal to the pressure within the systemic circulation and any left to right shunt that is present before is reversed—Eisenmenger's syndrome.

8. **The pulmonary hypertension can be classified into 4 types:**

Pulmonary arterial (or precapillary) hypertension:

1. Hyperdynamic (or hyperkinetic) pulmonary hypertension.

   This is due to increased pulmonary blood flow. This is usually associated with congenital heart diseases with left to right shunt, e.g. ASD,VSD, PDA or it may occasionally occur in hyperdynamic circulatory states, e.g. thyrotoxicosis, severe anemia, beriberi with heart disease, Paget's disease.
2. Vasoconstrictive pulmonary hypertension.

   This can be either vasoconstrictive due to arterial spasm or organic and truly obliterative.
3. Pulmonary venous (or post capillary) hypertension.
4. Primary pulmonary hypertension.

9. There are 4 causes of arteriolar vasoconstriction due to spasm.

1. Secondary to increased pulmonary blood flow, e.g. congenital heart disease with left-to-right shunt.
2. Hypoxia.
3. In response to certain drugs i.e. acetylcholine.
4. Secondary to pulmonary venous hypertension.

10. Causes of obliterative pulmonary hypertension (organic obstruction).

Common causes:

1. As a primary condition in congenital heart disease with a left to right shunt leading to reversal of shunt.
2. Secondary to vasoconstriction due to increased pulmonary flow
3. Thromboembolism
4. Tumor embolism

Less common causes:

1. Bilharziasis.
2. Various forms of pulmonary arteritis:
   i. Polyarteritis
   ii. Disseminated lupus erythematosus.
3. Diffuse interstitial pulmonary fibrosis.
4. Idiopathic pulmonary hypertension rarely.

11. There are 4 probable mechanisms which may cause primary pulmonary hypertension (exact etiology is not known).

1. Neurohumoral mechanism: It is evidenced by sudden reduction of pulmonary vascular resistance after the injection of intrapulmonary vasodilators or by breathing oxygen.
2. Thromboemboli :
   a. Thrombus b. Parasitic
   c. Blood cells d. Tumor cells.
   - It may be an end stage of unrecognised thromboemboli originated from leg or pelvic veins.
   - Emboli from unrecognised amniotic emboli during pregnancy, commonly occurs in young women of 20–40 years.
   - Emboli of parasites in diseases such as filariasis or schistosomiasis.
   - Thrombi of sickle cells in sickle-cell disease.
   - Emboli from tumor cells.
3. Collagen vascular diseases, for example
   a. Arteritis, polyarteritis.
   b. Systemic lupus erythematosus.
   c. Scleroderma.
   d. Rheumatoid arthritis.

   Some immunological factor may be responsible, as the primary pulmonary hypertension may present from birth as reported in some families for more than two to three generations.
4. Iatrogenic: Drugs/poisons—e.g. cobalt.

   Use of oral contraceptives bear a relation particularly in families with history of primary pulmonary hypertension or systemic lupus erythematosis.
   - Association of increased occurrence observed in Europe between 1967 and 1970 in patients who used anorectic agent aminorex fumarate (Menocil) which is structurally similar to ephedrine.

12. The following symptoms are present in pulmonary hypertension.

The patient is usually a young female with recent onset of:

1. Dyspnea, fatigue and weakness are the main symptoms.
2. Precordial pain on exertion is seen in 25–50% of patients due to the load on the right ventricle and also effort syncope due to low cardiac output. Occasionally, comes with severe chest pain when associated with dissection of the main pulmonary artery. Cardiac pain, syncope, giddiness and death may occur when the coronary arterial branch supplying SA node is involved.
3. Hoarseness in some cases is due to compression of recurrent laryngeal nerve by the enlarged pulmonary artery.
4. Cyanosis—peripheral cyanosis occurs secondary to reduced cardiac output.

Central cyanosis occurs at the end stage from right to left shunt through a patent foramen ovale.

Hyperventilation results in hypocapnea and decreased bicarbonate concentration.

13. The following 4 signs are present on physical examination in pulmonary hypertension.

1. J V P shows prominent 'A' wave due to the right atrium contracting against the increased resistance to fill of the hypertrophied, stiff, non-compliant right ventricle.
2. Palpable P_2 from an enlarged pulmonary artery.
3. Left parasternal heave either from hypertrophied right ventricle or from an enlarged pulmonary artery or both.
4. Auscultation reveals—loud pulmonary second sound with narrow split—loud pulmonary component of the second sound is due to high pressure in the pulmonary circulation causing high velocity closure of the pulmonary valve.

Pulmonary regurgitation gives rise to a decrescendo diastolic murmur along the left sternal border resembling the murmur of aortic regurgitation. This can be easily distinguished by a small pulse volume and absence of hyperdynamic peripheral circulation.

When pulmonary regurgitation is associated with pulmonary hypertension due to mitral stenosis, the pulmonary diastolic murmur is known as the 'Graham Steell murmur'. The tricuspid regurgitation due to dilatation of atrioventricular ring on the right side is associated with systolic murmur. If the foramen ovale is not closed throughout patients' life, the high pressure in the right atrium results in right to left shunt. Ejection click at pulmonary area, often S_4, right atrial gallop at the lower left sternal border may be heard.

14. There are 4 roentgenogram findings.

1. Cardiac enlargement with right ventricular prominence. The heart is usually of a normal size until right ventricular failure occurs. Right atrial prominence on the right border.
2. Left atrial enlargement is good evidence of rise in left atrial pressure. The left atrial appendage is visible on the left border. It widens the angle between right and left main bronchus. Enlarged left atrial shadow may be visible within the right atrial shadow.
3. Marked enlargement of pulmonary artery and its main branches. The dilated main pulmonary artery may appear as a bulge to the left of the mediastinum between the aorta and left border of the heart. The main branches of left and right pulmonary arteries are also enlarged in the proximal parts, only to be pruned in periphery due to severe vasoconstriction.
4. Oligemic lung fields—some ischemia of the peripheral lung fields. The severe peripheral vasoconstriction results in abnormally translucent peripheral lung fields.

15. ECG may show the following 4 signs:

1. Right axis deviation.
2. Right ventricular hypertrophy.
3. Right atrial overload.
4. Inverted T waves over the right precordium—RVH with strain pattern.

16. Echocardiography shows the following 4 signs:

1. Dilated pulmonary artery.
2. Dilated right ventricle.
3. Dilated right atrium.
4. Pulmonary valve shows absent 'A' wave with midsystolic notch and flutter indicating significant pulmonary hypertension.

17. Treatment of primary pulmonary hypertension consists of 4 groups of drugs which are useful in some patients.

1. Vasodilators—act directly on vascular smooth muscle, e.g. sodium nitroprusside, diazoxide, hydralazine.
2. β-agonists, e.g. sublingual isoproterenol, oral terbutaline.
3. α-adrenergic blockers, e.g. phentolamine, phenoxybenzamine.
4. Calcium channel blockers, e.g. nifedipine, amlodipine (Immunosuppressive agents, prostaglandin antagonists (indomethacin) are rarely used).

18. The following 4 measurements are advised before instituting long-term treatment with the above group of drugs to assess the efficacy and to detect unfavorable effects.

1. Arterial pressure.
2. Cardiac output.
3. Pulmonary vascular resistance.
4. Pulmonary artery pressure and its response to oxygen breathing or intrapulmonary injection of vasodilators.

(Normal pulmonary artery pressure does not exceed 30/15 mm Hg. However, it may reach levels of systemic blood pressure in severe pulmonary hypertension)

19. Specific treatment of pulmonary hypertension.

1. Mitral stenosis when present should be relieved surgically before pulmonary hypertension develops.
2. Any shunt should be closed before the development of pulmonary hypertension. If pulmonary hypertension develops, it indicates delay in closure of the shunt.
3. When the cause of the pulmonary hypertension is obscure, and if it is suspected to be due to occult emboli, anticoagulants are often given.
4. Rest, cardiotonic agents and diuretics are to be given for right heart failure. Oxygen is given for hypoxia.

PULMONARY EMBOLISM

It is estimated that as many as 3,00,000 Americans have fatal PE each year and as many as 34% of affected individuals present with sudden death. The majority die because of the failure in diagnosis. The mortality rate for PE without treatment is approximately 30%, whereas only 2–8%with adequate treatment.

PE is the third most common cause of hospital related deaths in the US. PE is one of the most common preventable complications in high-risk hospitalized patients and may be fatal if untreated. Only one-third of all hospitalized patients at-risk for venous thromboembolism (VTE) receive adequate prophylactic treatment. Venous thromboembolism (VTE) deep vein thrombosis and pulmonary embolism (PE) represent different manifestations of the same clinically entity. It recurs frequently, is often overlooked, and can result in long-term complications including chronic thromboembolic pulmonary hypertension (CTPH) and the post thromboembolic syndrome (PTS).

20. 4 sites of deep vein thrombosis (DVT) are:

1. Lower extremities are the major common sites. Other less affected are:
2. Upper extremities.
3. Mesenteric.
4. Pelvic veins.

The main goal in the management of DVT is the prevention of PE and PTS.

Proximal lower extremity DVTS (popliteal vein and above) have an estimated risk for PE is 50%. If not treated, approximately 25% of calf muscle vein thrombi propagates (in the absence of treatment) to involve popliteal vein and above.

21. The most common inherited risk factors are 4:

1. Factor V Leiden and prothrombin gene mutation.
2. Deficiency of the natural anticoagulants' proteins C, S, and antithrombin.
3. Hyperhomocysteinemia.
4. Increased levels of factor VIII.

22. Acquired risk factors for PE are:

1. Immobilization (includes immobilization in POP).
2. Surgery (includes major surgery, total knee or hip replacement /thoracic surgery CABG, neurosurgery).
3. Trauma without intracranial hemorrhage, acute spinal cord injury).
4. Pregnancy/postpartum.
5. Oral contraceptives.
6. Hormone replacement.
7. Malignancy.
8. Antiphospholipid syndrome (lupus anticoagulant and or/anticardiolipid autoantibodies).
9. Heparin induced thrombocytopenia (HIT).
10. Obesity (BMI > 30).
11. Myeloproliferative disorders.
12. Inflammatory bowel disease.
13. Central venous catheters.
14. Pacemakers.
15. Nephrotic syndrome.
16. MI, ischemia, stroke with lower extremity paralysis, congestive heart failure, pulmonary infections.

Stasis, hypercoagulability and injury to the vessels wall (Virchow's triad) are the main causes of pathogenesis.

23. Pulmonary embolism may present as on of the following 4 conditions:

1. Generalized symptom of dyspnea, chest pain and malaise in majority of patients.
2. Leg swelling and pain if a patient of DVT C/O dyspnea, chest pain suspect PE.
3. Acute cor pulmonale as manifested by sudden development of dyspnea, cyanosis, shock or syncope usually have a massive PE leading to cardiovascular collapse.
4. Pulmonary infarction usually present with pleuritic chest pain, dyspnea and hemoptysis and an audible friction rub.

Symptoms of cough, hemoptysis, palpitation, wheezing, angina like chest pain tachypnea (> 20/min). Tachycardia (> 100/min). S_4, $P_2\uparrow$, cyanosis.

(See Table E2 for D/D of Acute Chest Pain)

24. Investigations.

1. Biochemical tests

i. Troponin levels are raised; higher mortality in elevated levels. Troponin are elevated with or without CAD. Correlate with RV pressure overload.

ii. Brain natriuretic peptide (BNP): Raised levels in the absence of renal dysfunction, is also a marker of RV dysfunction in patients with PE. The elevated BNP levels are adverse predictors in acute PE.

iii. Arterial blood gases: Hypoxia is present (PaO_2 < 80 mm Hg). A normal PaO_2 does not rule out PE. Hypoxia in the absence of cardiopulmonary disease should rise the suspension of PE. In patients with cardiopulmonary collapse, a normal PaO_2 suggests that PE is an unlikely cause (PaO_2 > 80 mm Hg).

iv. D-dimer, ELISA test has sensitivity 88–100, specificity 10–68 positive and negative predictive values vary with different assays. D-dimer levels of < 500 mg/mL as determined by ELISA and < 200 mg/mL by whole blood agglutination assay have a high negative predictive value. The later is useful to exclude PE. It is less useful in patients with malignancy, recent surgery or trauma or liver disease. Useful to exclude acute venous thrombosis and PE.

2. Chest X-ray: More helpful in establishing other diagnosis. Nonspecific findings include pleural effusion, atelectasis and consolidation. The classical signs are uncommon. They include Westermark sign (regional oligemia).
   Hampton's hump (plural based wedge-shaped shadow).
   Palla's sign (enlarged right inferior pulmonary artery are uncommon).
3. ECG: Mostly useful to rule out other major conditions such as AMI:
   i. Specific findings is the classic S_1 Q_3 T_3.
   ii. Nonspecific ST-T changes— sinus tachycardia, AF and RBBB are common. The patients with acute PE and increase RV end-diastolic volume and TR may show three or four of the following abnormalities in three-fourth of the patients.
   iii. Incomplete or complete RBBB.
   iv. S wave > 1.5 mm in LI and AVL.
   v. Shift of transitional zone to V_5—clockwise rotation.
   vi. Q in LIII and AVF but not in LII.
   vii. RAD > 90° or indeterminate axis.
   viii. T↓ in LIII and AVF or leads V_1 to V_4.
4. Echocardiography: More than 50% of patients who are hemodynamically stable do not show RV dysfunction on transthoracic echocardiography (TTE). Patients who are hemodynamic collapse generally show RV dysfunction.
   - TTE can provide rapid bedside assessment in these critically ill patients.
   - TTE findings include RV dilatation, RV hypokinesia. TR, septal flatting, paradoxical septal motion, diastolic LV impairment secondary to septal displacement.
   - PA hypertension, reduced inspiratory collapse of the inferior venae cava and occasionally direct visualization of the thrombosis.

   Mc Connell's sign: In large PE with moderate or severe RV free wall hypokinesia, there is a relative sparing of the apex—this Mc Connell's sign has a specificity of 94% and a positive predictive value of 71% for PE. This is helpful in differentiating RV dysfunction due to PE versus other causes.
   This is mostly useful to evaluate acute cardiopulmonary syndrome, to help diagnosis or to exclude pericardial tamponade, aortic dissection, AMI, valvular dysfunction and myocardial rupture.
5. Ventilation perfusion (V/Q) scanning:
   This is useful in patients who have normal X-ray chest and who are not suitable for CT scanning—such as those with renal insufficiency, contrast allergy or pregnancy.
6. CT scanning: It can directly visualize the thrombus so it has become the standard technique for diagnosing PE. Useful in evaluating central PE thrombus (seen as intraluminal filling defect), direct in aging of inferior venae cava, pelvic and leg veins ventilation perfusion scan is useful.
7. MRI may be alternative to CT in patients who have contrast allergy. Cardiolinium enhanced MR angiography has 75–100% sensitivity 95–100% specificity.
8. Pulmonary angiography remains the gold standard in diagnosing PE; it has 97% sensitivity and 99% specificity. The event of noninvasive CT has regular HIE test.

25. Differential diagnosis of pulmonary embolism.

(see Table E-2—Acute Chest Pain)

1. Myocardial ischemia, infarction and myocarditis-associated with specific ECG and echocardiography changes.
2. Pericarditis and pericardial tamponade—associated with specific ECG and echocardiography changes.
3. Aortic dissection—diagnosed by TTE, CT with contrast, MRI or angiography.
4. Acute pulmonary edema—diagnosed by cardiac evaluation and chest X-ray.
5. Excerebration of primary and secondary pulmonary hypertension—h/o of pulmonary HT is helpful, however, worsening should prompt consideration of PE as a precipitating factor.
6. Pleurisy—diagnosed by exclusion.
7. Pneumothorax—plain X-ray chest, CT establishes the diagnosis.
8. Acute bronchitis and pneumothorax, h/o chest X-ray, sputum examination, and culture help to differentiate infection from PE.
9. Excerebration of asthma and COPD, h/o these disorders with a compatible course of illness is helpful.
10. Musculoskeletal pain—includes osteoarthritis, rib fractures, muscle strain. Pain is more reproductive. It is a diagnosis of exclusion.
11. Primary or metastatic lung cancer—associated with specific radiographic and histopathologic findings.
12. Subdiaphragmatic processes—ultrasonography, upper abdomen CT or MRI.

26. Treatment of PE.

Drug therapy of PE
Anticoagulants:
1. Heparin
2. LMWH

3. Fondaparinux
4. Addition of VKA.

For patients with nonmassive PE, subcutaneous LMWH IV, UFH or fondaparinux are recommended. Should be continued for 4–5 days and until INR is stable and ≥ 2.0. Unfractionated heparin enhances the activity of antithrombin (factor II a) and factor Xa activity. Anti Xa to anti IIa ratio 1:1. IV infusion of intermittent or subcutaneous administration to keep APTT at a level that corresponds to a plasma heparin level between 0.2–0.4 μ/mL. By protamine titration or 0.3–0.7 μ/mL by anti factor—Xa assay (103:104).

Nomogram should be used for dose adjustments. Treatment should be given for at least 5–7 days with an overlap with warfarin for at least 4–5 days until INR is therapeutic for 2 consecutive days.

2. LMWH: Antithrombin mediated inhibition of factor Xa, also inhibits thrombin (factor IIa). Anti–Xa to anti IIa ratio of 2–4:1. Dose varies depending on LMWH type, weight-based dosing is used. For example,

- Daltaparin—100 μ/kg SC every 13 hr or 200 μ/kg SC every 24 hr
- Enoxaparin—1 mg/kg SC every 12 hr or 1.5 mg/kg SC every 24 hr
- Nadroparin—86 μ/kg SC every 12 hr or 171 μ/kg SC every 24 hr
- Tinzaparin—175 μ/kg SC every 24 hr

Routine monitoring of anticoagulation treatment is not necessary.

Danaparoid sodium is mixture of glycosaminoglycans with predominant anti-factor Xa activity loading dose of 250 μ IV bolus (adjusted according to weight) 400 μ/h for 4 hours. 300 μ/h for 4 hours (adjusted according to weights). Maintenance 150–200 μ/h.

Not recommended in USA.

Direct thrombin inhibitors.

Recombinant hirudin—direct inhibition of thrombin activity—not routinely used).

Anti Xa Inhibitors

Fondaparinux: Antithrombin mediated selective inhibition of factor Xa 5–10 mg SCQD.

As safe and effective as unfractionated heparin in the initial treatment of hemodynamically stable patients with PE.

Warfarin: Inhibits hepatic V-carboxylation of glutamic acid residues of vitamin K dependent coagulation factors II, VII, IX and X; also inhibits production of antithrombotic protein C and S

Dosage varies to keep the INR between 2.0–3.0.

It may be guided by nomogram on day 1 of heparin; alternatively, initial warfarin dosing may be guided by the results of pharmacogenomics testing if available.

Heparin and warfarin should be overlapped for 4–5 days until INR becomes therapeutic for 2 consecutive days and continue for at least 3 months. Using 10 mg starting dose may achieve therapeutic INR more quickly without an increase in bleeding than 5 mg staring dose.

27. Thrombolytic therapy: It is highly individualized because of favorable results with anticoagulation for PE.

Thrombolysis should be reserved for hemodynamically unstable patients, with acute massive PE and low-risk of bleeding.

i. Streptokinase.
ii. Urokinase.
iii. Recombinant tissue plasminogen activator (rt-PA).
iv. Reteplase are the drugs available.

Local administration of thrombolytic therapy through the catheter is not advised owing to the risk of hemorrhage at the insertion site. (Refer: Thrombolytic treatment in AMI for dosage and others)

PULMONARY EMBOLECTOMY

Surgical embolectomy or catheter assisted or aspiration, fragmentation, or rheolytic therapy is indicated when anti-coagulation or thrombolytic therapy is contraindicated or unsuccessfull.

N Pericardial Disease

The normal pericardium is distensible and permits unimpeded expansion of the ventricles during diastole. Normally, it transmits intrathoracic pressure changes to the heart, resulting in increased venous return to the right side of the heart with inspiration and increased pulmonary venous return to the left side of the heart with expiration.

1. The functions of pericardium are:

1. It helps to maintain the shape of the heart within the chest cavity.
2. Reduces friction during the cardiac cycle by its two layers. Innervisceral layer is adherent to the myocardium about 35 mL of serous fluid is present between the inner visceral and outer fibrous layer.
3. It acts as a barrier to infections and inflammations.
4. It secrets prostaglandins that can modulate cardiac reflexes and coronary tone.

2. The causes of pericardial disease are:

(Etiologic classification)

1. Infective:
   - i. Viral: The specific viruses are:
     - Coxsackie A or B
     - Influenza
     - Echo 8
     - Herpes simplex
     - Chicken pox
     - Adenovirus

     When a virus is suspected, but could not be proved by isolation or serology and when no other cause is evident, the condition is often referred to as acute idiopathic pericarditis.
   - ii. Bacterial:
     - a. Specific: Tuberculosis. It may present as acute, subacute or chronic pericarditis. May persists as a chronic condition. There may be no other evidence of tuberculosis but in some cases early symptoms of systemic illness such as fever, anorexia, lethargy and weight loss may be present.
     - b. Non-specific: Usually secondary to cardiac surgery, immunosuppression, rupture of the esophagus or pneumococcal pneumonia, *Staphylococcus*, *Streptococcus*, gram-negative septicemia, *Neisseria gonorrhoeae*.
   - iii. Mycotic:
     - a. Histoplasmosis
     - b. Blastomycosis
     - c. Aspergillosis
     - d. Candidiasis.
   - iv. Other infections (syphilis, parasitic):

     Parasitic:
     - a. Amoebiasis
     - b. Toxoplasmosis
     - c. Echinococcosis
     - d. Trichinosis.
2. Vascular:
   - i. Myocardial infarction: It can occur either during the acute phase of the illness due to involvement of the pericardium in the infarcted area or as part of the postcardiac injury syndrome.
   - ii. Aortic aneurysm (with leakage into pericardial sac).
   - iii. Cardiac surgery (with leakage into pericardial sac).
   - iv. Hemorrhage within the pericardium during anticoagulant therapy.
3. Hypersensitivity or autoimmune reaction
   - i. Rheumatic fever: Pericarditis is usually associated with evidence of rheumatic carditis.

ii. Collagen vascular disease (collagenoses):
   a. Systemic lupus erythematosus (SLE)
   b. Rheumatoid arthritis (RA)
   c. Scleroderma
   d. Polyarteritis nodosa (PAN).
iii. Drug induced: Causing SLE-like syndrome, e.g:
   a. Hydralazine
   b. Procainamide
   c. Isoniazid
   d. Minoxidil
   e. Phenytoin
   f. Phenylbutazone
   g. Penicillin.
iv. Post cardiac injury:
   a. Postmyocardial infarction (Dressler's syndrome).
   b. Postpericardiotomy.

4. Metabolic:
   i. Uremia: It can also occur occasionally in patients receiving hemodialysis.
   ii. Myxedema: Rare, usually asymptomatic. Invariably resolves with treatment of hypothyroidism.
   iii. Hypercholesterolemia.
   iv. Hypoprotenemia with severe chronic anemia.
5. Traumatic:
   i. Penetrating chest wall injuries.
   ii. Non-penetrating chest wall injuries.
   iii. Surgical trauma.
   iv. Posti-rradiation: As a side-effect of irradiation of tumors within the thorax, especially tumors within the mediastinum.
   v. Post MI pericardial injury syndromes.
   vi. Post MI Dressler's syndrome.
   vii. Postpericardiectomy syndrome.
   viii. Dissecting aortic aneurysm.
6. Neoplastic:
   Primary
   i. Benign.
   ii. Malignant.
   iii. Invasion from the adjacent primary carcinoma of the bronchus, or from secondary deposits due to leukemia or tumors such as carcinoma of breast or lymphoma.
   iv. Tumors from distant metastasis to pericardium.
7. Congenital—rare. For example,
   i. Associated with atrial septal defect.
   ii. Familial pericarditis.
   iii. Mulibrey nanism pericarditis (autosomal recessive syndrome).
8. Miscellaneous: For example,
   i. Chylopericardium
   ii. Infectious mononucleosis
   iii. Sarcoidosis
   iv. Severe chronic anemia.

3. There are 4 common causes of pericarditis:

1. Myocardial infarction.
2. Viral infections (common with Coxsackie-B).
3. Rheumatic fever.
4. Tuberculosis.

4. There are 4 types of pericarditis:

1. Fibrinous, e.g. tuberculosis—acute fibrinous deposits show characteristic 'bread-and-butter appearance'.
2. Serous, e.g. rheumatic.
3. Hemorrhagic, e.g. malignancy, trauma.
4. Purulent, e.g. pyogenic infections.

5. There are 4 main clinical conditions of the pericardium:

Clinical classification
1. Acute pericarditis (< 6 weeks)
   a. Fibrinous.
   b. Effusive (or bloody).
2. Subacute pericarditis (6 weeks to 6 months)
   a. Constrictive.
   b. Effusive-constrictive.
3. Chronic pericarditis (> 6 months)
   a. Constrictive.
   b. Effusive.
   c. Adhesive (non-constrictive).
4. Pericardial effusion/tamponade.

6. Clinical presentation in acute pericarditis varies from patient-to-patient depending on the cause and underlying pathology and can be grouped into the following 4 categories:

The clinical manifestations are due to the fall in cardiac output and to systemic venous congestion.
1. Chest pain.
2. Dyspnea and other symptoms resulting from compression of heart and other organs. Symptoms of acute circulatory failure may be seen.
3. General symptoms of underlying disease.
4. Atrial arrhythmias.

7. There are 4 points to note in chest pain.

1. Site of pain: Retrosternal or parasternal. It may be at the lower end of chest in xiphoid area and may be confused with acute abdomen.
2. Character of pain: It may be so mild that it may be forgotten by the patient or may be very sharp and severe and uncomfortable with deep inspiration.
3. Radiation: Posterior and anterior to cervical region
   - Over either side of trapezius or
   - Over either shoulders (usually left)
   - Pain radiating down the arm (is very rare).
4. Precipitation or aggravation of pain: Often pain is pleuritic, i.e. made worse by deep inspiration, coughing, lying flat, exercise, swallowing, often

relieved by sitting up and leaning forward or adopting some other particular position.

8. Pain is often absent in a slowly developing pericarditis in conditions like:

1. Tuberculosis.
2. Postirradiation.
3. Neoplastic.
4. Uremic.

9. There are 4 important signs to look in pericarditis.

1. A pericardial rub: It is the main diagnostic sign of pericarditis. It consists of:
   a. Superficial scratching sound like the rubbing of sand paper and sound is best heard to the left of the lower sternum.
   b. Usually systolic but may consist of presystole, systolic and diastolic components.
   c. 'To and Fro rub' is the most common and is due to ventricular systolic and atrial systolic components. It is best heard over the 2nd, 3rd, intercostal spaces over the bear area of the heart.
   d. Better heard when stethoscope diaphragm is pressed firmly on the chest and the breathing is held in inspiration than in expiration. Because of its high pitched quality, it often sounds 'nearer' to the listener than a murmur.
2. If effusion develops, heart sounds become quieter. Hepatosplenomegaly ascites comes early than peripheral edema. Jugular venous pressure is raised and systemic venous congestion results.
3. If effusion is rapid and large cardiac tamponade develops. It interferes with diastolic filling. Patient may show signs of acute circulatory failure due to fall in cardiac output.
4. Pulsus paradoxus—change in pulse volume with breathing in which systolic pressure diminishes with inspiration—It is only a physical exacerbation. (The word paradox is misnamed).

10. There are 4 investigations:

1. X-ray chest: This is not specific. There is overall enlargement of cardiac silhouette and the lung fields are less congested than in cardiac failure. Heart shadow is like pear-shaped like a 'water-bottle' configuration of cardiac silhouette.
   Rarely the pericardium and cardiac edge can be distinguished separately along the left border.
   Pericardial calcification may be seen in chronic pericarditis.
   Diminished pulsation of cardiac silhouette are seen on fluoroscopy in large perfusion.
2. ECG.
3. Echocardiogram: It is particularly useful in detecting even small pericardial effusions. It is the most sensitive and specific test.
4. Paracentesis of pericardial effusion for diagnostic and therapeutic purpose.

11. There are 4 points to be noted in ECG in acute pericarditis not due to myocardial infarction.

The ECG changes are due to diffuse epicardial injury caused by associated epicardial epimyocarditis which are seen as:

1. Concave ST elevation like the back of a saddle, occurs in most leads involving two or three standard limb leads and V_2 to V_6.
2. ST elevation resolves after few days to be replaced by inversion of the T wave. The symmetrical T inversion is due to epicardial ischemia. Abnormal T waves may be permanent or they may revert to normal. Average resolution time is nearly two weeks.
3. Reciprocal depression is seen only in aVR and V1 and without significant changes in QRS complexes, except occasional diminution in voltage.
4. Depression of PR segment (below the TP segment) in V_2 to V_6 seen in many cases of pericarditis. This is an useful sign to differentiate from early repolarization variants.

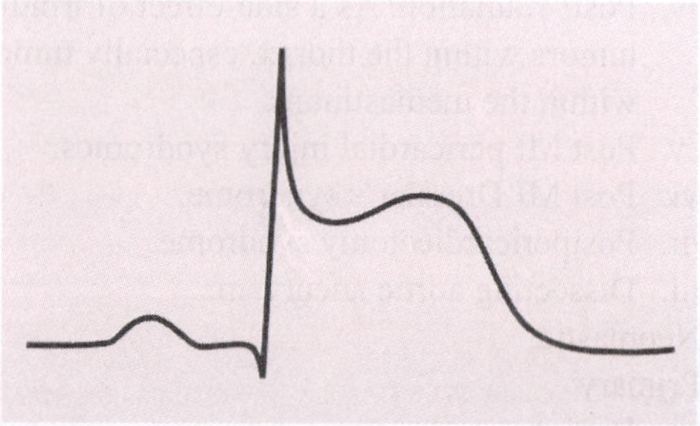

Fig. N-1: Typical concave ST elevation in pericarditis

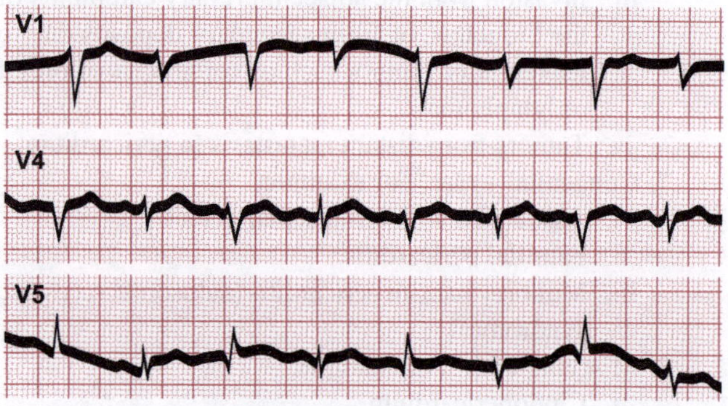

Fig. N-2: ECG showing low voltage and electrical alternans of the QRS in pericardial effusion

12. There are 4 points to be noted in ECG in pericardial effusion.

1. Sinus tachycardia is the commonest finding.
2. QRS complexes are of low voltage due to fluid within the pericardium inhibiting the conduction of impulses to the recording electrode.
3. QRS electrical alternans may occur. It consists of alternating complexes of differing morphology due to the heart swinging freely within the pericardial fluid.
4. Atrial ectopics or actual fibrillation may sometimes accompany.

13. The 4 differentiating points of ECG of acute pericarditis from acute myocardial infarction.

Table N-1

Pericarditis	*Myocardial Infarction*
1. ST segment is elevated with concavity upward like the back of a saddle	ST segment is elevated with convexity upward
2. Reciprocal changes may be only in aVR and V1	Reciprocal changes are usually more prominent
3. No significant QRS change except occasional diminution in voltage. No Q waves	QRS changes occur particularly the development of Q waves
4. T wave inversion occurs usually after ST segment returns to normal	T wave inversion occurs before the ST segment returns to isoelectrical

14. There are 4 causes of postcardiac syndrome.

1. Postmyocardial infarction when it is known as Dressler's syndrome.
2. A stab wound to the heart.
3. Postsurgical trauma.
4. Postirradiation.

It is presumed that the underlying mechanism of the postcardiac injury syndrome is an antigen-antibody reaction resulting from release of cardiac antigen into the circulation during the original illness. Usually, it manifests itself within one to three weeks after the original illness.

15. There are 4 clinical characteristics of postcardiac injury syndrome.

1. Pyrexia
2. Pericarditis
3. Pleurisy
4. Raised ESR.

Arthralgia may also develop.

16. Treatment of pericardial disease: It depends on the cause, duration and complications.

Drugs:

1. Non-specific treatment of viral or idiopathic pericarditis: Aspirin suffices for the control of pain 900 mg qid or 4th hrly. Indomethacin 25–75 mg qid 4th hrly.
   - Ibuprofen 400 mg qid.
   - Corticosteroids—Prednisolone 20–80 mg/day, in divided doses.
   - Corticosteroids are given in postpericardiectomy, and in idiopathic pericarditis. They are also given in purulent pericarditis as a complication of septicemia or diseases that spread from intrathoracic infections or from penetrating injury. Corticosteroids are not given unless the non-steroidal treatment has failed. When given, they should be tapered and discontinued as rapidly as the clinical condition improves.
   - Antibiotics are given.
   - Surgery is needed, if necessary.
2. Specific treatment is given in conditions like tuberculous pericarditis, amoebiasis, hydatid cysts, collagen diseases, etc.
3. Paracentesis is advised in pericardial effusion.
   Cardiac tamponade is diagnostic as well as therapeutic. This must be done if there is rapid accumulation of fluid or cardiorespiratory embarrassment.
   Pericardial fluid should be sent for complete analysis to differentiate transudate from exudate—hematocrit, TWBC, differential count, glucose protein, cytology, culture and sensitivity, grams staining, AFB staining, etc.
4. Surgical resection of pericardium or pericardiectomy is indicated:
   - For chronic constrictive pericarditis
   - For chronic recurrent effusions
   - For thick pyogenic effusions.

CARDIAC TAMPONADE

Cardiac tamponade is a clinical condition resulting from effusion into the pericardial space interfering with filling of the ventricles during diastole. Any cause of acute or chronic pericarditis may lead to the development of pericardial effusion.

17. The development of critical cardiac state depends on:

1. The amount of fluid—may be as small as 250 mL when the fluid accumulates rapidly.
2. It may be 1000 mL when the fluid accumulates slowly. The pericardium has time to stretch and adopt to the increasing fluid volume.
3. Volume of fluid required to produce tamponade varies directly with the thickness of the myocardium.
4. Inversely with the thickness of the pericardium.

18. The clinical features of cardiac tamponade results from the following mechanism:

The tightly contained layer of fluid around the heart interferes with filling of the ventricles during diastole. It causes:

1. Low cardiac output with a small stroke volume.
2. Compensatory tachycardia.
3. Reduced output of urine.
4. Restricted venous return resulting in venous congestion.

19. Common causes of pericardial effusion/cardiac tamponade.

1. Bleeding into pericardial space during cardiac surgery or during diagnostic procedures (including cardiac perforation during diagnostic procedures, perforation of the heart with a pacemaker catheter).
2. Tuberculosis.
3. Active viral or idiopathic pericarditis.
4. Rheumatic.
5. Postmyocardial infarction.
6. Tumors—most commonly carcinoma of lung, breast and lymphoma from the mediastinum.
7. Uremia and during dialysis.
8. Amoebic abscess rupturing into the pericardium.

20. Less common causes:

1. Trauma.
2. Pyogenic.
3. Postradiation therapy.
4. Acute pericarditis while on treatment with anticoagulants.
5. Collagen diseases.
6. Blood dyscrasiasis: Leukemia, purpura.
7. Myxedema.
8. Scurvy.
9. Postpericardiotomy syndrome.
10. Ruptured aneurysm of aorta into pericardium.
11. Fungal: actinomycosis, histoplasmosis.
12. Secondary to inflammation of surrounding tissue, e.g. pleurisy.

21. Clinical features: Classical signs of falling arterial pressure, rising venous pressure and a small quiet heart with faint heart sounds usually occur within minutes in conditions such as cardiac trauma. More frequently the cardiac tamponade develops slowly and signs and symptoms similar to that of heart failure, include dyspnea, orthopnea, hepatomegaly, raise in JVP are seen. The main signs are:

1. *Inspection:* JVP is markedly elevated with exaggeration of the 'X' descent. Often the 'Y' descent is absent. Sometimes venous paradoxus or Kussmaul's sign is also present. Apex beat is not visible.
2. *Palpation:* Apex is usually impalpable or very feebly felt. If palpable it is typically inside the lateral border of cardiac dullness.
   - Pulse is of small volume with sinus tachycardia.
   - Pulsus paradoxus is present.
   - Blood pressure is below 100 mm Hg.
   - Hepatomegaly.
3. *Percussion:* Increased cardiac dullness. Upper border in the second space, right border parasternal and left border outside the apex.
4. *Auscultation:* Heart sounds are faint and muffled. The fluid in the pericardial sac interferes with the conduction of sound to the stethoscope. As a result of low cardiac output, the heart valves close with a low velocity that generates very little sound.

22. There are 4 points to know about arterial pulsus paradoxus.

1. This is an exaggeration of the normal variation of systemic blood pressure during respiratory cycle and is not in anyway paradoxical. The fall of systolic blood pressure more than 10 mm Hg during inspiration is an important clue to the diagnosis of cardiac tamponade.
2. It may be found in one-third to half the cases of cardiac tamponade. It can also occur in other conditions.
3. In majority of cases, it can be easily detected while recording the blood pressure by using sphygmomanometer. Occasionally, it may be so marked that it can easily be felt at the radial artery.
4. The main mechanism of it is that the tightly contained fluid in the pericardial sac obstructs venous return to the heart and thereby cardiac filling. The pressure within the thorax and its contents falls in the normal way during inspiration. This fall of pressure in the pulmonary veins may result in abnormal fall of pressure that is less than the abnormal pressure within the heart as it sits in the tightly contained pericardial sac. As a result the flow of blood from the pulmonary veins to the heart is reduced or even reversed during inspiration causing a temporary reduction of cardiac output and blood pressure. Increased pressure that occurs in the thorax and pulmonary veins during expiration is sufficient to drive blood forward into the heart, restoring cardiac output and blood pressure.

23. Arterial pulsus paradoxus occurs in one-third to half of the patients with constrictive pericarditis or pericardial effusion. It is not pathognomonic of pericardial disease alone. It can also occur in:

1. Airway obstruction—For example:
   Asthma, chronic obstructive pulmonary disease (COPD).

2. Restricted cardiomyopathy.
3. Hypovolemic shock.
4. Cardiac failure.

24. There are 4 investigations of cardiac tamponade.

1. *X-ray chest/fluoroscopy:* This shows a typical large globular-shaped heart that may be indistinguishable from the heart of a cardiomyopathy. In pericardial effusion, the lung fields are characteristically clear whereas lung fields are typically congested with left ventricular failure due to cardiomyopathy.
   Fluoroscopy shows diminished pulsations of cardiac silhouette.
2. *ECG:* ECG shows sinus tachycardia often with low voltage QRS and sometimes QRS electrical alternans.
3. *Echocardiography:* This a very important investigation in the diagnosis of pericardial effusion. The echo free space between the visceral and parietal layers of the pericardium is occupied by the fluid.
   Even very small amount of fluid can be demonstrated. With large effusions, similar space may be demonstrated in front of the heart.
4. *Cardiac catheterization:* It is not routinely performed. If performed, it shows that the end-diastolic pressure within each of the four chambers of the heart is the same to within 5 mm Hg.

25. The following 4 points are noted in cardiac catheterization.

1. Right atrial pressure is raised with a prominent 'X' but no 'Y' descent.
2. Pericardial pressure is also elevated and equal to the right atrial pressure.
3. Pulmonary artery wedge pressure is equal or close to right atrial, right ventricular and pulmonary artery diastolic pressure.
4. The 'square root' sign of constrictive pericarditis is usually absent.

(In addition, injection of contract medium demonstrates the increase in distance between the outside of the cardiac silhouette and the outline of the left or right ventricular cavities).

26. Management of pericardial effusion/cardiac tamponade.

1. All the patients with pericarditis should be observed carefully for any development of effusion. If effusion is already present, one should look for signs of cardiac tamponade.
2. In the presence of effusion: Continuous monitoring of arterial and venous pressures and heart rate should be done. Serial radiograms of chest should be noted.
   Serial echocardiographic findings should be noted.
3. Resuscitation: If the tamponade is severe causing cardiorespiratory embarrassment with severe arterial hypotension, the patient should be immediately resuscitated by giving intravenous fluids to increase the cardiac output.
4. Pericardiocentesis by needle aspiration is done by using the apical or xiphisternal approach. If the needle is connected to an ECG lead, ST elevation on the cardiograph will indicate that the needle has touched the myocardium in which case the needle should be withdrawn a little.

The aspirated pericardial fluid that is blood stained can be differentiated from the left ventricle by its dark color and its failure to clot.

27. Paracentesis of pericardial effusion.

Withdraw few milliliters of fluid for diagnostic purpose. The needle is passed to the left of xiphoid process, inserted deep to the left costal margin and then directed toward left shoulder or the needle is inserted medial to the cardiac apex as seen in the echocardiography where a layer of fluid is lying infront of the heart. For therapeutic purpose it is safe to use a plastic cannula inserted over a needle or guide wire than to attempt aspiration at a time.

Dangers of paracentesis:

1. Sudden collapse due to aspiration of large effusion at a time.
2. Arrhythmias.
3. Injury to coronary artery.
4. Exacerbation of tamponade due to injury to right ventricle.

CHRONIC CONSTRICTIVE PERICARDITIS

Chronic constrictive pericarditis is a clinical condition caused by scarring and contraction of the pericardium interfering with filling of the ventricles during diastole. All causes of acute or chronic pericarditis can lead to chronic constrictive pericarditis.

28. Chronic constrictive pericarditis is:

1. Common in tuberculosis.
2. Frequent in rheumatoid arthritis.
3. Less frequent in hemopericardium.
4. Rare with acute pericarditis.

29. Pathophysiology.

1. The healing of an acute fibrinous or serofibrinous pericarditis follows obliteration of the pericardial cavity by the formation of granulation tissue that contracts resulting in scar formation. The obliteration of the pericardial cavity interferes with the filling of the ventricles during diastole. The hallmark of

constrictive pericarditis is the equalization of end-diastolic pressures in all 4 cardiac chambers that raise in both systemic and pulmonary pressures and thus progress to signs and symptoms of right and left heart failure.

2. Stroke volume is diminished. End-diastolic pressures in both the ventricles as well as the mean pressures in the atria, pulmonic veins and systemic veins are elevated to about the same levels. The clinical features are mainly due to the low cardiac output and restricted venous return causing venous congestion. This is augmented by sodium retention.

   Despite these hemodynamic affects, myocardial function may be normal, instead the ventricles may be considered to be underloaded.
3. Central venous pressure and right and left atrial pressures show an 'M'-shaped contour with prominent constrictive pericarditis unlike in cardiac tamponade. The pressure contour of cardiac tamponade differs in that the most prominent deflection is the 'X' trough whereas the 'Y' descent is usually absent. These changes are recognized by JVP and can be recorded.
4. Both ventricular pressure pulses exhibit characteristic 'square root' sign during diastole which is not seen in cardiac tamponade.

30. Clinical features:

1. Weakness, fatigue, weight loss and anorexia are common. Patient often presents with decreased muscle mass, protuberant abdomen and edema feet. Marked wasting of the muscles is often present and combined with the ascites may be mistaken for malignancy.
2. Ascites rather than breathlessness is prominent. Ascites is mainly due to increased venous pressure and partly due to sodium retention. Breathlessness is often present with exertion and orthopnea is common. Attacks of acute left ventricular failure causing acute pulmonary edema practically never occurs in chronic constrictive pericarditis.
3. Edema of the legs present but not marked.
4. Heart size is usually normal or only slightly enlarged. In about half the cases, there may be systolic indrawing of the anterior chest wall due to adhesions from the pericardium to the chest wall.

   Other features of the condition are generally similar to those of cardiac tamponade.
5. A small volume pulse with sinus tachycardia occurs compensate for maintaining cardiac output. However, the pulse is irregular due to atrial fibrillation in one-third of cases.
6. Slight arterial pulsus paradoxus may be present but is usually less prominent than in cardiac tamponade.
7. A markedly raised jugular venous pulse is seen—often with prominent 'X' and 'Y' descents and sometimes with a paradoxical increase on inspiration—(Kussmaul's sign). 'Y' descent is usually absent in cardiac tamponade.
8. The heart sounds are quiet and distant in contrast to cardiac tamponade. There may be an early third heart sound, i.e. pericardial knock occurring 0.06–0.12 sec after aortic closure is often present.

31. There are 4 other organs affected by chronic constrictive pericarditis.

1. *Liver:* Hepatomegaly is due to venous congestion. It impairs hepatic function. Anorexia, jaundice are often seen.
2. *Spleen:* Spleen is enlarged due to congestion. In the absence of infective endocarditis or tricuspid valve disease, splenomegaly in a patient with congestive heart failure should rise the suspicion of constrictive pericarditis.
3. *Kidney:* Nephrotic syndrome or sometimes only marked proteinuria or hypoalbuminemia occurs. This will augment the ascites and may complicate chronic constrictive pericarditis.
4. *Gut:* Protein-losing gastroenteropathy due to impaired lymphatic drainage from the small intestines may complicate chronic constrictive pericarditis. This can occur as a result of venous congestion.

32. The 4 investigations in chronic constrictive pericarditis are:

1. *Chest X-ray:* Heart size is usually normal or slightly increased. Pericardial calcification may be seen on lateral film or with fluoroscopy. The lung fields are usually clear.
2. *ECG:* Shows sinus tachycardia, voltage is often low. Atrial fibrillation is seen in some cases. T wave may be flattened or inverted.
3. *Echocardiogram:* May show pericardial fluid or thickened pleura. It has got a limited value.
4. *Cardiac catheterization:* The end-diastolic pressure within each of the four chambers is same to within 5 mm Hg. This is characteristic of chronic constrictive pericarditis. In addition, it may demonstrate thickened pericardium.

33. Treatment consists of:

1. Treatment of the cause, e.g. antituberculous treatment during the effusion stage may prevent constriction. It should be given in the pre- and postoperative periods.

2. Diuretics may be given before surgery. They should be given continuously so that drastic reduction of venous pressure is prevented. The reduction of high venous pressure is required to maintain cardiac output.
3. Digitalis may be beneficial to prevent the heart failure.
4. Pericardiectomy: When once the thickened pericardium is resected, there will be increased inflow of blood into the ventricles that may result in increased burden on the atrophic myocardium. It is the definitive treatment for chronic constrictive pericarditis. Complete cardiac decortication shows dramatic improvement.

O Acquired Diseases of the Aorta and its Branches

1. Introduction

Aorta is the principal conductance vessel in the body and is divided into 4 parts

1. Ascending aorta: It includes the aortic root, which contains the sinuses of Valsalva. The left and right coronary arteries arise from the left and right sinuses respectively.
2. The aortic arch gives rise to the great vessels of the head and upper limbs. These include innominate (brachiocephalic), the left common carotid, and the left subclavian arteries.
3. The descending aorta: Gives intercostal vessels as it courses through the posterior mediastinum. The vascular supply to the anterior spinal artery is included among these vessels.
4. The abdominal aorta begins just after the aorta crosses the diaphragm. It provides splanchnic ad renal arteries before bifurcating to become the common iliac arteries.

ANEURYSMS

Aortic aneurysm is defined as a pathologic dilatation to more than 1.5 times the normal diamater of the aorta. This can be either fusiform (symmetric dilatation or saccular (asymmetric outpouching) or pseudoaneurysm.

2. The walls of the aorta must stand against the pressure of each systolic thrust of blood. Aorta is under high tension than the rest of the arterial system because the wall tension depends on both diameter and pressure. In addition, the aorta is prone to diseases due to 4 causes:

1. Arteriosclerosis—which has replaced syphilis as the most common disease of the aorta.
2. Necrosis of the media.
3. Trauma.
4. Infection.

3. 4 major diseases arise out of stresses.

1. Arteriosclerotic occlusive disease.
2. Aneurysm.
3. Dissection.
4. Aortitis.

4. The causes of aneurysm are 4:

1. Arteriosclerosis—the commonest cause.
2. Cystic medial necrosis.
3. Trauma.
4. Syphilis and other infections.

5. Aneurysms of the aorta are divided into 4 varieties according to the site of affection.

1. Aneurysms of the abdominal aorta just below the renal arteries—most frequent—atherosclerosis is the common cause of aneurysm of abdominal and thoracic aorta.
2. Aneurysms of the descending thoracic or aorta distal to the origin of the left subclavian artery.
3. Aneurysms of the aortic arch.
   The most common aneurysms are fusiform, in which total circumference is involved and become diffusely dilated. Saccular aneurysms involve a portion of the wall and result in outpouching from a portion of the wall. Three-fourth of all aneurysms occur in the abdominal aorta just below the renal arteries.
4. Aneurysms of the ascending aorta—syphilis and cystic medial necrosis have predilection for the ascending aorta.

6. Aneurysms of the abdominal aorta commonly occur in 4 situations.

1. Men (Male to female ratio is 9:1)
2. Over sixty years of age with arteriosclerotic changes.
3. Association with hypertension (more than 50%) —persistent systolic hypertension further enlarges aneurysm and may predispose to their rupture.
4. Cigarette smokers.

Majority of the abdominal aortic aneurysms are caused by arteriosclerosis.

7. Aneurysm of the ascending wall caused by syphilis, was common before the introduction of penicillin. The causes of aneurysm of the ascending aorta at present are 4:

1. Cystic medial necrosis which may present along with Marfan's syndrome.
2. Hypertension.
3. Aging of the aorta.
4. Idiopathic.

8. When the aneurysm of the ascending aorta is due to cystic medial necrosis, it may result in aortic regurgitation leading to ventricular failure.

There are 4 ways in treatment.

1. Resection of the aneurysm.
2. Replacement of the ascending aorta.
3. Replacement of the aortic valve.
4. Coronary reimplantation.

9. Clinical manifestations are mainly caused by pressure on the adjacent structures. They depend on the site and size of the aneurysm. The following clinical features are seen.

1. Aneurysm of the ascending aorta or arch of the aorta causes pulsatile anterior chest wall swelling.
   Aneurysm of the arch of aorta. Causes pulsatile swelling near the manubrium sternum or parasternal region.
   Aneurysm of the descending thoracic aorta. Causes pulsatile swelling in the paraspinal region posteriorly aneurysm of the abdominal aorta. Causes pulsatile swelling in the midepigastric area.
2. Aneurysm of the aortic arch can exert pressure on the trachea and bronchus and produce cough with or without expectoration, stridor, dyspnea, segmental lung collapse or bronchiectasis.
3. Pressure on the superior vena cava caused by either aneurysm of the ascending aorta or arch of the aorta — produces venous congestion of the face, neck and upper limbs and dilatation of superficial chest veins. Headache or vertigo is due to increased intracranial tension.
4. Pressure on the main pulmonary trunk or pulmonary artery caused by aneurysm of either arch of aorta or descending thoracic aorta—produces acquired pulmonary stenosis or cor pulmonale.
5. Pressure on the esophagus can be caused by either aneurysm of arch of the aorta or descending thoracic aorta—produces dysphagia.
6. Pressure on the left recurrent laryngeal nerve produces paralysis of left vocal cord resulting in hoarseness of voice.
7. Pressure on stellate ganglion produces Horner's syndrome.
8. Aneurysms of the descending thoracic aorta tend to erode adjacent ribs, vertebrae and even the spinal cord at an advanced stage. They produce dull pain due to erosion of the ribs, sternum or vertebrae or sharp shooting pain of segmental distribution due to compression of nerve root or intercostal nerve. Compression of the spinal cord or impaired blood supply to the spinal cord can produce paraplegia.
9. Chest pain: It is an anginal pain due to coronary stenosis—caused by aneurysm of ascending aorta.
10. Tracheal deviation or 'tug' can be caused by aneurysm of aortic arch.
11. Features of aortic regurgitation: A loud aortic second sound with a ringing tambour-like' quality is heard in a normotensive young man.
12. Features due to embolic phenomenon can be caused by dislodgment of mural thrombi at the aneurysmal site.

10. However, there is much overlap with regard to clinical manifestations of the aneurysms—for example:

1. Pulsatile anterior chest wall swelling can be caused by aneurysm of the ascending aorta, or aortic arch.
2. Dysphagia can be caused by either aneurysm of arch of aorta descending thoracic aorta.
3. Superior venacaval obstruction can be caused by either aneurysm of ascending or arch of the aorta.
4. Pulmonary artery compression can be caused by either aneurysm of arch or descending thoracic aorta.

11. Roentgenography in aortic aneurysm.

They are often diagnosed by routine fluoroscopy or radiography in asymptomatic patients.

PA and oblique views with barium swallow is advised.

The 4 following sites can be diagnosed on X-ray:

1. Aneurysm of the ascending aorta: It produces a bulge on the right cardiac border near the hilar region. If it involves the right sinus of Valsalva, the bulge may appear at a lower point on the right cardiac border.
2. Aneurysm of the arch of aorta: It produces widening of superior mediastinum and a spherical protuberance. May appear at upper left or upper right mediastinal contour. Indirect evidence is obtained by distortion or displacement of trachea, left bronchus, or esophagus.

3. Aneurysm of the thoracic descending aorta is outlined well in barium swallow. Erosion of the adjacent vertebrae or ribs may be seen.
4. Aneurysm of the abdominal aorta may show curvilinear calcification in the walls of the aneurysm.

Sometimes, aneurysm is calcified, outlining the entire aneurysm.

Fluoroscopy is very useful in detecting expansile pulsations, which differentiate mediastinal shadows due to aneurysm from those caused by other tumors of mediastinum.

12. The 4 steps in investigations consist of:

1. Roentgenography.
2. Ultrasound: It determines the size of the aneurysm, thickness of its walls and detects any intraluminal clot.
3. Computed tomography: It actually delineate the abdominal aneurysm and detect the aneurysms that are at-risk or danger.
4. MRI/MRI Angiography.

13. The surgical treatment consists of resection of the aneurysmal segment followed by replacement with Dacron graft. Prognosis depends on 4 parameters:

1. *Size of the aneurysm:* The diameter of the normal abdominal aorta is 2.5 cm. When the diameter is more than 6 cm, the risk of rupture is great.
2. *Site of the aneurysm:* About 50% have 5 years and 70% have 10 years mortality rate for patients with thoracic aneurysm.
   Operative procedures on thoracic aortic aneurysm are more difficult than abdominal aortic aneurysm.
3. *Associated arteriosclerotic cardiovascular diseases:* About 50% of patients may have associated coronary disease.
   Severity of aortic regurgitation in aneurysm of ascending aorta.
4. *Associated diseases of other systems:*
   - Presence of pulmonary disease.
   - Systemic diseases like diabetes, collagen diseases, etc.

14. The usual course of an aneurysm is to rupture sooner or later. Hemoptysis may herald fatal hemorrhage. Aortic aneurysms may rupture:

1. Externally through the chest wall.
2. Into the mediastinal connective tissue.
3. Into the esophagus.
4. Into the trachea or left bronchus.
5. Into the pleura.
6. Into the pericardial cavity producing fatal cardiac tamponade or hemopericardium.
7. Into the stomach or duodenum.
8. Into another large vessel producing arteriovenous fistula.

15. Aortic aneurysms may rupture into 4 other large vessels.

1. Superior vena cava.
2. Inferior vena cava.
3. Pulmonary artery.
4. Pulmonary vein.

This may result in the formation of large arteriovenous fistula. A loud bruit or murmur and a palpable thrill is usually present over the fistula.

16. Rupture of superior vena cava is 4 times as common as rupture of an abdominal aortic aneurysm into inferior vena cava.

17. The incidence of aortic dissection is approximately

1. 2000 cases per year in the U.S.
2. Male to female ratio is 2:1
3. The peak incidence is in sixth and seventh decades.
4. Mortality in untreated cases of acute aortic dissection is 1% per hour in the first 48 hours.

18. It occurs approximately

1. 65% in ascending aorta.
2. 20% in descending thoracic aorta.
3. 10% in aortic arch.
4. Remaining in abdominal aorta.

DISSECTION OF THE AORTA

19. Pathogenesis 4 stages:

1. Supposed to be initiated by rupture of vasa vasorum within the media of the aortic wall or by cystic medial necrosis of the media.
2. Tear in the intima allows formation of intramural hematoma. Hematoma enlarges by a process of dissection—splitting the media longitudinally. Longitudinal cleavage of the aortic media by a hematoma is the characteristic feature of aortic dissection.
3. Hematoma can only be relieved by rupture—either externally or internally. External rupture through aortic adventitia results in immediate death. Internal rupture is fortunate to the patient and may lead to spontaneous cure. This 'cure' is only partial and often short-lived.
4. This 'cure' leads to 'double barrelled' aorta with an inner 'true' lumen and an outer false lumen—the outer wall of such a double walled aorta is not strong enough to withstand the systemic blood pressure. It progressively expands to become thinner and wider until it finally ruptures.

20. There are 4 common predisposing factors.

1. Congenital aortic stenosis and coarctation of the aorta, post-stenotic weakening of the aortic wall occasionally leads to aortic dissection.
   Marfan's syndrome—is an inherited genetic disorder of connective tissue with ocular, skeletal and cardiovascular manifestations. It is the major cause of death in patients affected with this disease. Ehlers-Danlos Syndrome.
2. Pregnancy: Aorta is supposed to be affected by the hormonal changes in the ground substance of connective tissue throughout the body, which occur in normal pregnancy.
3. Hypertension is commonly associated with dissection of the aorta.
4. Trauma—sometimes triggers dissection.
   It may be external as in blunt non-penetrating chest injury of an automobile accident.

Iatrogenic vascular trauma may produce aortic dissection: cardiac catheterization, coronary bypass surgery, cardiopulmonary bypass, or intra-aortic balloon counter pulsations may rarely cause dissection.

21. There are 4 rare predisposing causes.

1. Syphilis
2. Giant-cell aortitis
3. Atherosclerosis
4. Tuberculosis.

22. Site: The following 4 sites are more common.

1. Ascending aorta is commonly affected.
2. Intimal tear is usually located a few centimeters above the aortic valve. Medial dissection may confine to aorta or extend beyond the aortic arch.
3. 1/4th of cases occur in descending aorta.
4. Proximal limit of the medial hematoma is near the left subclavian artery and cleavage plane extends down to varying distance.

23. Clinical features:

The patient is usually a middle aged hypertensive man—However, known exceptions to this general rule are pregnant women and young individuals of both sexes with Marfan's syndrome.

Sudden onset of severe chest pain with obvious agony and sweating profusely resembles that of acute myocardial infarction. It is worthwhile to compare the characteristics of both conditions.

The 4 similarities between dissecting aneurysm and myocardial infarction are:

1. Both are most frequent in middle aged males.
2. Sudden and severe chest pain is the main symptom in both.
3. Onset is sometimes preceded by unusual strenuous exertion.
4. Sudden death within few hours of the onset is frequent.

24. Differences between dissecting aneurysm and myocardial infarction.

Table O-1

Dissecting aneurysm	*Myocardial infarction*
1. Pain radiates to the back, lumbar region and legs, also sometimes to arms and neck	Pain radiates mainly to shoulders, arms or jaw, rarely to back and never to lower half of the body
2. Discrepancy between the carotid pulses. Absence or inequality of one or more peripheral arterial pulsations	Peripheral arterial pulsations equal and normally present
3. Difference of BP in the two arms	BP is same in both the arms
4. Aortic diastolic murmur often present	No murmur of aortic regurgitation
5. Pulsus paradoxus due to cardiac tamponade is frequent	No pulsus paradoxus
6. Neurological manifestations are common	Neurological manifestations are not present
7. X-ray chest may show widening of mediastinum and perhaps unusual or bizarre mediastinal contour	X-ray chest does not reveal mediastinal abnormalities
8. ECG may show nonspecific ST-T changes. Infarction pattern is seen if coronary artery is obstructed by dissecting aneurysm	ECG shows classical infarction pattern, sometimes, 'coronary insufficiency' may cause non-specific ST-T changes

25. Obstruction to the vessels by dissecting aneurysm gives rise to the following 4 manifestations:

1. Obstruction of carotid and basilar vessels may occur singly or in combination resulting in neurological manifestations.
2. Obstruction to intercostal or lumbar arteries which feed spinal arteries can cause paraplegia due to spinal cord infarction.
3. Obstruction to coronary artery can cause typical myocardial infarction. More commonly cardiac failure may supervene as a result of aortic incompetence.
4. Obstruction to renal arteries result in anuria and uremia.

26. Investigations.

1. X-ray—widening of the superior mediastinum. Ascending aorta is enlarged out of proportion to the descending aorta. Descending aorta is larger than ascending aorta in dissection of descending aorta. Intimal calcification in the aortic knob may be seen.
2. ECG to differentiate from acute MI
3. 2D echo
4. TTE (Trans Thoracic Echocardiography)
5. MRI: It gives the highest accuracy, sensitivity and specificity for all acute aortic syndromes but it is rarely used as the first imaging due to various factors including non-availability at all places.

6. Computed CT
7. Cineangiography
8. Aortography.

27. Treatment of aneurysm of aorta and dissection of aorta.

1. Vigorous antihypertensive treatment temporarily prevents progress of the disease, i.e. from rupture and other complications. It helps to reduce the aortic pressure and left ventricular contraction.
   IV nitroprusside and IV propronolol are currently used. Labetalol Esmolol Metoprolol can be given.
   Hydralazine, minoxidil and diazoxide are not advised since they produce reflex inotropic stimulation of the left ventricle.
   Surgical treatment: It consists mainly of replacement of the aneurysmal segment with a Dacron graft attached to relatively normal aorta proximally and distally.
2. Aneurysm of ascending aorta.
   Total cardiopulmonary bypass is required. Resection of aneurysm is followed by Dacron graft. When aortic incompetence is present, prosthetic valve replacement is required.
3. Aneurysm of arch of aorta.
   Cardiopulmonary bypass is required. Resection and replacement by Dacron graft.
4. Descending thoracic and abdominal aorta.
   Do not require cardiopulmonary bypass.

Sometimes surgery is contraindicated by advanced age, severe associated disease or severe neurological manifestations. Immediate surgery is required in hypotensive patients who have aortic leak. Late death may be due to severe hypertension, heart failure or from severe aortic regurgitation or rupture of saccular aneurysm.
Others have choice between 'medical' and 'surgical' treatment.

ARTERIOSCLEROTIC OCCLUSIVE DISEASE

28. Majority of adults have some degree of arteriosclerosis. It is usually silent until it causes aneurysm or occlusive disease. Longitudinal elevated plaques appear in the intima. Occlusive diseases of the aorta occur if these plaques are complicated by any of the following 4:

1. Hemorrhage
2. Ulceration
3. Calcification
4. Thrombus formation.

29. Sites of occlusion of arteriosclerotic disease are 4:

1. Most frequent in the abdominal aorta.
2. Less common in arch of aorta.
3. Rare in ascending aorta.
4. Rare in descending thoracic aorta.

30. Atherosclerosis accounts for more than 90% of occlusion. When it affects the arch of aorta—it is one of the causes of 'aortic arch syndrome' or 'pulseless disease' and it should be differentiated from 4 other diseases.

1. Takayasu's arteritis
2. Syphilitic arteritis
3. Neoplasm
4. Trauma.

31. Nature and severity of clinical manifestations depend on 4 factors.

1. Location and severity of occlusion.
   The lesions tend to occur at the bifurcation of arteries so they are common at the origin of aortic arch vessels and at bifurcation of common carotids, iliac arteries, etc. The proximal left subclavian artery is commonly affected. These include subclavian steal syndrome, renal artery stenosis, mesenteric artery stenosis, aortoiliac insufficiency (Leriche's syndrome).
2. Adequacy of collateral circulation
3. Presence of previous occlusive lesions in the same or in neighboring arteries.
4. Affection of important target organs such as heart, brain, kidney, and when they have already suffered significant ischemic changes.

32. Clinical manifestations are mainly 4.

1. Men are affected more often than women in the fifth to seventh decades.
2. Claudication in lower extremities is common. Men commonly complain of inability to maintain a penile erection.
   Occurrence of cerebral ischemia suggests that more than one lesion is present. 'Steal syndromes' are common. Subclavian steal syndrome is triggered by vigorous movements of the arms—resulting in cerebral ischemia. Renal hypertension is common.
3. Bruits are heard over the carotids in the neck. Subclavian artery bruit in the supraclavicular fossa. Renal artery bruit is heard above the umbilicus. Bruits over the femorals are commonly heard.
   Absence or weak femoral pulses and distal pulses in the legs in Leriche's syndrome.
4. Ischemia of the lower limbs finally leads to gangrene. Ischemia of the upper extremities is unusual because of many collaterals.

33. Investigations are mainly 4.

1. X-ray to see any calcification of the vessel walls.
2. Occular pneumoplethysmography is useful to estimate the pressure in the opthalmic artery. It is particularly useful to evaluate a patient with carotid bruit. The pressure distal to the carotids is estimated.
3. Ultrasound technique by Doppler method gives information regarding the blood flow in the obstructed artery and may demonstrate reversal of flow in steal syndromes.

4. Arteriography identifies the location and severity of obstruction.
   Treatment is same as for any obstruction to the vessels—as angioplasty, bypass graft, or resection followed by graft.

Syphilis of the Aorta

The incidence of tertiary syphilis has fallen after the introduction of penicillin but to a lesser extent in the developing Asian countries than in the developed Western countries. Earlier to 1940, syphilis was treated with arsenic and bismuth injections which were not acceptable to many. Prime manifestations of tertiary syphilis of cardiovascular system are limited to the large vessels in which blood supply is provided by vasa vasorum. End-arteritis obliterans of vasa vasorum causes necrosis of tunica media with destruction of elastic tissue.

34. Syphilis of the aorta and its main branches can be described under 4 headings.

1. Syphilitic aortitis (uncomplicated) and syphilitic involvement of arteries arising from it.
2. Aneurysm of the aorta—most common complication.
3. Incompetence of the aortic valve—less common.
4. Coronary osteal stenosis.

35. The syphilis of the aorta is affected in the following descending order:

1. Ascending aorta—most commonly affected.
2. Aortic arch—next common.
3. Descending thoracic aorta.
4. Abdominal aorta.

The susceptibility of proximal aorta is probably due to its rich vascular and lymphatic supply.

36. The 4 regions of the aorta that are particularly susceptible to syphilitic aneurysm formation are:

1. Sinus of Valsalva just above the aortic valve.
2. Anterior right aspect of the ascending aorta.
3. Anterior portion of the aortic arch—saccular type.
4. Posterior portion of the descending thoracic aorta.

2 and 4 are either fusiform or saccular type.

37. The 4 less common affections of cardiovascular syphilis are:

1. Distal aortic involvement.
2. Pulmonary arteritis.
3. Myocarditis.
4. Myocardial gummata.

38. Pathology.

The proximal aorta is most commonly affected in contrast to more usual atheromatous involvement.

1. Microscopically—the vasavasorum of the aorta shows 'end arteritis obliterans' which:
2. Results in intimal proliferation and perivascular accumulation of lymphocytes and plasma cells.
3. Patchy destruction of muscular elastic tissue is characteristic.
4. The intima shows wrinkled 'tree-bark' appearance with plaque formation and thickening of the aortic wall.

39. Clinical manifestations of cardiovascular syphilis may be divided into 4 categories:

1. Those secondary to aortitis.
2. Those secondary to aneurysm formation.
3. Those secondary to aortic regurgitation.
4. Those secondary to coronary osteal stenosis.
   There can be combination of these.

40. Syphilitic aortic incompetence may not be differentiated from rheumatic aortic incompetence on clinical grounds—but the following 4 points favor the syphilitic etiology.

1. Presence of angina.
2. Presence of aortic aneurysm.
3. Involvement of other valves favor rheumatic origin. Whereas involvement of aorta alone favors syphilitic origin. Associated aortic stenosis favor rheumatic origin than syphilitic etiology.
4. Positive serological test.

41. Syphilitic coronary osteal stenosis.

Narrowing of the origin of one or both coronary arteries may occur frequently as a complication of aortitis. Syphilitic coronary osteal stenosis is suspected in young men or women suffering from angina in whom physical signs of aortic regurgitation are present. A positive serological test for syphilis strengthens the suspicion.

The 4 main symptoms/signs are:

1. Patient may complain of typical angina pectoris of effort indistinguishable from that caused by coronary atherosclerosis. The chest pain may be much prolonged for half an hour or more. Frequently, occurs at night when the patient is in recumbent position.
2. Signs of aortic regurgitation.
3. Flattening or inversion of T wave.
4. Diagnosis is confirmed by selective coronary artery catheterization and angiography.

42. Investigations mainly 4.

1. Serological tests for syphilis: They vary from less specific tests like venereal disease research laboratory (VDRL) test to the highly sensitive and specific fluorescent treponemal antibody absorption test (FTA-ABS).
2. X-ray chest: Prominence of the ascending aorta. Bulge of the aneurysm or widening of superior mediastinum. Linear 'egg-shell' calcification of the ascending aorta. Calcification of the walls of the aneurysm.

3. Echocardiography: This is useful to estimate the degree of aortic regurgitation to detect the size of the aneurysm and follow-up to identify the diastolic mitral valve flutter that cause Austin-Flint murmur in aortic regurgitation.
   To assess the left ventricular function.
4. Angiography and coronary arteriography reveal and localize the aortic aneurysm and the anatomical basis for angina pectoris.

NONSPECIFIC AORTITIS

43. This has been described under 8 (eight) different names.

1. Takayasu's syndrome.
2. Pulseless disease.
3. Aortic arch syndrome.
4. Young female aortitis.
5. Reversed coarctation.
6. Primary arteritis of the aorta.
7. Middle aortic syndrome.
8. Stenotic aortitis, etc.

44. The pathogenesis has been described under 4 steps:

1. Nonspecific inflammation of the aorta and its major branches.
2. Followed by constricting fibrosis or aneurysm formation.
3. Superimposed by intimal thrombosis or emboli formation.
4. Characterized by segmental or patchy distribution.

45. According to the site of stenosis or aneurysmal lesions, the aortitis clinically manifests as following syndromes:

Table O-2

Site of aortitis	*Clinical syndrome*
I. Ascending aorta	Aortic regurgitation Aneurysmal dilatation Coronary occlusion Coronary steal syndrome
II. Arch of aorta	Pulseless syndrome (Takayasu's disease) Cerebrovascular insufficiency Subclavian steal syndrome Aneurysmal dilatation
III. Descending thoracic	'Atypical' coarctation aorta Aneurysmal dilatation Hypertension
IV. Abdominal aorta including its bifurcation	Abdominal coarctation Renal artery stenosis (Renovascular hypertension) Mesenteric artery insufficiency (Abdominal angina) Aneurysmal dilatation Leriche's syndrome Thromboarteritis obliterans

46. Geographical, racial, age and sex incidence 4 points.

1. Common in South-East Asia.
2. Commonest among Mongolian races followed by Indo-Aryans.
3. Usually a disease of young females.
4. Sex-incidence:
   - Female: Male ratio
     - 7:1 in Japan
     - 5:1 in Mexico
     - 3:1 in India
     - 1.2:1 in Israel.

   Exact statistical data is not available in India.

47. Classification: There are 4 types:

1. Type I (Shimizu-Sano): Involvement localized to aortic arch and its main branches.
2. Type II (Kimoto): Involvement of thoraco-abdominal aorta and its branches, sparing the arch.
3. Type III (Inada): Contains features of type I and II
4. Type IV: Involvement of pulmonary artery and its branches.

48. Etiology and pathophysiology: Exact cause is not known.

The 4 possible factors are:

1. Immuological (Autoimmune disease). It has been occasionally reported in association with rheumatoid arthritis, systemic lupus erythematosus, which probably has an autoimmune basis.
   High prevalence of tuberculosis in Asian countries may be the cause of frequent association of the two diseases which is not seen in Western countries.
   Strongly positive Mantoux test is reported in 75–90% of cases. Delayed hypersensitivity to the tuberculosis may result in toxic injury to the vessel wall.
2. HLA typing suggests the possibility of genetic basis.
3. Viral infection: The high incidence of nonspecific aortitis in certain tropical countries and its rarity in colder climates suggests, the possibility of an insect vector such as the mosquito that carries the 'arteriotropic' virus. There is little evidence in favor or against this theory.
4. Atherosclerosis: It is claimed that Takayasu's disease in young persons especially in males is really an extreme and premature form of atherosclerosis (i.e. noninflammatory). This disease may be seen in elderly or middle aged persons. This claim has not yet received confirmation.

49. Clinical manifestations are:

More than 50% develop systemic illness characterized by:

1. Fever
2. Anorexia
3. Malaise
4. Weight loss

5. Headache
6. Night sweats
7. Arthralgia
8. Fatigue, etc.

50. Following 4 are the specific features:

1. Diminished or absent radial pulse in 96%.
2. Bruits in 94%.
3. Hypertension in 74%.
4. Eye changes described by Takayasu's are seen only in 25%.

51. Signs and symptoms depend on the stenosis or occlusion of one or more of the three great vessels.

Eye signs were described by Takayasu in 1908, a Japanese ophthalmologist in a young woman whose radial pulses were absent. Eye signs may range from a defective vision to the complete blindness.

They include the following 4 manifestations:

1. Conjunctival or retinal detachment.
2. AV anastamosis, retinal hemorrhage, microaneurysms, sometimes ring like vascular anastamosis surrounding the optic disk.
3. Cataracts.
4. Iris atrophy, etc.

AORTIC ARCH VARIETY (TAKAYASU'S DISEASE)

52. The 8 neurological manifestations of Takayasu's disease include:

1. Hemiplegia or hemiparesis.
   - Unilateral carotid obstruction is commonly associated with contralateral hemiplegia.
   - Aphasia, if the dominant hemisphere is infarcted.
   - Bilateral carotid obstruction involves bilateral pyramidal signs of upper motor neurone lesion.
2. Blindness or vertigo often heralds hemiplegia by months or years. It may be due to diminished carotid or vertebral flow or to the subclavian steal syndrome.
3. Transient or permanent unilateral blindness—affecting the ophthalmic artery. It may be associated with hemiplegia on the side opposite to the blind eye.
4. Convulsions—may be focal or general.

   Other less common neurological findings include.
5. Hemianesthesia.
6. Hemianopia.
7. Mental changes.
8. Cranial nerve palsies, etc.

   Often these neurological deficits coexist with hemiplegia.

53. Detailed examination of palpable arterial pulsations in all the 4 extremities is important. Palpate the pulsations in:

- Upper extremity
  1. Radial
  2. Brachial
  3. Axillary
  4. Subclavian.
- Lower extremity
  1. Dorsalis pedis
  2. Posterior tibial
  3. Popliteal
  4. Femoral.

The pulsations in the upper extremities may be feeble or absent on both sides though not to the same extent when bilateral subclavian artery obstruction is present. Normal strong femoral arterial pulse refutes the diagnosis of vascular shock.

54. Examine the blood pressure in all the 4 extremities.

BP may be identical in both upper limbs.

1. BP is unrecordable in severe subclavian obstruction.
2. Difference between right and left upper limb may not exceed 5 to 10 mm Hg.
3. The difference of BP in upper limbs is much greater in unilateral subclavian obstruction.
4. BP in the lower limb is usually high-'reversed coarctation'.

55. Auscultate over the following 4 arteries to detect a bruit.

1. Carotid arteries
2. Subclavian arteries
3. Renal arteries
4. Abdominal aorta.

Bruits are indicative of arterial disease.

Pulmonary artery involvement has been found in 50% of cases. Clinical manifestations are rare or absent as with primary pulmonary hypertension.

56. Hypertension in this disease can be due to many causes, but the 4 main causes are:

1. Renal artery stenosis—present in 35–85% of cases.
2. Involvement of baroreceptors by aortitis.
3. Loss of elasticity of aorta.
4. Coarctation like lesions.

The presence of hypertension in lower limbs with absent pulses in the upper extremities has caused this syndrome as 'reversed coarctation'.

DESCENDING THORACIC AND ABDOMINAL VARIETY

57. Clinical manifestations.

The 4 symptoms:

1. Chest pain—angina pectoris—is not a rare complaint. It is due to stenosis of the aorta or proximal segment of the coronary arteries. Myocardial infarction also has been reported.

2. Abdominal pain—abdominal angina—pain in the umbilical region after meals due to stenosis of superior mesenteric artery. It is not common.
3. Intermittent claudication—or tropical changes—when the stenosis of aortitis is at the aortic bifurcation (Leriche type). It is usually misdiagnosed as thromboangitis obliterans (TAO) or Buerger's disease especially when it occurs in young men who smoke heavily.
4. Local pain over the affected arteries in acute inflammatory stage. It is worth palpating the main arteries in young adults who complain of vague rheumatic pain. These patients usually have constitutional symptoms such as fever, malaise, etc.

58. The 4 signs.

1. Hypertension is the rule in 'middle aortic' type affecting the descending thoracic or abdominal aorta. Patient may present with severe hypertension of renal artery stenosis (unilateral or bilateral). These patients may present with hypertensive complications such as congestive heart failure or hypertensive encephalopathy.
   Arterial pulsations in the upper limbs are much stronger than in the lower limbs and this difference in pulse pressure is confirmed by taking BP in upper and lower limbs. The diagnosis of aortic hypertension may be missed if the blood pressure is estimated in an upper limb wherein the subclavian artery is stenotic.
2. Audible and palpable bruits over stenotic arteries. Auscultate over the spine from fourth dorsal to fourth lumbar (D4 to L4) vertebrae.
   Bruits of descending thoracic and abdominal aorta are also heard over the lower sternum and anterior abdominal wall. The site of maximal intensity indicates the location of stenotic aortic segment. Bruits over the upper abdomen are commonly caused by renal arteries and less commonly other large arteries such as the superior mesenteric or splenic arteries.
3. Cardiac findings: Heaving apex beat of left ventricular hypertrophy and a loud aortic second sound are usually secondary to hypertension.
   High pitched early diastolic murmur best heard at the lower sternal border is present in aortic incompetence.
   Signs of acute left ventricular failure or congestive failure with features of combined left and right sided failure.
4. Fundoscopy: This shows signs of hypertensive retinopathy in the 'middle aortic' stenosing aortitis or the renal artery stenosis type. The incidence of severe retinopathy including papilledema is much more common in renovascular hypertension due to stenosis of aortitis than in renal hypertension of other causes.

59. Stenosing aortitis of thoracic or abdominal aorta is often mistaken for congenital coarctation of the Aorta. Clinical differences are as follows:

Stenosing aortitis of escending thoracic or abdominal aorta	Congenital coarctation
1. BP may have been normal some years before	BP is elevated since birth
2. Palpable collaterals are less common	Palpable collaterals are common (Sussman's sign)
3. One or more of carotid or upper limb arterial pulsations are often feeble or absent (Takayasu's disease)	Carotid and upper limb pulsations are well palpable and equal—except in rare cases of coarctation proximal to subclavian origin
4. Bruits are heard over epigastrium and lower dorsal or lumbar spine	Bruits are heard at the level of upper sternum anteriorly and mid dorsal spine posteriorly
5. Hypertensive retinopathy including papilledema is quiet common	Severe hypertensive retinopathy is extremely rare
6. ESR is often raised	ESR is normal.
7. No rib notching in X-ray	X-ray chest usually shows rib notching
8. Aortography shows intimal irregularity with stenosis, poststenotic dilatation, aneurysm or even complete obstruction. A rat-tail appearance of the affected thoracic aorta is characteristic	Shows narrowing of the coarctation segment

60. Investigations: routine blood counts may show mild leukocytosis and anemia.

I. *ESR:* Shorter the duration of symptoms more likely the ESR is raised. It is moderately raised in early active phase of arteritis. A normal ESR does not exclude the diagnosis of nonspecific aortitis.

II. *Immunological tests:*
1. C-reactive protein.
2. Antistreptolysin titer.
3. Rheumatoid factor.
4. Antinuclear antibodies.
5. IgG or IgM.

6. GK α I2 globulin and gamma globulin.
7. Fibrinogen.
8. Mantoux test —strong positive is reported in 75–90%

These are elevated in more than half of the patients.

III. *Roentgenography and ECG:* These may show signs of pulmonary hypertension and right ventricular hypertrophy. X-ray chest is usually unrevealing. Sometimes, it may show a rim of calcification in the walls of the affected vessels.

IV pyelography in renal artery stenosis. It may show a non-functioning or small kidney on the affected side. Arteriography shows irregularity of intimal surface with stenosis of aorta or its branches, poststenotic dilatations, aneurysms or even complete obstruction. The affected thoracic aorta has been described as having a 'rat-tail' appearance.

IV. *Specific tests:* Noninvasive vascular laboratory studies are useful to confirm suspected reduction in arterial flow to the head and upper extremities.

Arterial biopsy may be positive in 20–35% of cases. Biopsy confirmation is not necessary and is a rare possibility in a living subject. Biopsy of diseased segment of aorta or artery is taken by a vascular surgeon during operation to establish the proof of arteritis. It is useless to take biopsy of a peripheral non-pulsative artery such as the radial or posterior tibial artery.

61. Medical treatment.

I. Steroids: Steroids are particularly useful in those patients who;
   i. Have systemic symptoms such as fever, malaise, weight loss, etc.
   ii. Are in the first or second decade.
   iii. Have a high ESR.
   iv. Do not have severe hypertension.

   Steroids are useful in relieving constitutional symptoms as well as arresting the disease to a large extent. Cyclophosphamide is given when it fails to respond to steroids. 2 mg/kg/day is adjusted to maintain the total leukocyte count more than 3000/cu mm.

II. Antiplatelet agglutination drugs like aspirin and dipyridamole are indicated in the treatment of transient ischemic attacks and to prevent progress.

III. Antihypertensive drugs: Hypertension is present in almost all patients with descending aorta or renal artery stenosis. It is only refractory or partly responsive to powerful antihypertensive drugs.

IV. Antituberculous drugs are useful in cases of strongly positive Mantoux or where there is family history of tuberculosis. It is only of empirical use.

62. Surgical treatment.

1. Endarterectomy.
2. Bypass surgery—is useful in renal artery stenosis.
3. Resection of a localized coarctation followed by surgical reconstruction by a graft.
4. Percutaneous transluminal balloon angioplasty for dilatation of stenotic lesion in the carotid, subclavian, renal and mesenteric arteries.

63. Prognosis.

It is a progressive disease, though the rate of progression varies considerably.

The cause of death is usually due to any of the 4 following complications.

1. Heart failure.
2. Renal failure.
3. Rupture of aneurysm.
4. CNS complications like:

   Thromboembolism/Infarction/Hemorrhage Encephalopathy.

GIANT-CELL ARTERITIS

64. Synonyms: Temporal arteritis, cranial arteritis.

Pathophysiology

1. It is a rare inflammatory arteritis affecting both sexes equally in old age. The cause of it is not known. This entity is different from Takayasu's disease which occurs in young women.
2. Large and medium sized arteries are affected. Arterioles and capillaries are not involved. Classical type of giant-cell arteritis occur in the temporal artery but other arteries may be affected, e.g. aortic arch, innominate, carotid, subclavian, occipital, ophthalmic, axillary, femoral, popliteal, vertebral, hepatic, coronary, etc.
3. Intima is thickened to more than expected to the age. Media shows inflammatory reaction when the internal elastic lamina is broken. The cellular infiltration consists of mononuclear cells and giant cells which may contain as many as thirty peripheral nuclei. Adventitia contain mononuclear inflammatory cells but no giant cells. It shows increase in fibrous tissue.
4. The lesions tend to be patchy or of segmental distribution.

   Polymyalgia rheumatic syndrome is associated with giant cell arteritis but without clinical evidence of arteritis.

65. When it affects the aorta, it may produce 4 complications.

1. Occlusion of aortic vessels.
2. Aneurysm of ascending aorta or arch of aorta.

3. Aortic regurgitation.
4. Aortic dissection.

66. Clinical features:

1. Temporal headache associated with fever, weakness, anorexia, weight loss and anemia.
   Pyrexia of unknown origin in an elderly person with high ESR should rise the diagnostic possibilities of giant-cell arteritis.
2. Painful tender nodules along the course of temporal arteries soon become pulseless and cord-like. Further, these patients may complain of intermittent claudication of the jaws, tongue during mastication or talking.
3. Rise in total WBC, ESR, α-2 globulin and fibrinogen are seen in giant-cell arteritis or polymyalgia rheumatica. Mild-to-moderate aneurysm may be present. Serum alkaline phosphatase may be slightly elevated. Important negative findings include normal muscle enzymes, normal electromyogram even in the presence of severe polymyalgia and normal muscle biopsies. The diagnosis of giant-cell arteritis or polymyalgia rheumatica depends on clinical findings or a positive muscle biopsy.
4. Higher incidence of severe visual impairment leading to loss of vision if not treated with high doses of corticosteroids. Salicylates, indomethacin or phenylbutazone are helpful but corticosteroids give remarkable dramatic response.

P Roentgenology

1. Before proceeding to read the X-ray chest, one should verify whether it is taken properly or not.

Properly taken X-ray should satisfy the following 4 points:

1. *Size:* It should include some portion of the neck above and some portion of the abdomen below to find cervical rib and gastric bubble respectively. The sides should include costophrenic angles on both sides.
2. *Inspiration:* It should be taken while breath is held during deep inspiration, not too deep inspiration.
   This is known by finding the costophrenic angles at or below the 7th or 8th rib. If the angles are at 4th or 5th space, one may see pseudocardiomegaly.
3. *Symmetry:* Both sternoclavicular joints should be in the same line. Scapula should be out.
4. *Penetration:* Normally some vertebrae should be visible behind the cardiac shadow, but not everyone. Every vertebra is seen in overexposed film. No vertebra is seen behind the heart shadow when it is underexposed.

The plain chest radiogram remains as an useful screening or initial test as it is a non-invasive procedure and relatively less expensive.

2. X-ray chest for cardiovascular system provides the following 4 informations:

1. Pathoanatomic changes in the size and shape of the heart.
2. Pathoanatomic changes in the size and shape of great vessels.
3. Pathophysiological changes in the pulmonary arterial pressure and flow.
4. Pathophysiological changes in the pulmonary venous pressure and flow.

The final conclusion should be drawn after correlating the radiological findings with clinical and laboratory findings.

3. There are 4 views of cardiac series:

1. Posteroanterior view.
2. Lateral view.
3. Right anterior oblique view at 45°.
4. Left anterior oblique view at 60°.
   Each view has got its own importance.

4. The 4 useful points in posteroanterior view. It is a commonly taken view and most familiar of all the views.

It is particularly useful in the assessment of 4 parameters.

1. Overall cardiac size.
2. Evaluation of pulmonary vasculature.
   Barium filled esophagus helps to outline the:
3. Aorta
4. Left atrium.
   Erect inspiratory PA radiographs are ideal to study the heart and great vessels.

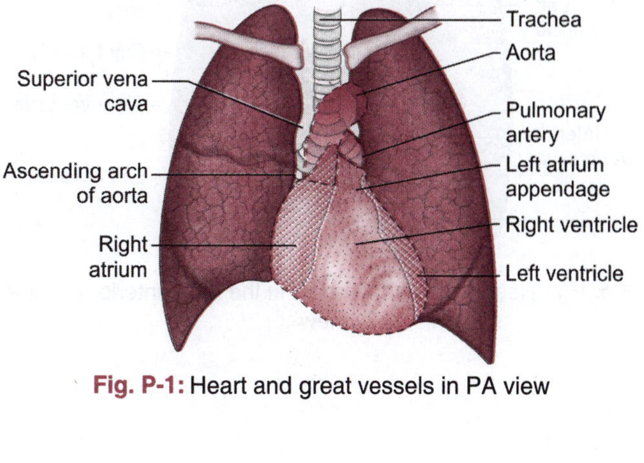

Fig. P-1: Heart and great vessels in PA view

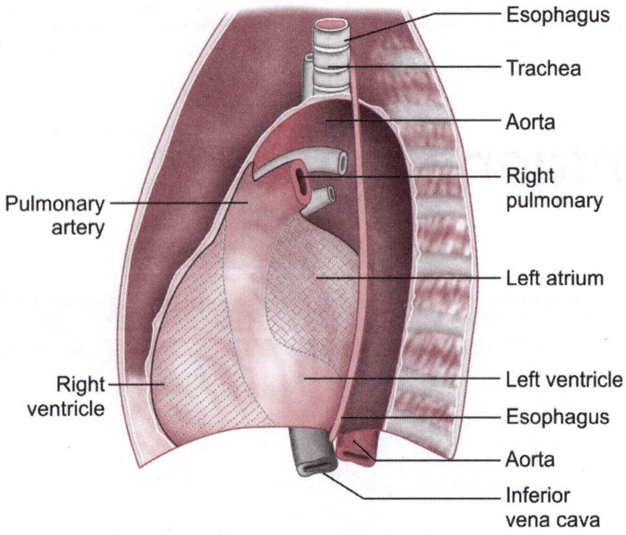

Fig. P-2: Heart and great vessels in lateral position

5. The 4 useful points in left lateral view are:

It is particularly useful in the evaluation of:

1. Pericardial disease—pericardial calcification.
2. Right coronary artery calcification.

   Barium filled esophagus helps to diagnose:

3. Aortic arch anomalies.
4. Left atrial enlargement.

6. The 4 useful points in right anterior oblique view at 45° are:

It is particularly useful to see the 4 cardiac chambers separately because each chamber enlarges in a different direction.

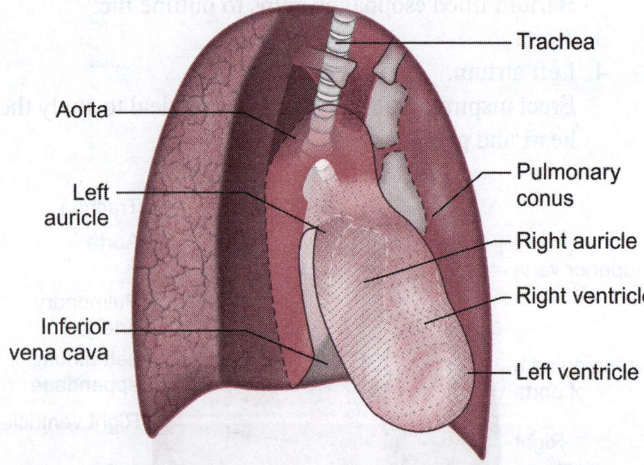

Fig. P-3: Heart and great vessels in the right anterior oblique view

1. Right ventricle expands anteriorly, superiorly and leftwards.
2. Left ventricle expands inferiorly and leftwards.
3. Left atrium expands posteriorly, rightwards and superiorly.
4. Right atrium expands rightward posteriorly and inferiorly.

   Barium filled esophagus in this view clearly shows the left atrial enlargement.

7. RAO is also useful in studying the following 4 structures:

1. Left atrium
2. Pulmonary conus
3. First part of the aorta
4. Barium filled esophagus.

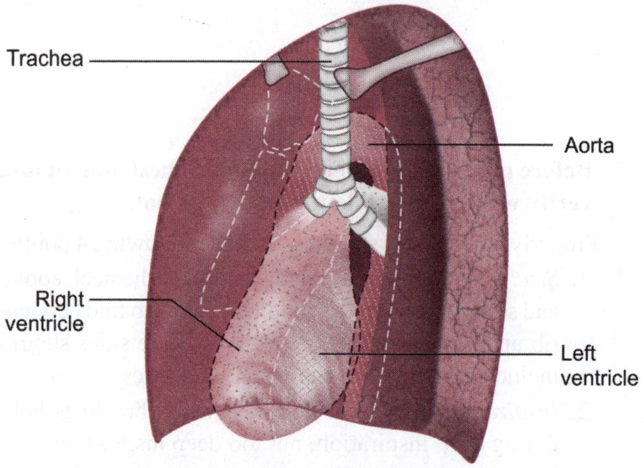

Fig. P-4: Heart and great vessels in the left anterior oblique view

8. The 4 useful points in studying left anterior oblique view at 60° are:

It is particularly useful in the assessment of:

1. Ventricular enlargement.
2. Left coronary artery calcification.
3. Thoracic aorta which is seen entirely.
4. Tracheal bifurcation—it evaluates the effect of enlarged left atrium on left bronchus.

Barium is usually taken in this view in order to see the tracheal bifurcation clearly and to evaluate the effect of left atrial enlargement on left bronchus.

9. The 4 chambers of the heart are better seen in 4 views.

1. PA view for left ventricular enlargement.

   When it enlarges it moves downwards, posteriorly and to the left.

   Measure the cardiothoracic ratio. Maximum diameter of the cardiac 'silhouette' is divided by maximal internal thoracic diameter. Normal ratio is less than 0.5.

2. Right anterior oblique (RAO) view with barium swallow for left atrial enlargement. Seen as an indentation of barium filled esophagus. Left atrium enlargement is suspected when a bulge is noticed beneath the pulmonary artery in PA view.
   When left atrium dilates further it is seen as a second border or 'double density' shadow behind the right atrium.
3. Right lateral view for right ventricular enlargement. Anterior wall of the right ventricle is directly behind the lower-third of the sternum.
   Radioluscent lung lies between the sternum and right ventricle in the retrosternal space. When right ventricle enlarges, it occupies the retrosternal space displacing the lung tissue.
   Dilated right ventricle passively displaces the other chambers particularly left ventricle. So, it is difficult to assess the size of the left ventricle when the right ventricle is enlarged.
4. Left anterior oblique (LAO) for right atrial enlargement. It is seen as a bulging of the cardiac silhouette to the right along with increase in curvature of right border. Estimation of the right atrial size is the least reliable of all the cardiac chambers by X-ray chest.
   Nowadays, cardiac series are not taken as it is mostly replaced by other investigations like echocardiography that provides a comprehensive assessment of the size of individual chambers.

10. There are 4 step-like convexities to be noted on left border from above downward.

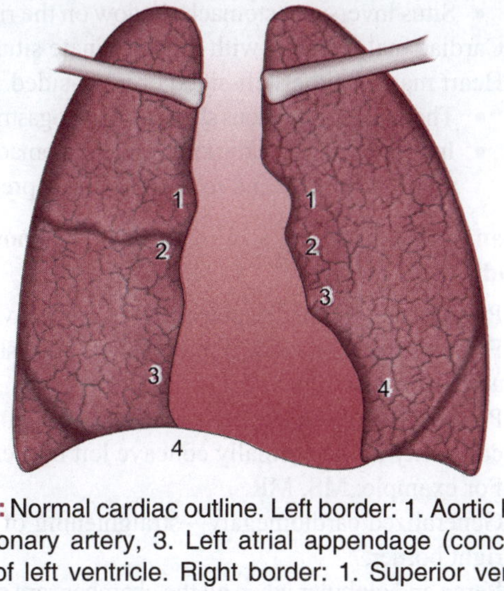

Fig. P-5: Normal cardiac outline. Left border: 1. Aortic knuckle, 2. Pulmonary artery, 3. Left atrial appendage (concave), 4. Sweep of left ventricle. Right border: 1. Superior vena cava (parallel to the upper mediastinum), 2. Arch of ascending aorta, 3. Border of right atrium, 4. Right cardiophrenic angle

1. Aortic knuckle prominence.
2. Straight line of pulmonary artery (left branch of the pulmonary artery).
3. Left atrial appendage seen especially if enlarged in penetrated PA view.
4. Wide sweep of the left ventricle ending at the apex on the diaphragm.

Left heart sits posterior to the right heart.
On frontal view, left atrial appendage is normally concave.

11. There are 4 points to be noted on the right border of the chest X-ray from above downward by two curves.

1. Superior vena cava shadow—slightly curved position—outer edge of SVC—with arch of ascending aorta.
2. Arch of ascending aorta.
3. More convex position formed by the outer border of right atrium.
4. Right cardiophrenic angle.
   On frontal view, right border is right atrium only:

12. There are 4 points to be noted about the heart in chest X-ray.

1. Position of the heart.
2. Size and shape of the heart and great vessels. Heart size is expressed in ratio of the maximum transverse diameter of the heart to the maximum transverse diameter of thoracic cage, i.e. the cardiothoracic ratio.
3. Calcified shadows.
4. Cardiovascular circulation reflected in the pulmonary circulation.

13. X-ray chest in an obese individual looks as any/all of the following 4:

1. The heart is transverse.
2. The diaphragm is raised.
3. The intercostal spaces are narrowed.
4. The chest is broad and short.

14. X-ray chest in a thin and tall individual looks as any/all of the following 4:

1. The heart is vertical.
2. The diaphragm is low.
3. The intercostal spaces are wide.
4. The chest is long and narrow.

15. Cardiac mensuration (estimation of cardiac size). The 4 measurements are:

1. Transverse diameter of the heart:
   This is the sum of the maximum projections of the right and left borders of the heart from the midline.
   Cardiothoracic ratio expressed as a percentage is the ratio between the maximum diameter of the heart and the maximum width of the thorax. Maximum width of

the thorax is measured from the inner edges of the rib above the costophrenic angles. Heart is enlarged if it is more than half

- Normally, the cardiothoracic ratio is < 0.5. An increase of > 1 cm of cardiac diameter from a prior film is a more reliable index.

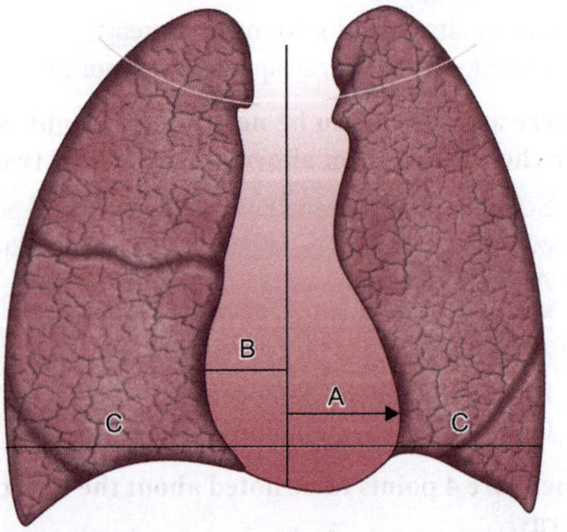

Fig. P-6: Measurement of transverse diameter of the heart and cardiothoracic ratio
A+B = Maximum diameter of the heart
C = Maximum transverse diameter of the chest
Normally the cardiothoracic ratio is < 0.5
An increase of > 1 cm of cardiac diameter from a prior film is a more reliable index.

2. Long diameter of the heart: This is the distance between the small notch on the right border of the heart between the right atrium and superior vena cava and the left ventricular apex.
3. Broad diameter of the heart (oblique diameter of the heart): This is the greatest diameter of the cardiac shadow perpendicular to the long diameter.
   From diaphragm-right atrial junction to pulmonary trunk-left atrial appendix junction.
4. Aortic arch diameter: This is the sum of the maximum extension to the right and to the left of the aortic shadow from the midline as projected above the base of the heart.

16. The following 4 points are to be noted in the over penetration of P-A view of the chest.

1. Left atrium—this is seen especially when it is enlarged.
2. Aorta—this is particularly well seen.
3. Calcification in the pericardium.
4. Calcification in the heart valves.

17. Screening of the heart.

This is of value in visualizing the following 4:

1. Calcification of valves.
2. Degree of pulsation in the pulmonary artery.
3. Degree of pulsation in the aorta.
4. Differentiation of pulsatile from non-pulsatile shadows.

18. There are 4 non-cardiac conditions where the heart is displaced.

1. Displacement to the opposite side, e.g. seen in pleural effusion, pneumothorax.
2. Displacement to the same side in fibrosis, collapse and hypoplasia of the lung.
3. Upward displacement is seen in obesity, distension of abdomen.
   Heart is raised with the diaphragm—unilateral diaphragmatic elevation.
   Apex is tilted upward.
4. Thoracic deformity—displaced to the left in scoliosis.
   - Common type of scoliosis is convexity of the curve to the right.

19. The 4 cardiac malpositions described are:

1. Dextrocardia:
   - This is a mirror image of the heart and the abdominal viscera (situs inversus)
   - Dextrocardia—apex on the right side
   - Situs inversus—stomach shadow on the right side.
2. Dextroversion:
   - Right-sided heart—apex on the right side
   - Situs solitus—aortic knob and the gastric air bubble are on the left side.
3. Levoversion:
   - This is a mirror image of dextroversion
   - Left-sided heart
   - Situs inversus—stomach shadow on the right side.
4. Cardiac malpositions with indeterminate situs:
   Heart may be either left-sided or right-sided.
   - The situs is ambiguous showing aorticogastric bubble
   - Indifference, i.e. aortic knob and the stomach are not on the same side and so the situs is not predictable.

20. Change in shape and size of the heart is noted in 4 conditions.

1. Prominence and undue convexity of the left ventricle:
   For example: AR, AS, hypertension, boot-shaped in advanced cases.
2. Prominence of left atrium is seen as a straightening or convexity in the normally concave left border.
   For example: MS, MR.
3. Generalized cardiomegaly—straightening of left and right border.
   Large and globular when all the chambers are enlarged.
   For example: Advanced MS upto atrial fibrillation, combined MS with aortic disease, multivalvular

disease, dilated or congested cardiomyopathy, anemia, thalassemia, myxedema, etc.

Cardiophrenic angle is obliterated in pericardial effusion.

PA view film should be taken 6 feet distance—Taking the film at 3 feet or 4 feet distance by 50 mA or 100 mA may show apparent enlargement.

Check—6 feet X-ray distance.

The heart size is overestimated in anteroposterior (AP) view also. So, PA views are accurate.

Concentric cardiac hypertrophy produces thickening of the ventricular wall at the expense of the chamber cavity and produces only slight cardiac enlargement or alteration of the cardiac silhouette.

4. Box or shelf-like projection in left ventricular aneurysm. Bulge on the right side in congenital aneurysm of right ventricle.

False negative results may be seen in aortic regurgitation because the heart enlarges downwards and laterally and the ratio does not increase.

False positive results may be seen in sternal depression, flat chest, or if diaphragm is high due to obesity or if the exposure is done during expiration.

21. There are 4 factors that influence the shape and size of the heart.

1. In infants: Transverse type and appears very large. Increase in size due to high position of the diaphragm which is raised normally—by large liver and gas distended infantile stomach. Conus and pulmonary artery are prominent on the left border and there is no aortic knuckle in infants.
2. In adults—heart decreases in size during full inspiration and increases in size during full expiration.
3. In pregnancy—transverse type of heart due to marked elevation of diaphragm. Enlargement of pulmonary conus is seen in late pregnancy.
4. In obese short-necked individuals—transverse type of heart.

22. Mediastinal and cardiovascular structures are frequently affected by each other because of their close spatial interrelationships.

The following 4 are some of the effects:

1. Enlarged left atrium displaces esophagus and descending aorta, elevates and compresses the left bronchus.
2. Double aortic arch compresses both trachea and esophagus.
3. Malignant lesion may invade the heart resulting in cardiac tamponade.
4. Malignant lesion that invades great vessels may cause superior vena caval syndrome.

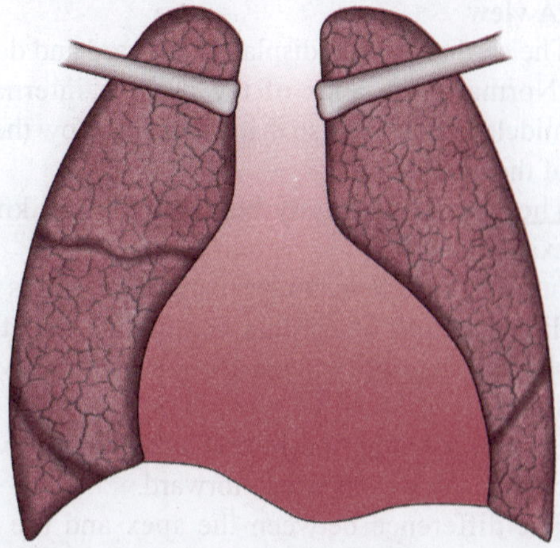

Fig. P-7: Cardiac outline in generalized cardiomegaly, e.g. pericardial effusion

23. Causes of generalized cardiomegaly on chest X-ray are:

4 Common causes

1. Congestive cardiac failure.
2. Multiple valve lesions.
3. Pericardial effusion.
4. Dilated (congestive) cardiomyopathy.

4 Less common causes

1. Myocarditis, e.g. rheumatic carditis.
2. Endocrinal disturbances, e.g. myxedema.
3. Hyperdynamic circulation, e.g. severe or chronic anemia, beriberi.
4. Ebstein anomaly—lung fields are normal in pericardial effusion, Ebstein anomaly and tricuspid regurgitation.

X-rays do not differentiate between the cardiac enlargement and pericardial fluid. Many prefer the term 'cardiac silhouette' to 'heart size'.

24. The 4 common causes of small cardiac shadow are:

1. Constrictive pericarditis.
2. Emphysema, chronic obstructive pulmonary disease (COPD).
3. Addison's disease.
4. Wasting diseases—malnutrition, dehydration, starvation, anorexia nervosa.

A smaller heart than average heart is difficult to define unless it is seen in a retrospective manner when it returns to normal size following successful treatment, e.g. heart response to steroid treatment in Addison's disease results in enlargement of the heart significantly.

25. Left ventricular enlargement.

In this condition, the heart rotates in a counter clockwise direction when viewed from above so that the following 4 findings are seen in different views.

In PA view

1. The cardiac apex is displaced outward and downward (Normally the apex of the heart is internal to the midclavicular line) so that it may lie below the shadow of the diaphragm.
2. The normal concavity below the aortic knuckle is exaggerated.
3. In LAO, the left ventricle enlargement causes posterior displacement of cardiac contour so that the heart shadow may project far enough back to overlie the spine.
4. On fluoroscopy, the interventricular groove at the cardiac apex is displaced forward.
   The difference between the apex and the point of opposite pulsations is increased.

Left ventricular enlargement in a PA film is seen as inferolateral protrusion of the cardiac apex. On a lateral film, cardiac apex protrudes inferoposteriorly.

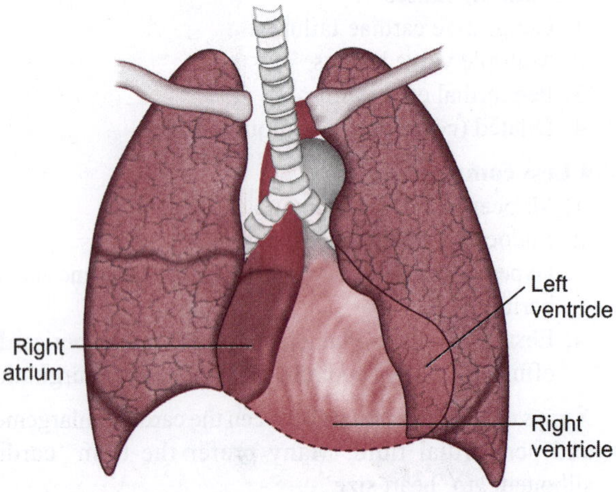

Fig. P-8: Cardiac outline in left ventricular enlargement

26. The common causes of left ventricular enlargement are:

1. Hypertension
2. Mitral regurgitation
3. Aortic regurgitation
4. Aortic stenosis
5. Coronary arteriosclerosis
6. Cardiac aneurysm
7. Coarctation of aorta
8. Aorta-pulmonary shunts.

The nature of cardiomegaly can be determined by the specific roentgen abnormalities.

Cardiac lesions with volume overload tend to present a greater degree of cardiac enlargement than with pressure overload.

Patients with aortic stenosis shows an increased convexity of left ventricle but very little enlargement. This is due to concentric hypertrophy of the left ventricle without dilatation of the cardiac lumen.

On the other hand, left ventricle hypertrophies and dilates in aortic incompetence resulting in much larger heart even before the development of congestive heart failure.

Both right-sided and left-sided heart failure can cause gross cardiac enlargement, the associated pulmonary vascular abnormality in each case is widely different.

27. Right ventricular enlargement.

In this condition, the heart rotates in a clock wise rotation when viewed from above so that the following 4 findings are seen in different views.

In PA view

1. The cardiac apex rises above the level of the diaphragm.
2. Enlargement of the ventricular outflow tract causes filling in and results in convexity of the normal concavity of the left heart border below the aortic knuckle.
3. In LAO view, anterior displacement of cardiac outline is considered to indicate right ventricular enlargement.
4. On fluoroscopy, the enlarged right ventricle is said to cause backward displacement of the interventricular groove at the cardiac apex.

The distance between the cardiac apex and the point of opposite pulsations on the left heart border diminishes.

The point of opposite pulsations is defined as that point on the left cardiac silhouette where the left ventricle and pulmonary artery are adjacent and where their pulsations being asynchronous can be distinguished from one another.

Right heart is normally located anteriorly and superiorly. Enlarged right heart contacts the lower-half of the sternum. Normally, the right heart contacts only the lower one-third of the sternum.

28. The 4 common acquired causes of right ventricular enlargement are:

1. Mitral stenosis.
2. Congestive heart failure.
3. Chronic pulmonary disease—cor pulmonale.
4. Tricuspid regurgitation.

29. The 4 common congenital causes of right ventricular enlargement are:

1. Fallot's tetralogy.
2. Atrial septal defect.
3. VSD.
4. PDA.
5. Pulmonary stenosis.
6. Primary pulmonary hypertension.
7. Aortopulmonary window.
8. Atrioventricular canal.

30. Left atrial enlargement.

It is the easiest to detect because of 4 reasons:

1. Left atrial appendage is seen as a localized projection between the shadows cast by the left ventricle and pulmonary artery on the left border. This gives rise to straightening of left border so-called mitralization of the heart.
2. As the left atrium enlarges it may dilate upward causing splaying of the tracheal bifurcation by elevation of the left main bronchus and rarely compression of this bronchus occurs.
3. When enlargement occurs, the right border of the left atrium can be identified through the shadow of the right atrium to the right of the spine forming a double density (double contour).
4. RAO with barium swallow demonstrates even slight degree of left atrial enlargement which cannot be identified by PA view. In this position, the left atrium projects backward and causes a localized displacement of the esophagus backward and to the patient's right (rarely to the patients left).

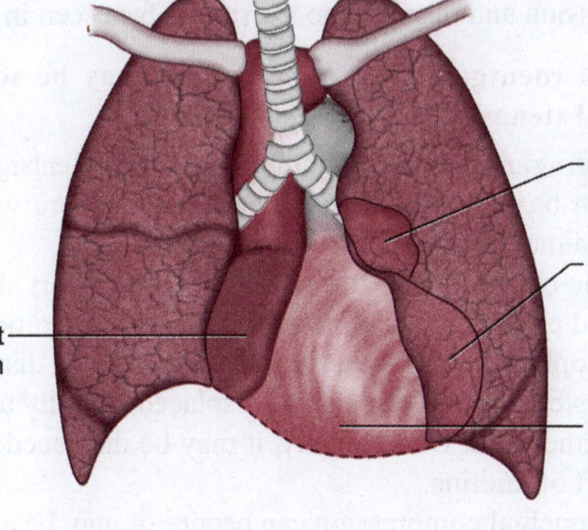

Fig. P-9: Cardiac outline in mitral stenosis showing prominence of left atrial appendage at left heart border (Marked dark)

31. The common causes of left atrial enlargement are:

1. Mitral stenosis.
2. Mitral regurgitation.
3. Aortic stenosis.
4. Aortic regurgitation.
5. Systemic hypertension.
6. Ischemic heart disease.
7. Cardiomyopathy.
8. Left atrial tumor/myxoma.

32. Double density shadow cast by left atrial enlargement may be found within the confines of the heart in some other conditions also indicating a variety of dilated vascular structures such as these 4.

1. Tortuous descending aorta.
2. Aortic aneurysm.
3. Coronary artery aneurysm.
4. Pulmonary varix.

33. Bulge on left heart border is seen in 4 conditions.

1. Enlarged left atrial appendage.
2. Ventricular aneurysm.
3. Pericardial cyst.
4. Myocardial mass.

34. The common causes of right atrial enlargement are:

1. Tricuspid stenosis.
2. Tricuspid regurgitation.
3. Pulmonary stenosis.
4. Pulmonary regurgitation.
5. Atrial septal defect.
6. Right atrial tumors.
7. Right-sided cardiomyopathy (right-sided endomyocardial fibrosis).
8. Ruptured aortic sinus into right atrium.

35. The 4 common causes of increased venous or right atrial pressure are:

1. Congestive cardiac failure.
2. Tricuspid obstruction.
3. Restrictive cardiomyopathy.
4. Tumors—right atrial or mediastinal tumor.

36. Prominent ascending aorta is seen in 4 conditions:

1. Aortic unfolding
2. Aortic regurgitation
3. Aortic aneurysm
4. Post stenotic dilatation.

37. Enlarged aortic knuckle is seen in 4 conditions:

1. Systemic hypertension
2. Aneurysm of aorta
3. Aortic regurgitation
4. Patent ductus arteriosus.

38. Small aortic arch is seen in 4 conditions:

1. Decreased cardiac output.
2. Mitral stenosis.
3. Coarctation of aorta.
4. Intracardiac left to right shunts.

39. The 4 common causes of pulmonary trunk enlargement are:

1. Pulmonary hypertension
2. Left to right shunts
3. Pulmonary regurgitation
4. Idiopathic dilatation.

40. Prominence of the pulmonary trunk is a reliable secondary sign of right ventricular enlargement with the following 4 exceptions:

1. Tetralogy of Fallot with hypoplasia of pulmonary trunk.
2. Idiopathic dilatation of the pulmonary artery.

3. Patent ductus arteriosus earlier to the development of Eisenmenger's complex.
4. Straight back syndrome, pectus excavation and scoliosis with narrowed anteroposterior diameter of the chest. In these conditions, heart is compressed, displaced, rotated to the left giving falsely enlarged pulmonary artery shadow.

41. Standard X-ray chest may be supplemented by image intensification fluoroscopy to detect the calcification.

Calcification may be seen in the following 4 areas:

1. Endocardium:
   - Mitral annulus
   - Mitral valve
   - Tricuspid valve
   - Aortic valve—bicuspid or tricuspid valve calcification, syphilis, old age, idiopathic hypercalcemia
   - As a rule, the extent of valvular calcification is proportionate to the severity of valve stenosis.
2. Myocardium:
   - Left atrial wall calcification.
   - Calcified thrombi in left atrium.
   - Old myocardial infarction calcification.
   - Calcification of left ventricular aneurysm.
   - Calcification of hydatid cyst.
3. Pericardium: Calcification—following pericarditis in
   - Tuberculosis
   - Purulent
   - Tumor
   - Rheumatic
   - Idiopathic
   - Postoperative
   - Post-traumatic
   - Uremia.
4. Vessels:
   - Calcification of aortic knob
   - Calcification of hematoma in dissecting aneurysm
   - Pulmonary artery calcification in mitral stenosis
   - Calcification of coronary arteries
   - Calcification of aneurysm of coronary artery.

Inverted 'Y'-shaped calcification just below the aortic knob in patent ductus arteriosus (PDA).

Calcification in coronary vessels below the age of 40 years is significant. Calcification above 40 years age is not significant. Coronary calcification is correlated with major vessel occlusion in majority of patients with chest pain.

Large calcifications are easily seen particularly in lateral and oblique views, small calcifications are verified and ruled out by fluoroscopy.

42. There are 4 X-ray signs of left atrial hypertrophy which is a good evidence of increased left atrial pressure.

(Over penetrated grid film is particularly useful)

1. Left atrial appendage seen on left border as a straightening or convexity of the normally concave left border below the pulmonary artery.
2. When left atrium further dilates it will be visible within the right atrium shadow on the right border. 'Double density' behind the right atrium.
3. Widening of the angle between right and left main bronchi. The desk shadow of left main bronchus is displaced upwards by the enlarged left atrium and lies more horizontally.
4. RAO barium swallow shows the indentation displacement of esophagus backward and to the right —'sickle-shaped' esophagus.

43. Esophagus is impressed by 4 structures in its thoracic course which is seen in RAO barium swallow from above downwards.

1. Aortic arch
2. Left bronchus
3. Left atrium
4. Descending aorta.

Abnormality of these structures causes alteration in the barium swallow.

The left atrial enlargement in mitral stenosis causes deep depression and displaces to the right—best seen in RAO.

44. The 4 roentgen abnormalities that may be seen in mitral stenosis are:

1. Left atrium is particularly affected—left atrial enlargement can be minimal, slight, moderate or severe when it assumes aneurysmal proportions.
   The chamber may form the bulk of the heart shadow and produces rather bizarre cardiac configuration.
2. Esophagus in RAO barium swallow may be displaced posteriorly and can also be displaced laterally usually to the right. Occasionally, it may be displaced to the left of midline.
3. Bronchial compression can occur—it may be a cause of stridor and if complete it may lead to lobar collapse particularly in the lower base.
4. Mitral stenosis with back pressure leads to the development of pulmonary hypertension followed by right ventricular enlargement.
   Pulmonary vascularity may show cephalization with decreased flow in severe mitral stenosis.
   Aorta and left ventricle are of normal size.

45. The 4 roentgen abnormalities that may be seen in mitral incompetence are:

1. Left ventricle enlargement is common.
   So, it is important to exclude:
   - Aortic valve disease
   - Hypertension
   - Ischemic heart disease.

2. Usually considerable left atrial enlargement is seen.
3. The degree of right ventricular enlargement depends on the presence or absence of pulmonary hypertension which is not as common as in mitral stenosis.
4. Paradoxical expansile pulsation of the left atrium during left ventricular systole is often seen on fluoroscopy. However, it may be frequently seen in mitral stenosis and is therefore not a diagnostic sign.

Accurate assessment of the severity of predominant mitral stenosis or incompetence is difficult on routine chest X-rays.

46. Accurate diagnosis is essential when they are selected for mitral valve surgery. So the following 4 other investigations are to be done.

1. Echocardiogram.
2. Trans-septal left atrial catheterization by contrast injection of left atrium.
3. Retrograde left ventricular catheterization.
4. Cine angiocardiography, etc. are useful.

47. Roentgen abnormalities of the aorta are classified as the following 4:

1. Elongation and tortuosity (unfolding of aorta).
2. Increase in diameter—aneurysm formation.
3. Decrease in diameter—coarctation, atresia, etc.
4. Calcium sclerosis.

The aorta is an elastic organ and when it undergoes degenerative changes or when it is subjected to increased pressure—it elongates and finally dilates. This is often referred to as unfolding or uncoiling of the aorta.

48. X-ray diagnosis of aneurysm of the aorta depends on the study of the aorta in 4 views:

1. Oblique view.
2. Frontal view.
3. Lateral view.
4. Fluoroscopy.

If still doubt exists, retrograde aortography or angiocardiography is done.

49. Aneurysm of the arch of the aorta. The 4 points to be noted are:

1. Aortic knob shows considerable increase in its size.
2. Trachea and esophagus are displaced to the right and posteriorly.
3. Left bronchus is displaced downward and to the right.
4. Left ventricle is usually enlarged and boot-shaped. (See for marked pulsations in the supraclavicular notch, and recurrent laryngeal nerve palsy).

50. Aneurysm of the descending aorta. The 4 important points are:

1. A double contoured shadow may be seen behind the heart due to dilated aorta.
2. There may be concave erosion of the vertebral body anteriorly (sparing the intervertebral cartilages) due to intermittent pulsating pressure.
3. Left ventricle also becomes enlarged.
4. Esophagus is displaced to the right and anteriorly, superiorly and on the left, inferiorly.

This is seen by taking esophagograms.
This is due to the fact that esophagus closely approximates the aorta.

51. Dissecting aneurysm of aorta. The 4 main points are:

1. Changing appearance of the aorta on serial examinations.
2. Calcifications which are laminated within the lumen of the aorta.
3. Sometimes double contour of the aorta may be identified.
4. Angiography may assist in the diagnosis.
   - Clinically this condition is found with hypertension syphilis
   - Infectious necrosis
   - Trauma.

52. Calcification of the aorta is seen at 4 sites.

1. Ascending aorta—it is frequent with leutic aortitis than with arteriosclerotic changes.
2. Thoracic and abdominal aorta—arteriosclerotic origin.
3. Occasionally in the intrapericardial portion of the aorta.
4. Over the aortic valves.

Calcification in the aortic valve area should be differentiated from calcification in mitral valve areas in the LAO view. In this mitral area falls in the posterior 1/3rd of the cardiac silhouette whereas aortic area falls in the middle 1/3rd.

53. There are 4 X-ray findings in coarctation of the aorta.

There is a congenital stenosis just distal to the origin of the left subclavian artery in the region of the ligamentum arteriosum.

1. A relative absence of shadow in a sector of the descending thoracic aorta—immediately below the aortic knob, giving the aorta a 'notched' appearance.
2. Appearance of an inverted '3' of the esophageal impressions—the upper being due to aortic knob, the lower to the poststenotic dilation.
3. Notching of the under surfaces of the ribs—caused by the hypertrophied, tortuous, kinked intercostal arteries. Notching is best seen in 4th to 8th ribs posteriorly and it is rare for third or higher ribs to be involved.

These changes are best seen in adults (past 10 years of age) and are rarely recognized in a child.

4. The left subclavian artery may be prominent.

The heart as a whole may be moderately enlarged due to left ventricular hypertrophy caused by hypertension and sometimes by the associated aortic valvular disease.

54. Rib notching is seen in the following 4 conditions:

1. Coarctation of aorta.
2. Superior vena caval obstruction.
3. Pulseless disease (Takayasu's disease).
4. Aortic stenosis.

Sometimes in generalized neurofibromatosis.

Rib notching is seen in the lower border of posterior parts of the ribs. Rib notching is not seen in children upto 10 years of age because collateral circulation is not properly developed.

Rib notching can be caused by any of the three major intercostal structures—intercostal arteries, veins and nerves, which can enlarge, compress and erode the lower border of the ribs.

In coarctation of the aorta—the rib-notching is due to dynamic dilatation and tortuosity of the arteries.

In superior vena caval obstruction—it is due to dilatation and tortuosity of the veins.

In neurofibromatosis—it is due to multiple intercostal neurofibromas.

55. There are 4 roentgen abnormalities in aortic valve disease.

1. In predominant aortic stenosis—90% is of congenital origin—left ventricular enlargement occurs rather late and the heart is often of normal size.

   Marked left ventricular hypertrophy occurs first later followed by dilatation. Calcification of the valve in males over 40 years is almost invariable.
2. In predominant aortic incompetence, left ventricle enlargement develops very rapidly and is generally very severe than in aortic stenosis.

   If left ventricle fails, functional mitral incompetence develops and this gives rise to left atrial enlargement. Calcification of the valve is less common.

   Left ventricular failure of other causes such as hypertension, ischemic heart disease will also produce functional mitral incompetence.
3. Dilatation of ascending aorta is common in aortic valve disease.

   It is slight in aortic stenosis where the ascending aorta is only affected. Whereas in aortic incompetence, the ascending aorta, aortic arch and even the descending aorta may be dilated.
4. On fluoroscopy, slow rising pulse of aortic stenosis can be recognized along the aortic contour so also the fast rising water hammer pulse of aortic incompetence.

   It is not always possible to differentiate between predominant aortic stenosis and incompetence on conventional X-ray films. So, other investigations like echocardiogram, contrast studies of aortic valve, retrograde catheterization, etc. are to be done.

56. There are 4 roentgen abnormalities in tricuspid valve disease.

This is rare as a primary lesion but functional incompetence is common secondary to right ventricular failure.

A. In tricuspid stenosis:
   1. Right atrial enlargement is seen as displacement of right cardiac border.
   2. Distension of superior vena cava is seen as widening of the upper mediastinum along its right upper border.

B. In tricuspid incompetence:
   3. Right atrial enlargement.
   4. Right ventricular enlargement seen as lifting of apex upward.

57. There are 4 roentgen abnormalities in ischemic heart disease.

1. Generalized cardiac enlargement is the main feature, the left side being more frequently affected than the right in chronic ischemic heart disease.

   Cardiac enlargement may persist for months but can regress even after a long period.
2. A cardiac aneurysm appears as a separate protrusion from the normal cardiac contour usually along the left cardiac border or slightly anterior or posterior to it depending on the side of the cardiac infarction.
3. Calcification of coronary artery is frequently visible on routine chest films of elderly patients and is not necessarily related to ischemic heart disease. It is significant in patients below 40 years age.

   (Coronary occlusion is demonstrated by arteriography).

   On fluoroscopy:
4. Absence of adequate ventricular contraction or even paradoxical pulsation with systolic expansion over the infarcted area of the heart may be visible but is usually difficult to see unless a cardiac aneurysm develops.

   Once cardiac aneurysm is fully developed, pulsation over it will be definitely abnormal and expansile during ventricular systole. This abnormal pulsation usually disappears with the improvement of the patient. (This is well seen in echocardiogram).

58. There are 4 roentgen abnormalities in hypertension.

There may be no change or minor degrees of change in recent hypertension.

The changes in heart shadow are seen well in long-standing cases of hypertension.

1. Left ventricular enlargement: 'Boot-shaped' heart is seen in the long-standing cases of hypertension with left ventricular enlargement.
   There is hypertrophy in the beginning followed by dilatation.
   Left ventricular enlargement due to functional mitral incompetence will also be seen.
2. Ascending aorta, aortic arch and descending aorta dilate and elongate and become more and more prominent—bulging slightly into right and left lung fields.
   Aortic dilatation and elongation sometimes appear as aortic unfolding.
   The degree of aortic dilatation largely depends on the severity of co-existing atherosclerosis.
3. Lateral view: As the aorta further dilates it tends to become tortuous, thus being clearly demonstrated on the oblique and lateral films.
   The barium filled esophagus may take a tortuous course tending to follow the thoracic aorta.
   Long-standing cases of systemic hypertension leads to gross cardiac enlargement particularly of left ventricle. Finally left ventricular failure supervenes.
4. Barium swallow: Aortic impression on a barium swallow becomes well-pronounced and widened.

59. There are 4 roentgen abnormalities in infective endocarditis.

1. Evidence of early congestive heart failure. This helps in the assessment of management and prognosis.
2. Presence of multiple small patchy infiltrates in the lungs of parenteral drug abusers with fever strongly favors the diagnosis of septic emboli of right-sided infective endocarditis.
3. Calcification on previously abnormal valve.
4. Aorta may show mycotic aneurysm.

Fluoroscopy: Abnormal motion of prosthetic valve indicates the presence of vegetations or partial dehiscence of the valve from aortic root. This helps to decide whether the valve replacement is needed during the management of prosthetic valve endocarditis (PVE).

60. Roentgen abnormalities in heart failure.

Pulmonary vascular abnormalities clearly show the underlying pathophysiology of heart failure in addition to specific chamber enlargement. It is studied separately in 4 headings:

1. Acute left-sided heart failure.
2. Chronic left-sided heart failure.
3. Acute right-sided heart failure.
4. Chronic right-sided heart failure.

61. There are 4 roentgen findings in acute left-sided heart failure: It is most common with acute myocardial infarction.

The pulmonary vascular abnormalities in acute left ventricular failure are usually not clear because:

1. The resultant pulmonary edema obscures the pulmonary vasculature.
2. The redistribution of pulmonary flow secondary to acute left ventricular failure is relatively mild.
3. Alveolar type of pulmonary edema shows 'Bat's-wing' appearance. The reason for this is not clearly understood.
4. Normal-sized heart.

Alveolar pulmonary edema with a normal-sized heart is the hallmark of acute left ventricular failure.

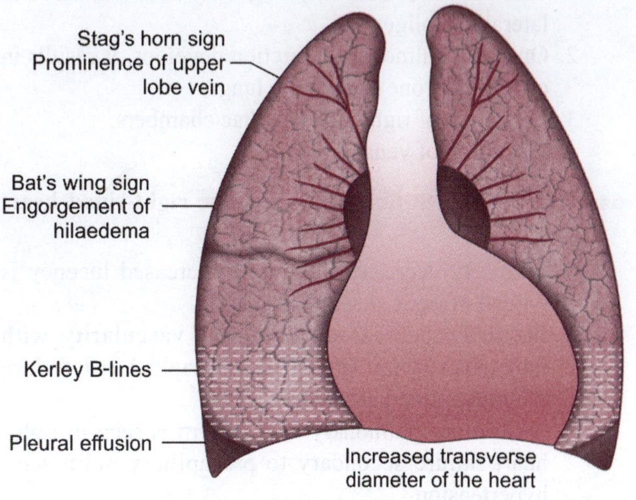

Fig. P-10: Roentgen findings of lungs associated with heart failure

62. The 4 roentgen findings of lungs in chronic left-sided heart failure are:

1. *Stag's horn sign (cephalization)*: Prominence of the upper lobe veins often likened to Stag's horns. This is due to increased pulmonary venous pressure in left

ventricular failure causing a relative diversion of blood from the lower to the upper zones in the erect posture.
2. *Bat's wing sign*: Enlargement of the hila and a ground glass appearance of perihilar region often likened to a Bat's wing. It is due to frank pulmonary edema or rarely uremic lung.
3. *Septal lines or Kerley B-lines:* Most commonly seen in the lower lobes near the costophrenic angles. They are fine dense lines thought to be due to edema in the lymphatics. When horizontal, they are known as Kerley B-lines.
4. *Pleural effusion:* Seen as obliteration of costophrenic angles in mild effusion.

Pulmonary hemosiderosis, ossification or both seen in long-standing severe postcapillary pulmonary hypertension.
It is associated with gross cardiomegaly. Transverse diameter of the heart is increased.
As a rule, heart size is never normal in chronic congestive heart failure. (VS see C-73).

63. The 4 roentgen findings in acute right-sided heart failure are:

This condition most commonly results from massive pulmonary embolism. It shows:
1. Rapidly developing centralization of the pulmonary vasculature. In addition, lungs may show localized or lateralized oligemia.
2. Once the pulmonary infarction develops, it results in opacities in one or both the lungs.
3. Dilatation of right-sided cardiac chambers.
4. Dilatation of vena cavae.

64. The 4 roentgen findings in chronic right-sided heart failure.

1. Diffusely decreased flow with increased lucency is typical of right-sided heart failure.
   Diffusely decreased pulmonary vascularity with unusually lucent lungs seen in right-heart failure without pulmonary hypertension.
2. Centralized pulmonary flow pattern is seen in right-heart failure secondary to precapillary pulmonary hypertension.
3. Cephalized flow pattern with unusually lucent lungs in right-heart failure secondary to left heart failure.
4. The degree of right-sided chamber enlargement is proportional to the severity of tricuspid incompetence.

65. The 4 common causes of chronic right-heart failure are:

1. Congenital pulmonary stenosis.
2. Ebstein anomaly.
3. Severe chronic obstructive pulmonary disease.
4. Recurrent pulmonary thromboembolic disease.

66. There are 4 signs to be looked in X-ray in atrial septal defect (ASD).

1. RAH.
2. RVH.
3. Dilatation of pulmonary artery and its branches dynamic pulsations—'Hilar dance' on screening.
4. Increased pulmonary vascular markings.
   - Pulmonary plethora versus mitral stenosis—redistribution of the vasculature with narrowing of the vessels at the lung bases and dilatation of those in upper lobes.

67. Hilar dance is an expansile pulsations of Hilar vessels, i.e. dilatation of pulmonary artery and its branches.

This occurs in any of the 4 lesions leading to left to right shunts.
1. ASD—most common.
2. PDA—more common.
3. VSD—less common.
4. Anomalous drainage of pulmonary veins to right atrium or superior vena cava—rare.

68. There are 4 X-ray findings in large-sized VSD.

1. LAH.
2. Biventricular hypertrophy.
3. Prominent pulmonary artery segment.
4. Increased pulmonary vascular markings.

69. Check for the following 4 changes in X-ray in tetralogy of Fallot (TOF).

1. Cardiac size is normal or even smaller than normal unless there is failure. Apex is above the diaphragm.
   - Concentric hypertrophy of left ventricle.
   - Boot-shaped heart in a cyanosed child is diagnostic of Fallot's tetralogy. Deep concavity in the waist of the heart differentiates from Eisenmenger's complex, pulmonary stenosis and others producing similar symptoms.
2. Pulmonary concavity.
3. Widening of superior mediastinum.
4. Oligemic lung fields.

70. Fluoroscopy for pulsations helps in recognizing the following 4 conditions:

1. 'Dynamic pulsations'—Hilar dance on screening in ASD. Dilatation of pulmonary artery and its branches.
2. Abnormal degree of aortic pulsations in aortic regurgitation.
3. Saccular aneurysm of the aorta seen as a rounded outgrowth from some part of the aorta. Its relation to

the aorta and its pulsations help to distinguish from an intrathoracic tumor.

4. In mitral regurgitation—the dilated left atrium is seen in anteroposterior view to expand markedly during ventricular systole.

71. The roentgen findings in patent ductus arteriosus are:

It is an arterial communication between the distal part of the aortic arch and left pulmonary artery. The shunt is from left to right resulting in increased pulmonary flow. There is a volume load on left atrium and left ventricle. There may be pulmonary hypertension in large shunts.

1. Pulmonary trunk dilatation is the rule.
2. Aortic knuckle is larger than normal in 50% of cases. There is filling of the angle between the knuckle and the pulmonary trunk.
3. Left border of the heart suggests left ventricular dilatation.
4. Left atrium is slightly enlarged in 25% of cases.
5. Calcification around the ductus may be seen.
6. Pulmonary plethora is variable.
7. Pulmonary edema where there is heart failure.
8. In older patients with Eisenmenger's complex central pulmonary arteries are prominent with rapid tapering to the periphery.

72. There are 4 sites of calcification that may be seen in X-ray of patent ductus arteriosus.

1. Aortic wall.
2. Orifice of the ductus.
3. End of the main pulmonary artery.
4. Ductus arteriosus especially when it is dilated to aneurysmal stage.

73. There are 4 roentgen abnormalities in constrictive pericarditis.

1. Pear-shaped heart. Heart is usually central in position and small.
2. A continuous convex right border from diaphragm to aorta is the constant finding. Above it, there is dilated superior vena cava.
3. Angles are free while in triangular-shaped heart these angles are usually obliterated.
4. Calcification of the pericardium is the hallmark of constrictive pericarditis.

74. There are 4 roentgen abnormalities in pericardial effusion.

1. General enlargement of the heart and distension of superior vena cava. All the cardiac contours are obliterated. Minimum amount of 300–500 mL is needed to detect radiologically. Fluid gravitates to the left side posteriorly. Hence, there is no increase in density of heart shadow due to effusion.
2. Cardiophrenic angle remain acute till sudden failure and secondary pulmonary changes occur.
3. The retrocardiac space is obliterated and the esophagus is displaced backward and to the right.
4. When pericardial effusion is associated with chronic failure, there is obvious pulmonary congestion and obliteration of right cardiophrenic angle. Patchy areas of atelectasis may also blunt the left cardiophrenic angle.

Radiology of the Pulmonary Circulation

Study of the radiological appearances of the lungs is of greatest value in the diagnosis and prognosis of disordered lung function in both heart diseases and lung diseases.

75. The 4 radiological features of hyperkinetic (or hyperdynamic) pulmonary hypertension.

The most distinctive appearance on plain X-ray chest is:

1. Dilatation of the main pulmonary artery—its main branches as well as smaller peripheral divisions producing a picture of pulmonary hyperemia which is uniform throughout the lungs.
2. Right ventricular enlargement is always seen with significant left to right shunt.

   The degree of pulmonary hyperemia is proportional to the magnitude of the left to right shunt.

   When surgical correction of a left to right shunt is done—the reduction of blood flow through the lungs will eventually result in.
3. A decrease in size of the pulmonary artery and its smaller branches. The appearance of pulmonary hyperemia will disappear.
4. Right ventricular enlargement also disappear once the shunt is closed.

   Regression of the pulmonary vascular distension and cardiac enlargement will begin slowly after successful surgery but may take many months.

   From the radiological point of view—pulmonary arterial hypertension should be distinguished from pulmonary venous hypertension. Pulmonary edema is the main feature to distinguish these two conditions. Pulmonary edema occurs very frequently in pulmonary venous hypertension and not in pulmonary arterial hypertension.

   By evaluating pulmonary vasculature, the diagnostic possibilities can be narrowed down, e.g. a uniform dilatation of the pulmonary vessels is suggestive of left to right shunt, then a left-sided obstructive lesion, later typically shows a cephaled pulmonary blood flow pattern.

76. When the pulmonary vasculature is considered in relation to the size of the aorta, the 4 following can be differentiated:

A. With pulmonary oligemia:
1. A dilated aortic arch associated with oligemic lung fields and right ventricular hypertrophy is practically diagnostic of tetralogy of Fallot.
2. A small aortic arch in the same circumstances is strongly suggestive of pulmonary stenosis with closed ventricular septum.

B. With pulmonary pleonemia:
3. It is often noticed that if the aortic arch is large the situation implies L to R shunt.
It indicates that the shunt is extra cardiac—usually through a persistent ductus.
4. If the aortic arch is small, it indicates the shunt is intracardiac.

In most of the left to right shunts, the size of the aorta is not a very reliable sign as to whether the shunt is intra or extra-cardiac until late childhood by which time in most cases the situation of the defect has already been accurately identified. In the persistent truncus arteriosus and aortopulmonary window—there is often a disparity between aortic root where the shunt is occurring and the aortic arch which is small.

Note: Pulmonary vascularity is normal in coarctation of aorta and aortic stenosis.

77. Causes of pulmonary oligemia may be described in 4 groups:

1. Obstruction to right ventricular outflow with a right to left shunt
   - Fallot's tetralogy.
2. Obstruction to right ventricular outflow without shunt
   - Pulmonary valve stenosis.
   - Pulmonary atresia.
   - Constrictive pericarditis.
3. Obstruction to right ventricular inflow
   - Tricuspid atresia—Ebstein malformation of tricuspid valve with pulmonary stenosis.
   - Tricuspid stenosis.
   - Underdeveloped right ventricle.
4. Right ventricular failure.

78. Causes of pulmonary plethora without cyanosis.

Left to right shunt only.
1. Atrial septal defect.
2. Ventricular septal defect.
3. Patent ductus arteriosus.
4. Aortic sinus fistula.
5. Partial anomalous pulmonary venous return.
6. Aorticopulmonary window.
7. Atrioventricular canal.
8. Left ventricle to right atrium.

79. Causes of increased pulmonary vascularity with cyanosis.

Bilateral shunt
1. Single ventricle.
2. Truncus arteriosus.
3. D-transposition of the great vessels.
4. Total anomalous pulmonary venous return.
5. Tricuspid atresia without pulmonary stenosis.
6. Double outlet right ventricle.
7. Hypoplastic left heart syndrome.
8. Eisenmenger's syndrome.

(Increased pulmonary venous vascularity is seen in scimitar and stenosis of individual pulmonary veins, total anomalous pulmonary venous return with obstruction, hypoplastic left heart).

Alteration in the pulmonary vessels

While studying the pulmonary vascularity, not only the abnormalities in pulmonary blood flow (plethora or oligemia) but abnormalities in distribution also should be noted.

Normally, in erect posture, gravity causes majority of the blood to flow to the base and upper lobe vessels are smaller than the lower lobe vessels. In supine position, blood flow in the apex is equal to the base.

80. Abnormal distribution of pulmonary blood flow pattern can be described in the following way. This is the result of change in pulmonary vascular resistance either locally or diffusely.

1. *Cephalization*: If the upper lobe vessels are larger than the lower lobe vessels, it is called as cephalization or vascular redistribution pattern. This is useful in the diagnosis of increased left heart pressure.
It occurs in postcapillary pulmonary hypertension when total intravascular pressure exceeds the oncotic pressure of the blood resulting in leakage of fluid out of the vessels and collects in the interstitium before pouring into the alveoli.
Pulmonary edema interferes with exchange of gases resulting in hypoxia which intern causes constriction of pulmonary vessels at the bases where there is greater pressure than the apices and so forces the blood flow upward. This is actually reversal of the normal physiology resulting in redistribution or cephalization of the pulmonary vascularity.

a. Left-sided obstructive lesions.
- Mitral stenosis
- Aortic stenosis.

b. Coronary artery disease with left ventricular failure.
c. Cardiomyopathy with left ventricular failure.
d. Mitral insufficiency even before the left ventricular failure.

The diagnosis of cephalization should not be made unless there is constriction of lower-lobe vessels. Dilatation of upper-lobe vessels is of secondary importance as they can be found without narrowing of the basilar vessels in many conditions as found in left to right shunts.

Left heart failure and mitral valve stenosis are the most frequent causes for the above said pattern.

The other radiological features are—cardiothoracic ratio > 0.5 and the vessel margins are distinct (in mild LHF).

In severe LHF, there is edema; hence the vessel margins become indistinct and the peripheral interstitial markings become more prominent.

In moderate LHF with large, indistinct upper lobe vessels and prominent interstitium, fluid may thicken the interlobular septa causing short lines perpendicular to the pleural surface. These are Kerley B-lines which indicate interstitial edema.

Cephalization → Interstitial edema → Alveolar edema
(Mild failure) (Moderate failure) (Severe failure)

Lateral X-ray findings in a congestive heart failure patient:

a. Plural effusion (thick fissure).
b. Edema.
c. Big left ventricle.
d. Vascular redistribution:
- With cephalization, lung auscultation is usually normal.
- With interstitial edema, crackling rales are audible.
- With alveolar edema, rales (wet crackles) are audible.

Marked enlargement of cardiac silhouette with no or mild signs of LHF indicates pericardial effusion or cardiomyopathy or multivalvular heart disease.

2. *Centralization*: It occurs in precapillary pulmonary hypertension. The pulmonary trunk and central pulmonary arteries dilate. The distal pulmonary arteries constrict in a concentric way from the periphery of the lung towards the hilum (centripetally). This phenomenon is called centralization. It is seen in idiopathic pulmonary hypertension, Eisenmenger syndrome, severe obstructive emphysema.
3. *Collateralization*: The numerous small and tortuous bronchial collaterals develop in the upper and medial lung zones close to their origin from the descending aorta in markedly decreased pulmonary flow. Severe pulmonary oligemia is seen in tetralogy of Fallot because of pulmonary stenosis. The pulmonary arteries are very small, smooth and branch gracefully. Marked reduction in pulmonary blood flow is seen in right sided heart failure without a right to left shunt. The lungs are more radiolucent.
4. *Lateralization and localization*: Uneven distribution of blood flow between the two lungs in favor of one lung, e.g. massive pulmonary embolism obstructing the main pulmonary artery on one side, the blood flow favor the opposite side of obstruction, i.e. through healthy lung only. The paucity of the pulmonary vascularity in the affected lung is termed as 'Westermark sign'. Localized abnormal vascular changes in a cyanotic child is an example of large pulmonary arteriovenous fistula.

Volume of the pulmonary flow is estimated by the degree of pulmonary arterial enlargement as long as the flow pattern remains normal. The distribution is assessed by abnormal flow pattern. Volume and distribution of pulmonary flow may change singly or combinedly depending on the nature of the underlying heart condition.

81. Unilateral difference in vessel pattern is seen in 4 conditions.

1. Massive embolism.
2. Central shunts.
3. Pulmonary artery stenosis or absence of one pulmonary artery.
4. Extrinsic pressure from right aortic arch, tumor, mediastinitis.

82. Uneven vascularity of a patchy nature is seen in 4 conditions.

1. Peripheral pulmonary arterial stenosis.
2. Pulmonary atresia.
3. Multiple pulmonary emboli.
4. Multiple pulmonary arteriovenous fistulae.

Bronchial Artery Circulation

83. Bronchial arteries are too small to be seen on the plain X-ray chest. However, in some congenital anomalies where the pulmonary circulation is affected with severe pulmonary oligemia, the bronchial collaterals become tortuous (collateralization) and develop in the medial and upper zones close to their origin from the descending aorta. Bronchial vessels are therefore occasionally seen in plain X-ray chest particularly in such congenital disorders such as the following 4:

1. Anomalies of the pulmonary artery:
   a. Pulmonary atresia.
   b. Severe hypoplasia of the pulmonary arteries.
   c. Pulmonary stenosis.
   d. Absence of pulmonary artery.
2. Tricuspid atresia.
3. Pseudotruncus arteriosus.
4. Fallot's tetralogy.

84. There are 4 radiological appearances of lung parenchyma in pulmonary venous hypertension.

The recognition of the radiological signs of pulmonary venous hypertension is of the greatest importance for the clinical management of patients as they may be the first indication of incipient left sided heart failure.

These are due to pulmonary edema and this can be either intra-alveolar or interstitial.

A. Intra-alveolar edema:
   1. Uniform density of the lung fields affecting the central areas and often leaving a clear periphery, the so-called 'Bat's wing' or 'butterfly shadows' in intra-alveolar edema. The confluent shadows of pulmonary edematous consolidation are commonly symmetrical and bilateral but they can be unilateral and even apical. They often affect the posterior segment of the lungs.

   The patient's posture at the time when he develops cardiac failure plays a part in the distribution of edema which sometimes accumulates in the most dependent parts of the lungs.

B. Interstitial pulmonary edema:

   It occurs more frequently particularly in mitral stenosis and left-sided cardiac failure.
   2. The so-called horizontal septal lines or Kerley's B-lines are seen at the edges of the lungs in the lower mid zones as short fine linear shadows.
   3. Excessive accumulation of interstitial pulmonary edema leads to blurring of details of vascular shadows particularly around the hila and bases. This makes interpretation of the pulmonary vascular pattern difficult and gives rise to poor definition of pulmonary arteries and veins.
   4. Occasionally, large draining lymphatics in the septal planes are seen as fine straight linear shadows 'lines A' crossing the normal arterial pathways connecting the more superficial lymphatics with the hilum and hilar lymph nodes.

Peribronchial cuffing with perihilar peripheral haze are additional findings of interstitial edema.

In right-heart failure, the lungs becomes unusually radiolucent because of decreased pulmonary blood flow whereas in left-sided heart failure, it is characterized by pulmonary edema and cephaloid blood flow pattern.

85. Septal lines or Kerley's B-lines are seen in the following 4 conditions:

1. Left-sided heart failure—they may persist after the regression of the heart failure and this is usually due to fibrosis or hemosiderin in the septa.

   Occasionally seen in non cardiac diseases such as:
2. Pneumoconiosis.
3. Lymphangitis carcinomatosa.
4. Lymphatic obstruction due to malignant disease at the hilum.

86. The 4 features of the pleural effusion in the cardiac condition are (There may be associated persistent basal pleural effusion in addition to the other signs of pulmonary venous hypertension):

1. Pleural effusions are common in left-sided cardiac failure being more frequently seen on the right side than on left side.
2. The volume of the pleural fluid varies considerably.
3. The effusion usually disappears with the improvement of the heart failure.
4. Occasionally, some pleural thickening remains.

87. The following 4 features are recognized when the pulmonary artery pressure rises secondary to the pulmonary venous congestion.

1. The main pulmonary artery and its main branches and the first and second division branches will appear dilated and the smaller peripheral arterial branches will at first retain their caliber. There is a correlation between the height of the pulmonary artery pressure and the size of the main pulmonary artery and its main branches.
2. As the pulmonary artery pressure further increases—the smaller arterial branches in the lower lobes will appear constricted, whereas in the mid and upper zones they will be of normal size.

   The narrowing of the pulmonary arteries in the lower zones of the lungs occur in response to the elevated pulmonary venous pressure, i.e. the venous pressure is already elevated to a critical level above the plasma osmotic pressure and this added the difference of the hydrostatic pressure between the bases of the lungs and the apices.

   This differential vasoconstriction at the bases lead to a deviation of blood flow from the lower zones of the lungs to the upper zone. This response of the pulmonary vasculature is directly opposite of the normal physiology where the blood to the upper zones is smaller than the lower zones of the lungs.

3. There is a good correlation of the radiological appearances with pathological findings showing selective vascular constriction at the bases of the lungs in contrast to the normal caliber of the small artery in the upper lobes.
   The vasoconstriction affecting the smaller pulmonary arteries at the bases is demonstrated by selective angiographic studies.
4. The basal arterial constriction is more marked in patients with severe mitral valve disease and is less marked in heart failure due to other causes such as hypertension, aortic valve disease and ischemic heart disease.

88. There are 4 features of the pulmonary ossification.

1. The ossified nodules are true lamellar bone and radiologically appear as very dense nodules widely scattered throughout the lower and mid zones of the lungs. They vary in size from tiny pin heads to sharply-defined calcified shadows of the size of a pea.
2. Pulmonary ossification occurs in mitral heart disease. They can appear within a few years of onset of cardiac lesion.
3. They are associated with pulmonary hypertension and with repeated episodes of interstitial pulmonary edema.
4. There is no association between hemosiderosis and pulmonary ossification.

89. Radiological appearances of 'Cor Pulmonale'.

(Heart disease secondary to pulmonary disease)
Chronic bronchitis is the most common cause of 'cor pulmonale'. Bronchitis will give rise to pulmonary arterial hypertension mainly due to vasoconstriction produced by hypoxia.

Plain X-ray chest film shows 4 features:

1. Right-sided cardiac enlargement associated with:
2. Marked dilatation of the pulmonary artery and its main branches.
   Arterial dilatation may be so marked that the appearance can simulate a septal defect with increased pulmonary blood flow.
   During the recovery phase.
3. Pulmonary vascular distension disappear rapidly and this is often followed by:
4. Diminution in right-sided cardiac enlargement.
   Persistence of right-sided cardiac enlargement with persistent dilatation of the main pulmonary artery indicates irreversible right ventricular failure.

90. 'Cor Pulmonale' may occur in more chronic diseases of the lungs associated with extensive pulmonary fibrosis or parenchymal destruction due to obliterative reduction of the pulmonary vascular bed. This is seen in 4 conditions:

1. Pneumoconiosis.
2. Advanced fibrocaseous tuberculosis.
3. Scleroderma.
4. Malignant infiltration such as lymphangitis carcinomatosa.

Right-sided cardiac enlargement is often associated with those disorders but the pulmonary vascular changes seen in chronic bronchitis are rarely visible since they are overshadowed by the extensive lung disease.

Q Electrocardiography

Electrocardiogram is a graphic representation of electrical activity of the heart—depolarization and repolarization. Interestingly, the machine recording the electrical activity is called electrocardiograph, and the record, the electrocardiogram.

ECG is an abbreviation of the English word.

EKG is an abbreviation of the German word Electrokardiogram. Some prefer to use EKG to avoid possible confusion with EEG (electroencephalogram).

The machine is called an electrocardiograph.

The tracing is called electrocardiogram (compare telegraph with telegram).

1. The 4 great scientists who contributed to the evolution of ECG:

1. *Augustus desire Waller:* British Physiologist of St Mary's Medical School, London published the first human electrocardiogram in 1887. It is recorded from Thomas Goswell, a technician in the laboratory.
   Waller AD. A demonstration on man of electromotive changes accompanying the heart's beat. J Physiol (London). 1887;8:229-34.
2. *Willem Einthoven:* Dutch physiologist attended when Waller demonstrated his technique at the First International Congress of Physiologists in 1889. Einthoven introduced the term 'electrocardiogram' at a meeting of the Dutch Medical Association. (Later he claims that Waller was first to use the term).
   Einthoven W: Nieuwe methoden voor clinisch onderzoek (New methods for clinical investigation). Ned T Geneesk. 1893;29II:263-86.
   He distinguished five deflections which he named P, Q, R, S, T. At this time, all the letters in English up to O were already in use for various other types of recordings in vogue like arterial waves, venous waves, etc. Hence, Einthoven chose next five unused letters of the alphabets for ECG waves.
   Noble prize winner in 1924.

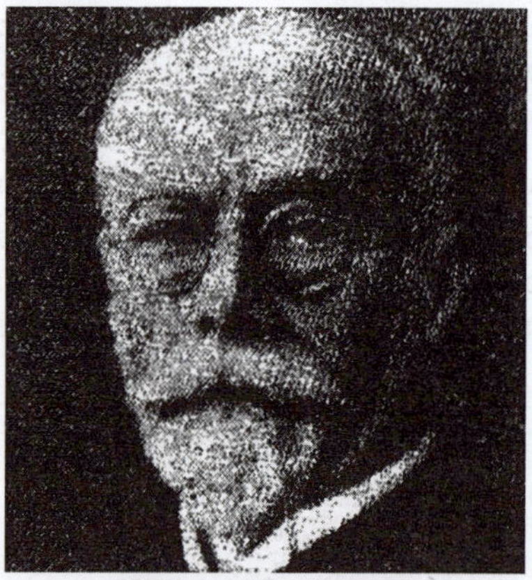

Willem Einthoven
(1860 - 1927)

Fig. Q-1

Einthoven W. Ueleber die Form des menschllichen Electrocardiograms. Arch f d ges Physiol. 1895;60:10-1-123.

Einthoven published the first organized presentation of normal and abnormal electrocardiograms recorded with a string galvanometer. Left and right ventricular hypertrophy, left and right atrial hypertrophy, the U wave (for the first time), notching of the QRS, ventricular premature beats, ventricular bigeminy, atrial flutter and complete heart block are all described in 1906.

Einthoven W. Le telecardiogramme, Arch Int de Physiol 1906:4:132-164 (translated into English. Am Heart J. 1957:53:602-15).

Einthoven addressed in 1912, the Chelsea Clinical Society in London and described an equilateral triangle formed by his standard leads I, II and III later called 'Einthoven's triangle'. This is the first reference in an English article to the abbreviation 'EKG'.
Einthoven W. The different forms of the human electrocardiogram and their signification. Lancet. 1912;(1):853.
Willem Einthoven got the Nobel Prize for inventing the electrocardiograph in 1924.
Electrocardiography is second only to the discovery of X-rays by Roentgen in importance among the physical methods used in clinical medicine.

3. *Wilson:* Recorded the complexes that represented electrical activity at a particular point in 1934.
4. *Emanuel Goldberger:* Improved the complexes of electrical activity at that particular point by improving to augmented limb leads aVL, aVR, aVF to Einthoven three limb leads and adding the six chest leads making the 12-lead electrocardiogram that is used today.

There are many other scientists besides them who contributed to the development of ECG to the present day knowledge. One of them to mention is Italian physicist Carlo Matteucci, in 1842, shows that an electric current accompanies each heartbeat.
Matteucci C. Sur un phenomene physiologique produit par les muscles en contration. Am Chim Phys. 1842:6:339-41.
Electrocardiography developed empirically and its basic diagnostic criteria remains empirical—DJ Rowlands.

BASIC ELECTROPHYSIOLOGY OF THE HEART

Electrocardiographic changes occur due to diseases which affect the electrical activity of the heart. Such diseases occur both within and outside the heart. As the electrocardiogram records only the electrical activity of the heart, it cannot give any idea about the mechanical function of the heart, and is therefore, limited in giving information about the status of the heart. However, ECG still remains the simple and very useful noninvasive technique in conditions like ischemias, infarctions, heart blocks, bundle branch blocks, arrhythmias hypertrophies, etc. No other investigation can give such an information that the ECG can provide with such clarity and accuracy. In spite of development of echocardiography, cardiac catheterization, nuclear studies, etc. The simple ECG investigation has its own important place in cardiac evaluation.

Electrical currents are produced during contraction of the heart—depolarization or cardiac impulse. These electrical currents spread into the tissues surrounding the heart and are distributed throughout the body. A small proportion of these spread all the way to the surface of the body, i.e. to the skin. If electrodes are placed over the body on opposite sides of the heart, the electrical potentials generated by the heart can be recorded by a galvanometer. Connections in the ECG are described as being made to the two terminals of a galvanometer.

Electrical Changes in a Single Cell

Resting cell is electrically positive on its surface and electrically negative inside relative to the outside of the cell (It is remembered as that both words _inside_ and _negative_ contains an *n*, _Outside Positive (OP)_ this is said to be in polarized state.

The resting cell has an excess potassium inside and an excess sodium outside and is thereby in a state of ionic imbalance (It is remembered that during evolution, plenty of sodium is freely available in the ocean and so it is available outside, whereas potassium is less and so it is kept locked inside the cell). The selectively permeable cell membrane maintains the balance by allowing potassium and sodium to pass through it only at certain times when energy is available.

2. **Chemical composition of extracellular and intracellular fluids.**

Table Q-1

	Extracellular	*Intracellular*
1. Na^+ (136–145)	142 mEq/L	10 mEq/L
2. K^+ (3.5–5.0)	5 mEq/L	141 mEq/L
3. Cl^- (98–106)	103 mEq/L	4 mEq/L
4. HCO_3^- (24–32)	28 mEq/L	10 mEq/L
5. Ca^{++}(4.5–5.5)	5 mEq/L	<1 mEq/L
6. Mg^{++}(1.5–2.5)	3 mEq/L	58 mEq/L
7. Glucose (80–120)	<100 mg%	0 – 20 mg%
8. pH (7.35–7.45)	7.4	7.0

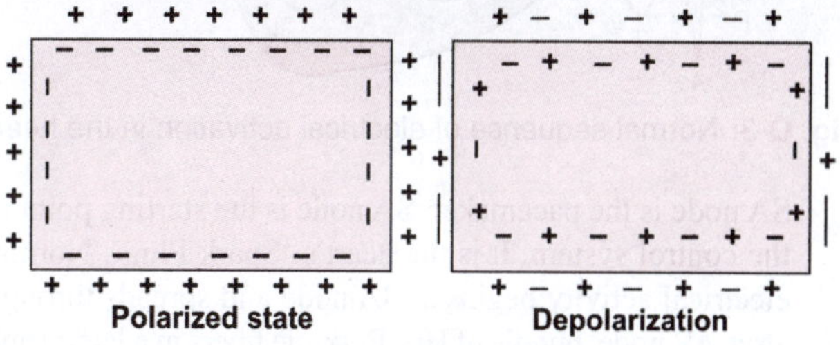

Fig. Q-2

The outer and inner surfaces of the cell can be compared to the two poles of a battery. When a cell is stimulated by connecting outer and inner surfaces to a battery, the negative interior becomes positive and the positive exterior becomes negative temporarily, and the cell is said to be depolarized. This phenomenon is called *depolarization.* When the stimulation passes off, the cell returns to its normal state of positive charge outside and negative charge inside and the cell is said to be repolarized. This phenomenon is called *repolarization.*

These complexes of electrical activity always precede contraction of the heart. Mechanical functions of the heart are achieved when this electrical activity gets converted into mechanical activity by very complex electromechanical coupling. However, it must be remembered that no mechanical activity of the heart takes place in the absence of electrical activity.

(*Note:* Biochemical changes occur earlier to electrical changes)

3. The sequence of changes that occur in a normal cell

1. Biochemical
2. Electrical
3. Mechanical
4. Functional.

4. Normal sequence of cardiac activation:

Depolarization and repolarization

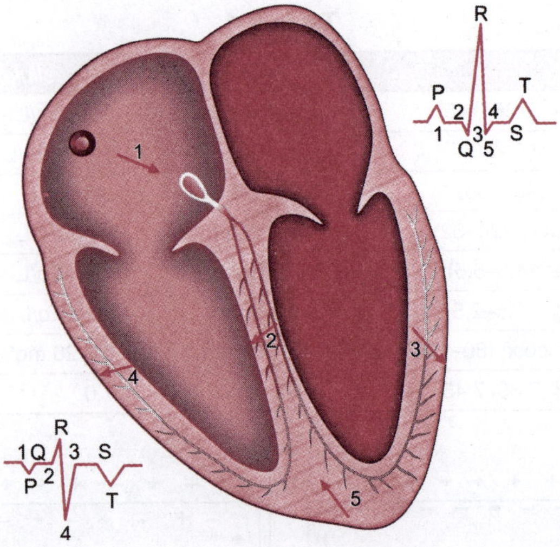

Fig. Q-3: Normal sequence of electrical activation in the heart

SA node is the pacemaker. SA node is the starting point in the control system. It is the heart's 'Spark Plug'. Normal electrical activity begins at SA node and spreads through atria, AV node, bundle of His, Purkinje fibers in a lateral and downward direction toward the apex (Fig. Q-3 arrow 1). The electrical stimulus originating from SA node proceeds away concentrically in all directions similar to a pebble dropped in a pool of water. The electrical activity is picked up by external skin electrode (Skin Sensors) and records an ECG. This cycle of electrical stimulation is known as normal sinus rhythm (NSR), which describes a form of orchestrated synchrony between the atria and the ventricles of the heart, producing the familiar (lub-dub) heart sounds.

1. Atria are thin-walled structures, little electrical activity is seen compared to the ventricles. P wave is the result of depolarization of atria. An electrode placed on the left side of the body records an upright P wave, whereas an electrode on the right side records a negative P wave.

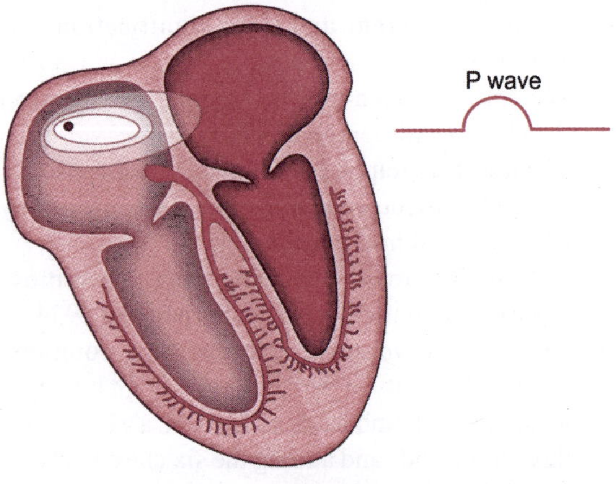

Fig. Q-4

0.04 sec is the appropriate time taken for the impulse to travel from SA node to AV node through the internodal pathway.

The depolarization wave passes from SA node to AV node where there is a 1/10th second delay. The electrical current moves very slowly in the AV node, and then into the bundle of His and electrical activity is not detected; hence, the ECG shows isoelectric PR interval. AV mode funnels these impulses from the atria and leads them to the start of the specialized 'electrical wires' in the ventricles. AV node plays major role in controlling the heart. PR interval is measured from the beginning of P wave to the beginning of the QRS complex. PR segment is the time taken by the AV node (slowest conducting tissue in the heart) to conduct impulse. PR segment does not include a wave.

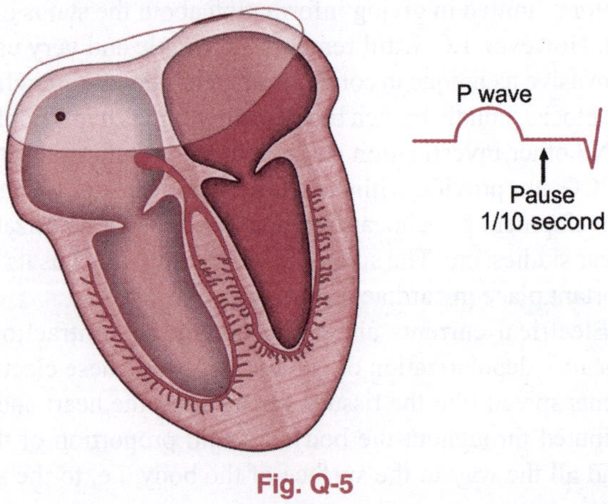

Fig. Q-5

AV node is named for its position between the atria and the ventricles.

Impulses spread later into the main ventricular mass from the subendocardial surface to pericardium by Purkinje system. Electrocardiographically, the ventricles consist of three muscle groups, right ventricle, interventricular septum which behaves like left ventricle and the left ventricle.

2. The first part of ventricular depolarization is Q wave (Fig. Q-3 arrow 2). It is the first negative wave of QRS complex which is relatively small, results from septal depolarization from left to right.
3. The thick left ventricular mass produces more current than right ventricle. The depolarization spreads outward simultaneously from both ventricles from endocardial surface to epicardial surface. Left ventricular electrical force overtakes the right ventricular electrical force. A large R wave is thus produced by depolarization of the left ventricle in left sided electrode (Fig. Q-3 arrow 3).

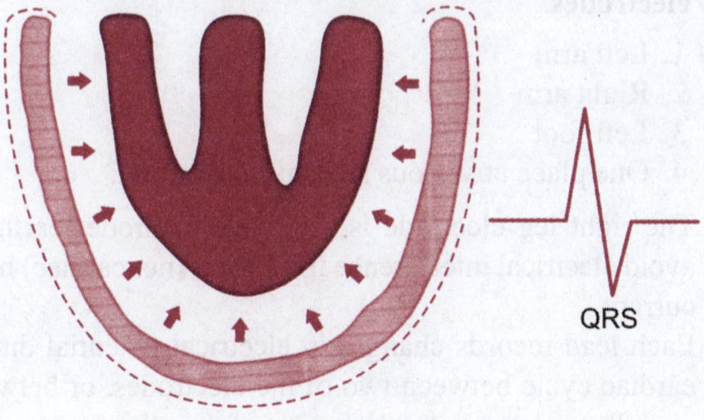

Fig. Q-6

R wave is the first positive wave of QRS complex, usually represents the electrical activity of the ventricle lying under the recording electrode and the S wave represents the activity of other ventricle. For example, in V1,V2, R wave represent right ventricular activity and S wave, the left ventricular activity.

In V5,V6, R wave represents left ventricular activity and S wave represents right ventricular activity.

4. Sometimes late activation of an upper part of the right ventricle produces a late negative deflection S wave (Fig. Q-3 arrow 4).

In the normal heart, the current flows primarily in the direction from the base toward the apex during almost the entire cycle of depolarization except at the very end—because the last part to be depolarized is the anterior walls of the ventricles near the base of the heart. So, immediately before the depolarization wave is completed it courses through the ventricles, the direction of flow reverses for about 1/100th second flowing from the apex towards the base, because the very last part to become depolarized is the anterior walls of the ventricles near the base of the heart.

There is no electrical activity for sometime, after the depolarization of ventricles until repolarization begins, which represents as isoelectric ST segment. Hence, ST segment represent the time gap between depolarizatioin and repolarization in the ventricles.

Repolarization process proceeds from endocardial to epicardial surface. Ventricular repolarization results in T wave. The repolarization is much slower than depolarization. The T wave is generally broad and in the same direction as a rule to the main wave of **QRS** complex—upright in left sided electrode.

In about 20–30% of cases, a positive deflection follows the T wave, called U wave appears. This is due to late ventricular repolarization.

After the repolarization, there is again a period of electrical inactivity and remain isoelectrical until the next impulse starts producing next P-QRS-T complexes.

The ECG machine is arranged in such a way that when a depolarization wave spreads towards a lead, the stylus of the machine moves upwards and when it spreads away from the lead the stylus moves downwards.

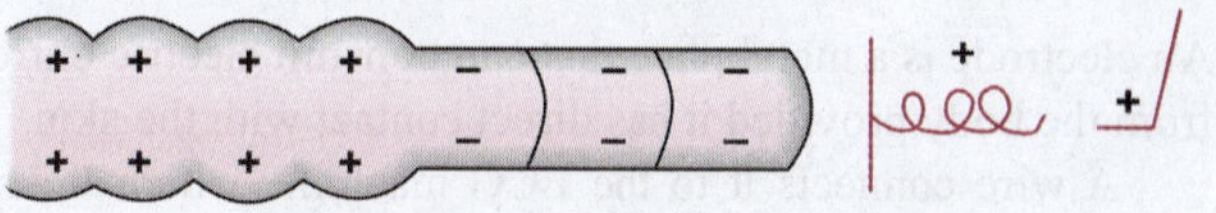

Fig. Q-7: Wave of depolarization: Skin electrode on ECG

When a wave of depolarization within the heart muscle, cells move towards positive (+) skin electrode, there will be positive (+) upward deflection recorded on ECG.

One should remember, that a positive depolarization wave moving towards a positive electrode, records a positive deflection (upward) on the ECG tracing. Similarly, depolarization moving away from a positive electrode records negatively (downward).

The ECG machine is designed in such a way only to show the direction and magnitude of the electric current produced by the heart. Therefore, if one masters a method of recognizing the direction of the heart's current, interpretation of ECG is simplified. It is understood, then, that anyone who reads ECGs must be able to tell the direction of current at any given point in the cardiac cycle. Depolarization can spread in all directions at a time in the heart but the deflection of QRS complex shows the average direction in which the wave of depolarization is spreading.

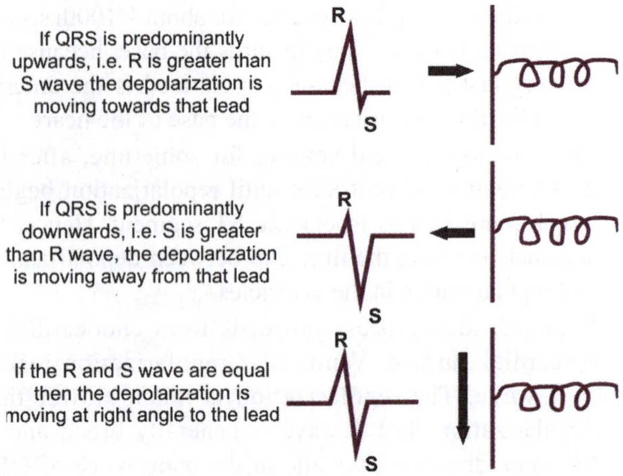

Fig. Q-8

If the current is going parallel to the electrode—no electrical activity is recorded (i.e. zero activity).

Einthoven put forward the concept that the human body represents a large volume conductor having the source of cardiac electrical activity at its center. Heart is the theoretical electrical center of the body. AV node is the center of the heart. Though this is not strictly correct, it still provides practical point for the clinician to work.

LEAD SYSTEMS

An electrode is a metal plate that can transmit electric current from the body provided it has direct contact with the skin.

A wire connects it to the ECG machine, which links it with one or more other electrodes. Therefore, a lead is an arrangement of two or more electrodes joined by wires that pass through the galvanometer of ECG machine.

The galvanometer is a current meter that provides a needle to move to-and-fro depending on the direction of current passing through it. This galvanometer needle movement is directly responsible for the up-and-down movement of the stylus.

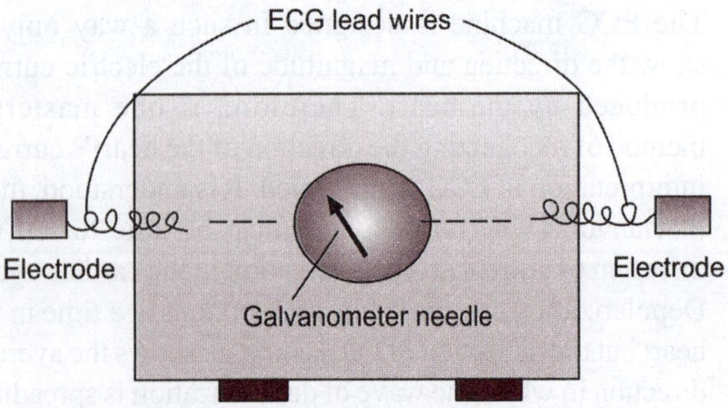

Fig. Q-9: An ECG lead = Electrodes + Lead wires + Galvanometer

If the stylus moves upward on ECG paper, the current is flowing towards a positive electrode. If the stylus is moving downwards, the current is flowing away from the positive electrode. The stylus is really an extension of the galvanometer needle, which is placed in the machine in such a way that it rotates up-and-down rather than right to left.

The electronic engineers have arranged lead's electrodes arbitrarily designated as positive. They have arranged in such a way that the movement of current towards this arbitrary electrode causes an upward deflection on ECG paper. This is the most important concept to be remembered in electrocardiography.

The term lead is used to denote the connection of the electrodes by wires to the galvanometer for record tracing. Proper meaning of 'lead' in ECG is an electrical picture of the heart. Although two electrodes can be connected to any part of the body 'to lead the current' from the heart to the galvanometer, it is customary to connect both forearms, the left leg and the precordium.

5. **Thus, the ECG lead system is composed mainly of 4 electrodes.**
   1. Left arm
   2. Right arm
   3. Left foot
   4. One place at various sites of precordium.

The right leg electrode is a ground electrode (earth) to avoid electrical interference from other (noncardiac) body current.

Each lead records changes in electrical potential during cardiac cycle between two of the electrodes, or between one electrode and a combination of the others.

Einthoven arbitrarily selected the three leads and their relationship between positive and negative electrodes in order to have major positive deflection of the QRS complex moving in an upward direction in normal individuals.

How to remember the origin of the leads?

It can be easily remembered by keeping a pointer directing from SA node toward the apex.

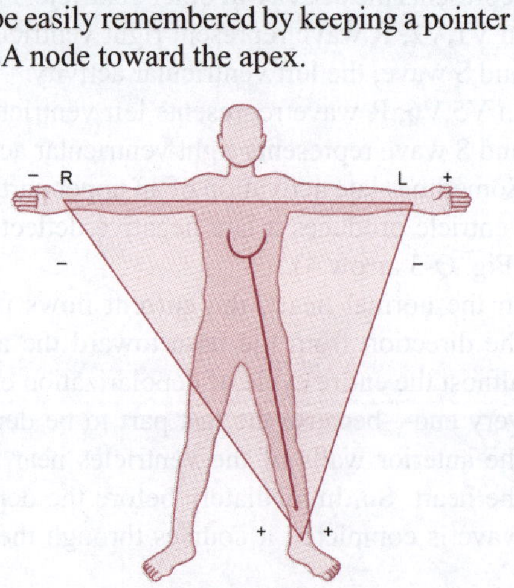

Fig. Q-10: Lead systems

The current is passing from SA node to AV node, bundle of His and Purkinje fibers toward the apex, i.e. the current is passing from right arm side toward left foot in a lateral and downward direction.

The electricity (current) that is liberated in the heart is measured by connecting with positive and negative poles. Which side is positive and which side is negative?

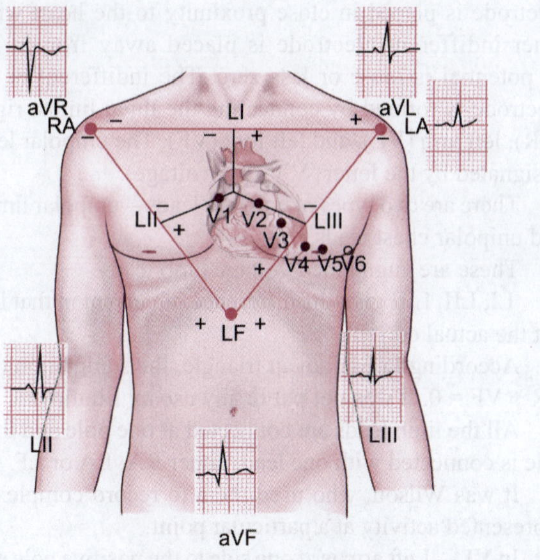

Fig. Q-11: Lead systems

LI—connects the leads left arm and right arm.

Current is passing from right arm to the left arm side, i.e. from SA node toward apex.

Therefore, left arm is positive
right arm is negative.

LII—connects the right arm and left foot.

Current is passing from right arm side to left foot side, i.e. from SA node to apex.

Therefore, left foot is positive
right arm is negative.

LIII—connects left foot and left arm.

Current is passing more towards left foot than left arm.

Therefore, left foot is positive
left arm is negative.

Thus, the positive side and negative side of each lead is known.

SUMMARY

LI = Left arm positive, Right arm negative:

It records the potential difference between the LA and RA.

VL (Left arm) – VR (Right arm)

LII = Left foot positive, Right arm negative:

It records the potential difference between the LF and RA.

VF (Left foot) – VR (Right arm)

LIII = Left foot positive, Left arm negative:

It records the potential difference between the LF and LA.

VF (Left foot) – VL (Left arm)

Thus, the right arm is always negative because the current is passing away from right arm.

Left foot is always positive because the current is passing always toward left foot.

Whereas, left arm is- positive in LI
negative in LIII

These are called Bipolar limb leads or standard leads. Here, two electrodes are placed on two extremities and both record particular pattern of the heart facing these extremities.

(The term standard leads was applicable only when there were no unipolar leads, there is no place for it in modern nomenclature.)

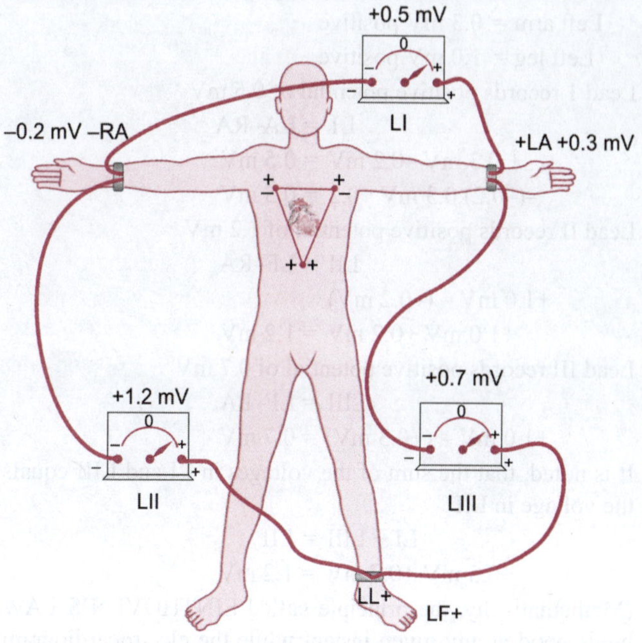

Fig. Q-12: Conventional arrangement of electrodes for recording the standard electrocardiographic leads. Einthoven's triangle is super imposed on the chest

EINTHOVEN'S LAW

If electrical potential of any two of the three standard leads are known at any given instant, the third one can be determine mathematically from the first two by simply summing up the first two.

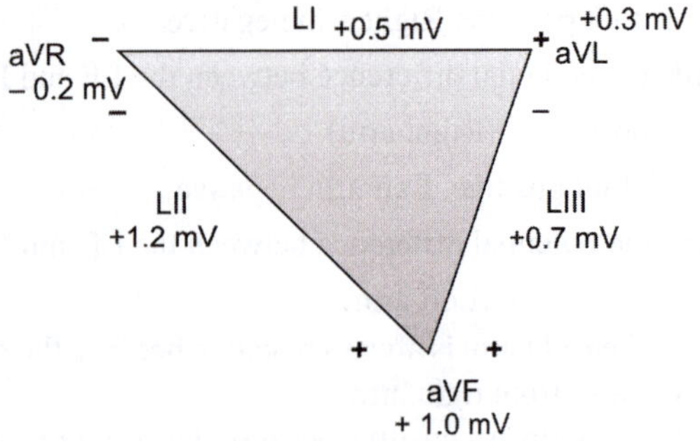

Fig. Q-13: Einthoven triangle

It is an imaginary triangle drawn around the heart by connecting the two arms and left leg.

The two apices at the upper part of the triangle indicates the points at which left arm and right arm connect electrically with the fluids around the heart, and lower apex is the point at which the left leg connects with the fluids.

Right arm = –0.2 mV negative with respect to the average potential of the body

Left arm = 0.3 mV positive

Left leg = 1.0 mV positive

Lead 1 records positive potential of 0.5 mV

LI = LA–RA

+ 0.3 mV –0.2 mV = 0.5 mV

–(–0.2) 0.3 mV +0.2 = 0.5 mV

Lead II records positive potential of 1.2 mV

LII = LF–RA

+1.0 mV – (–0.2 mV)

+1.0 mV +0.2 mV = 1.2 mV

Lead III records positive potential of 0.7 mV

LIII = LF–LA

+1.0 mV – (+0.3 mV) = 0.7 mV

It is noted, that the sum of the voltages in LI and LIII equals the voltage in LII

LI + LIII = LII

+0.5 mV +0.7 mV = 1.2 mV

(Mathematically, the principle called EINTHOVEN'S LAW holds good at any given instant while the electrocardiogram is recorded).

It is deduced as follows:

Lead I = LA – RA

Lead II = LF – RA

Lead III = LF – LA

Hence,

LI + LIII = (**LA** – RA + LF – **LA)**

= LF – RA

= LII

Unipolar Limb Leads

The bipolar limb leads record the potential difference between the two leads but it does not measure the actual current at the particular point. It was Wilson in 1934, invented unipolar limb leads. He measured the absolute electrical force at the site of positive electrode.

In unipolar limb leads, one electrode, called the exploring electrode is placed in close proximity to the heart while the other indifferent electrode is placed away from it so that its potential is more or less zero. The indifferent or neutral electrode is formed by connecting the three limbs; right arm (VR), left arm (VL), and left foot (VF). The unipolar leads are designated by the letter 'V'(V for voltage).

There are two types of unipolar leads—unipolar limb leads and unipolar chest leads.

These are augmented voltage limb leads.

LI, LII, LIII give the difference of current in that lead but not the actual current.

According to Einthovan triangle, the summation of VL + VR + VF = 0. It was not put to any use by Einthoven.

All the limb leads are connected at one pole and the other side is connected with one lead, either RA, LA or LF.

It was Wilson, who used them to record complexes that represented activity at a particular point.

In **VL**—Left arm is at one side to the positive pole and VL, VR, VF which is zero is, on the other side, to the negative pole.

This gives the actual amount of current at left arm.

In the same way

In **VR**—Right arm is at one side, connected to the positive pole and VL + VR + VF which is zero is on the other side, connected to the negative pole. This gives the amount of current at right arm.

In **VF**—Left foot is at one side connected to the positive pole and VL + VR + VF which is zero is on the other side, connected to the negative pole. This gives the amount of current at left foot.

The voltage at left arm, right arm and left foot are measured in this way. The complexes recorded by these leads were small.

VR, VL, VF unipolar leads, chest leads 'V' and esophageal leads are introduced by Wilson in 1934.

Further improvement was made by Goldberger to increase the actual voltage, that is at the right arm, left arm, left foot. It is called augmented voltage—so named as aVR, aVL and aVF.

Goldberger changed the connection of central terminal of Wilson. If aVL is being taken, aVL's negative wire is automatically disconnected by the ECG machine from the central terminal. This augments the voltage by a factor of 1.5.

What are aVR, aVL and aVF?

It is 1 1/2 times the actual current at that particular lead.

Augmented voltage at right arm is called aVR: It reflects the potential variation of atrial and ventricular cavities.

Augmented voltage at left arm is called aVL: It reflects the electrical potential from left lateral cardiac wall.

Augmented voltage at left foot is called aVF: It reflects the potential of the diaphragmatic or inferior surface of the heart.

VR—for VR, positive terminal is connected to right arm on one side and all other on other side to the negative pole, i.e. VR, VL, VF = 0.

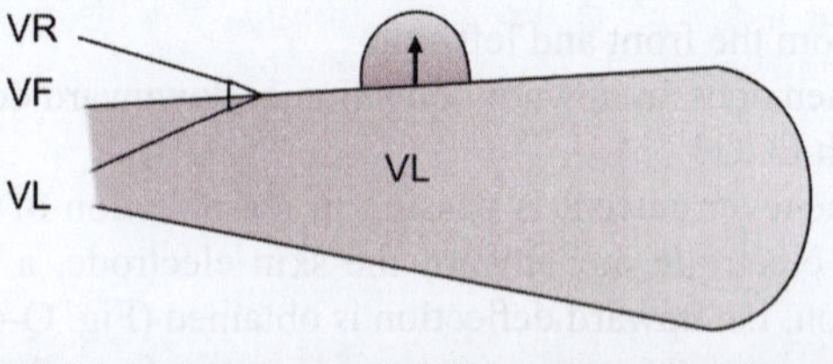

Fig. Q-14: Unipolar lead of Wilson: Positive VL terminal connected to the left arm and negative terminal to both arms and left foot

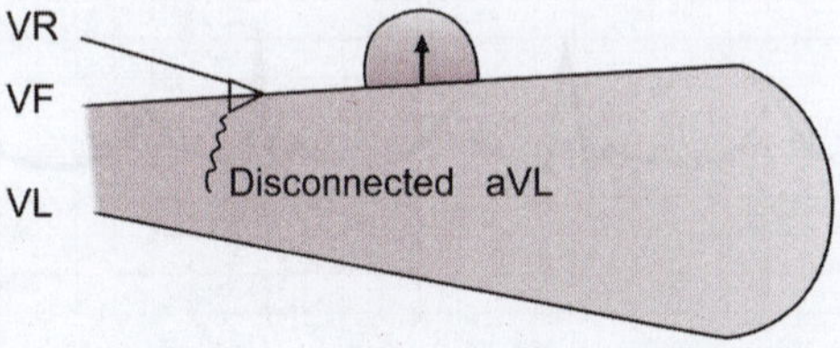

Fig. Q-15: Augmented unipolar lead of Goldberger: Positive terminal connected to the left arm and negative terminal connected to the right arm and the left foot

In augmented leads

aVL is connected at one end to the positive terminal and VR, VF are connected at the other negative pole end, disconnecting the VL

----| aVL ---- VR + VF |--------- negative

positive omitted VL

VR + VF gives the difference of LII.

----| aVR ---- VL + VF |---------- negative

positive omitted VR

VR + VF + VL = 0

VL + VF gives the difference of lead III.

---| aVF ---- VR + VL |---------- negative

positive omitted VF

VR + VL gives the difference of LI.

By connecting this way, the actual voltage at the limb is increased to 1½ times—so, it is named as augmented voltage at that particular limb—aVR, aVL, aVF.

SUMMARY

Wilson's VL = VL – [(VR + VLVF)/3] (whenever more than one lead is connected through the same terminal, the output is the average of the individual potentials)

Goldberger's aVL = VL – [(VR + VF)/2]

But, VL + VR + VF = 0 (indifferent or neutral electrode)

Therefore, VR + VF = – VL

And hence, aVL = VL – [(–VL)/2]

= VL + (VL/2)

= 1½ (VL)

Information obtained from these unipolar limb leads is basically same as (standard) bipolar leads. The six limb leads provide a round the clock view of cardiac electrical activity in the frontal plane of the body.

UNIPOLAR CHEST LEADS OR PRECORDIAL LEADS

6. The proximity of the heart to anterior chest wall is taken as basis to result in precordial leads. The six unipolar chest leads are selected in such a way that a direct lead is primarily influenced by the tissue immediately under the electrode. Normally, six standard chest leads (V1 – V6) are recorded in practice by positioning the chest electrode as follows. V7, V8 leads are recorded occasionally.

V1: 4th intercostal space of right sternal border
V2: 4th intercostal space of left sternal border
V3: Midway between V2 and V4
V4: 5th intercostal space in midclavicular line
V5: 5th intercostal space in anterior axillary line
V6: Midaxillary line at level of V4
V7: Posterior axillary line
V8: Posterior scapular line.

These positions are fixed irrespective of the condition or build and approximately represent the areas over the RV, IVS, and LV, respectively. Hence, V1, V2, record the electrical activity of the right ventricle, V3, V4 of the interventricular septum, and V5,V6 of the left ventricle. V7, V8 also represent the left ventricle but they are not used routinely.

7. Additional leads sometimes recorded are 4 types.

1. V3R, V4R: Position on right side corresponding to V3, V4.
2. V3(4), V4(4): V3 and V4 in higher interspace (4th).
3. Ve: Inferior border of sternum slightly to the left of ensiform process.
4. VSc: Below the inner end of the left clavicle.

The positive terminal connects the chest terminal, and the negative electrode called the indifferent or neutral electrode connects the left arm, right arm, and left leg simultaneously. Since the heart surfaces are close to the chest wall, each precordial lead mainly records the electrical potential of the cardiac tissue immediately below the electrode.

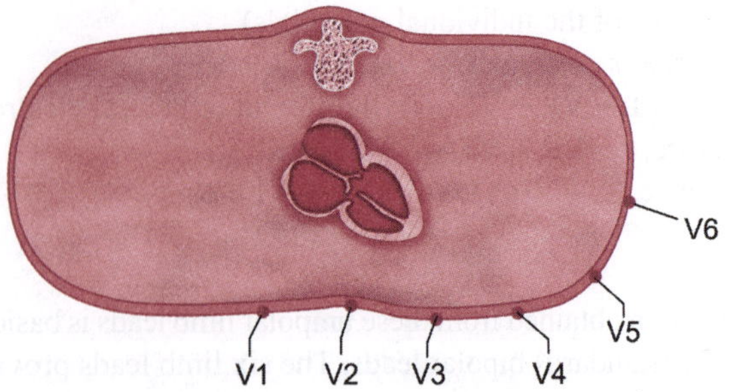

Fig. Q-16: The six unipolar chest leads look at the heart in a horizontal plane from the front and the left side

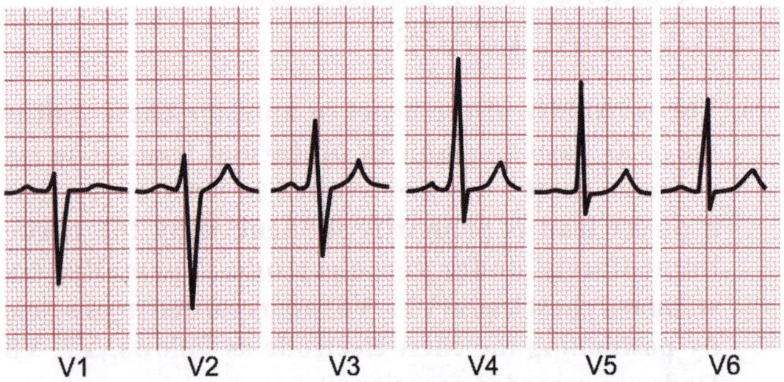

Fig. Q-17: Normal ECG recorded from six chest leads

The V_1 and V_2 are nearer the base of the heart than the apex. During the ventricular depolarization, the electrical current passes away from the V1 and V2, which results in negative deflection. V5 and V6 are mainly positive because the chest electrodes are near the apex, which is the direction of electropositivity during ventricular depolarization.

V3 and V4 represent transition between right and left sided patterns.

These six positions (V1 to V6) are selected to give round the clock view of the horizontal plane of the heart.

The mark on the knob of ECG machine select the lead, which makes the appropriate connection internally.

An electrode is also connected to the right leg to avoid interference from other (noncardiac) body currents. In addition to these connections, the ECG machine is earthed to avoid interference from its surroundings.

8. Thus the leads that are usually recorded can be analyzed as follows.

3 Bipolar limb leads
3 Unipolar limb leads
6 Unipolar chest leads
12 Total

For the purpose of analysis these fall into three groups.

Left sided leads: LI, aVL, V5 and V6

Right sided leads: aVR, V1 and V2

Inferior or diaphragmatic leads LII, LIII, aVF

Interpretation of ECG is easy if the directions from which the various leads 'look at' the heart is remembered. The six limb leads are said to be looking at the heart in a vertical plane, i.e. from the sides of the heart.

Thus leads LI and aVL look at the left lateral surface of the heart, LII, LIII and aVF at the inferior surface and aVR look at the right atrium.

The six precordial leads look at the heart in a horizontal plane from the front and left side.

When does an upward deflection or downward deflection occur on ECG?

Whenever current is passing in the direction of positive surface electrode, i.e. toward the skin electrode, a positive deflection, i.e. upward deflection is obtained (Fig. Q-4).

Whenever the current is passing away from the surface electrode a negative deflection, i.e. downward deflection is obtained.

The deflections in the limb leads are seen in the following way.

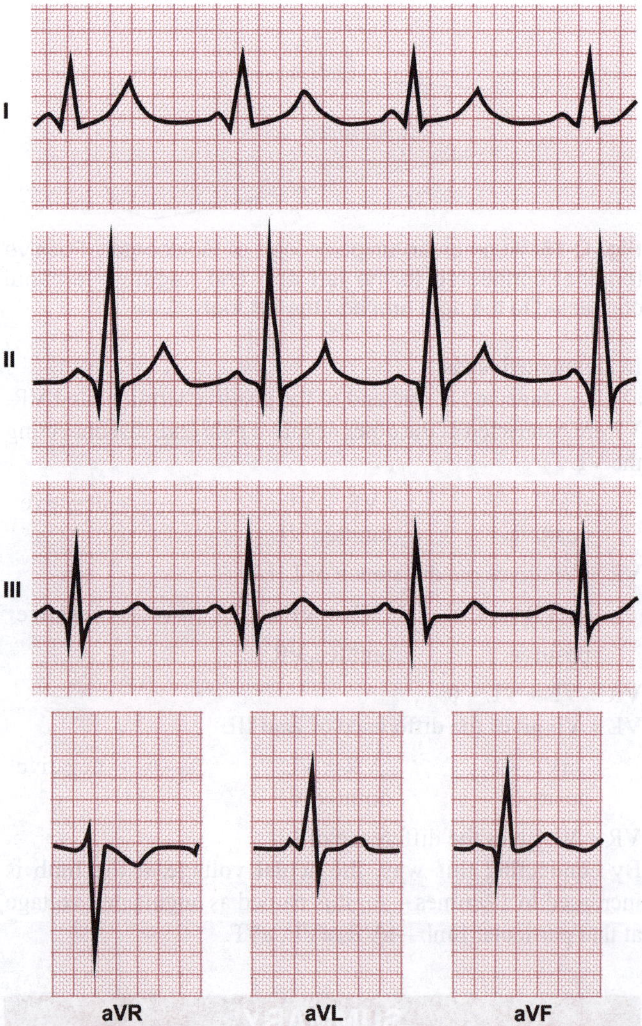

Fig. Q-18: Normal electrocardiograms recorded from the three standard limb leads and three augmented unipolar limb leads

In LI, i.e. left arm positive, right arm negative. In recording LI, the positive terminal of the electrocardiograph is connected to the left arm and the negative terminal is connected to right arm. The current is passing from SA node to AV node side. The current is passing in the direction from right arm to left arm side which is positive, i.e. from negative to positive side.

This results in positive wave.

Therefore, QRS is positive in LI.

In LII, i.e. right arm negative, left foot positive. In recording LII, the negative terminal of the electrocardiograph is connected to the right arm and positive terminal is connected to the left foot. The current is passing from right arm to left foot, i.e. from negative to positive side.

This results in positive deflection.

In LIII, left foot positive, left arm negative: In recording LIII, positive terminal of the electrocardiograph is connected to the left foot and negative terminal to the left arm. Current is passing more toward positive left foot side than left arm.

This results in positive upward deflection.

In aVR, the positive electrode is on right arm. The current is passing from right arm to left foot side, i.e. away from right arm.

This results in negative deflection.

Therefore, QRS is downward in aVR

In aVL, the positive electrode is on left arm. The current is passing from right arm to left arm side, i.e. toward positive side.

This results in positive upward deflection.

In aVF, the positive electrode is on left foot side. The current is passing from right arm to left foot side only, i.e. toward positive pole.

This results in positive upward deflection.

Thus, it can be concluded—in normal ECG there is positive, i.e. upward deflection in LI, LII, LIII, aVL and aVF, and downward deflection in aVR only.

To remember it easily, a pointer is kept in the direction of SA node to AV node, bundle of His, apex, i.e. from base to the apex, i.e. from right arm to the left foot side to get the answer in an easy way (see Fig. Q-7).

Always it is to be remembered that the direction of current flow in the heart is from SA node toward the apex, i.e. from right arm to left foot side.

Einthoven has measured the difference in the current from one pole to another. He connected the electrode of left arm, right arm, as lead I.

Lead I—Left arm and right arm

= VL (Left arm) – VR (Right arm)

Lead II—Right arm and left foot

= VF (Left foot) – VR (Right arm)

Lead III—Left foot and left arm.

= VF (Left foot) – VL (Left arm)

Lead I—He found the difference of current of left arm – right arm. Positive left arm from negative right arm.

Lead II—Positive left foot from negative right arm

Lead III—Positive left foot from negative left arm

Heart is the center of an electrical field that generates. The field diminishes rapidly with distance from its center. However, once the distance is > 12 cm the decrement is insignificant. Therefore, all electrodes placed more than 12 cm from the heart can be considered to be equidistant from the heart even if physically they are not.

An electrode placed over 12 cm distance from the heart is said to be at electrical infinity.

If an electrode is placed closer to the heart, less than 12 cm, the amplitude of the deflections will be influenced by the proximity to the heart. Thus, the closer the electrode to the heart, the greater the amplitude. This tells us that the deflections of precordial leads, which are placed on the chest wall are affected by their proximity to the electrical center of the heart. If, on the other hand, an electrode is placed farther than 12 cm from the electrical center of the heart, no matter how much farther it is placed, the amplitude of the deflection of that lead will not change significantly. This infers that the deflection in limb leads are not affected significantly by their distance from the heart.

This concept of electrical infinity from the heart help us to decide whether or not electrodes can be placed on a shoulder or amputated limb. There would be no difference whether an extremity electrode is placed on shoulder or wrist, thigh or ankle because that all are at infinity from the heart. For example, for an above knee amputated patient, the electrode is placed over the thigh. For practical convenience, the electrodes are placed over the wrists and ankles.

COMPLEXES, INTERVALS AND SEGMENTS

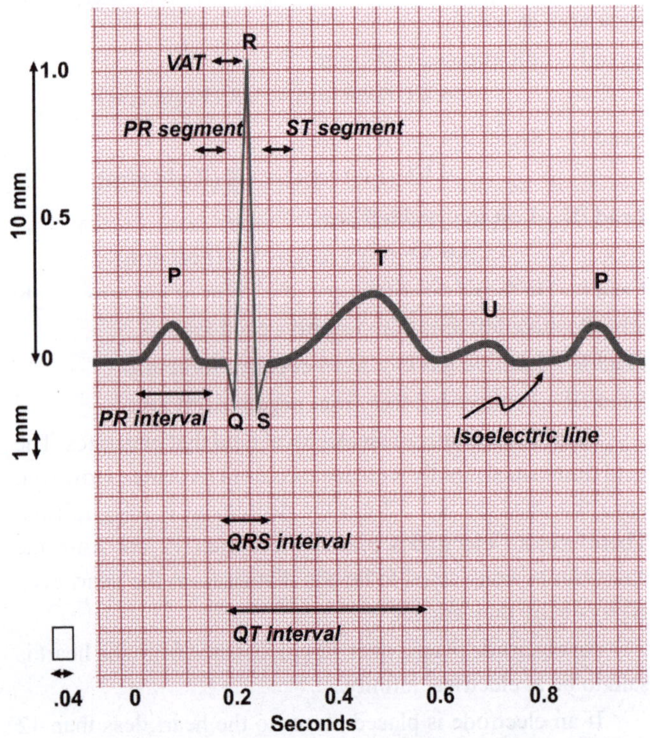

Fig. Q-19: Diagram of normal electrocardiographic complexes, intervals and segments

9. A normal ECG pattern shows 4 waves.

1. *P wave:* It represents atrial depolarization. It is usually an upright small rounded deflection.
2. *QRS complex:* It represents ventricular depolarization. Q wave is an initial negative area of the QRS. It is not the initial downward or negative deflection, since a wave cannot be made merely by one direction.

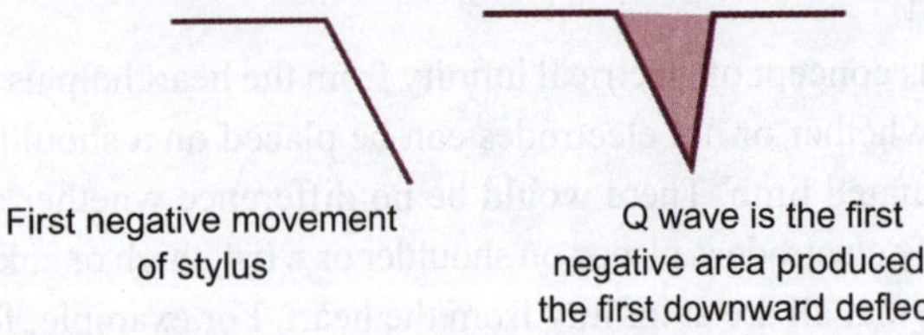

Fig. Q-20

A negative area can be produced only by a downward movement + a movement back to the baseline, i.e. isoelectric line.

R wave is a second upward deflection after a Q wave and S wave is a second downward deflection after R.

R wave is the second upward deflection produced by ventricular depolarization. R wave may or may not be preceded by Q wave

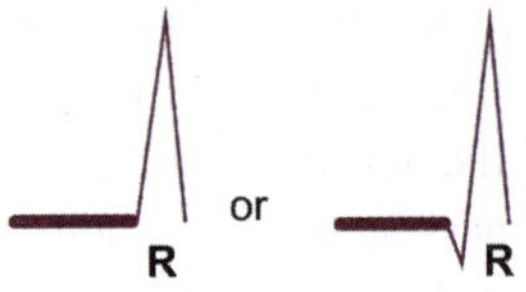

Fig. Q-21

S wave is the second downward deflection (negative) following R wave during depolarization of the ventricles.

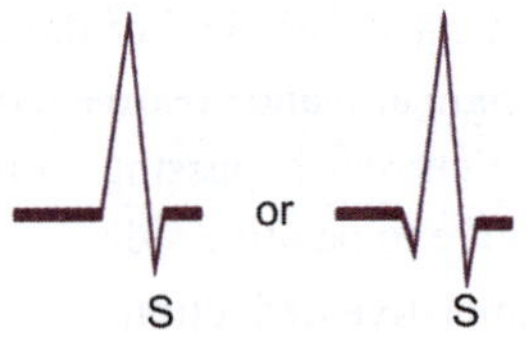

Fig. Q-22

When there is a upward deflection (positive) following the S wave, still during the depolarization of the ventricles is called R prime written as R'

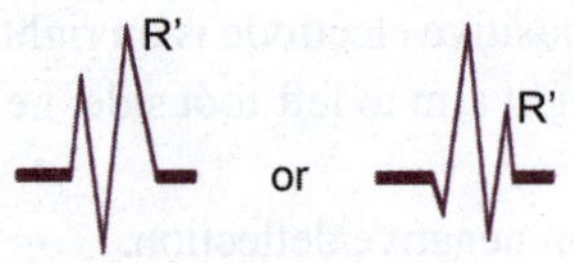

Fig. Q-23

When there is a downward deflection after an R', it is called S prime written as S'

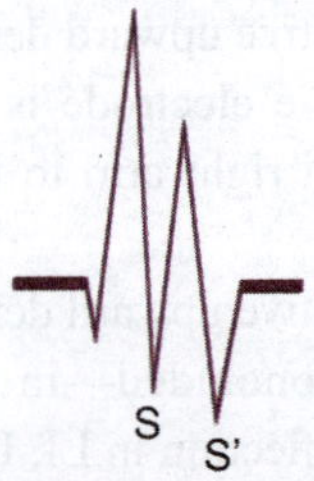

Fig. Q-24

A deep notch on R wave differ from S wave by not going below the baseline

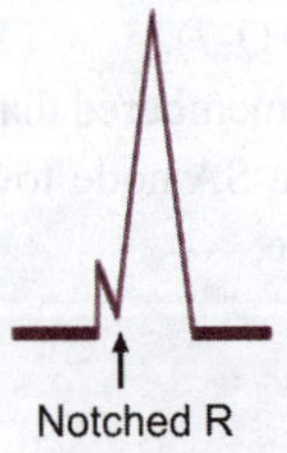

Fig. Q-25

A completely negative depolarization of ventricular complex is called QS.

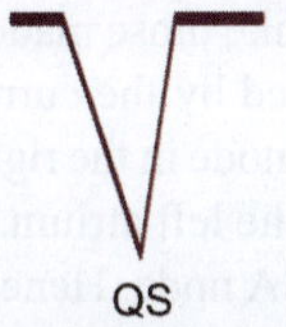

Fig. Q-26: No R wave

3. *T wave:* It represents ventricular repolarization in the same direction of QRS complex. T wave is the relatively long wave that follows a QRS. The T wave may be low, high, negative, positive or biphasic.

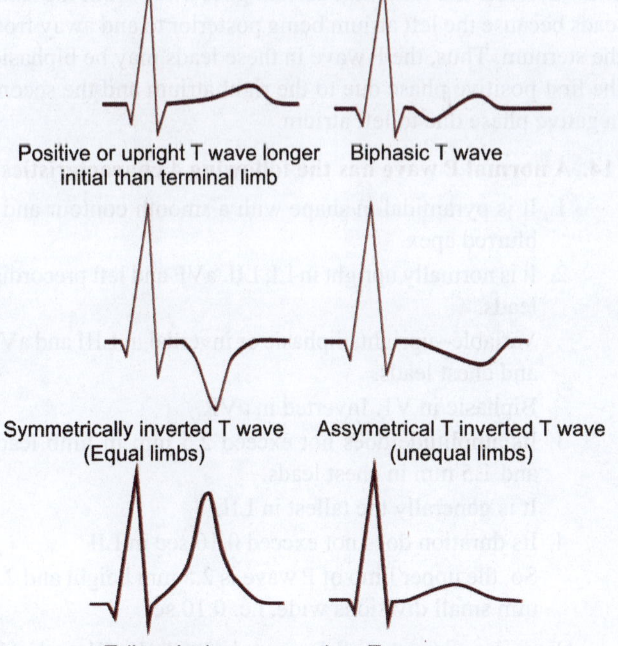

Fig. Q-27

Upward or positive T wave with longer initial than terminal limb
Biphasic T wave
Symmetrically inverted T wave (Negative or inverted T wave with equal limbs)
Asymmetrical T inversion (T inversion with unequal limbs)
Tall peaked T wave
Low T wave
Tall peaked T and low T are possible normal variant but may also be abnormal.

4. *U wave—following T wave:* It is not uniformly present, not clear. This may be due to late ventricular repolarization. It may represent papillary muscle repolarization.

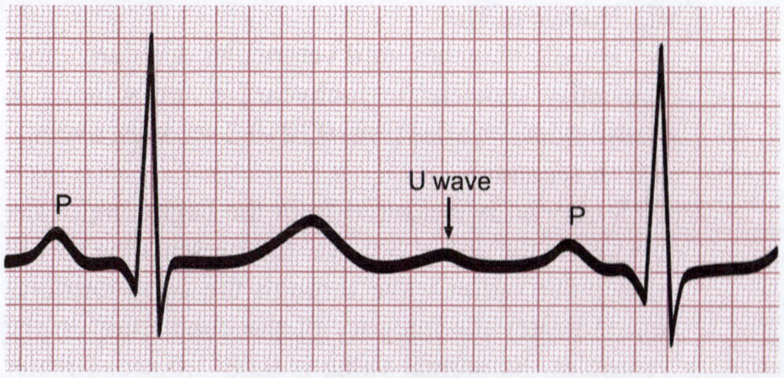

Fig. Q-28

Isoelectric line: It is the baseline or isoelectric level or the zero position of the record in normal person.
All upward deflections above the isoelectric line are called positive and all downward deflections are called negative.
A Q or S wave is always negative and an R wave is always positive.
A Q wave must always be in front of R and S wave always follows R wave.

10. The 4 normal time intervals:

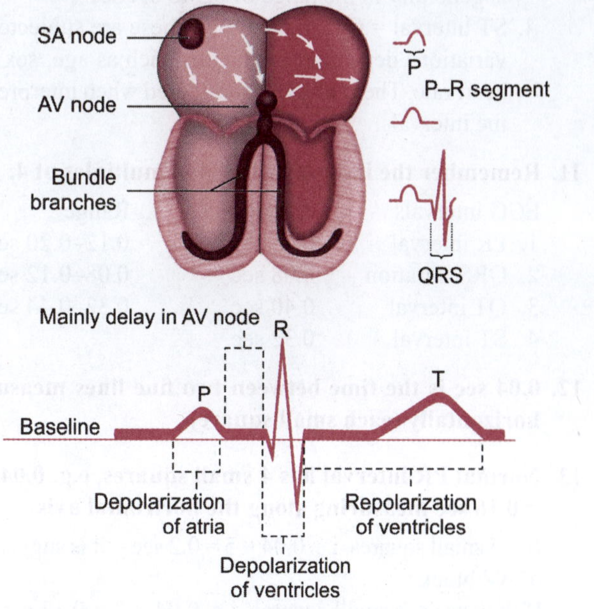

Fig. Q-29: The whole electrocardiogram can be summarized as shown in the diagram

1. PR interval is measured from the beginning of the P wave to the beginning of QRS complex.
   It represents atrioventricular conduction time of the impulse to travel across the:
   i. Atria
   ii. AV node

iii. Bundle of His

iv. Bundle branches until ventricular depolarization.

It usually shortens in tachycardia and widens in bradycardia. It varies from 0.12–0.2 seconds, average is 0.16 seconds.

2. QRS interval is measured from the beginning of the Q wave to the end of S wave. It represents the spread of depolarization wave through the two ventricles and indicates the integrity of the conduction in the ventricles. Its normal value is 0.08–1.0 sec. Greater than 0.12 second indicates intraventricular conduction disorder. It should be measured in the lead showing the longest interval.
3. QT interval is measured from the beginning of the Q wave to the end of the T wave. It represents the total electrical activity of the ventricles—depolarization and repolarization. It is markedly affected by the heart rate. It shortens in tachycardia and widens in bradycardia. The formula for corrected QT interval:
   QTc is by dividing the QT interval by the square root of the preceding RR interval
   (Normal 0.44 sec) QTc = QT √RR
   With a normal heart rate of 60–100 min. QT interval is generally in the range of 0.3 to 0.4 sec.
4. ST interval = QT minus QRS. These are subjected to variations depending on factors such as age, sex and heart rate. These must be considered when interpreting the intervals.

11. Remember the interval timings in multiples of 4.

ECG intervals	Average	Range
1. PR interval	0.16 sec	0.12–0.20 sec
2. QRS duration	0.08 sec	0.08–0.12 sec
3. QT interval	0.40 sec	0.32–0.44 sec
4. ST interval	0.32 sec	

12. 0.04 sec is the time between two fine lines measured horizontally (each small square).

13. Normal PR interval has 4 small squares, e.g. 0.04 × 4 = 0.16 sec measuring along the horizontal axis.

If > 5 small squares, i.e. 0.04 × 5 = 0.2 sec—it is suggestive of AV block.

If they are < 3 small squares, i.e. 0.04 × 3 = 0.12 sec—It is suggestive of abnormal pathway.

Normal variation: PR interval of more than 0.22 sec is seen in athletes and vagotonic individuals.

P WAVE

It represents atrial depolarization. The usual concept is that depolarization spreads from SA node toward AV node readily in concentric wave forms like those made by a pebble thrown into a pond. P wave is formed by the current traveling in the atria from SA node to the AV node in the right atrium and through the Bachmann's bundle to the left atrium. It is directed downward and leftward from the SA node. Hence, the current goes away from lead aVR and towards lead aVL and aVF. Therefore, P wave is negative in aVR and positive in aVL and aVF. The precordial leads, being over the ventricles, are at a lower level than the atria and current of P wave comes toward them from above. Therefore, P wave is positive in all chest leads. There is a special situation in V1 and V2 in relation to the P wave. The right atrial current comes from above downward toward V1 and V2, while the left atrial current goes away from the same leads because the left atrium being posterior to and away from the sternum. Thus, the P wave in these leads may be biphasic, the first positive phase due to the right atrium and the second negative phase due to left atrium.

14. A normal P wave has the following 4 characteristics.

1. It is pyramidal in shape with a smooth contour and a blurred apex.
2. It is normally upright in LI, LII, aVF and left precordial leads.
   Variable--upright, diphasic or inverted in LIII and aVL and chest leads.
   Biphasic in V1. Inverted in aVR.
3. Its amplitude does not exceed 2.5 mm in limb leads and 1.5 mm in chest leads.
   It is generally the tallest in LII.
4. Its duration does not exceed 0.10 sec in LII
   So, the upper limb of P wave is 2.5 mm height and 2.5 mm small divisions wide, i.e. 0.10 sec.

Normal variation: Tall P wave in leads II, III and aVF (Pseudo P pulmonale) may be seen in normal individuals with tall, asthenic built with low placed diaphragm and vertical heart, especially during tachycardia.

15. Abnormalities of P wave that should be looked for are:

1. *Inversion* in leads where P wave is normally upright. These changes are usually seen in conditions where the impulses through the atria pass in an abnormal way as in atrial ectopic or AV nodal rhythm.
2. *Upright* P wave in aVR is always abnormal.
3. *Increased amplitude:* Usually indicates hypertrophy or dilatation of atria.
4. *Increased width (duration):* Usually indicates left atrial enlargement.
5. *Diphasicity:* It is a important sign of left atrial enlargement where the second half of the P wave is significantly negative in LIII or V1.

6. *Notching*: P wave is widely notched and is taller in LI than in LIII. 'P mitrale'. Notching is considered significant when the distance between peaks exceeds 0.04 sec (Fig. Q-61B).
   It was first called P 'Mitrale' by Winternitz in 1935. Notched P waves can also result from an intra-atrial conduction defect between the right and left atrium and also from conditions other than mitral disease that cause left atrial overload. Although, it is commonly used as specific for mitral disease, the wide, notched P wave is not. A widely notched P wave is best called as intra-atrial block. If the left atrium is enlarged, the terminal part is late in depolarization and so the P wave widens. Widely notched P waves that are usually seen in diabetic patients with a normal sized left atrium and therefore represents intra-atrial block that is probably due to coronary artery disease.
7. *Peaking* is seen in right atrial strain. Tall pointed P waves are seen in LIII than in LI – 'P pulmonale' (Fig. Q-61A).
8. *Absence* of P waves.

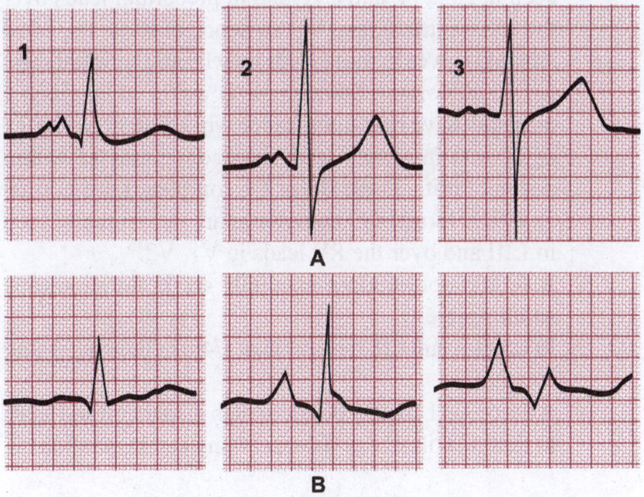

Fig. Q-30: A: P mitrale - Note wide, notched P waves taller in LI than in LIII; B. P-pulmonale : Note tall pointed P waves in LII and LIII and flat P in LI

16. Recognition of normal and abnormal P waves form the basis for diagnosing the arrhythmias.

Any P inversion in LI, LII or aVF indicates that it has its origin other than the SA node. Thus, the change in the morphology of P wave points toward a change in the sight of impulse formation.

P is upright in LI, LII, aVF and V6.

Biphasic in VI

Morphology of **P** waves are changed in—

Inverted P waves

1. Mirror image dextrocardia: P is inverted in LI along with other complexes.
2. Atrial premature beats
3. Nodal tachycardia
4. Junctional rhythm
5. Non-sinus (coronary sinus) rhythm
6. Wrongly attached limb leads

Changing shape

7. Wandering pacemaker
8. Atrial ectopics.

17. P wave amplitude and duration is changed in the following 4 conditions. See in LII or VI for P wave.

1. 'P pulmonale'—or 'P congenital'—in RAH
   Tall peaked P more than 2.5 mm height. (Fig. Q-30B and 61A)
2. 'P mitrale' in LAH
   P is notched. M' shaped (Fig. Q-30A and 61B) more than 2.5 mm wide.
3. Bifid P wave—
   P is taller and wider—more than 2.5 mm height and width—in biatrial hypertrophy
4. In hyper- or hypokalemia
   P is flattened in hyperkalemia.

18. P wave amplitude and duration increased in

1. Left atrial hypertrophy, e.g. mitral stenosis. The only common condition in which left atrium overload occurs without left ventricular overload is mitral stenosis. (The only common condition of the left ventricular volume overload that is not necessarily be associated with left atrial overload is aortic regurgitation).
2. Right atrial hypertrophy, e.g. pulmonary stenosis.
3. Cor pulmonale.
4. Congenital heart disease—giant P wave in Ebstein anomaly.

(See Fig. L-21)

19. The 4 conditions where the P waves are partially or wholly buried in QRS and T waves.

1. AV block
2. Paroxysmal atrial tachycardia (PAT)
3. Supraventricular extrasystoles
4. Hyperkalemia.

20. Causes of small P wave:

1. Atrial tachycardia
2. Atrial ectopic
3. Nodal rhythm (high nodal)
4. Nodal ectopic (high node).

21. Causes of inverted P wave:

1. Dextrocardia
2. Incorrectly placed leads (reversed arm electrodes—technical dextrocardia)
3. Nodal rhythm with retrograde conduction
4. Low atrial and high nodal ectopic beats.

22. The conditions where the P waves are absent.

1. Atrial flutter—replaced by flutter waves
2. Atrial fibrillation—replaced by fibrillary waves
3. SA block or sinus arrest
4. AV nodal rhythm (junctional rhythm)
5. Supraventricular tachycardia (P is hidden in QRS due to tachycardia)
6. Ventricular ectopic or ventricular tachycardia
7. Hyperkalemia
8. Idioventricular rhythm.

23. Rate and regularity of the P wave.

Irregularity of the sinus P wave rate is seen in sinus node diseases such as:

1. Sinus pauses
2. SA blocks
3. Extreme sinus bradycardia
4. Intermittent escape beats.

24. P and QRS relationship.

1. Each P is followed by QRS
2. Each QRS is preceded by P wave
3. PR interval is 0.12 to 0.2 sec.
   Prolongation of PR interval indicates AV conduction delay.
4. Absence of any relationship of P and QRS is diagnosed as AV dissociation.

Tp wave: It is formerly called Ta wave. It represents repolarization of atria. It is invisible, because atrial repolarization occurs during QRS complex, that is, ventricular depolarization. It can be best seen in complete AV block where P waves are not followed by QRS and are independent. Hence, there is a chance for the Tp wave to show itself.

Q WAVE

Small Q waves in the left ventricular leads results from depolarization of the septum from left to right—septal Q waves.

25. The significance of Q wave is one of the most important and sometimes most difficult to read. Q waves must be viewed in the light of the overall picture and must take into account of their:

1. depth < 2 mm (2 small squares)
2. width—1 small squares
3. leads in which they appear
   and the most important is the
4. clinical correlation.

26. A normal Q wave has the following 4 characteristics.

1. A small narrow Q wave of 1 to 2 mm deep is normally seen in LI, aVL and aVF and in precordial leads over the left ventricle, e.g. V5. Absence of these expected small Q waves in these leads may be an abnormal sign. Size is important. Sometimes, Q waves of less than 1 mm may have real significance while thin qS complex of 10 mm in certain leads may sometimes be within normal limits. Deep QS or Qr complexes are normal in aVR. Normal QS complexes are occasionally seen in LIII and over the RV leads in V1, V2.
2. It should not be more than 0.04 sec in duration (one small square).
3. In lead LI, and LII, it is less than 1/4th of the succeeding R wave.
4. A deep Q in LIII may be due to high diaphragm and tends to diminish in size or disappear on deep inspiration.

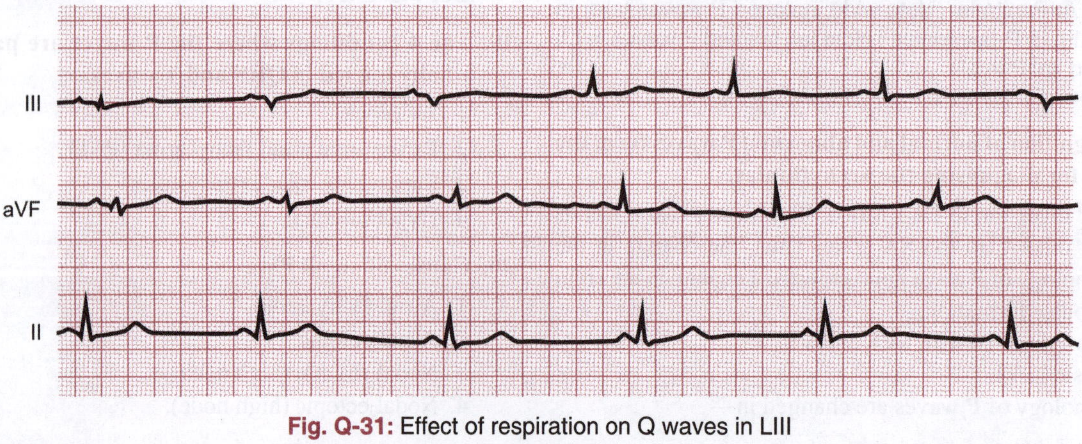

Fig. Q-31: Effect of respiration on Q waves in LIII

Old inferior infarction are often difficult to diagnose. Q waves in inferior leads should be viewed with suspicion particularly of lead III. Deep inspiration will often abolish them in LIII, indicating their benign character. In the Figure Q-31, the subject has taken a deep inspiration after the third complex

27. Q waves are pathological:

If they are more than 2 mm deep or more than 0.04 sec wide.

Of slightly less significance is its depth, 1/4th or more of the R wave in the same complex provided the R wave itself exceeds 5 mm.

Pathological Q waves are present in:

1. Myocardial infarction
   For example,
   i. Anterior septal—V1, V2, V3, V4
   ii. Anterolateral—aVL, V5, V6
   iii. Lateral infarction—LI, aVL
   iv. Inferior infarction—LII, LIII, aVF
   The relative or absolute depth of Q wave in LIII has no relationship to infarction. It usually indicates the presence of LVH. A deep Q in L III suggests LVH rather than infarction. The Q wave must be wide, i.e. at least 0.4 sec (40 msec) before it is considered to be due to infarction.
2. Hypertrophy
   LVH—V5, V6
   RVH—V1, V2
   Deep broad Qs in LI, aVL,V5,V6 in hypertrophic cardiomyopathy are not due to old MI but abnormal depolarization of asymmetrical septal hypertrophy.
3. In LBBB, Q waves appear in V1, V2 but Q in V5, V6 signifies myocardial infarction.
4. Pulmonary infarction
   Wide S in LI, Large Q in LIII
   Abnormal Q wave may be found in pulmonary embolism.
   Abnormal Q in LIII and AVF may be found in WPW syndrome (confuses with old inferior MI).

R WAVE

28. Tall R wave in V1 and V2 can occur in

1. Occasionally as a normal variant
2. Right ventricular hypertrophy
3. True posterior myocardial infarction
4. Sometimes lateral myocardial infarction.
5. Wolff-Parkinson-White syndrome (WPW syndrome)
6. Diastolic overloading of left ventricle
7. RBBB
8. Dextrocardia.

29. Poor progression of R wave—The amplitude of R wave is progressively reduced in V5 and V6.

Causes are:

1. Normal variant
2. Deformity of the chest wall
3. Left sided pneumothorax
4. Left sided plural effusion (massive)
5. Anterior and antroseptal MI
6. LBBB
7. Marked clockwise rotation
8. Incorrectly placed chest leads.

QRS COMPLEX

It is the most important complex in ECG. It represents depolarization of the two ventricles.

As mentioned earlier, the Q wave is produced by activation of the interventricular septum, by the septal branches of the left bundle branch at its origin (Fig. Q-3). Thus the current flows the septum from left to right direction. Hence, a negative Q wave is present in left sided leads V4 to V6 because the current is going away from left to right and not in V1,V2. Positive R wave in V1,V2 represents the right ventricular activity and the negative S wave denotes left ventricular activity. It is written as rS as the R wave is smaller than the S wave as the right ventricle being less muscular than the left. Similarly, R wave in V5, V6 represent the left ventricular activity and is larger than the S wave that represents right ventricular activity. Hence, it is written as qRs. This results in study progression from rS pattern to an Rs pattern from V1 to V6 and that there is a zone of transition where R and S are almost equal in magnitude in V3 or V 4.

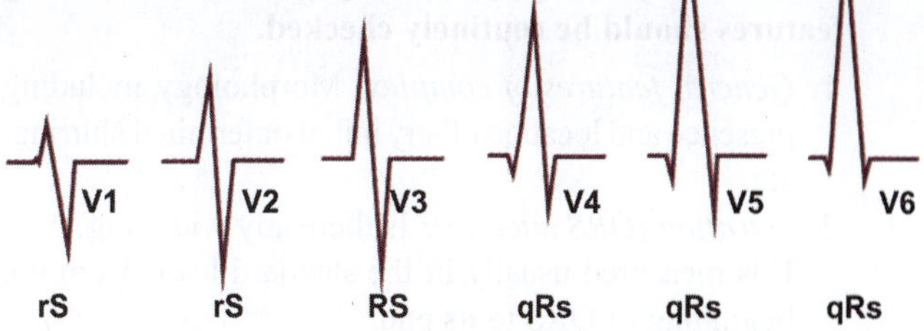

Fig. Q-32: Normal progression of QRS pattern in the chest leads

30. Different parts of the QRS complex are arbitrarily labeled in the following way:

1. If the first deflection is downward it is called as Q wave.
2. A deflection upwards is called as R wave. It may be preceded by Q or not.

3. A deflection below the baseline following an R wave is called S wave.
4. Any deflection below the baseline following Q wave without R wave is called as QS wave.

If the first deflection is downward, it is called as Q wave

A deflection upward is called as R wave. It may be preceded by Q or not. Subsequent deflection above the line are labeled successively as R', R"

A deflection below the base line following an R is called S wave. Subsequent negative deflection below the baseline are labeled as S', S"

Any deflection below the baseline following Q wave without R wave is called as QS wave.

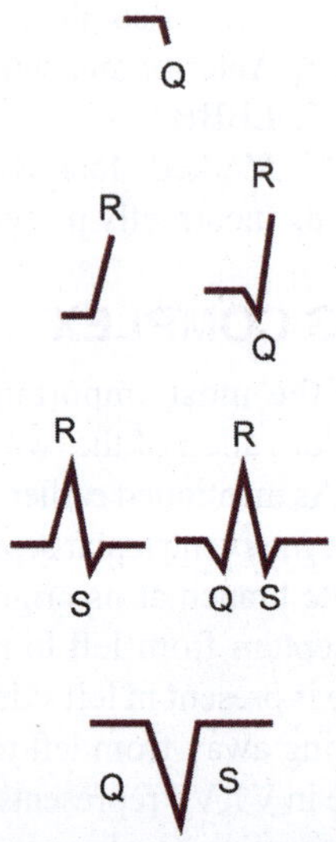

Fig. Q-33: Normal variation: Normal Q is seen in LII, LIII and aVF in obese individuals. Abnormal Q in LII, LIII and aVF with tall R wave is also seen in tall and asthetic individuals with vertical heart

A QS complex in V3R and V1, sometimes in V2 and very rarely in V3 may be seen in individuals with low lying diaphragm due to relatively higher chest electrode position. This can be rectified by recording precordial complexes one or two interspaces below.

31. While interpreting QRS complexes, the following features should be routinely checked.

1. *General features of complex:* Morphology including presence and location of any initial or terminal slurring, etc.
2. *Duration (QRS interval):* Is there any widening?
   It is measured usually in the standard leads from the beginning of QRS to its end.
   It is usually 0.05 to 0.10 sec. The precordial leads show a slightly longer QRS (0.10 or 0.12 sec) than the standard leads, the explanation for this is not clear.
   More than 0.12 sec indicates delayed conduction in the ventricle usually means a block of one of the bundle branches or a ventricular arrhythmia.
3. *Amplitude (or 'Voltage'):* Is there any variation?
   Accepted lower limits are 5 mm in standard leads and 10 mm in chest leads (total amplitude measured above and below the isoelectric line).
   Accepted upper limit in chest leads is 25–30 mV.
   Alternate large and small beats are seen in 'Pulsus alternans'.
4. Presence of Q waves (or equivalents).
5. Electrical axis in the frontal plane (limb leads).
6. *Transitional zone:* Relative prominence of the component waves in the precordial leads V1 to V6.
7. The timing of any intrinsicoid deflections in leads V1 and V6.
8. Presence of any R', R" or S', S" pattern.

QRS complex reflects depolarization of the two ventricles. A typical left ventricle lead complex is qRs. A typical right ventricle lead complex is rS.

32. A normal QRS has the following 4 characteristics.

1. The duration should not exceed 0.12 sec.
2. Total amplitude should be > 5 mm in standard leads. If the total amplitude above and below the isoelectric line is 5 mm or less in all three standard leads, it is abnormal (low voltage). Amplitude up to 20 or 30 mm are occasionally seen in LII in normal hearts. Maximum amplitude of 25 to 30 mm in precordial leads is accepted.
3. In lead V1, R wave is usually small and becomes progressively taller from V1 to V6. Failure of R wave progression to increase its amplitude while it moves across V1 to V6 is abnormal.
4. S wave has maximum amplitude in V1 and V2. It gradually decreases in size from V1 to V6. The intermediate or transition zone is seen at V3 to V4 where a combination of deflections obtained on either side of the precordium is present.

Normal variation: A tall R wave in V1 may be rarely seen in normal individuals in the absence of other signs of right ventricular hypertrophy or posterior myocardial infarction. In young thin individuals, left ventricular hypertrophy by voltage criteria may be observed despite abnormal heart. Poor R wave progression in precordial leads is seen in 38% of individuals.

QRS duration of between 0.10 sec and 0.12 sec is normal in athletes.

33. Ventricular depolarization—QRS complex duration and amplitude can be abnormal in:

1. Premature ventricular beats
2. Myocardial infarction
3. Initial depolarization
   For example, prolongation of initial depolarization in Wolff-Parkinson-White syndrome—delta wave with slurring of initial QRS.
4. Mid and late depolarization

For example, prolongation due to mid and late delay in LBBB.

5. Terminal depolarization

For example, prolongation due to terminal delay in RBBB.

Diffuse ---

6. Ventricular tachycardia
7. Minor uniform prolongation in left ventricular hypertrophy
8. Uniform prolongation in electrolyte abnormality, e.g. high serum potassium
9. Prolongation with total distortion in cardiomyopathy
10. Drugs/electrolytes—Digitalis, verapamil
11. Myocarditis, fibrositis
12. Pacemakers.

34. QRS complex changes can occur in local loss of muscle mass (MI) or in local conduction blocks as:

1. Prolongation of QRS
2. Bizarre pattern of QRS
3. Prominent Q waves
4. Decreased voltage.

35. There are 4 points to be checked in BBB where QRS is more than 0.12 sec.

RBBB	LBBB
1. R-R' in V1 or V2 (Right chest leads)	3. R-R' in V5 or V6 (Left chest leads)
2. Wide S in V5 or V6	4. Wide S in V1 or V2.

PR INTERVAL

PR interval results from AV delay.

This is measured from the beginning of the P wave to the beginning of the QRS complex (see Q-74).

Normal PR interval is 0.12 to 0.20 sec (3 to 5 small squares). It is customary to examine several intervals and mention the longest of all. If the conducting system is diseased or affected by digitalis, the PR may lengthen as the rate increases. PR interval is proportionately shorter in children and increased with age to normal. Sometimes, difficulty may arise when P is merging with QRS. In case of difficulty PR is calculated from top of P to the top of R instead of beginning of P to the beginning of QRS.

PR interval changes occur in the following conditions.

36. PR interval

1. In children—upper limit is 0.6 sec
2. In adolescents—upper limit is 0.18 sec
3. In adults—upper limit is 0.22 sec
4. PR is short if it is < 0.10 sec and long if it is > 0.22 sec.

37. Prolongation of PR interval occurs in

1. AV block: Due to coronary artery disease, rheumatic disease, etc. (1° block), IHD, occasionally inferior MI
2. Hyperthyroidism: In some cases
3. Digitalis, quinidine, occasionally beta-blockers, calcium blockers (verapamil)
4. Hypokalemia.

38. Shortening of PR interval occurs in:

1. AV nodal rhythm
2. AV dissociation
3. Wolff-Parkinson-White syndrome
4. Lown-Ganong-Levine syndrome
5. Type II glycogen storage disease (Pompe's)
6. Hypertrophic obstructive cardiomyopathy (HOCM)
7. Duchenne muscular dystrophy
8. Some hypertensive patients.

39. Variable PR interval occurs in

1. AV blocks—Mobitz type 1, where there is progressive lengthening of PR interval
2. Complete heart block
3. 2:1 AV block—Alternate P wave is not followed by QRS
4. Wandering pacemaker.

Normal variation of prolongation (upper limit) or shortening (lower limit) of PR interval can occur.

ST SEGMENT

It is the most important. ST segment is the gap between depolarization and repolarization.

ST segment follows immediately succeeding the QRS complex. It lies between the QRS complex and T wave. It is the part of the T wave between the end of the QRS and the point at which the slope of the T wave appears to become steeper abruptly.

It represents the middle part of the repolarization process of the ventricles.

The beginning of repolarization is inside the QRS.

ST segment is from the end of depolarization to the beginning of repolarization—no amplitude, no duration.

Normal ST segment is isoelectric—no depolarization or repolarization wave.

The ischemia or infarction can destroy the "Dielectric properties" of a cell membrane, so that potassium may flow out both during depolarization and repolarization. Sodium may continue to flow in during depolarization, i.e. ionic flow may be changed so that it can effect the baseline of ECG (Dielectric property of a membrane is the ability of the membrane to keep ions more on one side of membrane than on the other).

The T is sometime simply called as ST, T to show that the ST is really just an arbitrary division of the repolarization wave. In many leads, there is no obvious ST segment because there is no point at which the slope changes abruptly.

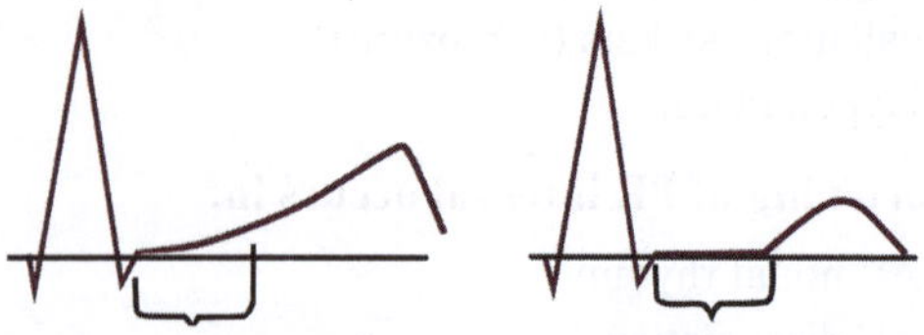

Fig. Q-34: Normal isoelectric ST segment

In shape, ST segment normally curves gently and imperceptibly into the proximal limb of T wave. It need not form a frankly horizontal course or sharp angle with the proximal limb of T wave.

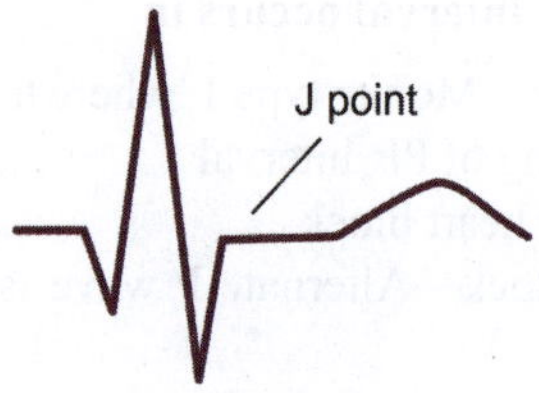

Fig. Q-35

The point at which it "takes off" from the QRS is called J or junctional point.

Its level in relation to baseline whether it is elevated above or depressed below the TP segment and its shape should be observed.

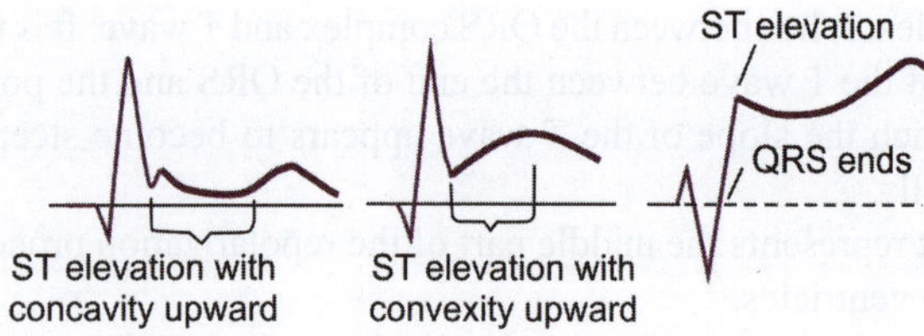

Fig. Q-36

ST elevation with convexity upward is a sign of myocardial infarction (See Fig. Q-135, 136).

The figure shows only ST elevation but not terminal R' because the QRS always finishes at or toward the baseline. An R' must have an area. It cannot be a deflection above the baseline. The ST segment begins at the baseline, and that is also, where the QRS ends when there is ST deviation.

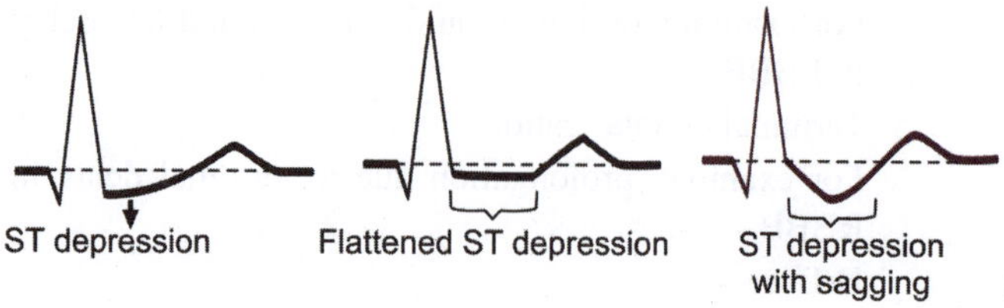

Fig. Q-37: Depression of ST segment

Horizontal depression of ST segment has been called "plane depression" which is highly suspicious of myocardial ischemia.

When ST segment is below the baseline with upward concavity is called "sagging".

40. A normal ST segment has the following 4 characteristics.

1. It is isoelectrical: It is on the same level as TP segment or slightly above or below.
2. It is sometimes normally elevated not more than 1 mm in standard leads and even 2 mm in some chest leads. ST elevation in the anterior chest leads is a normal variant when it follows an S wave. It is then referred to as 'high take off' ST segment.
3. It is not depressed by more than half a millimeter (0.5 mm).
4. In shape, the ST segment normally curves gently and imperceptibly into the proximal limb of the succeeding T wave.

It has no amplitude, no duration

Normal variation: Early repolarization syndrome: ST elevation with concavity upward is sometimes seen in normal individuals in leads II, III, aVF and V6. In such cases, it is important to rule out pericarditis and early phase of myocardial infarction especially in elderly individuals. Exercise abolishes the "Sikling Pattern". Serial ECGs and clinical correlation is helpful. (Refer Fig. Q-164, 165). ST elevation of 1–2 mm with concavity upward is more marked in some leads than others. See concave ST segment and T wave upright. This is a normal variant. It is common in some races than others.

The appearance resembles those of acute pericarditis. However, in pericarditis, the ST elevation is usually more marked and progresses to T wave inversion.

Similar ST changes may be transiently seen in the earliest hours after acute myocardial infarction or Prinzmetal angina but the distribution of changes and the reciprocal ST depression changes are of helpful in avoiding error.

41. ST deviation from isoelectrical line occurs in the following 4 conditions:

1. Injury to cardiac muscle, e.g. myocardial infarction.
2. Changes in the synchronization of ventricular muscle depolarization.
3. Due to drugs.
4. Due to electrolyte changes.

42. There are 4 points to be noted in ST segment changes.

1. ST segment elevation signifies an acute injury and returns to the level of the baseline in time. (*Note*: ST elevation seen in ventricular aneurysm does not return to the baseline in time).
2. If T wave also is elevated off the baseline suspect pericarditis.
3. The leads in which ST elevation or depression occurs to determine the location of infarction.
4. ST depression is suggestive of
   - angina
   - sub endocardial infarction
   - digitalis toxicity
   - the presence of ventricular hypertrophy—ST depression is indicative of myocardial ischemia but not coronary artery disease.

43. ST elevation occurs in (see Fig. Q-135–136)

1. *Acute myocardial infarction—fresh infarct:* ST elevation of more than 1 mm with convexity upwards is the characteristic finding in fresh myocardial infarction in leads over the affected area. Reciprocal ST depression in opposite leads is seen.
2. *Prinzmetal angina or variant angina:* ST elevation results from severe myocardial anoxia in contrast to ST depression with angina resulting from lesser degree of anoxia. No reciprocal ST depression.
3. *Pericarditis:* ST and T wave are usually elevated of the baseline with concavity upward in many leads (because the pericardium is all around) without reciprocal changes. ST is depressed in aVR, the lead which faces the uninjured surface (cavity of the heart). No abnormal Qs.
4. *Ventricular aneurysm:* ST elevation does not return to the baseline in time (present for many years—see old ECGs).
5. *Early repolarization syndrome:* It is a normal variant: ST segment is sometimes normally elevated with concavity upwards but not more than 1 mm in standard leads and 2 mm in chest leads. Sometimes, the T wave rises almost immediately after the end of the S wave and it appears as though there is no ST segment at all. This is called 'early repolarization syndrome' or 'sickling pattern', e.g. 'athletic heart', 'Edeiken pattern', 'high-take off'. This condition is not uncommon in healthy young adults. It does not require any treatment and must not be confused with changes of infarction.

   Less common causes

6. Myocarditis.
7. Hypertrophic obstructive cardiomyopathy (HOCM).

   Rare cause

8. Anomalous origin of left coronary artery from pulmonary artery (ALCAPA).
9. Cardias tumors.
10. *False positive:* LBBB, WPW syndrome, Cor Pulmonale, Drugs (Digitalis, quinidine effect, hyperkalemia, hypothermia).
11. *Noncardiac lesions like:* CVA—cerebral hemorrhage, dialysis, carcinoma lung with secondaries in the myocardium, GI bleeding, blood transfusion, intravascular coagulation.
12. DC Cardioversion.

44. Persistant ST elevation after the treatment of myocardial infarction is seen in:

1. Reinfarction
2. Local pericarditis
3. Aneurysm—(after 3 to 4 weeks)
4. Prinzmetal or variant angina—due to coronary spasm.

45. Horizontal or down sloping of ST segment depression of 1 mm or more at 80 msec beyond the J point is an accepted and highly specific evidence of myocardial ischemia. ST depression either horizontal depression or down sloping of ST—depression merging into T wave occurs in

1. Angina
2. Subendocardial infarction
3. Changes in the pattern of ventricular depolarization
4. Drugs and electrolytes.

46. ST depression commonly seen in the following 4 conditions can be easily differentiated.

1. *Myocardial ischemia (Angina):* Types of ischemic ST segment changes.
   a. Flatening: Normal sloping of ST segment is flattened so that it forms an angle of at least 90° with the descending limb of R wave. This horizontal or 'plane' depression of the ST segment makes a sharp angle with the proximal limb of still upright T wave.
   b. Subendocardial injury: The more severe the ischemia, the more ST depression. Horizontal or downward sagging with downward T waves in leads overlying the affected area.

2. *Left ventricular strain:* ST is depressed with concavity upwards with asymmetrical T inversion in left precordial leads. Similar changes are seen in aVL and LI with horizontal heart, in aVF and LIII in vertical heart.
3. *Right ventricular strain:* It is similar to left ventricular strain but changes are seen in right ventricular leads, LII, LIII and aVF.
4. *Drugs like digitalis effect:* ST segment shows depression and sagging with a downward slope and ending in a terminal rise to isoelectric line. It is compared to the hockey stick pattern or mirror image of a correction mark. The digitalis effect is best seen in leads with tallest R waves.

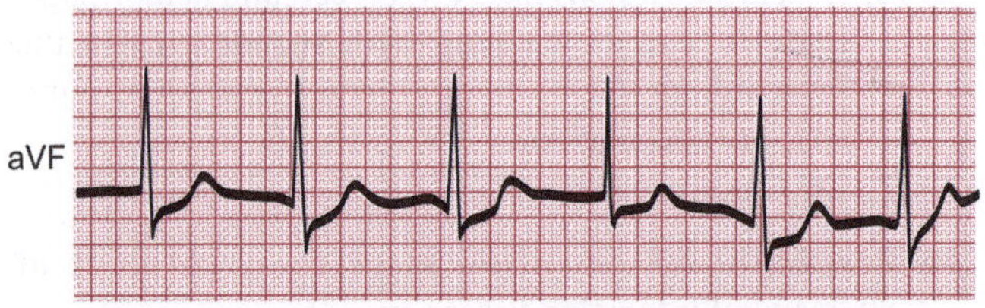

Fig. Q-38: Horizontal ST segment depression

Note: Pseudo depression of ST segment is associated with tachycardia/anxiety. ST segment assumes a continuous ascent with upward concavity. Prominent Ta (or Pt) deflection produced by atrial repolarization persists

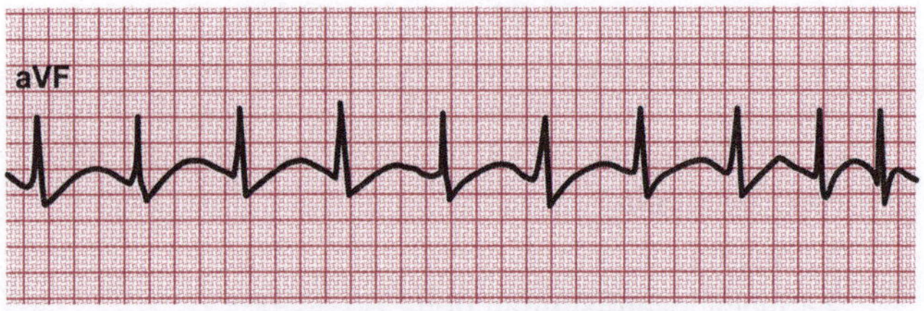

Fig. Q-39: Pseudo depression

47. Transient ST depression and T wave inversion may occur in (common in L I, II, III, AVL, AVF, and/or V4 to V6).

1. During pain in angina
2. Shock
3. Pulmonary embolism
4. Secondary to acute CNS lesions.

48. ST-T changes in a single ECG is not pathognomonic of coronary insufficiency because similar conditions can be produced by variety of conditions like

1. Left ventricular hypertrophy
2. Drug effect
3. Hypokalemia
4. Myocarditis

Diagnosis depends mainly on the clinical history and ECG changes during angina. Careful history is more valuable than ECG.

T WAVE

It represents ventricular repolarization. It is the recovery period of the ventricles when they recruit their spent electrical energy. Repolarization takes in the same direction of repolarization. So, T wave should be in the same direction of QRS. T waves in opposite direction to that of QRS waves indicate abnormality. For example, if QRS in V1 to V4 are negative and T waves are upright—it is suggestive of ischemic changes. Normal or abnormal T waves are determined more accurately by noting the frontal plane axis of QRS and T waves. Normal T wave axis does not differ from the frontal plane QRS axis by more than +45°.

Normal T wave height should not be more than 40% of preceding QRS wave and should be at least 20% of the previous QRS. So it should be 20–40% of preceding QRS wave.

49. A normal T wave has the following 4 characteristics.

1. It is normally upright in LI, LII and over the left precordial leads V3 to V6.
2. It is normally inverted in aVR.
3. Variable in LIII, aVL, aVF, V1 and V2. Certain general rules govern the variability. The T wave is normally upright in aVL and aVF if the QRS is > 5 mm tall. It may be inverted in the presence of smaller R wave in these leads. In the chest leads, the tendency to inversion over the left ventricle, V5, V6 rapidly decreases with increasing age and the T waves are considered abnormal in adults if they are inverted as far as to the left as V3.

   In the precordial leads T in V1 may be inverted normally at any age and in V2 also sometimes normally inverted. When the T wave is upright in V1 in normal heart, it is almost never as tall as T wave in V6.
4. The shape of the T waves is normally slightly rounded and slightly asymmetrical. When the T waves are sharply pointed or grossly notched, they should be regarded with suspicion, though it may be normal variant in precordial leads. A sharply pointed symmetrical T wave, upright or inverted is suspicious of myocardial infarction.

50. T waves are considered abnormal when they are

1. Low voltage
2. Flat
3. Inverted

} in which they are normally upright

4. Abnormally tall and peaked.

Flat or inverted T waves are quite frequently found on routine ECG examination and do not always signify abnormality or ischemia. Before final conclusion on abnormal T wave, it is worthwhile considering other factors which could lead to the changes.

Artefactual changes in the ECG are to be excluded as flat T wave may be produced by weak batteries and/or improper lead application. Batteries need to be checked for proper voltage and good patient preparation is always rewarding.

51. Physiological causes of T wave changes include

1. *Age and sex:* Flat or inverted T wave in young people especially in right sided chest leads is a normal variant. T inversion upto lead V3 may be present in persons below 35 years of age, usually in females. The diagnosis of ischemia should be made only after further investigation. Precordial T waves may be inverted during pregnancy.
2. *Post-prandial ECG:* T wave inversion may follow a large meal or after drinking ice cold water, usually in anteroseptal leads. ECG repeated on empty stomach may show normal pattern.
3. *Anxiety state:* Young individuals with chest pain and panic may show ECG changes highly suggestive of ischemia. Severe anxiety, fear, neurocirculatory asthenia, hyperkinetic circulatory syndrome show. T wave changes together with tachycardia. ECG repeated after administration of beta-blocker or sleep reverts to normal.
4. *Hyperventilation:* Young, hysterical, hyperventilating females often with chest pain show abnormal T wave in multiple leads. T wave changes similar to anxiety, fear are not infrequently seen in hyperventilation and lead to diagnostic dilemma.

52. Pathological causes of T wave changes include ischemic and nonischemic cardiac diseases and extra cardiac conditions.

Cardiac causes

1. *Ischemia/Infarction:* Symmetrically inverted T wave is seen in coronary artery disease and anoxia. Acute MI may give rise to tall T wave with wide blunt tip (apex)/(Vs hyperkalemia). Nonischemic cardiac conditions
2. *Myocarditis:* Asymptomatic myocarditis has been reported with viral fevers presenting with myalgia and fever such as echo virus, influenza virus, Coxsackie virus, etc. T wave inversion may be present for long time after the infection has been subsided. Diagnosis of coronary artery disease is made if clinical correlation is missing.
3. *Pericarditis:* Chronic constrictive pericarditis may present with localized ST-T wave changes and pose a diagnostic difficulty. Chest X-ray and echocardiographic study may be needed for reaching a definitive diagnosis.
4. *Cardiomyopathies:* Giant T wave inversion in the left ventricular leads is a rare form of apical hypertrophy in hypertrophic obstructive cardiomyopathy (HOCM).
5. *Ventricular hypertrophy:* Asymmetrical T wave inversion is commonly seen in left ventricular leads in hypertrophy with strain pattern in conditions, such as hypertension, aortic stenosis, etc. Clinical correlation is helpful.
6. *Post-tachycardia syndrome:* In about 20% of patients with paroxysmal tachycardia normal T wave becomes inverted for hours or days after the termination of acute attack. These changes are frequently seen in left sided chest leads and usually associated with prolonged QT interval. This phenomenon is not related to patients age or underlying disease. In ventricular tachycardia, T wave is in opposite direction to main QRS deflection.
7. Premature ventricular beats.
8. Bundle branch block.

53. Noncardiac causes of T wave changes include

1. *Endocrinal diseases:* Hypothyroidism, adrenal and pituitary hypofunction can all produce flat or inverted T waves. Early suspicion of these diseases must be kept in mind as they present with vague symptoms and unexpected ECG changes.
2. *Electrolyte Imbalance:* Hypokalemia and hypocalcemia produce marked T wave changes which are usually obvious. Tall T wave in K↑ with sharp apex (Vs AMI).
3. *Drugs:* Digitalis is notorious for causing various changes and T wave may show similar pattern of ischemia. As digitalis induce changes pronounce on exercise, this can further complicate the interpretation. Quinidine, procainamide and phenothiazine can also produce ST-T changes and a proper history of drugs ingested can avoid unnecessary investigation.
4. *Acute abdominal conditions:* Acute pancreatitis, cholecystitis can produce flat or inverted T wave.
5. *Raised intracranial tension:* Stroke, subarachnoid hemorrhage and similar conditions can lead to T wave changes in lateral chest leads. These changes are temporary and revert to normal once the actual disease has improved.
6. *Chest trauma:* Blunt nonpenetrating chest injuries can produce significant T wave changes. Sports injuries like kick on the chest, road traffic injuries, fall from a height, etc. may all cause abnormal T wave changes. These incidents may be forgotten and the ECG changes may suggest the ishemic diagnosis at a later date.
7. Shock.
8. Hiatus hernia.

54. T wave inversion commonly occurs in

1. Symmetrically inverted T—Infarction, IHD, coronary artery disease, anoxia.
2. Asymmetrically inverted T in V5 or V6—left ventricular hypertrophy.
3. Deeply inverted T—waves in left ventricular leads in apical hypertrophy of hypertrophic obstructive cardiomyopathy.
4. Downward sloping of ST segment merging into deeply inverted T wave in ventricular conduction abnormality —primary muscle disease.
5. Premature ventricular beats.
6. Bundle branch block.
7. Pericarditis.
8. Myocarditis.

55. Height of T wave is normally not above 5 mm in any standard lead, and not above 10 mm in any precordial lead.

Increase in amplitude of T wave occurs in

1. Normal
2. Inferior infarction (tall T in V1,V2)
3. True posterior infarct
4. Myocardial ischemia without infarction
5. Hyperkalemia
6. Certain forms of heart strain (ventricular overloading)
7. Cerebrovascular accidents
8. In psychotics.

Unusually tall T wave suggests myocardial infarction or potassium intoxication.

56. Low or flat T waves occur in

1. Thick chest wall
2. Emphysema
3. Myocardial ischemia/infarction
4. Myocarditis
5. Pericardial effusion
6. Digitalis effect
7. Hypothyroidism
8. Hypokalemia
9. Hypocalcemia
10. Non-penetrating chest injuries
11. Hyperventilation
12. Anxiety states.

Physicians interpreting ECGs are frequently confronted with unexpected finding of T wave flattening or inversion. Large number of these individuals will show normal record if artefactual and physiological causes are excluded and a record is repeated in fasting state.

Noncardiac causes should be considered and only after confirmation and support of other investigations including stress test and echocardiography the diagnosis of ischemia should be entertained.

QT INTERVAL

This is measured from the beginning of QRS to the end of T wave. It represents sum of depolarization and repolarization Calculate the corrected QT interval QTc by dividing the QT interval by the square root of the preceding RR interval. (Normal = 0.44 sec). QTc = QT/$\sqrt{RR}$

It represents total duration of ventricular depolarization and repolarization. It varies with heart rate, sex and age. Usually QT interval should be less than half of the preceding RR interval. This holds good for normal sinus rates.

57. Relation of heart rate and QT interval

QT	Heart rate/min
0.31 – 0.41	70
0.29 – 0.38	80
0.28 – 0.36	90
0.27 – 0.35	100

58. QT duration changes occur in the following conditions.

1. QT interval falls below half of the preceding RR interval if the heart rate falls below 65 bpm.
2. QT interval exceeds half the preceding RR interval if the heart rate increases above 90 bpm.
3. QT interval increases in congestive heart failure, myocardial infarction, hypocalcemia and by quinidine and procainamide, sometimes lengthened in rheumatic fever, myocarditis, and by phenothiazines.
4. QT interval is decreased by digitalis, calcium and potassium excess.

59. QT interval is prolonged in

1. Diffuse myocardial disease, congestive heart failure
2. Myocardial infarction
3. Rheumatic fever and other causes of acute myocarditis
4. Congenital QT syndrome
   i. Torsedes de pointes
   ii. Romano-Ward syndrome (autosomal dominant)
   iii. Jervill + Lange-Nielson syndrome (autosomal recessive) associated with sensorineural deafness
   iv. Syncope—always check QT interval in syncope.
5. Hypocalcemia
6. Hypothyroidism
7. Drugs like quinidine, procainamide, sotalol, amiodarone, and phenothiazine
8. Cerebrovascular accident
   i. Subarachnoid hemorrhage
   ii. Intracerebral hemorrhage.

Recurrent syncopial attacks are treated as epilepsy. May give family history of syncope. Grape juice increases QT interval, so do not take drugs with grape juice.

Careful observation shows that QT interval is not prolonged in hypokalemia unless there is associated hypocalcemia. It should not be more than half of RR interval.

60. Congenital long QT syndrome

1. T wave may be very close to the next P wave with which it may some times coinside and look like bifid P wave. Close observation can reveal that T waves and P waves are separate.
2. Respiratory sinus arrhythmia is common.
3. It may present with congenital sensory neural deafness referred to as) Jervill + Lange-Nielson syndrome (autosomal recessive).
4. This may suddenly go in to torsades de pointes leading to sudden cardiac death.

U WAVE

61. Normal characters of U wave.

1. Genesis is not clear. It may represent papillary muscle repolarization/Purkinje repolarization?
2. Not always present. The normal U wave is often best detected in V3.
3. Its polarity is the same as that of T wave.
4. Normally of low voltage. The amplitude does not exceed 2 mm or 1/4 the preceding T wave.

62. U wave changes are seen in the following 4 conditions.

1. Polarity is often reversed in myocardial ischemia, left ventricular strain, hypertension, etc.
2. Electrolyte disturbance, e.g. hypokalemia, hypercalcemia. It is more prominent.
3. Drug affects: Digitalis, quinidine, epinephrine. It is more prominent.
4. Miscellaneous conditions, e.g. thyrotoxicosis, exercise. It is more prominent.

63. U wave is transiently inverted during

1. Angina
2. Acute pulmonary embolism
3. LV overload
4. Digitalis effect.

It tends to be inverted in L II,L III,V1, and V2. In myocardial infarction most of the changes may revert to normal and yet inverted U wave may persist.

RECORDING OF A GOOD ECG TRACING

64. Follow the 4 principles while making the ECG records.

1. The patient must lie down properly and relax fully in a quiet room to prevent muscle tremor.
   Attendees if any, should not touch the patient.
   The patient's feet or hands should not touch any part of the cot or walls other than mattress.
   Muscle tremors and alternating current interference may result in abnormalities resembling atrial flutter and fibrillation in otherwise normal individuals.

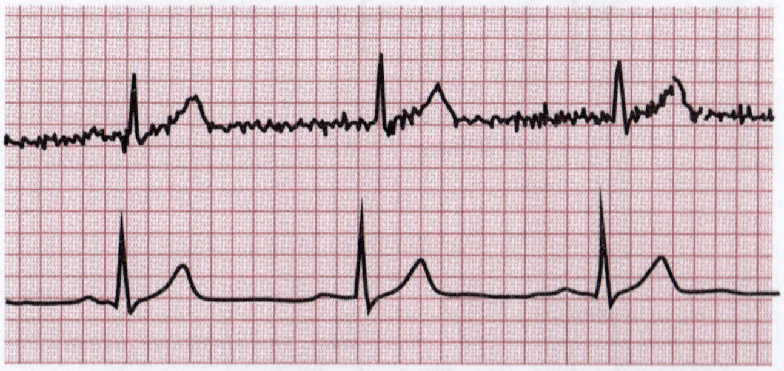

Fig. Q-40: Recording fault muscle tremors

   Electrical disturbance of baseline occurs if the patient is not relaxed properly as shown in the upper figure. Correct tracing is shown in the lower figure. It is difficult to find P waves in upper figure and atrial fibrillation may be diagnosed by mistake.
   For some reason or other if the patient has to be in any other position it is mentioned so that a note to this effect is made. Lying on either side, or sitting up alters the axis and transitional zone.
2. Connect the limb leads correctly. There should be no loose contact.
   Rubber straps over the limbs should be tied without much pressure to hold the electrode to a limb. Surprisingly, too tight rubber strap pressure is the commonest cause of muscle tremor artifacts. Rubber strap should be neither too tight nor too loose.
   Make sure that each lead is applied to the correct limb.
3. Verify the voltage. Calibrate with 1 mV signal (standardization).
4. Record the six limb leads and six precordial leads total 12 leads. Three or four complexes are sufficient for each lead.

65. There are 4 points to follow while screening the entire record to know whether it is properly taken or not.

1. Check the standardization.
   10 mm vertical height is equivalent to 1 mV. Should be straight, rectangular with 90° angle at all the corners. The stylus should move vertically 1 cm, i.e. 2 large squares = 1 mV and this calibration should be included with every record.

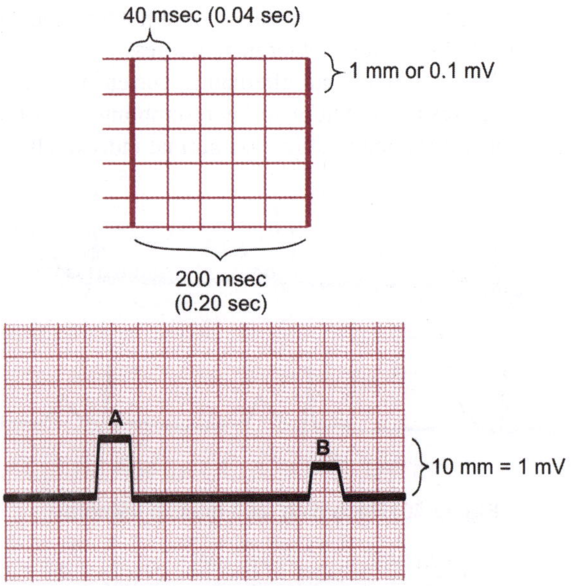

Fig. Q-41

A. Normal standardization of 10 mm—1 mV
B. Half-standardization. This expression is often shortened to 1/2 S. It is used when the QRS complexes are too large to fit on the paper. Here 1 mV = 5 mm.

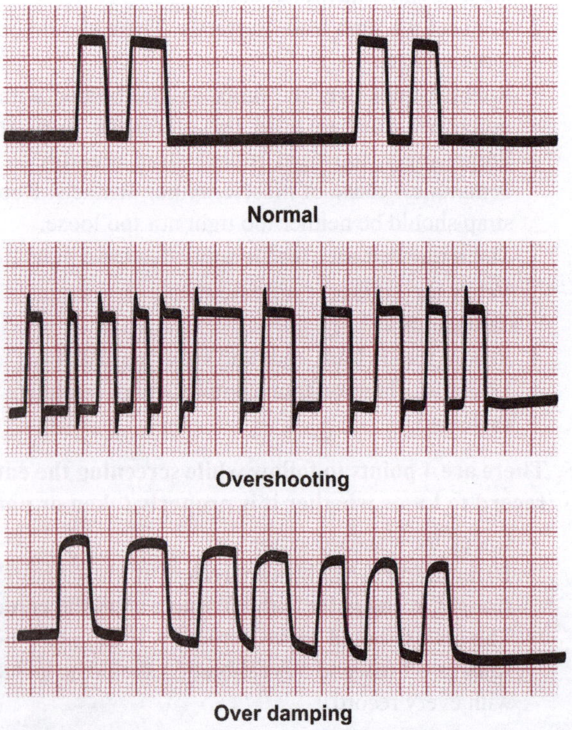

Fig. Q-42: A. Normal; B. Overshooting; C. Over damping

If it is not vertical, not showing 90° means that the needle is not moving properly.

A. Normal
B. Overshooting (under damped)
C. Over damping.

An over damped stylus will not respond to rapid changes in direction. Whereas an under damped stylus over responds. That means, under damped stylus will overshoot with each movement and so the amplitude of each movement is increased. If it is over damped, the amplitude of each movement will be decreased. The term 'critically damped' means normal.

Most machines are designed for quick and easy adjustment of damping. A slight increase in stylus heat intensity can decrease damping. It is also adjusted by the screw until the shape of the standardization pulse is square. If it is not corrected, the service engineer is contacted.

If the needle is tight, it moves with difficulty at some parts of the QRST complexes.

For example, abnormality due to tight needle. See Fig. Q-43B.

The needle moves normally upto QRS, but while returning it comes down slowly with difficulty showing ischemic changes.

(It is the ischemia of the machine but not the patient). Many patients with these false ECG go round and round to the consultants with an apprehension of ischemia. But really it is not.

In some cases, the needle may be loose and deflect more than normal. Q-43C

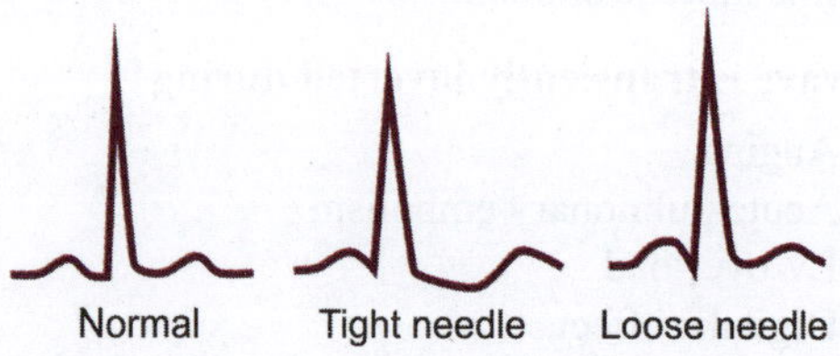

Fig. Q-43: A. Normal B. Tight needle C. Loose needle

This loose needle may deflect freely to show more voltage than normal. If the needle drops down too fast, it can produce abnormally deep S waves and false ST segments that move in an opposite direction to the QRS. It can even reverse the direction of a T wave.

Paper speed also should be correct. A paper roll that is too heavy will slow the paper movement, where a paper roll that is too light will speed it up. So, using a paper roll that is not manufactured for a particular model machine can change the paper speed.

2. Free of electrical disturbance
   Electrical disturbance is more common in our areas due to changes in voltage fluctuations in AC.
   Proper earthing should be maintained.
   There should be no loose electrical wiring in the room.
   Any electrical apparatus near to or touching the bed should be removed. Mere turning off an electrical appliance near the bed is not sufficient to eliminate interference. It must be unplugged from the switch board.
   A power cable in the room running parallel to the bed may create AC interference. This can be eliminated by rotating the bed 90°. The power cable should never cross over the bed or the cable should never cross over the patient's electrode that connects with the ECG machine.
   Always disconnect the patient cable of a cardiac monitor before ECG tracing is taken. The monitor and ECG machine cable must go to a common ground. Otherwise, a static charge may travel from one machine to the other with the patient as unwitting connector which may result in ventricular fibrillation.
   In case, if a diathermy is used during surgery, the ECG machine should be disconnected from the switch board to prevent damage to the stylus and to avoid blowing out fuse.
   To prevent AC disturbance—you can have rechargeable batteries. They do not cause such disturbance. They may cause some disturbance when the batteries become weak.

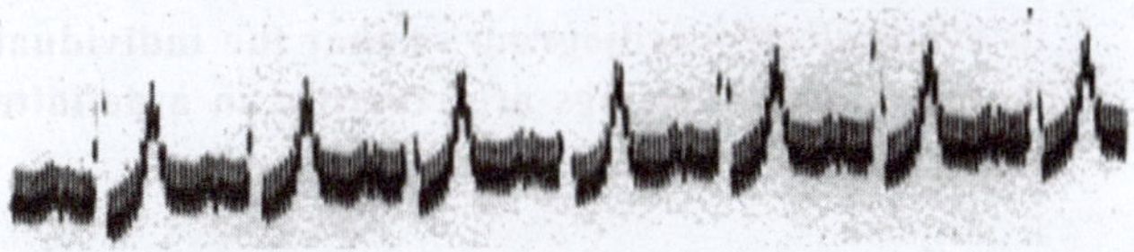

Fig. Q-44

Recording fault, AC interference. P waves are obscured and minor ST segment shifts are present.

3. Skin contact should be proper. Electrode jelly contains electrolytes and an abrasive. The abrasive is intended to break down the horny layer of the skin to form a continuous conductor. They lower the skin resistance and ensure better electrical contact between skin and electrode. Therefore, the jelly should be rubbed briskly and not delicately smeared on the skin before the electrode is applied.
   Apply jelly properly to have good contact. Special care is taken in chest leads. Jelly should be applied to the space where it is needed only. The jelly should not have continuity from one area to the other in chest leads. If the jelly is touching one area to the other, the electrical changes in one area will interfere with the other area. Small amount s of jelly should be applied. Large quantities tend to produce wandering baselines by allowing slight movements of the electrodes on the slippery paste.
   Dry paste does not lower skin resistance as well as moist paste.
   Chest area should be shaved if necessary before applying jelly.
   Suction bulb, called suction electrode of chest leads should be in proper contact and the connecting needle with the bulb should maintain good contact. Suction electrode can be used on amputated limb stumps or on limbs in plaster caste where only a shoulder or groin is exposed.
4. Leads should be properly attached.
   i. LA–connected to left arm.
   ii. RA–connected to right arm.
   iii. LF–connected to left leg.
   iv. RF–connected to right leg.
   Often the placement of the precordial is casual. It should be placed in exact position. Bony landmarks should be used in locating precordial points. Even minor displacement may produce considerable changes in the pattern.
   Check whether the leads are properly attached or not.
   For example, P is always upright in L1 except in dextrocardia—It becomes inverted in L1 if the limb leads are not attached properly. ECG as a whole cannot be interpreted if the electrodes are wrongly attached.
   A reversal of left and right arm connections could give rise to an error called technical dextrocardia; however, the precordial waves show a normal R wave progression. Abnormally high and lower lead placement can lead to wrong interpretation.

Recording fault, arm leads reverse by mistake: (Ref. Q-195, Fig. Q-154)

The QRS in lead I showed upside down, lead II and III are transposed, The lead aVR resembles aVL. Chest leads are unaffected. The limb leads suggest dextrocardia but the chest leads are normal. This is technical dextrocardia.
Faults in ECG machine: Over or understandardization, over damping, excessive stylus inertia, stylus drag, loose stylus, improper paper speed due to faulty motor, wandering baseline due to loose electrode contact and poor skin preparation could all alter the electrocardiogram interpretation in some or other ways.

VOLTAGE

The voltage of upright deflections (upright P, R upright T) is measured from the upper portion of the baseline to the peak of the wave.

The voltage of negative deflections (inverted P, Q, S, inverted T) is measured from the lower portion of the baseline to the lower portion of the wave.

66. When the sum of the voltages of all the QRS complexes of three standard limb leads is greater than 4 mV—the ECG is considered as high voltage ECG.

(Normal range measured from the peak of R to the bottom of S in standard leads vary between 0.5 and 2.0 mV with lead III lowest and lead II with highest voltage).
Standard leads: LI, LII, LIII
Cavity leads: aVR, aVL, aVF
Chest leads: V1 V2 V3 V4 V5 V6

67. There are 4 common causes of high voltage.

1. Thin chest wall especially in children
2. Left ventricular hypertrophy
3. Wolff-Parkinson-White syndrome
4. Hyperthyroidism
   (Sometimes, BBB)

68. There are 4 noncardiac conditions that cause low voltage.

1. General condition: Thick chest wall, obesity, old age, cachexia
2. Respiratory causes: Surrounding the heart
   Emphysema—lungs tend to envelop the heart to a greater extent than normally. Lungs act as an insulator to prevent spread of current from the heart to the surface
   Plural effusion—causes short circuits to a lesser extent
3. Myxedema
4. Generalized edema.

69. There are 4 cardiac conditions which cause low voltage (less than 5 mV in standard leads and 10 mV in the chest leads).

1. Myocardial infarction, diffuse coronary heart disease, cardiac failure
2. Cardiomyopathy with decreased muscle mass
3. Primary amyloidosis
4. Pericardial effusion or constrictive pericarditis.

70. Changing voltage:

Alternate QRS complexes are large and small (and occasionally T waves). This is called ***pulsus alternans***. It is caused by less number of contractile units during weak contractions and/or by alteration in the ventricular end-diastolic volume.

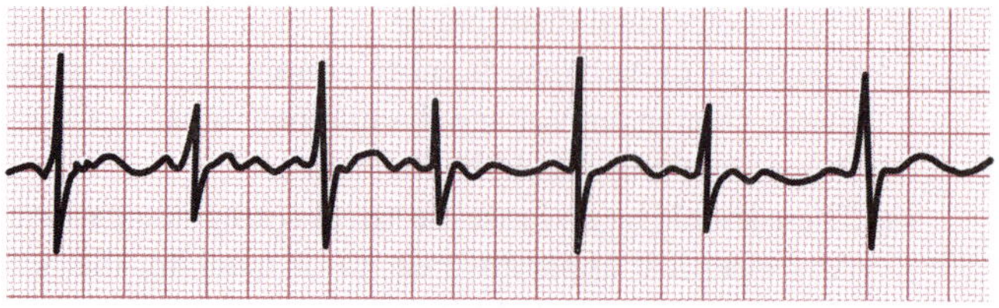

Fig. Q-45: Pulsus alternans

The heart beats strongly with one beat and then weakly with the next beat resulting in alteration of pressure amplitude, i.e. voltage despite regular or irregular rhythm.

This may be seen in following 4 conditions.

1. In severe left ventricular decompensation—where alternating left ventricular contractile force is usually seen.
2. Commonly seen in conditions with loud third heart sound.
3. Also seen during or following premature tachycardia.
4. May be seen after several beats following premature beat/extra systole—in patients without heart disease. This is most commonly observed in
   a. Heart failure
   b. Cardiomyopathy
   c. Hypertension
   d. Ischemic heart disease.

71. The following features should be examined systematically in every electrocardiogram so that the individual features of the tracings are recorded in a definite sequence to facilitate the diagnosis.

1. Rhythm
2. Rate
3. Voltage (Standardization)
4. Electrical axis — QRS axis
5. P wave — P axis
6. PR interval
7. Q wave
8. QRS complex (duration)
9. ST segment
10. T wave — T axis
11. U wave
12. QT duration.

Rhythm

A glance at ECG gives an idea whether it is regular or irregular. If it is regular, it should be noted whether it is sinoatrial—the commonest, AV nodal (junctional) or idioventricular. If it is irregular, know whether there is any definite pattern of irregularity, e.g. beats grouped in pairs, dropping of every third or fourth beat or whether it is irregularly irregular, etc. The rhythm disturbance will be discussed later in detail.

RATE

The ECG paper moves at a speed of 25 mm per second, i.e. 25 small squares.

Therefore, for one minute $= 25 \times 60$

$= 1500$ small squares/min

Measure the number of lines between two R–R.

1500/number of small lines of R–R interval = Heart rate.

The time between the two thin lines is 0.04 sec.

There are 5 lines between the two thick lines.

The time taken between 2 thick lines $= 0.04 \times 5 = 0.2$ sec.

Therefore, time taken for each thick line square is 0.2 sec. which contain 5 lines.

Suppose R – R interval is 5 lines, i.e. 1500/5 = 300/min, i.e. one thick square.

Suppose R – R interval is 10 lines, i.e. 1500/10 = 150/min, i.e. between 2 thick lines.

Suppose R – R interval is 15 lines, i.e. 1500/15 = 100/min, i.e. between 3 thick lines.

Suppose R – R interval is 20 lines, i.e. 1500/20 = 75/min, i.e. between 4 thick lines.

Suppose R – R interval is 25 lines, i.e. 1500/25 = 60/min, i.e. between 5 thick lines.

Suppose R – R interval is 30 lines, i.e. 1500/30 = 50/min, i.e. between 6 thick lines.

Thick lines can also be used to calculate the rate. A QRS complex coinciding with a thick line that should be selected. Number of large squares in between consecutive QRS complexes is estimated.

Rate is given by 300/n.

n = Number of large squares between two consecutive **QRS** complexes.

Memorise

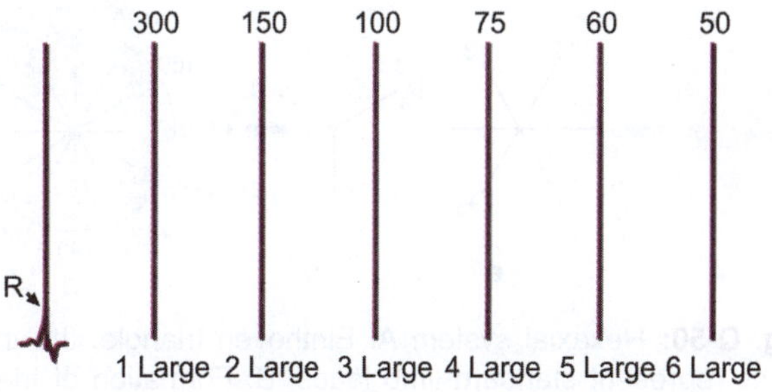

Fig. Q-46: Calculating rate from thick lines

Find a specific R wave that falls on a thick black line. Count off '300,150,100,75, 60, 50...' for each heavy thick line that follows. Memorize these numbers.

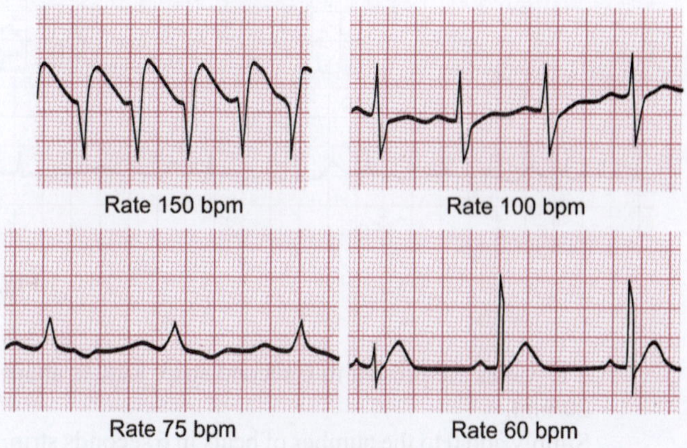

Fig. Q-47

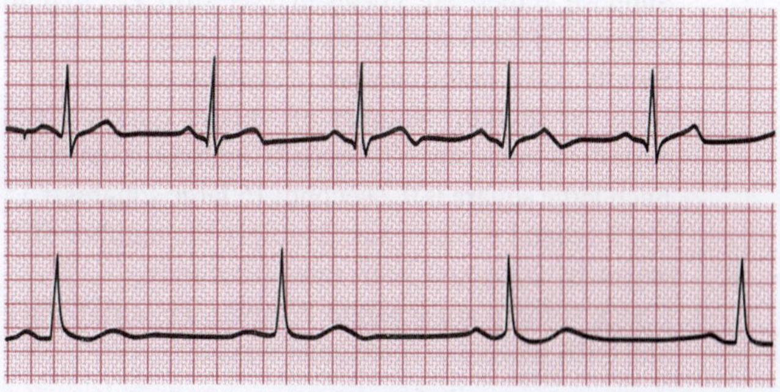

Fig. Q-48

72. The 4 factors to be followed while determining the rate.

1. Normal—1500/number of small lines between R–R. Memorize 300, 150, 100, 75, 60, 50—for making speedy calculation.

   This gives the distance between two thick lines containing 5 thin lines $= 0.04 \times 5 = 0.2$ sec.

   For every sec – 25 mm

   For every 3 sec – 75 mm

   For every 6 sec – 150 mm

   For every 60 sec – 1500 mm

   Normal rhythm— > 100 means sinus tachycardia < 60 means sinus bradycardia.

2. Bradycardia—Most of the ECG papers have markers at 3 seconds intervals. On such records, the simplest method is to count the number cardiac cycles (R) in 6 seconds and multiply by ten. Number of R waves per 6 sec strip × 10 cycles/6 sec strip × 10 = Rate.

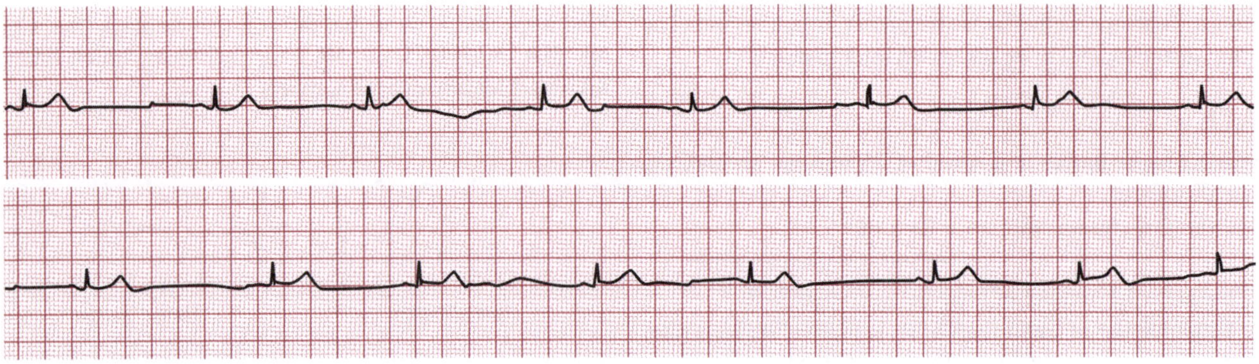

Fig. Q-49

2 R waves are present in 6 second strip. Rate is about 20/min.

Simply add 0 to the number of beats in 6 seconds strip.
Suppose, if there are 4 beats in 6 sec strip, i.e. 40 bpm
Suppose, if there are 3 beats in 6 sec strip, i.e. 30 bpm
Suppose, if there are 2 beats in 6 sec strip, i.e. 20 bpm
Simply add 0 to the number of beats in 6 sec strip.

3. Irregular rhythm: Number of squares over a given period of time, say 3.0 seconds interval is counted. Each large square is 0.2 second; 15 large squares = 15 × 0.2 second = 3 seconds. Multiply the number of R waves by 20 to give heart rate/60 seconds.
4. Check if there are separate P waves, i.e. atrial wave and QRS wave, i.e. ventricular waves.

If the rhythm is not of sinus origin describe both the atrial rate and ventricular rate separately.

AXIS

Electrical axis refers to the direction of depolarization (i.e. direction of total electrical activity) which spreads throughout the heart to stimulate the muscle fibers to contract.

73. The axis may be known for the

1. P wave
2. T wave
3. Initial and the terminal 0.04 second QRS
4. Entire QRS complex.

The entier QRS complex is in common use and others will not be specifically referred to.

Normal QRS axis +59°.

The average direction of spread of the depolarization wave through the ventricles as seen from the front is called cardiac axis. It is useful to know whether the axis is normal or not. It is the direction of electrical activity, i.e. vector. Vector is the direction of net result of cardiac impulse of RV and LV both depolarize. A vector is an arrow that points in the direction of current flow with the arrow point in the positive direction. Also by convention, the length of the arrow is drawn proportional to the voltage generated by the current flow. QRS vector gives an insight in ventricular hypertrophy, myocardial infarction, etc.

Depolarization of the ventricles are represented by a small initial deflection from left to right followed by a large deflection from right to left. The mean direction of these electrical forces can be represented by single force—the mean frontal plane QRS electrical axis.

Constitution of Hexaxial System

The axis can be known approximately from any two limb leads but it can be accurately known if all six limb leads are simultaneously inspected. One should know the hexaxial reference for exact calculation of axis in degrees.

Einthoven triangle is constituted by three standard limb leads. When they are rearranged to bisect each other, we obtain a triaxial reference system. If we join unipolar limb leads to bisect each other, we obtain hexaxial reference system—each line representing one of the six limb leads. By convention they are arranged in a circular fashion.

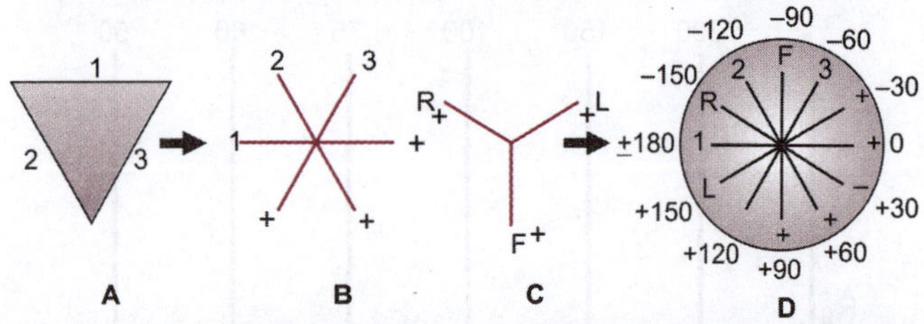

Fig. Q-50: Hexaxial system A. Einthoven triangle, the three sides represent standard limb leads. B. Formation of triaxial system the three sides of Einthoven triangle are rearranged so that they bisect each other. C. Unipolar limb leads D. The hexaxial system is derived from the lines of six limb leads (B + C) arranged in such away so that they bisect each other

Origin of Hexaxial System

Current is passing alround the heart—encircling the heart.

Draw an imaginary transverse line of LI, passing through the center of the circle and a vertical line passing through the center representing aVF.

The axis on the line representing lead LI pointing to the right = 0° and that pointing to the left = 180°. All axes above this line are negative and those below are positive. The axis on the line representing lead aVF—pointing to the lower pole is + 90° while that pointing to the upper pole is –90°.

A quick method of determining the axis approximately is by inspecting QRS deflection in LI and aVF. It depends on the fact that a positive QRS complex means that the axis is directed toward the positive pole of that lead, while a negative QRS complex means the axis is directed away from the positive pole of that lead.

74. Now there are 4 quadrants. Axis is determined by marking the QRS complexes in relation to the 4 quadrants.

Suppose—If QRS is positive in LI means it is in the left half.

If QRS is negative in LI, it means it is in the right half of the circle.

If the QRS is positive in aVF—it is in the lower half

If the QRS is negative in aVF—it is in the upper half.

Now let us deduce the axis by noting the positive or negative deflection in LI and aVF.

	LI	aVF	Quadrant	Axis
1.	Upright	Upright	0 to + 90°	Normal
2.	Upright	Inverted	– 0 to – 90°	LAD
3.	Inverted	Upright	+ 90° to + 180°	RAD
4.	Inverted	Inverted	– 90° to – 180°	Extreme RAD

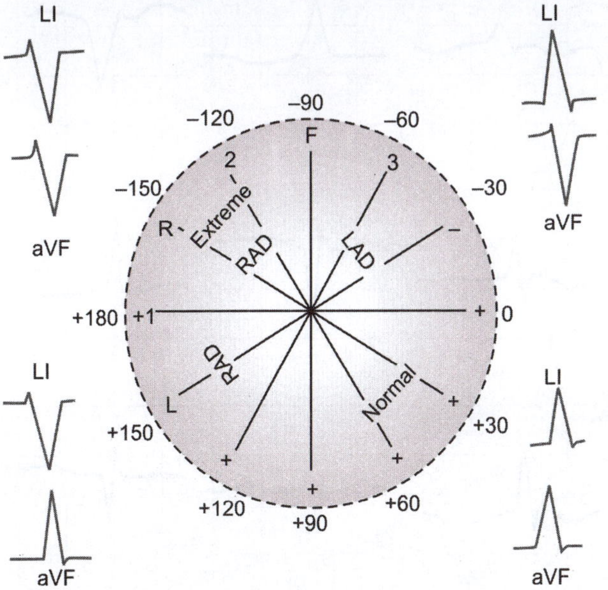

Fig. Q-51: The hexaxial reference system and range of axis

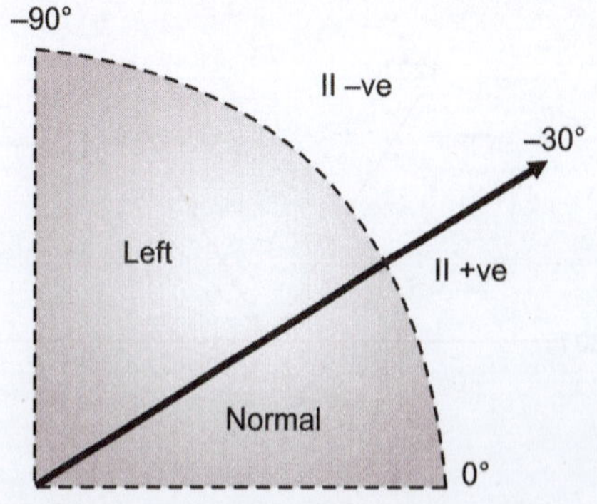

Fig. Q-52: If the axis is in the "left" quadrant take your second glance at lead II

If lead I and II +ve = Normal axis

If lead I +ve and lead II –ve = Left axis deviation

75. Determining the mean axis by seeing at the QRS complex in L1 and aVF.

Using leads 1 and aVF the axis can be calculated to within one of the four quadrants at a glance. If the axis is in the 'left' quadrant, take your second glance at lead II

1. Both I and aVF +ve = Normal axis
2. Both I and aVF – ve = axis in he Northwest territory
3. Lead I –ve and aVF +ve = right axis deviation
4. Lead I +ve and aVF – ve
   – lead II +ve = **normal axis**
   – lead II –ve = **left axis deviation**

Axis 0° to – 30° may occur normally in obese, pregnancy and ascites. The axis normally shifts progressively leftward with age.

Other method of determining the axis is by seeing the QRS complexes in LI and LIII. In general, when the R wave shows highest upward deflection in LI and lowest downward deflection in LIII, it signifies left axis deviation. When S wave is dominant in LI and R wave is dominant in LIII, it signifies right axis deviation.

Triaxial Vectoral System

The axis can be more precisely determined from any of the two limb leads.

For example, Lead I and Lead III

These are plotted along the axis of each lead. Perpendicular lines are dropped from these plotted points. A line is drawn from the center of the triaxial system to the point of intersection of the two perpendiculars. This gives mean QRS axis or vector.

For quick inference of the axis, the electrical principle should be followed. Electrical impulse is largest on the lead whose line of deviation is parallel to its path and smallest deflection is seen on the lead perpendicular to it. For example, an impulse traveling parallel to L1 will produce maximal deflection on L1 and minimal deflection in aVF which is at right angle to L1.

For easy method—see the lead with smallest deflection.

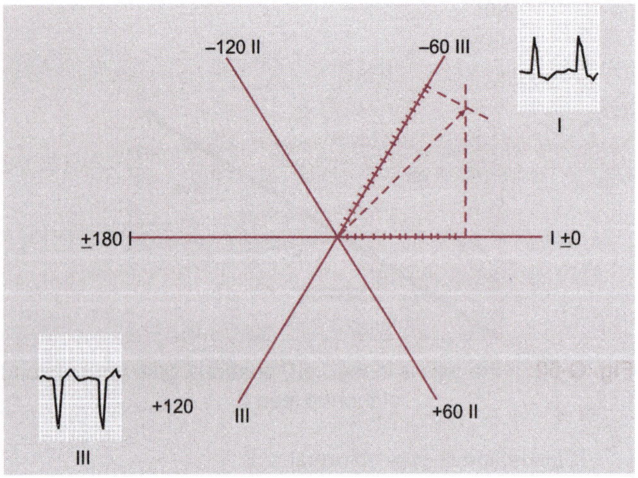

Fig. Q-53: Left axis deviation

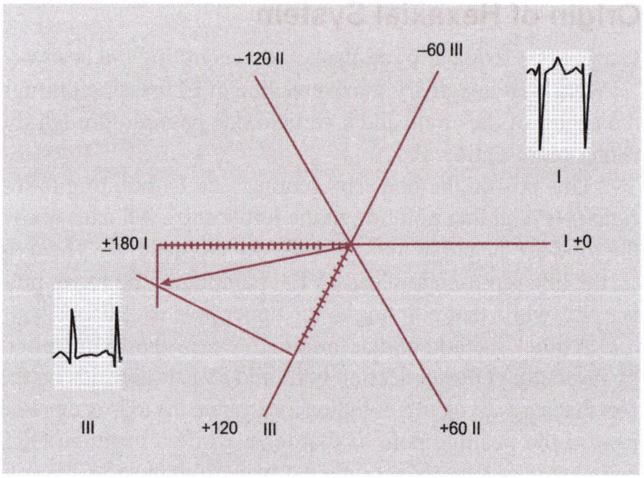

Fig. Q-54: Right axis deviation

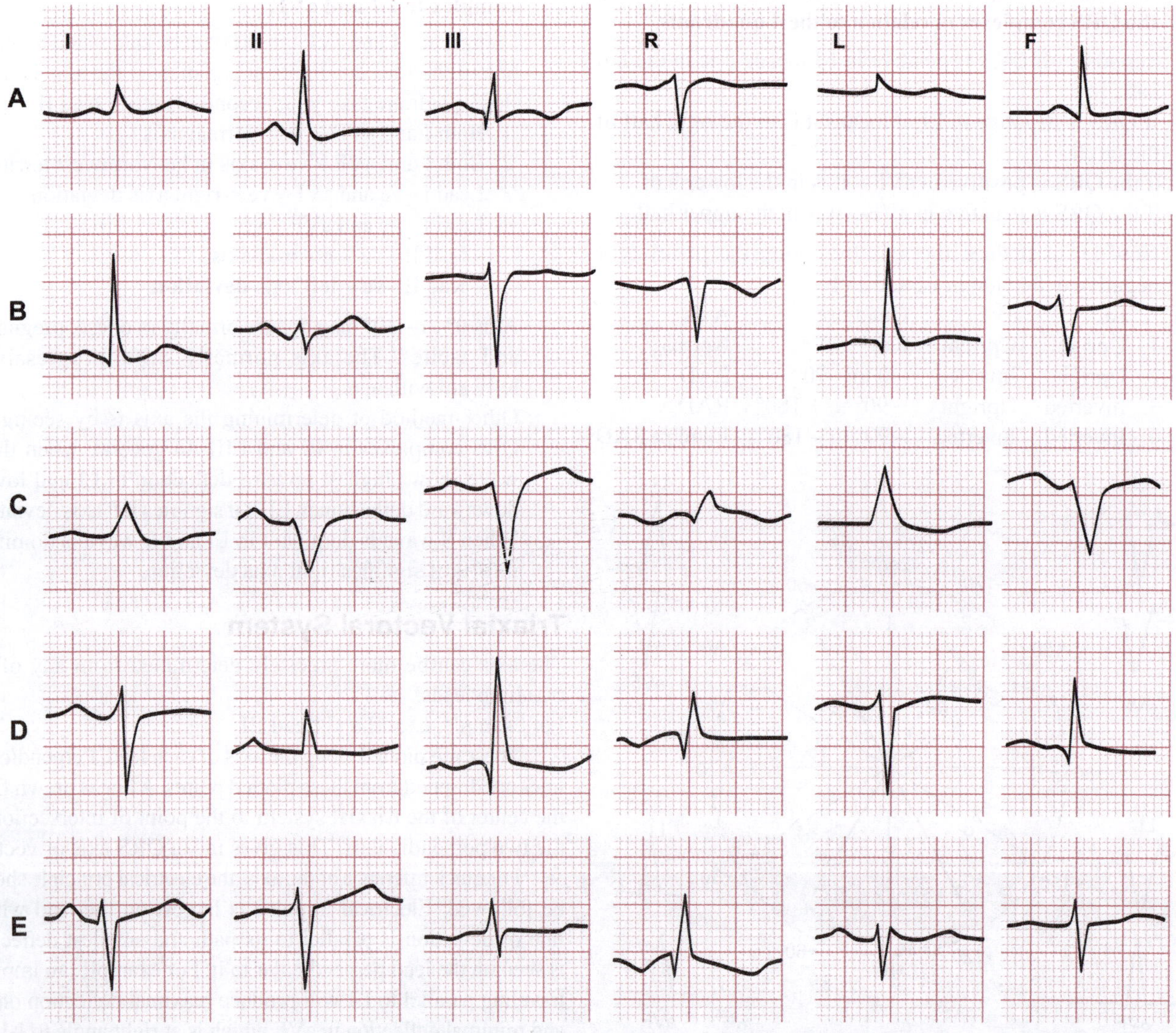

Fig. Q-55: Illustration of axis in the frontal plane: QRS axis in each tracing is as follows: A+60°, B −30°, C −70° D+135°, E −150°

The QRS is small in aVL, the lead perpendicular to it is LII. LII has the highest deflection than any other lead. Therefore, the axis should be parallel to LII. As the deflection in LII is positive, the deflection must be pointing toward the positive pole of LII, i.e. +60°.

In the similar way, others can be calculated at a glance.

The same principles and methods are applied to know the axis of T wave, and of the P waves. The QRS is indicated by the long arrow and T axis is indicated by the short arrow. The T wave axis is normally in the same direction of QRS. If they diverge by more than 60°, it indicates myocardial abnormality.

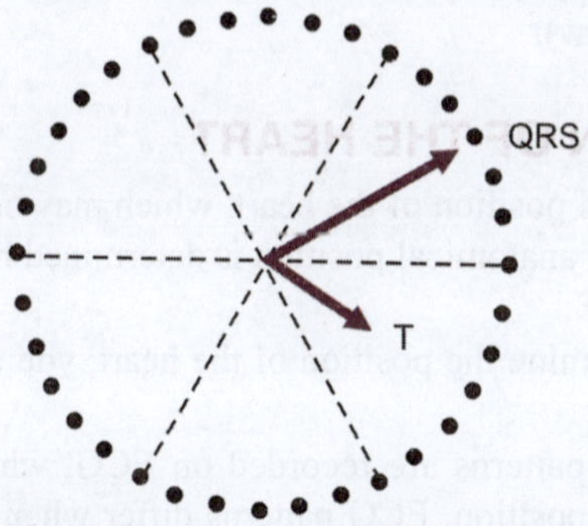

Fig. Q-56: QRS long arrow (minute hand) and T short arrow (hour hand) on the clock face of the frontal plane

We can locate the mean QRS vector as pointing forward or backward. The mean QRS vector may point toward the front or back of the patient. This is to know whether the ventricular depolarization proceeds forward or backward from the AV node.

Imagine the heart is at the center of the body and AV node is the center of the heart.

Lead V2 is obtained by placing the electrode on the chest just over the AV node.

The electrode for chest leads is the suction cup which is moved at different positions on the chest from V1 to V6 leads, but in each case the suction cup sensor is positive.

The position of the sensor cup for lead V2 places directly in front of the AV node.

Considering a sphere for lead V2, we can see that front half is positive and the back half is negative.

When a depolarization proceeds in direction perpendicular to the given lead, the deflection is minimal and/or isoelectric.

76. There are 4 ventricular conditions that cause axis deviation.

1. Change in the position of the heart.
   Shift to left, for example,
   i. Expiration
   ii. Supine position
   iii. Stocky fat persons.
   Shift to right, for example,
   i. Inspiration
   ii, Standing position
   iii. Tall lanky persons.
2. Hypertrophy of one ventricle—excess current on the same side.
   LAD in LVH—e.g. AS, AR, HT.
   RAD in RVH, e.g. PS, Fallot's tetralogy, increased pulmonary vascular resistance.
3. Bundle branch block (BBB)
   LAD in left anterior hemiblock (LAHB).
   RAD—in left posterior hemiblock (LPHB).
   RBBB or LBBB alone do not shift axis. Only hemiblocks shift axis – LAHB or LPHB.
   RBBB + LAD means – LAHB.
   RBBB + RAD means – LPHB.
4. Muscle destruction causes axis deviation to the opposite side because of scar tissue or fibrous tissue replacement, small quantity of muscle mass is available for conduction on one side than the other.
   Blockage of the smaller branches of the Purkinje fibers cause blockage of the conduction.
   Note: Muscular destruction causes the axis to shift to the opposite direction, but conduction block causes the axis to shift to the same side.
   Thus, the two effects may or may not neutralize each other. Consequently, the infarction do not produce consistent changes in axis deviation.
   Therefore, when the signs of old infarction are present in ECG such as
   i. Low voltage
   ii. Prominent Q wave
   iii. Increased duration of QRS
   iv. Bizarre spiking patterns of QRS complex.
   The diagnosis is usually definite and it is generally unimportant to determine the axis of the heart.
   Old infarctions do not show consistent changes in axis deviation.

77. Causes of left axis deviation (LAD).

1. Normal variation—horizontal position of heart
2. Mechanical shifts—abdominal tumors, obesity, ascites, abdominal distension
3. Physiological—expiration, high diaphragm from pregnancy
4. Q waves of inferior myocardial infarction
5. Left anterior hemiblock (LAHB)
6. WPW syndrome type B—right sided accessory pathway
7. Congenital lesions—both cyanotic, and acyanotic, e.g. tricuspid atresia, endocardial cushion defects, ostium primum ASD, univentricular heart

8. Artificial cardiac pacing (Right apical pacing)
9. Emphysema
10. Hyperkalemia
11. Right ventricular ectopic rhythm
12. Injection of contrast medium into left coronary (transient).

Note: left ventricular hypertrophy need not be a cause of left axis deviation.

78. Causes of right axis deviation

1. Normal finding in children and tall thin adults
2. Mechanical shifts—inspiration, emphysema, clockwise rotation
3. Chronic lung disease even without pulmonary hypertension
4. Pulmonary embolus
5. Right ventricular hypertrophy or dilatation
6. Anterolateral myocardial infarction
7. Left posterior hemiblock (LPHB)
8. Congenital heart diseases—Dextrocardia, ASD, VSD, PS, Fallot's tetralogy
9. WPW syndrome type A—left sided accessory pathway
10. Left ventricular ectopic rhythms
11. Some right ventricular ectopic rhythms
12. Injection of contrast medium into right coronary artery (transient).

While considering mechanical shifts in diseases like pneumothorax and plural effusion, usually cause a wholesale shift of the mediastinum, heart and all, pushing toward the opposite side, without necessarily rotating and do not necessarily affect the heart axis.

79. Causes of a extreme right axis (Northwest axis—no man's land) deviation.

1. Emphysema
2. Lead transposition
3. Artificial cardiac pacing
4. Ventricular tachycardia
5. Complex congenital heart diseases
6. Myocardial infarction
7. Aneurysm of ventricles
8. Rarely other conduction defects.

The QRS axis lies in right upper quadrant between – 90° to – 180°. Leads I, II and III all have dominantly negative S waves. (This is exactly opposite of normal ECG where all the leads have a dominantly positive R wave). It is called as S1 S2 S3 syndrome which indicates a very abnormal electrical axis occurring in congenital heart diseases.

80. The 4 features of S1, S2, and S3 syndrome are:

1. Prominent S waves in all 3 standard leads with S >R in at least one standard lead.
2. S wave in LII > S in LIII
3. QRS axis between – 90° to –180° (northwest axis)
4. A normal QRS duration (to rule out RBBB).

81. The causes of S1, S2, S3 syndrome include:

1. Complex congenital heart diseases including complete common AV canal, TGA, DORA, truncus arteriosus, single ventricle, etc.
2. Cor pulmonale
3. Anterior wall myocardial infarction
4. Straight back syndrome, etc.

(Cardiomyopathy, bifascicular or trifascicular blocks also may show).

POSITION OF THE HEART

The electrical position of the heart, which may or may not be related to the anatomical position is determined by two leads, aVL and aVF.

To determine the position of the heart, you see aVL and aVF.

Normal patterns are recorded on ECG, when the heart is in normal position. ECG patterns differ when the position of the heart varies. The augmented limb leads are useful in demonstrating the position of the heart. The aVR lead is little influenced by the position of the heart. Therefore, aVL and aVF are examined.

aVL is the cavity lead of left arm.

aVF is the cavity lead of left foot.

Normally, current passes to both sides, left arm and left foot. Therefore, normally—intermediate.

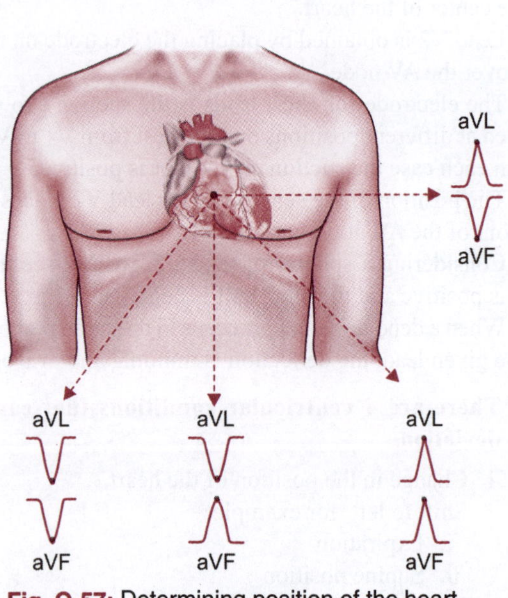

Fig. Q-57: Determining position of the heart from aVL and aVF

82. 4 positions of the heart are determined from aVL and aVF

Intermediate Position

Normally current passes to both left arm and left foot equally. So, left arm aVL upward.
Left foot aVF upward.

Horizontal Position

Current passes more toward the left arm. The left ventricle looks at left arm and right ventricle towards the left foot. Therefore,

Left arm aVL upward.
Left foot aVF downward.

Verticle Position

Current passes more toward the left foot. The left ventricle looks at left foot and right ventricle at the right arm.

Therefore,
Left arm aVL downward.
Left foot aVF upward.

If both aVL and aVF are negative, the direction of the current must be away from both the left arm and left foot which will be in rightward and upward direction indicating either dextrocardia or some very abnormal condition.

Indeterminate Position

aVL negative, aVF negative

ROTATION OF THE HEART

We can locate mean QRS vector as pointing forward or backward—i.e. to locate the 3 dimensions to the sphere.

Imagine, the heart is at the center of the body. AV node is the center of the heart.

Placing of chest lead V2 corresponds that the electrode is on the AV node.

Considering sphere for lead V2, we can imagine that the front half is positive and the back half if negative.

The QRS in V2 is usually negative, the mean QRS vector points backward because the thick LV is posteriorly located in the chest, so it draws the vector posteriorly. A positive QRS in V2 means that the mean QRS vector is positive forward which is not normal.

Rotation on longitudinal axis: Imagine, that an iron bar is driven in superior vena cava in a straight line down to the inferior vena cava. The heart could rotate around the bar. This can be recognized from the precordial leads V1 to V6.

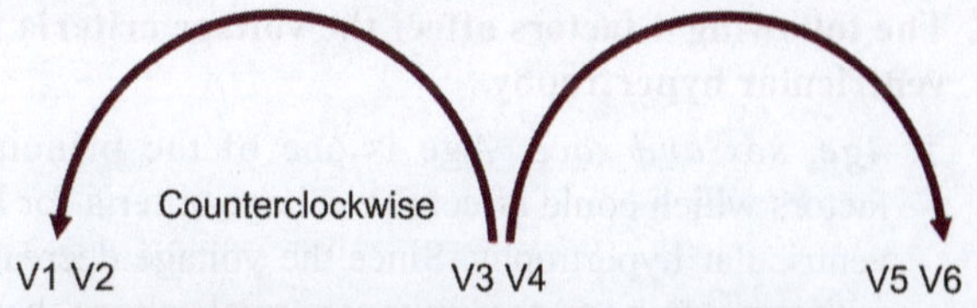

Fig. Q-58: Rotation in the horizontal plane

RS is normally equal in V3 or V4

When R is bigger or equal of S in V1 or V2, the transition is shifted from V3 or V4 to V1 or V2. Therefore, it is called anticlockwise rotation. When the transition appears in V5 or V6 it is called clockwise rotation.

V3 and V4—Normal transitional zone
V5 and V6—Clockwise rotation
V1 and V2—Counterclockwise rotation.

Rotation is in the horizontal plane whereas axis deviation is in the frontal plane.

SUMMARY

83. Leads to determine axis, position, rotation of the heart

1. The electrical axis indicates the direction of cardiac current in the frontal plane of the heart and is determined from leads LI and aVF
2. The electrical position of the heart is determined from leads aVL and aVF
3. Rotation of the heart is decided from the chest leads and is described as being normal, clockwise or counterclockwise
4. All the above features contribute to the ECG diagnosis but by no means are confirmatory of any condition. Very rarely, a correlation of axis, rotation or position of the heart can indicate or determine a specific condition with a fair degree of accuracy.

ECG IN HYPERTROPHIES

Cardiac hypertrophy is an increase in the mass of heart owing to enlargement of the existing muscle fibers. It may be localized or diffuse. The diffuse form is subdivided into concentric hypertrophy and eccentric hypertrophy. The terms systolic overload and diastolic overload have been used as an alternative to pressure overload as in aortic stenosis, and volume overload as in aortic regurgitation, respectively.

ECG relies on electrical changes to make inference about anatomy and it is quiet possible that changes which might occur in voltage have only a moderate relationship with ventricular mass.

84. The following 4 factors affect the voltage criteria for ventricular hypertrophy.

1. *Age, sex and race:* Age is one of the principle factors which could affect the voltage criteria for left ventricular hypertrophy. Since the voltage decreases with increasing age, the limits of normal voltage should be stratified by age.
   In the same way, there is considerable difference between male and female in the limits of normality of ECG measurements particularly in young adults. Criteria should also be sex dependant.
   High voltages may be commonly seen in young people under the age of 30, thin elderly women and emaciated individuals.
   Black individuals have a higher voltage in the ECG than white individuals, while the later have a higher voltage than oriental individuals.
2. *Hypertrophy and dilatation:* Left ventricular hypertrophy resulting from an enlarged chamber (aortic regurgitation) plays a bigger role in augmenting electrical potential than a thickened myocardium (aortic stenosis). In a case of increased muscle thickness with increased cavity size, there is an increase in voltage. On the other hand, an increased muscle thickness with same or reduced cavity size is associated with same or decreased voltage. This could explain the not uncommon situation of a grossly thickened heart muscle such as is found in cardiomyopathy with normal ECG voltage.
3. *Distance of heart from the surface electrode:* Precordial leads record better because they are strongly influenced by the distance of left ventricle from the electrode. Both left ventricle size and the heart from V5 or V6 interact as determinants of R wave voltage in left precordial leads.
4. *Associated diseases:* Coronary artery obstructive disease may be linked with development of left ventricular hypertrophy. Low voltages have been found in patients with congestive heart failure. In chronic obstructive airways disease, lungs tend to reduce the surface voltage. Pericardial disease can also affect surface voltage on account of an increased compression of the heart by excessive amount of pericardial fluid as in pericardial effusion. Thus, myocardial infarction, chronic lung disease, pericardial effusion may all result in reduced R waves, masking voltage criteria for left ventricular hypertrophy.

In routine practice, the voltage criteria is taken for chamber enlargement.

For all hypertrophies—see LII and VI.

Atrial Enlargement

P is the atrial wave. It is best seen in LII and VI. QRS is the ventricular wave, best seen in LI and precordial leads.

Lead V1 is directly over the atria. So, the P wave in V1 is the best source of atrial enlargement.

Atrium is well depicted in LII. The current passes from SA node to atria in the positive left foot direction. So, the atrial P wave is always positive and well seen.

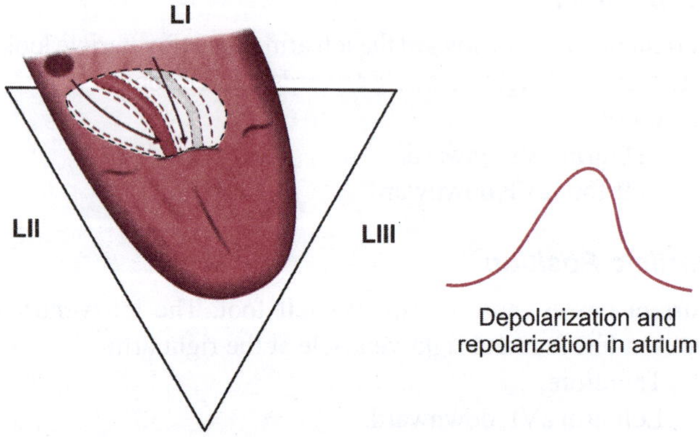

Fig. Q-59: Wave of depolarization in atria

(In aVR—the current passes away from the right arm. Therefore P, QRS, T are all negative. Any positivity in the aVR is abnormal).

Let us deduce the P wave.

The current passes first in the right atrium giving a positive upward deflection and then passes to left atrium which also gives positive upward deflection.

The first part of the upward deflection is caused by right atrial wave.

If the right atrium is hypertrophied more current passes in the right atrium and first part of it becomes taller > 2.5 mm.

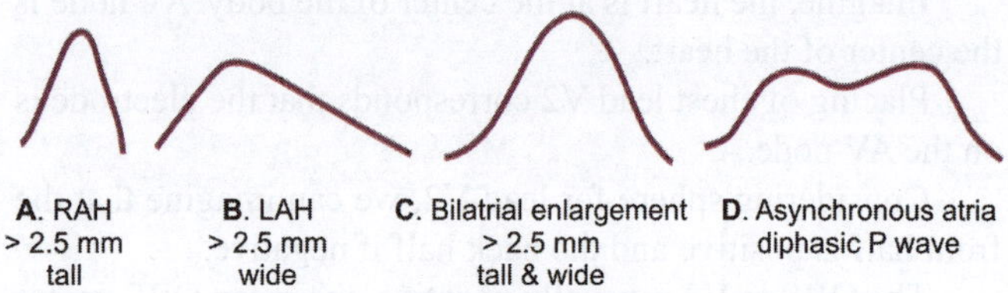

Fig. Q-60

If left atrium is hypertrophied, the wave comes down slowly and the P wave becomes wider. Width > 2.5 mm.

Thus in RAH—P is taller than 2.5 mm, in LAH P is wider than 2.5 mm.

If both atria enlarge—P wave is taller and wider than 2.5 mm. See Fig. Q-60C-Biatrial enlargement.

If the atrial contraction is not synchronous—the P wave will be diphasic. See Fig. Q-60D-Asynchronous atria.

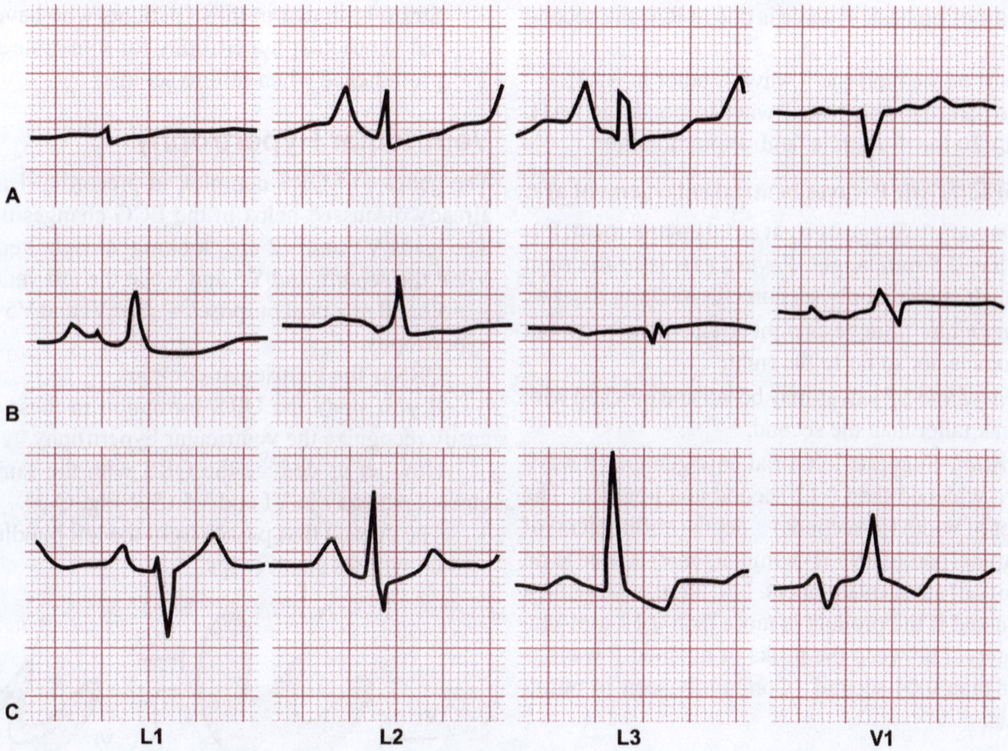

Fig. Q-61

A. *Right atrial hypertrophy:* Tall, peaked P wave manifested by right axis deviation. ECG from a patient with chronic obstructive lung disease

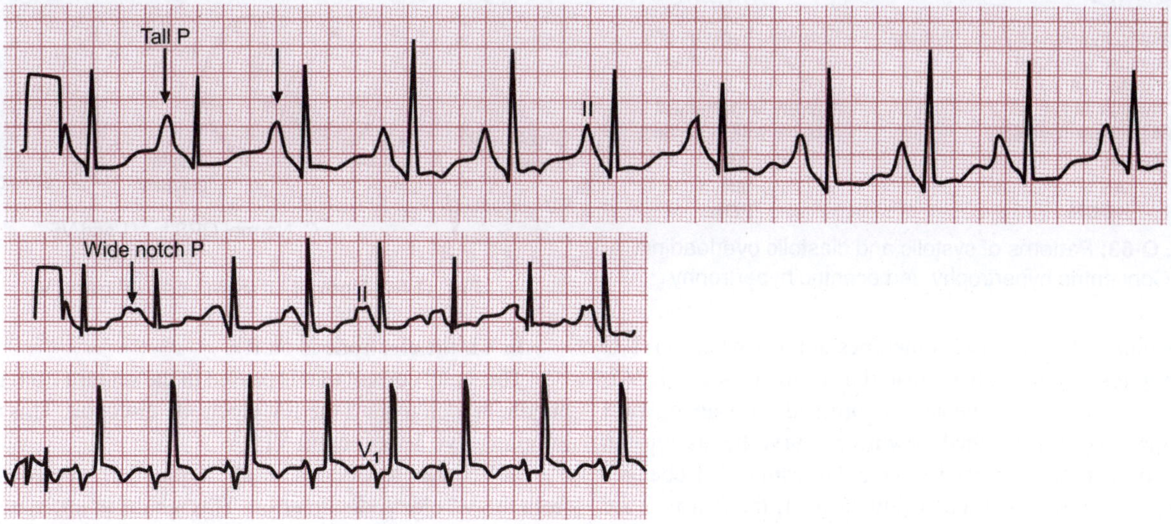

Fig. Q-62

B. *Left atrial hypertrophy:* Notching and prolonged duration of the P wave manifested by left axis deviation of the P wave. Note, M shaped P wave in LII, P wave duration > 0.11 second, terminal negative component of the P wave in lead V1. ECG from a patient with mitral stenosis.

C. *Biatrial enlargement:* Manifested by a tall P wave in V1. ECG from a patient with mitral stenosis.

The first part of biphasic P wave is due to RA, the second part is due to LA.
The first part of the biphasic P wave is taller in RAH.
The second part of the biphasic P wave is broader in LAH.
(See Fig. Q-30 for 'P-mitrale' and 'P-pulmonale)

85. The 4 characteristic P waves in atrial enlargement are:

1. *'P-pulmonale':* Suggests right atrial enlargement. P is taller than 2.5 mm height. P wave axis is to the right of +70°. It is commonly seen in chronic lung disease.
2. *'P-congenitale':* Suggests right atrial enlargement but the P axis is not so far to the right.
3. *'P-tricuspidale':* P waves may be tall and notched with first peak taller than the second.
4. *'P-mitrale':* Suggests left atrial enlargement. P wave is more widened than 0.12 second and notched. The product of width (in seconds) × depth (millimeters) of the terminal part of PV1 (P-terminal force) is used as an index of left atrial enlargement. Left atrial enlargement is indicated if the product is more than 0.14 mm-sec. The interval between the peaks of notched P wave is greater than 0.04 second . Commonly seen in mitral stenosis.

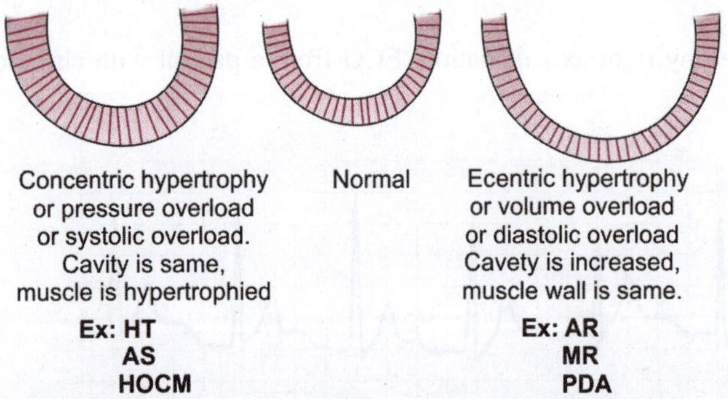

Fig. Q-63: Patterns of systolic and diastolic overloading. Concentric hypertrophy and ecentric hypertrophy

'Strain'—This term is sometimes applied when ST-T-U changes occur. Left ventricular strain is seen in V5, V6. The segments became depressed with an upward convexity and the final downward curve bends into an asymmetrically inverted T wave. The same ST-T changes are seen in left ventricular limb leads. If the R waves are tall in all three standard limb leads, the ST-T changes may be present in all the three leads. Often the earliest sign of left ventricular hypertrophy strain is inversion of U wave in left ventricular leads. Left ventricular hypertrophy need not be accompanied by left axis deviation. Significant left axis deviation with left ventricular hypertrophy suggests the presence of myocardial disease of left ventricle besides hypertrophy.

Strain is shown in those patients who have already have left ventricular hypertrophy for sometime and it becomes prominence when failure set in.

Ventricular Hypertrophy

The genesis of QRS complex in precordial leads which was already discussed helps in the ECG changes of hypertrophy. The leads V1 and V2 are 'looking' at right ventricle, V3 and V4 at the septum and V5 and V6 at the left ventricle.

For all practical purposes — See VI and V5 for ventricular hypertrophy.

QRS is the ventricular complex.

If you study the QRS formation in these leads you can easily recognize the ventricular hypertrophy.

Now let us deduce the QRS with the same principle of current pathway in VI and V5 (See Fig. Q-3).

The current first passes from the left bundle branch to the septum with its small twigs.

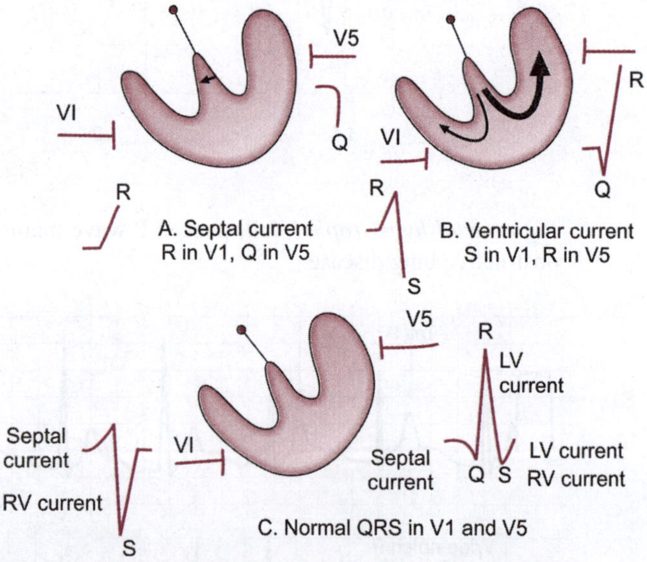

Fig. Q-64: Normal QRS waves in V1 and V5

In VI, the electrode is on RV.

The small current that is passed to the septum from the left bundle branch toward the RV electrode direction. This results in initial + ve deflection in VI.

In V5, the electrode is on LV. Septal current passes away from the V5 electrode direction. This results in initial negative wave in V5.

Thus +ve deflection starts in V1 resulting in R wave. –ve deflection starts in V5 resulting Q wave.

Therefore, Q waves are present in V5 and V6 but not in VI and V2.

In V3 and V4, which are septal, there is neutrality. So there may or may not be Q waves. If at all Qs are present, they are very small.

Now let us see again what happens in V1 and V5. The current then passes from right bundle branch to the right ventricle and left bundle branch to the left ventricle. After the septal current, slight current goes to the right side by right bundle branch giving slight increase in the positive deflection of the septal current, i.e. R wave is slightly lengthened by right ventricle current. But, the sum effect of RV +LV current is more toward the LV which is thicker and larger. Therefore, maximum current passes away from RV electrode toward the LV electrode. This gives maximum positive deflection in V5 and maximum negative deflection in V1. ECG returns to normal baseline when whole of the myocardium is depolarized. Thus, the QRS in chest leads shows a study progress of R wave from V1 to V6, where it is predominantly upward. The transition point where S and R waves are equal indicating the position of interventricular septum.

In V1 the positive R wave is formed by initial septal current followed by RV current. The negative S wave is formed by LV where the current is going away from the RV electrode. The negative S wave is due to more current of LV.

Now let us see again what happens in V5.

The positive V5 electrode is sitting on LV. The current first starts away from electrode to the septum from the LBB in the opposite direction giving a negative Q wave. Then the current passes both to the RV and LV and fast and more to the LV side because the LV is thicker and bigger in size. The sum effect is more toward the LV side giving rise to very big positive R wave. After the depolarization of LV, some current passes late in the opposite direction to the RV giving rise to a small negative S wave below the baseline.

Summary

In V5 negative Q is formed by septal current in opposite direction, positive R is formed by LV current, negative S is formed by RV current.

Now we have deduced the QRS in V1, V2 and V5, V6. In V3 and V4 the electrode is on the septum. So, the R and S are more or less equal or R wave may be slightly bigger because the LV is larger in size.

RIGHT VENTRICULAR HYPERTROPHY (RVH)

Always see V1 because the electrode sits on RV. R is smaller than S normally. But in RVH more current passes toward a right side giving rise to tall R wave. Therefore, R:S ratio is either equal or more than 1.

When RVH is present, there is a large R wave in V1 which becomes progressively smaller in the following chest leads. The progressive decrease in the height of R wave is gradual proceeding from the right chest leads to the left chest leads. The RVH adds more vector toward the right side, so there is often RAD (of the mean QRS vector) as well.

V5 in RVH - more current passes away from the V5 electrode because RV is enlarged. So, S wave in V5 is deeper, more than 5 mm. R waves are prominent in right precordial leads while deeper S waves develop in left precordial leads—this is the reversal of normal.

Left Ventricular Hypertrophy (LVH)

When the left ventricle is thicker than normal impulse will take longer time to traverse it. Therefore, QRS interval will increase toward or to the upper limit of normal.

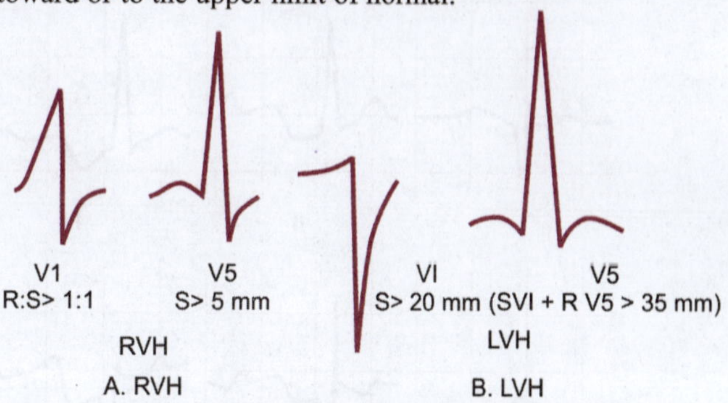

Fig. Q-65: RVH and LUH

Left Ventricular Hypertrophy (LVH)

In V1 more current is passed away from RV electrode. So more negative S wave. The S wave is deep more than 20 mm. In V5 the positive electrode is sitting on V5. More current passes toward the electrode because the LV is bigger and thicker in hypertrophy. Thus, the R wave is still taller than normal, more than 25 mm.

In LVH, the left ventricle is thicker than normal. So, the impulse takes longer time to traverse it and arrive at the epicardial surface. Therefore, the QRS interval increases toward or to the upper limit of normal. The intrinsic deflection may be somewhat delayed over the left ventricle and the voltage of the QRS complexes increases.

In LVH the normal LV features of QRS are exaggerated—tall R waves get taller and deep S waves get deeper. There may be LAD as the mean QRS vector moves leftward. There is a characteristic T weave which can usually be seen when LVH is present in V5 or V6. This inverted T wave has a gradual down slope and a very steep return to the baseline.

86. There are 4 points to be noted in V1 for hypertrophy of any of the 4 chambers.

Check V1 for hypertrophy

1. *Right atrial hypertrophy:* P more than 2.5 mm height. Large biphasic P wave with tall initial component.
2. *Left atrial hypertrophy:* P more than 2.5 mm wide. Large biphasic P wave with wide terminal component.
3. *Right ventricular hypertrophy (RVH):* Large R wave, R > S in VI, R:S > 1.

4. *Left ventricular hypertrophy (LVH)*
   Tall R wave more than 25 mm in V5.
   S in V 1 + R in V 5 is more than 35 mm.
   (S wave is normally larger than R in V1)

87. There are 4 points to be looked for RVH

1. R > S in V1, i.e. R : S > 1 in V1
   R wave becomes progressively smaller from V1 to V6
2. Deep S wave in V 5 and V 6—more than 5 mm.
3. RAD in the frontal plane indicated by a small R and deep S in L1, and abnormal anterior forces in the horizontal plane indicated by tall R in V1 and V2 with deep S in V5 and V6.
4. ST depression and T wave inversion in V1, V2 in RV strain pattern
   (QRS duration is within normal limits).

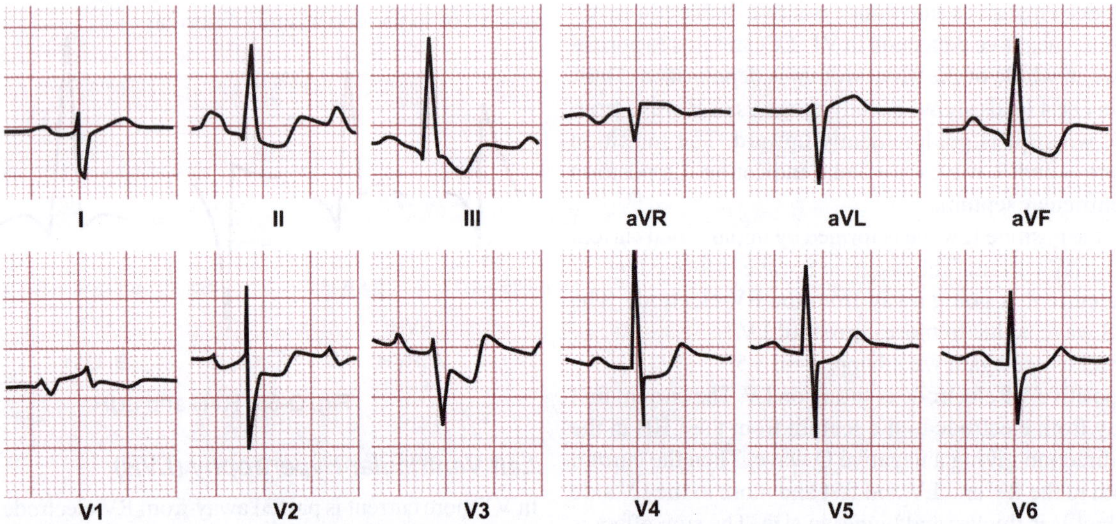

Fig. Q-66: Regular sinus rhythm; PR = 0.24 sec. QRS = 0.08 sec; Right axis deviation; Vertical position; Notched P waves of the P-mitrale type in LI and LII; ST depression and T wave inversion in aVF; Diphasic P wave with wide negative deflection is seen in VI; A prominent r is present in VI (R:S >1) and deep S present in V5-V6; There is ST depression in the precordial leads, most marked in V2-V3

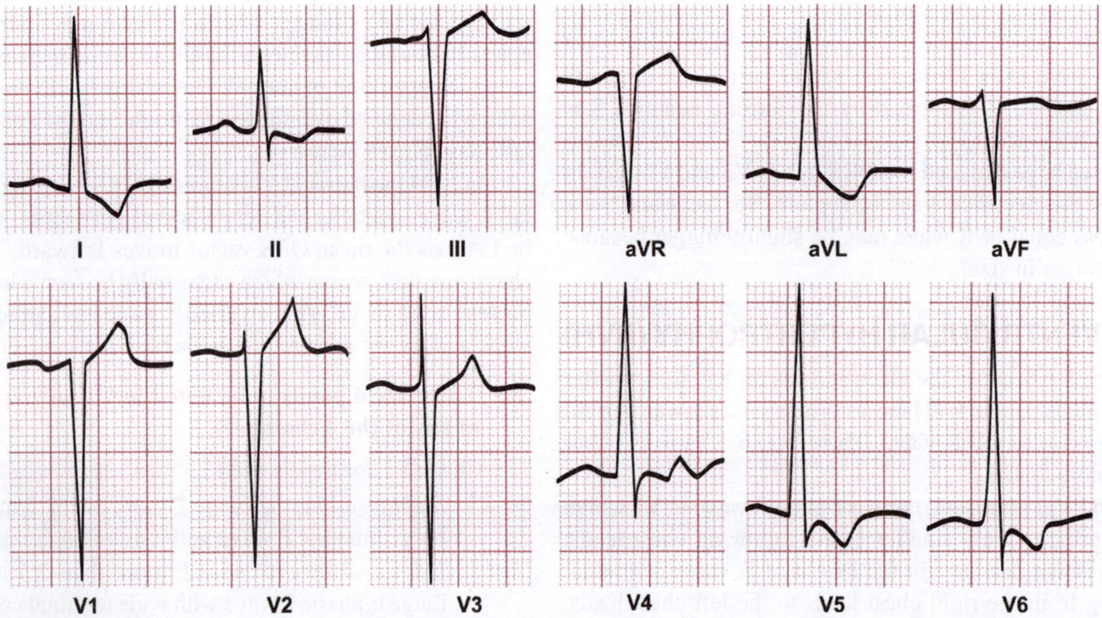

Fig. Q-67: Regular sinus rhythm. PR = 0.18 sec; QRS = 0.08 sec; Frontal plane axis = –18°; Horizontal position; There is ST depression and T inversion in LI, LII and aVL; R in LI = 20 mm (>15 mm); R in aVL = 18 mm (> 15 mm); S in V1 = 23 mm (20 mm); R in V5 = 26 mm; SV1 + RV5 = 49 mm (>35 mm); There is ST depression and T wave inversion in V5-V6; Note: T wave inversion is asymmetrical

Interpretation

Right ventricular hypertrophy, left atrial hypertrophy, first degree AV block, some of the ST-T changes are due to digitalis. Clinical diagnosis is mitral stenosis.

88. There are 4 points to be checked for LVH.

1. S in V1 + R in V5 > 35 mV.
   (or S in V1 > 20 mV or R in V5 or V6 > 25 mV).
2. LAD
3. Wide QRS
4. Asymmetrical T wave inversion in V5 or V6.

T wave slopes down slowly and returns up abruptly.

It should be remembered here that from each pair of leads the taller or deeper wave is taken into consideration. For example, if the RV2 is 20 mm tall and is taller then RV1 then RV2 has to be considered. Similarly, if the SV6 is 8 mm deep and is deeper than SV5, then SV6 has to be considered.

Interpretation

Left ventricular hypertrophy with strain;

Clinical diagnosis: Hypertensive cardiovascular disease.

89. There are 4 minimal voltage criteria for LVH.

The voltage criteria is not always reliable

1. Either R in LI or aVL > 13 mV
2. or R in V5 or V6 > 27 mV
3. or S in V1 > 20 mV
4. or S in V1 + R in V5 > 35 mV.
   provided the circulation is not hyperdynamic.

90. There are many different criteria for LVH. Following 4 are examples.

1. Sokolow + Lyon (American Heart J. 1949;37:161)
   – S V1 + R V5 or V6 > 35 mm
2. Cornell criteria (Circulation. 1987;3: 565-72)
   – SV3 + R aVL > 28 mm in men
   – SV3 + R aVL > 20 mm in women
3. Framingham criteria (Circulation. 1990; 81:815-820)
   – R aVL >11 mm, R V4-V6 > 25 mm
   – S V1-V3 > 25 mm,
   – R V5 or V6 > 35 mm, R1 + S III > 25 mm
4. Romhilt + Estes (Am Heart J 1986:75:752-58)
   – Point score system.

In the presence of left anterior hemiblock diagnostic criteria of LVH are changed. Rosenbaum suggested that an S wave in lead III deeper than 15 mm as predictive of LVH. Probably the best method is the Estes' scoring system for LVH.

1. R or S in limb lead 20 mm or more] S in V1,V2 or V3 25 mm or more] R in V4,V5 or V6 25 mm or more]	3
2. Any ST shift without digitalis	3
Typical "strain" ST-T with digitalis	1
3. LAD of—15° or more	2
4. QRS interval of 0.09 sec or more	1
5. Intrinsicoid deflection in V5, V6: 0.04 sec or more	1
Total	10

Score > 4 = LVH; 4 = probable LVH

91. Some causes of left ventricular hypertrophy.

1. Hypertension is the commonest
   less frequently
2. Aortic stenosis
3. Aortic insufficiency
4. Coarctation of aorta and some other conditions
5. Mitral regurgitation
6. Coronary artery disease
7. Cardiomyopathies
8. Congenital heart diseases—PDA, coarctation of aorta, tricuspid atresia.

In LVH, the left atrium may also be affected. In such cases the P-mitrale pattern with a leftward shift of the P wave axis, often combined to the terminal part of P wave may be seen.

92. Some causes of right ventricular hypertrophy:

1. Congenital lesions, e.g. Fallot's tetralogy, pulmonary stenosis and transposition of great vessels.
2. Mitral stenosis
3. Tricuspid regurgitation
4. Chronic lung diseases especially emphysema, COPD.

In RVH, the right atrium may also be affected. In such cases P-pulmonale pattern may be seen. If pure mitral stenosis is the causes of RVH, P-mitrale pattern may be seen.

93. Some causes of biventricular hypertrophy:

1. Ventricular septal defect
2. Cardiomyopathy
3. LV hypertrophy due to any cause with pulmonary hypertension and right ventricular strain with hypertrophy
4. Multiple valve lesion.

94. Some conditions associated with pressure or volume overload of the ventricles.

Table Q-2

	Pressure overload	*Volume overload*
Left Ventricle	1. Hypertension	Mitral regurgitation
	2. Aortic stenosis	Aortic regurgitation
	3. Hypertrophic obstructive cardiomyopathy	Patent ductus arteriosus
	4. Coarctation of aorta	Endocardial cushion defects
Right Ventricle	1. Pulmonary stenosis/ atresia	Tricuspid regurgitation
	2. Tetralogy of Fallot	Atrial septal defect
	3. Pulmonary hypertension	Partial anomalous pulmonary venous connection
	4. Chronic obstructive pulmonary disease (COPD)	Transposition of pulmonary veins

BUNDLE BRANCH BLOCK

Bundle branch block is most common and easily recognized out of all the different forms of intraventricular block.

Normal conduction wave spreads from SA node to AV node and bundle of His, and then to left and right bundle branches. Normal conduction wave from SA node to AV node gives rise to normal P wave and PR interval. However if there is delay in conduction of either right bundle branch or left bundle branch, there will be delay in ventricular depolarization. This results in widening of QRS. Normal time taken for depolarization to spread from interventricular septum to the farthest part of the ventricles is less than 0.12 second, i.e. 3 small squares on ECG paper. If the QRS is wider than 0.12 second, it is due to delay in the depolarization of ventricles. The block at the right bundle branch or left bundle branch causes delayed conduction resulting in widening of QRS.

A bundle branch block may be described as complete or incomplete depending on the total duration of the QRS, i.e. RSR' pattern in the chest leads. If the total duration is greater than 0.12 second, the bundle branch block is said to be complete whereas if it is less than 0.12 second, it is described as incomplete bundle branch block. Basically, these are expressions of conduction disturbance in the particular bundle.

Though the limb leads may be suggestive of a bundle branch block, it is always advisable to read from the chest leads only.

Normally, R and S waves in the chest leads have a single peak and nadir. In bundle branch block, there is an abnormal pattern described as RSR' pattern, implying two peaks instead of one. There can be a variety of these RSR' pattern as shown below.

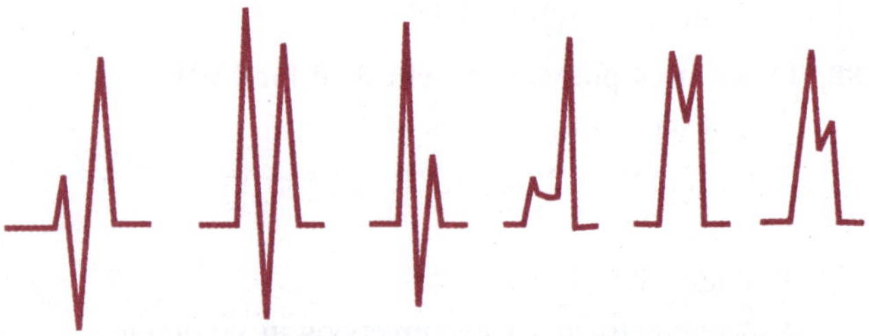

Fig. Q-68: Various RSR' patterns

A bundle branch can be easily recognized by observing which of the chest leads show RSR' pattern. If they are in right sided chest leads (V1,V2) then it is right bundle branch block; whereas if they are in left sided chest leads (V5, V6), it is left bundle branch block. Though it looks simple, it is a reliable method of diagnosing bundle branch block.

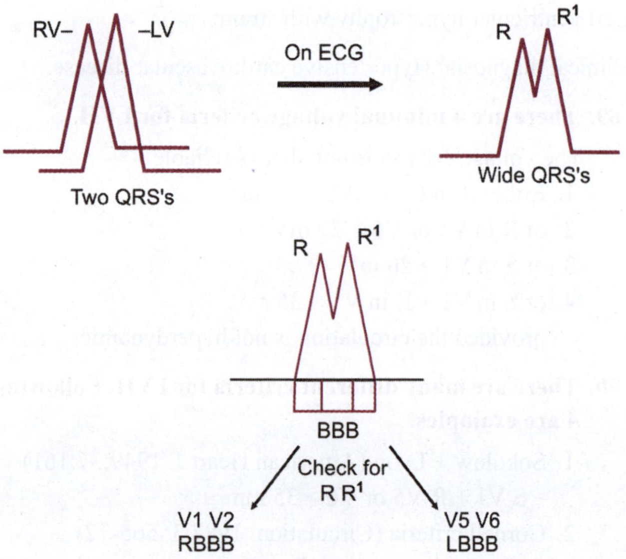

Fig. Q-69

The BBB can be explained in a simple way—the ventricles instead of firing simultaneously, they fire successively—one ventricle contracts slightly later then the other causing the "joined QRS's".

The ST-T changes, (ST segment depression and T wave inversion) accompanying RSR' pattern are directed opposite to the RSR' pattern in the respective leads. These ST-T changes are called secondary ST-T changes because they are secondary to the conduction disturbance in contrast to the primary ST-T changes due to ischemia and/or drugs.

The QRS widening also occur if the depolarization begins in the ventricular muscle itself , ectopic ventricular rhythm e.g. premature ventricular contraction.

P wave and PR interval are normal in sinus rhythm with bundle branch block, whereas it is not the case with rhythm beginning in the ventricles.

95. The genesis of QRS in right and left bundle branch blocks can be worked out by remembering the following 4 principles (See Fig. Q-57).

1. Normal depolarization of septum is from left to right.
2. The left ventricle has more muscle mass, so more current passes in the left ventricle because of greater muscle mass and gets more influence on ECG than the right ventricle.
3. Excitation spreading toward a lead causes an upward deflection.
4. Excitation spreading away from the lead causes a downward deflection.

Right Bundle Branch Block (RBBB)

When the impulse is blocked in right bundle branch, no conduction occurs down the right bundle branch. So, the only way of current to the ventricles is through the left bundle branch. The right ventricle is excited by the impulses from the left bundle branch to the right of the septum below the block. See Fig. Q-67

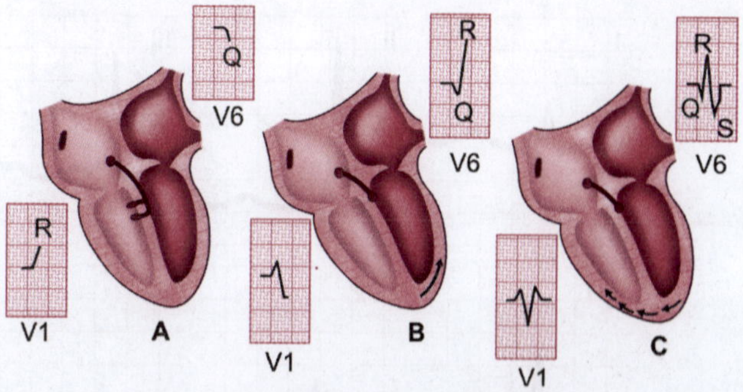

Fig. Q-70: Right bundle branch block

96. The 4 steps in the sequence of depolarization in RBBB.

1. Septum is depolarized as usual from left to right causing an R wave in right ventricular lead V1 or V2 and a small Q in left ventricular lead V5 or V6—See Fig. Q-70A—No change in initial vector.
2. Excitation spreads to the left ventricle causing S in V1 and R in V6—Fig. Q-70B
3. Right ventricle is excited after the left and it takes longer time for impulse to reach the right ventricle because of the failure of the normal conducting pathway. Therefore, there is a second R wave (R') in V1, broad and slurred S wave in left ventricular lead V5 or V6—Fig. Q-70C—terminal negativity.
4. Secondary ST-T changes in opposite direction of QRS.

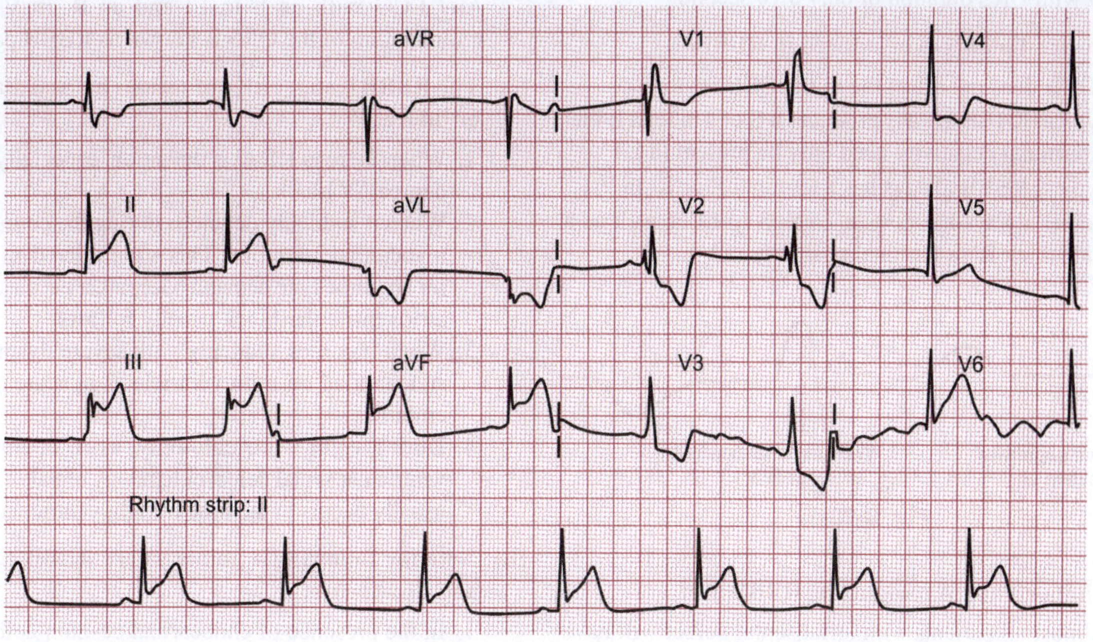

Fig. Q-71: Right bundle branch block: R and R' pattern in V1, V2; QRS > 0.12 sec; Secondary R wave in V1; Other features include slurred S wave in lateral leads and T wave changes in septal leads; also shows inferior wall MI and sinus bradycardia

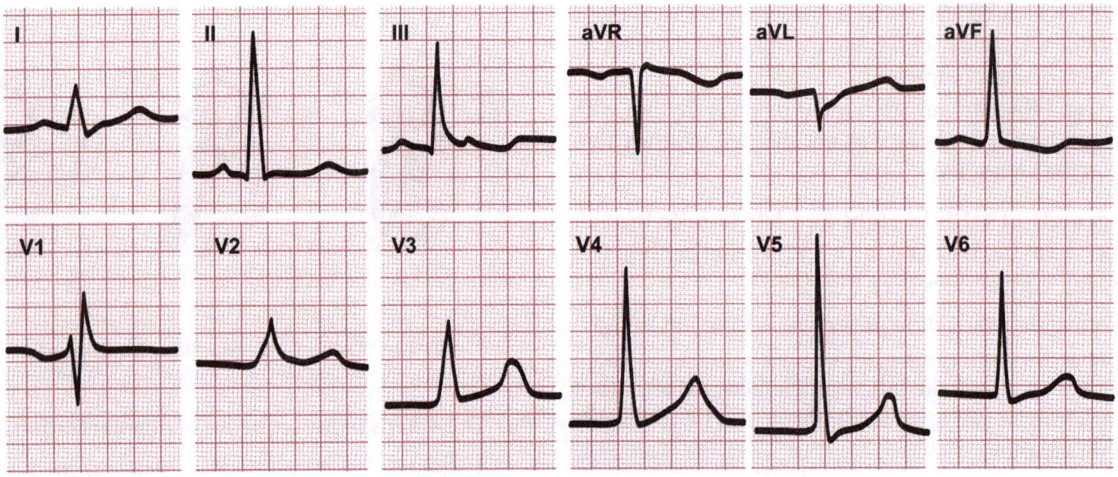

Fig. Q-72: Incomplete RBBB

97. Thus, the 4 ECG findings in RBBB are:

1. QRS is greater than 0.12 second.
2. R and R' pattern in RV lead V1,V2.
3. Broad slurred S wave in V5, V6.
4. Secondary ST-T changes opposite of RSR'

This figure shows acute inferior MI and sinus bradycardia also.

In incomplete RBBB—QRS is > 0.10 sec but < 0.12 sec.

Wide S in LI with late intrinsicoid deflection in V1 rsR pattern but with QRS duration of only 0.10 second.

98. There are 4 points to be noticed in RBBB.

1. RBBB does not affect the initial QRS vector
2. Typical RBBB always produces a S or s in lead I; that is terminal negativity need only be present in L I
3. Typical RBBB always has a terminal R or R' in V 1
4. RBBB always has a wide, thick S in LI as well as a wide thick R' or terminal positivity in V1.

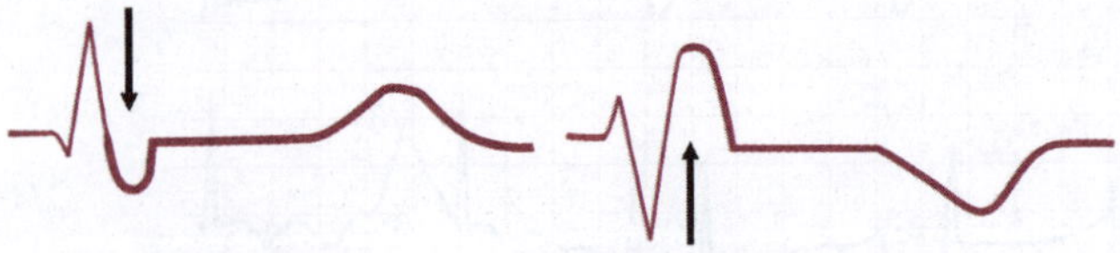

Fig. Q-73

99. The importance of recognizing RBBB are:

1. Almost all patients with atrial septal defect will have either RBBB or RBBB pattern. An ASD is unlikely without RBBB in ECG because of right ventricular volume overload which may cause stretching of the right bundle branch.
2. A RBBB or RBBB pattern may be the only sign of acute dilatation of right ventricle as in pulmonary embolism.
3. It may be the only sign of right ventricular hypertrophy, even though most patients with this pattern may have normal size.
4. It has significance in the presence of acute myocardial infarction.

A RBBB pattern may be a normal pattern and even with a marked left axis deviation, may be still a normal variant. Any ECG with an S in LI and an R' in V1 without prolongation of the QRS is known as RBBB pattern.

100. The RBBB is suggestive of serious myocardial damage or infarct—

1. When there is left axis deviation, especially with first degree AV block
2. When it suddenly develops during the course of acute myocardial infarction. This is considered an indication for an immediate demand pacemaker because complete atrioventricular block usually follows
3. When it comes suddenly with severe dyspnea due to sudden load on right ventricle as in acute pulmonary embolism
4. During right ventriculotomy, as in operation for a ventricular septal defect or tetralogy of Fallot. The block usually occurs at the time of right ventricular incision.

101. Note the following 4 points where RBBB can appear and disappears:

1. In the presence of endocardial cushion defect type of congenital heart disease, the RBBB is not indicative of myocardial damage.
2. RBBB is most common after operation on tetralogy of Fallot.

3. Various degrees of RBBB disappear after closure of ASD.
4. Disappear after decrease in size of right ventricle.

Left Bundle Branch Block (LBBB)

When the impulse is blocked in left bundle branch, no conduction occurs down the left bundle branch. So, only access to ventricular muscle is through right bundle branch. Therefore, the septum is depolarized first from right to left. Septal depolarization is the reversal of normal direction. It results in small Q in V1 and an R in V6. The right ventricle is depolarized before the left, so in spite of the smaller muscle mass there is an R in V1 and S in V6 often seen as a notch. Later depolarization of left ventricle causes S in V1 and another R in V6. Changes in left ventricular leads can be inferred from the sequence of depolarization. See Fig. Q-64 LBBB.

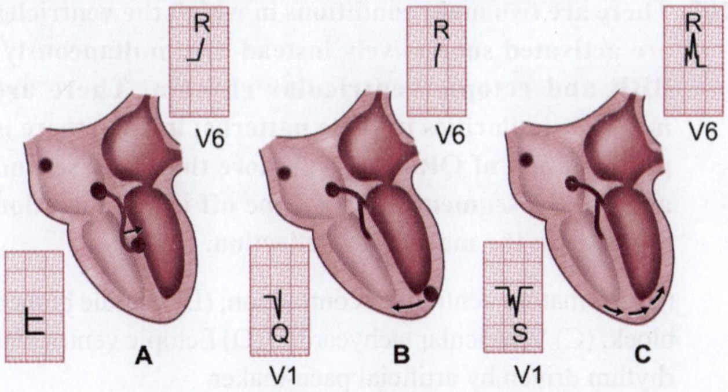

Fig. Q-74: Left bundle branch block

102. The 4 steps in sequence of depolarization in LBBB.

1. Septal depolarization from right to left—Q in V1, R wave in V5, V6; Fig. Q-74A. Note thechange in initial vector
2. RV depolarization from left to right—RV notch in V5, V6—Fig. Q-74B.
3. LV depolarization from right to left—LV—R' in V5, V6—Fig. Q-74C.
4. Secondary ST-T changes opposite of RSR'.

LBBB is best seen in V5, V6 where there is an opposite polarity of QRS, 'M' pattern. The 'W' pattern in V1 is not often fully developed. The absence of Q wave in V5 or V6 is one of the hallmarks of uncomplicated LBBB.

103. Thus, the 4 ECG findings in LBBB are:

1. Small Q in V1 and R in V6
2. R in V1 and S in V6 as a notch
3. S in V1 and another R in V6 giving an 'M' shape.
4. T is opposite of QRS in V5, V6.

104. There are 4 points to be noted in LBBB:

1. There should be no q wave or initial negativity in LI or V5,V6
2. There is a change in vector magnitude in the first half of the QRS, usually shown by a mid-QRS notch or slur.
3. In complete LBBB, the ventricular activation time is 70 msec (07 sec) or more.
4. In LBBB, the right precordial leads will not have terminal positivity

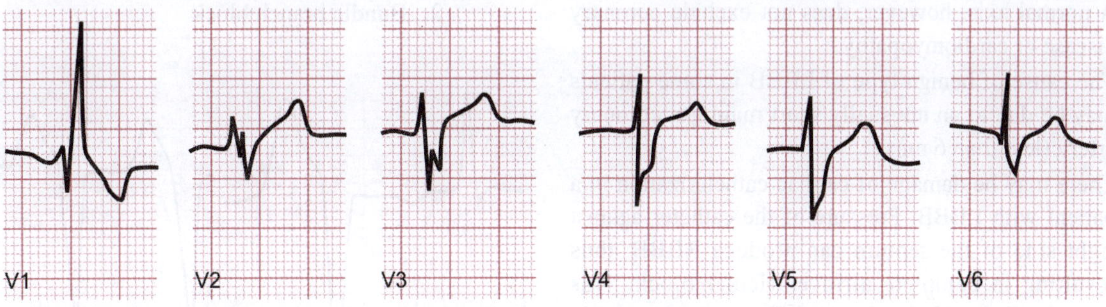

Fig. Q-75: Right bundle branch block best seen in VI, V2. See the RSR pattern in right precordial leads

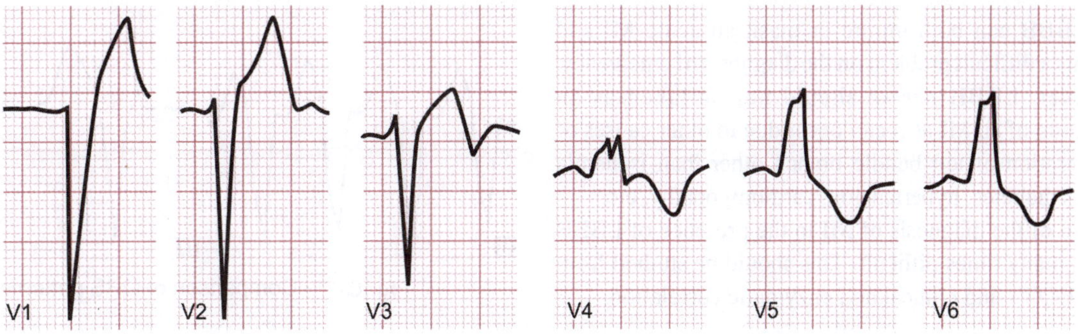

Fig. Q-76: Left bundle branch block: M pattern is best seen in left precordial leads—V5, V6

105. The importance of recognizing LBBB:

1. LBBB has a prognostic significance during infarction. When LBBB is present during acute myocardial infarction, the prognosis is worse than with no bundle branch block. But, there is no difference in infarction mortality whether LBBB developed during infarction or already present long before infarction. Surprisingly, it is RBBB that carries a worse prognosis than LBBB in AMI, in view of the dual blood supply to both bundle branches. The proximal part of the right bundle is supplied by a branch of left anterior descending artery as well as by the right coronary artery. The left bundle is supplied by septal branches of both right and left coronary arteries.
2. In patients with chronic LBBB with a left axis deviation of –30° or more, the incidence of myocardial dysfunction or cardiovascular mortality is more than those with a normal axis.

   For example, in aortic stenosis, a combination of LBBB with marked preoperative left axis deviation significantly increases the incidence of postoperative left ventricular failure and death after valve replacement. Combination of LBBB + LAD probably reflects diffuse myocardial damage since there is no increased incidence of coronary disease in such patients.
3. In chronic LBBB with or without normal axis, the prognosis is determined mainly by the degree of associated cardiovascular disease.

   A normal axis, however, does not exclude coronary disease or cardiomyopathy.

   The cause of benign type of LBBB in some patients may be due to an unusually short main left coronary artery (less than 6 mm).
4. There may be damage of cardiac catheterization in a patient with LBBB. Pressure of the catheter against right side of the septum can produce RBBB, thus resulting in complete atrioventricular block. This is more likely, if the right bundle is already partly blocked, as evidenced by long PR interval.

The LBBB can both mimic or mask an acute MI and presents a difficult problem on the diagnosis of emergency. However, LBBB *per se* should not be taken as an indication of an MI as it can occur due to other causes of degeneration of left bundle branch other than ischemia such as diabetes, hypertension, cardiomyopathy, etc. Beware of the diagnosis of MI in the presence of LBBB as it is many times difficult. This should be studied from serial ECG's and clinical and enzymatic correlation.

106. Usual width of QRS is 0.08 second but is occasionally as long as 0.9 msec (0.09 sec) and especially in young people, it is as short as 50 msec (0.05 sec). A wide QRS is due to conduction defect that has caused slowed or delayed conduction. The slowed conduction may be initial, middle or terminal third or uniformly throughout QRS. The following are 4 examples.

1. The most common conduction defect is bundle branch block
2. The next most common is divisional or fascicular block
3. The initial delay causing widening of QRS is pre-excitation
4. Uniform slowing of throughout QRS is caused by hyperkalemia, excessive dose of quinidine and tricyclic antidepressants.

107. There are two main conditions in which the ventricles are activated successively instead of simultaneously: BBB and ectopic ventricular rhythm. There are marked similarities in these patterns; in each there is prolongation of QRS interval more than 0.12 second and the ST segment finds a slope off in the direction opposite to the main QRS deflection.

(A) Premature ventricular contraction; (B) Bundle branch block; (C) Ventricular tachycardia; (D) Ectopic ventricular rhythm driven by artificial pace-maker.

The conditions where QRS is more than 0.12 second are:

1. Premature ventricular contraction
2. Bundle branch block

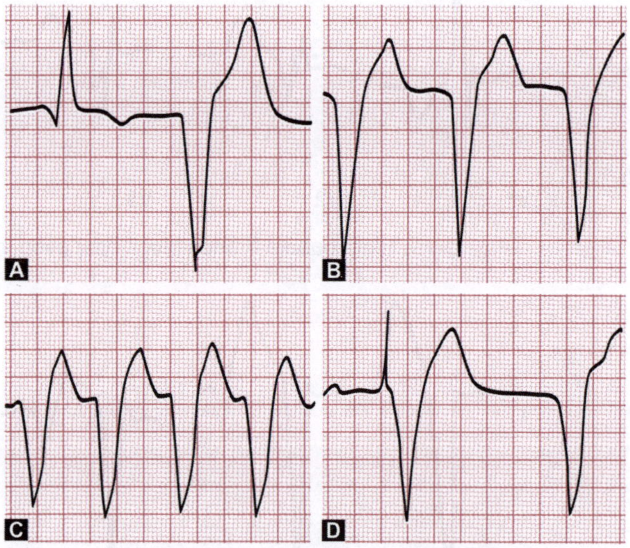

Fig. Q-77: Comparison of QRS patterns

3. Ventricular tachycardia
4. Ectopic ventricular rhythm driven by artificial pace-maker.

All these in common have prolonged QRS interval and ST segment sloping of T wave in direction opposite to main QRS deflection.
T wave polarity opposite to QRS is due to depolarization and repolarization disturbance produced by the block and the T wave changes are secondary.

108. Some other conditions where QRS is more than 0.12 second.

1. Coronary artery disease: Myocardial infarction/ ischemic heart disease
2. Drugs/electrolytes: Quinidine, tetracyclic anti -depressants, digitalis or verapamil, hyperkalemia
3. Cardiomyopathy
4. Myocarditis/fibrositis.

The RBBB is best seen in V1 or V2 where there is RSR pattern.
LBBB is best seen in V5 or V6 where there is notched 'M' pattern.
Remember, BBBs are diagnosed only from precordial leads. Do not attempt to diagnose from limb leads, sometimes it may go wrong.

Hemiblocks/Fascicular Blocks

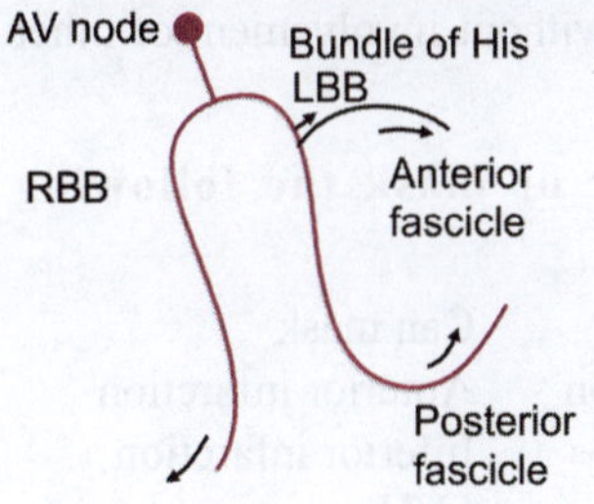

Fig. Q-78: Normal anatomy of bundle branches

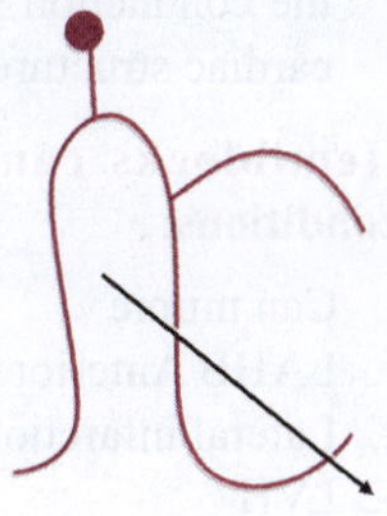
Fig. Q-79: Normal axis

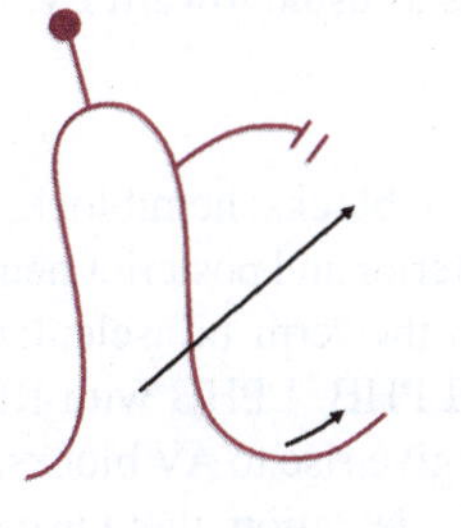
Fig. Q-80: Left anterior hemiblock

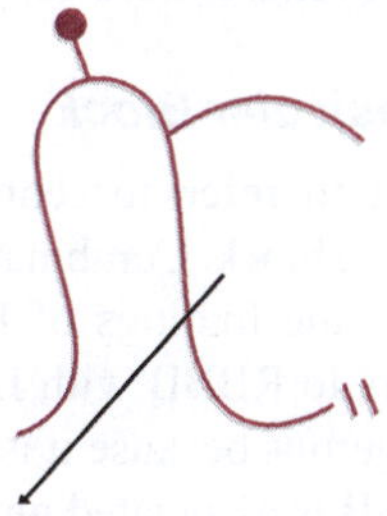
Fig. Q-81: Left posterior Hemiblock

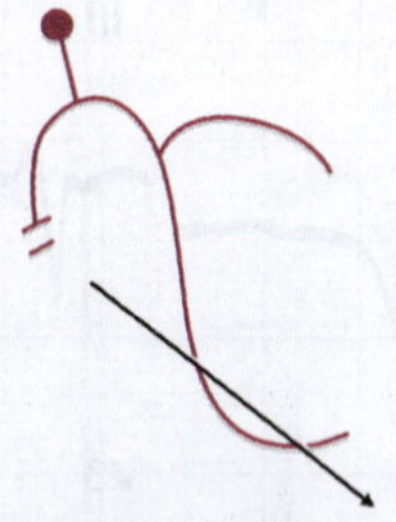
Fig. Q-82: RBBB

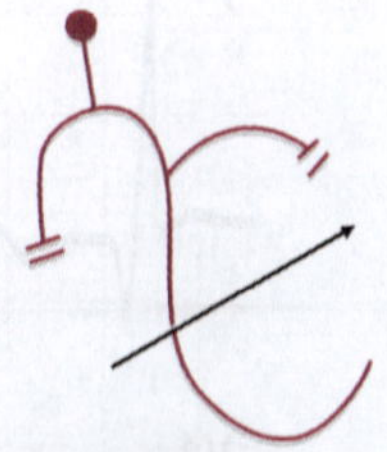
Fig. Q-83: RBBB + LAHB

Right Bundle Branch Block

Conduction problems in the distal parts of the left bundle branch gives rise to hemiblocks. A little detail anatomy of the branches of bundle of His is worth considering now.

The right bundle has no divisions but left bundle has two divisions—the thin anterior and thick posterior fascicle. The anterior division runs towards the base of the anterior papillary muscle of the left ventricle, the posterior division toward the posterior papillary muscle. The right bundle branch, anterior and posterior divisions of left bundle branch are considered as three fascicles from the atrioventricular division. The depolarization wave spreads into ventricles by these three routes—Fig. Q-78 Normal anatomy of bundle branches.

The cardiac axis depends on average direction of depolarization of the ventricles. Since the left ventricle contains greater muscle mass than the right ventricle, it has greater influence on the cardiac axis.
(Fig. Q-79 Normal axis).

Left Anterior Hemiblock (LAHB)

When the anterior fascicle of the left bundle branch blocks, the current cannot pass through it. Therefore, the current passes through the posterior fascicle which results in upward rotation of cardiac axis. LAD deviation is due to LAHB or left anterior fascicular block—Fig. Q-80 LAHB.

109. On the ECG, LAHB has the following 4 characters.

1. Left axis deviation (usually –60°) because the terminal forces are redirected leftward and superiorly.
2. Q1 S3 pattern
3. QRS normal or slightly widened (0.10 to 0.12 second)
4. Increase in depth of S waves in precordial leads.

The LAHB may mask the signs of LVH or lateral wall ischemia in left precordial leads. It may mask the signs of inferior wall infarct or ischemia.

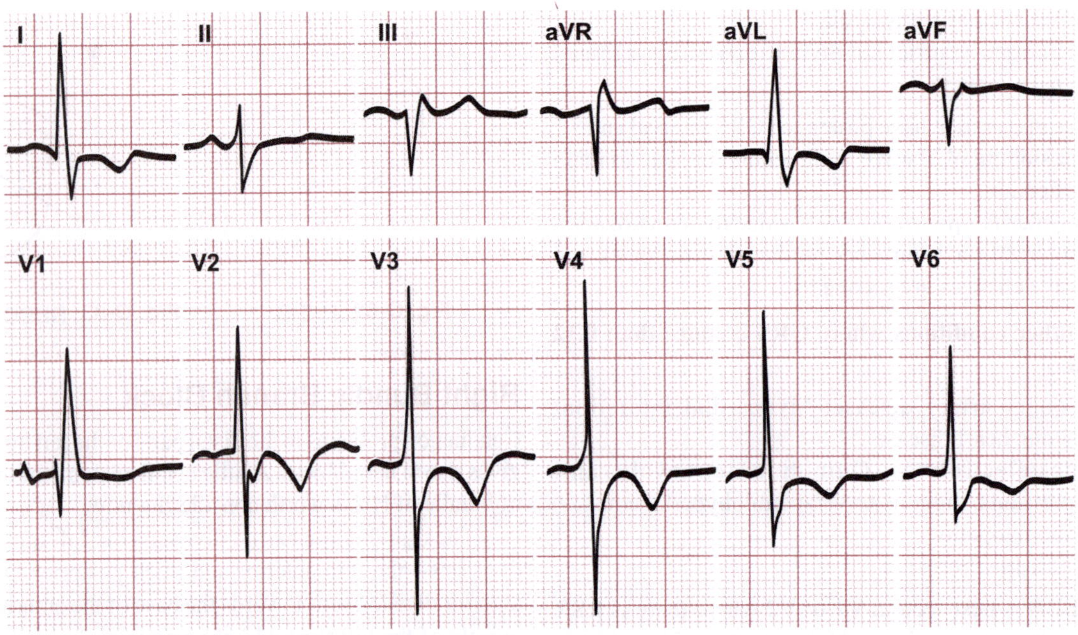

Fig. Q-84: RBBB with LAD = LAHB. See the wide S wave in V1 and V6 and rsR' pattern in V1. The T waves in LI, aVL and V2 to V6 are primary T wave changes

Left Posterior Hemiblock (LPHB)

The posterior deviation of the LBB is not often selectively blocked because the posterior division is thicker than the anterior division and has a double blood supply and hence it is less prone to damage. See Fig. Q-81 LPHB.

110. On the ECG, LPHB has the following 4 characters:

1. Right axis deviation (usually +120°) because the terminal forces are redirected rightward and inferiorly
2. Normal QRS duration
3. S1 Q3 pattern
4. No evidence of right ventricular hypertrophy.

RVH and vertical heart should be excluded before diagnosing the LPHB.

When RBBB is blocked the cardiac axis is normal because more current passes as usual toward left ventricle. See Fig. Q-82 RBBB

The left anterior hemiblock is common. Left posterior hemiblock is rare because it is thicker than anterior division and it has a double blood supply. It is an inflow-tract structure and thus avoids the stresses of outflow pressure and proximity to the danger area of the aortic valve.

111. The causes of hemiblocks are:

1. Commonly ischemic heart disease, acute myocardial infarction
2. Cardiomyopathy
3. Aortic valve calcification; it is possible for calcific lesions to impinge upon one, two or three fascicles (Lev's disease)
4. Lenegre's disease—sclerodegenerative changes within the conduction system without involvement of other cardiac structures.

112. Hemiblocks can mimic or mask the following conditions:

	Can mimic	Can mask
1.	LAHB Anterior infarction	Anterior infarction
2.	Lateral infarction	Inferior infarction
3.	LVH	LVH
4.	LPHB Anterior infarction	Anterior infarction

When RBBB is blocked, the cardiac axis usually normal, because more current passes as usual toward LV.

Bifascicular Block

The term refers to a combination of blocks; hemiblock, bundle branch block. Combination of anterior and posterior hemiblock gives the findings of LBBB, so the term bifascicular block refers to RBBB with LAHB or LPHB. LPHB with RBBB is dangerous because it is likely to give rise to AV blocks. When LBBB is associated with left axis deviation, there is evidence that the prognosis is less favorable than when the axis remains normal.

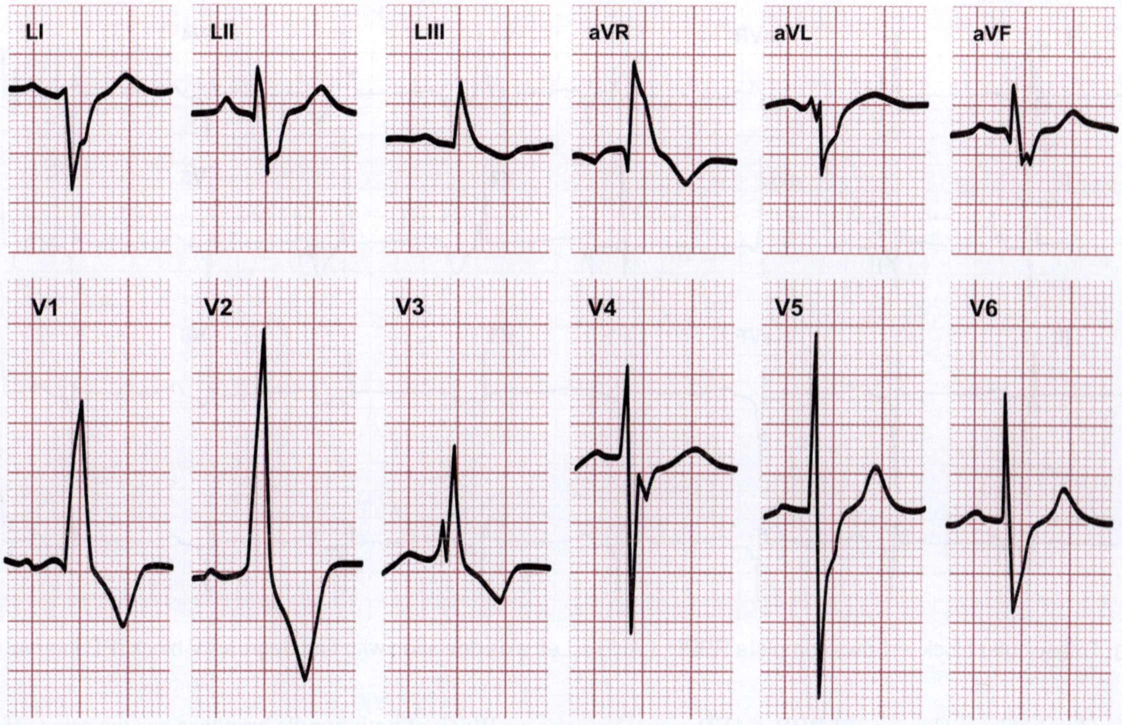

Fig. Q-85

In RBBB with LAHB, ECG shows LAD—Fig. Q-85
RBBB + LAHB
RBBB with marked right axis deviation (uncommon type of RBBB)
RBBB with RAD = LPHB
RBBB = LPHB – RAD.

These patterns obviously indicate widespread damage to the conducting system.

Trifascicualr Block

If the RBB and both fascicles of the LBB are blocked, complete heart block occurs. It gives the same findings of His bundle block. Block of three fascicles or bilateral bundle branch block (BBBB) is a life-threatening complication of anterior myocardial infarction. It may be indicated by LBBB with prolonged PR interval or RBBB with prolonged PR interval. Therefore, history of syncope in a patient with either LBBB or RBBB with marked axis deviation calls for thorough urgent assessment.

This figure shows complete right bundle branch block (RBBB), left anterior hemiblock (LAHB) and long PR interval. The combination of RBBB, LAHB and long PR interval has been called 'Trifascicular block'. It implies that conduction is delayed in the fascicle. A permanent pacemaker may be needed in this patient. However, there are other causes of a long PR interval such as delayed conduction in the AV node or atrium, so 'trifascicular block' is not a true ECG diagnosis.

Trifascicular block, this term can be appropriately applied to simultaneous block, complete or incomplete in any three out of five ventricular conducting fascicles—bundle of His, RBB, LBBB, anterior and posterior divisions of the LBB; but it is specifically mentioned to the three peripheral fascicles—RBB and the two divisions of the LBB. If all the three fascicles are blocked "complete AV block" results. Eight possible combinations of blocks can occur out of these three peripheral fascicular blocks.

Trifascicular block is a degenerative disease of the conducting system. This degeneration usually occurs below the AV node. Since RBBB and left anterior fascicles are thinner, they are commonly involve before another block supervenes in left posterior fascicle producing the complete heart block; this condition may be associated with degenerative disease of SA node also—"The sick sinus syndrome".

Trifascicular block is the most common form of complete form heart block in adults. The definitive treatment is permanent pacemaker implantation.

113. The possible 8 combinations are:

	RBB	LAD	LPD	ECG findings
1.	C	C	C	Complete AVB
2.	C	C	I	RBBB + LAH + AVB
3.	C	I	C	RBBB + LPH + AVB

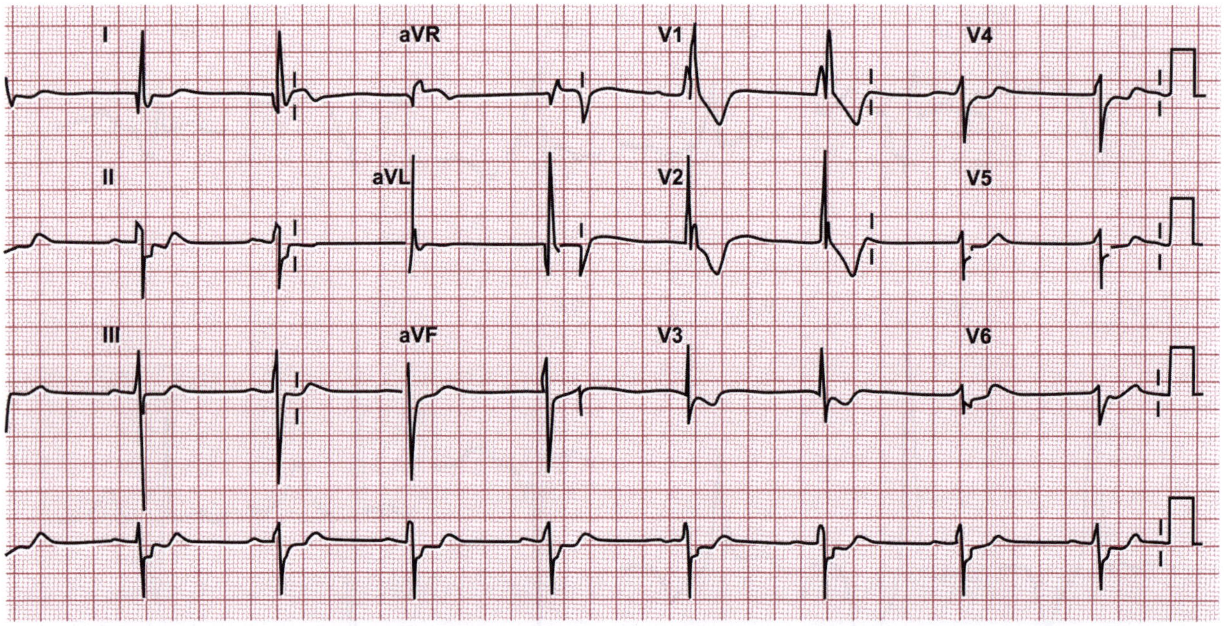

Fig. Q-86: Trifascicular block—shows complete RBBB, LAHB = Left axis deviation with first degree AV block (PR interval 0.12 sec)

4.	I	C	C	LBBB + AVB
5.	C	I	I	} various combinations
6.	I	C	I	] depending upon relative
7.	I	I	C	} degrees of incomplete
8.	I	I	I	] fascicular block

C = completely blocked; I = incompletely blocked; "AVB' = manifestations of 1st and 2nd degree AV block

Intermittent Bundle Branch Block

BBB may sometimes be permanent or intermittent or transient.

Bilateral Bundle Branch Block (BBBB)

If both bundle branches are completely blocked, no impulse can reach the ventricles. This results in complete AV block. If a branch is completely blocked and the other only partially blocked—results in either prolonged PR interval, i.e. first degree block of dropped beats or second degree block.

114. Therefore, the evidence of BBBB can be:

1. First degree block + BBB
2. Second degree block + BBB
3. Complete AV block
4. Sometimes RRBB sometimes LBBB.

This is an absolute evidence of that both bundle branches are involved. Since first, second and third degree blocks can be produced by other conditions also.

Block of both bundle branches has the same effect as the block of His bundle and causes complete heart block (3rd degree).

115. The following are the causes of RSR' variants in V1 to V2.

1. Occurs in 5% of normal people
2. Frequently occur in pectus or straight back deformities
3. Incomplete RBBB
4. RV enlargement
5. Acute cor pulmonale
6. Diastolic overloading of RV
7. WPW syndrome
8. Duchenne dystrophy.
   (See the point 24 for tall R waves)

116. Some notable points in bundle branch blocks:

1. Bundle branch blocks are diagnosed by RSR' pattern in the chest leads
2. If the RSR' pattern is in right chest leads V1, V2, then it is called right bundle branch block. If the RSR' pattern is in the left chest leads V5, V6 then it is called left bundle branch block
3. Bundle branch blocks are said to be complete if the RSR' pattern duration is more than 0.12 sec or incomplete if it is less than 0.12 sec
4. Intermittent bundle branch blocks, i.e. prolonged RSR' pattern present at times but not all times, probably

represents a transition stage before permanent block is established

5. Left bundle branch block and right bundle branch block occur with about same frequency (according to some RBBB is more frequent than LBBB)
6. Coronary disease is the most common cause of bundle branch block
7. In left bundle branch block, normal initial septal activation from left to right is disturbed, which results in the absence of Q waves in left precordial leads, which is one of the hallmarks of uncomplicated LBBB. Q waves in the left ventricular leads may be present or exaggerated in left ventricular hypertrophy, but in LBBB, these normal Q waves are absent
8. In bundle branch block, the ST is depressed with T wave directed to opposite of the terminal of the QRS complex. This opposite polarity is the natural result of depolarization-repolarization disturbance produced by the block and the T wave changes are therefore known as 'secondary'. They are no more than the block itself
9. Uncomplicated RBBB or LBBB do not show axis deviation
10. Bifascicular blocks are diagnosed by abnormal left or right axis deviation associated with RBBB
11. Trifascicular blocks are diagnosed in the presence of bifascicular block with prolonged PR interval of more than 0.2 sec, i.e. first degree AV block
12. LBBB causes less favorable prognosis than RBBB.

117. Causes of bundle branch blocks:

1. Coronary artery disease/acute MI
2. Rheumatic
3. Syphilis
4. Trauma
5. Tumor
6. Cardiomyopathy (HOCM, endomyocardial fibrosis)/ myocarditis)
7. Congenital
   a. Incomplete RBBB in ASD in 90%
   b. Ebstein's anomaly—RBBB is the rule
   c. Total anomalous pulmonary venous return
8. Aortic valve calcification/aortic stenosis (14% may have with severe aortic stenosis)
9. Lev's disease
10. Lenegre's disease
11. Drugs—digitalis
12. Following surgery for VSD, muscular subaortic stenosis

118. For exercise

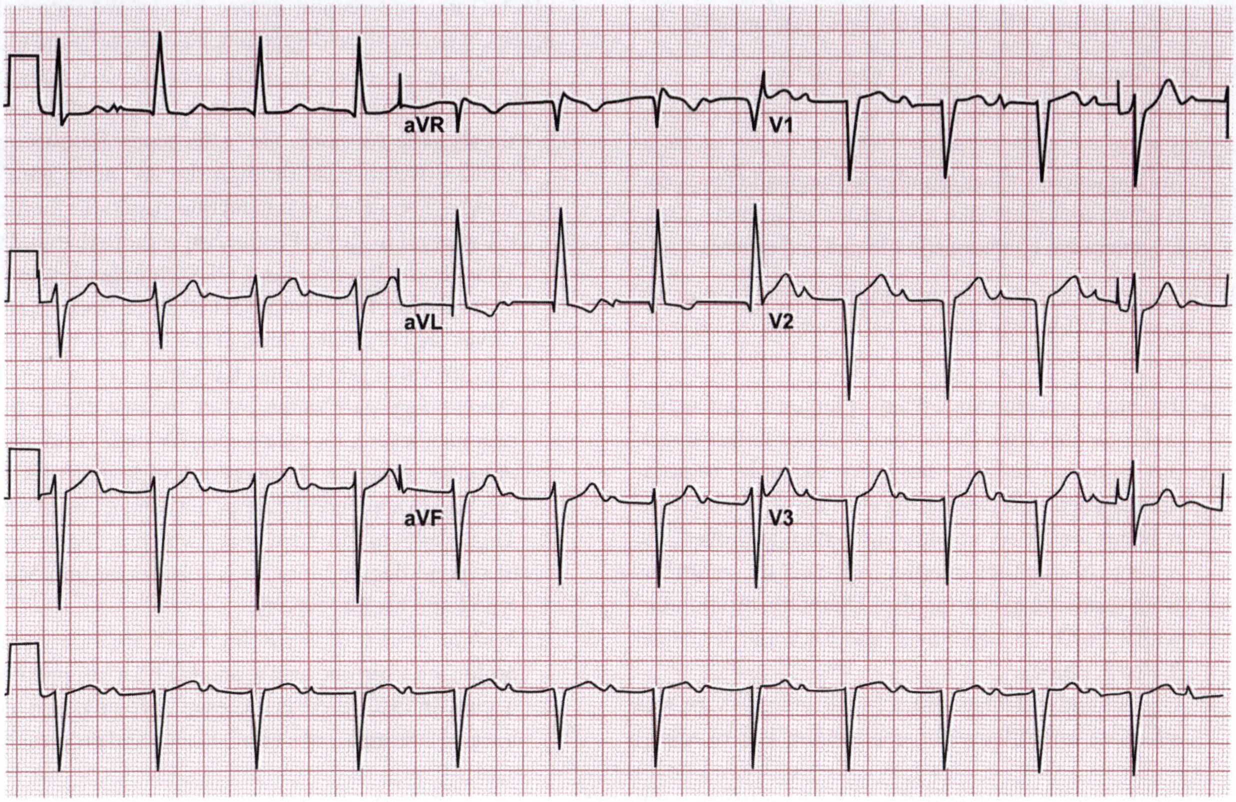

Fig. Q-87

Following are the abnormalities in the ECG

1. Left anterior hemiblock (LAHB)
   - LAD—QRS axis more than –30°
   - initial R wave in the inferior leads (II, III, aVF)
   - absence of any other cause of left axis deviation.
2. Left ventricular hypertrophy (LVH):
   In the presence of left anterior hemiblock the diagnostic criteria of LVH are changed. Rosenbaum suggested that an S wave in lead III deeper than 15 mm as predictive of LVH
3. Long PR interval (first degree AV block)
   PR interval longer than 0.2 sec
4. Left atrial hypertrophy (LAH)
   - M shaped P wave in lead II
   - P wave duration > 0.11 sec
   - Terminal negative component to the P wave in lead V1

Heart Block

Heart block usually means, the block at atrioventricular node (AV block). Atrioventricular junction is the only passage available for the current to travel from the atria to the ventricles as the rest of the AV ring and AV valves (mitral and tricuspid valves) are made of nonconducting fibrous tissue. AV node or bundle of His works as a "gatekeeper" to conduct the impulses from atria to ventricles. A delay in conduction through this juncture may be due to degeneration, fibrosis, destruction, inflammation, etc.

119. Thus, the heart blocks may be caused by:

1. Drugs like digitalis, beta-blocker, calcium channel blocker
2. Inflammation, such as diphtheria, rheumatic fever, etc.
3. Ishemic conditions like myocardial infarction
4. Degenerative conditions in old age and others.

120. The following 4 important points are to be known about the AV block in general before going into details of specific types.

1. The block is an abnormal delay or failure of conduction and is distinct from the normal delay or failure due to physiological refractoriness. For example, in atrial flutter, when atria are beating at a rate of 300 bpm—it is better for the AV conducting system to prevent the passage of impulses in order to protect the ventricles from receiving every impulse. Therefore, atrial flutter with 2:1 or 3:1 conduction is a more accurate term than 2:1 or 3:1 block.
2. One should not diagnose a block unless there was adequate opportunity for conduction. For example, if accelerated idioventricular rhythm develops and takes away control from the sinus node at a faster rate, the lower pacemaker may remain dissociated from the higher for many cycles—resulting with P waves traveling just behind the QRS with no chance of conduction to the ventricles. This is dissociation, yet no block.
3. Definition of degrees of block are only relatively accurate because the significance of block must always be assessed in the light of heart rate. Thus, 4 to 1 conduction when the atrial rate is 300 in atrial flutter is a satisfactory affair, but it is not a satisfactory affair with 4 to 1 conduction when the atrial rate is 80 bpm. Again the complications are far different if the atria is at a rate 70 bpm are dissociated from ventricles beating at 80 bpm.
4. Finally, it is now clear that block and dissociation are not synonymous. AV dissociation can be due to many causes, of which block is but one cause.

121. Classification of blocks (See Arrhythmias D 244-283)

From the ECG point, heart blocks or AV blocks are diagnosed in three degrees of severity.

(Second degree is subdivided into Mobitz type I and Mobitz type II = total 4)

AV block is also divided into incomplete and complete block. First and second degree blocks are incomplete blocks, whereas third degree block is the complete block.

1. *First degree AV block:* Here every P wave activity is conducted through AV junction to the ventricles but slowly. The AV node, the 'gatekeeper', allows every atrial wave to pass through the AV node gate but slowly. The delay in conduction results in increased PR interval in ECG. PR interval is more than 0.2 sec. Thus, every P wave has a QRS complex but the PR interval is prolonged more than 0.2 sec, because all the waves are conducted through the AV node but slowly. PR interval is greater than 0.2 sec.
   Second degree AV block: When the first degree block becomes severe, the gatekeeper, AV node conducts the impulses slowly with increasing time intervals from one beat to another till it drops out conduction of a beat. This results in 'dropped beat', which is characteristic of second degree block. It is subdivided into Mobitz type I and Mobitz type II.
2. *Mobitz type I:* The PR intervals are increasingly prolonged from one beat to another till a 'dropped beat' occurs. In ECG, there is successive prolongation of PR interval starting from a normal value and progressively

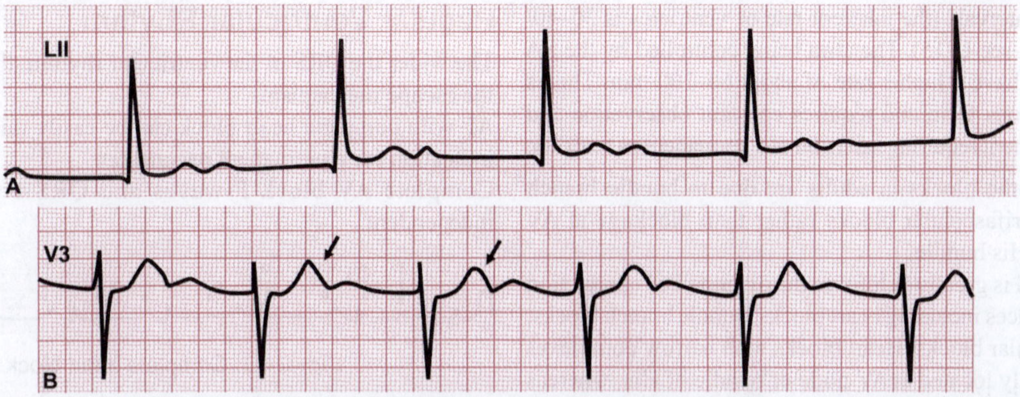

Fig. Q-88: A. Shows the PR interval is about 0.59 sec. B. Two of the P waves are indicated by arrows where the PR interval is about 0.46 sec

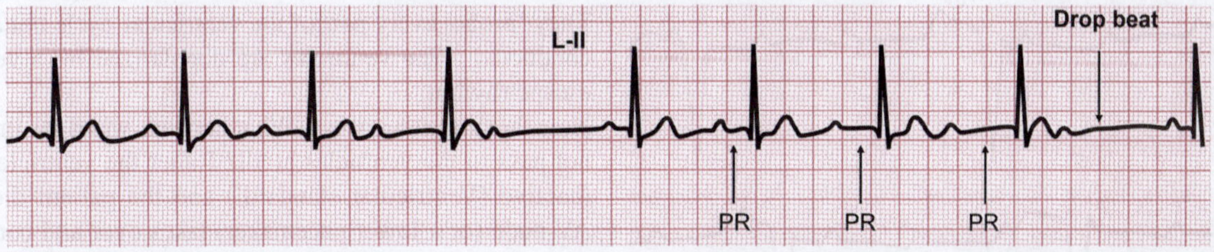

Fig. Q-89: Mobitz type I block (See also Fig. D-45): Progressive lengthening of PR intervals until a beat is dropped

increasing to abnormal values and ending in a dropped beat – with a pause- P without QRS.

In 1899, Wenckebach in Vienna, noticed dropped beats in jugular venous pulse tracing and observed in that dropped beat was preceded by a progressive prolongation of the interval between atrial and ventricular conduction. He described this before the advent of ECG (1902). Wenckebach again in 1906, without the help of ECG, observed dropped beats preceded by constant AV conduction intervals. It was 20 years later, that Mobitz proposed that these two forms of incomplete AV block be called type I and type II, respectively.

3. *Mobitz type II block:* In this, the AV node, gatekeeper, allows some waves to pass freely and some do not. When the P waves are followed by QRS regularly, some of the atrial waves are not allowed to pass through it. Some P waves have QRS complexes following them, while others do not have any apparent reason. This is a more serious type of second degree block as it may lead to slow heart rate of complete heart block. Depending in the number of P waves to the number of QRS waves following them, it is described as 2:1, 3:1 heart block.

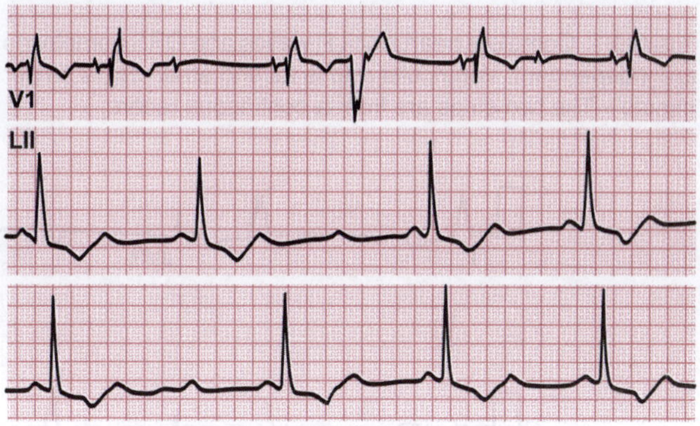

Fig. Q.90: Mobitz type II AV block (see also Fig. D-46)
Second degree Mobitz type II AV block

4. *Third degree heart block or complete heart block:* It is the most dangerous form of AV block where there is no relation between the P waves and the QRS complexes. AV node, the gatekeeper, does not allow any wave passing through it from the atria to ventricles. No P wave is conducted through the AV node and so the P wave and QRS wave are entirely independent of each other. In this condition, the QRS complexes are produced by the ventricles themselves at a slow rate with long

RR intervals (the inherent rate of ventricles is 30–40/min—see D-15). The atria being controlled by the SA node have a higher rate of about 60–100/min. This is a serious form and requires constant observation and treatment requiring insertion of a permanent pacemaker.

Most of the blocks in adults are due to bundle branch blocks, trifascicular blocks rather than blockage at AV node or His bundle.

The ECG is greatly helpful in the diagnosis of conduction disturbances including heart blocks, bundle branch blocks, trifascicular blocks. Heart blocks with narrow complexes are usually located at AV node or bundle of His, whereas a heart block with wide QRS complexes are usually fascicular blocks below the bundle of His.

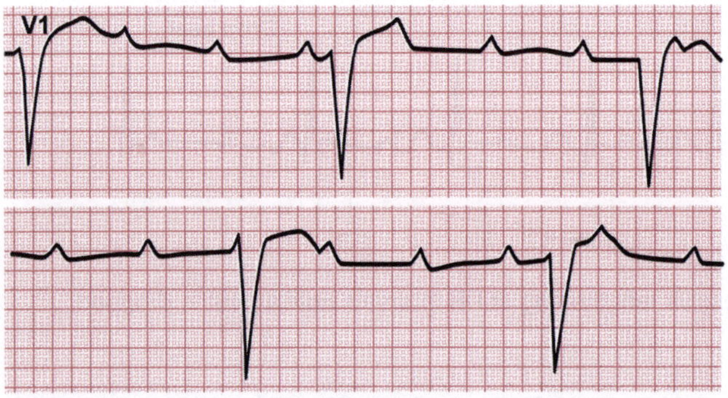

Fig. Q-91: Complete heart block P waves and QRS complexes are independent. Ventricular rate is 28 and atrial rate is 96 per minute—The two strips are from a continuous record

Regular Ventricular Rhythm

The wider the QRS of the ventricular rhythm, the less reliable the escape mechanism.

AF with complete heart block can be easily missed and is an indication for a permanent pacemaker.

Complete AV block P waves and QRS complexes are independent.

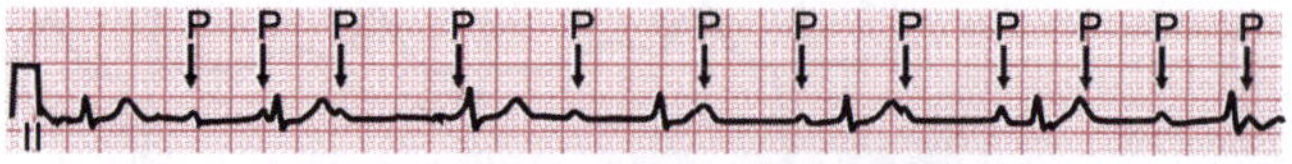

Fig. Q-93: Complete heart block

Complete heart block: P waves are not conduced to the ventricles because of block at the AV node. The P waves are indicated below and show no relation to the QRS complexes. They 'probe' every part of the ventricular cycle but are never conducted . The ventricles are depolarized by a ventricular escape rhythm.

Now the question arises—What happens when the impulse do not pass to the ventricles at all? Either the ventricles remain inactive (Ventricular standstill) and the patient dies or the AV node (or a lower pacemaker) takes over and controls the ventricles (nodal or ventricular escape). The result is that atria continue to beat in their own way and the ventricles beat in slower rate. The atria may continue to beat at a rate of 90/min, while the ventricles beat at a rate of 30 /min. This is easily recognized in ECG by the lack of relationship between the slow QRS ventricular rate and more frequent atrial P waves. Each has its own rhythm.

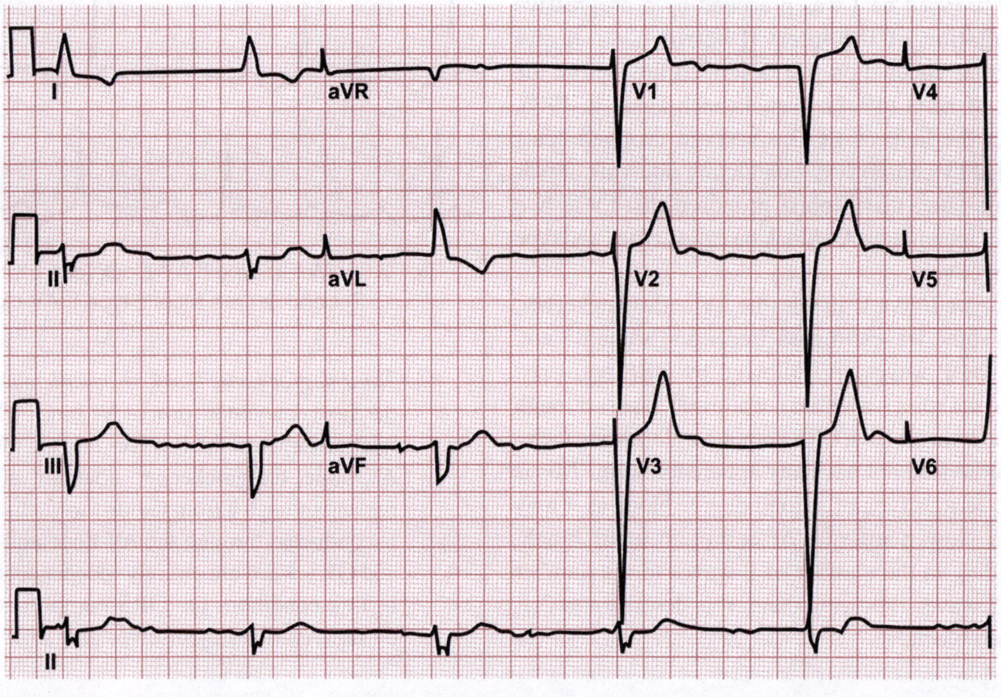

Fig. Q-92: Atrial fibrillation and complete heart block 'F' waves of atrial fibrillation and no P waves

122. Complete heart block (CHB) should be differentiated from atrioventricular dissociation (AVD).

Table Q-3

Atrioventricular dissociation (AVD)	*Complete heart block (CHB)*
1. It is a functional block of the AV node	It is an organic block
2. Temporary, reversible	Permanent, not reversible
3. Junctional or ventricular tissue fires at a faster rate than the sinus node so that AV node becomes refractory to the slower sinus impulse. Ventricular beat is faster than atrial beat	Ventricular beat is very slow than atrial beat. (The inherent rate of ventricle)
4. Antigrade conduction is intact as noticed by occasional passing of the sinus beat producing the 'capture beat' in the ventricle	As the defect is organic in the AV junction, there is no antegrade conduction—so there is no capture beat
5. Usually occurs in i. Digitalis toxicity ii. Inflammatory conditions like infectious endocarditis iii. MI iv. Postcardiac surgery In all these, there is increase automaticity, the ventricle with edema around the AV node causing a retrograde block	
6. Does not require a pacemaker as it is transient and reversible	Needs a permanent pacemaker
7. No hemodynamic consequences as the ventricular rate being faster	Hemodynamic consequences occur
8. Not serious	Serious

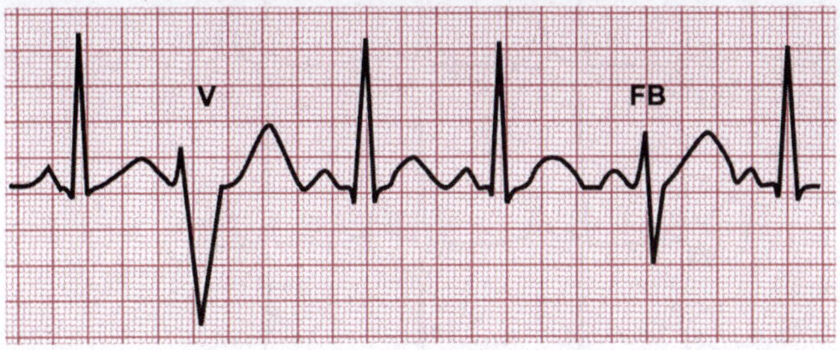

Fig. Q-94: ECG showing ventricular ectopic beat and fusion beat

123. Causes of marked bradycardia: Complete AV block is perhaps the most common cause of marked bradycardia. The conditions at a rate of 30 to 50 may occur in complete AV or SA blocks.

1. Blocks—SA block, second degree AV block, complete AV block and idioventricular rhythm
2. Sinus bradycardia
3. Tachycardias: Atrial flutter with high grades of AV block, e.g. 8:1 block with an atrial rate of 320 giving a ventricular rate of 40. Atrial fibrillation with marked AV block.
4. AV nodal rhythm

ACCELERATED CONDUCTION AROUND THE AV JUNCTION

There is an abnormal pathway of Kent – where the conduction bypass the AV node and directly goes from the atria to the ventricles. These conductions are diagnosed by short PR interval and abnormal notch in the QRS complex called delta wave. There are two well-known conditions—Wolff-Parkinson-White syndrome and Lown-Ganong-Levine syndrome, which are associated with clinical and ECG features of tachyarrhythmias.

Wolff-Parkinson-White Syndrome

Impulses originate from SA node and pre-excite peripheral conduction system and ventricles via an accessory pathway bypassing the AV node. This is thought to derive from incomplete separation of the muscular bundles of the atria and ventricles during the fetal development. After delay at AV node impulses also travel to ventricles via normal route to continue depolarization. A small portion of the ventricular myocardium is thus excited early, which results in early slurred upstroke of the QRS complex called (pre-excitation wave or delta wave). QRS appears prolonged not because it lasted longer but because it started earlier as a result of pre-excitation.

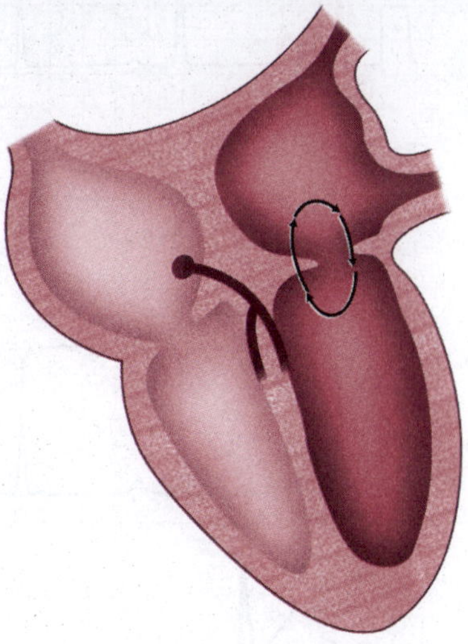

Fig. Q-95: Wolff-Parkinson-White (WPW) syndrome or pre-excitation syndrome

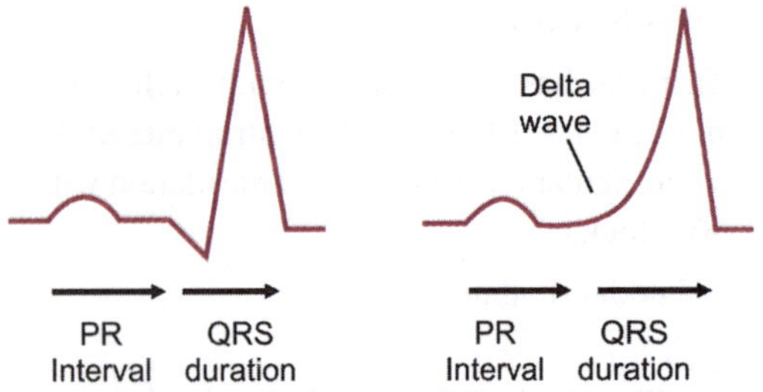

Fig. Q-96

The QRS is much longer than normal as the PR interval is shorter than normal. The PR interval usually measures 0.10 second. or less and the P wave is normal.

This purely electrocardiographic 'syndrome' has superficial resemblance to bundle branch block and therefore, sometimes been called as 'pseudobundle branch block'. In bundle branch block, the blocked ventricle is activated late so that the super added deflection is followed at the end of the normal QRS. PR interval untouched. In WPW syndrome the super added deflection is attached in front of the normal QRS, which results in shortening of PR interval by as much as lengthens QRS interval. In bundle branch block QRS is prolonged because one ventricle is activated late. Whereas in WPW syndrome one ventricle (or part of a ventricle) is activated abnormally early (pre-excitation).

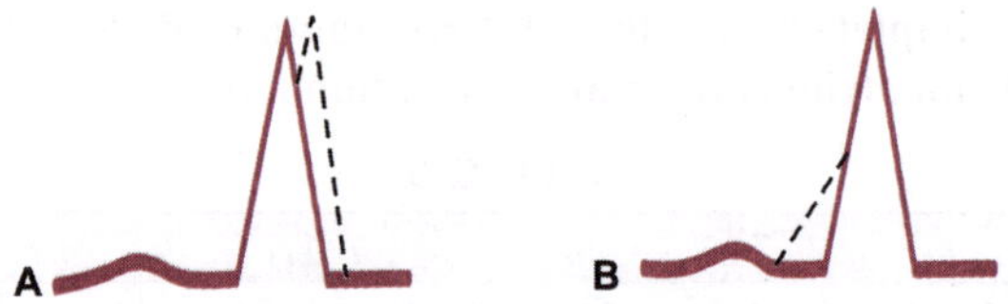

Fig. Q-97: A. Bundle branch block; B. Wolff-Parkinson-White syndrome, diagrammatic comparison (Ref. Fig. D-22)

124. WPW syndrome has the following 4 characteristics:

1. A shortened PR interval (< 0.12 sec) as the electrical impulse bypasses the normal delay produced by the AV node.
2. The presence of delta wave, a slurring of the initial upstroke of the QRS complex.
3. A widened QRS duration (> 0.12 sec) due to the pre-excitation of one ventricle and the asynchronous depolarization of both ventricles.
4. ST-T wave changes, with the direction of the T wave opposite to that of the QRS.

A Shortened PR interval may be the only ECG feature differentiating WPW syndrome from other conditions when the QRS > 0.12 second such as ischemic heart disease, left ventricular hypertrophy and bundle branch block.

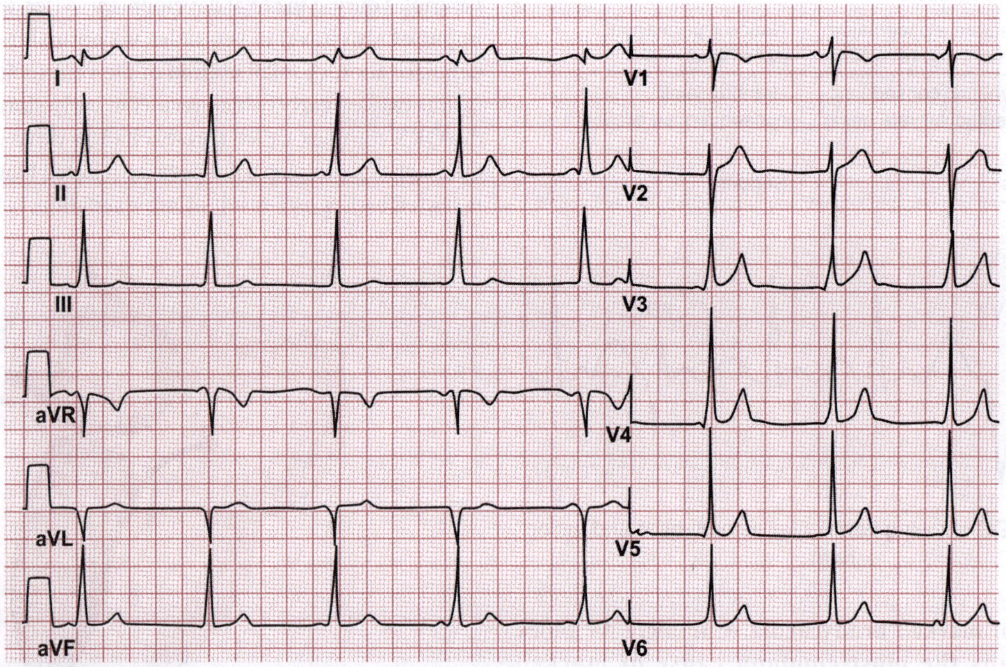

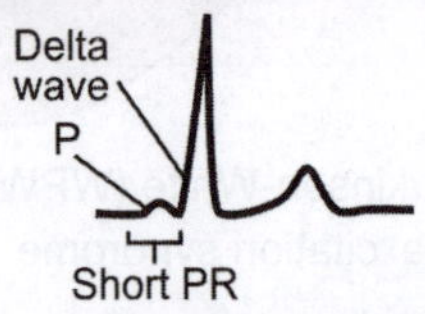

Fig. Q-98: Wolff-Parkinson-White syndrome. Short PR intervals with delta waves

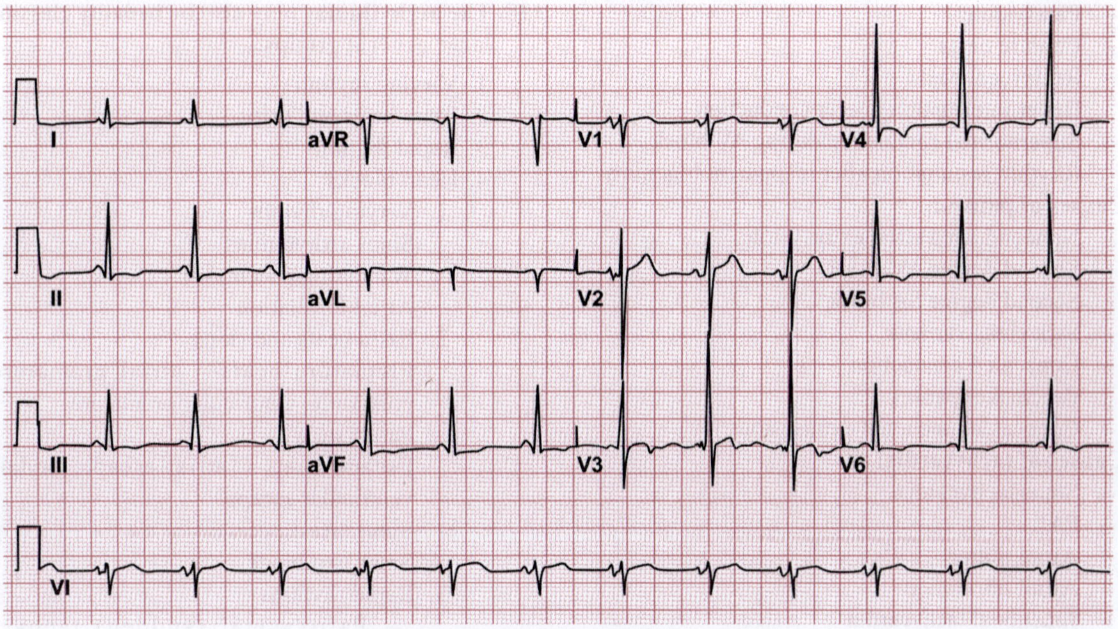

Fig. Q-99: Lown-Ganong-Levine syndrome

125. Localizing the accessory pathway of WPW syndrome: An accessory pathway of Kent, exists between atria and ventricles and causes early depolarization of the ventricle. The location of the accessory pathway may be deduced as follows:

Location	V1	V2	QRS axis
1. Left posteroseptal (type A)	+ve	+ve	left
2. Right lateral (type B)	–ve	–ve	left
3. Left lateral (type C)	+ve	+ve	inferior (90°)
4. Right posteroseptal	–ve	–ve	left
5. Anteroseptal	–ve	–ve	normal

WPW Syndrome

If the delta wave is positive in the right ventricular leads (V1 to V3) mimicking RBBB, it is called type A, whereas a negative delta wave in these leads mimicking LBBB pattern is called type B, WPW syndrome. Various forms of tachycardia, especially SVT with reentry occur frequently in these syndrome.

126. Lown-Ganong-Levine syndrome: It has the following 4 features:

1. Short PR interval of less than 0.12 sec (< 3 small squares)
2. No delta wave
3. Narrow QRS complex
4. Propensity to AV nodal reentry

Short PR without delta wave

It can be differentiated from the Wolff-Parkinson-White syndrome by the absence of delta waves and the normal QRS duration. The other features are same.

RHYTHM

(Refer the chapter on Cardiac Arrhythmias).

Many disturbances of rhythm and conduction are recognizable at first glance. For example, one can immediately recognize atrial flutter with 4:1 conduction, atrial fibrillation with rapid ventricular response or sinus rhythm with RBBB. There are, however, several dysrhythmias that defy immediate reorganization and it is for these we require a systematic approach:

127. Causes: Eight basic arrhythmias are – ECG wise

1. Early beats
2. Unexpected pauses
3. Tachycardia
4. Bradycardia
5. Bigeminal rhythms
6. Group beating
7. Total irregularities
8. Regular non-sinus rhythm at normal rates.

1. Causes of early beats:

- Extrasystole—atrial, ventricular, junctional

- Parasystole
- Capture beats
- Reciprocal beats
- Better interruption poorer conduction
- Supernormal conduction during AV block
- Rhythm resumption after inapparent bigeminy

2. Causes of pauses:
- Nonconducted atrial extrasystole
- Second degree AV block
- Second degree SA block
- Sick sinus variants
- Concealed conduction
- Pacemaker pauses
- Concealed junctional extrasystole

3. Causes of tachycardia:
- Sinus tachycardia
- PAT
- Atrial flutter
- Atrial fibrillation
- Junctional tachycardia
- Ventricular tachycardia
- Ventricular flutter
- Ventricular fibrillation

4. Causes of bradycardia:
- Sinus bradycardia
- SA block
- AV block
- Nonconducted atrial bigeminy

5. Skeleton classification of bigeminy:
- Extrasystoles—atrial, ventricular
- Parasystoles
- 3:2 conduction
- Reciprocal beating
- Fortuitous pairing in atrial fibrillation

6. Common causes of group beating:
- SVT with wencheback periods
- Atrial flutter with 2:1 fluttering
- Sinus rhythm with two or more consecutive extrasytoles
- Recurrent bursts of tachycardia with ventricular SVT
- Every third beat an interrupted ventricular extrasystoles

7. Common causes of chaotic irregularities
- Atrial fibrillation
- Atrial flutter with varying AV conduction
- Chaotic (multifocal) atrial tachycardia
  Shifting (wandering) pacemaker with atrial extrasystole

8. Sinus rhythm with multifocal extrasystole
- Mixed ventricular rhythm

128. The arrhythmias may also be broadly classified into 4 large general groups:

1. Varying rhythm
2. Extra beats and skips
3. Rapid rhythm
4. Heart blocks
   1. Varying rhythm
      Sinus arrhythmias
      Wandering pacemaker
      Atrial fibrillation
   2. Extra beats and skips
      Premature beats – atrial premature, nodal premature, ventricular premature
      Parasystole
      Escape beats – atrial escape, nodal escape, ventricular escape
      Sinus arrest
      Sinus exit block
   3. Rapid rhythms
      - Paroxysmal (sudden) tachycardia – Paroxysmal atrial tachycardia, paroxysmal nodal tachycardia, proxysmal ventricular tachycardia
      - Atrial flutter
        Ventricular flutter
        Atrial fibrillation
        Ventricular fibrillation
   4. Heart blocks
      - SA block
      - AV block

129. Following points are to be checked for rhythm, abnormal waves, pauses, irregularities, etc.

1. Check for P wave for its morphology—Chern the P waves
2. Check for QRS for its morphology—MILK the QRS
3. Check the relation between P wave and QRS waves. Is every P wave followed by QRS? Is every QRS preceded by P wave?
4. Measure the RR interval routinely for rate, rhythm. Is it regular or irregular?
5. Measure the PR interval. Normal 0.12 to 0.2 sec. (3 to 5 small squares). More than 0.2 sec is suggestive of AV block. Less than 0.12 sec is suggestive of abnormal pathway, or the atria have been depolarized close to the AV node.
6. Measure the QRS duration (normally 2 to 2.5 mm, i.e. 0.08 to 0.1 sec). If more than 3 squares, i.e. 0.12 sec, it is definitely abnormal—see for BBB.
7. Measure the QT interval for arrhythmias, drugs and electrolyte effects.

(Wave is present in the intervals. No wave is present in the segment. PR segment, ST segment, TP segment —have no waves—isoelectrical).

8. Check for any atrial or ventricular ectopics.

130. Following 4 simple observations help to diagnose arrhythmias.

1. P waves for atrial rhythm (cherchez le P).
2. QRS complexes for ventricular rhythm (MILK the QRS). Give priority to QRS behavior in the detection of arrhythmias.
   Measure the QRS duration in at least two leads because it may be that initial or terminal forces are isoelectric in a particular lead, causing QRS to appear narrow in that lead only.
   If the QRS is of normal duration, the rhythm is supraventricular, but if it is wide and bizarre, it may be supraventricular with aberrant conduction or ectopic ventricular. One has to distinguish between aberrant conduction and ectopy which will enable to get the most of the QRS milking process.
3. Relationship between P waves and QRS complexes for atrioventricular conduction (Who's married to whom ?)
4. Any abnormal complexes—early, late and unusual contour.
   When the depolarization begins in the SA node it is called 'sinus rhythm'. Depolarization can begin in other places also and then the rhythm is named after that part of the heart where the depolarization sequence starts.

131. ECG findings of arrhythmias can be described under 4 main headings.

1. Supraventricular rhythms
   A. Sinus rhythm
   B. Atrial rhythm
   C. Nodal rhythm
2. Ventricular rhythms
3. Unusual complexes or beats
4. Atrioventricular conduction variations.

The depolarization spreads to the ventricles in the normal way via the bundle of His and its branches. QRS complex is therefore normal and is the same whether depolarization starts from the SA node, atrial muscle or AV node.

132. Arrhythmias are classified in a simple way into 4 groups depending on their origin (see D-32, 33)

1. Sinus arrhythmias—arrhythmias in relation to the sinoatrial node
2. Atrial arrhythmias—arrhythmias of atrial origin
3. Nodal arrhythmias—arrhythmias arising in and around the AV junction
4. Ventricular arrhythmias—arrhythmias originating in the ventricles.

Supraventricular Rhythm

Sinus rhythm: P wave upright and regular in leads LII, LIII and aVF, unchanging in shape. The PR interval falls within normal limits. Each P wave is followed by a narrow QRS of normal contour.

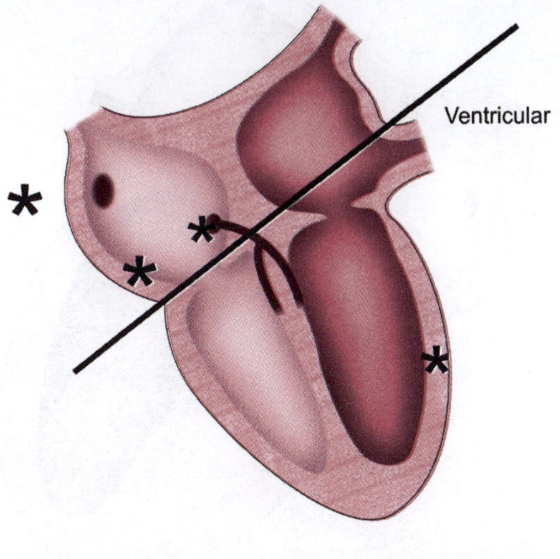

Fig. Q-101: Supraventricular and ventricular rhythms—their origin

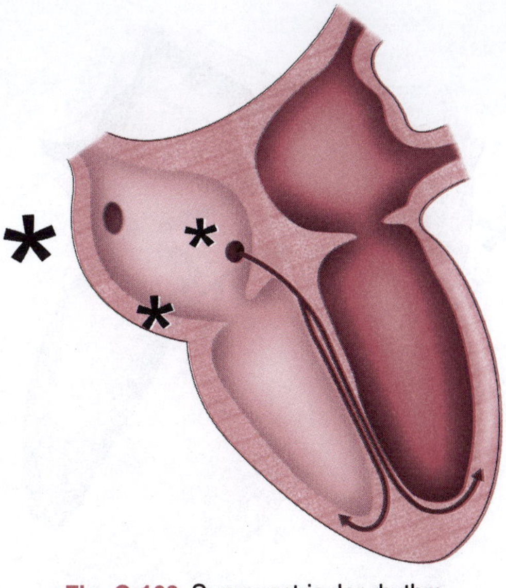

Fig. Q-102: Supraventricular rhythm

133. The 4 common sinus arrhythms are:

Normal sinus rhythm: Impulses originate at SA node at normal rate of 60–100/min with less than 10% variation

1. *Sinus tachycardia:* Rate more than 100/min (Ref. Fig. D-7)
2. *Sinus bradycardia:* Rate less than 60/min (Ref. Fig. D-8)
3. *Sinus arrhythmia:* P waves identical in morphology but rhythmically irregular. Variation is more than 10%. The most common form is during respiratory changes. Each P is followed by QRS with constant PR interval.
4. *Sick sinus syndrome:* Bradycardia alternating with tachycardia

Diseases involving the SA node may lead to marked bradycardia causing dizziness and syncope. In addition to periods of bradycardia, the patient may develop supraventricular tachycardia. Medical therapy may worsen bradycardia. Hence, these patients need pacing. (Ref.*226–229)

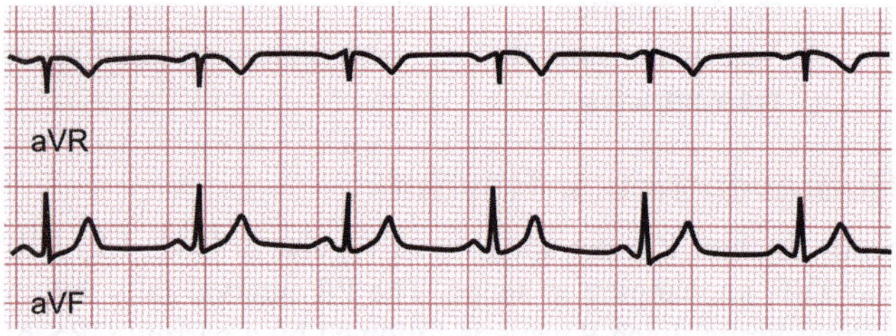

Fig. Q-103: Normal sinus rhythm PR = 0.96 sec; Rate = 63 bpm; P, QRS is normally inverted in aVR and normally upright in aVF. Each QRS is preceded by a P wave, rate, RR intervals regular

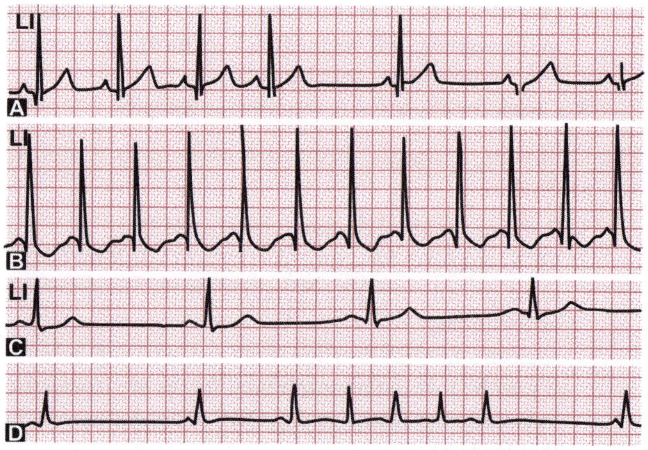

Fig. Q-105: A. Sinus arrhythmia B. Sinus tachycardia C. Sinus bradycardia D. Sick sinus syndrome

134. Atrial rhythm: The impulses originate somewhere in the atrium.

1. *Non-sinus (Coronary sinus) atrial rhythm:* P waves are identical and regular but inverted in LII, LIII and aVF signifying the origin other than SA node. Impulses originate low in the atrium, pass retrogradely and distally.

   These are associated with a normal (rather than short) PR interval. Such beats are likely to arise from the neighborhood of the coronary sinus, so the terms coronary sinus rhythm and coronary sinus extrasystoles are used. It is to be suspected that such a combination can also indicate left atrial origin.

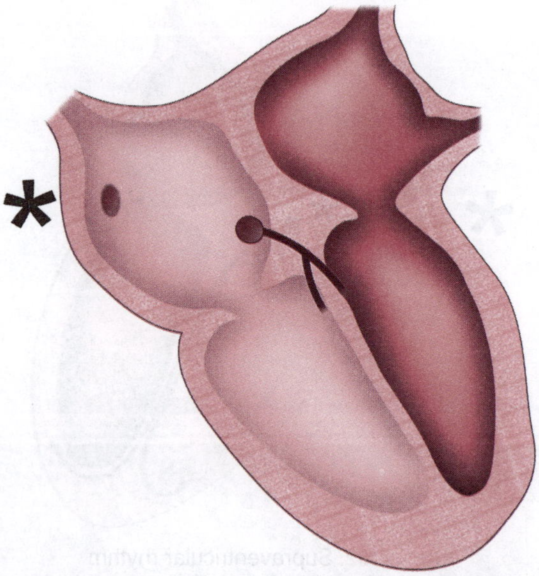

Fig. Q-104: Sinus arrhythmia (Ref.* Fig. D-7)

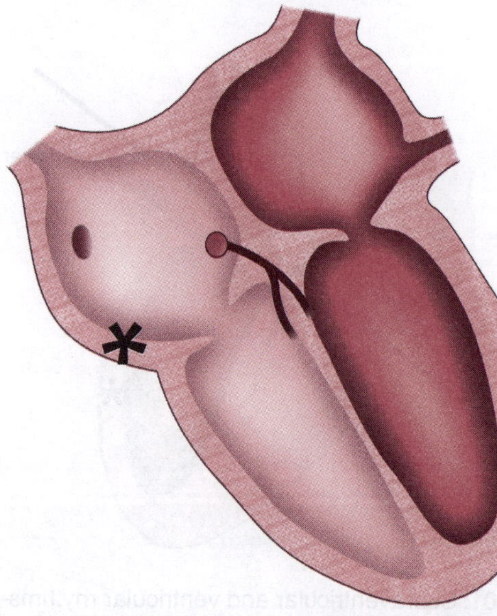

Fig. Q-106: Atrial rhythm: The impulse originates somewhere in the atrium

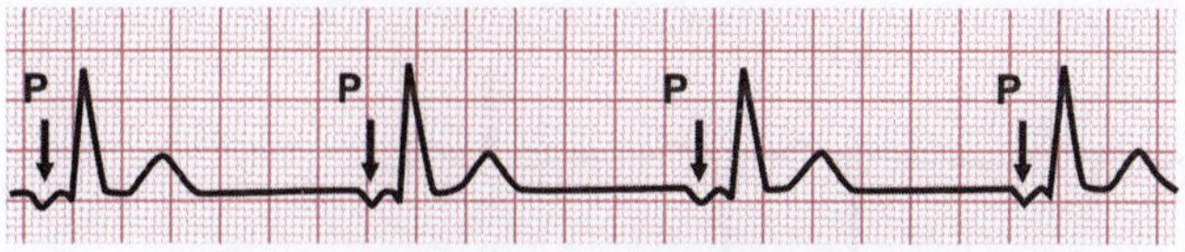

Fig. Q-107: Coronary (sinus) atrial rhythm

P waves are inverted but identical indicating origin of impulse from other than SA node.

If P ↓ is seen in LII, LIII, aVF, with normal QRS , one has to differentiate between the junctional rhythm coronary sinus and left atrial rhythm. If the PR interval is <0.12 sec it is in favor of junctional rhythm. If the PR interval is normal, see the precordial leads.

In coronary sinus rhythm, the impulse arises from neighbourhood of coronary sinus in the right atrium. So that P waves are positive in V5, V6 but negative in V1 V2.

In left atrial rhythm, the P waves are positive in V1 V2 and negative in V4V5V6. One has to see all leads before coming to conclusion.

(Note: P waves are always positive in L1 except in dextrocardia):

It is usually benign condition without clinical significance.

2. *Wandering atrial pacemaker:* The impulses originate from various foci in atria, so the morphology of P wave varies from beat to beat in a same lead often associated with variation of RR interval, PP interval (and hence RR interval).

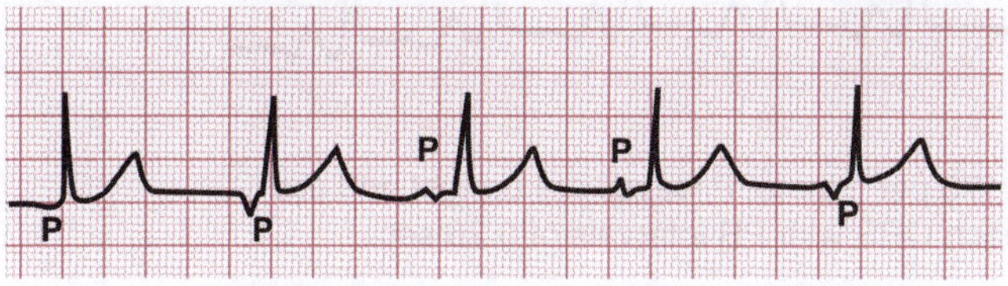

Fig. Q-108: Wandering pacemaker: P wave contour varies; indicates origin of P wave from various foci of atria. Variation of PR, PP, RR intervals

It is characterized by P waves of varying shape. P waves are upright in some, inverted in some, flattened in some. PR interval varies from 0.12–0.2 sec. When the pacemaker is higher in the atria, RR interval, heart rate is also higher.

If the PR interval is shorter as the pacemaker moves lower in the atria, the rate is slower. So wandering pacemaker is associated with variation of RR and PP interval. This is a benign arrhythmia and usually the patient is asymptomatic. Usually occurs in

i. Young individuals with high vagal tone
ii. Acute rheumatic fever
iii. Infective endocarditis
iv. Patients on digitalis.

It should be differentiated from multifocal atrial tachycardia where the heart rate is more than 100/min. Usually occurs in elderly and severe illness if the patient is on digitalis, the drug should be stopped. If the patient is symptomatic because of arrhythmias treatment as same that for sinus bradycardia.

3. *Multifocal atrial tachycardia:* Impulses originate from multiple foci in atria in an irregular and rapid way. It is different from wandering pacemaker as the heart rate is usually more than 100/min. It is usually seen in pulmonary disease with respiratory or cardiac failure.

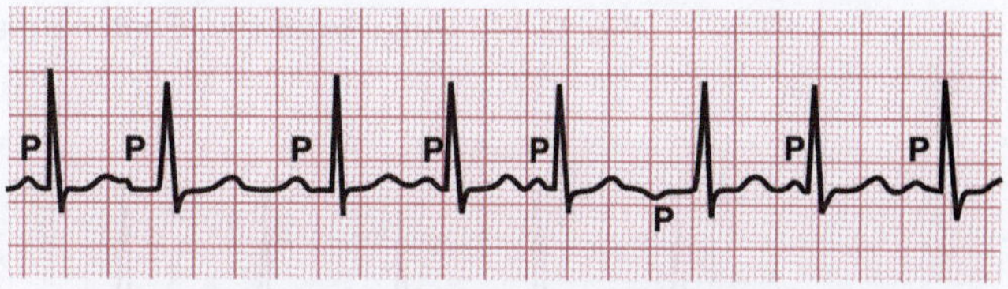

Fig. Q-109: Multifocal atrial tachycardia; P wave contour vary and rapid. PR, RP and thus RR intervals may vary

4. *Atrial ectopics:* (see D-52, Fig. D-10)

P waves are premature. P wave morphology is different from sinus P wave followed by QRS. Compensatory pause present but not full compensatory pause (one for ventricular premature beat)

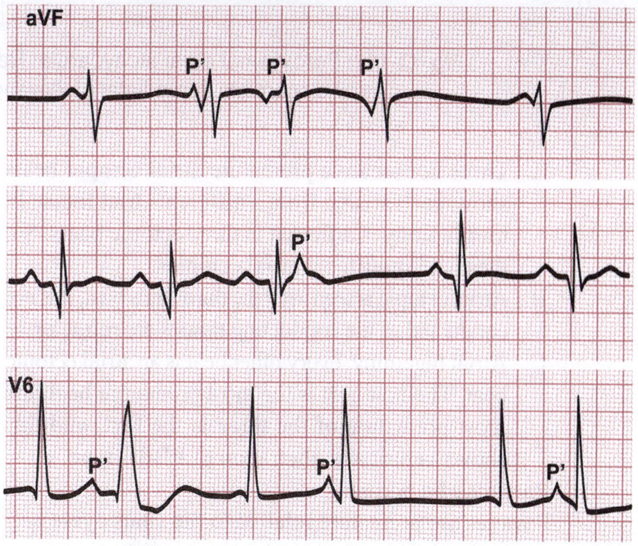

Fig. Q-110: Atrial ectopic beats labeled P'

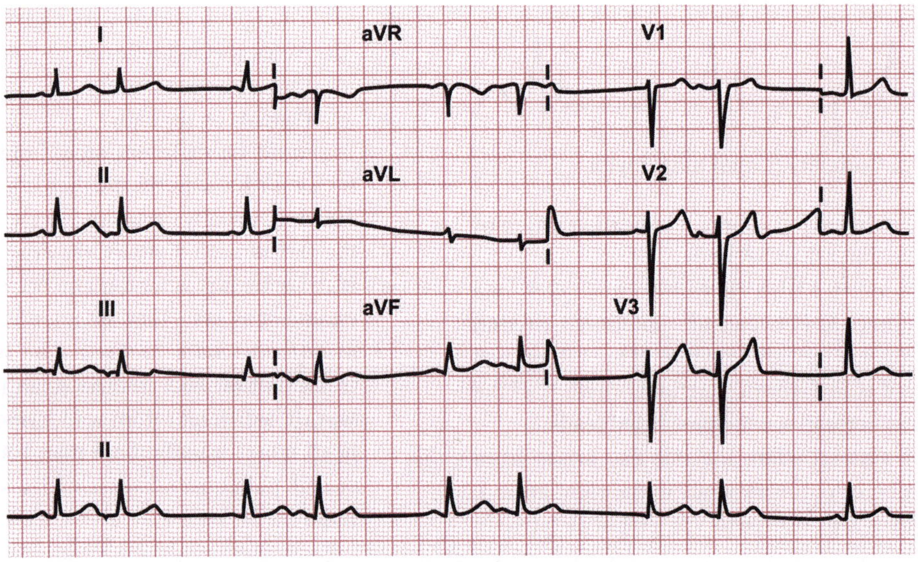

Fig. Q-111: Atrial bigeminy. Each normal beat is followed by atrial premature beat

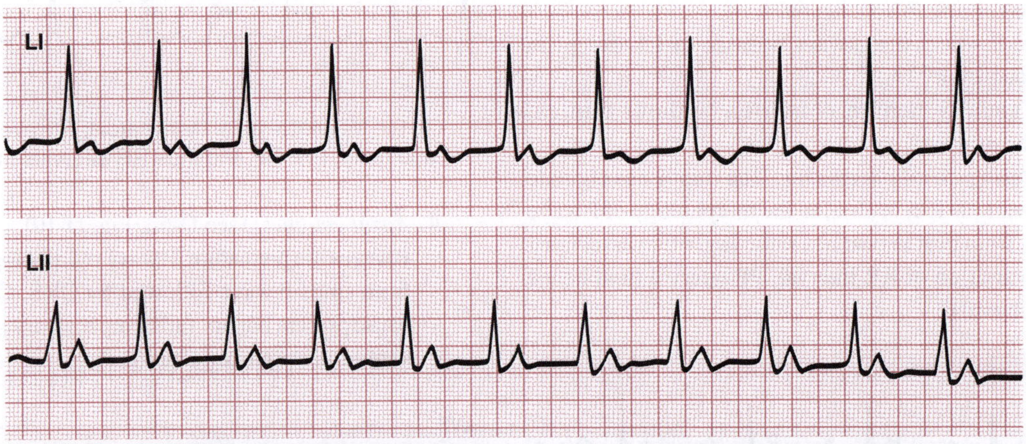

Fig. Q-112: Paroxysmal atrial tachycardia: Rate 170 per minute; P waves are upright and are clearly discernible immediately following each QRS with PR intervals of 0.26 sec

A. Three consecutive premature atrial ectopic beats show, each arising from a different atrial focus. P' morphology is different in three ectopic beats. So, these are multifocal atrial ectopics.

B. Atrial ectopic is seen after the third sinus beat, it is not conducted as the conducting tissues are refractory.

C. Atrial bigeminy; every other beat is an atrial ectopic beat. The first beat is the most premature beat; the most premature of the three is the first, and this shows ventricular aberration of LBBB type.

Rate may be normal.

P waves are premature relative to the sinus cycle. Morphology is different from sinus P wave.

Compensatory pause is present but not full compensatory pause.

5. *Paroxysmal atrial tachycardia (PAT):* (See D-58 Fig. D-11) It is a reentry tachycardia. Reentry of impulses occur in and around the AV node due to slowing in area of unidirectional block. P waves are regular and identical in LII, sometimes merged with T waves with very rapid rate of 160–220/min.

P waves occur at a faster rate 150–250 bpm; regular tachycardia with repeated firing of an ectopic foci.

PAT—P waves regular and inverted.

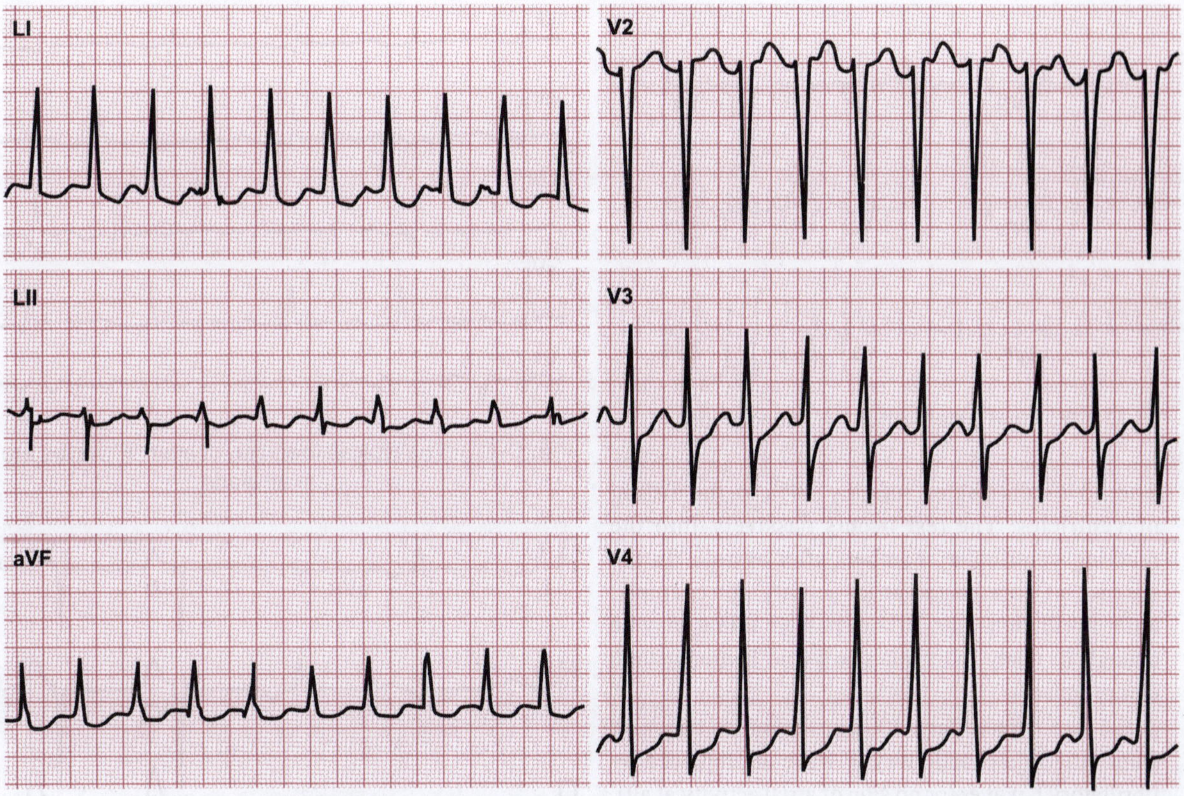

Fig. Q-113: Atrial tachycardia with a rate of 230 per minute. See normal QRS interval and ST depression

AV node cannot conduct atrial rate above 200/min. Thus, if the atrial rate is faster than 200/min. AV block occurs.

Irregular ventricular rate is frequent in atrial tachycardia with changing block.

6. *Atrial flutter:* (see D-66 Fig. D-12, 13, 14)

   When the atrial rate is above 250/min, the AV node cannot conduct. Impulses travel in a circular course in the atria resulting in rapid, regular 220–330/min flutter or F waves. Rapid, undulating, identical P waves (F waves) give a 'sawtooth' appearance. Depending on the AV block the rate may be 150 (2:1 block). 100 (3:1 block), or 75 (4:1 block)/min.

   See the characteristic 'sawtooth' or 'picket-fence' appearance. It is an intra-atrial reentry circuit usually at about 300 bpm. This patient is taking rather more digoxin and has a very slow ventricular response.

8. *Atrial fibrillation:* (see Fig. D-15, 16, 17)

   This is a common arrhythmia. RR intervals are irregularly irregular, and the pulse is irregularly irregular with pulse deficit.

   Atrial contraction occurs during ventricular relaxation (diastole) and its sole function is to fill the ventricles with blood in preparation for ventricular contraction.

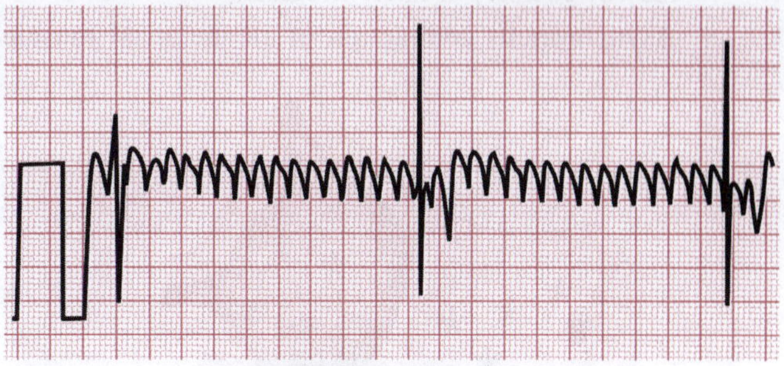

Fig. Q-114: Atrial flutter

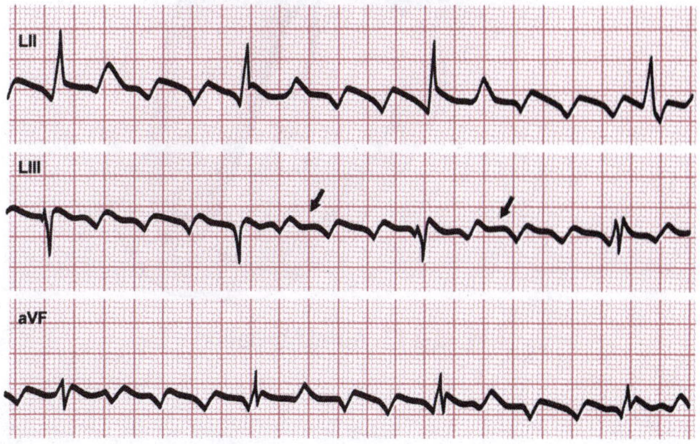

Fig. Q-115: Atrial flutter with 4:1 AV conduction—Sawtooth appearance, isoelectric line is seen clearly between F waves

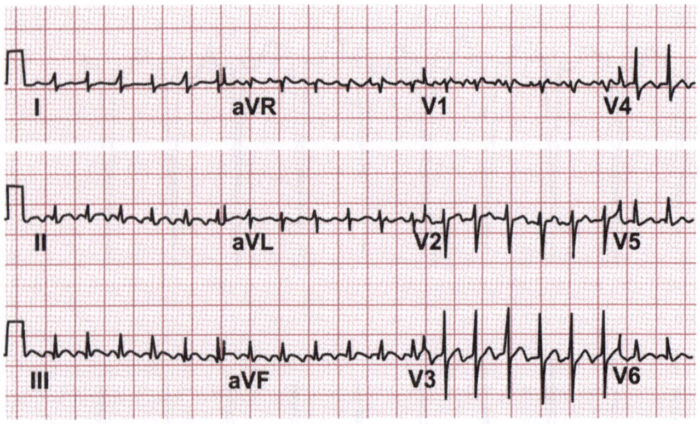

Fig. Q-116: Atrial flutter with 2:1 AV conduction

The atria contributes roughly 30% to the filling of ventricles. The rest occurs passively into the relaxing ventricular chambers after systole. In the absence of coordinated atrial activity, for example, atrial fibrillation—the 70% of passive filling may be enough in many individuals to avoid hemodynamic compromise.

Atrial rate is more than 300/min. Impulses originate from atria in a chaotic way. P wave are replaced by fibrillatory F waves (or no sign of atrial activity at all). QRS complexes are irregularly irregular. The baseline may be coarsely or finely irregular.

Asynchronous contraction of all the atrial muscle fibers. When the individual muscle fibers contract independently they are said to be 'fibrillating'.

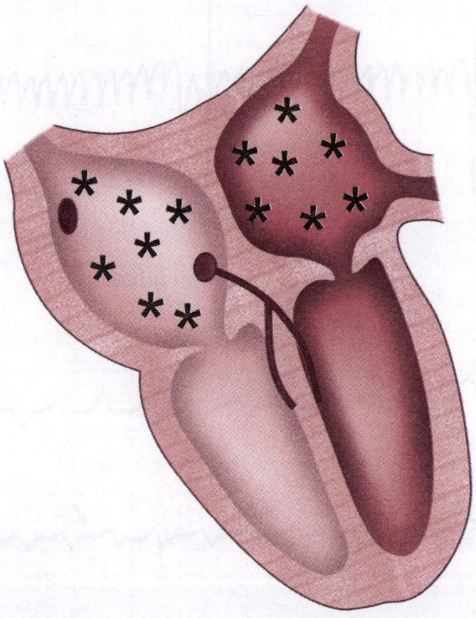

Fig. Q-117: Atrial fibrillation

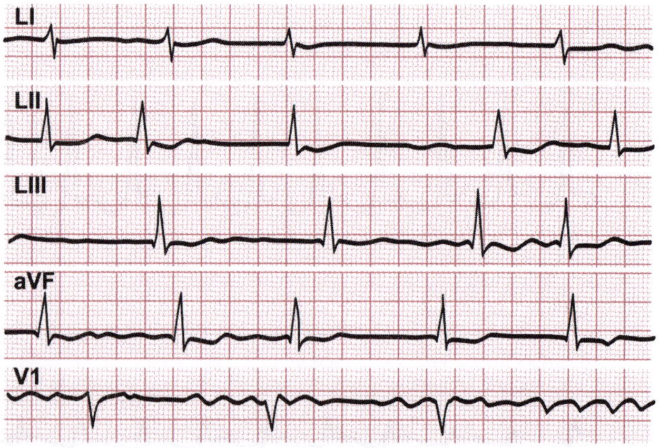

Fig. Q-118: The typical, irregular, uneven 'F' waves are seen in all leads

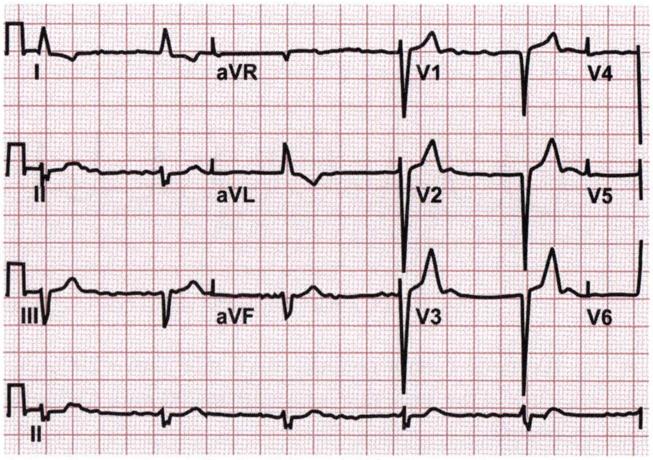

Fig. Q-119: Atrial fibrillation and complete heart block

- 'F' fibrillary waves of atrial fibrillation seen and no P waves
- Regular ventricular rhythm
- The wider the QRS of the ventricular escape rhythm the less reliable the escape mechanism
- Atrial fibrillation with complete heart block can be easily missed and is an indication for a permanent pacemaker.

9. *Atrial flutter/fibrillation:* (see D-59 Fig. D-15)

   Coarse atrial fibrillation may sometimes resemble atrial flutter and the rhythm with characteristics of both flutter and fibrillation are seen.

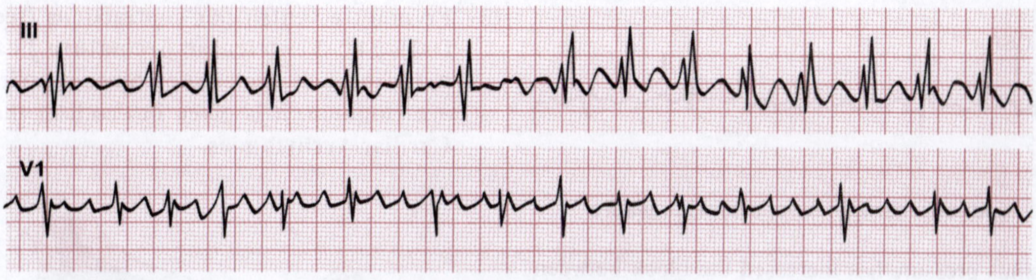

Fig. Q-120: Atrial flutter-fibrillation

Atrial waves are well formed and regular for not calling as fibrillation, yet not regular enough to be called as flutter.

135. Irregularity of the atrial fibrillation with pulse deficit may be clinically imitated by the following 4 arrhythmias.

1. Frequent ectopic beat: Atrial, nodal or ventricular. These ectopics often produce a pulse deficit. It is important to note that a pulse deficit is not diagnostic of atrial fibrillation alone.
2. Atrial tachycardia (flutter) with varying block.
3. Gross sinus arrhythmia or sinus rhythm with varying block.
4. Wandering pacemaker.

Nodal (or Junctional) Rhythm

(see D-164–167, Fig. D-19-20)

Nodal rhythms are diagnosed by a negative P wave either preceding, following or lost in a QRS complex.

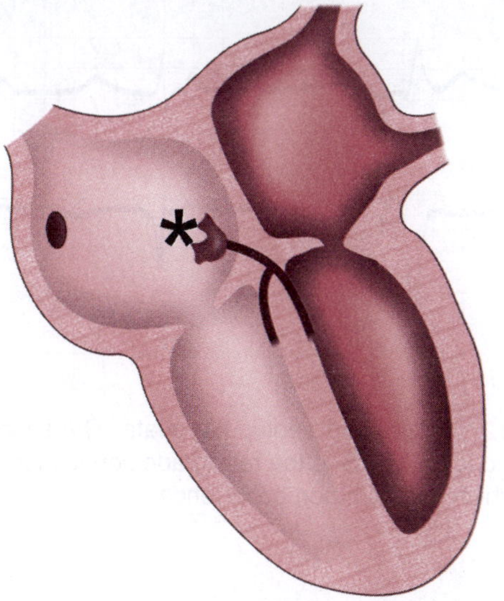

Fig. Q-121: Nodal (or junctional) rhythm

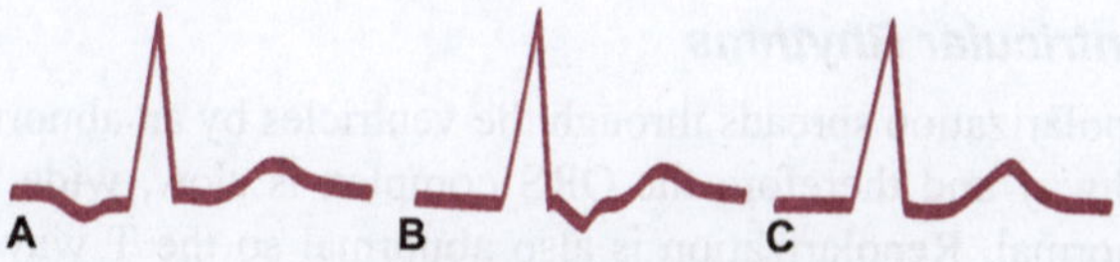

Fig. Q-122: AV nodal patterns

Impulses originate in AV node with retrograde and antegrade direction. P waves may not be identified and QRS complexes are regular and normal in shape because the ventricles are activated down the bundle of His in the normal pathway. Since the origin of impulse is AV node, the heart rate is usually 40–60/ min. P waves in LI, LII and aVF tend to be inverted because the impulses that originate in AV node are transmitted in a retrograde fashion to the atrium.

P waves may precede or bury or follow QRS complexes depending on whether the junctional rhythm reaches and depolarizes the atrium before, at the same time or after the ventricles contract.

A. Abnormal 'retrograde' P waves precedes QRS with short PR interval (upper nodal rhythm).
B. Abnormal P wave follows QRS (lower nodal rhythm).
C. No P waves—P wave coincides with QRS (mid-nodal rhythm).

Junctional (or nodal) Tachycardia

The AV node depolarizes frequently. The P wave may be seen very close to QRS or may not be seen at all. The QRS complex is normal shape as in other supraventricular arrhythmias. Paroxysmal AV junctional tachycardia at a rate of 185 bpm. **Carotid sinus pressure** this has both diagnostic and therapeutic usefulness in supraventricular tachyarrhythmias. It is always worth trying at bed side as it may make the nature of the arrhythmia more obvious.

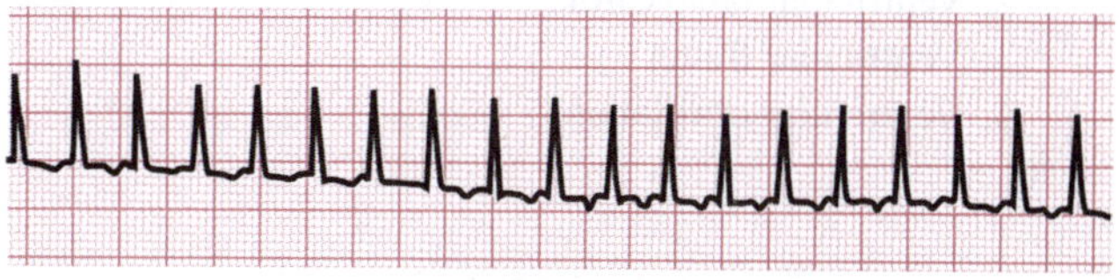

Fig. Q-123

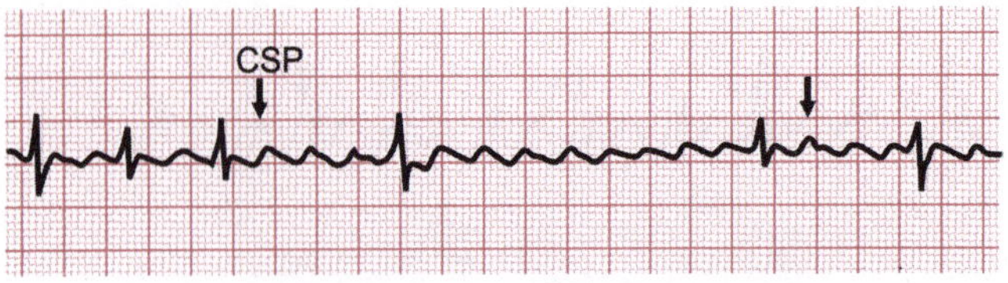

Fig. Q-124: Atrial flutter with carotid sinus pressure

Carotid sinus pressure has increased the block between atria and ventricle, and the diagnosis of atrial flutter is made easy.

Ventricular Rhythms

Depolarization spreads through the ventricles by an abnormal pathway and therefore the QRS complex is slow, wide and abnormal. Repolarization is also abnormal so the T wave is abnormal in shape.

Ventricles are activated from automatic cells within the ventricles. This can be due to irritability of the ventricles or malfunction of other potential rhythms. QRS complexes are wide (more than 0.10 sec) compare to supraventricular arrhythmias.

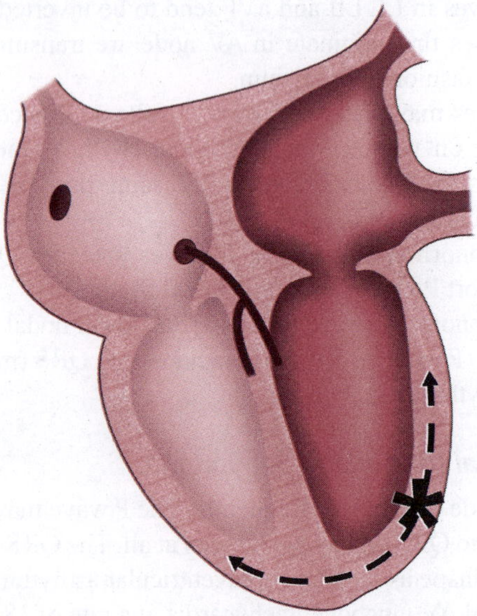

Fig. Q-125

136. There are 4 common ventricular rhythms:

1. Premature ventricular contractions
2. Ventricular tachycardia
3. Ventricular flutter
4. Ventricular fibrillation

137. Premature ventricular contractions (see D-179, Fig. D-25-31): Ventricular premature beats have the following 4 characteristics. Since ventricular ectopics are common, it is given in detail in the chapter on Cardiac Arrhythmias.

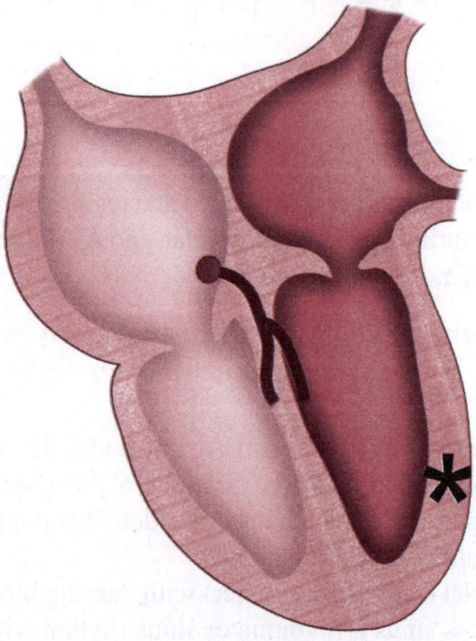

Fig. Q-126

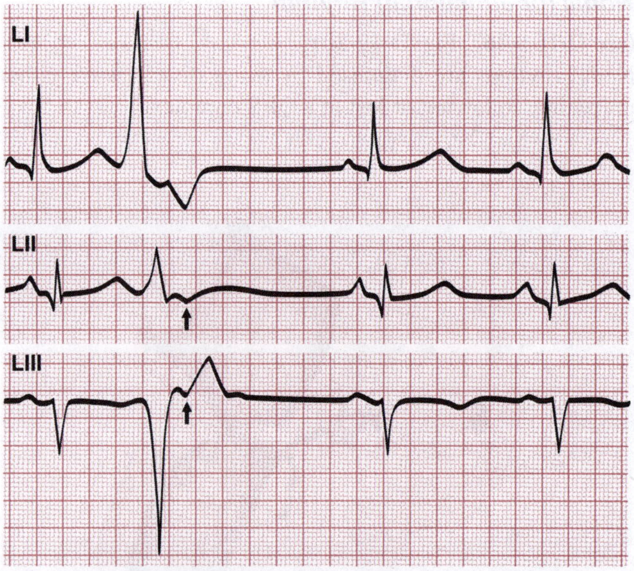

Fig. Q-127: Premature ventricular beats: The second beat in each lead is a PVB. See the retrograde conduction to the atria in this which is a common occurrence

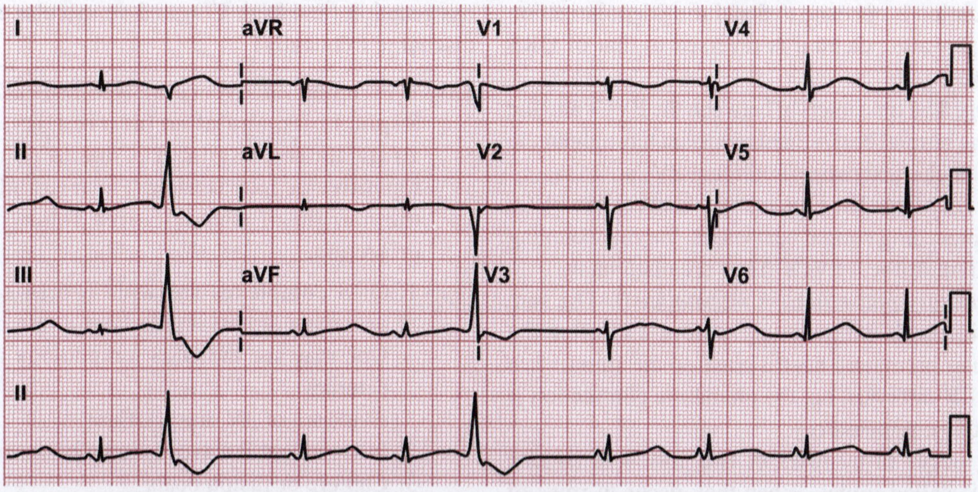

Fig. Q-128: Two ventricular premature beats are seen in each lead. They are premature, wide followed by full compensatory pause

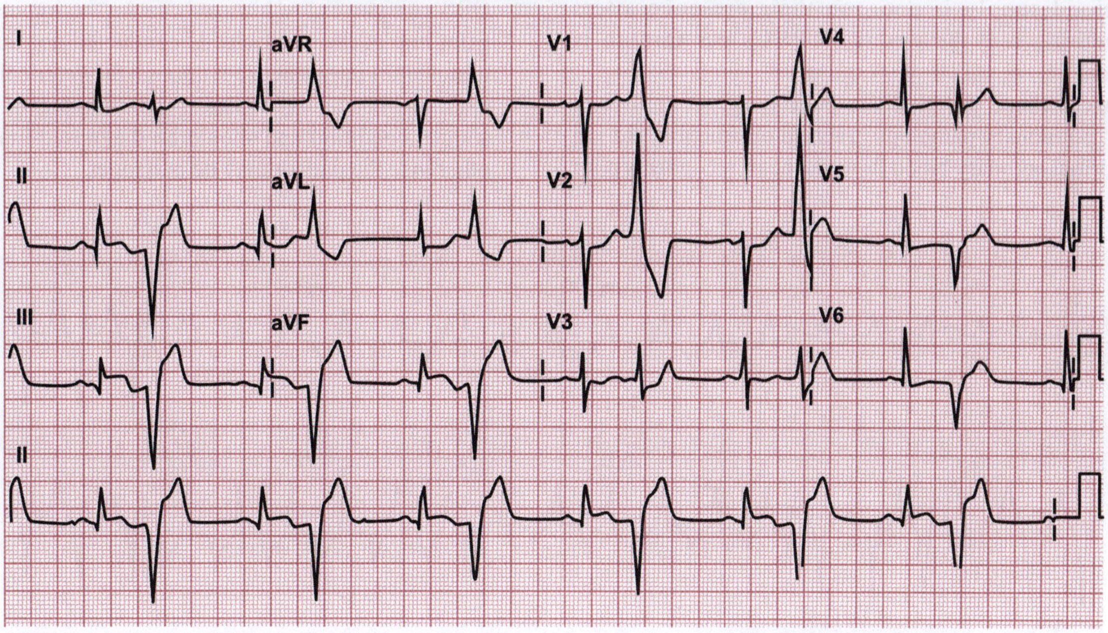

Fig. Q-129: Ventricular bigeminy or coupling. PVB follows each normal beat. There are also features of acute inferior myocardial infarction. This figure also shows ST elevation in LII, LIII and aVF which are features of acute inferior myocardial infarction

1. *Prematurity:* They are premature to the normally conducted beats. The QRS is not preceded by P wave (absence of P wave)
2. *Wide bizarre QRS contour:* It is wider than normal and distorted in bizarre shape. The cause is that the impulse is conducted mainly through the slowly conducting ventricular muscle rather than the Purkinje system.
   QRS complex has a very high voltage. A normal wave passes through both ventricles; consequently, the depolarization waves of the two sides of the heart neutralize each other. In PVBs the impulse travels only in one direction so that there is no such neutralizing effect. One side of the heart is depolarized while the other side is still polarized. This results in high voltage. It may arise from single focus or multiple ventricular foci. ST segment slopping of in the opposite direction of QRS. The T wave following premature ventricular beat is in the opposite direction to the main deflection of the QRS complex because the slow conduction of the impulse through the cardiac muscle causes the area first depolarized also to repolarize first. This results in the direction of current flow in the heart during

repolarization is opposite to that during depolarization and the T wave potential is reversed to that of QRS complexes.

3. *Coupling:* The time interval between the PVCs and the preceding normal beat remains constant throughout the ECG. It is characteristic of unifocal PVCs.
   Varying coupling: The time interval between the PVCs and the preceding normal beat varies. Varying coupling occurs in multifocal PVCs. They are malignant.
4. *Compensatory pause (unless interpolated):* The sum of RR intervals immediately before and after the ventricular premature beat is equal to the sum of two regular RR intervals, i.e. the premature contraction is completely compensatory.

When they occur in by rows of two followed by one normal beat, it is called triplet. When they occur in rows of three followed a normal beat, it is called quadruplet.

PVCs often gives a clue that the heart's own (coronary artery) blood supply is poor, so their presence alters that something may be wrong. 6 PVCs per minute is pathological.

In cases where the blood is poorly oxygenated (e.g. drowning, pulmonary pathology, tracheal obstruction, etc.) in spite of normal coronary blood flow, the heart recognizes poor oxygenation (and high CO_2 and ventricular ectopic foci will discharge frequently).

138. Ventricular tachycardia: (see D-192-205, Fig. D-34) Rapid, broad and often bizarre QRS complexes with a rate above 140/min. It is due to reentry with rapid repetitive depolarization. The irritability starts along the margin of ischemic area following myocardial infarction.

1. QRS complexes are wide (>0.14 sec) and bizarre occurring almost regularly at a rate of 150–200 bpm
   One may see the QRS morphology as in ventricular ectopics.
   Evidence of AV dissociation:
2. Independent P waves (shown by arrow)
3. Capture or fusion beats
4. Beat to beat variability of the QRS morphology

(Note the absence of rs, RS or Rs complexes)
QRS complexes are bizarre because the impulse arising from one of the ventricles is conducted not through the normal Purkinje system but through the ventricular muscle itself and hence, wide bizarre QRS complexes. This is a serious condition and should be diagnosed immediately otherwise the patient may be in danger.

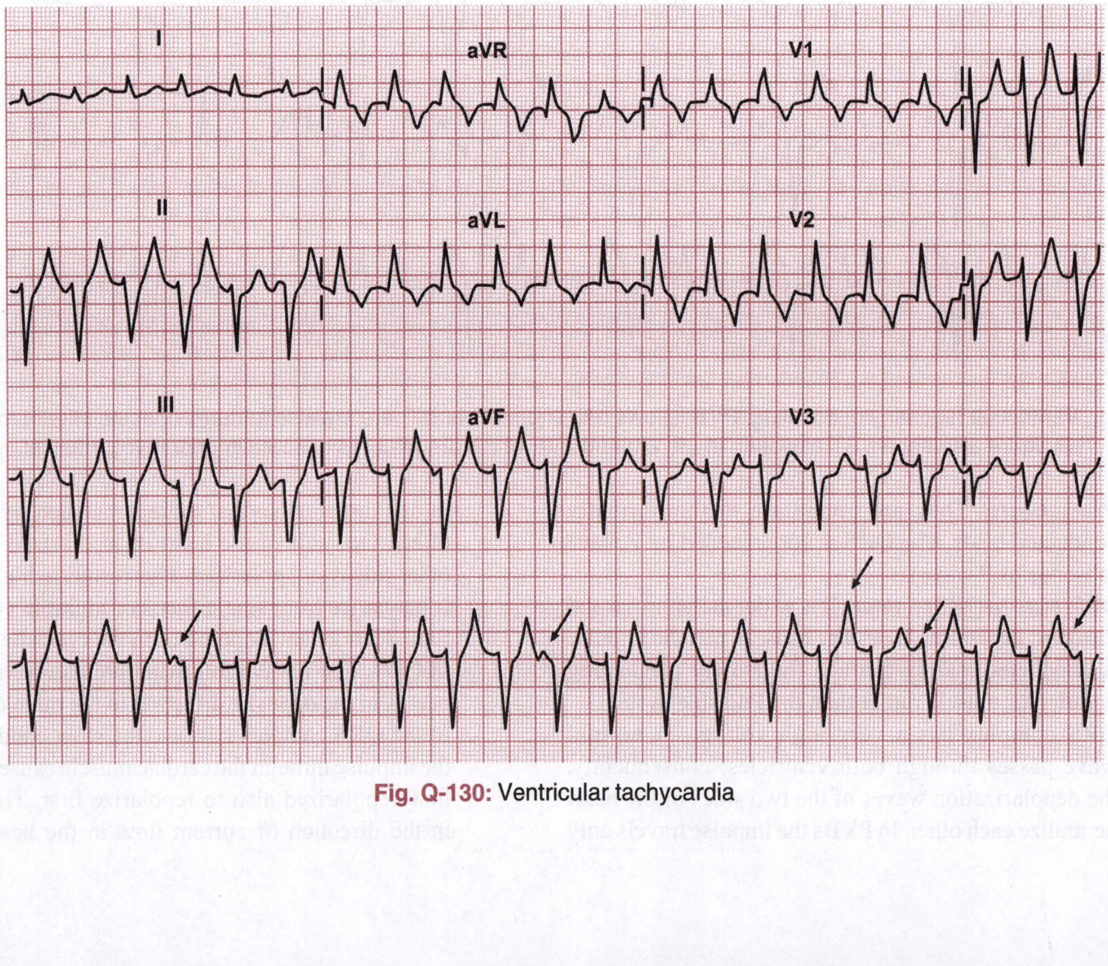

Fig. Q-130: Ventricular tachycardia

139. Ventricular flutter (see D-207, Fig. D-35): This is a rare terminal arrhythmia before going into fibrillation.

1. Regularly occurring QRS complexes at a rate of 180–250 bpm. QRS complexes are wide and bizarre.
2. No P waves.
3. No distinct T waves.
4. The amplitude of undulation may be large or small depending on the myocardial status. The amplitude is small in severely damaged heart.

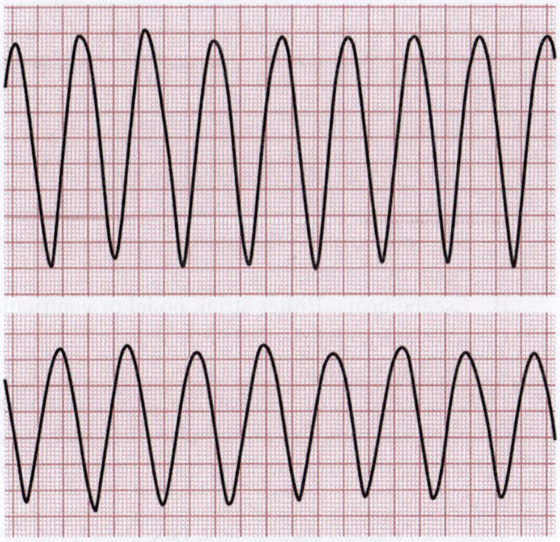

Fig. Q-131: Ventricular flutter

140. Ventricular fibrillation: (see D-208, Fig. D-36–37) Ventricular depolarization is chaotic. There are no true QRS complexes and the baseline shows chaotic undulations. ECG is totally disorganized.

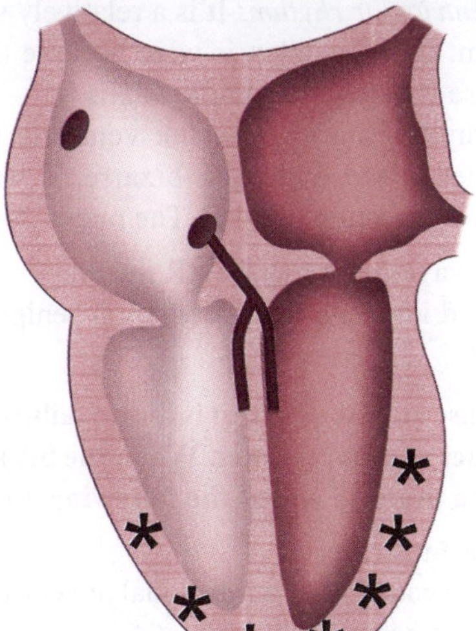

Fig. Q-132: Ventricular fibrillation

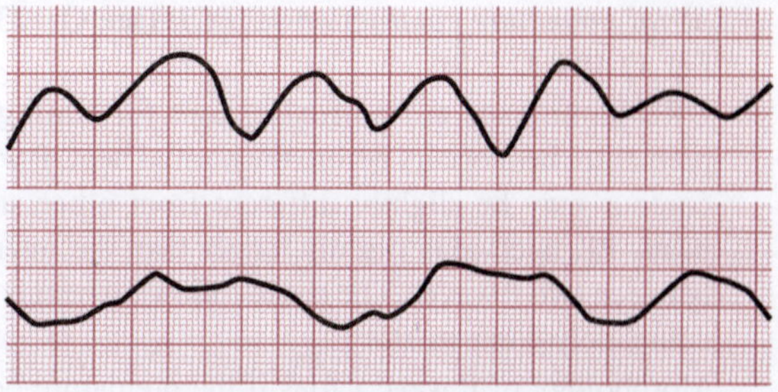

Fig. Q-133: Ventricular fibrillation

1. Irregularly irregular rhythm of varying configuration without any identifiable P, QRS, T waves
2. Ventriculaar rate may be as slow as 150 bpm or as fast as 500 bpm
3. P, QRS, T waves are replaced by fibrillary waves with sharp or rounded upper and lower ends
4. The amplitude of fibrillary waves progressively deteriorates immediately before asystole. When it is ended with cardiac standstill, it is represented by a straight line in the ECG without any electrical activity in the cardiac muscle.

These terminal arrhythmias are very serious and urgent treatment is needed for survival.

Unusual Complexes or Beats

The contour and timing of complexes vary. If the QRS morphology differs in the same lead, it should be differentiated whether this is from atrial, nodal or ventricular origin.

141. Ventricular fibrillation: (See D-208 Fig. D-36-37)

A. Early premature contractions:
   1. Atrial premature contractions
   2. Junctional or nodal premature contractions
   3. Ventricular premature contractions.

B. Escape beats:
   4. Sinus pause and sinus arrest
   5. Atrial escape beats
   6. Junctional escape beats
   7. Ventricular escape beats
   8. Idioventricular rhythm finally end in the cardiac standstill.

Any part of the heart can depolarize earlier it should, the following heart beat is called extrasystole or premature contraction. The premature contraction or extrasystole or ectopics may arise in the atrial muscle, junctional or nodal region or in the ventricular muscle—it is the same that of escape beats but the difference is that an extrasystole comes early and an escape beat comes late. Premature contractions occurring before next normal beat is expected in a regular rhythm.

1. *Atrial premature contractions (APC):* (see Q-123–4, Fig. Q-104, D-7-8)
   QRS complexes are normal except for timing. A premature beat occurs before the normal beat. P wave contour may be slightly different from other sinus beats. PR interval is slightly longer than the interval between two P waves. The pause following beat is not completely compensatory.
   Morphology of P wave varies if the premature beats arise from multiple foci.
2. *Junctional (Nodal):* There is no P wave before the premature beat, and the QRS complex looks normal. The compensatory pause is complete.
   The premature beat originate either in the AV node or in the bundle of His.
3. *Ventricular premature beats (Q-137, Fig. Q-125–126, D-181, Fig. D-26–31):* They originate from ectopic focus in the ventricles.

Escape Beats

Escape beats and dissociation are not primary. They are secondary to underlying primary disturbance. Escape beats are seen in SA and complete AV block. It is considered as a safety mechanism whereby the heart is protected when the higher pacemaker fails—usually the SA node. The different parts of the heart are able to initiate depolarization sequence, for this gives the heart the series of "fail-safe" mechanisms, that will keep the heart going if the SA node fails. The escape beat is indeed 'a friend in need'. Usually the escape maker is in the AV node (nodal escape), but when it fails, a focus in the ventricle may take over (ventricular escape). Escape may be for a single beat ending with an unusual long pause, or but a few beats or may be more or less permanent idioventricular rhythm.

Escape beats are commonly seen in AMI when they may be associated with sinus bradycardia. It is important not to try to suppress an escape rhythm, because without it the heart might stop altogether.

4. *Sinus pause and Sinus arrest:* (See. Fig. D-41–43)
   There is a block at SA node normal sinus beat is missed and the next beat may resume with another sinus beat. If the pause is longer, it is called sinus arrest (SA block). When the SA node fails to initiate an impulse any of the following may occur.
   A. SA node resumes:
      The SA node again takes over to resume normal rhythm. The resulting pause is not an exact multiple of the cycle.
      A beat is omitted and PP interval is the normal length.

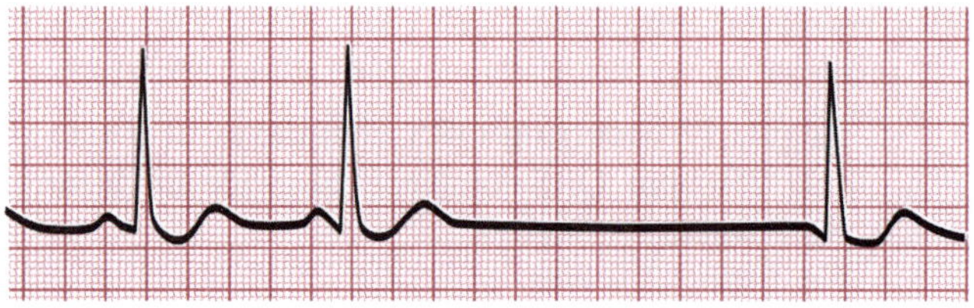

Fig. Q-134

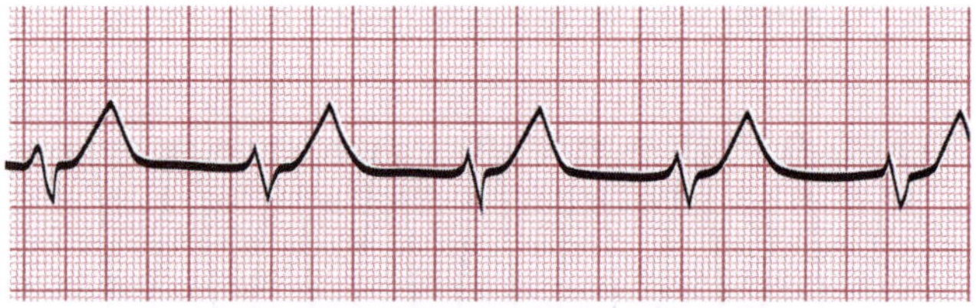

Fig. Q-135: Idioventricular rhythm

      SA node arrest—the normal rhythm is restored again by SA node.
   B. Escape beats: Either atrial, nodal or ventricular.
   C. Idioventricular rhythm
   D. Cardiac standstill
5. *Atrial escape beat:* Following a pause, an atrial ectopic focus may fire an impulse after such a pause stimulating the atria. Impulse travel through AV node normally.
6. *Junctional (nodal) escape beat:* (see D-244, Fig. D-42) SA node failure results in take over by depolarization by AV node usually after 1.2–1.6 sec.
7. *Ventricular escape beat:* When the SA node and AV node fail, automatic cells in the ventricle will take over, usually after 1.8–2.3 sec. Wide QRS complexes with a different contour from that of a normal sinus beat is seen. (see D-244, Fig. D-44)
8. *Idioventricular rhythm:* It is a relatively slow regular rhythm. QRS complex is wide because the origin of impulse is below the bundle of His.
   The rhythm starts from the ventricle itself. QRS complexes are wide and bizarre. T waves are in opposite direction of QRS. The rate is 20–40 /min.

Absent P waves with regular RR intervals.

Accelerated idioventricular rhythm is benign should not be treated.

142. Sinus pause and sinus arrest is due to failure of the sinus node to act as a pacemaker. When the SA node fails to initiate an impulse one of the following 4 may occur:

1. SA node resumes
2. Escape beats: Either atrial, nodal or ventricular escape beats can occur.
3. Idioventricular rhythm
4. Cardiac standstill.

143. The 4 salient features of SA block are:

Incomplete

1. Occasional absence of PQRST sequence
2. P waves absent
3. QRS sequence at slow rate
4. QRS interval normal or prolonged, depending on site of ventricular pacemaker.

144. Prolonged QRS duration. Now we can summarize the conditions associated with delayed intraventricular conduction time.

(see Q-108, Fig. Q-77)

1. When the impulse is initiated in an ectopic ventricular focus.
   i. Ventricular premature beat
   ii. Ventricular escape beat
   iii. Ventricular tachycardia
   iv. Idioventricular rhythm (from a low pacemaker)
   v. Accelerated idioventricular rhythm
   vi. Ventricular parasystole.
2. When intraventricular conduction is slowed:
   i. Intraventricular block (bundle branch block)
   ii. Ventricular aberration.
3. When conduction to one ventricle is accelerated:
   i. Wolff-Parkinson-White syndrome—initial slurring of QRS (delta wave)
4. Artificial pacemaker (See D-319)
5. Coronary artery disease—Myocardial infarction/ ischemia
6. Drugs and electrolytes—digitalis/verapamil, hyperkalemia
7. Cardiomyopathy – total distortion
8. Myocarditis/fibrocytic

   (5, 6, 7, 8 are also due to delayed intraventricular conduction).

Pacemaker rhythm: Transvenous pacemaker initiates beat in right ventricle but not in SA node, so the QRS is wide. The pacemaker discharge gives rise to a narrow ventricle line at the onset of QRS complex known as pacemaker 'spike'. The usual heart rate setting of permanent pacemaker is 72 per minute.

145. Differentiation between supraventricular and ventricular tachycardias:

Accurate diagnosis of regular tachycardia can be surprisingly made at bed side with close observation to clinical detail. One should follow some principles, and misconceptions and false theories are to be taken out of the mind. Apply stethoscope to the precordium and eyes to the neck veins simultaneously. Search for presence or absence of cannon 'a' waves or flutter waves in the jugular pulse, variation in the intensity of first heart sound and splitting of the second heart sounds.

Following 4 points help to differentiate supraventricular and ventricular tachycardia:

1. Splitting of the second sound is due to ventricular asynchrony whereas irregular cannon waves in the neck and variation in intensity of the first sound is due to dissociation between the atria and ventricles.
2. Signs of dissociation are easily found at the bed side than in the tracing because the independent P waves are more often than not lost in the ventricular complexes.
3. Dissociation does not prove ventricular tachycardia, but it excludes atrial tachycardia and therefore; it is likely to be more ventricular. Dissociation can occur between atrial and AV pacemakers. When ventricular aberration is also present, the imitation of ventricular tachycardia may be perfect both clinically and electrocardiographically.
4. Regular cannon waves with every beat may be seen in atrial tachycardia or ventricular tachycardia with 1:1 retroconduction. If there are irregular cannon waves in the neck or the first sound varies in intensity from beat to beat it is in favor of dissociation, and this suggests ventricular tachycardia. If there is no varying intensity of first sound and cannon waves are regular, this is against dissociation and the tachycardia is probably supraventricular with the exceptions of ventricular tachycardia with retrograde 1:1 conduction and ventricular tachycardia with concurrent atrial fibrillation.

Summary of differentiating tachyarrhythmias.

146. Clinically 4 points:

1. Wide splitting of heart sounds
2. Variation in intensity of first sound
3. Cannon waves in jugular pulse
4. Effect of carotid sinus stimulation.

147. Electrocardiographically—(in ECG that look like ventricular tachycardia) 4 main points.

(see Chapter D - Arrhythmias—tachyarrhythmias)

1. Study of QRS morphology
2. Study of P waves
   a. in conventional leads especially II and V1
   b. in esophageal lead
   c. intracardiac—His bundle electrocardiogram
   d. during administration of procainamide or acetylcholinic
3. Look for Dressler beats
4. Look for isolated extrasystoles in previous tracings.

Administration of procainamide intravenously with precautions: If the tachycardia is ventricular, the response is good. If it is supraventricular, the drug may momentarily block AV conduction and reveal the atrial rhythm disturbance between the now more widely spaced ventricular complexes. Acetylcholine also have similar effect.

Arrhythmias may be recognizable in any lead but as a general rule V1 is the best of all 12 leads because the pattern of aberrant ventricular conduction and ectopic ventricular beats are distinctly recognizable. It reveals the P wave character as well. It is a mistake to depend on a single lead and at times it is necessary to search every lead.

V1 is an excellent single lead for recognizing bundle branch pattern. We know that bundle branch block and ventricular ectopics could produce remarkably similar complexes. Bundle branch block causes one ventricle to be activated ahead of the other. Similarly ventricular ectopic causes activation in one ventricle ahead of the other. So, both of them cause activation 'in series' but not in 'parallel' (cause activation successively but not simultaneously).

In left bundle branch block and in right ventricular ectopic, excitation begins in right ventricle earlier than left ventricle, i.e. general direction of depolarization is from right to left. Since the excitation is away from V1 electrode, LBBB and right ventricular ectopic will produce predominantly a negative complex in V1.

In contrast, RBBB and left ventricular ectopic produce a predominant left-to-right activation and will therefore produce positive complexes in V1.

When the PVCs are from right ventricle, i.e. when it looks like LBBB. The qR or QR is seen in the left pericardial leads. When PVC is from left ventricle, i.e. when it looks like an RBBB. The qR or QR is seen in right pericardial leads.

QRS + ve in V1	–	RV ectopic
QRS - ve in V1	–	LV ectopic

148. Therefore V1 is the best single lead to distinguish between—

1. right and left bundle branch block.
2. between right and left ventricular ectopic beats.
3. between the left ventricular ectopic beats and ventricular aberrations of right bundle branch block type.
4. Also best for distinguishing atrial activity.

149. Some more practical points:

Watch the tracings while it is coming out of the machine with a trained and alert eye. For some more practical observations, pattern in the following **4** leads should be checked.

1. *Lead I:* If the complexes are inverted, check your arm electrode—they are almost certainly changed.
2. *Lead III:* If the Q wave is present, ask the patient to take a deep breath and hold it for a few heart beats. This helps to distinguish between important and unimportant Q waves.
3. *Lead VI:* If tall R waves are seen in right ventricular complexes instead of the usual down stroke, take a lead or two further to the right V3R V4R to get QRS complexes with major deflection downward.
4. *Lead V6:* If deep S waves are seen in left ventricular complexes instead of the usual tall upright wave, take a lead or two further to the left V7, V8 to get a pattern with the major deflection upward.

Atrioventricular Conduction Variations

AV conduction is known by observing the relationship between P waves and QRS complexes. The basic principle is to observe whether the P waves are always related to QRS complexes or sometimes related to QRS complexes or never related to QRS complexes. Do the P wave is followed by QRS or each QRS is preceded by P wave.

(Intraventricular conduction defects include right and left bundle branch block, which is discussed separately).

150. The following are AV conduction variations:

1. Fixed normal PR interval: Each QRS is always preceded by P wave with normal fixed PR interval—Normal sinus rhythm.
2. Fixed but short PR interval
   a. Wolf-Parkinson-White syndrome
   b. Lown-Ganong-Levine syndrome
   b. Non-sinus (or coronary sinus) atrial rhythm
   d. Nodal rhythm
3. Each QRS is always preceded by P but with PR interval varies.
   a. Wandering atrial pacemaker
   b. Multifocal atrial tachycardia.
4. Each QRS is always preceded by P but PR interval is fixed and prolonged (>0.2 sec). First degree AV block. First degree heart block: PR interval > 0.20 sec.
5. Mobitz type I second degree AV block or Wenckebach phenomenon.
   PR interval is normal in the first beat but lengthens progressively till a P wave fails to conduct and so the QRS is dropped. Thus, there is progressive lengthening of PR interval with intermittent dropped beats.
   After a pause the next AV nodal conduction begins with again normal PR interval with progressive lengthening of PR interval till a QRS beat is dropped.
6. Mobitz type II—second degree AV block.
   Some Ps are preceded by QRS and some are not.
   PR intervals constant and then a P wave suddenly fails to conduct.

The block is lower, nearer the bundle of His, bundle branches or at the level of the three fascicles.
PR intervals constant but the ventricles respond to every second or third beat in the heart. 2:1, 3:1 or 4:1 block, 3:1 or 4:1 block is formed high-grade AV block.
Pulse slow and regular.

7. Third degree heart block
Complete heart block
Ref. Fig. Q-91-92
No relationship between P wave and QRS complexes. P and QRS are independent of each other. QRS complexes are regular but at a slower rate than the P waves. Third degree (complete) AV block is a high AV block.
If complete AV block occurs above AV node, a junctional (or nodal) rhythm takes over and conduct the impulse producing narrow QRS complexes at the intrinsic rate of AV node, usually 40–55/min.
Low AV block: If the block is below the AV node (i.e. bundle of His, bilateral bundle branch or trifascicular), the QRS are wide and the rate is of intrinsic of a ventricular pacemaker, i.e. about 20–40/min.
8. The relationship between P waves and QRS are independent of each other but the QRS rate is more rapid than P wave rate - AV dissociation.
AV dissociation—P and QRS are independent of each other, ventricles beat independently at a slightly faster rate than the atria and the PR interval becomes shorter and the last P wave is seen to have walked through QRS.

ECG IN MYOCARDIAL INFARCTION

Whenever occlusion of a coronary artery occurs, the portion of the myocardium that is supplied by that particular vessel is affected. The damage progresses through stages of ischemia, injury finally infarction.

Ischemia means reduced blood supply. It is always reversible, infarction is always irreversible and injury is potentially reversible depending on the type of condition and treatment.

All the effects of three zones are seen in ECG.
A central—dead or necrotic zone—Infarction Q/QS
A middle—Injury zone—ST elevation
An outer—Ischemic zone—T inversion or ST depression.

The "three I" is the basis for recognizing and diagnosing the signs of myocardial infarction.
Ischemia, literally means reduced blood supply. T wave inversion is the characteristic sign of ischemia and may vary from a slightly flat or depressed wave to deep inversion (symmetrically inverted).

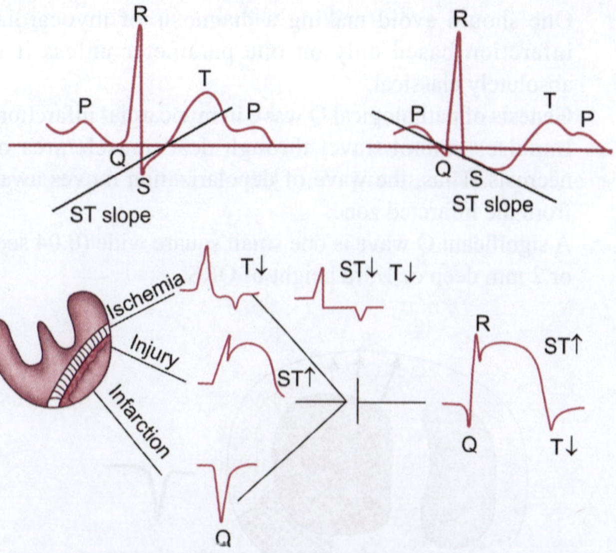

Fig. Q-136: ECG patterns of ischemia, injury and infarction

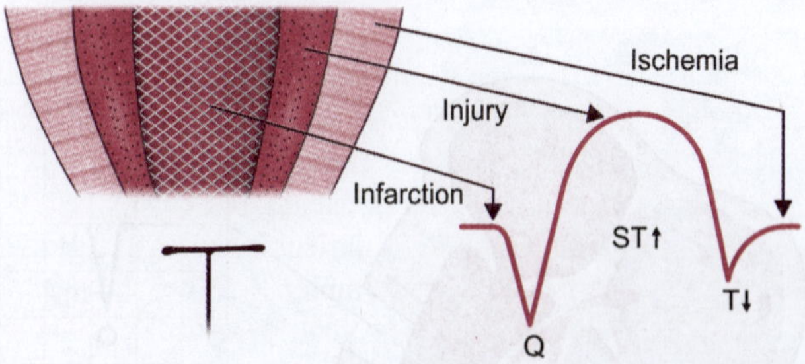

Fig. Q-137: Zone of ischemia injury and infarction—QRS and T waves changes

Since the chest leads are nearest the ventricles, T wave changes are most prominent in these leads. Always check V1 to V6 for T wave inversion to see if there is diminished coronary blood flow (early changes).
ST elevation means that the infarction is fresh (acute or recent).
Ischemia manifest in the ECG as symmetrically inverted T wave and/or ST segment depression. ST segment depression can be horizontal, down going or upgoing from the J point (the point marking the end of QRS complex and the beginning of the ST segment).
The horizontal and down going ST segments are relatively more specific for ischemia than the upgoing one's (symmetrical T inversion is seen in ischemia, asymmetrical T inversion is seen in LV hypertrophy).

151. It should be emphasized that diagnosis of myocardial infarction is usually based on the following 4 points:

1. History
2. Clinical findings
3. ECG
4. Cardiac enzymes.

One should avoid making a diagnosis of myocardial infarction based only on one parameter unless it is absolutely classical.

Genesis of pathological Q wave in myocardial infarction: Impulses cannot travel through dead muscle/area of necrosis. Thus, the wave of depolarization moves away from the infarcted zone.

A significant Q wave is one small square wide (0.04 sec) or 2 mm deep or 1/3rd height of QRS.

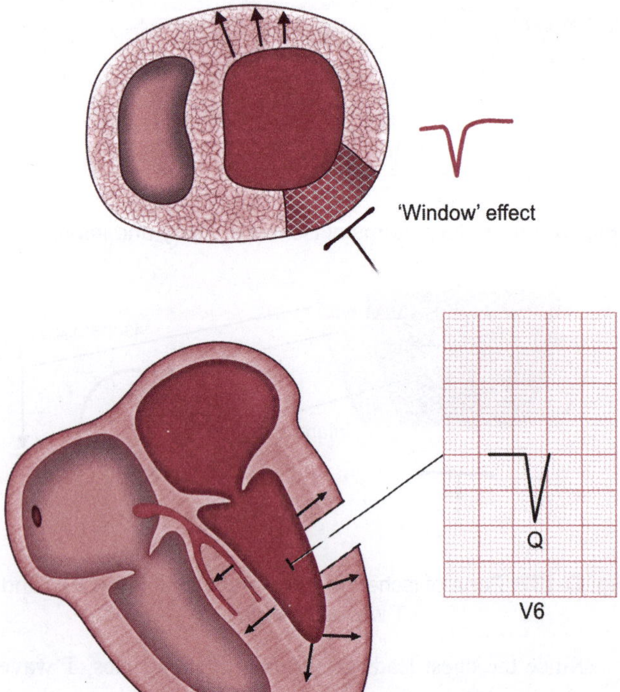

Fig. Q-138: Depolarization moving away from the electrode on the side of infarcted area. 'Window effect' results in Q wave formation

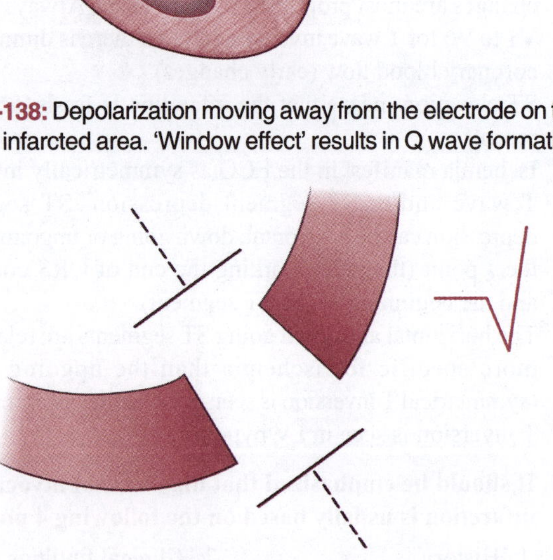

Fig. Q-139: Window effect, significant wave

Though the current passes toward the electrode, it cannot pass or travel in that direction because the tissue is infarcted. The electrode placed outside will have window effect and behaves like the electrode that is placed on the other direction, i.e. opposite side, because the tissue is dead. Since the electrode behaves as if it is placed on the other side—the current passing on the opposite direction gives negative Q wave.

The area of infarction extends from endocardial surface to epicardial surface of the myocardium in transmural infarction. Normally, the impulses travels from endocardial to epicardial surface, i.e. the ventricles are depolarized from inside outwards. Whenever there is infarction, there will be an 'electrical hole' between the ventricular cavity and the exploring electrode through which impulses cannot travel. Thus, the impulses or electrical forces travel away from the exploring electrode resulting in negative Q/QS wave. This is the 'window' effect of transmural infarction. An electrode looking at the heart over the window will record a cavity potential, i.e. a Q wave. Since the dead tissue cannot conduct the impulses, the overlying electrode behaves like the electrode that is placed on the other direction in the opposite side records a negative QS deflection and the neighboring electrode an abnormal Q wave (> 0.04 sec, i.e. more than one small square across and/or more than 2 mm deep).

The depth of Q wave depends on the location of the exploring electrode in relation to the site of infarction and the amount of tissue involved from endocardium to epicardium.

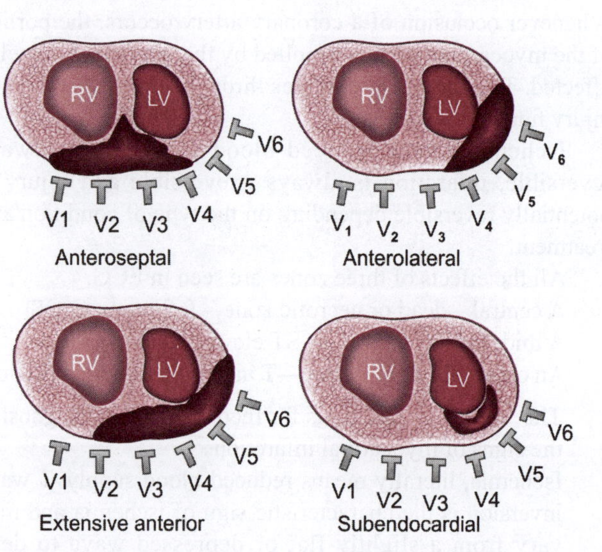

Fig. Q-140: Diagrammatic representation of site of infarction

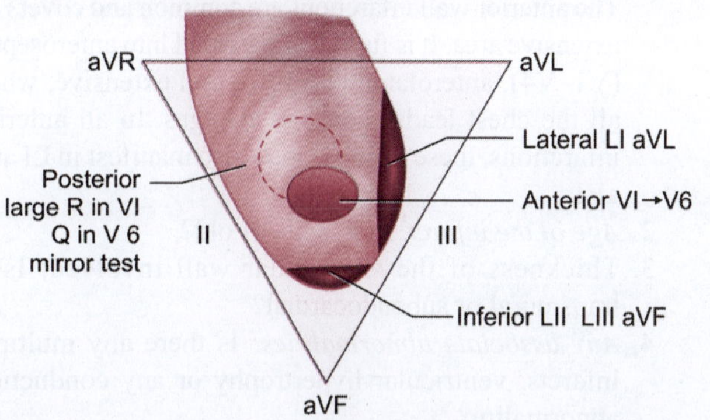

Fig. Q-141: Diagrammatic representation of site of infarction and leads

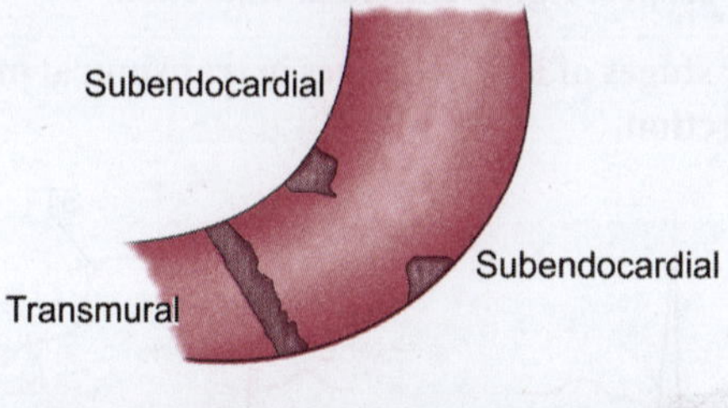

Fig. Q-142: Subendocardial infarction

Subendocardial infarction: In subendocardial infarction, the current pass away from the electrode. So ST depression there is no Q wave because the infarcted area affected is only the endocardial portion of the myocardium. The epicardial region is not affected. There is ST depression with T wave inversion in several of the limb leads and precordial leads.

Subendocardial infarction is less common because it has double blood supply. Subepicardial is more prone to MI.

Ischemia }
Injury } The "three I" triad is the basis for
Infarction } diagnosing MI

High lateral wall infarction: The changes are seen sometimes only in aVL. They may be demonstrated by placing the precordial leads higher up on the left side in 3rd and 4th intercostal space.

152. There are 4 general locations in the left ventricle where infarction commonly occurs:

1. Anterior infarction	V1 to V6	Q/ST↑, T↓
2. Lateral infarction	LI, aVL	Q/ST↑, T↓
3. Inferior infarction	LII, LIII, aVF	Q/ST↑, T↓
4. Posterior infarction	large R in V1,	ST↓

Mirror image test:

Infarction can occur in more than one area in left ventricle. One may be very old and one may be acute, so correlate the ST elevation with reciprocal ST depression in appropriate leads for the location of an infarct.

Always take right chest leads, i.e. V3R, V4R when posterior or inferior infarction is suspected. Presence of QS in V3R or V4R and/or an ST elevation of even 1mm not only suggest involvement of the septum but also indicates that AV block of varying degrees probably develop.

153. Relation of coronary arteries with myocardial infarction (See Fig. E-1)

1. Left anterior descending artery occlusion—causes anterior and anteroseptal infarctions and often responsible for infarction of the apex.
2. Left circumflex artery occlusion causes lateral infarctions—anterolateral, inferolateral, or high lateral.
3. Right coronary arteries supplies the right ventricle.
4. Posterior descending artery from right coronary artery occlusion is responsible for true posterior and inferior myocardial infarctions.

In 10% of the hearts, the left circumflex artery crosses and supplies the posterior descending artery—Its occlusion causes infarction of the inferior and true posterior walls as well as the lateral wall of the left ventricle.

Left ventricle has greater power, so two vessels of left coronary artery—left anterior descending artery (LAD), and left circumflex artery, where as right ventricle has lesser power, so one vessel—right coronary artery (RCA).

LI, aVL	– left circumflex artery
LII, LIII, aVF	– right coronary artery
V1	– proximal right coronary artery
V2,V3,V4	– left anterior descending artery (LAD)
V5, V6	– left circumflex artery (LCX)

ECG tells which coronary artery is affected.

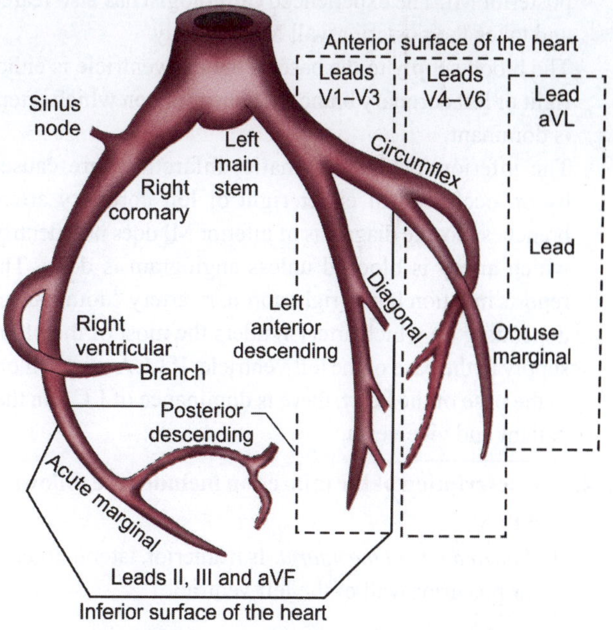

Fig. Q-143: Relation of coronary arteries and ECG leads

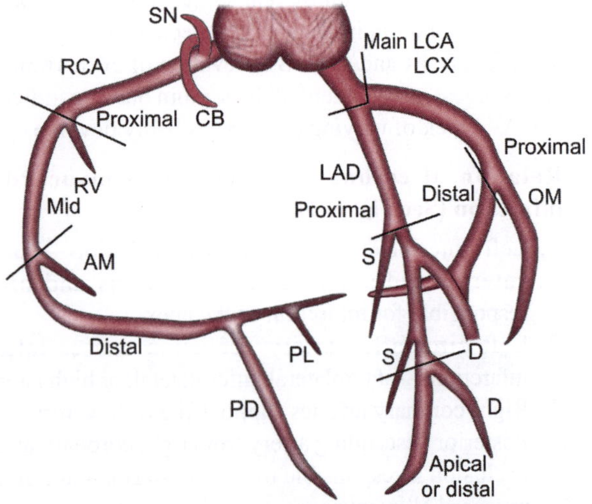

Fig. Q-144: Schematic diagram of coronary artery branches **RCA:** right coronary artery SN: sinus node branch: CB, conus branch; RV: right ventricular branch; AM: acuts marginal branch; PD: posterior descending branch; PL: posterolateral branch of left ventricel
LCA: left coronary artert
LAD: left anterior descending branch; S: septal branches; D: diagonal branches
LCX: left circumflex coronary artery; OM: obtuse marginal branch

For many years, right coronary artery (RCA), consider to play a minor role, in the blood supply of the heart. Development of coronary angiogram has demonstrated that RCA supplies blood to SA node, AV node and bundle of His. So, one can expect dangerous arrhythmias in acute posterior MI. The experienced cardiologist has also feared and takes the posterior wall MI seriously.

The blood supply to the base of the left ventricle is either right or left coronary branches depending on which artery is dominant.

The inferior (or diaphragmatic) infarctions are caused by on occlusion of either right or left coronary artery branches. So, the diagnosis of inferior MI does not identify, which artery is blocked unless angiogram is done. The reports mention left or right coronary artery "dominance" depending on which artery renders the most of the blood supply to the base of the left ventricle. If LCA supply more to the base of the heart, there is dominance of LCA in that patient and vice versa.

154. The description of the infarction includes the following 4 points:

1. *Site and size of the infarct:* Is it anterior, lateral, inferior or posterior wall of the left ventricle?

   The anterior wall infarctions are common and covers an extensive area. It is further subdivided into anteroseptal (V1–V4), anterolateral (V5,V6) and extensive, when all the chest leads show the changes. In all anterior infarctions, these changes may also manifest in LI and aVL.
2. *Age of the infarct:* Is it acute or old?
3. Thickness of the ventricular wall involved: Is it transmural or subendocardial?
4. *Any associate abnormalities:* Is there any multiple infarcts, ventricular hypertrophy or any conduction abnormality?

MI usually means: Infarction in the left ventricle.
In inferior wall infarction if there is rise in JVP and fall in BP—suspect right ventricular infarction.

155. Four stages of ECG changes in transmural myocardial infarction.

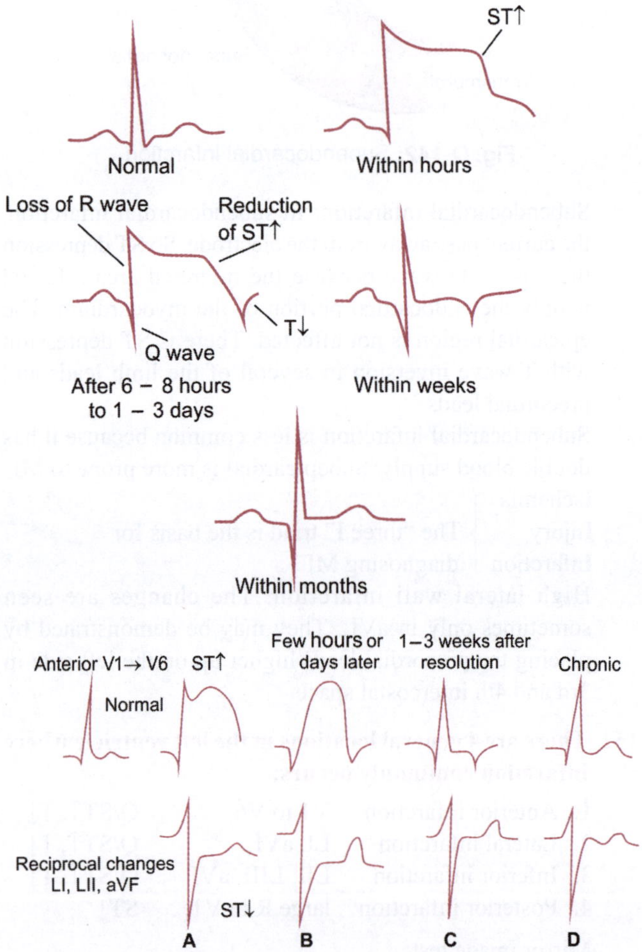

Fig. Q-145: Schematic representation of 4 stages of ECG changes in transmural myocardial infarction

Table Q-4

A. Acute or fresh infarct	ST elevation – Hyperactive, ST concavity is lost ST depression in opposite leads—reciprocal changes
B. Few hours or few days	ST elevation with convexity upward, T inversion, abnormal Q as the infarction establishes Q is bigger and deeper after few hours or days. Posterior leads show ST depression—reciprocal changes
C. One to three weeks after	ST comes to normal or almost normal level but T is still inverted Abnormal Q remains
D. Old or healed infarct. One to few months after	Only abnormal Q remains. Q is the footprint of old MI. ST, T otherwise becomes normal

156. The ECG changes in myocardial infarction undergoes serial changes as time passes from hours to days to weeks to months. This is called evolution of infarct. It is therefore, obvious that serial—

ECGs, 2–3 times per day for the first few days and then once a day per week or so is important. It is useful to know the age of infarction and prognosis. There are 4 stages of evolution of infarction.

These stages can be demonstrated by taking serial electrocardiograms:

Stage I: Acute phase or fresh infarct: In the first few hours—ST segment is raised with convexity upwards—Q may or may not appear.

Stage II: Q waves appear ST segments slowly returns to isoelectric line. T becomes inverted.

Stage III: Q waves are present, ST isoelectrical, T wave symmetrically inverted (arrowhead inversion).

Stage IV: The T wave gradually becomes shallower and returns to normal. The only evidence of previous infarction is the presence of pathological Q waves.

Sometimes with good collateral circulation, the necrotic area shrinks and the Q waves may disappear and no evidence of infarct may be seen.

157. Infarction usually means it is in the left ventricle. It can also occur in right ventricle. There are 4 common sites of infarction where ECG shows definite localization (left ventricle):

1. *Anterior septal infarction:* (Fig. Q-146)
   Q and/or ST elevation and T inversion in
   LI, aVL, V1 to V4
   (Ref. Chapter-F Acute MI, Fig. F-3)
2. *Anterolateral infarction:*
   Q and/or ST elevation and T inversion in
   LI, aVL and V4 to V6
   (Remember: Lateral Infarction—for LI and aVL)
3. *Inferior or diaphragmatic infarction:* (Fig. Q-148)
   Q and/or ST elevation and T inversion in
   LII, LIII and aVF
   Reciprocal ST depression inV2–V5
4. *True posterior infarction:* (Fig. Q-149)
   Tall R in V1 and V2
   may be Q in V6.

Mirror image test:

The posterior wall infarction may be associated with inferior wall infarction manifesting only as reciprocal change with ST-T changes in opposite direction in anterior leads V1–V4, which usually indicates a posterior wall infarction in addition to the inferior wall infarction. Posterior wall infarction is uncommon and best diagnosed by an esophageal ECG or echocardiogram.

Note ST elevation with upward convexity in leads LI, aVL and V1–V5; reciprocal ST depression in LII, LIII and aVF; T wave inverted in LI and aVL.

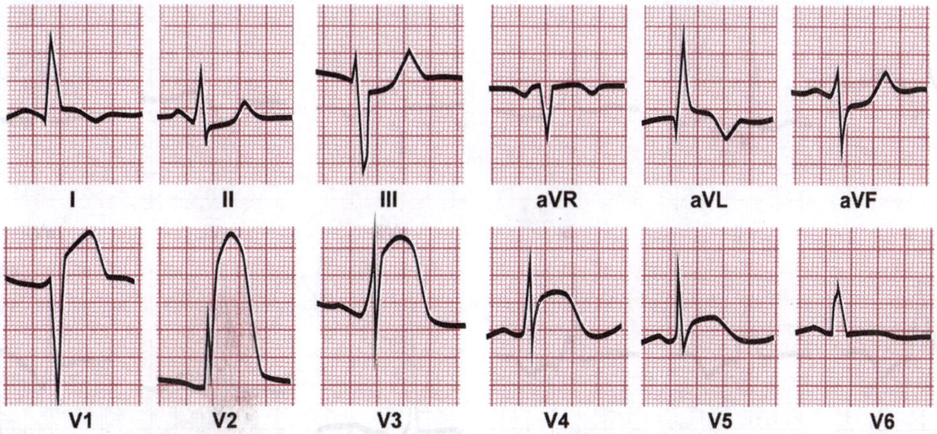

Fig. Q-146: Acute anterior myocardial infarction (recent in six hours): Regular sinus rhythm, PR = 0.14 sec; QRS = 0.06 sec; Frontal plane axis = –10º ; Horizontal heart position;

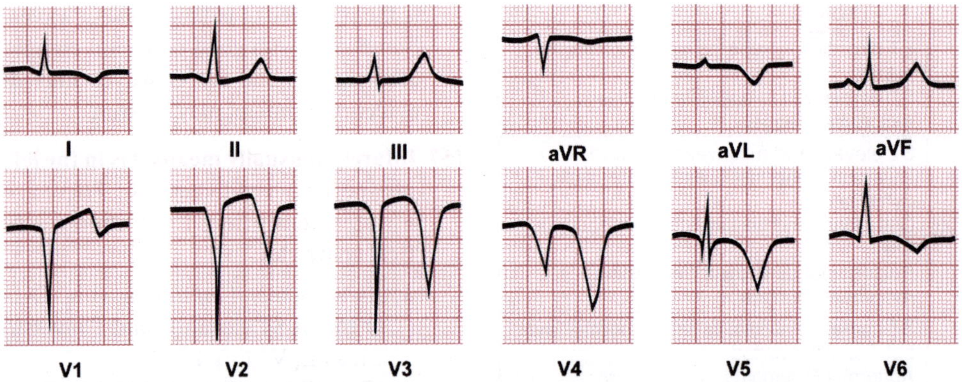

Fig. Q-147: Anterior myocardial infarction (late pattern—6 months old): Regular sinus rhythm; PR = 0.14 sec; QRS = 0.08 sec; Frontal plane axis = +60°; Note QS complexes in V1–V4 and deep symmetrically inverted T waves in LI, aVL, V2–V6

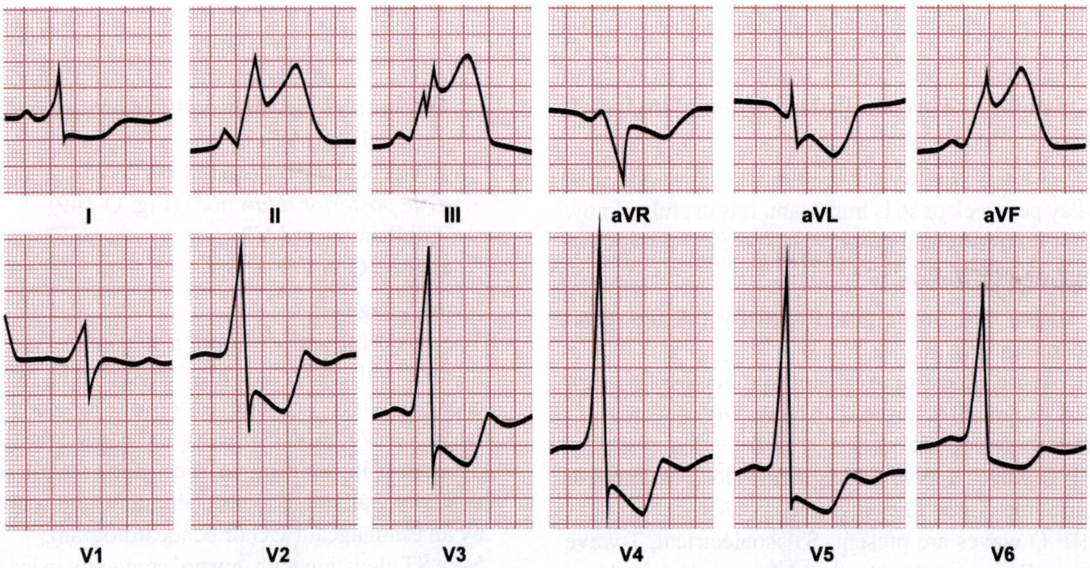

Fig. Q-148: Recent inferior myocardial infarction; Wolff-Parkinson-White syndrome; Regular sinus rhythm; PR interval = 0.1 sec; QRS = 0.12 sec; Note marked ST elevation in LII, LIII and aVF with reciprocal ST depression in LI, aVL and all precordial leads. There is slurring of the upstroke of the R wave in LI, LII, LIII, aVL and in all precordial leads

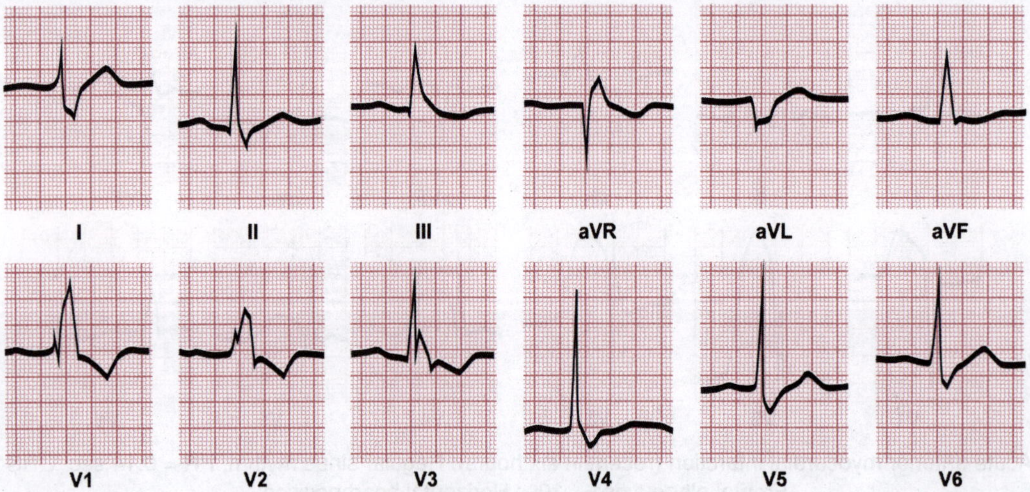

Fig. Q-149: Posterior myocardial infarction

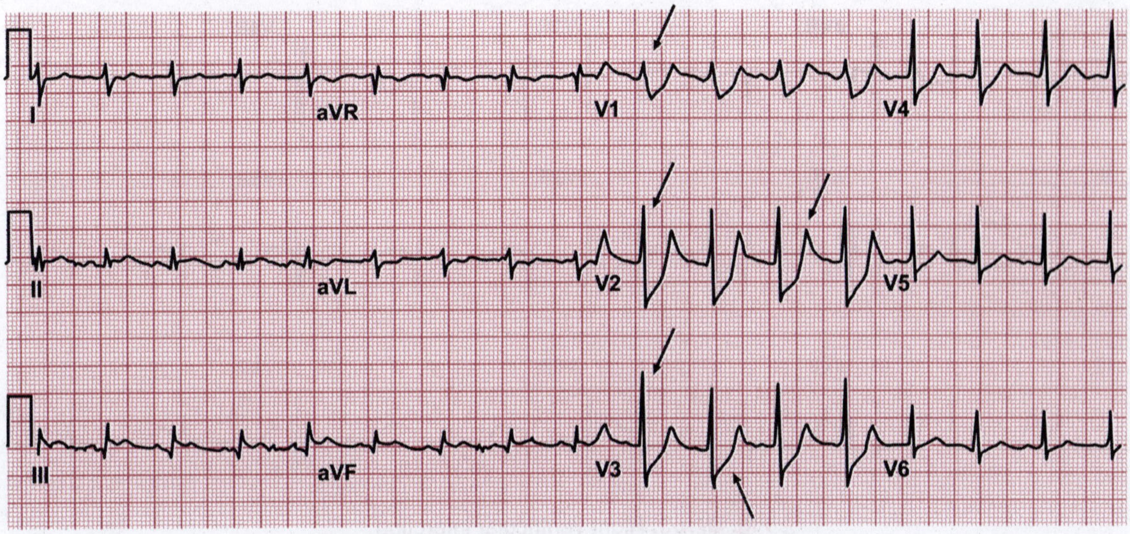

Fig. Q-150: Acute posterior myocardial infarction

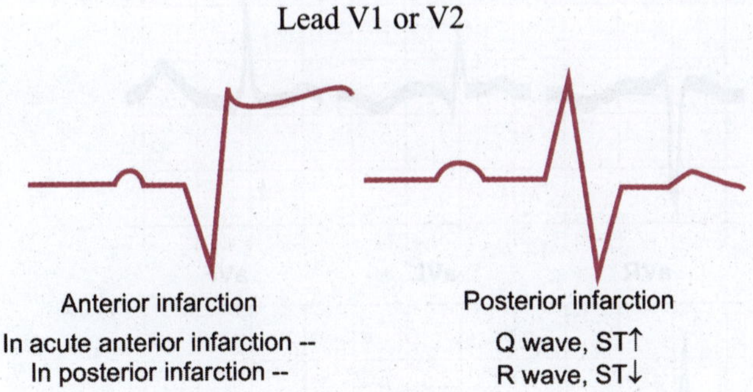

Fig. Q-151

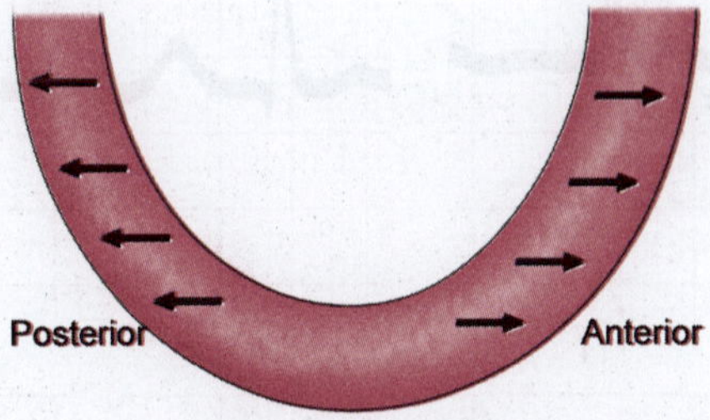

Fig. Q-152

Regular sinus rhythm; PR 0.24 sec, QRS 0.14 sec, ventricle position, A wide S wave is present in leads LI, V4–V6, a wide R in aVR, rSR' (with a very small s) in V1; Notched and wide R in V2–V3, ST depression and T inversion in V1–V3, ventricular activation time (VAT) in V1 = 0.11 sec.

Note prominent R wave in right precordial leads (reciprocal of posterior Q wave) right bundle branch block; first degree AV block.

Q wave and ST elevation occur in V1 and V2 in anterior infarction. So, posterior infarction could appear as opposite— Prominent R wave and ST depression.

In lead V1, if Q wave turned upside down—would appear like an R wave (mirror image).

When you see a large R wave in V1 or V2 suspect posterior infarction even though right ventricular hypertrophy can cause them.

History and clinical examination would help.

Electrical activity of anterior and posterior wall of left ventricle is in opposite direction.

Depolarization of anterior wall of ventricle starts from inside to outside of left ventricle anteriorly. Depolarization of posterior wall of left ventricle start from inside to outside of left ventricle posteriorly. Thus, the depolarization of anterior and posterior wall of left ventricle point in opposite direction.

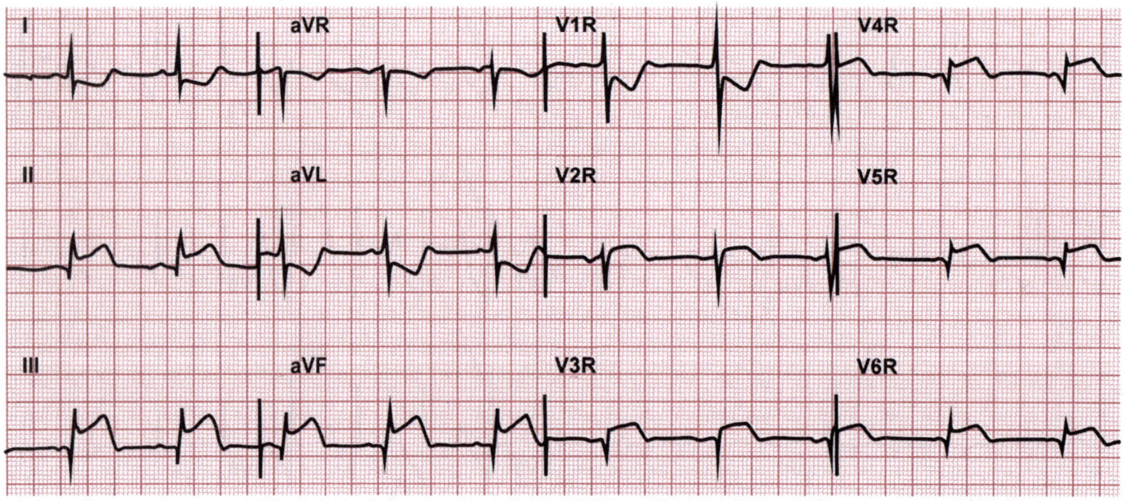

Fig. Q-153: Right ventricular infarction

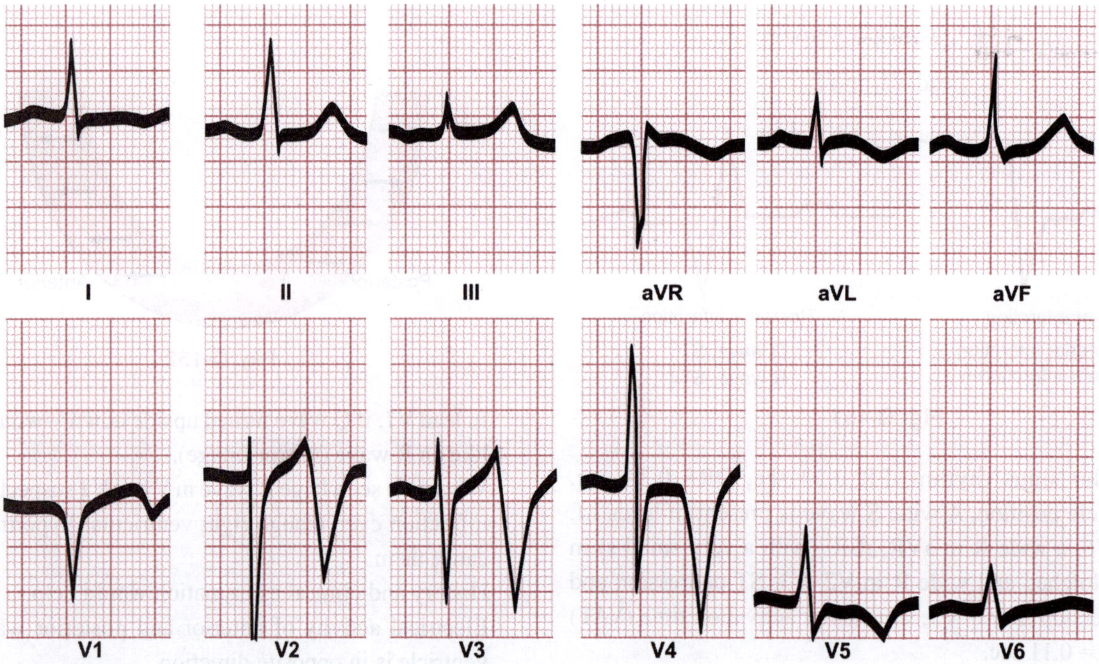

Fig. Q-154: Subendocardial infarction; Left ventricular hypertrophy: Regular sinus rhythm; PR = 0.16 sec; QRS = 0.08 sec; intermediate heart position; Note T wave inversion in leads LI and aVL; Very deep, symmetrically inverted T waves in V2-V4. No abnormal Q waves are present. Note tall R waves in V5-V6; R in V5 = 30 mm

Always take right chest leads V3R, V4R, when posterio-inferior infarction is suspected. Presence of QS in V3R or V4R and/or an ST elevation of even 1mm not only suggest involvement of the septum but also indicates that AV block of varying degress will probably develop.

Remember:

Q indicates infarction or necrosis

ST elevation indicates injury

T inversion indicates ischemia

Subendocardial infarction involves only small area of myocardium. They cause flat (horizontal) ST depression and T inversion in overlying leads.

158. Subendocardial infarction involves only the endocardium. Causing ST ↓.

The causes of ST depression are:

1. Subendocardial infarction
2. Positive Master's test—when a patient of ischemic coronary diseases exercised, ST depression occurs

3. Digitalis
4. Posterior infarction in V1 and V2 (opposite of ST ↑ of anterior infarction—mirror image).

Always exclude nonspecific ST-T changes.

159. Atrial infarction: It indicates involvement of large area. It is suspected when atrial arrhythmia, e.g. atrial fibrillation develops in the presence of ventricular infarction.

1. Widespread depression of the PR segment in the presence of atrial arrhythmia.
2. Elevation of PR segment in left chest leads with reciprocal depression in right chest leads.
3. Elevation of PR segment in LI with reciprocal depression in LIII.
4. Abnormal P wave contour.

160. The 4 important general points to be noted in ECG of acute myocardial infarction.

1. Time relationship: Usually ST segment changes appear early within the first few hours and progress, later T waves become inverted. Rarely, no changes are seen in ECG for several days or even for 2 to 3 weeks.
   ST changes are usually the most transitory;
   the T changes are more lasting;
   the Q waves are most likely to remain as permanent footprint of infarction.
   Sometimes T waves instead of becoming inverted, actually become taller and appear as an upward extension of the rising ST segment. This early tall T wave may be confused for the later tall T wave of reciprocal leads. Similar persistent T waves are not uncommon with angina. T waves become shallower and finally returns to normal.
   Well established Q waves may sometimes completely disappear. Persistent ST elevation or the presence of an rSR in V6 suggest possibility of ventricular aneurysm.
   Persistent elevation of ST segment in several leads suggests pericarditis.
   In acute infarction, changes of evolution must be in evidence. Progressive changes from day-to-day are the conclusive evidence of an active acute process.
2. The ECG should be considered supportive and confirmatory of the clinical diagnosis, and should not supersede it. If the patient is strongly suspected of acute infarction clinically, he should be treated accordingly even if the ECG is normal. The ECG changes may appear late or rarely they may appear in the routine leads, although infarction is a clinical certainty. Other investigations like enzyme estimation can help in the diagnosis.
3. The Q waves of infarction may be better revealed in premature ventricular beats than in the sinus conducted beats.
4. Appearance of other abnormalities besides changes specific for acute myocardial infarction. The ECG tracing often shows low voltage and the QT interval is prolonged reaching its maximum in the second week. Any arrhythmia or block may develop. Continuous monitoring reveals arrhythmias in 75–95% of patients. Commonest arrhythmias are premature ventricular beats, next supraventricular premature beats, atrial fibrillation, ventricular tachycardia, accelerated idioventricular rhythms and supraventricular tachycardia. AV blocks develop often with inferior infarction than anterior infarction.

161. It is estimated that with 12 lead ECG, only 80–90% infarctions are diagnosable. The remaining can be missed. The probable causes of missed diagnoses are:

1. Failure to take serial tracings. This can occur when there is long interval between the appearance of pain and delayed electrical changes in ECG.
2. Failure to take additional exploratory chest leads in doubtful cases. Small area of infarction can be missed.
3. Anterior infarction in the presence of left bundle branch block. Loss of QRS amplitude over the left ventricle is a clue to infarction in the presence of left bundle branch block.
4. Simultaneous infarction in opposite direction neutralizing each others pattern.
   If the patient is taking digitalis, it neutralizes ST elevation.

162. Following are some of the conditions in which ECG is falsely positive or falsely negative with respect to the changes of infarction (see Q-39).

Table Q-5

False positive	*False negative*
1. Prinzmetal angina	ECG taken too early
2. Pericarditis	Abnormal locations or small infarctions
3. Ventricular aneurysm	Bundle branch blocks (especially LBBB)
4. Early repolarization syndrome	WPW syndrome
5. Myocarditis	Multiple infarcts (diagonally opposite)
6. LBBB and WPW syndrome	Atrial or right ventricular infarctions
7. Cor pulmonale	Presence of arrhythmias
8. Digitalis effect	Digitalis effect
9. HOCM	
10. Quinidie therapy	
11. Cardiac tumor	
12. Noncardiac lesions like CVA	

ECG IN CORONARY ARTERY DISEASE/ ISCHEMIC HEART DISEASE

(Refer the Chapter-E on Coronary Artery Disease/Ischemic Heart Disease)

Electrocardiographogenic Disease

Abnormalities in ECG do not necessarily indicate cardiac disease, much less coronary insufficiency. When deviation of ST-T from normal occur in the middle-aged and elderly they are simply interpreted as coronary insufficiency/ischemic heart disease. Many patients are becoming cardiac disease oriented and unnecessarily becoming cardiac crippled. This may be true statistically but each case should be analyzed before labeling it as coronary insufficiency.

163. The normal range is wide and limits cannot be satisfactorily defined. The changes seen at times are normal variants. The following 4 are some examples.

One should remember the following facts before attaching them 'cardiac' or 'coronary' label.

1. Persistent 'juvenile' precordial pattern in young healthy Negroes. Unusual ST elevation is common in Negroes.
2. ST-T depression in suspended hearts.
3. Precordial T inversion during pregnancy.
4. RBBB pattern in marathon runners is a typical example —whose heart is hardly be doubted.

164. Extracardiac factors that mimic myocardial disease.

Many factors influence the repolarization, which are reflected in ST segment and T wave alterations. The T wave and to a lesser extent ST segment are unstable and they can be easily altered by many major or minor provocations.

I. Physiological stimuli that can affect:
   a. Eating, drinking ice water, grape juice
   b. Posture
   c. Hyperventilation
   d. Emotional disturbance—fear or anxiety
   e. Neurocirculatory asthenia, hyperkinetic circulatory syndrome together with tachycardia

II. Electrolyte disturbance : Hyperkalemia, hypocalcemia

III. Drugs: Including digitalis, quinidine, procainamide, adrenaline, isoprenaline, insulin, phenothiazine

IV. Systemic diseases
   a. Acute abdomen—acute pancreatitis, cholecystitis
   b. Shock
   c. Hiatus hernia
   d. Cerebrovascular accidents—stroke, subarachnoid hemorrhage
   e. Psychosis
   f. Endocrine disturbance.

165. The heart may be a victim of many diseases—that is not primarily cardiac—particularly coronary artery disease the CVS changes that are seen secondary to other diseases.

1. Pulmonary embolism
2. Anemia
3. Hyperthyrodism
4. Myocarditis from infections (pneumonia, infective mononucleosis)
5. Connective tissue disorders—sarcoidosis, amyloidosis, scleroderma, disseminated lupus erythematosis.
6. Friedrich's ataxia
7. Progressive muscular dystrophy
8. Myasthenia gravis.

These can produce changes in electrocardiogram indistinguishable from changes of coronary artery disease.

166. Therefore, before labeling as coronary insufficiency for IHD one should ask the following 4 questions.

1. Could this be a normal variant?
2. Could this be physiological?
3. Could this be due to extracardiac cause?
4. Could these changes be due to heart disease other than coronary?

The chances of 1 and 2 branding them as coronary is pitiable. From the above statements, one should know that an 'Abnormal' ECG tracing does not mean an abnormal heart.

Remembering this will save many from cardiac invalidism.

EXERCISE STRESS TESTING

167. Stress test is employed in ischemic heart disease to measure the coronary blood flow in response to increased myocardial oxygen demand.

ECG stress testing is ideal because

1. It is ideal to perform in large number of patients
2. It is the stress produced to increase the myocardial oxygen demand in a safe and reproducible manner
3. The changes are easily observed in ECG that are specific in alteration of CVS function

   ST segment depression is taken as the end point to define ischemia in standardized exercise test.
4. The risk of exercise test is very small.

   One fatal and two nonfatal complications for 10,000 tests.

   A physician should always be present throughout the exercise test to observe the patient, to evaluate the ECG, BP, during the exercise and to decide whether the test can be continued or not.

168. Four forms of stress test:

1. Physical exercise—commonly performed test
2. Pharmacological—dobutamine, adenosine, dipyridamole, atropine
3. Electrical—pacing
4. Nuclear studies—e.g. thallium scintigraphy.

169. The information content of stress testing is enhanced by adding the following 4 techniques.

1. Metabolic gas analysis
2. Radionucleide imaging
3. Echocardiography
4. Myocardial contrast Echo.

170. Metabolic Equivalent (Met): It is the resting total body oxygen consumption (VO_2) in a 70 kg 40-year-old male. It is the unit to calculate work activity.

1. It is the requirement of 35 mL/kg/min oxygen at basal metabolic rate.
2. (VO_2) It is arteriovenous (AV) oxygen difference multiplied by cardiac output (CO)
3. (VO_2 max) It is the index of maximal exercise capacity or functional capacity
4. Exercise testing protocols—Two major protocols are commonly used—Treadmill and Bicycle ergometry.

171. Four modes of physical stress tests are used.

1. Steps: Either single or multiple.
   Two step system of exercise developed by master is an example of tests with standardized external workloads. Master's stairs have become standardized during the past many years.
2. Motor driven treadmill—Speed and inclination are controlled by the operator.
   Bicycle ergometer and treadmill tests are standardized by heart rate response and designed to reach the maximal possible exercise load. They differ in the method of determining the end point of the exercise.
3. Bicycle ergometer—Controlled by the patient.
4. Stress test in recumbent position during the course of cardiac catheterization.
   Leg exercise is performed with a bicycle device or isometric handgrips by squeezing an ergometer.
   Pacing stress test—by pacing induced tachycardia.
   1, 2, 3 are commonly done.
   Fourth is done only in special circumstances in specialized units.

172. Test procedure: 4 safety measures.

1. Plan the duties of each member of the team—all the members of the team should have training in cardiopulmonary resuscitation (CPR).
2. Defibrillator within cable reach of treadmill, turned on charged (200 J) during test and paste applied.
3. Emergency drugs including IV fluids, etc.
4. Facilities for endotracheal tube, ventilation, suction, etc.

173. Four indications of stress test.

1. For the detection of asymptomatic silent myocardial ischemia (SMI) or early coronary heart disease.
   or screening test for SMI.
   It can be used as a first screening test in persons with risk factors like smoking, hypertension, dyslipidemia and family history of heart attacks.
   Second screening test—Maximal exercise test:
   Men 40–50 years with > 2 risk factors.
   Men above 50 years with 1 risk factor.
   Women above 50 years with > 2 risk factors.
   Individuals working as pilots, railway and bus drivers and persons with similar job of responsibilities for the safety of others and expensive machinery they handle.
   Useful in evaluation of sports medicine.
   This is being done as a routine medical check-up in many developed countries.
2. For confirmation and documentation of angina: A diagnostic procedure—30–50% of patients with typical history of angina have normal resting ECG or have equivocal changes. Producing anginal pain by treadmill stress test not only confirms the diagnosis but also helps to assess the complete disability. This helps in the management and avoidance of multi-therapy and to take decision about coronary artery bypass graft surgery. It may also help to assess which vessels are involved.
   Patients developing angina or ST-T changes early in exercise protocol are either have multiple vessel disease or have a block higher up in one of the major vessels. Stress test helps in deciding the severity of coronary artery disease.
3. For evaluation of postmyocardial infarction patients.
   To assess the functional capacity before permitting to start normal work, sexual activity and recreational activity after myocardial infarction. Activity is permitted depending on the functional capacity.
   Patients developing angina or ST-T changes during exercise test in postmyocardial infarction period are likely to have two or three vessel disease. Sudden deaths are common in postinfarction patients with positive stress test and are very less in number with negative stress test.
   In one study the mortality in the first year after myocardial infarction was 27% in those with exercised induced ST changes, and only 2% in those without ST changes.

The indication is relatively stronger in young patients than in elderly.

4. For evaluation of prognosis during therapy or after bypass surgery.
   Response to drugs in coronary artery disease (CAD) after coronary artery bypass graft (CABG) can be documented.

174. Treadmill exercise test today has become an essential test in evaluation of patients with CAD. It should be a screening test on an annual basis for all high-risk groups. The following points must be remembered.

1. It does not tell about the percentage of coronary blockage.
2. It is contraindicated in unstable angina. Therefore one should be careful in doing this test in patients with doubtful history of anginal pain.
3. Symptom limited or heart rate limited depend on case to case.
4. False-positive and false-negative cases do occur.
5. Should be done fasting in the morning.
6. If the indication is to "rule out CAD", then it should be done without medicines for 2 days before.
7. If the indication is CAD evaluation then it should be done 'with morning medicines taken'. Often helpful in deciding need for a bypass surgery. In fact, it is often a more important investigation than angiography.
8. If cases are selected properly, it carries negligible mortality.

175. Patient preparation and precautions before procedure.

1. No drinking, eating or smoking—2 hours before
2. No strenuous physical activity at least 12 hours before testing
3. Off the drugs—for diagnostic TMT—digitalis 1 to 2 hours before and other drugs 3 to 5 half lives before testing
4. On the drugs—for prognostic TMT
5. Detailed explanation and demonstration of the procedure
6. Adequate skin preparation and special electrodes
7. Room temperature between 64° and 72°F and humidity of less than 60%
8. Do the clinical examination and resting ECG.
   Re-examine after TMT.

176. Master's 'two-step' exercise test is very simple and can be done in any clinic. It has:

1. 'Two-steps'
2. Each step is 9 inches height
3. 8–10 inches deep
4. 18–27 inches wide.

Procedure

A resting ECG is taken first. Patient is instructed to walk up and down the steps for a definite number in 1 to 1 1/2 minutes. (The number of trips is known from the Master's table—it varies by age, sex, weight.)

An ECG is taken immediately after the exercise.

If normal, it may be repeated at intervals of several minutes to find out the presence of abnormality.

If ECG remains normal in a patient with angina, the double two-step test is done. It should not be done within one hour of the simple two-step test.

The patient walks double the number of times of single test in 3 minutes.

The criteria for a positive double two-step test is same as the single test.

It is preferable to take leads V3 to V6, aVR, aVL, aVF, LI, LII, LIII in that sequence after exercise. This allows speed and is sufficient for evaluation.

The 12-lead ECG is always better to have less false-positive results.

177. Choice of exercise can be made by comparing treadmill and bicycle ergometry mode.

	Treadmill	*Bicycle Ergometry*
1.	Maximum oxygen uptake	Less oxygen uptake
2.	Uses legs, arms and chest	Uses legs and arms Immobile chest
3.	Controlled by operator Minimum cooperation is required from the patient	More cooperation from the patient is needed
4.	Distorted ECG	Better ECG

These are not suitable for stress echo or stress hemodynamics.

178. TMT protocol—comparison.

	Modified Bruce	Naughton Bruce
1.	Low workload can be performed in	High workload
2.	Post-MI	Useful in stable angina pectoris
3.	Post-CABG	
4.	Post-PTCA	

179. Consequences of myocardial ischemia during exercise test.

1. Chest pain—not sensitive
2. Arrhythmias—not specific
3. Pump dysfunction—stress echo is done
4. ST segment shift—hallmark of ischemia.

180. Ischemic ST segment response is generally defined as

1. A flat depression of ST segment 1 mm or more below the baseline in LI, LII, LIII, aVL, aVF, and V5–V6. (Isoelectric line is taken as the level of the PR segment and the TP level.)
2. ST should be inscribed horizontally or obliquely downward and should last for more than 0.06–0.08 sec. The depression is like square or plateau type.
3. T wave changes from an upright T to a flat or inverted T in any leads except L III or the reverse in any lead.
4. Appearance of arrhythmias which were not present in the resting ECG.

If the threshold of positivity is seen at 0.05 mV, there will be more false-positive tests and fewer false-negative ones.

A. Regular sinus rhythm; Flat T wave in aVL may be evidence of some lateral wall abnormality

B. After exercise; Note the horizontal ST depression in V3–V6; This is 4 mm in V4. There is slight ST elevation in aVR; T has become inverted in aVL

The changes after exercise are consistent with coronary insufficiency.

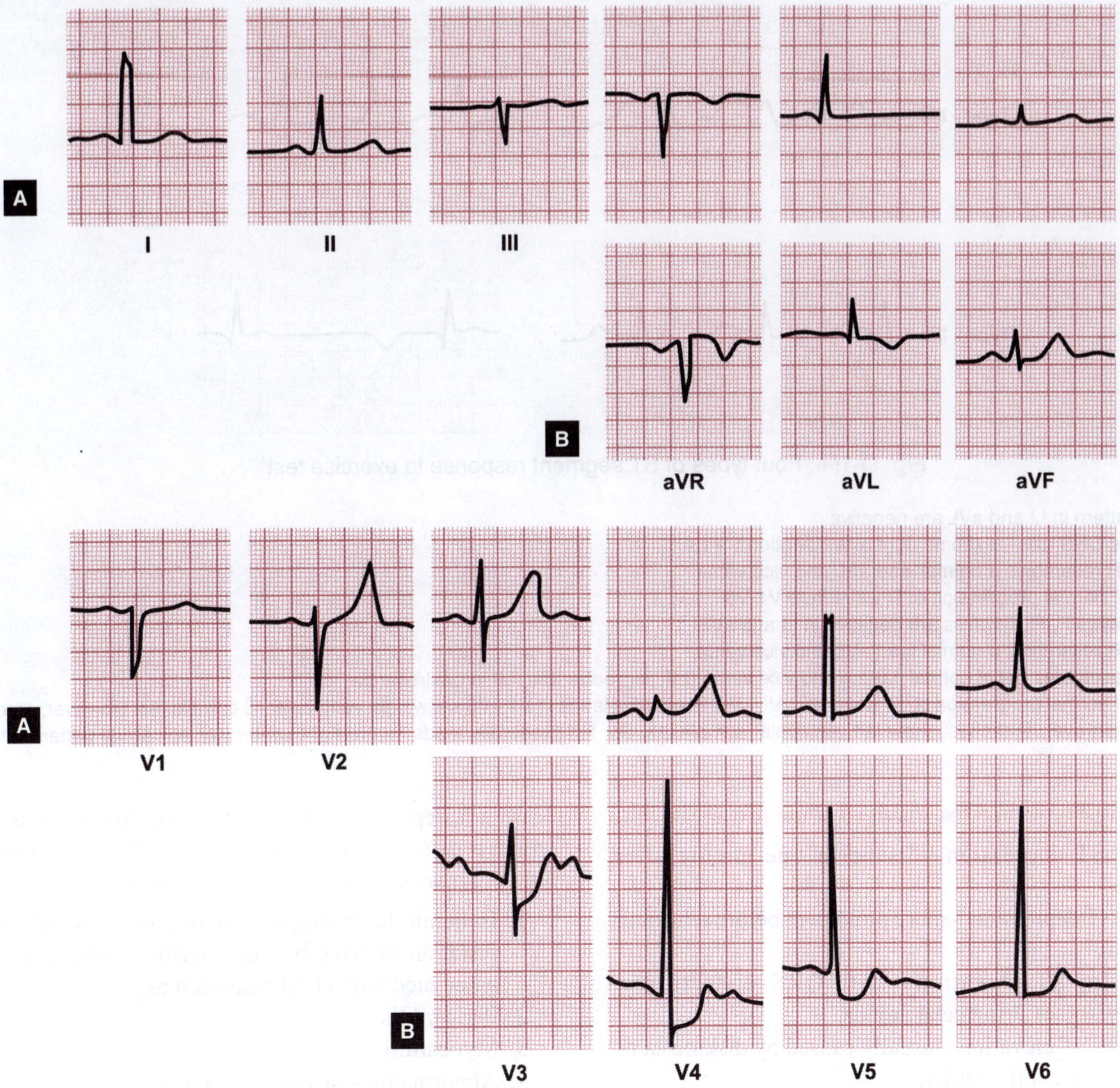

Fig. Q-155: Ischemic heart disease

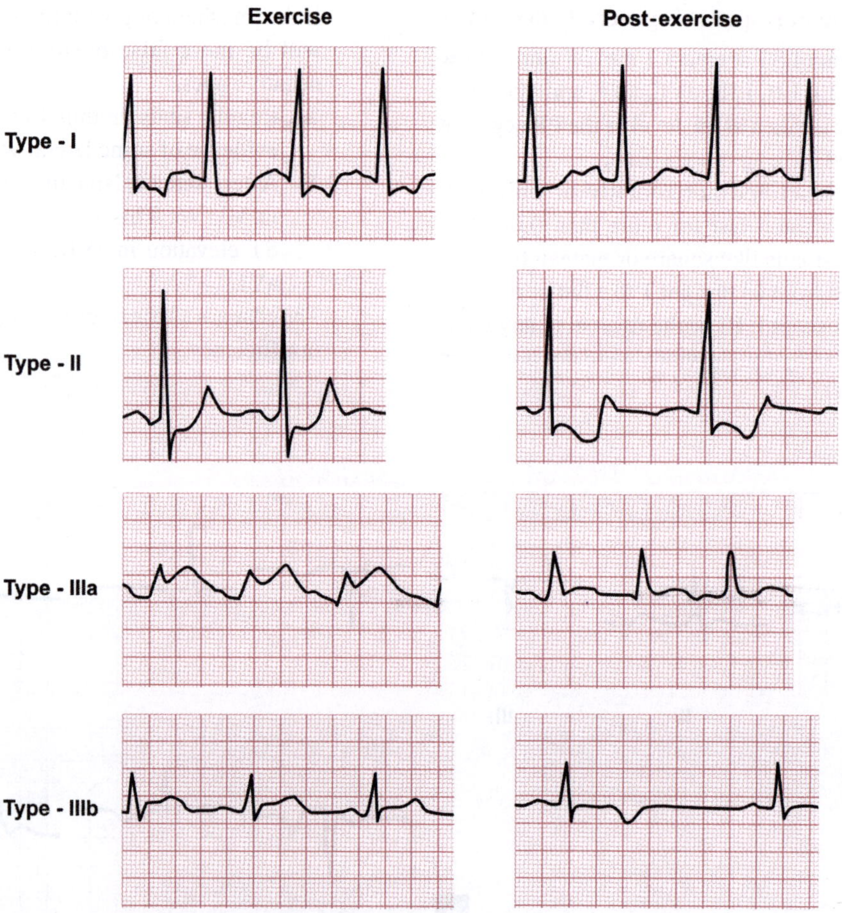

Fig. Q-156: Four types of ST segment response to exercise test

1. Entire pattern in LI and aVL are negative
2. Abnormal QRS axis—extreme right axis deviation > +180°
3. Lead aVR resembles a normal lead aVL and vice versa
4. Failure of normal progression of R wave from V1-V6
5. All the waves P, R, T waves are negative in LI and aVL
6. Lead aVR resembles a normal lead aVL and vice versa
7. Lead II resembles LIII of normal pattern and vice versa (LIII is greater than LII in dextrocardia)
8. Failure of normal progression of 'R' wave from VI – V6. Precordial leads in V1 –V6 show right ventricular rS complexes. However, precordial leads taken over right chest show left ventricular complexes. So, left precordial leads record right ventricular epicardial pattern and vice versa.

181. There are 4 types of ST segment response to exercise test.

Type I: ST depression—disappear one minute after exercise.

Type II: ST depression—more prominent before returning to normal.

Type IIIa: ST elevation—with QRS distortion—characteristic of Prinzmetal angina.

Type IIIb: ST elevation—usually caused by diskinesia or scarring of the left ventricle.

182. Do not depend on T-wave changes alone—as they are more difficult to interpret as evidence of coronary heart disease. Inverted T wave may occur in:

1. Ischemic heart disease—may appear as only manifestation of IHD, but also occur in other conditions associated with chest pain such as:
2. Pericarditis
3. Myocarditis
4. Abnormalities of vasoregulation.

183. False-positive results are least likely in those

1. Who shows ST depression early in the test and in whom the changes remain for more than 5 minutes after stopping the exercise
2. Who experiences typical angina during the test
3. Who shows minimal increase in heart rate
4. Who shows minimal decrease in BP. (Compared to the control values)

184. A positive exercise ECG test results indicate the likelihood of coronary artery disease in:

1. 98% of patients with typical angina
2. 88% of patients with atypical angina
3. 44% of patients with non-anginal chest pain
4. 25–33% in asymptomatic patients—silent myocardial ischemia. (The percentage is always variable from place to place)

185. False-positive ST changes can occur in

1. Endocardial disease—e.g. mitral valve prolapse
2. Myocardial—Left ventricular hypertrophy, cardiomyopathy, myocarditis, WPW syndrome (Pre-excitation variant), LBBB
3. Pericardial disease
4. Drugs and electrolyte disturbances, e.g. digitalis, diuretics, potassium. (*Note*: RBBB does not interfere with ischemic changes.)

186. General causes that give false-positive ST changes are:

1. Anemia
2. Systemic hypertension
3. Hyperventilation
4. Vasoregulatory abnormalities.

Nonfasting state, sudden exercise, technical errors can give rise to false-positive ST changes.

187. False-negative TMT can occur in (coronary artery disease is present but no ST segment shift).

1. When ischemia is in silent area
2. Infarcted segment
3. Using drugs like beta-blockers, vasodilators.
4. When stress is inadequate—< 85% of heart rate and physical incapacity, etc. also give false-negative result.

188. The following data is to be collected for interpreting the exercise test.

1. Duration of exercise
2. Heart rate response
3. BP response—BP should be recorded every 3 minutes—fall of BP can cause cold, clammy skin and sweating
4. Presence of anginal symptoms—Angina, dyspnea, fatigue, claudication. 12-lead exercise test is 90% sensitive.

189. Acute conditions that are contraindicated for stress test are:

1. Acute myocardial infarction
2. Unstable angina
3. Acute myocarditis or pericarditis
4. Known ominous coronary artery disease, e.g. left main artery or triple vessel disease.

190. Chronic conditions that are contraindicated for stress test are:

1. Uncontrolled severe congestive heart failure
2. Uncontrolled severe systemic hypertension (200/110)
3. Uncontrolled arrhythmias
4. Uncontrolled intracardiac conduction abnormalities e.g. high-grade AV block, tachy-brady arrhythmias.

191. Relative contraindications for stress test are:

1. Severe aortic stenosis—idiopathic subaortic stenosis. Stress test can be done in mild to moderate aortic stenosis
2. Suspected left main coronary artery stenosis
3. Severe hypertension
4. HOCM and other forms of outflow tract obstruction
5. Acute aortic dissection
6. Moderate stenotic valvular lesions
7. Acute PTE/pulmonary infarct
8. Electrolyte abnormalities.

192. General causes that are contraindicated for stress test are:

1. Acute systemic illness
2. Physically or mentally handicapped
3. Drug toxicity—e.g. digoxin, quinidine, adriomycin
4. Unwillingness to give consent.

193. When do you terminate the stress test?

In the target heart rate, exercise is continued until the patient attains 80–90% of his expected maximal heart rate (available from tables).

In the maximal exercise test, exercise is progressively increased until the maximum workload is achieved.

Both tests are terminated at a lower level of work, if the patient develops

1. Chest pain—progressive anginal pain, dyspnea/severe fatigue
2. Signs of cerebral insufficiency or CNS symptoms—ataxia, vertigo, visual or gait problems, confusion—or signs of poor perfusion—pallor, cyanosis, cold and clammy skin.

3. Raise in BP—systolic more than 250 mm Hg, diastolic more than 120 mm Hg or progressive fall in systolic BP.
4. Significant ECG changes
   ST elevation >1 mm in non-Q leads
   Marked ST depression changes 2 mm or more.
   Sustained ventricular arrhythmias, ventricular tachycardia.
   Proximal supraventricular tachycardias—AF, AV block.
   Axis deviation or LBBB or hemiblock.

194. Other potentially important observations to terminate the exercise test are:

1. ST elevation
2. Severe angina pectoris
3. Exercise induced U wave inversion
4. Exercise induced ventricular tachycardia.

195. Following parameters are monitored to assess an exercise test. The occurrence of chest pain during stress test is more likely to be due to ischemic heart disease in a 60-year-old hypertensive male smoker with high levels of serum cholesterol than a 30-year-old normotensive female non-smoker with normal serum cholesterol. Keeping this example in view, the following parameters are assessed.

1. Development of anginal pain at lower than normal workloads or at lower heart rates are specific of coronary artery disease.
   It is positive in about 80% ischemic heart diseases. Though pain is a subjective phenomenon and it varies with individuals and cannot be measured directly.
   Poor exercise tolerance: The test may have to be stopped early because of dyspnea or exhaustion. It may indicate diseases of other systems such as respiratory system or psychological feeling of inability to continue.
   Clinical features of new S3, apical pansystolic murmur (papillary muscle dysfunction), pulmonary basal rales.
2. Heart rate: Target heart rate
   Normal THR = 220, ... Age in years. This is the normal expected increase in heart rate with increasing exercise from stage 1 to 3 or 4. THR may not indicate adequacy of effort as it is influenced by many factors.
   Chromotropic incompetence: Less than normal response per stage of exercise and may plateau at submaximal workloads.
   Accelerated response: inappropriate for low workloads
3. ECG changes:
   Normal response: PR, QRS and QT shortening as heart rate increases. P amplitude increases, PR segment slopes down and J-point depresses.
   A. Development of ischemic ST depression.
      i. Horizontal depression > 1mm
      ii. Downsloping depression of > 1mm with T inversion
      iii. Upsloping with > 1 mm depression of JT 80 msec.
      iv. ST elevation in Q or non-Q wave leads—> 1 mm of J-point elevation, persistently elevated > 1 mm at – JT 80 msec.

      Sensitivity of the test may be increased from minor ST depression of 1 mm (0.1 mV). Specificity of the test is increased by stricter criteria of ST depression of 2 mm (0.2 mV) or more.
   B. T wave flattening or inversion: Symmetrical T wave inversion of ischemia with sharp pointing arrow edge or flattening.
   C. Increase in R wave amplitude: Height of R wave reflects left ventricular size. In normal person, the left ventricle empties completely with exercise, becomes smaller, as a consequence produces a smaller R wave. In ischemic heart disease, the volume of the left ventricle and size of the R wave usually increases on exercise because it could not empty completely. It may be effected by other factors.
   D. Development of ectopic beats or life-threatening arrhythmias: Sinus tachycardia during exercise suppresses any such activity in a healthy person.
4. Blood pressure: Normal response is increase in systolic BP with increasing workload of peak of 160–200 mm Hg; diastolic may remain same or decrease or increase by 10 mm Hg. Abnormal response is failure to increase systolic BP by > 120 mm Hg (or) sustained decrease of > 10 mm Hg (or) a fall below standing rest values.

196. Safety and risk of treadmill test: In general the test has an excellent safety record provided all the necessary safety precautions are taken. The test can be safely performed in compensated congestive heart failure with no major complications.

1. The mortality and morbidity rates are < 0.01% and 0.05%, respectively among nonselected population.
2. In myocardial infarction, the mortality is 0.03% within 4 weeks of its onset.

3. The risk of a major complication is twice when a symptom limited protocol is used against a low-level protocol.
4. In patients with life-threatening ventricular arrhythmias—2.2% developed sustained ventricular tachyarrhythmias.

ECG IN CHILDHOOD AND CONGENITAL HEART DISEASE

197. Many important points are to be considered while interpreting ECG in children because the normal variants are more diverse than in adults. It is important to reserve ECG diagnosis of abnormality without clinical data. Following 4 are examples:

1. The rate is relatively faster.
2. PR interval and QRS duration are relatively shorter.
3. Right ventricular wall is almost the same thickness of the left ventricular wall at birth; and this leads to different findings when compared to adults. QRS mean axis about +90°, which is normal at this age. Right axis deviation and right ventricular dominance are the rule in newborn infant.
   R wave in right precordial leads and S wave in left precordial leads is a normal finding. The pattern may resemble right ventricular hypertrophy or right bundle branch block of the adult, which is normal in the child.
4. Inversion of T waves in the anterior chest leads is a normal finding in childhood. T waves may be normally inverted further to the left of the precordium.

198. Many congenital heart diseases show a normal ECG. Normal tracings are more commonly seen in lesions where there is primary stress on the left ventricle such as:

1. Aortic stenosis
2. Coarctation of aorta
3. Ventricular septal defect
4. Patent ductus arteriosus.

A normal ECG, therefore, by no means excludes a congenital lesion.

199. The ECG may show difference depending on the stage of the disease. There may be differences between the tracings from different patients with the same deformity. See the examples of VSD or PDA.

1. The tracing will probably be normal in the beginning when it is mild.
2. Ventricular diastolic overloading pattern may develop later.
3. When pulmonary hypertension develops, right ventricular hypertrophy is added to the left ventricular diastolic overloading.
4. Finally, when pulmonary hypertension is marked, pattern of right ventricular hypertrophy may be evident.

Therefore, it is quiet evident, that the tracings depend on the stage of the disease, whether it is mild, moderate or severe.

200. Some rarer congenital lesions are associated with diagnostic pattern. Following 4 are examples.

1. Anomalous origin of left coronary artery from the pulmonary artery. Q wave, ST elevation and T wave inversion are present in LI, aVL and left chest leads, a pattern similar to anterolateral infarction.
2. Dextrocardia with situs inversus.
3. Ostium primum/common AV canal group—endocardial cushion defect.
4. Ebstein's anomaly.

201. The tracing in congenital lesions seldom gives the correct diagnosis. It often helps as a guide. It is better to study the tracing under the headings of the 4 main components.

1. P waves	2. QRS complex
3. T wave	4. U wave.

202. P waves:

1. Dextrocardia with situs inversus. P is inverted (left-sided venous atrium and vena cava). All complexes in LI are inverted.
2. P congenitale: Tall and peaked P waves in LI and LII with tall, mainly positive P waves in right chest leads. P congenitale is seen mainly in cyanotic congenital lesions but also in pure pulmonic stenosis.
   The frontal plane axis of P is generally between +30° and +45°. It differs from P-pulmonale where the frontal plane axis is to the right of to +60°.
3. Tall P waves occur in tricuspid disease (stenosis or atresia).
4. Tallest P waves (Himalayan P waves) occur in Ebstein's anomaly.

QRS Complexes

203. Determination of the 4 features of QRS complex.

1. Mean axis
2. Hypertrophy
3. Bundle branch block

4. Pre-excitation are helpful in giving clue to the diagnosis.

1. *Mean QRS axis:* Always study the mean QRS axis from hexaxial reference system.
   When left axis deviation is present in a cyanotic child, the most likely diagnosis is tricuspid atresia.
   Other possibilities are transposition of great vessels, single ventricle and some other lesions.
   When the initial portion of the QRS complex shows marked left axis deviation, while the terminal part shows right bundle branch block; the possibility is ostium primum or endocardial cushion defect. Such pattern may sometimes be seen with secundum defect also.
2. *Ventricular hypertrophy:* The diagnostic importance of hypertrophy patterns is quiet obvious. Right ventricular hypertrophy is seen in pure pulmonary stenosis, atrial septal defect and most of the cyanotic heart diseases. Dominant R wave in V1 in tetralogy of Fallot is usually changes to RS or rS by V2, whereas it remains dominant in V1–V4 in pure pulmonic stenosis.
   Left ventricular hypertrophy is seen in aortic stenosis, coarctation of aorta, ventricular septal defect and patent ductus arteriosus. R/T ratio of more than 10 in V5 or V6 in aortic stenosis indicates severe obstruction.
   Remember, that ventricular hypertrophy need not be associated with axis deviation. In fact left axis deviation is seen in 25% cases of left ventricular hypertrophy; and right axis deviation is seen in less than 66% cases of right ventricular hypertrophy.
3. *Bundle branch block:* Right bundle branch block is commonly present as hemodynamic changes of right ventricular diastolic overloading.
   a. Atrial septal defect is a typical example where 90% of patients with this lesion manifest with RBBB.
   b. Total anomalous pulmonary venous return—RBBB is frequently seen.
   c. Ebstein's anomaly: RBBB is a rule but the QRS complexes of the right precordial leads are typically of quiet low voltage.
   d. After surgery of VSD—a well-known postoperative complication.
   The LBBB is rare but occasionally seen in conditions where there is predominant strain on the left ventricle such as aortic stenosis. It is a common postoperative complication of muscular subaortic stenosis.
4. *Pre-excitation:* WPW syndrome has been associated with many congenital lesions, but most common associations are Ebstein's anomaly and primary cardiomyopathy.

Katz-Wachtel phenomenon: It is described where there is equiphasic complexes in two or more limb leads, often with similar equiphasicity in the mid-precordial leads. This is present in many congenital heart diseases but is perhaps most common in ventricular septal defect. Prominent Q waves in the right precordial leads are in favor of right atrial hypertrophy. Prominent Q waves in left chest leads, or in LII, LIII and aVF, sometimes reaching a depth of 10 mm are mostly in favor of ventricular septal defect. Prominent Q waves in limb and left chest leads are significant of muscular subaortic stenosis.

T Waves

It is helpful in differentiating tetralogy of Fallot from triology (pulmonic stenosis, atrial septal defect and right ventricular hypertrophy) or from pure pulmonic stenosis. T waves are usually inverted in right chest leads in tetralogy whereas in triology or pure pulmonic stenosis, the T waves are frequently inverted as far to the left as V4 or V5.

U Waves

These have been largely ignored in the description of tracings in congenital lesions. Inverted U waves in left chest leads are an early sign of left ventricular overloading, systolic or diastolic.

ECG IN SPECIFIC CONGENITAL CARDIAC DEFECTS

After the above discussion of ECG changes in congenital lesions, the ECG manifestations in the common congenital anomalies and in those with distinctive features are described below.

204. Few ECG patterns are diagnostic in congenital heart diseases and they are associated with rarer forms.

Four examples are:

1. True dextrocardia (Q-205, Fig. Q-156)
2. Ebstein anomaly (Q-216, Fig. L-21)
3. Osteum primum/common AV canal group
4. Anomalous left coronary artery arising from the pulmonary artery—pattern is similar to anterolateral myocardial infarction—Q waves, ST elevation, T inversion in LI, aVL and left precordial leads.

205. True dextrocardia: The 4 diagnostic features of dextrocardia in ECG are (See L-31, 32):

In this congenital anomaly, there is complete transposition of both ventricles and atria. The aortic knob is also to the right. Thus the P vector is pointed to the right, inferiorly and anteriorly resulting in inverted P wave in LI and an

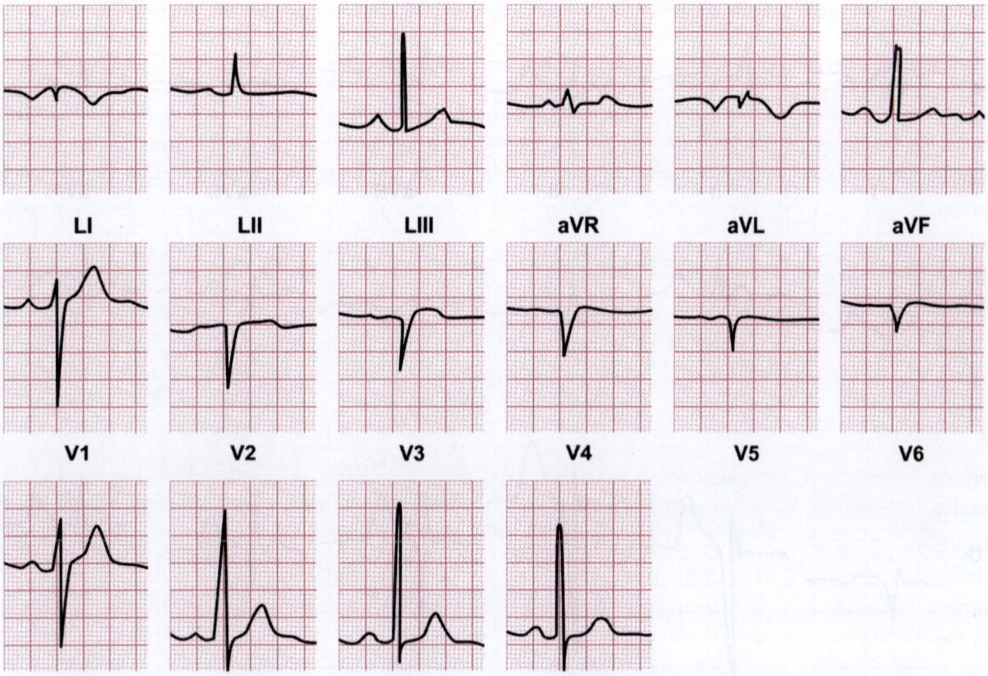

Fig. Q-157: True dextrocardia

upright P wave in aVR. The mean QRS vector is directed right, inferiorly and slight posteriorly. T vector is also pointed to the right, inferiorly and anteriorly.

In true dextrocardia, reversing the arm electrodes and using right precordial leads will produce a normal ECG provided there is no associated cardiac defects.

206. Technical dextrocardia (see Q-65): It is worth mentioning here.

In technical dextrocardia, the technician may interchange the right and left arm electrodes. This will produce dextrocardia pattern in standard and extremity leads but will not change the normal pattern in precordial leads and so the R wave progression is seen. This is not an uncommon technical artefact.

A. Shows
   1. All the waves in LI and aVL are negative.
   2. Lead aVR resembles aVL.
   3. LII resembles LIII and vice versa.
B. Standard and extremity leads are taken correctly
C. Precordial leads look absolutely normal with progressive increase in the height of R wave from V1 to V6. This is against the diagnosis of dextrocardia in which the R wave decreases in height while going toward the left chest leads. This confirms the diagnosis of 'technical dextrocardia' produced by the technician connecting the right arm electrode to the left arm and vice versa.
B. Shows the same patient when standard leads are taken correctly.

207. Four causes of rS complexes in all the precordial leads.

1. Dextrocardia
2. Cor pulmonale
3. Extensive anterior wall infarction
4. Congenital absence of left pericardium.

208. Ventricular septal defect (VSD): The 4 points in ECG.

1. Prominent Q waves in left chest leads or in LII, LIII and aVF.
2. High voltage equiphasic QRS complexes in mid-precordial leads in 50–75%.
3. Hypertrophy depending on severity and stage of the lesion. May be normal or show left ventricular hypertrophy or combined ventricular hypertrophy or right ventricular hypertrophy.
4. Pattern of BBB, complete or incomplete in 20–30%.

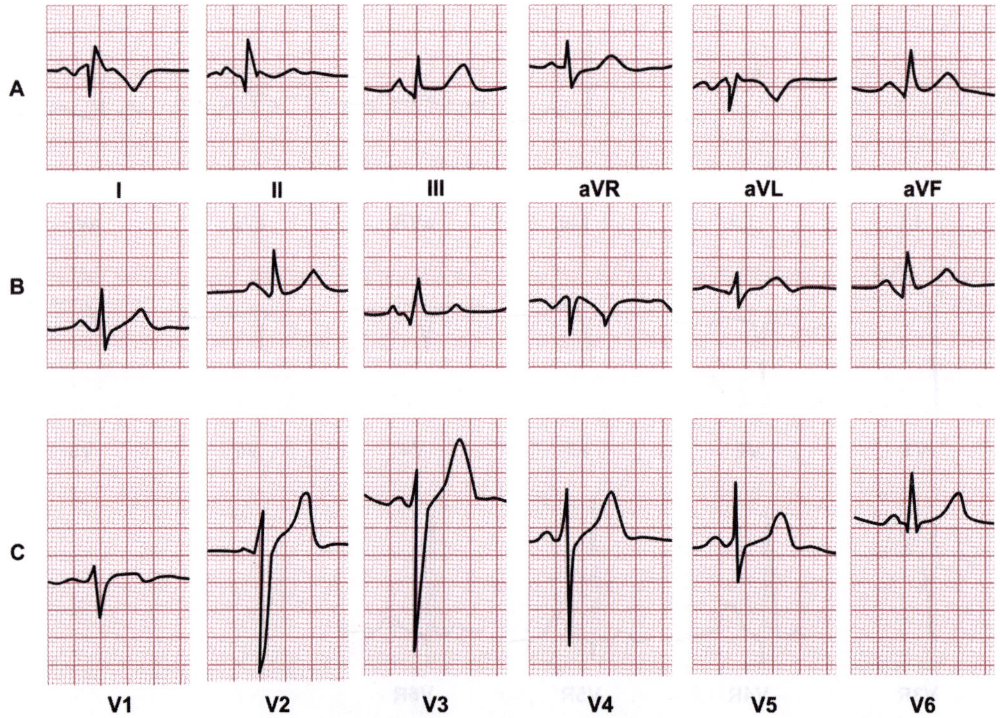

Fig. Q.158: Technical dextrocardia

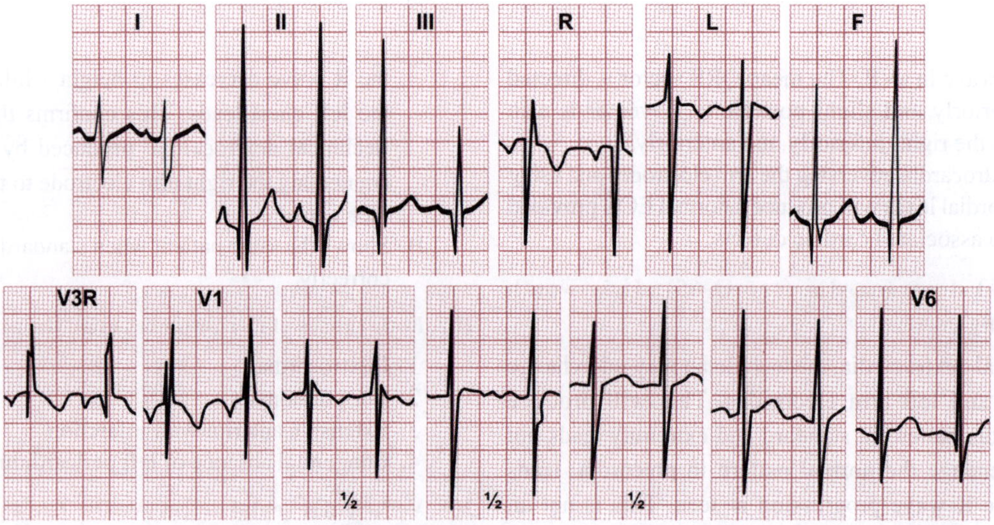

Fig. Q-159: From a child with VSD. See deep Q waves in LII, LIII and aVF. Incomplete RBBB pattern and equiphasic RS pattern in mid-precordial leads

209. Atrial septal defect (ASD): The 4 points in ECG.

1. Right atrial hypertrophy—P-congenitale in some.
2. Right ventricular hypertrophy; degree of right atrial hypertrophy and right ventricular hypertrophy depend on the severity of pulmonary arterial pressure.
3. Pattern of RBBB in majority—up to 90% in some series. Incomplete RBBB in osteum secundum (complete RBBB in 10% of cases).
   RBBB with LAD and prolongation of PR interval in osteum primum.
4. First degree AV block (common in sinus venosus type) and arrhythmias in few.

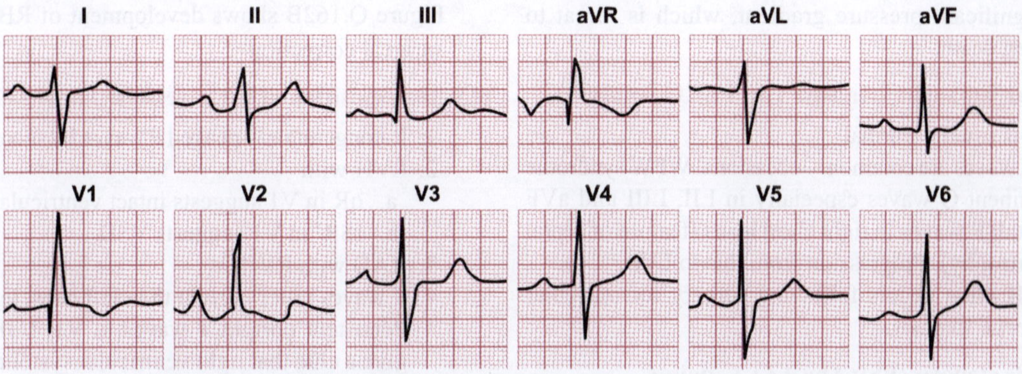

Fig. Q-160: Pointed right precordial P waves suggest right atrial hypertrophy; typical RBBB pattern of right ventricle and right ventricular hypertrophy with diastolic overloading

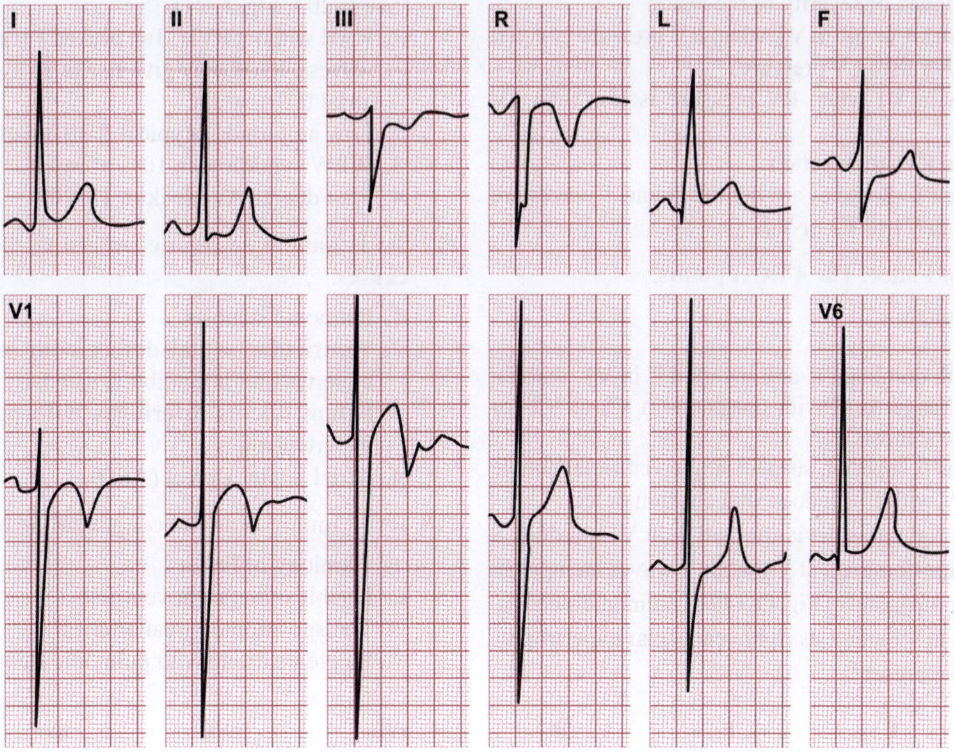

Fig. Q-161: Patent ductus arteriosus; High voltage QRS with tall upright T in V5, V6

210. Patent ductus arteriosus (PDA): The 4 ECG points.

Similar to VSD but differ in the following points:

1. Left atrial hypertrophy is probably the most common abnormality—P is notched and wide.
2. Left ventricular hypertrophy is often of diastolic overloading type. RVH is seen depending on the development of pulmonary hypertension.
3. RBBB pattern is seen but less common than in VSD.
4. Fist degree AV block is more common.

Left ventricular hypertrophy with diastolic overloading.

211. Aortic stenosis: The 4 ECG points.

1. Normal in 25% of cases.
   Various stages of LVH: Abnormally large posterior forces as S in V1 of 30 mm or more. LVH with strain pattern in severe cases.
2. LBBB in few.
3. Abnormal T wave. A superior T wave vector in the frontal plane is suggestive of severe obstruction.
4. Abnormal ST segment: Watch the ST segment in V5 through V7 during exercise to detect the development

of significant pressure gradient, which is threat to sudden death.

212. Muscular subaortic stenosis: The 4 ECG points.

1. Axis is usually normal
2. Delta waves are common—occasional WPW syndrome
3. Prominent Q waves especially in LII, LIII and aVF with tall R waves in right chest leads (feature of septal hypertrophy). Progression from this to LVH
4. LBBB often occurs following surgery for muscular subaortic stenosis.

213. Pulmonic stenosis (PS): The 4 ECG points.

1. P-congenitale
2. Right ventricular hypertrophy: The degree of RVH is a useful index of severity of the lesion
   RVH with rR or qR in V1 when RV pressure is equal to or higher than LV pressure.
   Rs or rS in V1 when RV pressure is less than LV pressure.
3. RAD and RV strain pattern
4. In severe PS, R waves are dominant and T waves are inverted in V1 to V3 or V4.

214. Tetralogy of Fallot: The 4 ECG points.

1. P-congenitale
2. RAD
3. RVH with dominant R and inverted T in V1, with an abrupt change to rS with upright T in V2 or V3 (of pulmonic stenosis).
4. If the axis is superior, suspect single ventricle, double outlet RV with PS, endocardial cushion defect.

See marked right axis deviation, tall R in V1and deep S waves become dominant at V2 while T waves are upright at V3 (for comparison of Fig. Q-149 of pulmonic stenosis. Tall R wave in V1 suggests right ventricular hypertrophy. P-congenitale present.

Figure Q.162B shows development of RBBB following surgical correction

215. Transposition of great vessels: The 4 ECG points.

1. P-congenitale—peaked P waves by second or third day
2. RVH with
   a. qR in V1 suggests intact ventricular septum
   b. rSR' in V1 suggests VSD
3. RAD with RVH
4. T waves taller in right than left chest leads.
   Persistent upright T waves in V1, V3R after 4 days give a clue that right ventricular systolic pressure is at systemic level.

216. Ebstein's anomaly: The 4 ECG points.

(See L-203, Fig. L-21)

1. RAH without RVH. Tall peaked P waves (Himalayan P waves). RAH may give rise to arrhythmias especially atrial tachycardia.
2. Low amplitude, atypical RBBB pattern.
3. WPW syndrome in 10% of cases.
4. First degree AV block in 15–20%.

217. RVH among acyanotic congenital heart diseases—4 causes.

1. Pulmonic stenosis
2. Ventricular septal defect with pulmonary artery hypertension/infundibular stenosis
3. Patent ductus arteriosus with pulmonary artery hypertension
4. Atrial Septal Defect (ASD).

218. RVH among cyanotic congenital heart diseases.

1. Tetralogy of Fallot
2. Double outlet right ventricle
3. Transposition of great arteries
4. Single ventricle with pulmonic stenosis

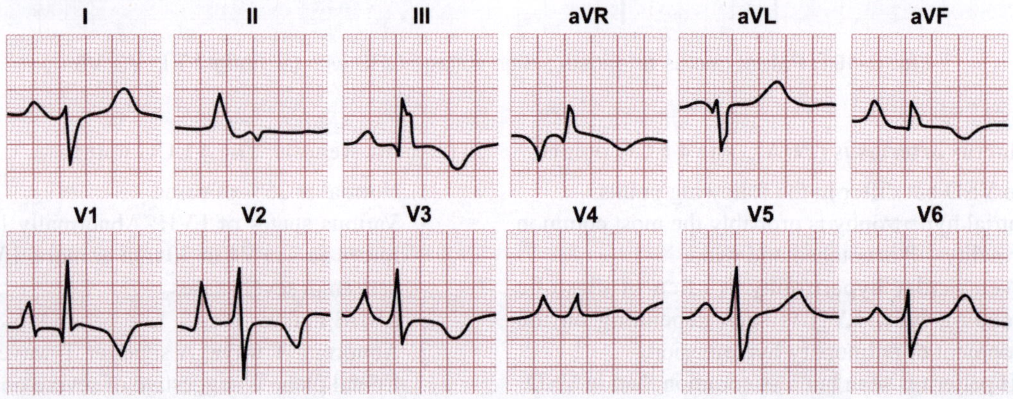

Fig. Q-162: Pulmonic stenosis: Shows right ventricular hypertrophy and strain pattern (systolic overloading). P-congenitale suggests right atrial hypertrophy. Marked right axis deviation and relatively low equiphasic complexes in V5, V6

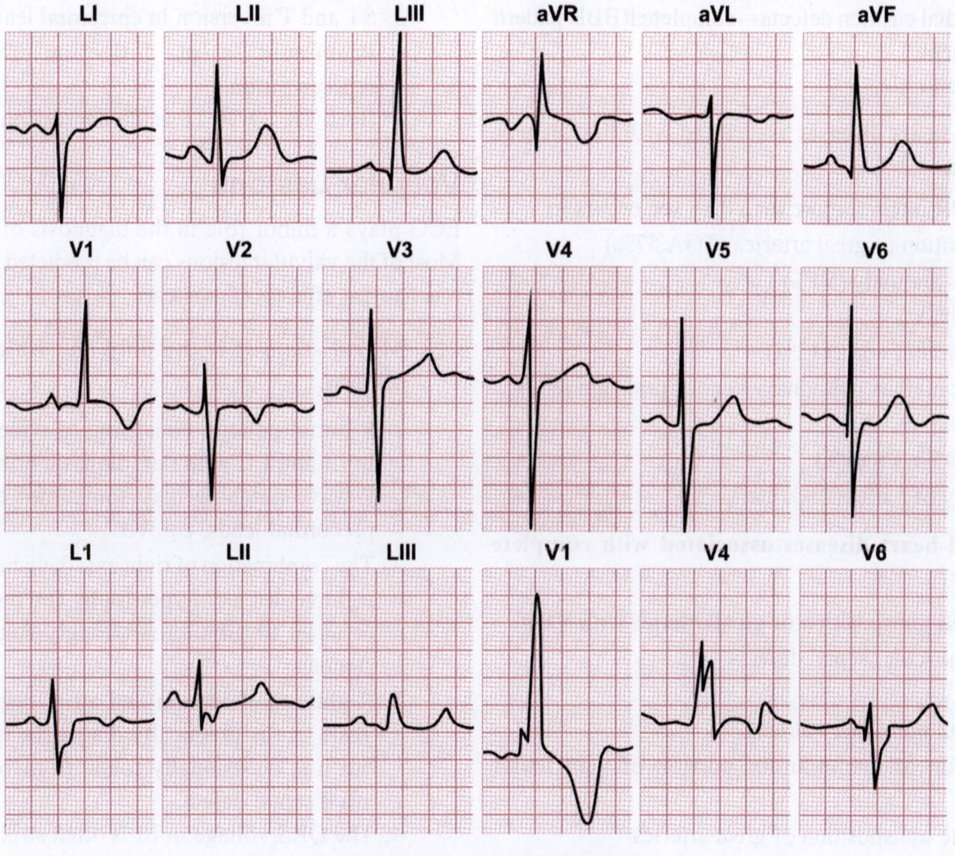

Fig. Q-163: Tetralogy of Fallot

5. Aortic atresia
6. Persistent truncus arteriosus
7. Severe pulmonic stenosis with RL shunt at the atrial level
8. Eisenmenger syndrome.

219. The 4 criteria for LVH are:

1. Voltage of R wave in V6 greater than maximum normal for age
2. Voltage of S wave in V1 greater than maximum normal for age
3. Secondary T wave inversion in V5 and/or V6.
4. Deep Q wave 4 mm over the left precordium.

220. LVH among acyanotic heart diseases.

First 6 months

1. Endocardial fibroelastosis
2. Left coronary artery from pulmonary artery
3. Glycogen storage disease
4. Coronary calcinosis
5. Aortic stenosis

After 6 months

6. Coarctation of aorta
7. Aortic stenosis
8. VSD
9. PDA
10. AP window
11. Isolated myocarditis
12. Systemic arterial hypertension.

221. LVH among cyanotic heart diseases

1. Tricuspid atresia
2. Transposition of great vessels
3. Anomalous systemic venous drainage
4. Truncus arteriosus.

222. Complete RBBB—Normal variant.

1. Ebstein's anomaly
2. Atrial septal defect with pulmonary artery hypertension
3. Double outlet right ventricle
4. Right ventriculotomy.
(Incomplete RBBB—Atrial Septal Defect).

223. Left axis deviation in a cyanotic child.

1. Tricuspid atresia—80–90%, most likely diagnosis. 'P-tricuspidale'
2. Transposition of great vessels—T waves tall in right chest leads than left

3. Endocardial cushion defects—complete RBBB pattern also present
4. Single ventricle.

224. Congenital heart diseases associated with first degree heart block.

Prolonged PR interval more than 0.18 sec occurs in

1. Transposition of great arteries (TGA 57%)
2. Ebstein's anomaly (50%)
3. ASD (43%)
4. Coarctation of aorta (12%)
5. Total anomalous pulmonary venous drainage (8%)
6. VSD (6%)
7. PDA (3.4%), PS (3%)
8. Tetralogy of Fallot (2%), etc.

225. Congenital heart diseases associated with complete heart block.

1. Corrected transposition of great arteries with VSD
2. Atrioventricular septal defects
3. PDA
4. VSD with pulmonary atresia
5. Aneurysm of membranous portion of ventricular septum
6. Complete transposition of great arteries
7. Tricuspid atresia
8. Coarctation of aorta
9. Hypoplastic left heart syndrome
10. Marfan's syndrome
11. Tumors of the AV node
12. Rubella heart block.

226. Tricuspid atresia: The 4 ECG points.

1. P-tricuspidale
2. LVH
3. LAD in 80–90%
4. LBBB in some.

ECG IN MISCELLANEOUS CONDITIONS

227. Anxiety reaction.

It is not uncommon to see ECG abnormalities in patients suffering from anxiety and hyperventilation with supposedly normal hearts. Following 4 ECG changes have been described.

1. Sinus tachycardia
2. Prolonged PR interval
3. ST and T inversion in epicardial leads
4. Prominent Ta (pt) deflection produced by atrial repolarization.
(Ref. Fig. Q-39 - Pseudo depression of ST segment)

Valvular Lesions

ECG plays a minor role in the diagnosis of valvular lesions. Most of the valvular lesions can be predicted from their known mechanical effects on the heart.

228. Mitral stenosis is the only one which has a specific pattern.

1. P-mitral pattern, consisting of wide notched P wave in LI and LII with flat, diphasic or inverted P in LIII. P wave notching may sometimes best seen in mid-precordial leads, e.g. V3.
2. The combination of right axis deviation with or without right ventricular hypertrophy and the P-mitral pattern or atrial fibrillation is strongly suggestive of mitral stenosis.
3. Right axis deviation and atrial fibrillation under 40 years age is practically diagnostic of mitral stenosis, but it is occasionally found in thyrotoxicosis and in atrial septal defect.
4. The QRS voltage in LI is often strikingly low.

229. The effects of other valvular lesions are produced from their known mechanical effects. Some of the useful points of ECG in valvular diseases are given below, which help to predict the diagnosis. These are of indirect help.

1. Aortic regurgitation or mitral regurgitation predominantly affects the left ventricle. Initially gives rise to a pattern of left ventricular diastolic overloading; later, like aortic stenosis they produce typical strain pattern.
2. Combined mitral and aortic lesions often produce patterns suggesting biventricular enlargement.
3. Tricuspid stenosis is suggested where right atrial enlargement is associated with first degree AV block without preponderance of either ventricles. Low voltage RSR' complex is not infrequently found in V1.
4. Pulmonic stenosis shows P-congenitale and RVH.

230. Electrical alternans.

The QRS complexes are in alternating direction, one upward and the other downward. It is much less than its mechanical counterpart, 'pulsus alternans'. Total alternans, that is, alternation of P waves as well as Q waves is almost

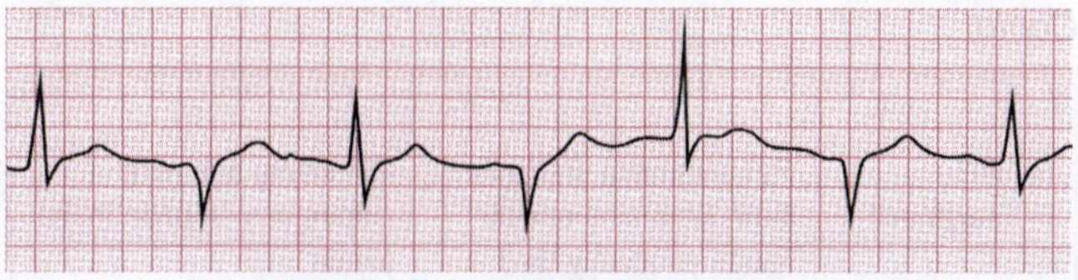

Fig. Q-164: Electrical alternans

pathognomonic and usually indicates pericardial effusion. In pericardial effusion, there will be low voltage and ST elevation besides electrical alternans. It is best seen in the chest leads where the QRS points in different directions! This is rarely seen and is due to the heart moving in the effusion.

1. QRS complexes are in alternate direction
2. Total alternans, that is alterations of P wave as well as QRS wave is almost pathognomonic of pericardial effusion
3. It is much less than its mechanical counterpart 'Pulsus alternans'
4. It differs from pericardial effusion as there is no low voltage and ST elevation.
(See Fig. N-2 – Electrical alternans in pericardial effusion)

231. Acute pericarditis.

Whatever is the cause of acute pericarditis, the characteristic finding is an elevation of ST segments in many leads with upward concavity including all three standard leads. The changes in pericarditis are probably due to short circulation of impulses by pericardial fluid or thickened pericardium, which causes low voltage and the spread of inflammation to the myocardial layer immediately subjacent, which causes ST and T wave changes. It should be differentiated from acute myocardial infarction.

The 4 most striking differences are:

Table Q-6

	Acute pericardias	Acute infarction
1. ST shape	Concave upward	Convex upward
2. ST reciprocity	Absent	Present Elevated in affected lead depressed in opposite lead
3. T wave	T will often not become inverted until the ST has returned to baseline	T usually becomes inverted, while the ST is still elevated
4. Q and QT	Q absent QT normal	Q present QT prolonged

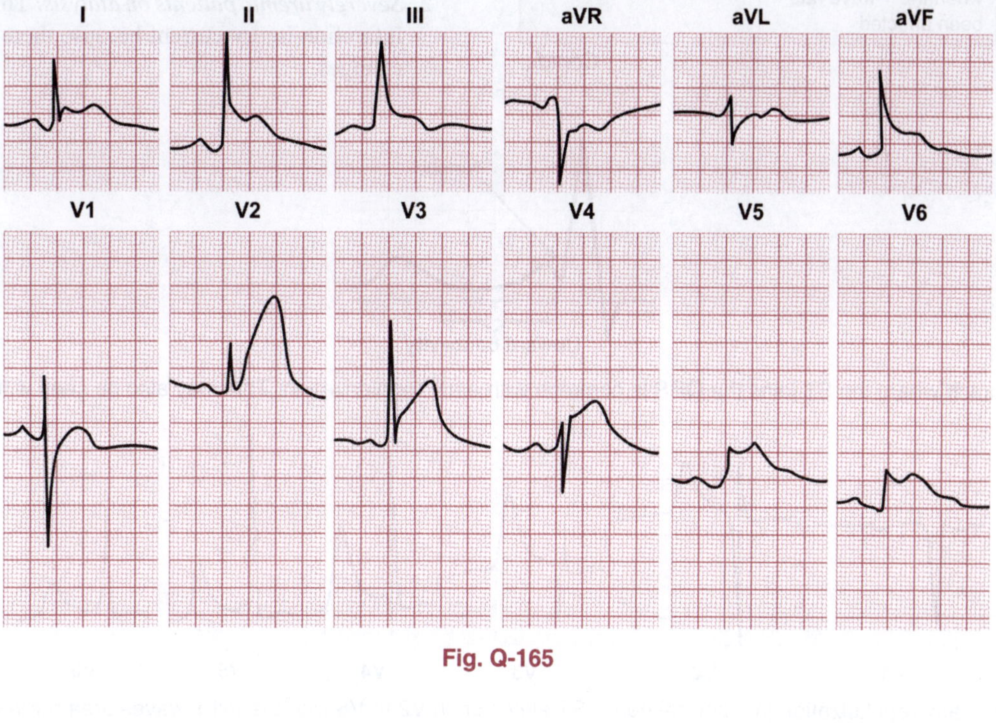

Fig. Q-165

232. The 4 salient features of chronic pericarditis are:

1. Low voltage
2. Flat or inverted T waves
3. Fixed axis
4. Possible P-mitral pattern or atrial fibrillation.

233. Early repolarization: It is common in athletes, young black males. Early repolarization may persist for decades. ST elevation of early repolarization should be differentiated from that due to pericarditis in which both have upward concavity.

There are 4 differentiating points pericarditis from early repolarization:

Table Q-7

	Pericarditis	Early repolarization
1. Leads present	ST elevation in both limb and chest leads in early pericarditis, ST elevation tends to be left of the frontal T wave	ST elevated in chest leads alone (Rarely seen in limb leads only ST tends to be to the right of both QRS and T in the frontal plane
2. T wave	T becomes lower as the hours pass. Therefore, they may look alike in the early hours of pericarditis when the T wave has been affected	ST is always associated with a tall T wave

Contd...

Contd...

	Pericarditis	Early repolarization
3. PR segment	PR segment shifts in both limb and chest leads probably due to subepicardial atrial injury. It is often best seen as an elevation in aVR	PR shifts are rare especially in precordial leads
4. Exercise	No affect	ST comes back to isoelectric line. This test is unreliable because exercise can sometimes exaggerate rather than normalize early repolarization

234. The conditions that can cause ST elevations that may mimic acute infarction, pancreatitis, pericarditis or early repolarization.

1. *Cerebral hemorrhage:* It has occasionally caused ST elevations of marked degree without reciprocal changes suggestive of pericarditis. Reciprocal ST depression can also occur and exactly look like acute myocardial infarction. The long QT interval, however, caused by the cerebral abnormality makes the diagnosis of pericarditis unlikely.
2. *Severely uremic patients on dialysis:* This looks like an infarction injury current because there are reciprocal changes.

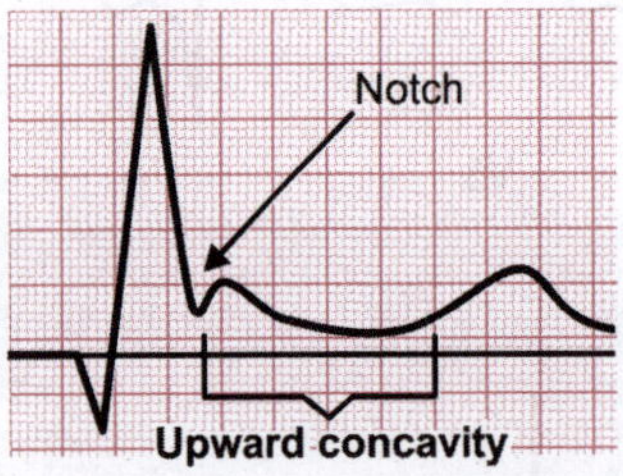

Fig. Q-166: A notch where the ST joins the QRS is common with early repolarization. This may also be seen with pericarditis

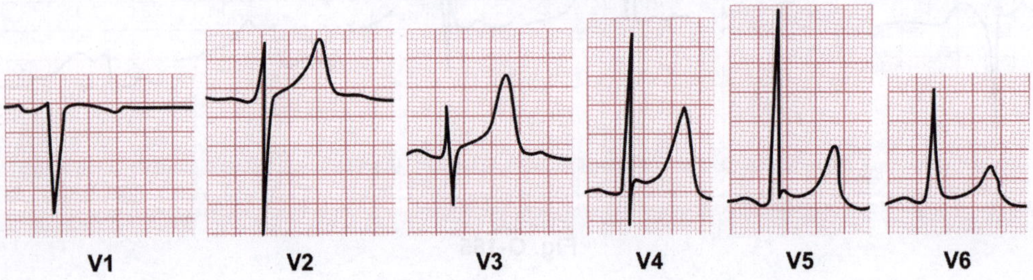

Fig. Q-167: Early repolarization in a normal heart. ST elevation in V2 to V6 with the tall T waves area normal variation

3. *Carcinoma lung with infiltration of the myocardium:* It can produce an infarction like injury current with characteristic reciprocal changes.
4. *In gastrointestinal hemorrhage or cancer with secondary anemia receiving blood transfusion:* Disseminated intravascular coagulation causing fibrin thrombi followed by lysis was assumed to be the cause in some reports.

235. Cardiomyopathy:

None of the ECG abnormalities is diagnostic of cardiomyopathy except the progressing pattern from septal hypertrophy to get generalized left ventricular hypertrophy—seen in the prolonged follow-up hypertrophic subaortic stenosis.

Therefore, however, a few points are to be noted which favors the diagnosis.

1. Bundle branch block pattern that is present is atypical and splintered. There is tendency to RBBB and RVH in endomyocardial fibrosis.
2. The association of WPW syndrome with familial cardiomyopathy. The dearth of significant arrhythmia or block in obstructive cardiomyopathy.
3. The combination of left ventricular hypertrophy with right atrial hypertrophy in muscular subaortic stenosis, obstructive or nonobstructive.
4. Glycogen storage disease tends to produce oversized QRS complexes in all leads with short PR interval.

236. Low voltage with inverted T waves in all or most of the leads are seen in:

Any diffuse myocardial involvement

1. Diffuse ischemic disease
2. Heart failure treated with digitalis
3. Myxedema
4. Myocarditis
5. Cardiomyopathy

Pericardial involvement

6. Acute ('T stage') pericarditis
7. Chronic constrictive pericarditis
8. Pericardial effusion.

237. There are 4 common ECG findings in myxedema.

1. Low voltage QRS in all leads
2. Sinus bradycardia
3. Increased PR interval
4. Flat or inverted T wave.

Sinus bradycardia helps to distinguish from similar appearance in constrictive pericarditis in which bradycardia is most unusual.

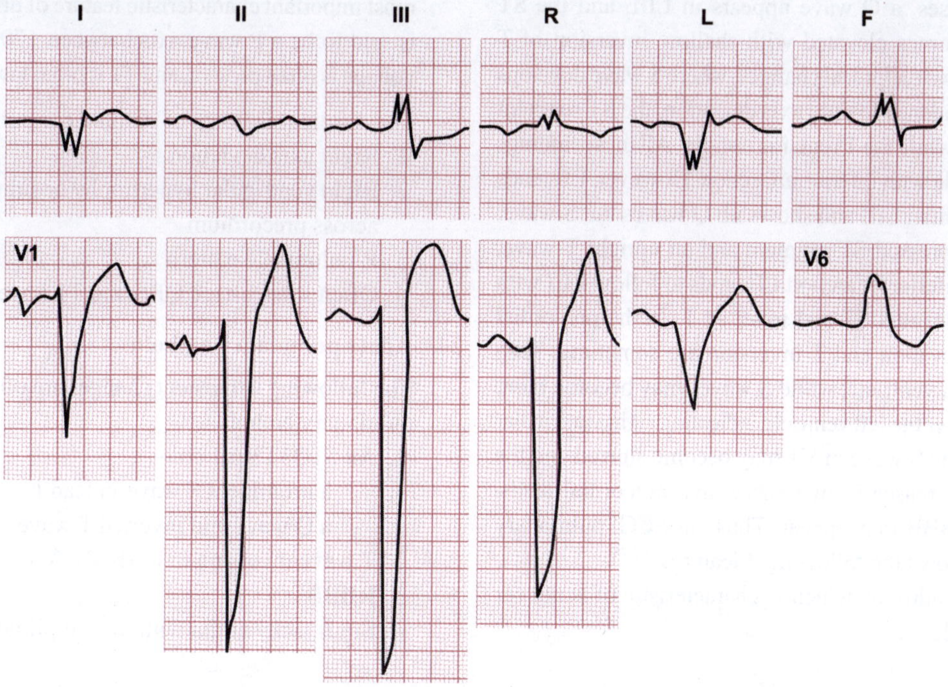

Fig. Q-168: Primary cardiomyopathy a typical pattern of intraventricular block with notching and blurring of the QRS is seen. P waves are also wide and notched suggestive of left atrial enlargement

238. Athletes heart syndrome consists of:

1. Sinus bradycardia
2. First degree AV block
3. Tall QRS
4. T wave inversion (2%).

Certain ECG changes are common in highly trained athletes.

239. There are 4 types of miscellaneous effects to be searched in ECG.

1. Pulmonary effects, e.g. emphysema, pulmonary infarction.
2. Electrolyte effects, e.g. potassium, calcium.
3. Patterns, e.g. strain, etc.
4. Drug effects, e.g. digitalis, quinidine, etc.

240. Acute cor pulmonale.

The pattern of cor pulmonale develops rapidly within few minutes of a massive pulmonary embolism and if the patient survives, the ECG pattern may revert to normal within hours to a day or two, or may persist for weeks.

The most important of it lies in its ECG pattern, which mimics inferior infarction and clinical picture also is serious to confuse with acute myocardial infarction. The distinction is difficult to make.

In typical cases, a Q wave appears in LIII, and the ST segment becomes elevated with shallow inversion of T wave. LI shows reciprocal changes, where S wave develops indicating tendency to right axis deviation, the ST segment is depressed while the T remains upright. All these findings are compatible with inferior infarction. However, LII tends to follow LI than LIII and shows no Q waves but S wave, a slightly depressed ST segment and an upright T wave, whereas in inferior infarction LII tends to follow LIII with a Q wave, elevated ST and inverted T. In the precordial leads, ST elevation and T inversion are sometimes seen over the right ventricle, while S waves may become more prominent over the left ventricle indicating right ventricular dilatation. The S wave in V1 may become slurred and the R/S ratio decreases in two successive precordial leads. Transient RBBB may appear. Thus, on ECG, pulmonary infarction shows the following **4** features.

1. S1 Q3 syndrome, which is characteristic of acute cor pulmonale
   Wide S in LI and large Q in LIII
2. ST depression in LII
3. T inversion in V1–V4
4. Transient or incomplete RBBB.

241. The differences between the acute cor pulmonale and inferior infarction may be summarized as follows.

1. LII tends to follow LI rather than LIII—shows no Q waves but S waves
2. The changes may evolve and recede in a matter of hours rather than weeks or months.
3. ST-T deviations in limb leads are slight, whereas they may be prominent in inferior infarction.
4. In right precordial leads, they resemble anteroseptal rather than inferior infarction.

Note: Think of pulmonary infarction while you are diagnosing inferior infarction from the limb leads and anteroseptal damage or infarction from the precordial leads.

242. Chronic cor pulmonale.

It is most often seen in emphysema characterized by right axis deviation and sometimes pattern of right ventricular hypertrophy with strain. Enlargement of right atrium is manifested by the P-pulmonale pattern consisting of low P in LI with tall, peaked P waves in LII, LIII and aVF. The most important characteristic feature of diffuse lung disease is said to be a P wave axis between +70° and +90°. Low voltage is often present, and T1 is often low voltage than T3.

The 4 salient features of chronic cor pulmonale are:

1. Right axis deviation
2. Right ventricular hypertrophy or simply rS complexes across precordium
3. P-pulmonale pattern
4. Often low voltage QRS and T1 lower than T3.

243. Acute pulmonary embolus.

The following 4 transient changes are often seen in a large pulmonary embolus.

1. An S1Q3T3 pattern—
   - a prominent S wave in lead I
   - a Q wave and inverted T wave in lead III
2. T wave inversion in leads V1–V3
3. RBBB
4. Sinus tachycardia with low amplitude deflections.

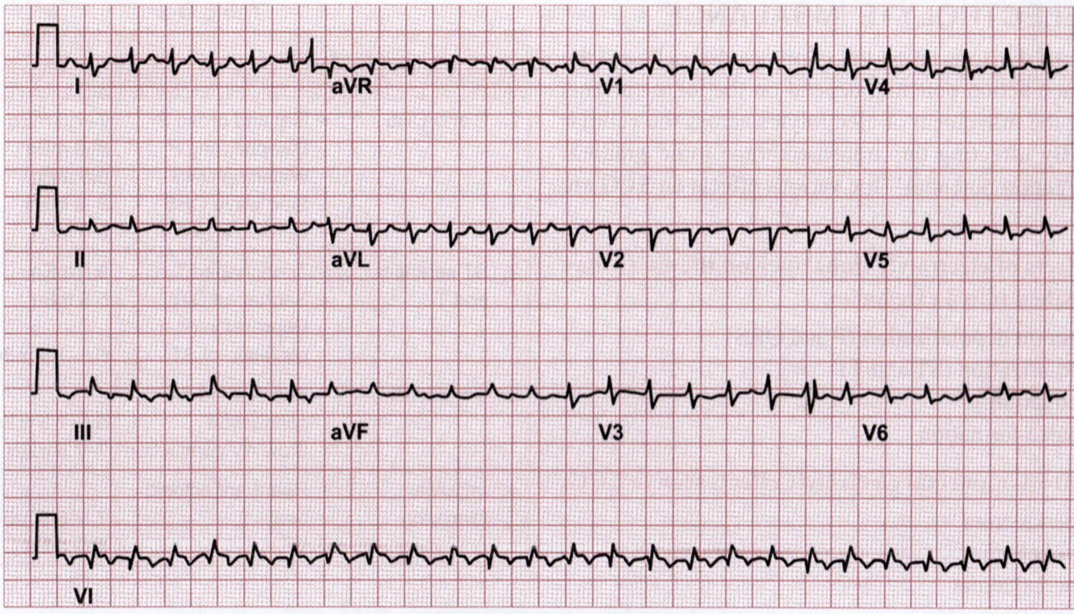

Fig. Q-169: Acute pulmonary embolus

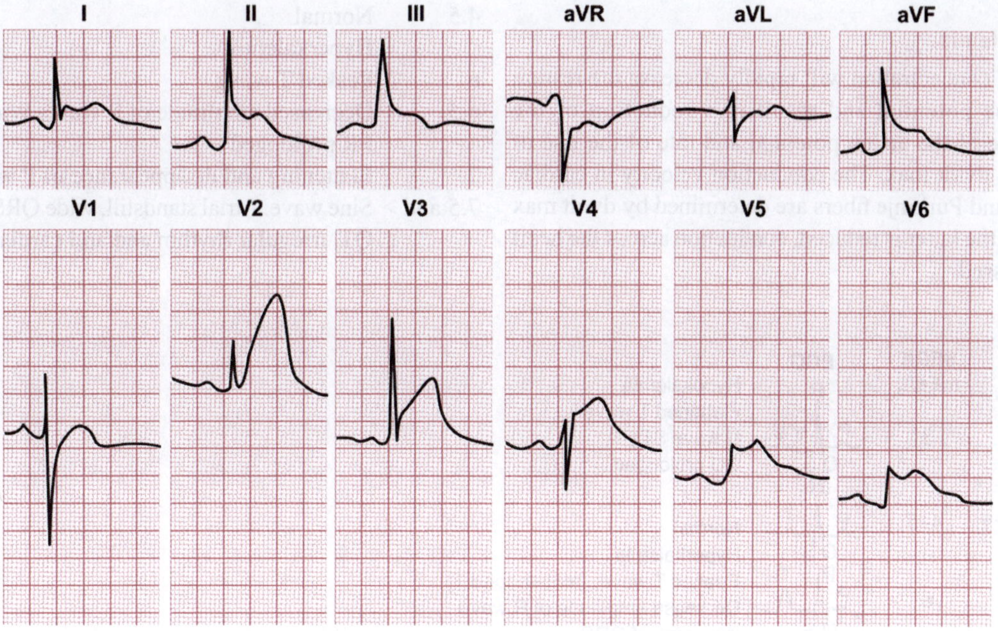

Fig. Q. 170: Intracranial hemorrhage

244. Intracranial hemorrhage.

Intracerebral or subarachnoid hemorrhage can produce sudden changes in ECG.

1. Wide and prominent T waves
2. T waves are usually inverted but sometimes upright
3. T waves are continuous with large U waves giving the effect of long TU complex
4. Frequent bradycardia.

ECG IN ELECTROLYTE IMBALANCE

The passive and dynamic properties of myocardial cells and the transmembrane action potential depend on the ionic currents produced by the movement of electrolytes across the cellular membrane. By affecting this transmembrane ionic gradient and thus the action potential—the various effects on ECG are produced.

245. The effects of electrolyte imbalance on the ECG may be classified into 4 categories.

1. Effect on depolarization (P and QRS)
2. Repolarization (ST and T)
3. Conduction
4. Impulse formation.

246. There are 4 important electrolyte effects seen in ECG.

1. Hyperkalemia
2. Hypokalemia
3. Hypercalcemia
4. Hypocalcemia.

POTASSIUM

247. Hyperkalemia.

Increased concentration will rapidly decrease the resting membrane potential and result in a reduction of the magnitude of the action potential and rate of the rise of phase 0 – dv/dt max. The conduction velocity in cardiac muscles and Purkinje fibers are determined by dv/dt max and since the latter is reduced, conduction across the heart is suppressed.

Table Q-8

	ECG changes	*Levels (normal 3.5–5.0 mEq)*
1. P and QRS	– Flat and broad P – Disappearing P – Widening QRS – Sine wave QRS – Cardiac arrest	7–7.5 mEq 8–9 mEq 6.5 mEq 8–9 mEq 8.0 mEq
2. ST segment and T	– Tent-shaped T – Shortened QTc – Depression or elevation of ST	5.5 mEq 5.5 mEq 6.5–7.5 mEq
3. Conduction	– Accelerated AV conduction – Slow AV conduction	5.5–7.5 mEq 7–7.5 mEq
4. Impulse formation	– Reentrant ectopic beat – VF	7.5–8.5 mEq 8–9 mEq

SERK mEq/L

3	Hypokalemia – Flattened T wave. U wave prominent
4.5	Normal
	Hyperkalemia
6	Peaked T wave
6.5	Decreased amplitude of R wave, Widening of QRS, PR prolonged
7	Flattening and disappearance of P wave
7.5 and >	Sine wave. Atrial standstill, wide QRS and prolonged QT, irregular rhythm and and cardiac arrest

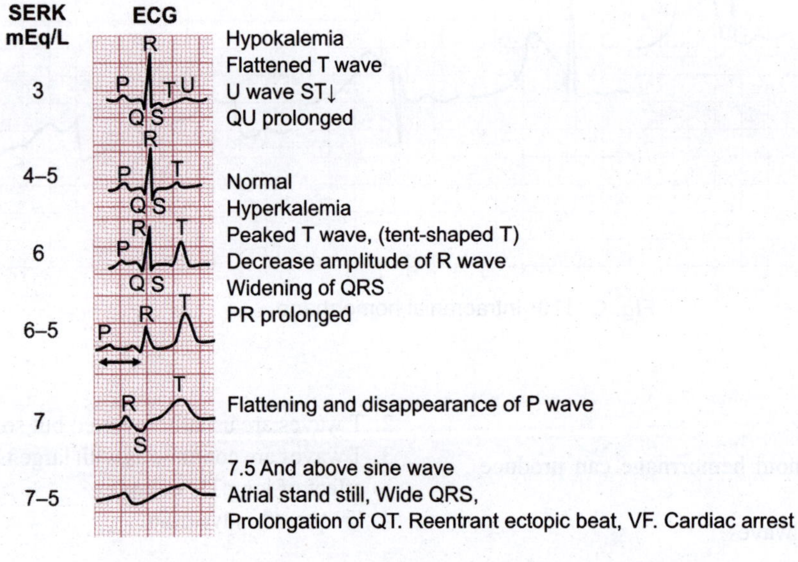

Fig. Q-171: Serial ECG changes in hyperkalemia

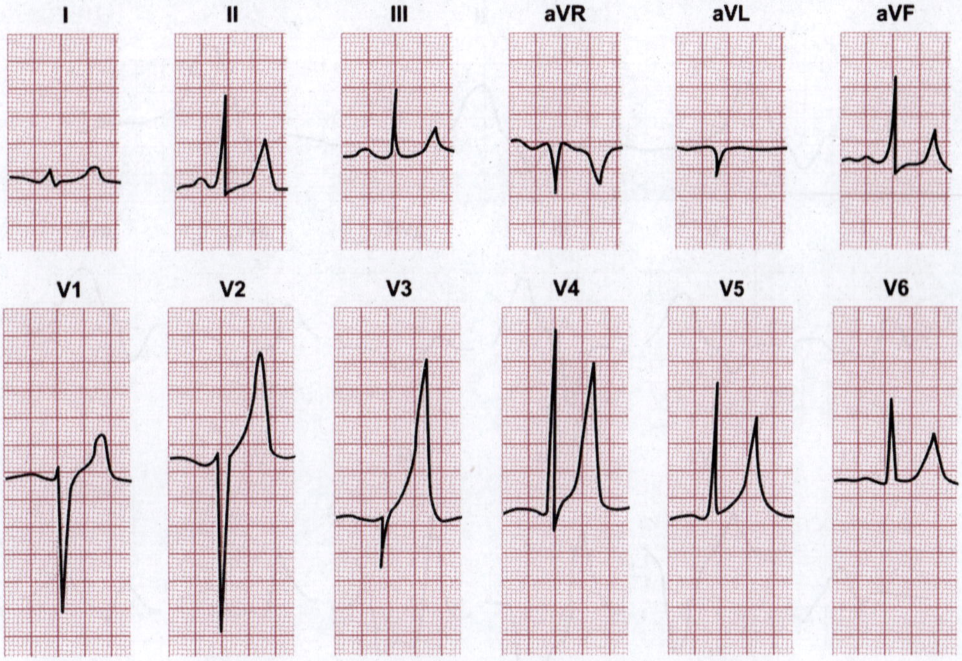

Fig. Q-172: Tall-peaked T waves due to hyperkalemia

Tall T waves can also occur in acute ischemic heart disease (IHD).

Tall T waves in IHD are blunt tipped.

Tall T waves in hyperkalemia are sharp tipped.

Tall peaked T waves are earliest changes.

T waves amplitude is usually greater in pericardial leads.

Atrial standstill may develop as serum potassium increases.

Hyperkalemia is one of the commonest causes of death in renal failure. Factors which contribute hyperkalemia are high dietary intake of potassium, impaired renal function, hypoaldosteronism, aldosterone antagonist (Aldactone, triamterene), and metabolic acidosis. Succinylcholine, a muscle relaxant can produce release of potassium from the cells, and should be used with caution in the presence of renal failure.

Absorption of potassium from blood during gastrointestinal hemorrhage and hypercatabolic states are other contributory factors.

'Pseudohyperkalemia' with elevated serum but not plasma potassium is seen in leukemias, polycythemia, and thrombocytosis and results from there release of potassium from platelets and WBC during coagulation. This type of hyperkalemia is not associated with toxicity and does need to be treated. Sometimes, false hyperkalemia may be seen if the blood specimen is hemolyzed or if the tourniquet is too tight causing release of potassium from tissue, and occasionally from sequestering blood through thin gauge needles with force (by producing hemolysis).

Note: Tall T can occur in early phase of acute MI. This should differentiate from the tall T of K↑. Tall T waves are sharp in K↑ whereas blunt in early acute MI.

HYPOKALEMIA

Progressive decrease of potassium below 2.7 mEq results in increased resting membrane potential and amplitude of the action potential. Widened QRS indicates slowing of conduction through the myocardium or peripheral conduction system. The repolarization abnormalities result from lowering of the extra-cellular concentration of potassium.

248. There are 4 important changes in hypokalemia.

1. Depressed ST by 0.5 mV.
2. Prominent U wave of 0.1 mV, U wave amplitude more than T in the same lead.
3. Small or flattened T wave.
4. Prolonged PR, bidirection tachycardia, ventricular fibrillation, arrhythmias like SVT, PVC, AV junctional rhythm.

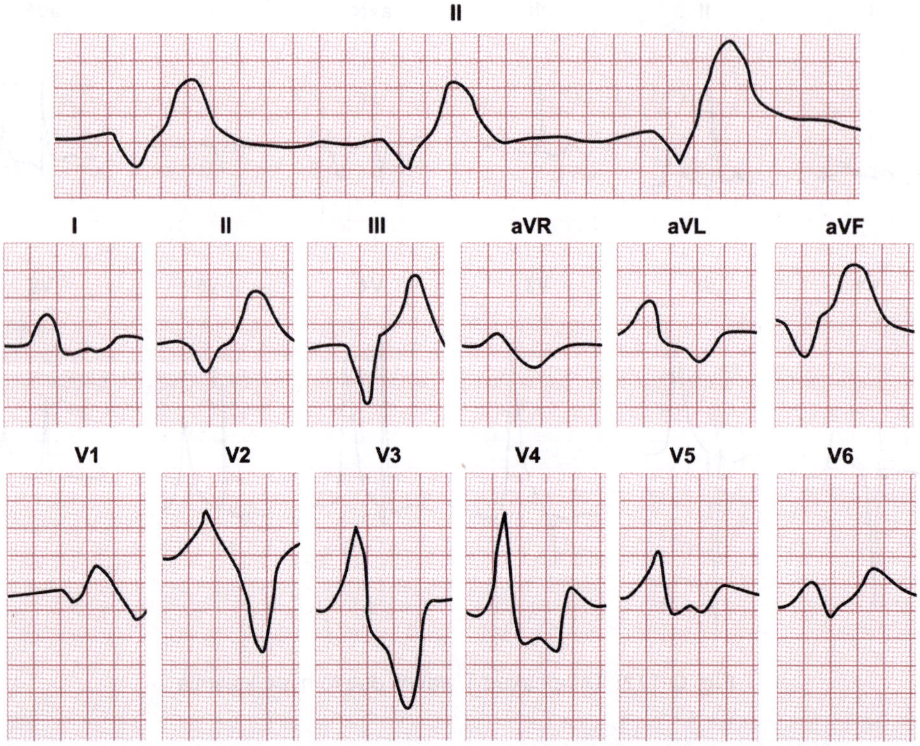

Fig. Q-173: Echocardiogram of hyperkalemia showing atrial standstill, wide QRS and prolongation of QT in hyperkalemia

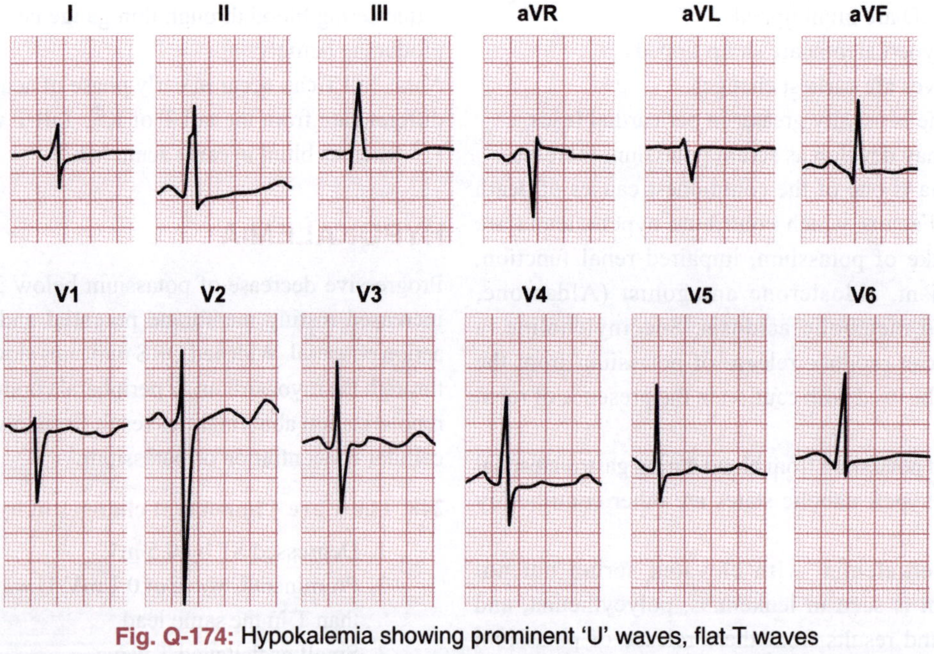

Fig. Q-174: Hypokalemia showing prominent 'U' waves, flat T waves

HYPERCALCEMIA

Serum calcium varying from 9–11 mEq that do not significantly affect either the resting potential, shape of phase 3 or the amplitude of the action potential.

249. ECG changes in hypercalcemia.

1. Calcium more than 12 mg/100 mL produces shortening of QTc.
2. Widening and rounding of T waves.

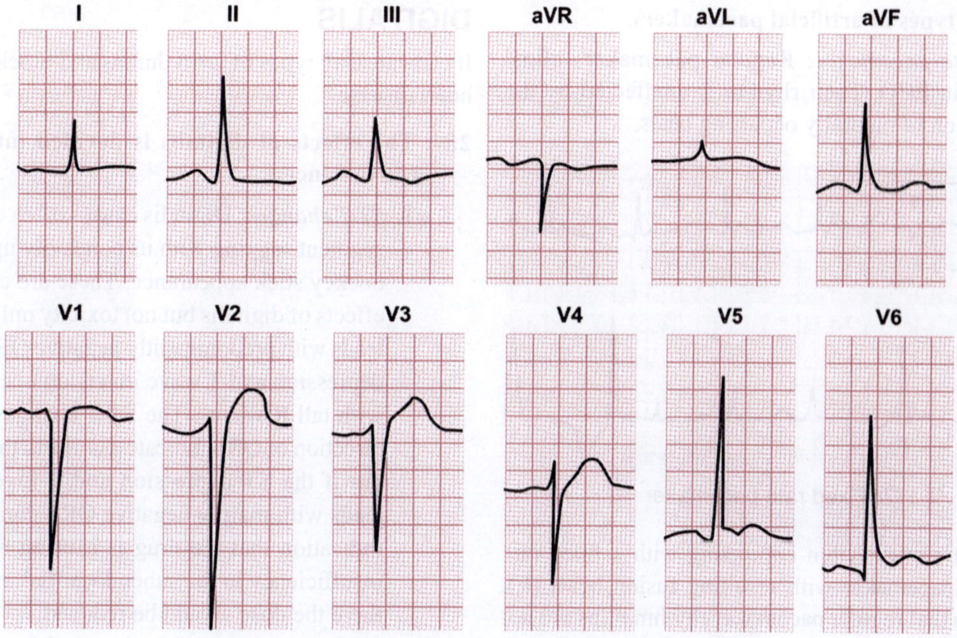

Fig. Q-175: Hypercalcemia showing shortening of QTc

3. Severe hypercalcemia of hyperparathyroidism can lead to sinus arrest, AV block.
4. Atrial fibrillation.

HYPOCALCEMIA

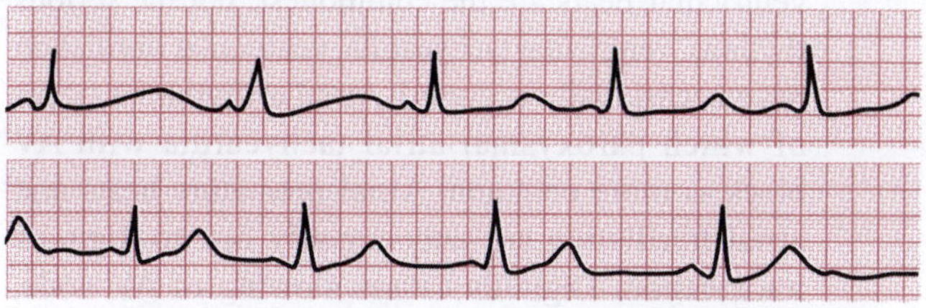
Fig. Q-176: Hypocalcemia showing prolongation of QTc

250. Results in:

1. Prolongation of QTc with no abnormality of T wave. QT prolongation results from lengthening of ST segment due to prolongation of phase 2 of the action potential curve.
2. T inversion.
3. Prolonged PR, sinus bradycardia, sinoatrial block, complete AV block.
4. VF.

MAGNESIUM

Isolated abnormalities of magnesium within the range encountered clinically do not have significant effect on the action potential.

Hypermagnesemia: Reduced AV conduction on magnesium infusion when the Mg level more than 3.5 mEq (normal 1.5–2.5 mEq/L).

251. Hypomagnesemia:

1. Widened QRS, QT
2. Peaked T
3. ST depression
4. Exacerbates digitalis arrhythmia.

252. There are 4 types of important patterns.

1. Strain pattern:
   Asymmetrically inverted T Wave
   See for LV strain in V5
   RV strain in V2
2. Artificial pacemaker:
   See for pacemaker spikes
3. Subendocardial infarction:
   Flat (horizontal) ST depression
4. Pericarditis:
   Flat or concave ST segment elevation
   (seen in where QRS is negative—Right chest leads) or ST segment elevation with T wave off from the baseline.
   (seen in leads where QRS is positive—LI or LII)

Artificial Pacemakers

(See D-319)

253. There are 4 types of artificial pacemakers.

1. *Fixed rate pacemaker:* Regular pacemaker 'blips' are seen in ECG. Their rhythm is unaffected by the intervention of naturally occurring beats.

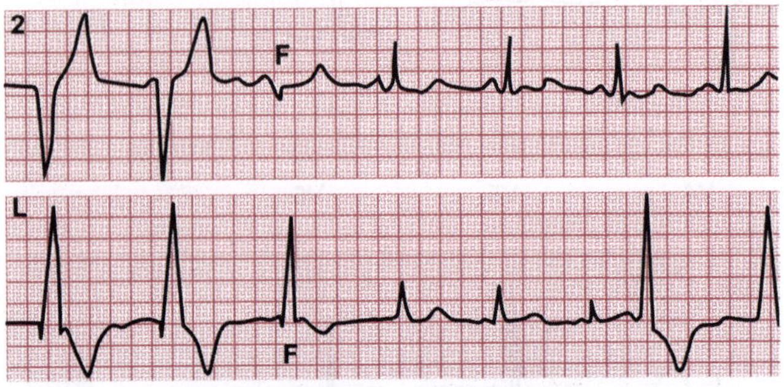

Fig. Q-177: Fixed rate pacemaker

Note that sinus rhythm competing with a fixed rate artificial pacemaker with resulting fusion beats (F). Note also that regular pacemaker rhythm blips are not disturbed by the natural beats.

2. *Demand pacemaker (Ventricular inhibited):*

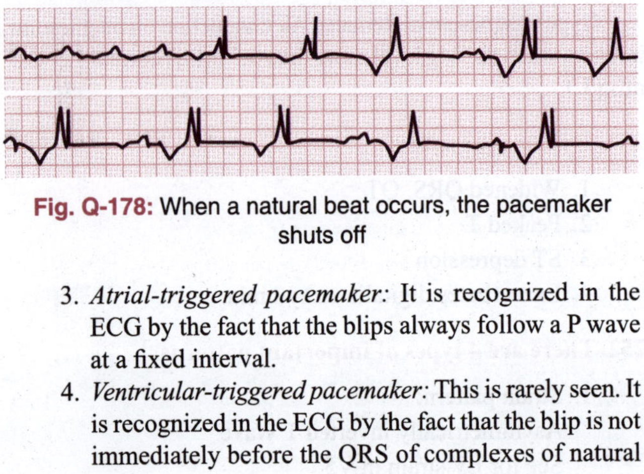

Fig. Q-178: When a natural beat occurs, the pacemaker shuts off

3. *Atrial-triggered pacemaker:* It is recognized in the ECG by the fact that the blips always follow a P wave at a fixed interval.
4. *Ventricular-triggered pacemaker:* This is rarely seen. It is recognized in the ECG by the fact that the blip is not immediately before the QRS of complexes of natural beats.

Caution

It is difficult to distinguish between a fixed rate and demand pacemaker, if there are no natural beats, because the demand pacemaker if it is not interrupted by natural beats will continue to fire regularly. The demand pacemaker works exactly like a ventricular escape rhythm, whereas the fixed rate pacemaker functions like ventricular parasystole; therefore, both can produce fusion beats.

Both atrial-triggered and ventricular-triggered pacemakers become demand pacemakers when there are no natural complexes to trigger them.

DIGITALIS

It can cause all types of arrhythmias and blocks and resembles heart disease.

254. The effects of digitalis is devided into 4 groups for convenience.

1. *ST-T changes:* Digitalis causes often characteristic ST segment sagging with its concavity upward. It gives a hockey stick appearance. These are considered as the effects of digitalis but not toxicity unless they occur in leads with predominantly negative QRS deflection. ST depression and T wave inversion occur in those leads with tall R waves. The ST-T changes in the opposite direction of QRS indicate a uniform therapeutic action, but if the ST depression and T inversion occurs in leads with mainly negative QRS complexes—it is an indication that the drug is causing relative coronary insufficiency in the subendocardial muscle layers and there the dose should be reduced.
2. *Ventricular premature beats:* Often multifocal and often proceeding to bigeminy. Though this is an arrhythmia, since it occurs much more often than any arrhythmia, it is described as a separate category. These are a definite sign of digitalis toxicity and are indication to revise dosage.
3. *Arrhythmias:* Almost all types of arrhythmias are encountered with digitalis complication. Premature ventricular beats are the commonest, but the serious rhythms, ventricular tachycardia, ventricular fibrillation have occasionally occurred. Atrial arrhythmias occur of which paroxysmal atrial tachycardia with AV block is more common. Atrial premature beats and atrial fibrillation are uncommonly due to digitalis intoxication. Digitalis causes slowing of AV node, AV nodal acceleration or both, which may sometimes cause AV dissociation. The digitalis in small doses depresses both SA and AV nodes, but in higher or toxic dosage it continues to depress SA node but increases AV nodal automaticity.
4. *Blocks:* Sinoatrial, atrioventricular and intraventricular blocks have occurred with digitalis toxicity. Simple PR lengthening first degree block is common and partly results from vagal stimulation. Complete AV block can occur without any warning symptoms. Prolongation of QRS interval occurs rarely with digitalis toxicity. Slowing of the heart in sinus rhythm is due to increased vagal effect on the SA node. In atrial fibrillation, slowing of the ventricle is a desirable result of AV block.

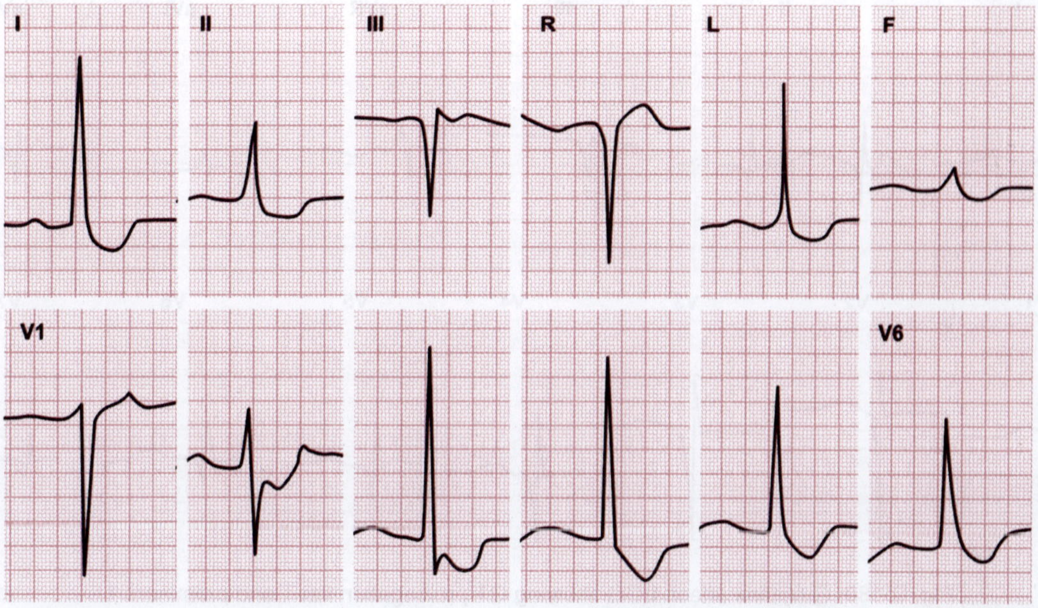

Fig. Q-179: Digitalis effects. Note sagging ST segment in most leads giving hockey stick appearance with short QT interval

255. Digitalis effects on normal ECG.

1. Downward displacement of ST junction
2. Decrease in amplitude of T followed by diphasic and total inversion of T
3. ST depression
4. Shortened QTc.

The changes are noted in II, III, aVF and left precordial leads. Hypokalemia also causes ST depression, but QT is shortened in digitalis effect.

256. Therapeutic effects of digitalis.

1. ST, T wave changes
2. Shortening of QT
3. Prolonged PR
4. Slowing of ventricular response in AF.

257. Toxic effects of digitalis.

1. PAT with block
2. Nonparoxysmal AV junctional tachycardia with AV dissociation
3. SA blocks
4. Second degree and third degree AV blocks
5. PVCs and bigeminy or trigeminy
6. Ventricular tachycardia
7. Bidirectional tachycardia
8. Ventricular fibrillation.

All conduction defects and arrhythmias except intraventricular conduction defects, second degree AV block, parasystole and multifocal tachycardia are known in digitoxicity.

QUINIDINE

258. Toxic effects of quinidine are :

1. AV blocks
2. Atrial slowing, intra-atrial blocks, atrial standstill.
3. QT prolongation—Torsades de pointes
4. PVCs.

259. EMETINE

The ECG changes persist for days to weeks after it is stopped and do not correlate with toxicity. Changes are:

1. ST depression
2. T inversion
3. Prolonged PR
4. Serious side effects are intraventricular conduction disturbances.

260. CISAPRIDE

It is a dopamine antagonist that does not cross the blood-brain barrier; represents an advance in prokinetic therapy in the central nervous system. Side effects are minimal. However, the following serious cardiac arrhythmias are reported.

1. Ventricular tachycardia
2. Ventricular fibrillation
3. Torsades de pointes
4. QT prolongation.

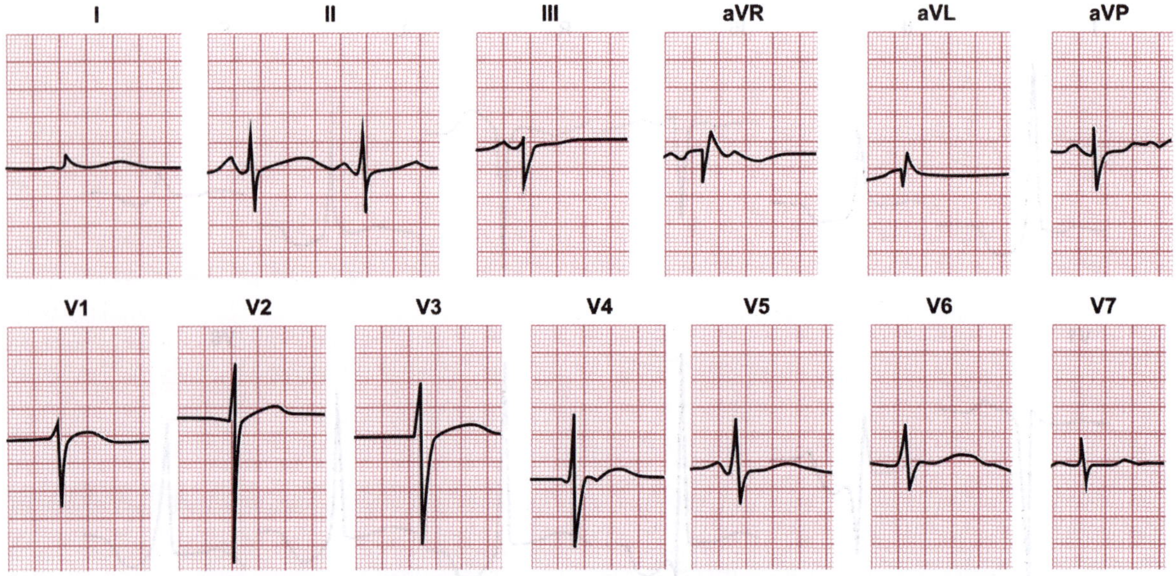

Fig. Q-180: Quinidine effect: ECG showing QT prolongation flat T and prominent 'U'

These have emerged most often with concurrent use of drugs that inhibit hepatic cytochrome P-450 metabolism. Cisapride is contraindicated when such drugs are being used. In addition, it should not be used in persons with a cardiac rhythm disorder underlying heart disease, renal failure, electrolyte disturbances or drugs that may be proarrhythmic. An ECG is obtained before cisapride is given and checked for arrhythmias and any prolongation of the QT interval.

PHENOTHIAZINE AND RELATED DRUGS

261. Most of the antipsychotic and antidepression drugs may alter the ECG pattern in 20–50% of patients receiving medication.

The 4 more frequent changes are:
1. Diminution of T wave amplitude
2. Appearance of prominent U wave
3. Depression of ST segment
4. Prolongation of QT interval.

262. When antipsychotic and antidepression drugs are used in high doses, they may cause the following arrhythmias.

1. At SA node—sinus tachycardia
2. At atria—atrial fibrillation
3. At AV node—AV nodal block
4. At ventricles—PVBs, VT, VF.

Baseline ECG before starting high doses is necessary—caution is taken to revaluation or discontinuation of therapy at the first sign of ventricular tachycardia.

263. Following are the normal variants of ECG:

1. Grusin pattern II or early repolarization syndrome. ST elevation with concavity upward. T-wave is tall and asymmetrical with gently sloped descending limb ending in a prominent U wave.
   It should not be mistaken for:
   a. Acute phase of myocardial infarction
   b. Acute pericarditis
   c. LVH
   d. Hyperkalemia.
2. Juvenile ECG pattern: T inversion in V1 to V4 usually present in children up to 14 years.
3. Isolated Q in lead III: Presence of isolated prominent Q in LIII may be found in normal people. The pathological Q in LIII should be more than 1/3 of R.
4. Flat or inverted T wave—Although suggestive of IHD, these changes are often nonspecific.

T inversion in LIII or V1 alone is not significant.
Normal variation: PR interval of more than 0.22 sec is seen in athletes and vagotonic individuals.

INTERPRETATION OF THE ECG

264. There are 4 diagnostic values of ECG to detect the following abnormalities:

1. Rate disorders, e.g. tachycardias, bradycardias.
2. Rhythm disorders, e.g. arrhythmias—tachyarrhythmias, bradyarrhythmias, blocks, etc.
3. Anatomical disorders, e.g. hypertrophy, myocardial infarction.
4. Cardiac involvement in other systemic disorders, e.g. rheumatic fever.

265. There are 4 limitations of ECG. It does not provide information regarding:

1. Mechanical events of the heart
2. Tone of the heart
3. Reserve power of the heart
4. Etiology of the heart disease.

266. There are 4 points to be observed while evaluating ECG.

1. History, clinical examination and laboratory tests are to be correlated with ECG.
2. Should be compared with previous ECGs, if any.
3. Borderline or doubtful cases should be observed with future ECG.
4. ECG can be repeated either before or after exercise, after giving drugs like pro-banthine to block vagal affects or propranolol to block sympathetic effect.

(*Note:* ECG may show false-positive or false-negative findings). *Caution to the beginner:* A patient with organic disease may have normal ECG or a normal person may show nonspecific abnormalities.

267. History: Note the following 4 points which are not modifiable.

1. *Sex:* Certain conditions are especially predominant in one sex.
2. *Age:* Normal pattern in pediatric practice is considerably different from adults.
3. *Race:* Certain ECG changes seen in young normal. Negroes may be an abnormal pattern rather than a white person of the same age.
4. *Height, weight, body fluid:* Obese and thick chest walled individuals have a low voltage.

268. Note the following 4 points in the history which are modifiable by the disease process.

1. BP and clinical impression.
2. Medication—Remember that digitalis can affect the ECG pattern for as long as 3 weeks after the drug has been stopped.
3. Associated pulmonary disease.
   Emphysema, plural effusion, postoperative chest surgery can affect the heart position and voltage of the complexes.
4. Provisional diagnosis and/or pertinent cardiorespiratory findings.

269. Study the standard leads (I, II, III) and extremity leads for:

1. Heart position (aVL, aVF)
2. Axis deviation (LI, aVF) or (LI and LII)
3. Note the
   i. PR interval
   ii. QRS interval
   iii. QTc—intervals—QT interval corrected to the rate
   iv. VAT—ventricular activation time.
   It is noted from the standard leads as a routine but it is not necessary.
4. Note any abnormalities in
   i. P wave—morphology, origin, etc.
   How much height for RAH
   How much broad for LAH
   Whether it is preceding every QRS or not.
   ii. QRS complex
   see for any abnormal Qs
   iii. ST segment—elevated or depressed: Ischemic changes
   iv. T wave—for hypertrophy, ischemia.

270. See the precordial leads for:

1. Degree of rotation on the long axis
   Normal, clockwise or counterclockwise rotation.
2. Hypertrophy—See in V1 for chamber hypertrophy.
   See in V1–V2
   V5–V6
3. Note any abnormality of P wave
   Q wave, QRS complexes
   ST segment
   T wave
   —for ischemic heart disease
4. Blocks—Arrhythmias.
   RBBB, LBBB
   V1–V2, V5–V6.

271. The following conclusions are made while interpreting ECG when it is abnormal.

1. Borderline—only minor changes are present that will be determined clinically and taking serial ECG at intervals
2. Abnormal ECG—typical of the diagnosis
3. Abnormal ECG—consistent with—(name the condition)
4. Abnormal ECG—not characteristic of any specific disease.

The ECG should always be interpreted in relation with the clinical findings. It is only like any laboratory test. Normal ECG does not mean normal heart and an abnormal ECG does not necessarily mean organic heart disease. A patient with an organic heart disease may have normal ECG or a normal person may show nonspecific ECG abnormalities.

ECG Report
A Systematic Approach to Early Stage Reading an ECG for a Beginner

Patients's Name: Sex: Male/Female Date:
Address: Age: Years Weight: Kg
BP: Urine: Albumin-Sugar

Relevant history
Clinical finding

Rate: Atrial /min
Ventricular /min position: aVL aVF
Voltage: LI + LIII – LII (L3 = aVF – aVL; L2 = aVF – aVR:L1 = aVL – aVR)
(N: > 5 mV in limb lead > 10 mV in chest leads: High voltage L1 + 2 + 3 = 5mV) Total amplitude is measured above and below the isoelectric line.

High voltage:		Noncardiac causes of low voltage	
1. Thin chest wall	Yes/No	1. Thick chest wall	Yes/No
2. LVH	Yes/No	2. Emphysema/Pleural effusion	Yes/No
3. Hyperthyroidism	Yes/No	3. Myxedema	Yes/No
4. WPW syndrome	Yes/No	4. Generalized edema	Yes/No
Cardiac causes of low voltage			
1. Acute ML/Diffuse LHD	Yes/No	5. HF treated with digitalis	Yes/No
2. Precordial effusion/		6. Myocarditis	Yes/No
Chronic constrictive pericarditis	Yes/No	7. Primary amyloidosis	Yes/No
3. Cardiomyopathy with decrease	Yes/No		
4. Anterior rotation of apex	Yes/No		

QRS Axis Frontal (or vertical): LI LII LIII aVF
Horizontal axis: S > R in V1 Posterior/Anterior
Rotation at
P in LI and LII (No dextrocardia/limb attached correctly)
Rhythm: Regular sinus rhythm Yse/No Each P is followed by QRS Yes/No
RR and RP intervals Regular/Irregular
P Wave morphology:
P ↓ APBs nodal, rhythms, non-sinus ( ) rhythm, wandering pacemaker, dextrocardia, technical dextrocardia
Amplitude/duration ↑: P-'Pulmonale' , P-'Congenitale', P-'Mitrale' , Bifid , K↑, K↓
Partially or wholly buried in QRS: AV block, PAT supraventricular extrasystoles, K↑
Absent P: Atrial flutter/fibrillation, SA block, sinus rurrest, Nodal rhythm
Irregular P: Sinus pause, SA block, sinus bradycardiac, intermittent escape beats
QRS wave morphology RSR' pattern Yes/No
Abnormal waves
PR intervals = sec (> 0.2 sec AV block, digitalis, hyperthyroidism, pacemaker
< 0.2 sec-WPW/LGI, syndrome, non-sinus (coronary sinus) atrial rhythm, nodal rhythm, some hypertensives)
QRS duration = sec (>0.2 sec) I. Impulse from an ectopic ventricular focus– i. PVB's, ii. VT iii. ventricular escape beat iv. Accelerated idioventricular rhythm v. idioventricular rhythm from a low pacemaker vi. ventricular parasystole;II Intraventricular conduction delay: i. BBB, hemiblock ii. Ventricular aberation; III. Conduction in one ventricular is accelerated: WPW syndrome (initial shurring of Q wave –delta wave); IV. Artificial pacemaker; V. CAD—M/Ischemia; VI. Drugs and Electrolytes i. Digitalis/Verapamil ii. Hyperkalemia; VII. CMP'-Total destruction VIII. Myocarditis/fibrositis (5,6,7,8, are also due to delayed intraventricular coordination)
QT interval: sec (N: 032–0.43 sec. Shorter in tachycardia, broader in bradycardia)
WPW syndrome Yes/No (short PR, pre-excitation delta wave, wide QRS,ST-T opposite of QRS)
Hypertrophy: See LII or V1

RAH	P wave	> 2.5 mm	P 'Pulmonale'	Yes/No
LAH	P wave	> 2.5 mm	P 'Mitral'	Yes/No

RVH	Yes/No	R:S in V1	1:1	R in V2	8 mm	
RAD	Yes/No	Wide QRS	YES/NO	S in V5 or V6	5 mm	
Progressively tall from		V1 to V4	Yes/No	ST ↓ in LIII, aVR, V1, 2, 3,		Yes/No
LVH : Yes/No						
S in V1	+ R in V5	–	> 35 mm	R in LI	R in V1	
S in V2	+ R in V6	–	> 40 mm			
LAD	Yes/No	wide QRS	Yes/No	Asymmetrical T↓ in V5 or V6		

Ischemia

Q Waves < 2 mm deep < 0.04 sec width < 1/4th of R Yes/No 1/3rd of R in LIII Yes/No

i. MI
ii. Hypertrophy (LVH-V5, V6; RVH-V1, V2 deep broad Qs in LI, aVL, V5, V6 in HOCM due to septal hypertrophy
iii. In LBB Qs appear in V1, V2 but Q in V5, V6 signifies MI
iv. Pulmonary infarction—wide S in LI and large Q in LIII.

ST segment elevation

i. Acute MI (ST↑at least in two consecutive leads with reciprocal ST↓ Yes/No
ii. Prinzmetal angina or variant angina Yes/No(severe spasm causes ST↑ but no reciprocal ST↓).
iii. Pericarditis Yes/No (ST-T elevated off the baseline in many leads with concavity upward. No abnormal QS or QS complexes).
iv. Ventricular aneurysm Yes/No (persistent ST↑for many years or RSR' pattern in V6, see old ECG)
v. Early repolarization syndrome (congenital)—a normal variant, ST↑off the baseline with concavity upwards (exercise abolishes the sickling pattern)
vi. Hypertrophic obstructive cardiomyopathy HOCM
vii. Myocarditis
viii. Normal variant: athlete heart, pattern, high take off
ix. Cardiac murmurs
x. False positive: LBBB, WPW syndrome, cor pulmonale, drugs (digitalis effect, quinidine), hyperkalemia.
xi. Noncardiac lesions like CVA: Cerebral hemorrhage, dialysis, carcinoma of lung with secondaries in myocardium, GI bleeding, blood transfusion, intravascular coagulation
xii. ALCAPA (abnormal origin of left coronary artery from pulmonary artery—very rare.

ST segment depression > 1 mm Yes/No

Normally the ST segment and T wave should merge smoothly and improbably. Horizontal or down slopping of ST segment 1 mm or more at 80 msec beyond continuous ascent with upward concavity. Prominent Ta (or Pt) deflection produced by atrial repolarization persists

i. Angina	Yes/No	v. Subendocardial MI	Yes/No
ii. Digitalis toxicity	Yes/No	vi. Changes in ventricular depolarization	Yes/No
iii. LV strain	Yes/No	vii. Hypokalemia	Yes/No
iv. RVH	Yes/No	viii. Hypomagnesemia	Yes/No

T wave T↓ in V1———→ V4 subendocardial infarction Yes/No

I. In the muscle
  i. Symmetrical T↓ = IHD, anoxia, ST with concavity upward followed by T wave (coronary T or Pardee T wave) Yes/No
  ii. Deeply inverted T ↓ = Apical hypertrophy or cardiomyopathy Yes/No
  iii. Asymmetrical T↓ = No LV strain or hypertrophy Yes/No
  iv. Downward slopping of ST segment merging into a deeply inverted T ventricular conduction abnormally Yes/No
II. Abnormal sequence of depolarization: PVBs, BBB, pericarditis, myocarditis Yes/No
III. Drug effects Yes/No
IV. Electrolyte disturbance Yes/No

Abnormal tall at waves in precordial leads—Myocardial ischemia/CAD Yes/No
Pulmonary effects: Low voltage of emphysema Yes/No
Pulmonary infarction:
S1 QIII (wide S in LI, Large Q in LIII) Yes/No
T↓ in V1 tp V4 Yes/No

ST↓ & T↓ in LIII		Yes/No	
Transient RBBB		Yes/No	
RAD		Yes/No	
After exercise	Heart rate		BP
ST segment	Depression/Elevation	Yes/No	
T wave	makening/inversion	Yes/No	
R wave height	decrease/increase/normal	Yes/No	
Arrhythmias		Yes/No	

Summery

Impression

Students are advised to practicing by filling these ECG reports at least 100 times.

R Echocardiography

The use of ultrasound waves to visualize intracardiac structures, their disposition and movements is termed as echocardiography. It records information in the form of echoes, i.e. reflected sonic waves. The frequency of sound is expressed as cycles per second or hertz (Hz).

Normal limit of the audible sound is 20000 cycles/second or 20 hertz (Hz).

High frequency ultrasound waves greater than 20000 cycles/second which are not audible to the ear are used in this diagnostic methods. The frequency in the range of millions of Hz or mega hertz (MHz) is used.

1. The following 4 basic principles are to be studied:

1. *Physics of piezoelectric crystal:* The transducer instrument has a piezoelectric crystal. It has got a peculiar character with two wires inside, one fiber is transmitting and the other is receiving the ultrasound waves. The transducer acts as a transmitter 0.1% of the time and as a receiver about 99.9% of the time.
   It transforms electrical energy into mechanical energy and an electrical signal is created which transform into mechanical sound energy. When the reflected sound energy is returned to the sensor which then function as a sensor (receiving), changes the mechanical information into electrical energy. High frequency waves are electrically generated at measured intervals by the piezoelectric crystal. The duration of the transmitted sound waves in a conventional echocardiographic transducer is approximately one microsecond with a repetition of about 1000 pulses per second.
2. *Velocity:* Velocity of ultrasound in human body is generally 1.540 meter/second. The velocity remains constant. So, increase in frequency is associated with decrease in wavelength and decrease in frequency is associated with increase in wavelength. Generally, higher frequencies are used in younger patients in whom the need for penetration is minimal and lower frequencies are needed for older patients. Higher frequencies penetrate less but have finer resolution whereas lower frequencies penetrate deeper but sacrifice resolution.
3. *Reflection:* Various organs in the body have varying density and as such have varying acoustic impedance. When ultrasound is passed, some are reflected and some are passed into the tissues further. Strong echoes are produced when a greater degree of reflection occurs. Sound waves pass through soft tissues until they encounter an interface with a substance of different acoustic impedance such as the myocardium blood interface. The change in the acoustic impedance causes that portion of the sound wave which is perpendicular to the interface to be reflected back to the transducer. These reflected echoes are then detected by the transducer. The received signals are displayed on an oscilloscope and can simultaneously be recorded by a strip chart recorder for permanent record. The resultant image is that of particular cardiac structure at their respective depth displaced across a time axis. This is called an M-mode recording.
   Amount of stress applied to the crystal is determined by measuring the strength of the reflected electric charge as a voltage, i.e. the echo strength.
   The speed of the sound wave is known by measuring the time taken for the sound impulse to travel from the transducer to the structure and back. The depth of the structure can be calculated as:
   Distance = Velocity × Time/2.

All the measurements can be made by utilizing this principle.

4. *Resolution:* It is the ability to differentiate structures which are physically close. The thickness of the structure must be at least 1/4th of the ultrasound wavelength before it can be recognized separately. The ultrasound of 2.5 MHz can recognize 0.6 mm thickness. The ultrasound of 7.5 MHz can recognize 0.02 mm thickness. Theoretically, 2.5 MHz transducer can resolve structures as close as 0.15 mm and a 7.5 MHz can resolve 0.05 mm apart, but practically this is not possible.

   Axial resolution error occurs if two surfaces lie one behind the other and the distance is not large enough for the returning signals to be identified separately. Structures above 1.5 to 2 mm difference is seen. Less than 1.5 to 2 mm distance between the two parallel lines (tissues) cannot be appreciated by ultrasound.

   Lateral resolution means separating the closely lying structures in a plane perpendicular to the beam. This depends on the stage of the ultrasound field across the width of the tissue. Less than 10 mm width is not appreciated by ultrasound. It can differentiate above 10 mm width. Axial resolution can be overcome if the direction of the pulse is less but not lateral resolution. The sound beam has the same width as the transducer near the transducer, but the same field diverges after a depth. Side lobes cause problem in lateral resolution. Lateral resolution occurs when side by side tissues are at the same distance from the transducer and within the beam.

2. There are 4 stages of progression in the development of echocardiography.

1. *A-mode (A for amplitude):* It is used to locate immobile surfaces. The amplitude or height of each peak of the echo is proportional to its intensity.
2. *B-mode (B for brightness):* It is the intermediate step between A and M mode. The amplitude of peak is indicated by the brightness of the dots; hence the term B (for brightness).

   A and B modes are good for static structures like pelvis, abdomen but not for moving structures like heart. Very useful in abdominal and gynecological disorders.
3. *M-mode (M for motion):* It is useful for moving organs like heart. It transmits and receives ultrasound waves along a single line. The resulting image has been termed as 'ice-pick' view of the heart. The transducer must be directed in different positions to visualize different parts of the heart.
4. *Two-dimensional or cross-sectional echocardiography (2D Echo):* It is a real time echocardiography. The transducer is moved rapidly by a small electric motor and provides continuous representation of cardiac structures. 2-4-further advances have come as 3 or 4-dimensional Echo, transesophageal echo (TEE), intracardiac echo, doppler flow velocity, tissue doppler, etc.

3. Echocardiographically, the heart is visible as a collection of acoustic interfaces by which you can distinguish 4 structures.

1. Myocardium, cardiac chambers (blood), anterior wall and posterior wall of each chamber, size of the cavity and their contents.
2. Valve leaflets.
3. Great vessels.
4. Pericardium, pericardial fluid.

All these have characteristic echoes.

4. Echocardiogram can show the:

1. Size and shape.
2. Relative position.
3. Direction.
4. Pattern of motion of each of the above structures.

5. Echocardiography is considered as an essential part of the routine check-up for a patient with heart disease. The indications for echocardiography in an adult are:

1. Complaints of chest pain (typical or atypical), shortness of breath, syncope, palpitation. It is especially helpful when the cause for the complaint is not evident.
2. Presence of cyanosis, congestive heart failure, cardiomegaly, arrhythmia, abnormal chest X-ray, abnormal ECG.
3. Heart murmurs including the 'innocent murmurs' or abnormal sounds (or clicks).
4. Pyrexia of unknown origin which may be caused by subacute bacterial endocarditis, pericardial effusion or myxoma.
5. Evaluation of families where one family member has had asymmetrical septal hypertrophy or sudden death.
6. Baseline evaluation in patients with high-risk heart disease as in hypertension, Marfan's syndrome, muscular dystrophy.
7. Presence of anterior mediastinal mass to rule out a cyst or unusual vascular anomalies.
8. Patients receiving treatment which can affect myocardial function such as chemotherapy or radiation.
9. Patients with atrial fibrillation who need cardioversion to evaluate left atrial size and clot.
10. Evaluation of all patients before cardiac catheterization or cardiac surgery.
11. Follow-up studies after cardiac surgery, trauma to the chest to rule out pericardial effusion or decreased contractility due to myocardial contusion. In general, follow-up studies of any known cardiac disease.

12. Non-cardiac disorders which may alter cardiac function such as AV fistula or airway obstruction.

6. The various factors that determine the final recording is governed by:

1. Properties of the sound.
2. Configuration of the ultrasound beam.
3. Piezoelectric element.
4. Properties of the medium.
5. The interface through which the sound passes.
6. The echo amplification.
7. Display.
8. Finally, the technically trained personnel.

7. Expertize is required to the examiner who interpret the echocardiographic readings. The principle problem is produced by poor transmission of ultrasound through bony structures or air-containing lungs. The examiner should avoid these structures. 4 methods have been developed to overcome the problem.

1. The patient is commonly placed in the left recumbent position to move the heart from beneath the sternum.
2. The subxiphoid or subcostal transducer position is used in patients with hyperventilated lungs and a low diaphragm.
3. The apical transducer position with two-dimensional echocardiography has greatly improved the success rate in problem cases.
4. The suprasternal notch position is useful especially for Doppler studies.

   The number of technically unsatisfactory recordings are minimized with the development of techniques like transesophageal echocardiography (TEE). Better instruments and examining techniques by the skilled persons minimized the false reports to less than 5–10%.

8. There are 4 advantages of echocardiography:

1. It is non-invasive and virtually harmless.
2. It is economical compared to other sophisticated imaging techniques.
3. It visualizes intracardiac structures directly, and is an useful diagnostic tool in congenital and acquired heart diseases.
4. 90–95% of heart diseases can be diagnosed by a skilled examiner.

9. There are 4 limitations of echocardiography:

1. *Echo drop:* Structures which lie parallel with ultrasound beam do not reflect sound waves well and so give a false reading. Thus fossa ovalis may give a false reading of atrial septal defect—false drop out.
2. *Lateral resolution:* Ability to differentiate two points side by side at a distance of 4–5 mm is much less than the X-ray.
3. *Off axis echoes:* A strong reflecting object gives more deep echoes than the structures lying in its axis at the edge of the beam.
4. *Chronic chest diseases like emphysematous lungs overlying the heart*: The sound waves are poorly transmitted through gas and air.

10. M-mode echocardiography is obtained in 4 planes from left parasternal region—three views are taken followed by 4th M-mode sweep.

1. Across the left ventricular cavity: Left ventricular wall thickness, its movements, thickness of interventricular septum are visualized.
2. At the level of the anterior leaflet of mitral valve: It gives a strong echo and is easily recognized by the formation of ABCDEF waves. The E to F slope indicates the speed closure of the mitral valve, normal value being 70 to 150 mm per second. It is of value in detecting rheumatic mitral valve diseases like mitral stenosis, mitral regurgitation, calcification or vegetations on mitral valve, mitral valve prolapse.
3. At the level of the aortic valve and left atrium. This is useful to measure the left atrial size, diameter of the aortic root and movements of the aortic valve.
4. M-mode sweep: The transducer is moved from aortic root to the apex and recording is made on. Normal relation of aortic root and septum and mitral valve is noted. The anterior wall of the aorta is in continuity with the echoes from the interventricular septum and the posterior wall of the aorta is in continuity with the echoes of the anterior leaflet of the mitral valve. This is an important feature of echo anatomy. Left atrium lies most posteriorly.

   M-mode gives an ice-pick view of the heart and is compared to entering a dark room with a pencil torch and only a small lighted area is visualized. On the other hand, two-dimensional echocardiography is like entering the same dark room with a search light and the whole room is lighted. Despite advancement of unidimensional M-mode technique of early 1970s to the two-dimensional technique of late 1970s, each has got its place. The ECG is recorded simultaneously and permits accurate measurement of the timing of cardiac events including the opening and closing of the valves. This information is presented graphically.

11. There are 4 methods which complement each other in diagnosing heart disease:

1. M-mode echocardiography.
2. Two-dimensional or cross-sectional real time echocardiography.
3. Doppler echocardiography, including color flow Doppler.
4. Contrast echocardiography.

   Two-dimensional echocardiography: In this, the resulting information is synthesized into a two-dimensional picture.

   It is also possible to produce a two-dimensional image of the heart either by electronically triggering a series of crystals in rapid succession or by mechanically sweeping a single crystal back and forth in an arc. The rapid succession of images produced are then electronically compiled into an image resembling slice through the heart. The transducers used are mechanical or electronic beam steering (phased array), sector or linear scanners. Two-dimensional Echo mainly offers spatial resolution. The ultrasound beam scans the cross sectional plane at high rate to yield time to time or instant information about two-dimensional geometry. Each form is composed of a number of lines and greater the number of lines the greater is the clarity of images. However, it should be adjusted with reference to the form and depth of imaging. The linear density is inversely proportional to the depth of interrogation.

12. Two-dimensional echocardiography studies are more frequently used clinically especially for the following 4:

1. Evaluating left ventricular function.
2. Evaluating valve orifice area.
3. Evaluating congenital heart diseases.
4. Evaluating further delineating the structures seen on M-mode.

Two-dimensional echocardiography is useful to obtain an infinite number of slices of the heart. All images could be categorized into three orthogonal planes. These are long-axis, short-axis and four-chamber planes. The long-axis plane is the imaging plane that transacts the heart perpendicular to dorsal and ventral surfaces of the body and parallel to the long-axis of the heart. Short-axis plane is perpendicular to the long-axis plane of the heart. The plane that transacts the heart approximately parallel to the dorsal and ventral surfaces of the body is the four-chamber plane. These planes are with reference to the heart and not to the thorax or body. The two-dimensional echocardiographic examination is planned according to the position of the transducer.

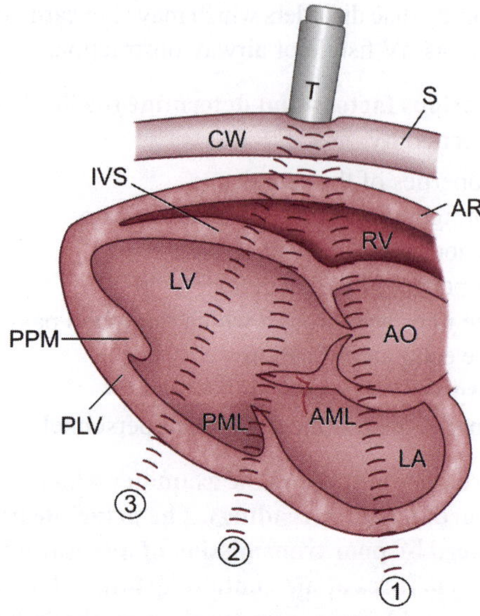

Fig. R-1: A diagrammatic presentation of the cardiac structures traversed by three echo beams.

T. Transducer; S. Sternum; CW. Chest wall; ARV. Anterior wall of right ventricle; RV. Right ventricular cavity; IVS. Interventricular septum; AO. Aorta; LA. Left atrium; LV. Left ventricle; AML. Anterior mitral leaflet; PML. Posterior mitral leaflet; PPM. Posterior papillary muscle; PLV. Posterior left ventricular wall.

13. There are 4 positions of the transducer by which images are studied in different planes in two-dimensional echocardiographic examination.

Imagine the patient lying in the left lateral position with head on the right side and feet on the left side. Transducer is placed on the chest wall—left sternal border at 3rd or 4th intercostal space.

I. **Parasternal long axis position:**
   i. Root of aorta—aortic valve, two sinuses are seen out of three (RCS—Right coronary sinus, NCS—Non-coronary sinus). Anterior wall of aorta continuous with interventricular septum. Posterior wall of aorta continuous with anterior mitral leaflet, left atrium, left ventricular outflow tract.
   ii. Body of left ventricle—Mitral valve, AML—anterior mitral leaflet, PML—posterior mitral leaflet with chordae tendineae. Mitral valve with its both leaflets is seen moving as 'Clapping Hands'. Left ventricle with its cavity, posterior wall of left ventricle, interventricular septum.
   iii. Left ventricular apex.
   iv. Right ventricular inflow tract—tricuspid valve: In the parasternal long-axis view, the patient's

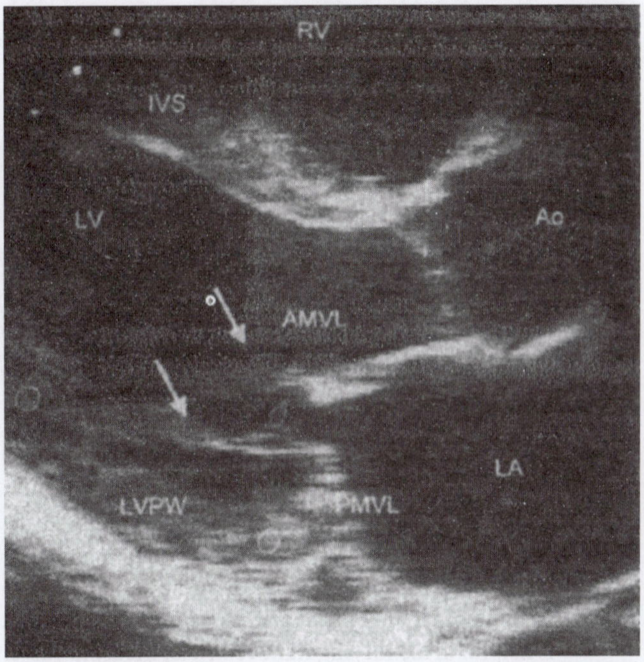

Fig. R-2: Parasternal long-axis view

head is to the right side of the screen, and the feet are to the left. The chest wall is at the top and the posterior left ventricular wall is at the bottom of the monitor. In this view, the aorta is on the right with its anterior wall continuous with interventricular septum and posterior wall continuous with mitral valve. The mitral leaflets are well-identified which resemble 'clapping hands' as they open and close. The leaflets open fully in opposite direction during diastole. The chordae tendineae and papillary muscle attachments are seen as an extension of the mitral leaflets. The left atrium lies posterior to the posterior aortic root. The right ventricle lies anterior to interventricular septum.

II. **Apical 4-chamber position:**
   A. Four-chamber plane
      i. Four chamber.
      ii. Four chamber with aorta.
   B. Long-axis plane
      i. Two chamber—left ventricle, left atrium.
      ii. Two chamber with aorta.

The apical four chamber view is very frequently studied. Depending on the transducer orientation, the left ventricle, and left atrium lie on the left side of the screen, and right ventricle and right atrium to the right side of the screen. Apex is located at the top of the picture while the base (atrial chambers) is at the bottom. The interventricular and interatrial septum lie in the midline and separate the chambers. The septal tricuspid leaflet inserted more anteriorly toward apical side as compared to anterior mitral leaflet. The posterior mitral leaflet is attached laterally.

This is again modified into apical 2-chamber, 3-chamber, 5-chamber views depending on positioning of the transducer.

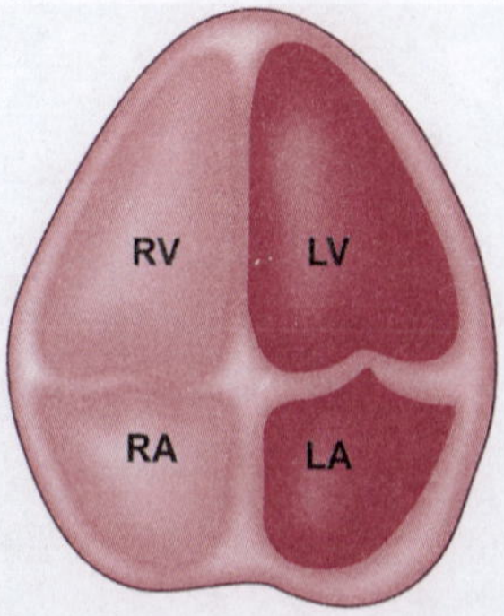

Fig. R-3: A diagrammatic presentation of apical 4 chamber view of the heart demonstrates all the 4 chambers

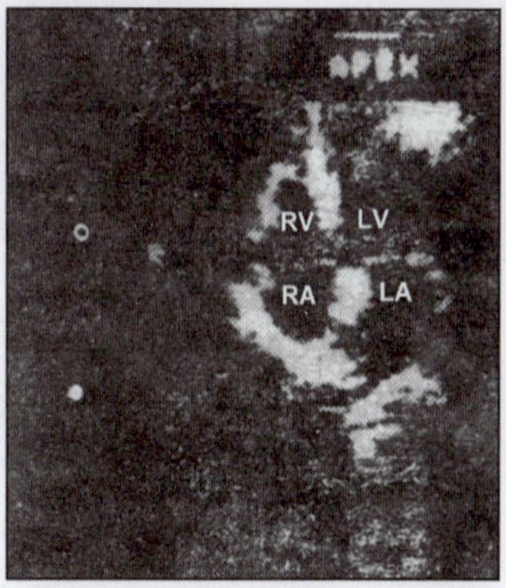

Fig. R-4: Apical 4 chamber view

III. **Subcostal position:**
   i. Four-chamber plane—all four chambers and both septa.
   ii. Short-axis plane—left ventricle, right ventricle and inferior vena cava.

IV. **Suprasternal position:**
   i. Four-chamber plane—arch of aorta, descending aorta.
   ii. Long-axis plane—arch of aorta, pulmonary artery, left atrium.

The subcostal and suprasternal views, though are very important in the study of pediatric practice are comparatively less significance in valvular heart diseases. There are many short-axis views at different tomographic levels of the heart.

14. Parasternal short axis plane are seen at 4 different levels by changing position of the transducer.

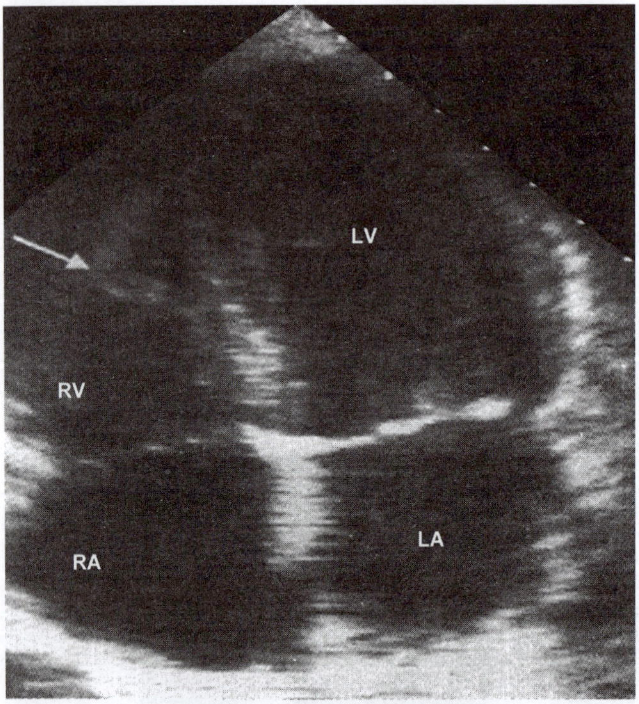

Fig. R-5: Subcostal 4-chamber view—pericardial effusion is seen

Position 1: Transducer is pointed towards apex of the heart—Left ventricular cavity at the level of posterior papillary muscle (PPM), small portion of the right ventricular cavity.

Position 2: Ultrasonic beam traverse through—Left ventricular chamber at the level of edges of mitral valve leaflets (AMV and PMV) and chordae tendineae.

Position 3: At the level of mitral valve: Transducer is directed superiorly and medially—'Fish mouth' appearance of mitral valve, left ventricle, right ventricle, left ventricular wall is seen well.

Position 4: At the level of aorta, transducer is further directed superiorly; medially—root of the aorta (AO), aortic valve leaflets, three sinuses of aorta—right coronary sinus, left coronary sinus, non-coronary sinus are seen, left atrium, interatrial septum, right atrium, tricuspid valve, right ventricle, right ventricular outflow tract, pulmonary valve, right pulmonary and left pulmonary artery, coronary arteries are seen.

There are many short-axis views at different tomographic levels of the heart like aorta, mitral valve, papillary muscles, etc. These views are mainly to see left ventricular walls, aorta and aortic cusps with slight variation in angulation. The short axis of the examination of the base of the heart can also record the pulmonary and tricuspid valves, right ventricular outflow tract, pulmonary artery, which can be traced upto its bifurcation, mitral orifice, etc. Ultrasound has the ability to pass through soft tissues but the bones (ribs and sternum) and air in the lungs present as barriers to the sound beam. Therefore, the echocardiogram must be performed along the left sternal border usually in the left third to fifth intercostal spaces. Additional information is obtained by scanning through the apical, subcostal and suprasternal area where the heart or great vessels are in direct contact.

15. Thus there are 4 positions at which the transducer is kept in two-dimensional echocardiography to obtain much information in 4 planes.

1. *Parasternal position:* Transducer is positioned over the left third to fifth intercostal spaces along the left sternal border and it is angled in various directions. It is helpful in identifying right ventricle, tricuspid valve, mitral valve, aortic ring, ventricular septum, posterior wall of the ventricles.
2. *Apical or 4 chamber view:* Useful in diagnosing very complex congenital heart diseases. All 4 chambers, atrial and ventricular septum are visualized.
3. *Subcostal view:* Heart is viewed from below. All the 4 chambers are visualized but in mirror image fashion.
4. *Suprasternal view:* Useful in identifying the diseases of great vessels like aorta, pulmonary artery, etc. So it helps in the diagnosis of coarctation of aorta, aortic arch syndrome, patent ductus arteriosus, etc.

All the defects in the heart can be demonstrated by 2D or cross-sectional real time echocardiography by its various long-axis and short-axis views.

Bare area of the heart is at left parasternal line where there is no lung tissue. When transducer is kept at this area, the image is appreciated.

16. Doppler echocardiography: M-mode and two-dimensional echocardiography mainly create ultrasonic images of the heart. Doppler echocardiography uses ultrasound to evaluate velocity and turbulence of blood flow within the cardiovascular system. So it is helpful in identifying abnormal blood flow patterns that occur in cardiac shunts and valvular regurgitations. This technique depends on the fundamental principle, that sound waves reflected from moving objects, such as intracardiac red blood cells undergo a frequency shift. The speed and direction of red cells and thus of blood can be detected in the heart chambers and great vessels.

Doppler and color Doppler echocardiography have a basic advantage of quantification, timing of events in the evaluation of cardiac disorders. It has an added advantage over 2D Echo. Except for coronary arteries, it can practically give all information about cardiac disorders. Many cardiac centers in the world are directly relying on the Echo findings. Today catheterization should be done only after this investigation has provided inconclusive results. It is useful in:

1. Evaluating valvular disorders.
2. Identifying and classifying congenital heart disease.
3. Fetal cardiac studies and fetoplacental studies.
4. Myocardial diseases such as cardiomyopathies.
5. Pericardial diseases.
6. Quantification of aortic and pulmonary pressures, shunts and gradients.
7. Evaluation of coronary artery diseases (CAD).
8. Preoperative and post-treatment follow-ups.

17. There are 4 points know about Doppler shift or Doppler frequency:

1. When the ultrasonic wave is reflected by a stationary object, the transmitted frequency (ft) and the reflected frequency (fr) are equal, i.e. ft = fr.
2. When the target reflecting the ultrasonic energy is moving toward the transducer, the reflected frequency (fr) is greater than the transmitted frequency (ft), i.e. fr > ft.
3. When the target is moving away from the transducer, the reflected frequency (fr) is less than the transmitted frequency (ft), i.e. fr < ft.
4. The difference between the reflected and transmitted frequency is known as Doppler shift or Doppler frequency.

It is possible to calculate the velocity of the moving target by the following formula:

$$fd = fr - ft$$

$$fd = 2\,ft\,\frac{v\cos\theta}{C}$$

$$v = \frac{fd.C}{2\,ft\,(\cos\theta)}$$

C—velocity of sound.

18. To determine the velocity of blood, it is necessary to know the following 4 factors:

1. Transmitted frequency (ft).
2. Receiving frequency (fr).
   1 and 2 gives the Doppler frequency (fd).
3. Angle (0) between the paths of ultrasonic beam and moving target.
4. Velocity of the sound in the medium.

Red cells are the targets in Doppler echocardiography. Moving blood is displayed within M-mode or two-dimensional Echo. The direction of the blood is displayed in color. The instrument displays the blood moving toward the transducer in yellow and red shades and the blood moving away from the transducer in blue shades.

19. Invasive echocardiography.

Although the main advantage of the echocardiogram is non-invasive, this can be used as an invasive procedure. Transesophageal echocardiography is used by placing a two-dimensional transducer at the end of a flexible endoscope. It is now possible to obtain high-quality two-dimensional images via the esophagus. It is also possible to combine with pulsed Doppler, color Doppler or contrast studies.

1. This is useful in patients in whom routine examination from the usual position is impossible technically.
2. Useful in those patients where the two-dimensional echocardiography findings are not well-appreciated as in cases of endocardial cushion defects (AV canal defects, aortopulmonary window).
3. The major application for transesophageal echocardiography is during cardiac surgery. The transesophageal probe can be used to monitor cardiac function throughout the surgical procedure. Surgeons are finding it very useful during open heart surgery. This is found very useful while doing transmyocardial revascularization (TMR) by laser beams. Bubbles of laser rays passing through the myocardium are well-visualized by TEE.
4. It is useful postoperatively in assessing cardiac morphology and function after surgical procedure.

20. Transesophageal echocardiography can be done in 4 ways. It is an outpatient procedure and requires no sedation. It is sometimes even better than angiography or CT scan in evaluating certain disorders.

1. Single plane.
2. Biplane.
3. Multiplane.
4. Contrast color flow studies.

21. Single plane transesophageal echocardiography is useful in evaluation of posterior heart structures.

1. Left atrial disorder.
2. Descending aorta.
3. Pulmonary veins.
4. Interatrial septum.
5. Endocardial cushion defects.
6. Early identification of thrombi/emboli.
7. Early identification of vegetations/tumors.
8. Pre- and postoperative evaluation of LV function.

22. Biplane transesophageal echocardiography has an advantage over the single plane in evaluating the following 4 structures:

1. Pulmonary valve.
2. Pulmonary artery.
3. Vegetations.
4. Right atrial appendage and interatrial septal defects.

23. Multiplane transesophageal echocardiography: It helps in evaluation of the heart in all planes and has a definitive advantage in total evaluation.

Routine indications of multiplane transesophageal echocardiography are:

1. Infective endocarditis.
2. Source of emboli for left ventricular appendage.
3. Evaluation of prosthetic valve.
4. Interatrial shunts, AV canal defects.
5. Mitral valve disease.
6. Masses.
7. Suspected atrial, subaortic lesions.
8. Aortic diseases.

24. Transesophageal contrast color flow studies: It is now possible with this technique by using Levovist contrast to evaluate.

1. Proximal coronary artery lesions.
2. First few cm of left main coronary artery (LMCA).
3. Left anterior descending (LAD) artery.
4. Left circumflex (LCX) artery lesions.

25. Contrast echocardiography.

Ultrasound detects intravascular bubbles with extreme sensitivity. The injection of any fluid into intravascular spaces results in many microbubbles that appear as a cloud of echoes on the echocardiogram. It is a sensitive method of detecting right-to-left shunt. When the contrast is injected, it is initially seen in the right ventricle. It then passes through the interventricular septum and appears in the left ventricle. Right-sided contrasts enhance right sided flow and left-sided contrast enhances both right and left-sided cardiac flow signals. Right-sided contrasts are agitated saline, blood, mannitol, echovist and left-sided contrasts are Levovist and Albunex. In few years, from now contrast Echo will become like contrast CT. About 20% of conventional echoes are incomplete because of poor window and will need proper contrast studies. It is necessary for proper evaluation of pulmonary artery pressure, intracardiac shunts, etc.

Following are some commonly used contrast agents:

1. Saline.
2. Dextrose in water.
3. Indocyanine green dye.
4. Hydrogen peroxide—It gives a strong contrast effect by producing tiny intravascular bubbles of oxygen.

Commercially manufactured microbubbles may be available soon.

There are good number of cases where contrast echocardiography can be used.

26. Echocardiography can be used with invasive procedures such as:

1. Monitoring for pericardiocentesis.
2. Monitoring for endomyocardial biopsy especially from right ventricle.
3. Therapeutic catheterization for balloon angioplasty.
4. Therapeutic catheterization for septostomy.

NORMAL ECHOCARDIOGRAM

27. M-mode echocardiogram of mitral valve: The echos from the mitral valve are readily visible in its full length.

1. The anterior leaflet of mitral valve has a downward motion in mid-diastole with a characteristic 'M'-shaped configuration while the smaller posterior leaflet is essentially a mirror image 'W' configuration except the amplitude of its motion is less.
2. The end of the systole just before the onset of diastole (i.e. before opening of mitral valve) is designated as "D" point.
3. The maximum opening position of the anterior mitral leaflet is designated as "E" point. The DE excursion is an indirect evidence of pliability of mitral valve but it is also directly affected by cardiac output.
4. The nadir of initial closing wave is designated as "F" point, following the E point, the anterior mitral leaflet tends to partially reclose and more posteriorly upto 'F' point and corresponds to the phase of diastasis in left ventricular filling. The diastole closing slope/rate or the E to F slope is frequently not straight but curved. The EF slope is affected by various conditions which will be discussed later.
5. In late diastole, the atrium contracts, blood is propelled through the mitral orifice and the leaflets reopen and reaches a peak at 'A' point. The height of A point is usually less than E point except in conditions with impaired diastolic relaxation. The valve begins to close again with atrial relaxation.
6. Ventricular systole begins during the downward slope and may produce a slight interruption of the closure wave at 'B' point. It is not always evident. At times there may be an exaggerated 'B' point. B-bump or notch is an indirect evidence of elevated left ventricular end-diastolic pressure.

7. Complete closure occurs following the onset of ventricular systole at 'C' point.
8. AC slope indicates the closure of the mitral orifice. There may be slight interruption of the closure wave at 'B' point.

28. There are 4 points to be observed about tricuspid valve in M-mode Echo:

1. It lies anterior to mitral valve.
2. It does not show any anatomical continuity with either of great vessels.
3. Normally only the longest anterior leaflet is recorded unless right ventricle is dilated or some pathological state exists.
4. The configuration and valve pattern is similar to the mitral valve.

29. There are 4 points to be observed about pulmonary valve:

1. It is the most difficult valve to image. It can be seen in about 85–90% of cases in children and in about 50-60% in adults.
2. Normally posterior cusp is usually seen anterior to atriopulmonary sulcus.
3. The diastolic motion is known as EF segment.
4. Almost coinciding with 'P' wave of ECG an 'A' dip is seen which has got hemodynamic explanation.

30. There are 4 points to be observed about aorta and aortic valve:

1. The aorta is represented by two parallely moving echoes which move anteriorly during systole, i.e. towards the transducer and posteriorly during diastole, i.e. away from the transducer. Left atrium lies posterior to the aorta.
2. Normal anterior wall of the aorta is in anatomical continuity with the echoes from the interventricular septum while the posterior wall of aorta is in continuity with the echoes of the anterior leaflet of mitral valve.
3. The aortic valve leaflets lie within the root of the aorta, only the anterior aortic valve leaflet is recorded. The right coronary cusp is the most anterior leaflet and non-coronary cusp is the most posterior leaflet. The aortic leaflets show a characteristic box like configuration within the aortic root in systole as the aortic valve opens. Very occasionally, the left coronary cusp may be seen in the center of the box.
4. As the leaflets come together during diastole, the closed valve is recorded as a center linear echo which is thinner than the either of the aortic root.

31. There are 4 points to be observed about left ventricular cavity and right ventricular cavity in M-mode Echo.

1. It is bounded anteriorly by interventricular septum and posteriorly by left ventricular wall.
2. Both walls are approximately 1 cm thick in diastole and the thickness increases during systole.
3. Both walls move toward each other during systole so that the diameter of the cavity decreases. Both walls move away from each other during diastole so that the diameter of the cavity increases. The left ventricular dimension should be measured just beyond the mitral valve or at the chordae tendineae. The end-diastolic dimension is measured at the onset of QRS complex while the end-systolic dimension is measured at the instant of maximum downward (posterior) position of the interventricular septum which usually precedes the peak upward (anterior) position of the posterior left ventricular wall. In abnormal septal motion, the instant of peak upward position of the posterior ventricular endocardium may be taken at end-systole.
4. A small portion of the right ventricular cavity lies anterior to the interventricular septum. The anterior wall of the right ventricle may not always be imaged especially in adults. Right ventricular dimension can be obtained only when the anterior wall of the right ventricle is clearly marked otherwise only an estimation is made.

Left ventricular dimensions have its own limitations especially in cases of regional wall motion abnormalities such as with coronary artery disease or left bundle branch block. Although M-mode measurements are still clinically used, they are slowly replaced by quantitative measurement of two-dimensional and Doppler echocardiography.

32. Some normal M-mode echocardiographic measurements in adults.

	Range (cm)	Average (cm)
1. Right ventricular dimension	Flat 0.7 to 2.3	1.5
2. Right ventricular dimension	Left lateral 0.9 to 2.6	1.7
3. Interventricular wall thickness	0.6 to 1.1	0.9
4. Left ventricular internal dimension	Flat 3.7 to 5.6	4.7
5. Left ventricular internal dimension	Left lateral 3.5 to 5.7	4.7
6. Left atrial dimension	1.9 to 4.0	2.9
7. Aortic root dimension	2.0 to 3.7	2.7
8. Aortic cusps separation	1.5 to 2.6	2.9

These are approximate measurements and are not identical in all conditions to the criteria developed by the American Society of Echocardiography.

Echocardiographic report consists of the following:

I. LV	End Systolic	Circ	:
		Area	:
		Length	:
		Volume	:
	End Diastolic	Circ	:
		Area	:
		Length	:
		Volume	:
Ejection Fraction:			
Aorta			
LA			
	Mitral	DE amplitude	:
		EF slope	:
		EPSS	:
LV		ESD	:
		EDD	:
PML moves posteriorly		ESD	:
		IVS	
Normal aortic opening		EDD	:
Tricuspid valve			
Pulmonary valve			
IVS and LVPW LVPW		ESD	:
		EDD	:

II. 2D

Ejection fraction

Global LV function segmental: any evidence of hypokinesia, akinesia or dyskinesia

Chambers

Valves

IAS and IVS

Any evidence of shunt

Any evidence of calcification and thrombus.

Any evidence of pericardial effusion.

III. Doppler study (Pulsed/continuous)

Aortic flow:

Mitral 'E' wave: 'A' wave:

Tricuspid flow:

Pulmonary flow:

Any evidence of spectral broadening to suggest obstruction.

Any evidence of turbulence.

Any evidence of shunt or regurgitation.

IV. Color Doppler flow imaging

Revealed normal laminar flow

Any evidence of variance to suggest any obstruction

Any evidence of shunt

Any evidence of regurgitation

DISORDERS OF THE MITRAL VALVE

MITRAL STENOSIS (MS)

The detection of mitral stenosis was the first clinical application of echocardiography.

33. The following information can be obtained from echocardiography in mitral stenosis:

1. Diagnosis of mitral stenosis:
   i. M-mode provides an assessment of motion and thickness of valve leaflets and calcification.
   ii. 2D Echo provides spatial image of the valve and direct measurement of valve orifice.
   iii. Doppler provides hemodynamic assessment of the stenotic orifice.
2. Assessment of severity of mitral stenosis.
3. A guide to surgeon whether the patient needs valvotomy or valve replacement.
4. In case of valve replacement, the left ventricular outflow tract dimensions may guide the surgeon for the type of prosthesis to be used.
5. Presence or absence of vegetation.
6. Left atrial thrombus.
7. Postoperative follow-up by serial echocardiograms.
8. Indirect assessment of mitral stenosis on various cardiac structures like pulmonary arterial hypertension, left ventricular function, other associated lesions, etc.

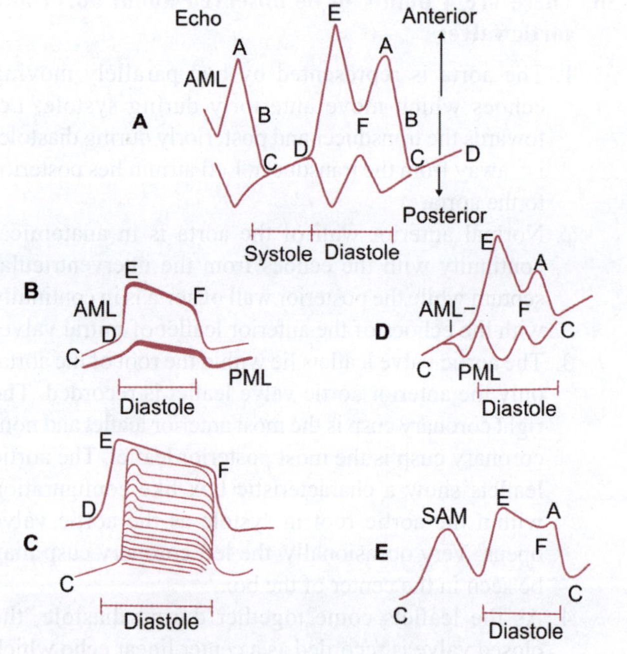

Fig. R-6: Diagrammatic representation of normal echo of anterior (AML) and posterior mitral leaflets (PML)

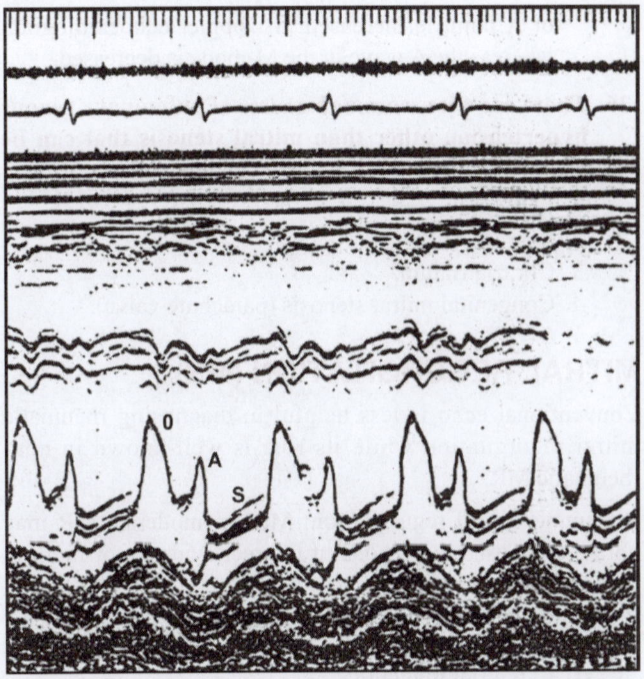

Fig. R-7: Echocardiogram of a normal mitral valve. The anterior and posterior leaflets are shown moving in opposite direction during diastole. The leaflets are seen as a series of parallel lines during ventricular systole moving gradually up the tracing

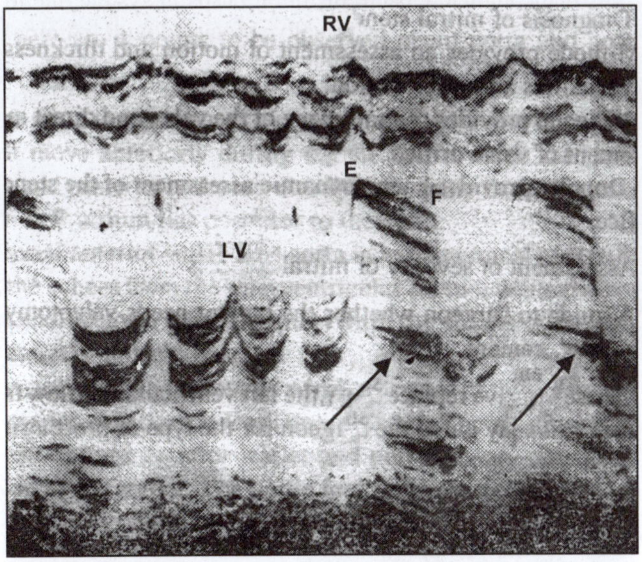

Fig. R-8: Mitral stenosis indicated by the diminished EF slope, abnormal motion of the posterior leaflet and the dense valvular echoes (arrows) which suggestive of fibrosis (see Fig. I-2, I-3, I-4)

1. Normal mitral valve.
2. Mitral stenosis.
3. Atrial myxoma.
4. Mitral valve prolapse.
5. Hypertrophic obstructive cardiomyopathy.

In the echo,

A - point indicates the end of anterior movement resulting from left atrial contraction. CD segment indicates the closed position of both mitral leaflets during ventricular systole; E is the end of anterior movement as the leaflet opens; the EF slope results from posterior motion of the AML during rapid ventricular filling. SAM indicates systolic anterior movement in hypertrophic obstructive cardiomyopathy.

34. There are 4 characteristic M-mode diagnostic features of mitral stenosis:

1. Decreased pliability of cusps (DE amplitude): The motion of the mitral valve is considerably altered. The normal 'M'-shaped configuration of mitral valve during diastole is no longer present since the presence of a holodiastolic atrioventricular pressure gradient (diastasis) prevents rapid closure of the valve in mid-diastole. There is increased thickness of mitral leaflets. In addition, the number of echoes originating from the valve are increased when the valve is fibrotic or calcified.
2. Diminution or absence of end-diastolic 'A' wave: Although sinus rhythm was present, there was no reopening of the valve with atrial contraction and no 'A' wave because of ineffective or insufficient atrial contraction or the valve is too rigid to respond to a small increase in left atrial pressure. Thus, the hallmark of mitral stenosis is the absence of valve closure in mid-diastole and of reopening in late diastole.

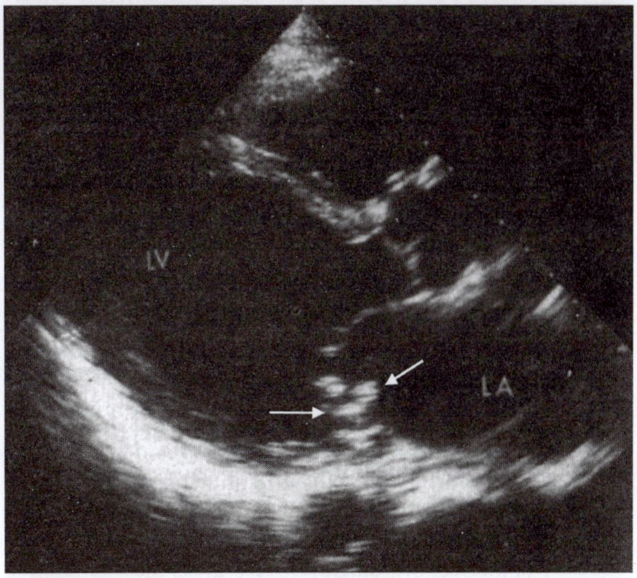

Fig. R-9: Echo showing calcification of mitral annulus. Mitral annulus calcification appears as echo dense mass

3. Decreased EF slope: This is because the left atrial/left ventricular pressure gradient remains constantly elevated throughout diastole. Though EF slope has a poor relation with the severity of stenosis, still it is seen in large number of cases of mitral stenosis. However, a reduced EF slope may be found in other conditions like reduced left ventricular compliance as found in cases of aortic stenosis, hypertrophic cardiomyopathy, coronary artery disease, rapid atrial fibrillation, etc. Decreased cardiac output also reduces the diastolic slope of mitral valve motion.
4. Inadequate separation of the anterior and posterior leaflets during diastole. This is a very specific sign of mitral stenosis. Normally the two leaflets move in opposite direction during diastole but when fused as in mitral stenosis they do not separate widely and may appear to move in the same direction. This may be occasionally seen in isolated chronic mitral insufficiency, and during rheumatic fever. This is possibly due to commissural fusion and valvular fibrosis which draws the smaller less mobile posterior leaflet forward in diastole.

35. Two-dimensional echocardiogram assists in the qualitative and quantitative assessment of mitral stenosis. There are 4 points to determine this as the procedure of choice:

1. Doming of any valve on two-dimensional echocardiogram is characteristic of stenosis of the valve. It is seen in the long axis examination. The doming differentiates the valve that is really stenotic from that opens poorly because of low flow. Doming of the anterior leaflet (AML) gives an arched appearance in diastole directed toward interventricular septum. The base of the AML is anchored and the lip is fixed by commissural fusion and chordal shortening. The mid-section is the only mobile part of AML which becomes domed.
2. Degree of mitral stenosis is seen in short-axis examination. It can visualize and measure the stenotic orifice restricting the blood flow. (Normal 4–6 cm^2).
3. It is the procedure of choice in assessing the pliability and fibrosis of the mitral valve especially when there is subvalvular adhesions. (Vs M-mode Echo is useful only to measure the amplitude of the anterior mitral leaflet.) It also helps to decide whether the commissurotomy is suitable or not by estimating the mobility and the degree of calcification.
4. The effects of mitral stenosis such as atrial fibrillation, pulmonary hypertension, etc. can be detected.

Doppler echocardiography also gives the quantitative measurement of mitral stenotic orifice. The atrial velocity or A point is increased in Doppler echocardiogram whereas the A wave in the M-mode is decreased.

36. There are 4 less common causes of pulmonary venous hypertension other than mitral stenosis that can be usually differentiated by echocardiogram.

1. Left atrial myxoma.
2. Supravalvular ring.
3. Cor triatriatum.
4. Congenital mitral stenosis (parachute valve).

MITRAL REGURGITATION (MR)

Conventional echo is less helpful in diagnosing rheumatic mitral regurgitation while its role is well-known in non-rheumatic MR.

Rheumatic mitral regurgitation: Mild to moderate MR may not be diagnosed by Echo. But indirect evidence of findings suggest the diagnosis.

37. There are 4 findings for indirect evidence of MR:

1. Left atrial dilatation.
2. Left ventricular dilatation. Hyperdynamic motion of left ventricle due to volume overload in severe cases of MR is seen. Left ventricular stroke volume is increased.
3. Incomplete closure of mitral cusps in systole due to severe MR. This is usually associated with left atrial and left ventricular dilatation.
4. Thickening of mitral valve and some minimal evidence of mitral stenosis in case of rheumatic etiology.

MITRAL VALVE PROLAPSE (MVP)

38. MVP can be diagnosed by 4 ultrasonic methods and each has its own advantages:

1. *M-mode echocardiography:* An abrupt posterior (downward) motion of the mitral valve apparatus in mid or late systole is the usual finding. It often corresponds with the mid or late systolic click corresponding to the auscultatory or phonocardiographic finding of this condition. It is reasonably positive finding though not specific of MVP. The prolapse is holosystolic in some of the patients, i.e. the posterior displacement of the valve is present throughout the systole. These findings may be absent in many patients of MVP.
2. *Two-dimensional echocardiography:* It is more sensitive and specific than M-mode Echo for MVP because it detects both superior and posterior displacement of mitral cusps into left atrium while M-mode Echo detects only abnormal posterior displacement.

i. There may be either a mid-systolic dip of mitral cusps into left atrium or bucking of one or both leaflets into left atrium during systole.

ii. There may be continuous bowing or hammocking of mitral leaflets throughout systole.

An intermediate form may be seen when mild posterior bowing begins at the start of systole followed by sudden mid or late posterior systolic collapse of mitral leaflets. The posterior displacement of mitral leaflets from the CD line should be 2 mm or more.

iii. Thickening of the mitral leaflets is common and is due to myxomatous degeneration.

iv. The leaflets may be redundant and fold on themselves in diastole.

Presence of thickening and redundancy are more in favor of MVP than the leaflets moving into left atrium during systole.

3. *Doppler echocardiography:* This is the ultrasonic procedure of choice for any valvular regurgitation. It detects high velocity jet during ventricular systole into the left atrium. Detection of high velocity systolic flow with sample volume near the back of the left atrial wall indicates more severe form of mitral regurgitation.
4. *Color flow Doppler:* This is another procedure in assessing and quantifying the valvular regurgitation. The regurgitant flow of blood into the left atrium is seen during ventricular systole. The velocity is very high, mosaic, multi-colored pattern. The location, direction and size of the regurgitant blood flow can be recorded. A multi-colored regurgitant flow is seen in the left atrium.

Technique for quantifying mitral regurgitation is to calculate stroke volume through two different orifices. The flow ejected from the left ventricle to the aorta and flow passing from left atrium to left ventricle are known first. The difference in the regurgitant volume and regurgitant fraction can be calculated. This needs correct measurement of stroke volume and it may not be possible in all patients. Parasternal long-axis and apical four-chamber views are equally sensitive in detecting MVP. The best technique for detection of MVP is to place two transducers at a site where it is perpendicular to the chest wall. If it is placed too much superiorly and angulated inferiorly, then a false-positive MVP may be produced because the heart moves away from the transducer during systole. The mitral valve which moves by both the motion of the heart and mitral annulus is then perceived as also moving posteriorly away from the inferiorly angulated transducer. If the transducer is placed too low on the chest wall, the posterior leaflet may not be seen well and a false-negative result may be given.

AORTIC STENOSIS (See Fig. L-8 2D ECHO)

39. There are 4 points to be observed in M-mode echocardiographic features of aortic stenosis:

1. It provides qualitative diagnosis of aortic stenosis, whether due to rheumatic fever, degenerative changes or advanced congenital bicuspid valve. It is almost impossible to identify the etiology when there is far advanced calcification.
2. Dense and multiple echoes within the aortic root especially during diastole due to calcification and/or fibrosis of the cusps. If aortic cusps are identified, they may appear thicker than the aortic wall.
   Vegetations from endocarditis can produce similar dense echoes. However, these echoes will be patchy with normal systolic openings of aortic cusps.
3. Decreased systolic excursion of opening cusps. This excursion will usually be below 16 mm but will depend upon the severity of the lesion.
4. Concentric left ventricular hypertrophy depending upon the severity of the lesion.

40. There are 4 points to be observed in 2D echocardiography:

1. This will be more diagnostic. It provides semiquantitative estimation of aortic stenosis. It is best carried out in the parasternal long- or short-axis projections.
2. Very echogenic and bright aortic cusps are seen due to thick lining. In follow-up cases, calcification is usually seen beginning at the base of the involved leaflets and progresses toward the free edges. Right coronary cusp is the most commonly affected cusp.
3. Systolic dome-like deformity is seen irrespective of the etiology. The leaflets tend to curve inward instead of lying parallel to the adjacent wall.
4. Decreased motility of the cusps is present by an absolute decrease in maximal separation and/or orifice size.

41. Generally aortic stenosis cannot be reliably quantified by conventional echo. A semiquantitative estimate of its severity can be made by the following 4 features by 2D Echo:

1. Maximum long-axis aortic separation less than 8 mm is seen usually in severe stenosis. It may be moderate upto 12 mm.
2. Short-axis measurement of aortic valve area: An area of less than 0.75 cm^2 is usually suggestive of critical stenosis.
3. Degree of calcification or fibrosis of the cusp.
4. Presence or absence of left ventricular hypertrophy. The more the LVH, the greater is the stenosis.

42. Doppler echocardiography has revolutionized the role of echo. Best technique is to utilize continuous wave Doppler. The 4 advantages of Doppler echo in patients with aortic stenosis are:

1. It provides the quantitative diagnosis of aortic stenosis and helps in the management of aortic stenosis patients. Whereas the M-mode gives qualitative diagnosis of AS and 2D Echo gives semiquantitative diagnosis of AS.
2. It is possible to measure the pressure gradient across the aortic valve by using the modified Bernoulli equation. It is obvious that the gradients depend on both the aortic valve area and flow across the valve. There will be a smaller gradient in a patient with severe aortic stenosis due to reduced cardiac output. Cardiac output can be measured by the use of one of the Doppler stroke volume measurement through an orifice that does not have a diseased valve. Increase in Doppler velocity occurs as the gradient increases.

   Modified Bernoulli equation to measure a pressure drop or gradient across an obstruction:

   $P = P1 - P2$ $P1$ = Pressure proximal to an obstruction.
   $P2$ = Pressure distal to an obstruction.

   $P = 4\ V2$ $V1$ = Blood velocity proximal to an obstruction.
   $V2$ = Blood velocity distal to an obstruction.
3. Aortic valve area can be calculated by 'Continuity equation'. This technique has been used with reasonable accuracy to calculate aortic valve orifice area in valvular aortic stenosis. Combining the Doppler principle for measuring blood flow and pressure gradient helps in calculating valve area utilizing the 'Continuity equation'. The continuity equation states that the blood flow proximal to an area of obstruction must be equal to the blood flow passing through the area of obstruction. The volume of the blood proximal to an obstruction and the velocity of blood through the obstruction are known. The velocity and the area of left ventricular outflow tract must be measured in order to calculate the blood flow proximal to a stenotic valve. By measuring the velocity of flow across the valve, the aortic orifice area can be calculated.

   Continuity equation for calculating the area of stenotic valve,

   $$A1 \times V1 = A2 \times V2$$

   $$A2 = \frac{A1 \times V1}{V2}$$

   A1 = area proximal to stenosis
   A2 = area of stenosis
   V1 = velocity proximal to the stenosis
   V2 = velocity through the stenosis.

   Probability of critical aortic stenosis is extremely high if a high velocity of greater than 4 m/sec is present and the patient is managed accordingly. If the velocity is within normal limits or mildly elevated, the possibility of significant stenosis can be excluded. If the velocity is in an intermediate zone, it would indicate a pressure gradient between 25 and 50 mm Hg and it needs additional hemodynamic information for proper management.
4. Secondary signs such as left ventricular hypertrophy with increased thickness of the left ventricular walls can be noted. Though the degree of left ventricular hypertrophy has been used to assess the aortic stenosis, this is not nearly as reliable as the use of valve gradients and valve area.

   There is an excellent correlation between the gradient measured both by Doppler technique and cardiac catheterization.

AORTIC REGURGITATION (AR)

43. The role of conventional echocardiography in aortic regurgitation comprises the following 4 features:

1. It helps in qualitative diagnosis of AR.
2. It helps in the assessment of possible etiology like vegetations, rheumatic mitral valve involvement, aortic root disorders, congenital anomalies, etc.
3. It helps in assessment of severity and guides for surgical intervention.
4. It helps in knowing about left ventricular function.

44. The following 4 features are observed by conventional echocardiography in aortic regurgitation:

1. Fluttering of mitral valve during diastole. This is because, the leaflet is caught between the antegrade flow from left atrium and retrograde diastolic flow of aortic regurgitation stream which is directed toward the mitral valve. Sometimes, not only the mitral leaflets flutter but also the interventricular septum and posterior wall of left ventricle may show fine diastolic oscillations during diastole. The fine fluttering of IVS and posterior LV walls assume importance in the presence of mitral stenosis with rigid cusps, which are unable to flutter.
2. Premature closure of mitral valve in the presence of severe, usually acute AR.
3. There may be even early opening of the aortic valve on M-mode recording due to elevated left ventricular diastolic pressure.
4. Secondary effects of AR on the left ventricle such as left ventricular dilatation and hyperdynamic motion due to LV volume overloading.

45. The following 4 signs of conventional echo helps as a rough guide for timing of surgery:

1. LV size greater than 5.0 to 5.5 cm.
2. LV shortening less than 25%.
3. LV diastolic dimension more than 7.0 cm.
4. The degree and duration of diastolic fluttering of mitral valve and the degree of excursion of IVS and posterior LV wall.

These factors operate even if the patient is not significantly symptomatic.

46. Color Doppler echocardiography.

It is the method of choice in AR as with all other valvular regurgitations. It can quantitate AR. The color Doppler provides a 2D display of AR jet. This is sensitive and specific for the presence of AR because of the following 4 reasons:

1. It shows a Doppler sample in the left ventricular outflow tract and the recording of high velocity flow during diastole.
2. The width of aortic jet at valve orifice identified by color (color M-mode) flow Doppler is used to judge the severity of AR. The validity of this has yet to be confirmed.
3. Continuous wave Doppler records the rate of decrease in the velocity of the regurgitant blood. It reflects the severity of AR. Severe AR produces a faster fall in velocity as the pressure difference between aortic and left ventricle falls rapidly.
4. It can know the difference between aortic flow and pulmonary artery flow or mitral flow by which AR can be judged.

TRICUSPID STENOSIS (TS)

Echocardiographic findings of tricuspid stenosis and regurgitation are similar to those of mitral stenosis and mitral regurgitation.

47. The 4 echo features of tricuspid stenosis are:

1. Reduction of diastolic closure slope.
   Paradoxical diastolic motions of posterior cusp.
2. Thickening of valve leaflet.
3. Doming of anterior leaflet in diastole due to commissural fusion in 2D Echo.
   It is invariably associated with mitral valve disease.
4. Gradient across TV > 2 mm → TS
   > 5 mm → severe TS.

TRICUSPID REGURGITATION (TR)

48. In majority of cases, TR is secondary to pulmonary hypertension, consequent to rheumatic heart disease (RHD) or any other cause. Rheumatic TR usually has an element of TS and invariably exhibits MS. Like MR, TR is also diagnosed by indirect echo signs in 2D. These signs include the following 4:

1. Dilated RV.
2. Dilated RA.
3. Paradoxical IVS motion due to RV volume overload where IVS moves posteriorly toward left ventricular wall in diastole and anteriorly in systole.
4. Contrast 2D Echo is more sensitive and specific method. About 3–5 mL of normal saline is injected into an antecubital vein. Microbubbles enter RA and RV and the contrast shows to and fro motion between RV and RA. Moreover, due to TR the microbubbles travel backward into the inferior vena cava and hepatic veins thereby opacifying these structures.

All the modalities available in echocardiography are complementary to each other. Though Doppler echo gives hemodynamic information, the anatomical and functional information is provided by the conventional echo.
Color Doppler shows TR jet.
(TR vel) 2 × 4 = RV Pr.
RV Pr + 10 = PA Pr.

CONGENITAL HEART DISEASE

Deductive echocardiography: After the advent of 2D echocardiography (2D Echo) and Doppler techniques, echocardiography is fast becoming a definitive diagnostic procedure for patients with congenital heart disease. This study provides critical morphological and functional information even in the most complicated cases. The cardiac catheterization requirement is lessened following adequate echocardiographic examination.

49. Deductive echocardiography: This term is used to the technique by which an attempt is made to deduct the anatomy systematically—the atria, atrioventricular valves, ventricles, semilunar valves and great vessels. Previously this has done by combining the X-ray chest and M-mode echocardiogram (MME). Now, the 2D Echo alone can provide the information of almost all the cardiac components. How helpful is this deduction approach to unfold the mystery of even the most complicated congenital malformation is seen below:

1. Locating the vena cava recognizes the atrial situs.

IVC (R) Aorta (L)	} Solitus	RA → R LA → L
IVC (L) Aorta (R)	} Invertum	

2. Pulmonary veins can be viewed in the apical four chamber view and signify location of the left atrium.
3. Bifurcation of pulmonary artery distinguishes this vessel from the aorta and its arch branches.
4. The tricuspid valve is recognized by the fact that it inserts into the interventricular septum closer to the apex than the mitral valve.
5. Distinguishing between the mitral valve and tricuspid valve helps to recognize the ventricles since they always accompany the appropriate atrioventricular valve.
6. The semilunar valves are identified as a part of the appropriate great vessels. Once these valves are recognized, the aorta and pulmonary artery are recognized.
7. Interatrial septum identifies both the atria.
8. Interventricular septum identifies both the ventricles.

ECHOCARDIOGRAPHY IN LEFT TO RIGHT SHUNTS

Ultrasound technique has shown development in non-invasive diagnosis of left to right shunts.

50. Recent development has evolved the 4 stages:

1. M-mode echocardiography (MME).
2. Cross-sectional or two-dimensional echocardiography (2D Echo).
3. Continuous and pulsed wave Doppler echocardiography.
4. Color Doppler/color flow mapping.

Color flow mapping is an exciting advance over the conventional Doppler. This technique is more sensitive, saves time and is helpful for detecting atypical multiple and postoperative residual shunts.

The other developments include invasive echocardiography, contrast echocardiography, transesophageal echocardiography, etc.

A complete anatomical and physiological diagnosis can be arrived with Echo and Doppler facilities and a diagnostic cardiac catheterization can be avoided in majority of patients with left to right shunts.

The left to right shunts encountered in clinical practice are at atrial, ventricular or aortopulmonary level.

51. The 4 shunts at atrial level include:

Commonly

1. Atrial septal defect.
2. Partial anomalous pulmonary venous connection.

Uncommonly

3. Rupture of sinus of Valsalva aneurysm into right atrium.
4. Coronary artery fistula into right atrium.

52. The 4 shunts at ventricular level include:

Commonly

1. Ventricular septal defect.
2. Endocardial cushion defects.

Uncommonly

3. Rupture of sinus of valsalva into right ventricle.
4. Coronary artery fistula into right ventricle.

53. The 4 shunts at aortopulmonary level include:

Commonly

1. Patent ductus arteriosus.
2. Aortopulmonary window.

Uncommonly

3. Rupture of sinus of valsalva.
4. Coronary arteriovenous fistula.

Others include persistent truncus arteriosus, anomalous pulmonary origin of coronary artery, aortic sinus aneurysm and fistula, etc.

54. It is worth mentioning certain general and technical considerations before proceeding to individual shunts.

The 4 important points of information needed in a patient with left to right shunt include:

1. Anatomical defect—site, size, number and magnitude of the shunt.
2. Presence or absence of pulmonary hypertension.
3. Associated anomalies.
4. Presence of any vegetations.

To achieve maximum information, echocardiography should be performed from parasternal, apical, subcostal and suprasternal windows. Subcostal views are particularly useful in infants and small children. Recent introduction of transesophageal echocardiography provides certain advantages over the conventional transthoracic approach for delineation of interatrial septum. Contrast echocardiography performed by injecting indocyanine green, agitated saline or 5% glucose through a peripheral vein has been used in the diagnosis of intra- and extra-cardiac shunts. The utility of contrast studies has decreased after the advent of Doppler echocardiography which provides excellent information regarding left to right or right to left shunts and about the magnitude of the shunt.

Color flow mapping is an exciting advance over the conventional Doppler. This technique is more sensitive, saves time and is very useful for detecting atypical multiple and postoperative residual shunts.

ATRIAL SEPTAL DEFECT (ASD) (See Fig. L-8)

55. The visualization of ASD by MME is possible but the technique is difficult. The MME features of ASD are indirect and non-specific and merely reflect right ventricular volume load pattern. Conditions which produce right ventricular volume overload such as tricuspid regurgitation, pulmonary regurgitation and anomalous pulmonary venous connection may show similar echo findings.

The following 4 Echo methods are useful in identifying ASD:

1. 2D Echo 2. Contrast Echo
3. Transesophageal Echo 4. Doppler Echo.

1. *2D Echo:* Subcostal four chamber view is preferred for visualizing ASD and the accuracy is almost 98%. False-positive diagnosis from subcostal view is uncommon.
   Artifactual dropouts are common in parasternal short-axis (50%) and apical four-chamber view (30%) and a false-positive diagnosis can be made.
   In ostium primum ASD, atrial septal dropout extends upto the ventricular septum. On the other hand, in ostium secundum ASD, there is always some residual atrial septal tissue in contact with the interventricular septum.
   2D Echo not only identifies ASD but is also an excellent means of differentiating a secundum from primum type of ASD. It can also detect more severe forms of endocardial cushion defects with a coexistent VSD. Sinus venosus type of ASD is the most difficult type of ASD and can be missed easily by 2D Echo in some cases.
   Associated anomalies such as mitral valve prolapse, anomalous pulmonary venous connection and left superior vena cava are common and can be detected by 2D Echo and contrast studies.
2. *Contrast Echo:* Contrast studies with 2D Echo enhances the diagnostic sensitivity. Contrast studies reveal positive contrast in patients with right to left shunt and negative contrast in left to right shunt. With the contrast examination, one can visualize an echo filled right atrium and right ventricle. The left atrium and left ventricle are echo free. Contrast studies from left arm are very useful for detecting associated persistent left superior vena cava.
3. Transesophageal echocardiography is claimed to visualize atrial septum in a better way and detect all varieties of ASD with improved accuracy.
4. Doppler studies are particularly useful in cases:
   i. Where ASD is suspected but not visualized on 2D Echo, e.g. sinus venosus defect.
   ii. In cases where a differentiation between a small ASD and a patent foramen ovale is needed.
   iii. Where decision regarding need and timing of surgery is needed.
   iv. In assessment of associated regurgitant lesions, if any. Doppler studies help in quantification of QP/QS, pulmonary artery pressure.

With Doppler study one can visualize the red encoded blood passing from left atrium to the right atrium through the defect.

VENTRICULAR SEPTAL DEFECT (VSD) (See Fig. L-11 for 2D Echo)

56. The 4 methods of echocardiography gives following information regarding VSD:

1. *MME:* Diagnosis of VSD by MME is unreliable. Features suggestive of left ventricular volume overload are present in cases with significant left to right shunt. Flutter of pulmonary valve and tricuspid valve can provide a clue to supracristal and Geriode defect, respectively. Flutter of mitral valve may be present in patients associated with aortic regurgitation. MME can also provide some information about pulmonary hypertension.
2. *2D Echo:* It explores large areas of the septum and defects as small as 3 to 4 mm. It is possible to delineate the site of VSD and categorization into subvalvular (inlet, subtricuspid, subaortic, subpulmonary, double committed subarterial) and muscular (apical, central, outlet) defects are possible. The localization of site of VSD helps the surgeon to decide surgical approach which can be transatrial or transventricular.
3. Contrast echocardiography is useful in diagnosis if the shunt is from right to left. The contrast echoes initially appear in the right ventricle and later in left vetricular outflow tract. In cases with left to right shunt through the VSD shunt produces negative echo-free effect in the right ventricle and can be seen on the right side of the septum. In a large VSD when the right ventricular systolic pressure exceeds 50% of the systemic pressure some right to left shunt may occur during diastole and contrast bubbles may be seen traversing the defect.
4. *Doppler studies:* Pulse Doppler is useful but the color Doppler has become the technique of choice. It is particularly useful:
   i. When multiple defects exist. It detects multiple VSD jets, and useful in diagnosing postoperative residual jets.
   ii. In diagnosis of small defects which have been missed on 2D Echo. It is sensitive (90%) and specific (98%) for diagnosis of VSD. However,

Doppler and 2D Echo should be studied together rather than in isolation.

iii. Doppler studies are very useful for estimation of QP/QS and pulmonary artery pressure.

iv. Doppler velocity across the VSD can reflect the pressure difference between the left and right ventricle during systole. Substracting the pressure gradient from the left ventricular systolic pressure provides an estimate of the right ventricular systolic pressure.

PATENT DUCTUS ARTERIOSUS (PDA)

57. The clinical diagnosis is easy when typical features are present. The diagnosis is difficult in neonates with respiratory distress. Echocardiography helps in the diagnosis.

1. *MME:* Dilatation of left atrium with increased left atrial ratio is the only indirect method of suspecting PDA on MME. Left ventricle is also dilated and shows excessive movement of the septum and the posterior left ventricular wall.
2. *2D Echo:* Direct demonstration of PDA on 2D Echo is sometimes possible by the suprasternal or high parasternal approach.
3. *Contrast Echo:* Umbilical artery contrast studies are useful for PDA in a sick newborn.
4. Doppler studies are sensitive (96%) and specific (100%) for the diagnosis of PDA. Demonstration of turbulence in pulmonary artery and descending aorta without pulmonary artery regurgitation and aortic regurgitation respectively is diagnostic of PDA.

The diagnosis of other uncommon left to right shunts can also be reliably made by Echo Doppler studies. Echocardiography diagnoses most of the cases with left to right shunts and enables the clinician to make a decision regarding operative or conservative management. The technique is invaluable in follow-up of patients who are awaiting surgery or undergone surgery.

TOTAL ANOMALOUS PULMONARY VENOUS CONNECTION

58. All the 4 pulmonary veins empty into a common pulmonary venous chamber behind the left atrium. They produce additional echoes posterior to the left atrium.

(See the chapter on congenital heart disease for echocardiographic findings of individual congenital lesions.)

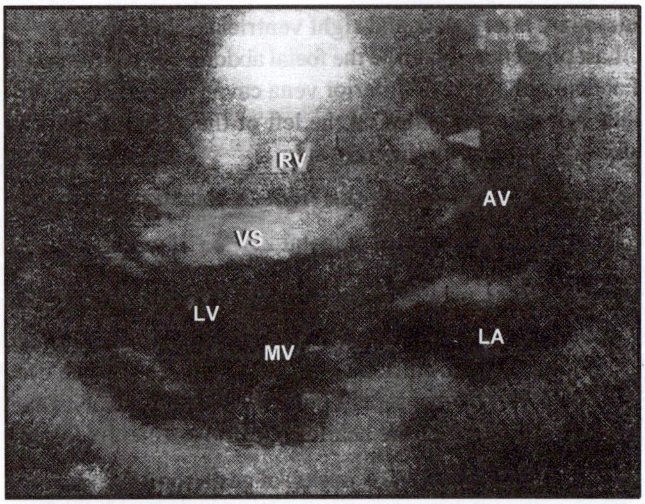

Fig. R-10: 2D Echo of tetralogy of Fallot. Loss of continuity between ventricular septum (VS). The dilated aorta overrides the ventricular septum (see Fig. L-20)

FETAL ECHOCARDIOGRAPHY

Basic difference between prenatal and postnatal echocardiography of the heart is that in fetal echocardiography there is no additional information like clinical signs, ECG, X-rays to assist the diagnosis. The diagnosis entirely depends on the operators interpretations of the echocardiogram which decides the result of pregnancy.

59. There are several factors which come in the way of proper interpretation. The important 4 are:

1. Gestational age.
2. Maternal obesity.
3. Oligo- or polyhydramnios.
4. Continuously changing position of the fetus.

60. There are 4 aims of echocardiographic evaluation of fetus:

1. Evaluation of cardiac structure.
2. Evidence of cardiac failure.
3. Evaluation of cardiac rhythm.
4. Evaluation of blood flow velocity at each cardiac valve.

61. There are 4 basic principles to understand which are extremely essential for orientation and interpretation in fetal echocardiography.

1. The four-chamber view is the easiest view to identify the heart. Due to more horizontal position of the fetal heart this view is achieved by a straight-cut across fetal thorax at the base of sternum.
2. The spine is the most important landmark in fetal echocardiography. The descending aorta lies on the

spine and left atrium lies on the aorta. The sternum is opposite of spine and right ventricle lies beneath the sternum. This basic principle helps in identification of all chambers of the heart in four chamber view.

3. Left and right heart connections are obtained by different angulations of the transducer. This will give four-chamber aortic root view, left ventricular long-axis projection, arch of aorta, pulmonary artery, duct and right ventricular connections.
4. Last projection should be the fetal abdomen to see the position of abdominal aorta and inferior vena cava which indicate atrial situs. Normally aorta lies on the left of the vertebral body and inferior vena cava on the right side.

62. There are 4 points to assess in the 4 chamber view.

1. Heart occupies one-third of fetal thorax. If more, it suggests fetal cardiomegaly.
2. Size of right and left atrium which should be the same.
3. Size of ventricular cavities which are approximately equal.
4. Opening of atrioventricular valves with each cardiac cycle. Atrial and ventricular septa and atrioventricular valves meet together at the crux of the heart.

63. From the 4th month (16 weeks) of gestation all findings can be noted in every pregnancy of gestation if the heart is normal.

64. There are 4 points to note about great arteries by 4 chamber aortic root view, left ventricular long-axis projection obtained by different angulations of the transducer.

1. There are two arterial valves. Pulmonary valve is anterior and cranial to aortic valve.
2. Size of pulmonary artery and aorta: Normally pulmonary artery size is greater than aorta in fetal life.
3. The two great arteries are at right angle at the origin.
4. The pulmonary artery arises from anterior ventricle and gives rise to duct while aorta arises from center of chest and gives rise to arch.

65. MME has an important role in the evaluation of fetal cardiac abnormalities. There are 4 advantages of MME.

1. It can detect intracardiac surface more precisely than frozen cross-sectional image.
2. Measurements can be timed more accurately within the cardiac cycle.
3. Motion of each cardiac valve can be examined.
4. Fetal arrhythmias can be noted.

66. There are 4 advantages of Doppler echocardiography.

1. It can identify cardiac valves better.
2. It can identify or record characteristics of blood flow.
3. It can note blood velocity and volume through each cardiac valve.
4. It can assess ratio between systolic and diastolic flow in umbilical artery. This is an important use because absence of diastolic flow indicates poor prognosis.

67. Fetal echocardiography has an important place in prenatal assessment of fetal heart. It is useful because of 4 advantages:

1. It can predict fetal cardiac anomaly with accuracy.
2. Termination of pregnancy of an inoperable lesion is an important application of the technique. Echocardiographic accuracy alone is not enough to decide operability.
3. Fetal arrhythmias can be detected early.
4. Fetal cardiomegaly can be detected and its sole effect on congestive heart failure can be treated prenataly.

ISCHEMIC HEART DISEASE
(See IHD/CAD E-101)

Detection of myocardial ischemia can be made by 2D Echo. It can identify ischemic myocardium by motion, thickening and thickness of various segments of the heart.

68. Echocardiography has the following 4 roles in IHD.

1. Diagnosis.
2. Prognosis.
3. Assessment of complications.
4. Role in secondary prophylaxis.

69. Diagnosis of IHD is useful in:

1. Transmural myocardial infarction
   – Acute
   – Chronic.
2. Non-Q wave MI.
3. Stable angina.
4. Screening for IHD—stress echocardiography.

70. Diagnosis is made by observing the:

1. Regional wall motion abnormalities (RWMA).
2. Wall motion thickening (WMT).
3. Changes in ventricular dimensions.
4. Correlation with ECG in localization of infarct.

A. **Regional wall motion abnormalities (WMA):** Regional WMA is one of the hallmark of AMI. Experimental studies have shown that WMA occur within seconds of ischemia (5–10 beats) following acute coronary occlusion. They are present in all cases

of transmural MI and can manifest even prior to ECG changes. The WMA are mainly:
- Akinetic (no inward motion with almost absence of systolic thickening). At times the wall segments may appear to move due to adjacent contracting segments.
- Dyskinetic (paradoxical systolic motion with no contractility).
- Hypokinesia (decreased amplitude and rate of endocardial excursion). This should be interpreted with caution. Hypokinesia is a less useful finding in AMI and can be seen in normal individuals without ischemia due to heterogenicity of normal functions. This is sometimes seen in very old people with other cachexia symptoms due to other causes. While assessing WMA, one determines the presence, extent and severity because they can be related to overall pump function.

Single vessel versus Multivessels disease:

Single vessel asynergy

The WMA is located in the territory of involved single vessel. The stress of infarction may induce compensatory hyperkinesia in single vessel disease.

Multivessel disease (remote asynergy)

A remote asynergy occurs when the stress of infarction exceeds the perfusion capacity of additionally stenosed vessel. This remote asynergy, which is not seen in single vessel disease can be easily visualized by 2D Echo.

There may be late improvement in remote asynergy. High CPK enzyme levels and unimproved remote asynergy may represent infarction at a distance.

Adjacent non-infarct asynergy

Segments contiguous with akinetic or dyskinetic segments may appear to be hypokinetic. This may overestimate the extent of infarct in acute MI.

B. Wall motion thickening (WMT): This is a very specific sign of IHD. A normal myocardial muscle increases in thickness with systolic contraction. In MI this systolic thickening is either absent or decreased. However, at times, in an acute ischemia, there may be systolic thinning and the thickening may increase in diastole. WMT abnormality is more accurate than WMA in assessing the presence and extent of infarction. This is because motion of non-infarcted and non-ischemic muscle can be influenced by adjacent muscle. Some myocardium may be stunned with decreased function, even though histologically there is no infarction. As such both the signs should be well-evaluated. Though the percentage of systolic thickening can be measured, but with experience, a visual impression gives adequate information. Moreover, systolic thickening produces better separation of normal from infarcted myocardium rather than endocardial motion alone.

C. Changes in Ventricular Dimensions: The majority of the evidence, to date, suggests that once the margins of an infarct are established, they remain fairly constant over a period of time in the absence of reinfarction. Significant expansion within the infarct, however, may occur in about 25% of patients. It may occur as early as 3 days after acute MI and once initiated appears to continue through the first week of survival. The regional and generalized dilatation are ominous signs of acute MI.

D. Correlation with ECG in localization of infarct: There is usually a good correlation of regional WMA with ECG location of infarct. This is especially true if all scan planes are meticulously examined. The parasternal long-axis view and apical 4-chamber views are ideal for the study of interventricular septum. Apical infarcts can be best-studied from apical views. Inferior infarcts can be well visualized from short-axis view and apical 2-chamber views.

M-mode Echo can visualize WMA in about 80% of patients with acute MI. The main limitation of M-mode Echo is that it samples only a relatively small portion of LV at any given time. Several areas like apex, lateral wall, etc. are inaccessible to M-mode Echo. The complex rotational and transitional motion of the heart is difficult to be appreciated by M-mode Echo and may influence wall motion abnormality. Most of these limitations are obviated by 2D Echo which can visualize practically all segments of the left and right ventricles. Various studies have shown a good correlation between 2D Echo WMA and angiography.

71. Echo in chronic IHD. It presents with:

Fixed segmental wall motion abnormalities, myocardial scar or LV aneurysm. The regional WMA may be a result of (a) single, small area of infarction (b) prior massive infarcts or may be seen if multiple small areas of ventricular damage are present. As such they may vary in severity, distribution and extent. Comparison of wall motion changes in areas that are adequately visualized by echo (87–95%) and angiograhy have been excellent. The major source of discrepancies relate to differences in definition of visual grade.

Following 4 changes are seen:

1. Fibrosis/scar formation is common following myocardial infarction. Scar tissue is typically more echo dense than surrounding muscle.

2. The ventricular wall is thinner than normal (less than 6 mm or 30% less than the surrounding normal area).
3. Systolic wall motion and thickening is significantly reduced in scarred area.
4. LV aneurysm may be seen.

72. Non-Q wave infarction and stable angina pectoris.

Echocardiogram records myocardial wall motion abnormalities which are either due to acute ischemia even though transient or damage due to acute or chronic infarction. As such echo can be normal in non-Q wave infarction or stable angina pectoris. The abnormality in wall thickening and motion can be visualized only if chest pain or myocardial ischemia is present at the time of study or within minutes of the episode of myocardial ischemia. Patients with isolated T wave inversion with mild ST segment changes in ECG usually show normal echo study. Greater the ST segment depression (more than 2 mm) and T wave inversion (more than 3 mm) better are the chances of getting an abnormal echocardiogram. However, there is no case-to-case correlation between ECG and Echo. As such a normal echo study does not exclude IHD and patient should not be carried away with the impression that the heart is perfectly normal. The possible reasons for low sensitivity of 2D Echo in non-Q wave MI or stable angina are:

1. Ischemia may be transient.
2. Infarct size may be too small to be picked up by Echo.
3. The ischemic injury may involve entire LV circumference giving an appearance of symmetrical LV contractility rather than localized wall motion abnormality.
4. The ischemia has not led to any injury to the myocardium.

73. Correlation of wall motion abnormalities with coronary artery lesions.

An attempt has been made to predict the location of arterial obstruction by correlating it with the site of abnormal contracting myocardium. However, all obstructed arteries may not produce wall motion changes due to the following reasons:

a. Obstruction may be partial with no ischemia at rest.
b. Collaterals may preserve the function of the myocardium despite a severe or even a total obstruction of the artery that normally perfuses the myocardium. Various workers have suggested the following scheme to correlate the 2D Echo abnormalities with arterial lesions.
   1. *Parasternal long-axis view:* The anterior interventricular septum seen in this view is almost invariably perfused by left anterior descending artery (LAD). Basal 1–2 cm of the IVS is perfused by first septal perforator branch, hence the lesion proximal or distal to this branch can be deduced. The posterior LV free wall is perfused by the left circumflex artery (LCA). It is not routinely involved in inferior wall MI that results from obstruction of posterior descending artery (PDA)
   2. *Short-axis view:* In this scan plane, the LAD supplies anterior portion of LV free wall + anterior half of IVS. The PDA supplies the posteromedial portion of LV free wall + posterior half of IVS. The LCA perfuses the posterolateral wall.
   3. *Apical four-chamber view:* The apex and the distal 1/2 or 2/3rd of IVS is supplied by LAD. The proximal 1/3rd of IVS is affected by lesions of posterior descending artery (PDA). The posterolateral free wall is perfused by LCA.
   4. *Apical two-chamber view:* The PDA supplies the basal 1/2 or 2/3 of inferior wall. The rest of the LV is supplied by LAD.

The above scheme is mainly an approximation because distribution varies from patient to patient.

74. Prognosis in IHD.

1. 2D Echo is an important tool for evaluating prognosis after MI. The short-term and long-term prognosis is related to the extent of myocardial damage which, in turn, contributes to the degree of LV dysfunction and hence to the overall morbidity and mortality. The overall prognosis, besides depending on other factors like status of non-infarcted myocardium or infarct expansion is mainly dependent on extent of functional infarct size. This is determined by:
   a. Qualitative evaluation
   This is done by seeing the extent of wall motion abnormalities (WMA). The extent and the severity of WMA recorded have been compared to both clinical and hemodynamic evidence of ventricular performance in various clinical studies. A clear-cut relationship has been established between the degree of WMA and patient's status.
   b. Quantitative evaluation
   This is done by estimating:
   – Wall motion score index
   – Percentage of non-contractile myocardium.
2. **Wall motion score index (WMI)**
   In this approach the LV is divided in a number of equal segments, usually nine (Heger et al) utilizing various scan planes. The wall motion within each segment is then determined, usually on a visual basis and assigned a numerical score.
   Hyperkinesia = 0

Normal motion = 1
Hypokinesia = 2
Akinesia = 3
Dyskinesia = 4
Aneurysm = 5.

3. WMI is calculated by dividing the total score by the number of segments examined. Thus, the normal WMI as per above scoring system is one. Higher the WMI, adverse is the prognosis.
4. Percentage of non-contractile myocardium: In this technique the apical 4-chamber and 2-chamber views are imaged. The normal and abnormally contracting myocardial segments are identified visually. A higher value has been related to adverse prognosis.

75. The following 4 points help to identify the ischemic heart disease:

In reversible ischemia:

1. The resting record shows normal septal and posterior ventricular motion.
2. With handgrip exercise, septal motion and thickening are absent due to ischemia. Total wall thickening remains normal. Posterior ventricular wall motion is unchanged. As long as the myocardium retains normal thickness, the damage is potentially reversible.
3. Following recovery from ischemia, septal motion and thickening returns to normal.
   Echocardiography using exercise, pacing or drugs is becoming increasingly popular because the septal wall motion and thickening are very good indicators of ischemia. Systolic motion of the interventricular septum is normal at rest. However, with exercise, the distal-half of the septum becomes ischemic and akinetic.

Irreversible ischemia:

4. In myocardial infarction, e.g. anterior myocardial infarction: The posterior left ventricular wall moves and thickens normally in systole. The anterior and septal walls fail to move or thicken from diastole to systole. Decrease in total thickness indicates irreversible damage. The loss of myocardial tissue is indicative of scar formation.

76. Assessment of left ventricular function in IHD.

There are many echocardiographic techniques for assessment of left ventricular performance in patients with ischemic heart disease. The following points are obtained from MME, 2D Echo, Doppler study and Color Doppler flow imaging for the assessment of left ventricular function.

1. Left ventricle:
   a. End-systolic circumference
      Area
      Length
      Volume
   b. End-diastolic circumference
      Area
      Length
      Volume
   c. ESD
   d. EDD.
2. Mitral valve:
   a. DE amplitude
   b. EF slope
   c. EPSS (E-point septal separation)
   d. MV Flow.
3. Global/segmental left ventricular motion for any evidence of hypokinesia, akinesia or dyskinesia.
4. Ejection fraction.
   MME—E-point septal separation (EPSS) increases when left ventricular ejection fraction decreases and abnormal closure of mitral valve occurs in patients with elevated atrial components of the left ventricular diastolic pressure.

2D Echo is best for assessment of regional wall motion abnormality. Assessment of motion of each segment provides a wall motion score for the entire chamber. Ejection fraction can also be calculated from the apical two chamber or four-chamber views in patients with ischemic heart disease. Frequently, the status of the base of the left ventricle is taken as a better predictor of prognosis than global ejection fraction especially in patients who have aneurysm of apex.

Doppler echocardiography can also be used for assessment of global left ventricular function. When global left ventricular function deteriorates, the acceleration and peak velocity are reduced. Mitral valve flow can reflect altered left ventricular filling. In ischemic patients, the early diastolic flow or E-point is reduced and the velocity of flow with atrial systole (A point) is increased. Thus E/A ratio is changed from a normal positive value to a negative one.

E>A normal
A>E abnormal.

77. The complications of acute myocardial infarction can be recognized by echocardiography.

1. Infarction extension

Wall motion score index increases. Percentage of normal muscle decreases. This can be an extension of original infarction or reinfarction at a new site. Occurs in 7–10% of cases of AMI during first 10 days. About 20% of thrombolyzed patients get it due to reocclusion. Serial Echo every 48 hours has detected that 50% of anterior wall myocardial infarction develop extensions. Common with non-transmural MI. Prognosis bad due to double the incidence of shock.

2. **Infarct expansion**
   Regional score index worsens but percentage of normal muscle is same. Infarcted area dilates and is functionally more abnormal. It is a part of "ventricular remodeling". The ultimate result will be LV aneurysm and this will impair LV function and prognosis.
3. **Left ventricular aneurysm**
   There is loss of myocardial thickness, scar formation, localized dilatation. Echo and angio correlation is good and Echo is the gold standard to detect and following LVA. End result of infarction expansion. The aneurysm can be:
   a. Anterior b. Posterior
   c. Lateral d. Apical.
   The behavior of aneurysm may be akinetic, hypokinetic; or dyskinetic.
   It may have a clot or not and may be small or large. Definite wide neck is seen between the functional segment and aneurysmal segment.
   Spontaneous Echo contrast—a precursor of LV thrombus often seen. When the LVA is large and the remaining muscle dilates the end result is ischemic cardiomyopathy.
4. **Pseudoaneurysm**
   It is a serious complication which represents the rupture of the free wall. It is an incomplete rupture of the myocardium and the sac is formed only by pericardium and no muscle tissue. The blood leaving from left ventricular cavity is trapped in the pericardium resulting in clot formation in the pericardium. An aneurysmal wall consisting of clot and pericardium is seen. The echocardiographic findings are characteristic with the neck of the aneurysm being smaller than the body. Doppler flow pattern can differentiate between a true and a false aneurysm. TEE is highly useful. When LV cavity contracts, the pseudo-aneurysmal cavity enlarges. Urgent surgery is indicated in pseudoaneurysm.
5. **Ventricular septal perforation**
   Aneurysmal dilatation and frequent perforation of the ventricular septum is another complication of acute myocardial infarction. 2D Echo can identify the septal aneurysm and perforation can be visualized occasionally. Color flow Doppler is the procedure of choice. The high-velocity systolic flow going from left to right ventricle through the perforation can be recorded.
6. **Mural thrombus**
   These clots often occur with aneurysms especially those involving the anterior wall and apex. The thrombi can be visualized in the cavity. They may be mobile and hence a greater chance of producing systemic emboli. Other thrombi may be layered along the wall and may be likely to break loose. Echo is the gold standard for picking up thrombi. Thrombi occur in 20–40% cases of MI 5% embolise. Mural thrombi occurring within 48–72 hours have a bad prognosis. Commonly seen in LV apex and can be seen in RV or LV. Seen attached to IVS also. The nearby segmental wall motion abnormality is another clue. Detection and follow-up of future course of thrombi is a great advantage with Echo. "Smoky echoes" seen in LV cavity are the precursors of thrombi and are due to Roular formation.
7. **Acute mitral regurgitation**
   – Papillary muscle dysfunction due to fibrosis of papillary muscles.
   – Rupture of papillary muscles.
   – Pseudo MVP with defective coapting beyond mitral annulus.
8. **Pericardial effusion and pericarditis**
   Seen in 15–17% of cases of myocardial infarction. Common in anterior wall MI and large MI. Pericarditis is seen in the first 3–4 days.

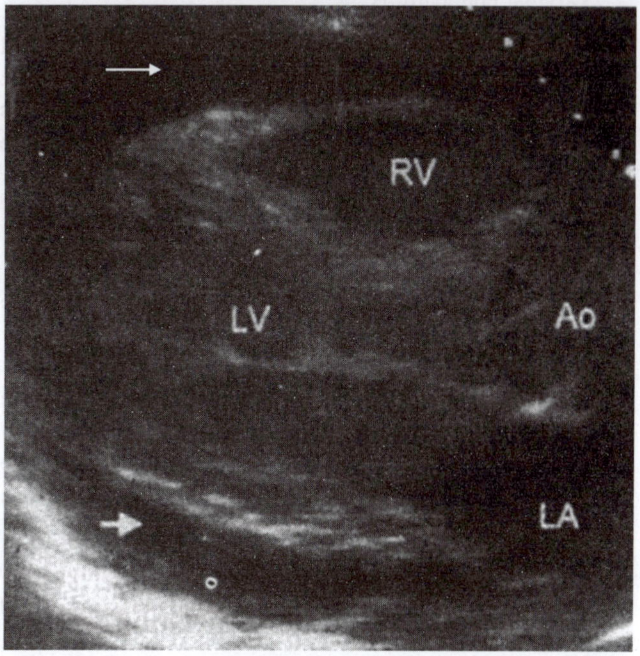

Fig. R-11: Parasternal long axis-view showing effusion anterior to right ventricle (RV) and posterior to left ventricle (LV)

Effusion can be due to:
- Pericarditis
- Anticoagulation – Tamponade and constriction can occur
- Congestive heart failure
- CPR
- Dressler's syndrome.

78. Echocardiography in acute myocardial infarction has the following 4 advantages:

1. 2D Echo carried out in the early course of the disease is helpful in establishing the diagnosis. It provides prognostic information as well. It can serve as a base line record for detecting future ischemic events such as expansion of infarction or its complications.
2. It can identify the high-risk patients experiencing complications. It can recognize the complications of acute myocardial infarction.
3. It is useful in the assessment of status of the myocardium not involved in the present myocardial infarction because unsuspected previous MI may be discovered.
4. It is an useful guide to know the efficacy of reperfusion therapy, angioplasty, etc.

A resting and stress 2D Echo before discharging the patient can provide future prognostic information.

Infective Endocarditis (IE)

Echocardiography visualizes vegetations of infective valvular endocarditis.

79. 4 mm is the minimum diameter of vegetations required to be appreciated by echocardiogram by transthoracic approach. Transesophageal echocardiogram is more sensitive and even smaller vegetations can be appreciated.

80. The characteristics of IE seen on echocardiography are mainly 4.

1. The vegetations appear as echoproducing masses attached to the infected valve.
2. They are usually asymmetrical.
3. They commonly involve one leaflet more than the other, but may be present on more than one valve.
4. If the vegetation is associated with destruction of the valve or if it is on a 'long stalk', its excessive motion can be appreciated on both M-mode and 2D Echo.

81. One of the major advantages of echocardiography is that it can detect the complications arising out of vegetations such as:

1. Hemodynamic effects of valvular regurgitation when the valve is destroyed and grossly incompetent.
2. Premature closure of the mitral valve is visualized because of the very high left ventricular diastolic pressure when aortic valve is involved.
3. Aortic abscess as a relatively echo-free space adjacent to the aortic root.
4. Mitral valve diverticulum by transesophageal echocardiogram.

82. Echocardiography is useful in identification of malfunctioning of the prosthetic valve:

Abnormal rocking motion of a ball or disc-type prosthetic valve usually results from a thrombus or from ball variance or may occur due to pulling of loose sutures from the annulus.

1. Malfunctioning of Bjork-Shiley valve in the mitral position shows rounding of the E-point on the M-mode echocardiogram.
2. A flail porcine valve in the mitral position can easily be detected by 2D echocardiogram. Thickening of porcine valve leaflets may indicate deterioration of the valve.
3. Doppler echocardiogram can identify the prosthetic valves which have a central orifice such as a tissue valve or St Jude mechanical valve.
4. Transesophageal echocardiogram can identify the regurgitation of mitral valve or deposition of small thrombi or vegetations.

CARDIOMYOPATHIES

Dilated cardiomyopathy (DCM): It is a syndrome characterized by cardiac enlargement with impaired systolic function of one or both ventricles. Because of the gradually increasing symptoms and often slow onset, dilated cardiomyopathy may remain undiagnosed or wrongly diagnosed for a long time. Sometime, one see a patient being treated as asthma or COPD referred for an echo because of cardiomegaly on X-ray turning out to be dilated cardiomyopathy. Echocardiogram is ideally suited for the diagnosis of DCM, and is very often gives prognostic value.

83. There are 4 important observations in echo of DCM:

1. *Ventricular size:* Normal adult left ventricle size is 5.2 cm. In dilated cardiomyopathy, one or commonly both ventricles are dilated and may be huge even upto 8 cm. Left ventricle dilates and normal or minimal thickening of walls (no hypertrophy). 2D Echo enables us to measure the end-systolic and end-diastolic volumes and also measure the ejection fraction. The ejection fraction is always reduced and end-diastolic volumes of 80 mL/m^2 MSA are abnormal.
   Left atrium may also be dilated.

2. *Wall motion:* Global hypokinesia of all the LV/RV walls is a diagnostic feature of DCM. Dilatation combined with reduced function causes the EPSS to increase on the M-mode Echo. EPSS of 2 cm is usually associated with left ventricular ejection fraction (LVEF) < 30%. Signs of reduced cardiac output includes a poorly moving aorta, reduced opening of the mitral valve and slow closure of aortic valve.
   The impairment of left ventricular wall motion in DCM is diffuse and includes the posterior wall whereas in ischemic heart disease or severe coronary artery disease, at least one portion of the left ventricle, usually the posterior wall continues to exhibit normal motion. So, in IHD, there is regional hypokinesia.
3. *Intracavitary thrombus:* This is a common complication and is often seen at the left ventricular apex or occasionally at the right ventricular apex. Thrombi may also be seen in left atrium and rarely in the right atrium.
4. *Mitral and tricuspid function:* Mitral and tricuspid incompetence is frequently associated and may be due to dilatation of the corresponding ventricles. Color and Doppler techniques are ideally suited for detection and quantification of these lesions. Presence of tricuspid regurgitation enables us to derive estimates of the peak pulmonary systolic pressure and assessment of pulmonary arterial hypertension.

Doppler evaluation of systolic and diastolic left ventricular function: The left ventricular outflow spectral trace is used to assess systolic function; the time to peak acceleration of aortic flow pulse shows prolongation with reduced pump function. The duration and magnitude of the flow velocity profile are decreased reflecting reduced stroke volume.

The mitral diastolic inflow provides a measure of left ventricular filling. The ejection fraction and fractional shortening have been used to predict outcome. The left ventricular size is not a indicator.

84. There are 4 Echo parameters associated with low annual mortality in DCM:

1. LVIDd
   LV wall thickness in diastole < 4.0 with EF = 28%
2. LVIDs
   LV wall thickness in systolic < 2.5 with EF > 28%
3. EPSS < 22 mm
4. EF 28%.

85. There are 4 Echo parameters associated with high annual mortality in DCM.

1. LVID
   LV thickness in diastole > 4.0
2. LVIDs
   LV wall thickness in systole > 2.5
3. EPSS >22
4. EF < 28%.

RESTRICTIVE CARDIOMYOPATHY (RCM)

86. There are 4 important findings in echo of RCM.

1. Thickening of left ventricular wall without dilatation with normal-sized left ventricular cavity and normal systolic function.
2. Diastolic relaxation is impaired with impairment of diastolic function.
   In amyloidosis: Early left ventricular filling is reduced. The doppler mitral E wave is decreased and A wave is increased. Later filling is restricted and E and A waves are reversed—'pseudonormalization'.
3. Valves may be uniformly thickened in addition to hypertrophy of ventricular walls. Interatrial septum may be uniformly thickened.
4. 'Speckled' appearance of myocardium is characteristic in amyloidosis. It is due to localized variations in echo density.

87. Hypertrophic obstructive cardiomyopathy (HOCM)

There are 4 important diagnostic signs of echocardiography in HOCM:

1. Systolic anterior motion (termed as SAM) of mitral valve is an early echocardiographic sign which is related to the left ventricular outflow obstruction. The shorter the distance between the septum and the anterior leaflet of the mitral valve and the longer the duration of apposition between these two structures, the more severe the degree of left ventricular outflow obstruction.
2. Mid-systolic closure of the aortic valve. It is not specific of HOCM alone. It occurs in discrete subaortic stenosis. When present it usually indicates a significant amount of obstruction.
3. Asymmetrical septal hypertrophy (ASH) with or without obstruction. The ratio of the hypertrophied septum to the posterior wall of the left ventricle exceeds 1.3/1.0 and the motion of the hypertrophied septum is reduced. ASH is frequently transmitted as an autosomal dominant trait. Patients with ASH who do not show systolic anterior motion (SAM) of the mitral valve do not have left ventricular outflow obstruction. 2D Echo helps in evaluating the effectiveness of myotomy and myectomy.
4. Doppler echo may show an abnormal pattern with abnormally high velocity occurring in late systole. The

systolic gradient can be estimated. Prognosis is poor if the gradient is more than 50 mm Hg. Left ventricular hypertrophy and reduced ventricular compliance alters the doppler recording of mitral valve flow. The early diastolic velocity or E point is reduced and the late velocity with atrial systole is increased.

88. There are 4 common conditions where systolic anterior motion (SAM) may be noted:

1. Anemia.
2. Hypovolemia.
3. Hyperdynamic left ventricle.
4. Hypertrophic cardiomyopathy (HOCM).

Therefore, it may be concluded that SAM is a non-specific sign. It can occur whenever the left ventricular systolic volume is reduced either because of hypertrophy as in HOCM or in the presence of hyperdynamic circulatory state.

89. 2D Echo helps in differentiating most of the suspected cases of HCM. Limitations of asymmetrical septal hypertrophy (ASH) in the diagnosis of HCM by echo are mainly 4.

1. Thickness of the septum may be difficult to measure correctly by echocardiogram since the left side of the septum is clearly identified but not the right side.
2. Septal hypertrophy is not pathognomonic of HCM alone. It can occur in other diseases like right ventricular hypertrophy.
3. Some patients may show concentric rather than asymmetric hypertrophy with HCM in which case the septum and posterior left ventricular walls are equal in thickness.
4. 2D Echo gives additional information by indicating the shape and location of hypertrophy. Variety of septal thickness are noted.
   i. Hypertrophy of the basal two-thirds of the septum while the apex is virtually free of hypertrophy.
   ii. Sometimes, there may be apical hypertrophy with proximal septum being relatively thin.
   iii. There can be concentric hypertrophy. Obliteration of the left ventricular cavity is almost always present.
   iv. Echoes from the diseased septum in HCM are more reflective or 'speckled' than those from the free posterior wall. Unusual 'ground-glass' appearance of hypertrophied septum may be seen due to changes in cellular architecture and fibrosis.

PERICARDIAL DISEASE

Pericardial Effusion

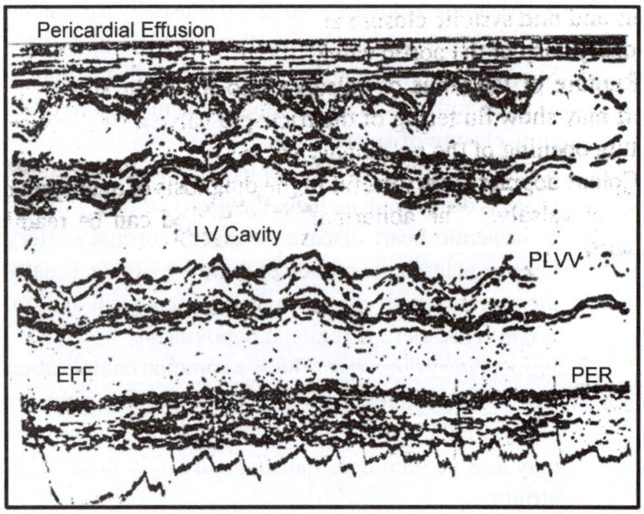

Fig. R-12: M-mode echocardiogram showing pericardial effusion (EFF). Relatively echo free space (EFF) is seen lying above the pericardium (PER). Both effusion and pericardium lie below the left ventricular cavity (LV cavity) and the posterior left ventricular valve (PLVV)

90. The detection of pericardial effusion is one of the first and the most useful applications of echocardiography. The principle underlying the use of ultrasound is simple. The acoustic properties of fluid are different from the cardiac muscle. The effusion surrounding the heart is less echogenic than the myocardium. The 4 points to be kept in mind while studying Echo are:

1. The echocardiogram can detect even as little as 20 mL of pericardial fluid which would be easily missed by other methods. There is a clear space between the posterior left ventricular epicardial echo and the surrounding pericardium. There is a clear space also between the anterior wall of the right ventricle and the chest wall.

   In large pericardial effusions, the anterior and posterior cardiac walls move in the same direction rather than in opposite directions and the amplitude of the anterior wall of the right ventricle is excessive and this is described as 'swinging heart'. The motion of all cardiac structures is distorted. The diagnosis depending on this pattern of motion can be misleading. Abnormal septal motion, false-positive finding of mitral valve prolapse, systolic anterior motion of the mitral valve were reported in such patients.

2. M-mode echocardiography can make the qualitative diagnosis of pericardial effusion. There can be conditions where the fluid collects in a non-uniform way surrounding the heart.
3. 2D echocardiography is more reliable in identifying the location and amount of fluid that is collected in the pericardial sac.
4. Both pleural effusion and pericardial effusion can be identified and differentiated. The pleural effusion can be identified since it is separated from the heart by the descending aorta. Pericardial effusion, on the other hand, is between the aorta and the heart.

CARDIAC TAMPONADE

Once an echocardiographic findings confirm the pericardial effusion, echo signs of cardiac tamponade should be searched for.

91. There are 4 Echo findings which favor the diagnosis of cardiac tamponade:

1. Compression of right ventricular free wall in early diastole.
   This is noticed by posterior displacement of the anterior free wall on the M-mode. This is confirmed by the diastolic collapse of right ventricular free wall on 2D Echo.
2. Diastolic collapse of right atrial free wall on the 2D four-chamber view.
   Both diastolic collapse of right ventricle and right atrium are very sensitive for detecting hemodynamic impairment secondary to tamponade and may precede the clinical signs of tamponade.
3. Exaggerated respiratory variation of transvalvular Doppler flow.
4. Altered hepatic venous flow is also characteristic of cardiac tamponade.
   Reduction of size of the right ventricular cavity, flat diastolic motion of the left ventricular wall and variations in the E to F slope of the mitral valve, although present are not reliable of cardiac tamponade.

CONSTRICTIVE PERICARDITIS

Echocardiography is of some use in constrictive pericarditis. The echo signs of constriction are not very sensitive and are certainly not specific. At best they arise the suspicion of this condition.

92. There are 4 Echo findings in constrictive pericarditis:

1. Lack of diastolic motion, i.e. a flat diastolic slope of the posterior left ventricular wall.
2. Abnormal motion of interventricular septum.
3. A very short and steep E to F slope of the mitral valve.
4. A dilated inferior vena cava that does not become smaller with inspiration.

Doppler studies of the pulmonary and systemic veins provide alternative approaches to the diagnosis of constrictive pericarditis.

CARDIAC TUMORS AND THROMBI

ATRIAL TUMORS

Left atrial myxoma is the most common cardiac tumor. Echocardiography is extremely useful for identifying these tumors.

93. 2D Echo can identify the 4 parameters:

1. Size.
2. Shape.
3. Site of attachment of the mass to the cardiac structure.
4. Obstruction to the flow.

Transesophageal echocardiography is extremely useful since it provides an outstanding view of the left atrium. Even further definition of atrial masses can be identified with this unobstructive view.

94. Echocardiogram can identify the 4 pathologies:

1. Left atrial tumors (myxoma) and thrombi.
2. Right atrial myxoma and thrombi.
3. Ventricular tumors and thrombi.
4. Invasion and metastasis of the heart.

DISEASES OF THE AORTA

95. The entire 4 portions of the aorta can be visualized by echocardiogram.

1. M-mode and 2D Echo visualizes the root and proximal portion of the aorta.
2. Suprasternal approach visualizes arch of aorta and proximal portion of the descending aorta.
3. 2D parasternal long-axis visualizes descending aorta posterior to left atrium and left ventricle.
4. Subcostal view or transducer over the abdomen visualizes the abdominal aorta.

Entire aorta can be visualized clearly by transesophageal echocardiogram.

96. The following 4 diseases of the aorta can be easily detected by echocardiogram:

1. Supravalvular aortic stenosis can be detected by 2D Echo or Doppler.
2. Dilatation of the aorta which occurs in Marfan's syndrome or cystic necrosis can be detected easily.
3. Coarctation of aorta.
4. Aneurysm of aorta.

AORTIC DISSECTION

97. The following 4 methods of echocardiography help to identify the aortic dissection:

1. 2D Echo can detect aortic dissection. In addition to usual position, the right parasternal position may be useful in detecting true and false lumina indicating systolic fluttering of the intimal flap.
2. Transesophageal Echo is more useful and is the procedure of choice.
3. Doppler identifies the flow characteristics in the false channel that are distinctly different from those in the true channel.
4. Color Doppler helps in correct diagnosis by indicating the difference between the false and true lumina and helps to identify the entry point of dissection.

98. Aneurysm of the sinus of valsalva.

2D Echo and transesophageal Echo are useful to image the sinuses because the root of the aorta can be imaged. The 4 important Echo features are:

1. Bulging of the sinus, usually anterior or right coronary sinus into the right ventricular outflow tract or interventricular septum is seen.
2. Rupture: There is discontinuity of the anterior wall of the sinus and mid-systolic closure and coarse fluttering of the right coronary cusp of the aortic valve.
3. Rupture of the sinus of valsalva into the right side of the heart may show fluttering of the tricuspid valve as well as premature opening of the pulmonary valve.
4. Color Doppler is very useful in the diagnosis of aneurysm of sinus of valsalva. The abnormal jets of blood can be readily visualized.

S Cardiac Catheterization and Coronary Angiography

It is the single most important investigation in the diagnosis of cardiac disorders. This investigation is the sheet anchor for the cardiologists.

Cardiac catheterization is not warranted in the great majority of patients with heart disease. It is indicated where more precise or detailed information is needed to decide on the need for surgery or which surgical procedure should be done.

1. Catheter is passed through a vein to the right side of the heart and through an artery to the left side of the heart. Femoral vessels are usually chosen. Following studies are done:

1. Blood sample withdrawal and oxygen studies.
2. Pressure recording in various chambers of the heart.
3. Abnormal path taken by the catheter.
4. Opaque dye studies or angiocardiography.

2. Cardiac catheterization is indicated in 4 groups of diseases.

1. Coronary artery disease
2. Valvular disease
3. Congenital heart disease
4. Cardiomyopathy.

3. The following information can be obtained from the cardiac catheterization:

1. Intracardiac and intravascular pressure measurements.
   Cardiac catheterization allows the direct measurement of intravascular and intracardiac pressures.
   Thus for instance, the pressure within the left ventricle at the end of diastole may be measured to assess the left ventricular functions.
   Normal Left ventricular pressure at the end of diastole is < 12 mm Hg.
   Pressure in left ventricular failure is >12 mm Hg.

   Pulmonary Wedge Pressure
   Pulmonary wedge pressure is measured by wedging the tip of the catheter in a main branch of the pulmonary artery so that the vessel is blocked. The pressure that is measured via the tip of the catheter approximates the back pressure from the left side of the heart.
2. Measurement of pressure gradient across the valve: The gradient across the stenotic valves can be recorded and the valve area is calculated. The wave form may be characteristic.
   Example of measuring the pressure difference between left ventricle and aorta during systole helps in assessing the severity of the lesion. A difference greater than 50–60 mm Hg indicates severity of the lesion.
3. Cardiac output, pulmonary vascular resistance and systemic vascular resistance and quantification of coronary blood flow.
   The oxygen content of the central venous blood taken by the catheter from the pulmonary artery or outflow tract of the right ventricle may be compared with the oxygen content of arterial blood and the difference is used to calculate the cardiac output by Fick principle as explained below:
   Total quantity of O_2 taken up by the lungs/minute = Cardiac output × Arterial content oxygen – Central oxygen venous content.
4. Detection and quantification of intracardiac shunts.
   Blood sample withdrawal and estimation of oxygen content.
   Abnormal shunts may be quantitated.
   Measurement of oxygen saturation on the right side of the heart provides information about the severity of the shunt. Thus, an increase of oxygen saturation in right ventricle as the catheter is withdrawn from the

pulmonary artery indicates ventricular septal defect, whilst an increase in right atrium indicates atrial septal defect.
5. Quantification of coronary blood flow.
6. Intracardiac electrograms, His bundle electrograms, electrical pacing studies and intracardiac phonocardiograms.
7. Acute effects (hemodynamic and electrophysiologic) of cardioactive drugs and experimental studies of newer drugs.
8. Cardiac biopsy: Endocardial biopsy of either left or right ventricle is occasionally performed in the diagnosis of cardiomyopathy. It is rarely done to detect the rejection following cardiac transplantation.

4. Postoperative cardiac catheterization is indicated when residual symptoms present. Such studies may reveal:

1. Loss of patency (Restenosis) in CABG surgery.
2. Restenosis of valve or malfunctioning of prosthetic valve.
3. Inadequate correction of a congenital defect.
4. Residual disease of ventricular myocardium.

5. Angiography: It is the most commonly used method of cardiac catheterization. It is the imaging of contrast medium injected into a large vessel or chamber of the heart for radiographic anatomy of the great vessels and chambers (aorta, pulmonary artery). It gives the information about both anatomy and severity of the lesion. Selective angiography demonstrates specific lesions.

1. The route taken by the catheter gives information about the anatomy of the lesion. Examples are passage of a catheter across a septal defect (ASD or VSD) or along an anomalous pulmonary venous system draining into the right side of the heart.
2. The difference in amount and density of contrast medium that passes an obstruction such as stenosed coronary artery or aortic valve. The surgical relief of angina demands precise definition of the coronary anatomy by selective arteriography. Radiographic anatomy of the coronary arteries and detection of coronary artery spasm can be demonstrated. So, it helps in refractory angina, angina at rest, objective evidence of ischemia at low workload, low heart rate. In patients with chest pain, maximum number of angiograms are done to determine the presence or absence of atherosclerotic coronary artery disease or coronary artery spasm.
3. Flow of contrast backwards into left ventricle or left atrium in aortic or mitral regurgitation.
4. Filling of an aneurysmal sac of left ventricle.

6. In patients with pulmonary arterial hypertension, cardiac catheterization should be done to search for lesions such as:

1. Mitral stenosis
2. Left to right shunt
3. Multiple pulmonary emboli
4. Peripheral pulmonic stenosis.

CORONARY ANGIOGRAPHY

It is the present day gold standard procedure for diagnosing the coronary artery diseases. It helps in refractory angina, angina at rest, objective evidence of ischemia at low workload, low heart rate. It gives precise information which is difficult to obtain by other noninvasive procedures like treadmill exercise tests which has serious limitations and stress thallium while less costly but still imperfect.

7. Indications for coronary angiography:

1. Symptomatic or asymptomatic (SMI) patients with evidence of severe inducеble ischemia.
2. Post MI angina.
3. Recurrent angina.
4. Post MI LV dysfunction.

Procedure: Right femoral route is preferred. Seldinger technique is used. Under local anesthesia. Cannulate the artery and vein with a hollow long needle. The vessel is punctured and guide wire passed through it. The needle is withdrawn having the guide wire inside. Vascular sheaths (preferably with valves to stop backflow of blood) are inserted with the vessel over the guide wire and wire taken out.

5000 IU of heparin IV is given routinely after the vascular access is obtained. Through the arterial sheaths coronary catheters are navigated through the aorta to the aortic root under fluroscopy. The arm catheters engage the coronary ostia with little manipulation. Coronary artery pressure must be checked to avoid damping of the pressure wave form. Radiopaque material is injected through the catheters to visualize the coronary anatomy and pictures are taken from various angulations to delineate the vessels. Both left and right coronaries are imaged sequentially. Left ventricular angiogram is done to assess left ventricular systolic function and mitral regurgitation. Catheters and the vascular sheaths are removed and pressure bandage is applied over the groin at the puncture site. Strict immobilization of the lower limbs is advised for at least 12 hours.

8. Local Complications (over the arterial puncture site).

1. Hematoma
2. Psudoaneurysm
3. Arteriovenous fistula
4. Limb ischemia.

Systemic complications

9. Minor complications:

1. Nausea, vomiting
2. Chills
3. Urticaria
4. Bronchospasm.

10. Major complications:

1. Anaphylaxis
2. Myocardial infarction (< 0.01%)
3. Arrhythmias:
   a. Tachyarrhythmias (VT, VF, (< 0.01%)
   b. Bradyarrhythmias: Blocks, asystole
4. Paralytic stroke (embolism < 0.01%).

11. Limitations:

1. Severity of stenosis may not be assessed accurately in borderline cases.
2. Morphology of lesion may not be obvious.
3. Eccentric lesions may be underestimated.
4. Occurrence of acute coronary events cannot be predicted from coronary anatomy alone.

12. Normal pressures in the 4 chambers of the heart are:

1. Right atrium 0–8 mm Hg.
2. Left atrium 8–10 mm Hg.
3. Right ventricle 15–30/0–8 mm Hg.
4. Left ventricle 80–120/4–12 mm Hg.

13. Normal pressures in the 4 great vessels near the heart are:

In mm of Hg

1. Superior vena cava 0–6 mm Hg (See RA Pr).
2. Pulmonary artery wedge pressure 6–10 mm Hg (See LA Pr).
3. Pulmonary artery 15–30/0–8 mm Hg (See RV Pr).
4. Aorta 80–120/60–85 mm Hg (See LV Pr).

14. Know the following pressures:

1. Jugular venous pressure not more than 2–3 cm.
2. Central venous pressure 0–2 cm low.
   a. With Louis angle as reference point 10 cm high
   b. With midaxillary point 0–5 cm low as zero 15 cm high
3. Partial pressure of O_2 PO_2 is (83–98 mm Hg) 11–13 kPa
4. Partial pressure of CO_2 PO_2 is of venous blood 4.8–6 (36–46 mm Hg)

(Normal pH is 7.30–7.44, HCO_3 = 21–28 mEq/L, SaO_2 = 97–100%)

Earlier, the cardiac catheterization is primarily done for diagnostic purpose only. It is now practised as a therapeutic procedure for various cardiovascular diseases. The new approach of catheterization based treatment is discussed in the chapter on interventions in cardiovascular diseases.

Cardiac catheterization findings of various diseases are given at the appropriate chapters.

T Interventions in Cardiovascular Diseases

From 1950s to 1970s cardiac catheterizations were performed mainly to evaluate the disease and the treatment. However from 1980s invasive cardiology has progressed from primarily diagnostic procedures to therapeutic procedures for various cardiovascular diseases. This new application of catheterization-based treatment is known as 'interventional cardiology'.

1. There are 4 groups of cardiovascular diseases where interventional techniques are used for treatment:

1. Opening of stenotic coronary arteries.
2. Dilatation of obstructed valves.
3. Dilatation of noncoronary arterial obstruction.
4. Closure of intracardiac defects:
   a. Rashkind double umbrella device for PDA.
   b. 'Button device' for ASD, PDA, etc.

2. The treatment is achieved by involving delivery of the following 4 modalities:

1. Mechanical
2. Thermal
3. Microsurgical
4. Light energy.

3. There are 4 interventional methods for opening of stenotic coronary arteries:

1. Percutaneous transluminal coronary angioplasty (PTCA)
2. Coronary atherectomy:
   a. Directional coronary atherectomy (DCA)
   b. Rotational atherectomy
   c. Transluminal extraction catheter.
3. Intracoronary stents
4. Laser angioplasty—
   a. Hot-Tip laser
   b. Excimer laser
   c. Holmium laser.

4. Dilatation of obstructed valves is performed by balloon valvuloplasty. There are 4 conditions where balloon valvuloplasty is performed:

1. Mitral stenosis
2. Aortic stenosis
3. Pulmonary stenosis
4. Tricuspid stenosis.

5. Dilatation of noncoronary artery obstruction is done by 4 methods:

1. Balloon angioplasty in coarctation of aorta, aortoarteritis
2. Balloon angiopalsty in renal and peripheral arteries
3. Laser angioplasty
4. Atherectomy.

6. Balloon angioplasty in noncoronary artery obstruction is useful in 4 conditions:

1. Coarctation of aorta
2. Aortoarteritis
3. Pulmonary artery stenosis
4. Peripheral and renal artery stenosis.

INTERVENTIONS FOR CORONARY ARTERY DISEASE

7. Percutaneous transluminal coronary angioplasty (PTCA):

PTCA stands for:
P - 'Percutaneous'—through the skin
T - 'Transluminal'—within the lumen of an artery
C - 'Coronary' artery
A - 'Angioplasty'—remodeling the artery.

As the name implies, it is a percutaneous technique. It is a technique to dilate the stenosed coronary arteries.

In 1977 in Zurich, Switzerland, a young physician named Andres Gruentzig inserted a catheter into a patient's coronary artery and inflated a tiny balloon, successfully opening a blockage and restoring blood flow to a human heart. Today over one million coronary angioplasties (PTCA) are performed each year throughout the world. It is recommended in the beginning for patients with angina pectoris refractory to maximal medical therapy and having a single vessel disease with proximal, discrete, subtotal noncalcific and concentric stenosis. Now, with improvement in balloon catheters, major technical improvements, the PTCA is indicated in the following 4 conditions:

1. Coronary artery stenosis with evidence of inducible ischemia or angina
2. Angina including unstable angina
3. Acute myocardial infarction (AMI)
4. Previous stenosis of coronary artery bypass graft (CABG)

8. The 4 definite indications of PTCA in acute myocardial infarction are:

1. Cardiogenic shock
2. Failed thrombolytics
3. Thrombolytics contraindicated
4. Post MI angina.

'Direct or primary' PTCA refers to angioplasty, which is undertaken as a primary reperfusion strategy without prior thrombolytic therapy.

9. Advantages of primary PTCA therapy are:

1. Early/late patency high
2. Low rate of recurrent ischemia
3. Few reinfarctions
4. Less intracranial bleeding
5. Survival in high-risk patients
6. Reperfusion check
7. Early relief of chest pain
8. Short hospital stay.

10. There are 4 complications of PTCA:

1. Acute occlusion within 24 hours after PTCA in 2–6% of cases and accounts for most of the morbidity and mortality.
2. Restenosis in one-third of patients over a six month period.
3. Need for emergency CABG to < 3%.
4. Death in < 1%.

11. Restenosis is common in:

1. Males.
2. Angina or unstable angina of less than 6 months duration.
3. Total occlusion or significant post PTCA residual stenosis.
4. Diabetes mellitus.

Fortunately, restenosis is most often present as recurrent angina and not as acute myocardial infarction or sudden death. Repeat PTCA has same success and complication rates comparable to first PTCA.

Procedure of PTCA

Arterial access is obtained and valved arterial sheaths with side arm is inserted as in diagnostic coronary angiograhy. Through the sheath, a guide catheter usually with an internal diameter of 0.84" is introduced under fluoroscopy. The catheter is advanced over a guide wire into the aortic root. Catheter is manipulated within the aortic root to engage the coronary ostium. After a stable engagement is done, coronary artery is filled with a contrast dye and stenotic segment visualized. A 0.014" soft guidewire is advanced across the coronary lesion. Care is taken to avoid internal dissection.

Once the wire is across the lesion, a suitably sized deflated balloon is advanced across the lesion over the guidewire. After confirming the placement of balloon across the lesion by angiography, the balloon is inflated 6–8 atmospheres of pressure. The balloon is kept inflated across the lesion as long as the patient tolerates or usually up to 5 minutes. The balloon is deflated leaving the guidewire across.

Stent

Stent implantation is preferred if smooth adequate dilation is not achieved or if the reference vessel diameter is 3 mm or more. Commonly used stents are metallic. They may be tubular or coiled in shape. They may be available as mounted on balloon or as bare stents. Bare stents can be crimpled upon a balloon. The stent, which present over the balloon is then advanced over the guidewire and positioned across the lesion. As the balloon is inflated, the stent expands and gets opposed to the vessel wall. Within the stent, the balloon is dilated to 12–14 atmospheres of pressure to get perfect opposition of the stent to vessel wall.

Once good dilatation of the stenotic lesion is achieved without any residual stenosis or dissection, the guidewire and the guide catheter are withdrawn.

Stents are useful in giving perfect dilatation with no residual lesion and bail out from any dissection flaps due to playing balloon dilation.

PTCA—restenosis—stent thrombosis.

12. Restenosis is the most important disadvantage of PTCA. Some facts:

1. Restenosis may be as high as 40–50% by 6 months following dilatation of complex lesions

2. Stent implantation decreases restenosis to 15–20%
3. Stent thrombosis can occur in 1% of patients within 1 month
4. Heparin coated stents still decreases the rate of restenosis.

The problem of immediate and late stenosis with PTCA or other methods posed a challenge. This is overcome in the past few years by the development of metallic intravascular stents, which is left within the vessel at the site of stenosis to ensure its patency and possibly to prevent restenosis. Another problem with PTCA and stent implantation is its high cost of disposables. Indegenous manufacture of balloons and stents is one way to decrease the cost significantly. But for the cost consideration, there should be no hesitation in advising PTCA and stent to all suitable patients. The advent of heparin coated stents and glycoprotein IIb-IIIa receptor antagonists further improved the safety of PTCA and decreased restenosis rates.

13. The 4 types of stents currently available are:

1. Gianturco-Roubin
2. Palmz-Schatz
3. Wiktor

(1–3: Balloon expandable)

4. Wallstent—self expandable.

14. Aggressive anticoagulation is given with the following 4 drugs to prevent immediate thrombosis at the site:

1. Heparin
2. Aspirin
3. Ticlopedine
4. Glycoprotein IIb-IIIa receptor antagonsts.

Heparin should be followed by oral anticoagulation for 8 to 12 weeks by which time the stent will be fully endothelialized.

CORONARY ATHERECTOMY

Atherectomy is a term, which denotes percutaneous catheter mediated removal of atheroma using catheters designed especially for this purpose.

New devices have been tried to overcome the major limitation of PTCA. New methods are aimed at removal of atheroma by scraping, shaving, abrading, burning or melting or modeling it by breaking, stretching and welding. Atherectomy would inflict less damage to the underlying vessel wall than with uncontrolled injury associated with balloon.

15. There are 4 types of atherectomy devices available currently:

1. Shaving and retrieval (directional coronary atherectomy (DCA)).
2. Microabrasion (rotational atherectomy)
3. Drilling
4. Suction

(3–4: Transluminal extraction endarterectomy)

16. The mechanism of directional coronary atherectomy (DCA) is excision of atheroma that protrudes into the catheter system through the window without damaging the vessel wall. This device is most suitable for lesions in the proximal arteries larger than 3 mm in diameter. It is preferred over balloon in the following 4 conditions when the stenosis is:

1. Eccentric
2. Ulcerated
3. Ostial
4. Bifurcation.

DCA is not suitable for distal stenosis, diffusely diseased artery and in severe angulation of the artery.

17. Directional coronary atherectomy (DCA) has been shown to be safe and effective with a success rate of 88%.

The major complications of DCA are 4:
1. Need for emergency CABG in 4.4%
2. Myocardial infarction in 4.8%
3. Restenosis over 6 months ranges approximately 23%
4. Mortality rate of 0.6%.

Percutaneous Transluminal Rotational Atherectomy (PTRA)

18. The PTRA method has the following 4 advantages:

1. It has air-turbine powered, guide-wire directed, high speed rotation of a small elliptically shaped stainless steel burr coated with abrading diamond particles.
2. It reduces the atheromatous plaques into millions of microparticles, which embolize into the distal circulation.
3. It selectively abrades the lesions by differential cutting of hard rather than soft, elastic tissue, which is reflected back.
4. It is considered to be suitable for hard calcified, long, diffuse lesions involving the middle or distal portions of relatively small sized vessels.

19. The overall success rate of PTRA procedure in a multicentric study is 95%. This has the following 4 major complications:

1. Acute myocardial infarction in 5.6%
2. Need for emergency CABG in 1.6%
3. Restenosis approximately (30%)—this is nearly that of PTCA
4. Death in 0.5%.

Laser Angioplasty

20. Recent multicenter studies reported procedural success rate of 85–93%. It has 4 major complications:

1. Acute closure—5.6%
2. Emergency CABG—3.4%
3. Myocardial infarction—3.5%
4. Death—0.4%.

This is not significantly different from conventional balloon angioplasty.

21. Angioplasty versus coronary artery bypass surgery

The superiority of one over the other is still undetermined. The technology of PTCA and CABG has been changed remarkably during the last decade. Trials like Randomized Intervention Treatment of Angina (RITA), German Angioplasty Bypass Surgery (GABI), Emory Angioplasty Surgery Trials (EAST) and Coronary Angioplasty versus Bypass Revascularization Investigation (CABRI). Lack of uniformity in the recruitment criteria and trial end points were some drawbacks. Therefore, the logic of superiority of one over the other is still under dilemma. Following points may be observed while deciding:

1. Angioplasty may be a better option than CABG in a single vessel disease. In a single vessel disease, PTCA, atherectomy with or without stent is an established indication.
2. Angioplasty may also be preferred in two-vessel disease with good left ventricular function. CABG is preferred in double vessel disease particularly involving left anterior descending artery in association with diabetes mellitus. For long-term results, left main stem disease should be dealt with CABG.
3. CABG is preferred in multivessel disease.

   With the continued technical advancements in angioplasty and CABG, there is no universal strategy in the management. Sometimes, both are complementary to each other. Cost is the major consideration in India. Choice should be made after proper evaluation of coronary anatomy underlying clinical condition, local experience, social and economic circumstances.

22. Single vessel disease patients faired well on drug therapy rather than CABG. In PTCA with single vessel disease patients showed 4 advantages:

1. More symptomatic relief
2. Increased effort intolerance
3. Less ischemic events
4. Less requirement of antianginal tablets after PTCA as opposed to drug therapy alone.

It is a common question asked by the patient to his family doctor to advise whether the PTCA is definitely needed or not. Angioplasty is advised in a single vessel disease if the patient remains symptomatic with angina. However, asymptomatic single vessel disease may be managed with drug therapy. There is evidence that single vessel disease without any angina fair well prognostically without any intervention. Sometimes, the lumen may become normal by controlling risk factors like smoking, reducing LDL, triglycerides, etc.

Transcatheter Balloon Valvuloplasty

Balloon mitral valvulopalsty (BMV): The first successful balloon valvuloplasty of the mitral valve was reported by Inoue in 1984 and in rheumatic mitral stenosis by Lock et al. in 1985.

Percutaneous mitral balloon valvuloplasty (PMBV): Use of balloon catheters for dilating the valve became a therapeutic alternate to surgical mitral valvotomy in mitral stenosis.

23. The 4 advantages of percutaneous mitral balloon valvuloplasty (PMBV) are:

1. Relatively low risk
2. General anesthesia is not required
3. Is done in cardiac catheterization laboratory
4. Can be discharged in 24 hours (usually discharged after 3 days).

24. The 4 factors of the valve should be considered echocardiographically prior to percutaneous mitral balloon valvuloplasty are:

1. Valvular rigidity, mobility of the leaflets
2. Valvular calcification
3. Valvular thickening
4. Amount of subvalvular disease.

25. The following 4 features are assessed by echocardiography before the procedure:

1. Mitral valve scoring is done according to the grading of characteristics of mitral valve morphology as proposed by Wilkins et al. before the procedure and patients with score < 8 were selected.
2. Mitral valve area is determined by pressure half time (T ½ method).
2. Pressure gradient across mitral valve is determined by Echo Doppler method.
3. Transesophageal echocardiography (TEE) is done to exclude left atrial thrombus.

26. The results of percutaneous transluminal mitral valvuloplasty (PTMV) is compared to the closed mitral commissurotomy (CMC).

1. Balloon valvuloplasty does not require thoracotomy. It is very much acceptable in young unmarried girls due to social reasons on account of the absence of thoracotomy scar.

2. Balloon valvuloplasty does not require general anesthesia.
3. Patient can be discharged in 3 days whereas surgery requires 10 days hospital stay.
4. Complications are less—no pulmonary complications related to anesthesia, no bleeding, etc.

Percutaneous mitral balloon valvuloplasty is an excellent alternative to surgery. Patients with mobile, minimal calcification, minimal thickening of valves, minimal subvalvular fibrosis are the best candidates. However, if there is associated regurgitation of valvular disease (of mitral, aortic or tricuspid) balloon valvotomy is not indicated, which can be repaired surgically.

PMBV is said to be successful when mitral valve area increases to more than 1.0 cm^2 or an increase in mitral valve area by 25% in patients with predilatation area of <1 cm^2. Primary success rate is about 95%.

Since this procedure has come recently, the long-term results are still awaited. The indications also may increase. It may replace surgery in future in some of the early valvular lesions. There will be definite encouragement while the technique is improving as it is a nonsurgical and needs less hospital stay.

However, main problem of PTMV is its financial constraints in a developing country like India. This problem can be overcome to some extent by reuse of balloon after proper sterilization. When a study was conducted in 22 Indian centers, noted that all institutions except one reuse their balloons. A balloon on an average of 7.2 times was used after sterilization with ethylene oxide. In spite of several advantages of PTMV, CMC is being practised in large numbers because of its lower cost.

27. The 4 major complications of PMBV are:

1. Cardiac perforation resulting in tamponade (1.6%)
2. Mitral regurgitation 1.43%
3. Left to right shunt which usually disappears in 80–90% within 3 months
4. Death 2%.

Mitral restenosis is defined as loss of 50% of the increase in mitral valve area achieved by PMBV. Incidence is 1–5%, which is comparable to that seen after surgical mitral commissurotomy.

AORTIC BALLOON VALVULOPLASTY (ABV)

Balloon dilatation of aortic valve relieves obstruction by opening of the fused commissures and fracturing the calcium deposits on the leaflets.

It can be performed retrograde from femoral artery or antegrade across the atrial septum. It is indicated when the peak systolic gradient is 50 mm Hg or more on catheterization with or without mild aortic regurgitation.

28. The 4 advantages of percutaneous aortic balloon valvuloplasty (PABV) are:

1. Relatively low risk
2. No general anesthesia
3. Performed in cardiac catheterization laboratory
4. Can be discharged in 3 to 4 days.

Patient can return to full activity immediately.

Should not be done in calcified, degenerative aortic valve stenosis. This should be limited to selected patients. The long-term results are still awaited.

29. Complications of PABV procedure are:

1. Aortic regurgitation
2. Transverse aortic wall tears
3. Femoral artery tear
4. Thrombosis
5. Left bundle branch block
6. Ventricular arrhythmias
7. Laceration and avulsion of the aortic cusps
8. Local hemorrhage

Procedural mortality may be as high as 5%.

PULMONARY BALLOON VALVULOPLASTY (PBV)

It is the treatment of choice for congenital valvular pulmonic stenosis. This is also used occasionally to alleviate cyanosis in children.

There is significant fall in gradient across the pulmonary valve in majority of the cases.

30. Pulmonary stenosis in the newborn may be a medical emergency. Infants who have the following 4 manifestations need emergency treatment:

1. Severely increased right ventricular pressure (measured at cardiac catheterization)
2. Cardiomegaly
3. Cardiac failure
4. Cyanosis.

31. Patients for percutaneous pulmonary balloon valvotomy are selected in children or adults by the following 4 criteria:

1. Right ventricular pressure, three-quarters or more of systemic pressure
2. Pulmonic valve gradient of 50 mm Hg or more

3. Mild to moderate pulmonary stenosis
4. Pulmonary valve dysplasia (cannot effectively be treated by balloon valvotomy).

Long-term follow-up data is necessary to come to any concluding recommendations.

32. The 4 complications are:

1. Pulmonary regurgitation
2. Reactive infundibular spasm
3. Perforation
4. Subepicardial hemorrhage in the right ventricular infundibulum.

PBV has replaced surgical valvotomy for valvular pulmonary stenosis by its high success rate and low incidence of complications.

BALLOON ANGIOPLASTY OF PULMONARY ARTERY STENOSIS

33. The angioplasty is considered successful if the diameter increases by at least 50%.

The 4 complications are:

1. Hemoptysis
2. Pulmonary edema
3. Aneurysm formation
4. Artery rupture.

BALLOON ANGIOPLASTY OF COARCTATION OF AORTA

34. The first successful balloon dilatation of the coarctation of aorta was reported in 1982. The dilatation is considered successful when the gradient across the stenotic segment is reduced by 50% and the diameter increased by at least 30%.

Complications include the following 4:

1. Early aneurysm
2. Late aneurysm
3. Aortic tears
4. Aortic dissection.

Because of significant incidence of aneurysm formation, the balloon dilatation is generally reserved for recurrent stenosis which develop after surgical repair.

Closure of the intracardiac defects like ASD, VSD, etc. are dealt in chapter on congenital heart disease.

U Role of Surgery in Cardiology

1. Landmarks in cardiac surgery:

1. The first cardiac surgery to be performed was ligation of patent ductus arteriosus (PDA) in 1938 by GROSS.
2. The first systemic-pulmonary shunt was successfully created in 1945 by Blalock and Taussig (BT shunt).
3. The first open heart surgery under cardiopulmonary bypass (CPB) was the repair of an atrial septal defect (ASD) in 1954 by Gibbon.
4. The first heart transplantation was done in 1967 by Dr Barnard.

2. The heroic attempts of cardiac surgery has advanced by leaps and bounds and even the pediatric surgery is acceptable with very low mortality rates with the advancements of 4 supportive techniques:

1. Cardiac anesthesia
2. Bypass techniques
3. Myocardial preservation
4. Total circulatory arrest.

3. Common cardiac operations that can be done when the heart keeps beating not requiring extracorporeal circulation are—(closed heart surgery)—the following 4:

1. Mitral commissurotomy in mitral stenosis
2. Correction of patent ductus arteriosus
3. Pericardiectomy in constrictive pericarditis
4. Correction in coarctation of aorta.

When the function of heart and lung is carried out extracorporeally by heart-lung machine while surgeon operates is known as open heart surgery.
(See Chapter-I on Valvular Diseases—Valvular Surgery)

4. Significant development has occurred in cardiac surgery particularly in 4 fields:

1. Coronary artery bypass graft (CABG)
2. Cardiac valvular surgery
3. Surgery for cardiac arrhythmias
4. Cardiac and cardiopulmonary transplantation.

Some procedures like dynamic cardioplasty for cardiomyopathy, etc. are not practised routinely.

CORONARY ARTERY BYPASS SURGERY (CABG)

When a road is blocked, we create a bypass. In the same way, when a coronary artery is blocked, we can create a bypass channel to carry blood beyond the block. The operation to provide bypass channel is called bypass operation. This operation requires heart lung machine as for the other open heart operations. The bypass channels are fixed precisely onto the blood vessels of a still, motionless heart. The surgeon may opt to bypass one, two, three or rarely more blocks.

5. The 4 goals of coronary artery bypass grafting (CABG) are:

1. Increase of blood flow to the myocardium
2. Increase of oxygen supply
3. Improvement of left ventricular function
4. Finally increase in longevity and improvement in the lifestyle.

6. The patient gets the following 4 benefits by achieving the above goals:

1. Relief of pain
2. Improvement in cardiac function, so increase in exercise tolerance
3. Prevention of impending myocardial infarction
4. Prolongation of life.

7. There are 4 indications for myocardial revascularization:

1. Chronic stable angina (disabling angina pectoris).

2. Preinfarction angina (synonyms—unstable angina, acute coronary insufficiency, intermediate syndrome, etc.)
3. Asymptomatic patients with signs of ischemia on treadmill exercise test with demonstration of occlusion in one or more vessels especially the left main coronary artery by coronary angiography.
4. In acute myocardial infarction, when the pain occurs after thrombolytic therapy or reinfarction occurs, demonstrated by coronary arteriogram.

Emergency bypass graft is done in acute myocardial infarction in highly specialized units when the decision is made after coronary arteriography.

An emergency bypass graft also can be done if a patient with unstable angina waiting for surgery develops myocardial infarction.

The only contraindication for coronary artery bypass graft is the presence of very diffuse arterial disease making bypass nonbeneficial or the presence of any other terminal disease.

8. Indications for coronary artery bypass graft varies from country-to-country, place-to-place depending on the facilities, expertise, economic status of the patient. Mere presence of coronary artery disease is not an indication for bypass surgery. However, bypass surgery is a must when the medical treatment has failed if the following 4 findings are present:

1. Left main stem disease (> 50%)
2. Triple vessel disease with left ventricular ejection fraction (LVEF) > 20%
3. Two vessel disease with proximal left anterior descending artery narrowing
4. Isolated proximal left anterior descending artery (LAD) (>50%) narrowing with nondominant right coronary artery (RCA).

9. There are 4 prerequisites for coronary artery bypass graft operation (CABG).

1. Demonstration of occlusive coronary vessels with adequate distal coronary arteries by coronary angiogram.
2. The myocardium distal to the coronary obstruction should be viable.
3. An adequate left ventricular function should be present.
4. Angina patients with adequate distal vessels but poor left ventricular function are also eligible.

10. The commonly used 4 types of grafts are:

1. Reversed long saphenous vein
2. Reversed short saphenous vein
3. Radial artery
4. Internal mammary artery.

11. The long saphenous vein is most commonly used because it offers 4 advantages:

1. It can be easily dissected.
2. It has large diameter—It allows high flow due to its large diameter even during peak demands.
3. The length of the vein is adequate to graft more than two vessels.
4. It avoids burdensome dissection in the chest especially in the very sick patients.

The advantage of coronary artery bypass graft (CABG) using long saphenous vein has been widely accepted since Favaloro's first clinical implantation of this conduit in 1967.

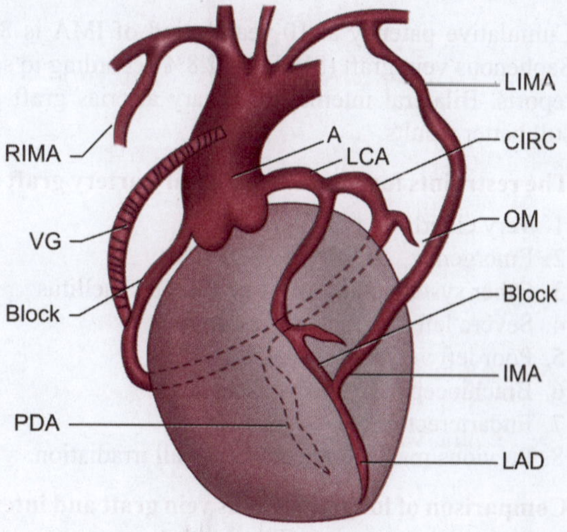

Fig. U-1: Use of vein and mammary artery as bypass channels. A=Aorta; Circ=Circumflex artery; IMA=Internal mammary artery grafted to left anterior descending artery; LAD= Left anterior descending artery; LCA=Left coronary artery; OM=Obtuse marginal artery; PDA= Posterior descending artery; RIMA=Right internal mammary artery; VG=Vein graft

12. Arterial grafts are used in some centers and found better results than venous grafts.

Arterial conduits for CABG are preferred because of 4 advantages:

1. Long patency
2. Easy to harvest
3. Associated with minimal or no complications
4. Minimal response to vasoconstrictors.

13. The 4 arterial grafts currently in use are:

1. Internal mammary artery
2. Right gastroepiploic artery
3. Inferior epigastric artery
4. Radial artery.

14. Initial attraction towards internal mammary artery (IMA) is because of its 4 advantages:

1. Proximity to left anterior descending artery
2. Similar diameter of the graft and coronary artery
3. Artery to artery anastamosis
4. The proximal anastamosis.

15. The internal mammary artery is durable due to the following 4 reasons:

1. Internal elastic lamina with few fenestrations, greater endothelial dependant relaxation.
2. Elastic tissue in the media.
3. Greater prostacycline production which prevents platelet agglutination.
4. Nourishment from the lumen.

Cumulative patency at 10-year-period of IMA is 84%. Saphenous vein graft (SVG) is 52.8% according to some reports. Bilateral internal mammary arteries graft give still better results.

16. The restraints for internal mammary artery graft are:

1. Very elderly
2. Emergency
3. Other systemic diseases like diabetes mellitus
4. Severe left ventricular hypertrophy
5. Poor left ventricular function
6. Brachiocephalic arterial disease
7. Endarterectomy
8. Previous mastectomy or chest wall irradiation.

17. Comparison of long saphenous vein graft and internal mammary artery graft. The 4 points are:

Table U-1

Long saphenous vein graft (LSV)	*Internal mammary artery graft (IMA)*
1. Its length is adequate to graft more than two vessels	Its length is limited to graft one vessel
2. It has a large diameter and allows high flow even during peak demands	Though its size matches with the host vessel, its maximal blood flow is limited by its internal diameter
3. Normally veins carry blood flowing under low pressure. When the veins are used as bypass channels they are subjected to high pressure which may cause thickening of bypass channels leading to graft occlusion. Currently, around 10% of vein grafts block off at 1 year and 50% by 10 years postoperatively	Can be affected by diffuse arterial disease. 90% remain patent even after 10 years
4. Can be easily dissected—however it leaves a scar over the leg	No scar over the leg

18. CABG procedure with other conduits have to be searched when situation in patients arise, such as the following 4:

1. Who had bilateral vein-stripping procedures
2. Who have extensive varicosities
3. Who have postphlebitic syndrome
4. Who required the use of these vessels in previous arterial reconstructive surgery and whose internal mammary arteries are too small in length and caliber and friable.

19. Approximately 15% of patients who underwent coronary artery bypass graft need alternate conduits. This percentage is likely to rise as the patients who underwent CABG procedures 10–20 years ago require reoperation because of the 4 factors.

1. Progression of the native disease.
2. Occlusion of a long-term graft secondary to athero-sclerotic infiltration or intimal hyperplasia.
3. Incomplete initial revascularization.
4. Combination of the above.

The growing need of absent or unsuitable IMAs and LSVs for grafts demands a search for newer alternate conduits. Right gastroepiploic artery (RGEA), inferior epigastric artery (IEA) radial and splenic artery, umbilical vein, synthetic grafts, LSV homografts are tried. Out of these RGEA and IEA from the abdomen have been found to be promising with more than 90% patency rates at short term follow-up of 1–2 years. Long-term results are awaited.

20. The 4 advantages of right gastroepiploic artery (RGEA) are:

1. It has similar size of internal mammary artery.
2. It has similar histology.
3. It has improved vasodilator properties as a pedicle graft instead of free graft.
4. It has good vessel length and caliber.

This can be brought retrogastric or antegastric through a small opening in the diaphragm. Early patency rates of free and pedicle internal mammary and right gastroepiploic arteries are similar.

21. The 4 disadvantages of gastroepiploic artery graft are:

1. It is a muscular artery.
2. Vasa vasorum punctate the media.
3. Spasm has been demonstrated when used as a free graft.
4. Long-term results are awaited.

(When the advantages and disadvantages are equal, those methods are not used.)

22. Inferior epigastric artery graft : The 4 disadvantages are:

1. Histology is similar to gastroepiploic artery but atheromatous plaques have been demonstrated
2. Only useful as a free graft
3. Limited length
4. Patency is not compatible.

Radial artery grafts are not encouraging as the patency rates are low.

23. Modes of surgery for resolving myocardial infarction (MI) and acute myocardial infarction (AMI).

1. Emergency coronary artery bypass graft (CABG) surgery for myocardial reperfusion during acute myocardial infarction.
2. Elective coronary artery bypass graft (CABG).
3. Reoperation for coronary artery disease (CAD).
   Coronary artery bypass graft is not a curative but a palliative operation. Reoperation for coronary artery disease is sometimes necessitated due to progression of the native disease (atherosclerosis) or due to graft occlusion or combination of both. In experienced hands it does not carry any higher mortality than the first operation.
   Restenosis occurs in about 5% of grafts per year. Thus after about 10 years, 50% of grafts get restenosed.
4. Intraoperative transluminal coronary angioplasty.

This is another development in the field of coronary artery bypass graft surgery. Specially designed coronary artery dilators are passed across the stenotic lesion and then gradual dilatation is done. More end arterectomies are needed in severe diffuse narrowing of the terminal vessels.
Intracoronary thrombolytic therapy with streptokinase or urokinase for myocardial reperfusion in acute myocardial infarction is a nonsurgical but invasive procedure.
Percutaneous transluminal coronary angioplasty (PTCA) for myocardial revascularization (perfusion) in acute myocardial infarction is also a nonsurgical but invasive procedure. The results are good in the hands of experienced cardiologists especially when the lesion is single, discrete and short.

24. Surgical results of coronary artery bypass graft (CABG) depends on 4 risk factors:

1. Age:
   – younger the age better the results
   – because of less atherosclerosis.
2. Chronicity and severity of the underlying disease.
3. Extent of myocardial damage.
4. Existence of other risk factors, such as diabetes, hypertension, obesity, smoking. CABG does not modify the natural history of coronary artery disease. Risk factors have to be modified and some form of medication has to be continued.

With an experienced surgical team, the surgical mortality is about 1% in otherwise fit persons with normal or near normal left ventricular function. The mortality increases with poor left ventricular function.

25. Current results of CABG surgery 4:

1. Mortality is less than 1% if the LV function is good. Mortality increases upto 10–12% if the LV dysfunction sets in.
   Morbidity: Definite complications, which are unavoidable and unpredictable are:
2. Stroke 2%
3. Acute renal failure 1–2%—usually transient
4. Major wound infection 1–2%.

Number of patients are now coming back who underwent saphenous vein revascularization practised in seventies for 2nd, 3rd or even 4th reoperation. Redo surgery is feasible with either no or little increase in mortality and morbidity. Results achieved with redo surgery are as good as primary surgery and the clock is set back roughly by another 10 years.
CABG has undergone 25 years of proven benefit. The emphasis is now in choosing CABG over medical therapy for the preservation of myocardium at jeopardy of infarction as well as relief of angina. After myocardial infarction the ventricular function gets impaired. CABG is also necessary to preserve remaining myocardium at jeopardy.

26. There are 4 complications of myocardial infarction where surgical intervention is required (Ref. F-202, Fig. F-9).

1. Left ventricular aneurysm—incidence is 3–20%. More than 80% are located in the anteroapical region.
   Most of these patients have associated coronary artery disease and coronary artery bypass graft (CABG) is advised along with left ventricular aneurysm resection.
2. Postinfarction ventricular septal defect (VSD)—
   It is one of the serious complications. It may need emergency surgery and intra-aortic balloon pump

(IABP) and vasopressor support. If the patient improves with medical management, surgery can be delayed. Surgery for anterior septal rupture carries better results than posterior septal perforation.

3. Postinfarction mitral regurgitation—It may occur due to:
   i. Infarcted papillary muscle.
   ii. Rupture of the head or body of papillary muscle.
   iii. Fibrosis of the papillary muscle.
   iv. Left ventricular wall motion abnormality.

   Even if the left ventricular function is good, patient may develop cardiac failure and cardiogenic shock. Emergency surgery may be needed. Valve is repaired or replaced.
4. Postinfarction left ventricular rupture.

It can cause sudden catastrophe or may lead to cardiac tamponade or psuedoaneurysm formation.

27. Surgery is indicated in any one of the 4 complications of left ventricular aneurysm:

1. Presence of angina
2. Left ventricular failure
3. Tachyarrhythmias
4. Thromboembolic episodes.

When the coronary artery block is localized and the rest of the artery is normal, bypass will be very effective. When the road beyond the block is narrow and crowded, even if the bypass channel is created the traffic is not likely to flow smoothly. Similarly, if the coronary artery beyond the block is not healthy, diffusely diseased, the bypass surgery may not be beneficial as when the distal artery is healthy. Likewise, when the heart muscle is irreversibly damaged by a severe attack and is badly scarred, a bypass operation may give varying results of varying degree of relief from pain depending on the extent of damage and amount of viable heart muscle.

In conditions where there is diffuse atherosclerosis of coronary arteries as in diabetes, hypertension, smoking after surgery aggravate the disease.

Are there any alterations to bypass operation when the coronaries are diffusely blocked ?

The basic problem is that bypass channels do not flow smoothly. In such cases, other methods to carry blood to the muscles should be searched.

28. One of the following 4 methods are tried in such diffuse atherosclerotic disease of the coronary arteries:

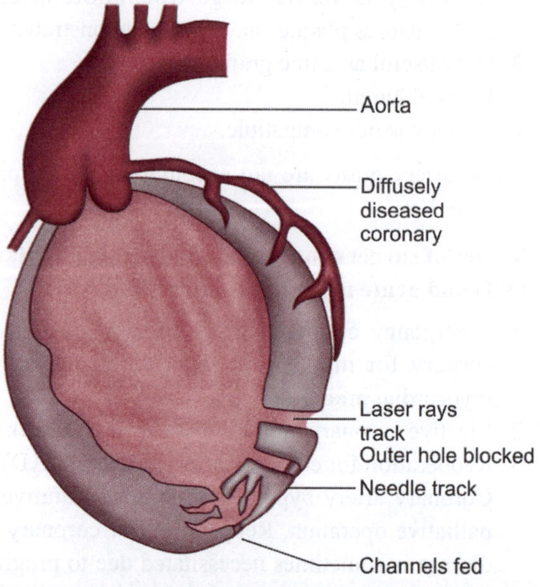

Fig. U-2: Blood flows from the lumen into heart muscle through needle/laser holes

1. *Needle/laser holes:* This technique is described by Dr PK Sen of Bombay in 1969. He created holes in the heart muscle using a needle while the other end of the holes got plugged. The inner needle tracks remained open and carried the blood from the chamber into the muscle. This is revived by others in US the holes being created by laser beams, not needles. This method is simple and safe and satisfying either *per se* or combined with bypass surgery. Further studies and long-term observations are needed.
2. *Myopexy:* Bringing a muscle from the chest wall (Latismus dorsi muscle) over to the heart to create a new source of blood supply to the heart. This operation is called myopexy (myo = muscle; pexy = fixation) (see Dynamic Cardiomyoplasty point No 49).
3. *Omentopexy:* Omentum is brought onto the heart to cover it. It provides an additional source of blood supply to the heart when it becomes adherent, when standard bypass operation is not safe. Omentopexy is used successfully in some cases.

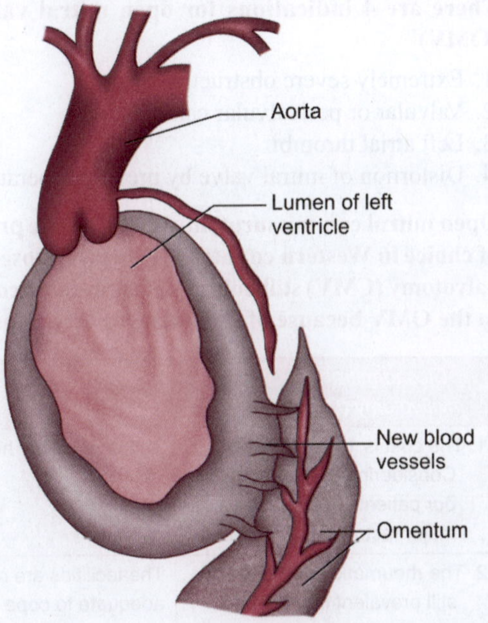

Fig. U-3: Vessels growing into the heart from omentum

4. *Embedding an artery:* When the standard bypass operation is not possible, the bleeding end of an artery is buried into the muscle of the heart.

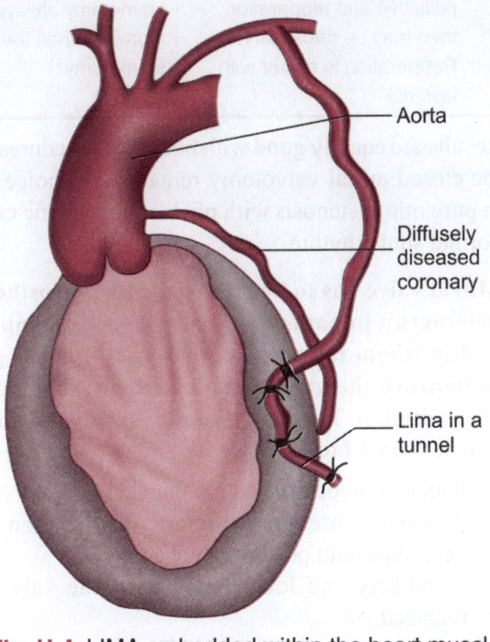

Fig. U-4: LIMA embedded within the heart muscle

Thus, when a bypass surgery is not possible, there are few surgical alternatives, which could indirectly improve the blood supply to the heart.

Transmyocardial revascularization (TMR) by laser beam: This latest technology has been finding place in cardiac surgery. So, it is worth mentioning now. This is based on the principle of early fetal circulation of the heart before the development of coronary arteries, i.e. before 5 to 6 weeks. The heart of viper and reptiles receive blood via the sinusoids in which blood within the chambers seeps into the heart muscle directly carrying oxygen and nutrients through naturally occurring channels.

Latest development is the use of laser beams for creating channels instead of using needles (described by Dr PK Sen). Heart laser machine is used—(40 joules, pulse—50 milli seconds).

29. Indications of TMR by laser:

1. Cardiac failure of class III or IV
2. Multivessel coronary artery disease
3. Diffuse coronary artery disease
4. Earlier CABGs
5. Multiple PTCAs
6. Conduits no longer available
7. Elderly with cerebrovascular accidents.
8. Diseases of other systems—Respiratory disease, renal disease, etc.

30. Contraindications of TMR:

1. Absence of angina or reversible ischemia.
2. LVEF < 25%.
3. Patients who cannot tolerate general anesthesia or thoracotomy.
4. Uncontrolled arrhythmias.

31. Preoperative screening—

1. Assess the revascularization—EF, viable myocardium.
2. Discontinue aspirin one week before.
3. Coagulation profile.
4. Antibiotic prophylaxis.

Intra-aortic balloon counter pulsations are used during the procedure to perfuse the heart.

32. Precautions:

1. Practice laser away from the patient
2. Wet towels
3. Wet surroundings
4. Fixing of head of the laser limb should be checked
5. Use safety glasses
6. Avoid inflammable anesthetic gases
7. All staff should be educated about laser
8. Fire extinguisher should be kept ready.

33. Transesophageal echocardiogram (TEE) studies are done while passing the laser. The following observations are made by TEE while using the laser.

1. Bubbles are seen
2. Transmural penetration of the bubbles
3. Bright red blood jet
4. ST segment changes on ECG.

The laser is released at the peak of R wave by computer control.

34. Laser beam is passed—through:

1. Anterolateral
2. Apical
3. Posterolateral
4. Diaphragmatic walls.

Less energy is needed for apex, more energy for lateral wall. Laser beam is passed to create channels at number of places about 20–30 or even 40 channels are created on the status of the myocardium. Avoid coronary arteries, fat, and scar tissue while passing the laser beam.

35. Bleeding channels are controlled by:

1. Compression with dry swabs
2. Hemostatic agents, e.g. surgical
3. Autologous blood coagulation
4. Suturing by 6 'O' suture material.

36. Results:

1. Chronic patency
2. Endothelialization
3. Capillary neoangiogenesis
4. Formation of anastomotic vessels
5. Thrombus do not form in the vessels
6. No fibrosis
7. No scarring
8. Early postoperative recovery.

37. Advantages:

1. Safe
2. Effective
3. Technically easy
4. No need of cardiopulmonary bypass.

VALVULAR SURGERY

(Refer valvular surgery in Chapter-I 244–261.)

38. There are 4 indications for closed mitral valvotomy (CMV):

1. Pure mitral stenosis
2. No valvular or perivalvular calcification (Shown by fluoroscopy and/or echocardiography)
3. No suspicion of left atrium thrombosis (Sometimes left atrial clots are missed in transthoracic echocardiography prior to closed mitral valvotomy. They are better visualized with transesophageal echocardiography).
4. No previous operation for mitral stenosis.

39. There are 4 indications for open mitral valvotomy (OMV)

1. Extremely severe obstruction
2. Valvular or perivalvular calcification
3. Left atrial thrombi
4. Distortion of mitral valve by previous operation.

40. Open mitral commissurotomy (OMC) is the procedure of choice in Western countries. However, closed mitral valvotomy (CMV) still holds its place in India compared to the OMV because of the following 4 reasons:

Closed mitral valvotomy (CMV)	*Open mitral valvotomy (OMV)*
1. The cost is 10 times less. Considering the economy of our patients, it becomes a major factor	The cost is very high.
2. The rheumatic heart disease still prevalent in India and majority belong to this group to undergo treatment. The facilities available can cope up with the load of the cases	The facilities are not yet adequate to cope with the number of cases of cardiac surgery. Open heart surgery needs more facilities
3. The time and blood requirements are less	Needs more operation time and more blood
4. The valve surgery is only palliative and reoperation then may be necessary. Reoperation is easier with less risk	Reoperation through sternotomy always carries more risk than the primary sternotomy

Results are equally good with both the procedures. Hence, the closed mitral valvotomy remains the choice in India in pure mitral stenosis with pliable, noncalcific cusps and normal sinus rhythm.

41. Mitral valve has to be replaced with a prosthesis or a heterograft in patients who are severely symptomatic and in whom the surgeon feels that it is not possible to improve the valve function in mitral stenosis and regurgitation. The results of mitral valve replacement depends on 4 factors:

1. Patient's myocardial function
2. Pulmonary artery pressure prior to operation
3. Technique and postoperative care
4. Durability and long-term use of the valve that is replaced.

Patients with a prosthetic valve must be maintained permanently on anticoagulants.

Increased mortality is associated with the degree of myocardial functional disability and pulmonary hypertension.

42. The 4 late complications of any valve replacement are:

1. Paravalvular leakage
2. Thromboemboli
3. Mechanical dysfunction of prosthesis
4. Infective endocarditis.

Bleeding due to anticoagulants is same as in any patient on anticoagulant therapy.

Advantage of tissue valve over prosthesis is the less thromboembolic complication and no necessity for anticoagulants.

(See Chapter-I Valvular Diseases - Valvular surgery - aortic, tricuspid, pulmonary valves.)

(See Chapter-L Congenital Heart Disease - Surgery in congenital heart diseases)

SURGERY FOR CARDIAC ARRHYTHMIAS

43. The 4 modes of treatment of cardiac arrhythmias are:

1. Drugs
2. Pacing
3. Surgery
4. Automatic implantable defibrillator.

44. Surgery is indicated mainly in 4 groups of arrhythmias:

1. Supraventricular arrhythmias
2. Intractable supraventricular tachycardia
3. Ventricular tachycardia
4. Ventricular arrhythmias with coronary artery disease.

45. The 4 supraventricular arrhythmias that need surgery are:

1. Wolf-Parkinson-White syndrome (WPW syndrome)—accessory atrioventricular connection
2. Enhanced atrioventricular nodal connection
3. AV node reentry
4. Conduction through Mahaim fibers.

46. Accessory pathway in WPW syndrome may be present at 4 sites:

1. Right free wall
2. Left free wall
3. Anterior septum
4. Posterior septum.

The diagnosis is made by His bundle recording and site is located by intraoperative mapping.

The technique is division of the tracts or cryoablation at 60°F for 2 minutes through midsternotomy.

47. The 4 intractable supraventricular tachycardias that may need surgery are:

1. Paroxysmal supraventricular tachycardia due to AV node reentry or concealed accessory AV connection.
2. Refractory atrial fibrillation (AF) or atrial flutter with fast ventricular response.
3. Direct AV tract from atrial muscle to His bundle.
4. Mahaim fibers.

Interruption of His bundle is done by cryoablation.

48. The 4 ventricular arrhythmias without coronary artery disease that need surgery are:

1. Idiopathic: It needs ventriculotomy and exclusive procedure or cryoablation.
2. Nonischemic cardiomyopathy—surgical exposure and cryoablation is helpful.
3. Arrhythmogenic right ventricular dysplasia—encircling ventriculotomy and excision is helpful.
4. Torsades de pointes—This syndrome is characterized by increased QT interval, congenital deafness and syncope.

Left stellate ganglion resection is helpful.

Ventricular arrhythmias with coronary artery disease that requires surgery.

These arrhythmias are the result of ischemia or post-myocardial infarction. They occur:

- when there is no uniform state of repolarization.
- when there is slow desynchronized conduction.
- when there is ventricular ectopic foci.

Two methods of treatment are available:

I. *Direct:* The patient is evaluated preoperatively with the help of programmed premature stimulation. The arrhythmogenic zone is identified and isolated by intraoperative mapping and ablated by:
   a. Cryoablation
   b. Encircling endocardial ventriculotomy
   c. Endocardial resection

II. *Indirect method:* Thoracic sympathectomy, coronary artery bypass grafting (CABG) and left ventricular aneurysmal resection.

DYNAMIC CARDIOMYOPLASTY

49. There are 4 indications of dynamic cardiomyoplasty:

1. Idiopathic cardiomyopathy (CM)
2. Idiopathic dilated-cardiomyopathy
3. Valvular myopathy
4. Ischemic myopathy.

In this procedure, latissimus dorsi is conditioned by electrical stimulation for few weeks before transferring to the heart. Muscle is raised as flap with its arterial supply intact and wrapped around the heart. It is electrically stimulated in synchrony with ventricular systole using an implant pacemaker. It improves about 30% of pump function. It reduces ventricular wall tension and limits cardiac dilatation. It should be preferably done when the patient is in NYHA class II or III and should not be delayed till NYHA class IV.

CARDIAC TRANSPLANTATION

The first cardiac transplant was done by Dr Barnard in 1967. Since then many transplants have been reported from various advanced centers.

The first successful cardiac transplant in India was done by Dr Venugopal and his team at All India Institute of Medical Sciences, Delhi on 3rd August, 1994, second on 8th July 1995, third on 20th July 1995.

50. Cardiac transplant is indicated as an end-stage in cases of severe advanced heart disease where the medical and surgical treatment have failed.

The recipient should be:

1. Preferably below 40 years of age.
2. Having less chances of infection and less chances of complications of immunosuppressant drugs.
3. Free from illness of other organs, diabetes mellitus, peripheral vascular diseases, pulmonary infection.
4. Mentally prepared for surgery.

51. The donor should be:

1. Free from cardiac or coronary heart disease
2. Free from any transferable disease
3. Compatible with the recipient
4. Free from diseases like diabetes, etc.

52. The 4 donor criteria are:

1. Brain death—No brain function, apnea
2. Age limit
3. No malignancy
4. ECG, Echo, enzymes, etc. normal.

53. Acute rejection of transplant is diagnosed by:

1. General features like fever, chest pain
2. Increased total leukocyte count, lymphocytes or T-cells
3. Decrease in the voltage of ECG
4. Cardiac failure.

The diagnosis is confirmed by transvenous right ventricular biopsy.

54. The early mortality is due to:

1. Mainly due to acute rejection
2. Infection in 50% of cases
3. Chronic rejection
4. Malignancy.

55. Morbidity is mainly due to immunosuppressants and their side effects. Malignancy can occur due to immunosuppression.

4 immunosuppressants which are in use are:

1. Cyclosporine-A
2. Steroids
3. Azathioprine
4. OKT 3 (Immuran)

Endomyocardial biopsy to see any refusal.
Medication for the rest of their life.

56. Postoperative physiology:

1. Normal left ventricular function
2. Normal exertion
3. Donor SA node activity
4. Survival >85% upto 1 year
   60% upto 5 years.

57. Total artificial heart (Jarvik).

The advantages and disadvantages are:

1. No rejection
2. A fewer medical complications
3. No immunosuppression
4. Disadvantages:
   i. Mechanical failure
   ii. Thromboembolism
   iii. Anticoagulants are necessary

CARDIOPULMONARY TRANSPLANTATION

58. The results are now encouraging because of 4 factors:

1. Improved selection of the patient.
2. Improved methods of graft preservation.
3. Use of cyclosporine-A—which is a better immunosuppressant.
4. Efficient management of postoperative complications.

59. Indications for cardiopulmonary transplantation:

1. Primary pulmonary arterial hypertension.
2. Acquired or congenital irreversible pulmonary arterial hypertension.
3. End-stage pulmonary disease with no medical or surgical treatment.
4. Rare pulmonary AV fistulae.
5. End-stage chronic obstructive airway disease.
6. Interstitial pulmonary fibrosis.
7. Cystic fibrosis.
8. Irreversible chemical/physical pulmonary damage.

60. Some facts about heart and heart-lung transplants:

1. Since the first human heart transplant in December 1967 by Dr Barnard, the procedure has been changed in the last three decades from an experimental operation to an established treatment.
2. Approximately about 2300 heart transplants are performed each year in the United States.

Combined heart and lung transplants began in 1981 to treat patients with conditions that severely damage both these organs. As of 1995, about 500 people in the United States and 2000 worldwide have received heart-lung transplants.

At any given time, about 3500 to 4000 patients are waiting for heart or heart-lung transplant.

3. First barrier to successful transplantation is rejection of the donor organ by the patient. This was overcome in 1983 by the introduction of the drug cyclosporine to suppress the rejection. Cyclosporine along with other medications like azathioprine, prednisolone have significantly improved the survival of patients.
4. Researchers are working on safer and more effective immunosuppressants for future testing. Some of the more promising drugs are FK-506 and mycophenolate mofetil.
   Research is underway to develop even better ways to control transplant rejection and improve survival.
   Work is under progress to make immunosuppressive drugs with fewer long-term side effects so that coronary artery disease development and lung destruction may be prevented.
5. A transplanted heart functions differently from the old one. Because the nerves leading to the heart are cut during the operation. The transplanted heart beats at faster rate about 100 to 110 bpm. The new heart also responds more slowly to exercise and does not increase its rate quickly as before.
6. A patients prognosis depends on many factors including age, general health, and immune response to the transplant.
   Recent figures shows that 73% heart transplant patients live at least 3 years after surgery. Nearly 85% of patients return to work or other activities they like. Many patients enjoy swimming, cycling, running or other sports.
   Sixty percent of heart-lung transplants patients survive at least one year. 50 percent live at least 3 years.
   Thirty to fifty percent of patients who had heart-lung transplant develop bronchiolitis obliterans.
7. Monitoring transplant patients for signs of heart rejection is done by biopsy by bioptone attached at the end of the catheter. If the biopsy shows damaged cells, the dose and kind of immunosuppressive drugs are changed. Biopsies of heart muscle are usually performed weekly for 3 to 6 weeks after surgery, then every 3 months for the first year and then yearly thereafter.
8. According to the United Network for Organ Sharing (UNOS) of United States, the estimated first year charges for a heart transplant is 209,100 US $ and annual follow up charges are $15,000. In most cases, these costs are paid by private insurance companies.
   During the patient's stay in the ICU he has been supervised while doing his breathing exercises and taught to do a little active or active assisted exercise, and wound splinting while coughing.
   After the patient being shifted to the ward from the ICU he has been ambulated and taught to do range of motions exercises for the rest of the stay in the hospital.
   On the day of discharge, the patient has been given a home exercise program and explained in detail about the do's and don'ts individually depending upon the surgery or the interventional procedures done upon him or her.

Rehabilitation program—Physiotherapy

Do's in common with all cases (surgical and procedures)

1. Breathing exercise has to be done once in 2 hours roughly about 10 times for a period of 3 months.
2. Walking once daily for a period of 3 months is compulsory.

Walking Protocol

No.of weeks	Slow phase warm up	Brisk walk (exercise)	Slow phase cool down	Total time
1st week	5 minutes	5 minutes	5 minutes	15 minutes
2nd week	5 minutes	7 minutes	5 minutes	17 minutes
3rd week	5 minutes	9 minutes	5 minutes	19 minutes
4th week	5 minutes	11 minutes	5 minutes	21 minutes

Gradually an increase of 2 minutes is made every week in the brisk walking phase till the end of 3 months, i.e 12th week 5 minutes + 30 minutes + 5 minutes → 40 minutes.

3. This is suggested to be continued for lifelong for CABG patients.
4. Stair climbing is suggested if needed, and when done both legs should be placed on the same step, while walking down the steps, stand, relax for 30 seconds and slowly walk down.

Don'ts for Sternotomy Patients

1. Avoid lifting heavy objects (more than 5 kg).
2. Avoid bending forward to restrict any movement of the sternum.
3. Avoid driving for a period of 8 weeks.
4. Avoid indulging in sexual activity for about 2 months.
5. Avoid outdoor games for children.

Arm Exercises

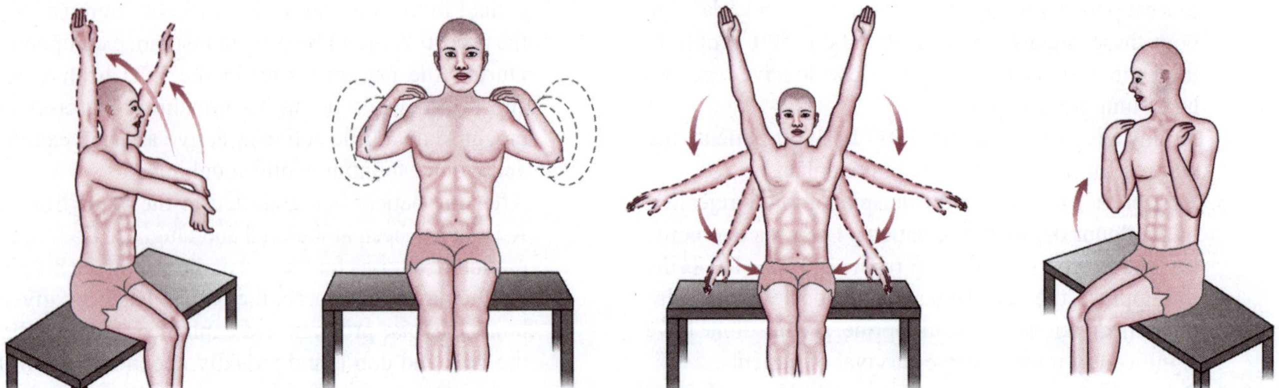

Leg Exercises

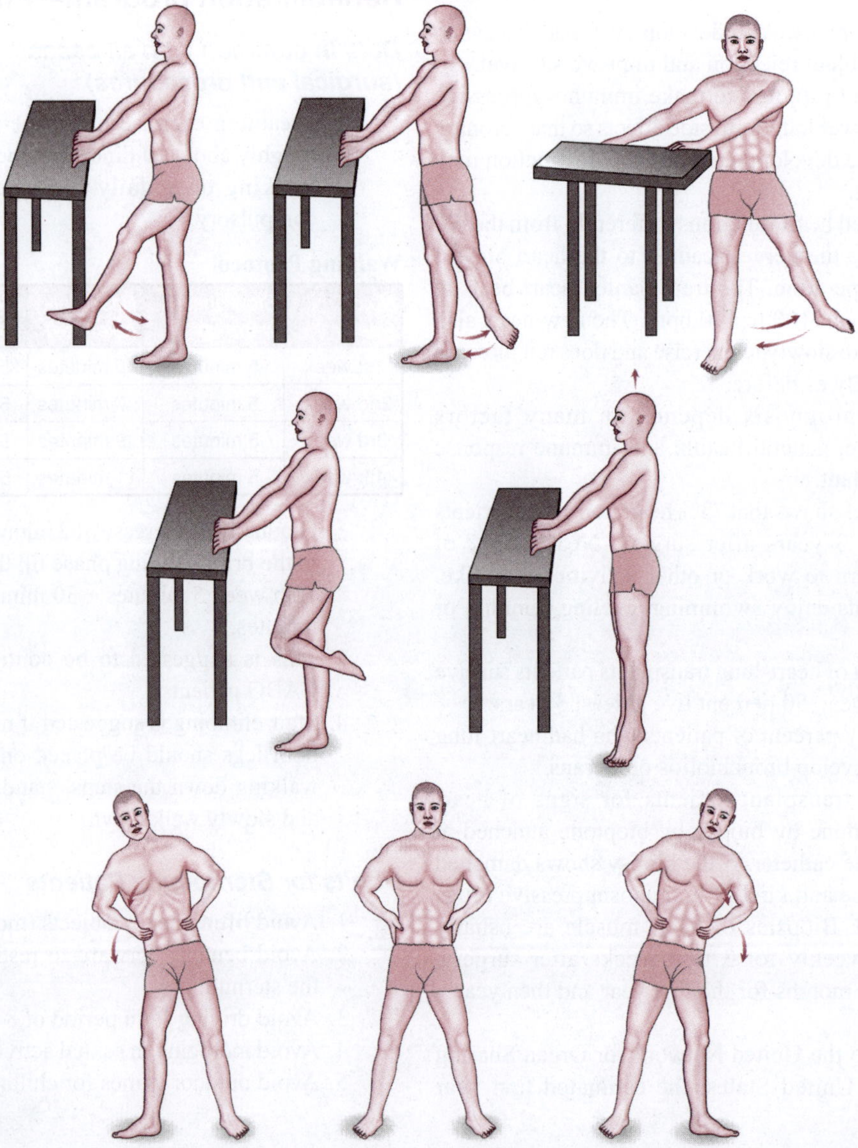

Neck Exercises

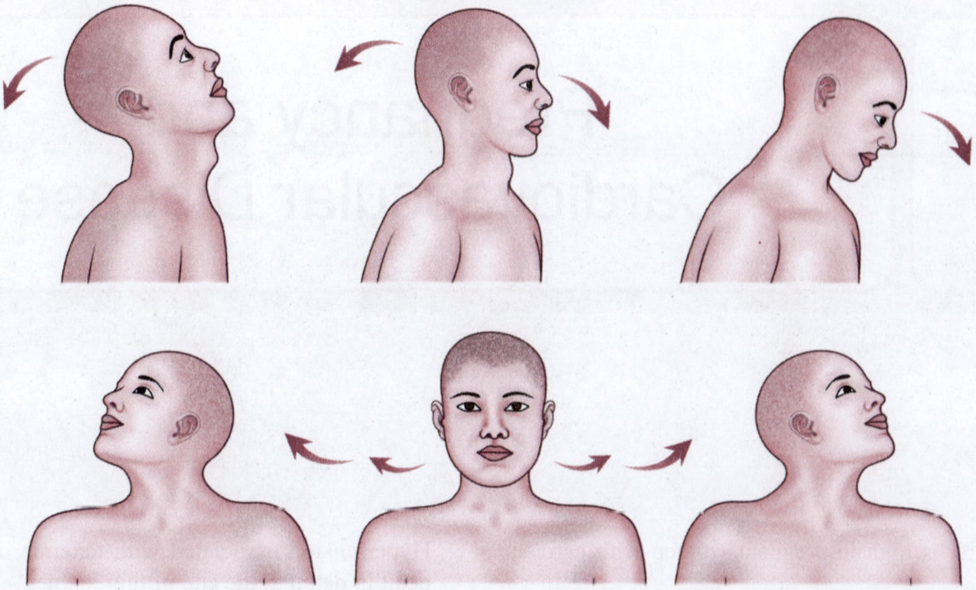

These exercises are done twice daily and each move is repeated 5 to 10 times.

This protocol helps in stretching the scar, mobilize your joints which helps in improving your physical status.

Try to do exercises slowly and at your phase but to their full range, do not exercise if you are tense, try to relax first and enjoy bringing your body to normal.

Exercising daily helps in getting back to normal life faster.

RECOMMENDATIONS OF ACTIVITIES

Patients is recommended to go back to his work after 12 weeks of surgery and has to complain to the local doctor if he or she has any breathlessness or pain in the chest while walking.

A gradual increase in the activity is suggested to children like participating in outdoor games and to entertain average walk of about 30 minutes by 12th week of surgery.

Guidelines to Check Upon the Improvements

Exercise tolerance test, i.e.

1. Distance walking: To check the distance covered by the patient in a given time at the end of every month.
2. Stair climbing: Number of steps climbing at the time of discharge compared with the steps climbing at each visit to the doctor.

Check List on Monthly Basis

Month 1: Walking covered by patients should be 21 minutes and steps of about 10 up and down.

Month 2: Walking of about 29 minutes and 20 steps.

Month 3: That is at the end of 12 weeks as we had discussed earlier patient should reach 40 minutes of walking, patient can climb upto 30 steps.

Ask for complaints of dyspnea, angina, or breathlessness, if yes, the patient should be immediately asked to consult the concerned doctor.

FEEDBACK

A regular feedback is taken so as to see if the patient is able to do his normal activities of daily life.

To be able to work and lead a productive life, and if not why?

To reassure.

V Pregnancy and Cardiovascular Disease

Maternal mortality is high in pregnant women with cardiac disease.

Cardiovascular disease (CAD), leading cause of deaths for woman in the US and the most developed countries. Women do not realize the risk of CVD as a problem and they still feel that cancer, especially the breast cancer is their common cause of risk. Actually one in 2.6 women, deaths are due to heart disease, stroke or other CVD, in contrast to one in 30 women who will die from breast cancer. CAD claims the lives of 2,83,886 women annually compared to 41,566 from breast cancer and 67,894 from lung cancer.

Recent advances in the treatment of congenital heart disease have allowed more women to survive into child bearing age and therefore attempt pregnancy. Congenital heart disease now represents a common cause of heart disease complicating pregnancy in the US. Advances in obstetrics have also allowed pregnancy in older mother in whom hypertension and acquired heart disease are more prevalent. Rheumatic heart disease, although less than in the past is still prevalent in the low economic groups in India and may manifest clinically for the first time in pregnancy. Because the cardiac disease has an important bearing on the health of the mother and fetus during pregnancy it is essential that obstetricians and cardiologists have a working knowledge in both the subjects so that impact of various cardiac diseases on pregnancy and postpartum period may be appropriately dealt.

1. Cardiac diseases that are encountered in pregnancy can be broadly classified into 4 groups:

1. Stenotic lesions.
2. Cyanotic diseases.
3. Regurgitant lesions.
4. Left to right shunts.

1 and 2 do not tolerate hemodynamic changes in pregnancy whereas 3 and 4 tolerate pregnancy well.

Hypertension associated with toxemia of pregnancy is dealt in detail at the end of this chapter.

2. In general:

1. NYHA Grade 0-2A—go through pregnancy well.
2. NYHA Grade 2B-4 must be advised not to become pregnant or correct the structural abnormality and take up pregnancy.
3. Stenotic lesions and cyanotic heart disease do not tolerate the hemodynamic changes of pregnancy.
4. Regurgitant lesions and left to right shunts tolerate pregnancy well.

3. Heart disease in pregnancy is estimated as follows:

1. About 84% are due to rheumatic valvular disease.
2. About 13% congenital heart disease.
3. About 1.8% hypertensive heart disease.
4. About 0.6% other cardiac problems.

The above figures are variable from country to country and place to place, more in underdeveloped countries and less and less in developed countries.

4. Maternal mortality rates are estimated as follows:

1. Maternal mortality averages 4.5% but varies very much with the severity of the cardiac problem.
2. In NYHA Grade I-IIA is 2%—similar to noncardiac pregnancies.
3. In Grade IIB-IV is 18%.
4. When atrial fibrillation is present, the MMR is 32%.

Infant mortality rate (IMR) also varies between 8.6% in Grade 0-IIA and 31% in Grade IIB-IV and 50% when there is atrial fibrillation.

The MMR and IMR are low in Kerala and high in Bihar and Uttar Pradesh states in India.

5. Normal physiological changes occur during pregnancy and postpartum period:

Table V-1

Parameter	Trimester ~1st	Trimester 2nd	Trimester 3rd	Labor and delivery	Postpartum
1. Heart rate	↑5–10%	↑10–15%	↑15–20%	↑20–30%	↓
2. Blood volume	↑	↑↑	↑↑↑	↑	↓
3. Stroke volume	↑5–30%	↑30–40%	↓20–30%	↑ 300–500 mL with each contraction	↓
4. Cardiac output	↑5–30%	↑30–40%	↑>40%	↑50%	Initial ↑ then ↓
5. Systolic BP	↔ to ↓	↓	↑		Baseline
6. Diastolic BP	↔ to ↓	↓	↓ to ↔	↑	Baseline
7. Pulse pressure	↑	↑	↑	—	—
8. Systemic vascular resistance	↓10–30%	↓30–40%	↓30–40%	↑	Baseline

Heart rate, cardiac output, and stroke volume: Cardiac output is estimated to increase by approximately 30–50% above the baseline. The increase is attributed to higher preload as a result of increased blood volume, decrease in systemic vascular resistance and resulting after load reduction and increase in maternal heart rate by 10–15 beats per minute. During the 3rd trimester stroke volume and cardiac output are depended on body position, and an increase in the lateral position and decrease in the supine position due to compression of inferior vena cava by the gravid uterus.

Blood volume increases in pregnancy is attributed to estrogen mediated stimulation of the renin aldosterone system, leading to salt and water retention along with various other and maternal and placental hormones. The blood volume expansion varies from 20–100% and an average around 50%. The relative increase in plasma volume as compared to RBC mass leads to physiologic anemia of pregnancy usually manifest around 30th week.

Blood pressure and systemic vascular resistance decline. BP falls about 10 mm Hg during pregnancy. BP starts falling in 1st trimester, reaches a nadir in mid pregnancy, and returns to baseline before term. Pulse pressure widen due to greater fall in DBP than SBP. About 11% of women develop the uterocaval syndrome of pregnancy with significant symptomatic reduction in BP when lying on their back due to venocaval compression from the gravid uterus.

Hemodynamic changes during labor and delivery: Every uterine contraction displaces about 300–500 mL of blood into the general circulation (auto transfusion), there is an increase in stroke volume, heart rate, and there by cardiac output, blood pressure, and oxygen consumption. However, these changes may be influenced by the type of delivery—vaginal versus cesarean and varies with the type of anesthesia and analgesia.

Hemodynamic changes in postpartum period: In spite of blood loss during delivery there is temporary increase in effective venous return due to relief of caval compression and auto transfusion. This may lead to increase in stroke volume, cardiac output, and filling pressure. In women with previous existing cardiac disease, these hemodynamic changes may lead to profound deterioration of clinical condition. The hemodynamic changes associated with pregnancy usually persist for a few weeks postpartum and may take up to 12–24 weeks to return to prepregnancy level.

In addition, a hypercoagulable state exists with decrease in protein S, increased stasis and venous hypertension.

6. Common cardiac lesions encountered in pregnancy are:

1. Rheumatic valvular heart disease	Obstructive or regurgitant lesions
2. Congenital heart failure	Left to right shunts right to left shunts
3. Cardiomyopathies	Dilated, postpartum dilated, hypertrophic
4. Patients with prosthetic valves	Commonly mitral, aortic
5. Myocarditis	Infective, toxic, chemical induced
6. Primary pulmonary hypertension	—
7. Aortic disease	Aortitis, coarctation, Marfan's syndrome
8. Coronary artery disease	Unstable angina, myocardial infarction

7. Cardiovascular evaluation in pregnancy:

Findings in normal pregnancy:

I. Common symptoms
1. Fatigue, dyspnea/orthopnea
2. Palpitation
3. Reduced exercise tolerance
4. Lower extremity edema.

II. Signs: Physical examination
1. Lower extremity edema
2. Increased heart rate and wide pulse pressure
3. JVP↑ with prominent A and V waves and brisk X and Y descent
4. Upward and left ward deviation of apex
5. Flow murmur (pulmonary and aortic)
6. Mammary scuffle (left sternal border continuous murmur) and cervical venous hum may be present
7. Increase S1 and exaggerated splitting of S2
8. Hyperventilation/pulmonary basal rales.

III. ECG findings
1. Sinus tachycardia
2. Left axis deviation
3. Increased R/S ratio in V1 and V2
4. Repolarization change.

IV. Echocardiographic findings:
1. Increased LV diastolic dimension, LV wall thickness, and mild increase in contractility
2. Moderate increased in size of right atrium, right ventricle and left atrium
3. Functional pulmonary, tricuspid, and mitral regurgitation
4. Small pericardial effusion.

8. Other investigations:

1. X-ray chest should be performed only when it is absolutely necessary and with shielding of the pelvic area with protective lead.
2. MRI: is sometimes needed to diagnose cardiac disease, its safety profile is unknown and it should be avoided if possible.
3. Invasive testing: Pulmonary artery catheterization with fluoroscopy is useful for patients with hemodynamic deterioration especially during labor, delivery, and the early postpartum period.
4. Cardiac catheterization in pregnancy is rarely needed except in AMI or to allow ballon valvuloplasty. Vascular access from the arm is preferred to the leg wherever feasible.

9. Risk assessment and general principles of management. This involves multidisciplinary approach with—

1. Preconception counseling.
2. Contraception.
3. Potential maternal and fetal risk.
4. Long-term morbidity and mortality.

10. Risk assessment is mostly guided by:

1. Baseline functional class (NYHA class).
2. Severity of cardiac disease.
3. LV function.
4. Pulmonary pressure.

11. Maternal New York Heart Association (NYHA) class II or higher symptoms and left sided obstruction were predictive of neonatal complications. In one study includes:

1. Premature birth
2. Intrauterine growth retardation (IUGR)
3. Respiratory distress syndrome
4. Death.

12. Preconception risk assessment includes:

1. Thorough history of cardiac symptoms and arrhythmias.
2. Baseline exercise tolerance and functional class.
3. Baseline ECG and echocardiography with ventricular function and pulmonary pressures.
4. Detailed discussion with the patient about the risk to the mother and fetus.

Prophylactic intervention for cardiac disease that significantly increases the risk of pregnancy should be performed where appropriate and feasible before the pregnancy is contemplated.

13. Pregnancy is definitely discouraged in conditions such as:

1. Cyanotic heart disease
2. Eisenmenger syndrome
3. Severe pulmonary hypertension
4. Severe stenotic lesions.

These patients cannot tolerate the hemodynamic changes in pregnancy.

14. Risk predictors of adverse maternal and fetal outcomes:

1. Prior cardiac events.
2. Prior arrhythmias.
3. NYHA class II or higher.
4. Cyanosis.
5. Ejection fraction <40%.
6. Pulmonary hypertension (pulmonary artery systolic pressure >50% of systemic pressure).
7. Severe AS (valve area < 1.5 cm^2, Doppler jet velocity >4 m/sec).

8. Symptomatic or severe MS
9. Severe aortic or MR with NYHA class III or IV symptoms
10. Hypertrophic obstructive cardiomyopathy (HOCM)
11. Maternal anticoagulation
12. Other severe systemic diseases.

15. General principles of treatment of risk pregnancy.

Preconception

1. Effective contraception until pregnancy is desired.
2. Consider valve repair or correction of anomaly prior to conception if pregnancy poses a risk.
3. Avoid drug that cause adverse fetal side effects.

During Pregnancy

4. Use only those drugs which are absolutely indicated and discontinue or replace the drugs which are contraindicated in pregnancy.
5. If symptoms worsen, and if indicated, consider correction of anomaly or valve repair or replacement.

During Labor and Delivery

6. Invasive monitoring if needed.
7. Cesarian operation for obstetric indication.
8. Monitor for decompensated heart failure and pulmonary edema and treat accordingly.

16. Postpartum: General principles of treatment:

1. Adjust and optimize medications.
2. Consider correction of a normally or valve replacement if indicated.
3. Treat postpartum anemia.
4. Counseling and contraception for future pregnancies.

17. NYHA grade 0-2A—Tolerate pregnancy and go through well. Grade 2B-4 must be advised not to become pregnant or correct the structural abnormality and then take up pregnancy. Conservative management of cardiac decompensation during pregnancy is usually as safe but watchful expectancy is desired.

Following 4 groups of drugs are judiciously chosen:

1. Anticongestive therapy (digoxin and diuretics)
2. Antibiotic prophylaxis
3. Anticoagulants
4. Antiarrhythmic.

18. There are 4 critical periods of danger of cardiac decompensation in pregnancy:

1. 12–32 weeks of pregnancy.
   The most critical period is between 28–32 weeks. About 50% of those patients who develop congestive:
   1. Cardiac failures are in class I or II of NYHA classification.
   2. During labor and delivery.

   Uterine contraction are increased during labor which in turn increases cardiac output by 15–20%. During second stage, venous return decreases, there by decreasing cardiac output which is also critical.
3. Immediately after delivery. The obstructive effect of uterus on IVC (inferior vena cava) is lost and there is a sudden transfusion of blood from the lower extremities and the uteroplacental tree. This result in large and abrupt increase in cardiac output.
4. 4–5 days after delivery.

Pulmonary embolus from silent iliofemoral thrombus can result in sudden death.

19. The patients with the following disease are particularly at danger:

1. Primary pulmonary hypertension
2. Eisenmenger's syndrome
3. Aortic stenosis
4. Cyanotic heart disease.

20. Management of some congenital heart diseases during pregnancy:

1. *Atrial septal defect (ASD) and patent foramen ovale (PFO):* Isolated atrial septal defect and patent foramen ovale is usually well tolerated in pregnancy and considered low risk in general. Paradoxical pulmonary embolism (PE) during pregnancy has been reported. Correction of significant shunt (> 1.5:1) should be corrected prior to pregnancy. Secundum atrial septal defect that is repaired is not associated with an increased risk of complications.
2. *Ventricular septal defect (VSD):* Ventricular septal defect without pulmonary hypertension is usually well tolerated during pregnancy. Correction of ventricular septal defect before pregnancy and prior to the development of pulmonary hypertension eliminates the risk of pregnancy. In pregnant patient with ventricular septal defect and pulmonary hypertension, a drop in blood pressure during or after delivery may result in reversed of shunt. This may be prevented by close monitoring of blood pressure, volume replacement and by use of vasopressors.
3. *Patent ductus arteriosus (PDA):* Patent ductus arteriosus without pulmonary hypertension usually is tolerated and has a favorable outcome. Management principle is same as in ventricular septal defect.
4. *Congenital aortic stenosis:* Congenital bicuspid valve is one of the most common cause of aortic stenosis. (See in valvular disease).

5. *Pulmonary stenosis:* Isolated pulmonary stenosis is usually well tolerated in pregnancy. It should be corrected before pregnancy if severe (peak gradient of >60 mm Hg) percutaneous ballon valvuloplasty during pregnancy may be needed in patients with severe right ventricular failure.
6. *Ebstein anomaly:* Noncyanotic Ebstein anomaly is usually well tolerated in pregnancy. Cyanotic patients are at very high-risk of maternal heart failure and fetal prematurity or death. Care should be taken to prevent drop in blood pressure during labor and delivery and close hemodynamic monitoring is required along with rest, oxygen, antibiotic prophylaxes and blood gas monitoring. It is sometimes associated with Wolf-Parkinson-White (WPW) syndrome and pregnancy may precipitate supraventricular arrhythmia.
7. *Tetralogy of Fallot (TOF):* Women who have undergone successful repair during childhood with little or no residual outflow tract gradient, without pulmonary hypertension and preserved ventricular function usually tolerate pregnancy well.
   The result of pregnancy is very poor for both mother and fetus once cyanosis occurs.
   In women with uncorrected or only partially corrected tetralogy of Fallot, increased blood volume during pregnancy with increased venous return and decreased systemic vascular resistance may result in right to left shunt and cyanosis. A similar change may also occur with a fall in blood pressure during labor and delivery. It is also associated with high rate of premature labor, spontaneous abortion and fetal growth deterioration. The risk of fetus developing cardiac defects ranges from 3–17%.
   Patients with partial correction may have residual lesions such as pulmonary regurgitation right ventricular outflow obstruction, and right ventricular dysfunction and/or at risk of heart failure and arrhythmia during pregnancy.
   Poor signs include—maternal hematocrit > 60%, arterial saturation below 80%, right ventricular hypertension and syncopal attacks. Close hemodynamic and blood gas monitoring during labor and delivery and antibiotic prophylaxis is recommended.
   Patients with cyanosis should be discouraged pregnancy as the resulting outcome is poor.
8. *Coarctation of aorta:* Coarctation of aorta has favorable outcome when it is not associated with hypertension, congestive heart failure, or aortic dissection seen in some cases. It is also associated with Circle of Willis aneurysms and cerebral hemorrhage from rupture of aneurysm during pregnancy is possible.
   Strict bed rest, controlling of blood pressure and prevention of cerebral hemorrhage and aortic dissection is important. β-blockers are usually the antihypertensive drug of choice but care should be taken not to lower the blood pressure unduly which may compromise uteroplacental circulation. Fetal asphyxia is another complication of β-blocker, which should be kept in mind.
   Coarctation of aorta with systemic hypertension, heart failure, or peak gradient of >20 mm Hg should be corrected prior to pregnancy.
   Women with prior surgical repair of coarctation of aorta remain at risk for aortic dissection as the aortic valve is still abnormally weak. Correction of coarctation aorta during pregnancy is indicated in patients with severe uncontrollable hypertension or heart failure.

21. Valvular heart disease in pregnancy:

Valvular diseases generally associated with high-risk of maternal and/or fetal risks include:

American College of Cardiology and American Heart Association (ACC/AHA) guidelines:

1. Symptomatic mitral stenosis.
2. Severe aortic stenosis with or without symptoms.
3. NYHA class III or IV symptoms with mitral or aortic regurgitation.
4. Valvular diseases associated with pulmonary hypertension.
5. Valvular diseases associated with left ventricular dysfunction.
6. Hypertrophic obstructive heart myopathy (HOCM).
7. Marfan's syndrome.
8. Mechanical prosthetic valve requiring anticoagulants.

1. Mitral stenosis (MS): It is one of the most common rheumatic valvular diseases seen in pregnancy. Management depends upon the severity of stenosis, symptoms, and time of diagnosis.

i. MS diagnosed before pregnancy—MS with valve area of <1cm^2 or moderate symptomatic stenosis should be offered percutaneous mitral ballon valvuloplasty (PMBV) or valve repair if PMBV is not possible.

ii. In patients with mild MS (valve area > 1.5 cm^2) pregnancy is usually tolerated with a favorable result.

iii. In patients of MS with already pregnant is aimed at reducing heart rate and left atrial pressure. β-blockers are the drug of choice. Selective β-blockers are preferred over nonselective β-blocker to avoid β-mediated uterine relaxation. Left atrial pressure may be controlled by salt restriction and diuretics (excessive use of diuretics can lead to reduction in uteroplacental circulation).

iv. In patients with atrial fibrillation (AF):

a. Digoxin, a selective β-blocker, or a non-dihydropyridine calcium channel blocker used to control the ventricular rate response in atrial fibrillation.

b. Direct current cardioversion: In patients we have hemodynamically unstable due to AF in spite of optimal medical therapy.

c. PMBV may be necessary during pregnancy but it should be avoided in first trimester if possible and should be done with proper abdominal and pelvic shielding.

In severe MS, refractory to medical therapy and where not amenable to PMBV, mitral valve repair or replacement may be necessary.

d. Protection against thromboembolism is recommended throughout pregnancy for all patients with AF (except with lone AF and/or low-risk for thromboembolism).

Therapy with anticoagulant or aspirin should be chosen according to stage of pregnancy.

Most patients with MS can safely undergo vaginal delivery. The rapid increase in venous return during labor and delivery may cause significant decompensation and so requires very close monitoring with guidance of pulmonary artery cauterization during labor and delivery and immediate postpartum period (12–24 hours) during which time relief from uterocaval obstruction can cause increased venous return and pulmonary edema.

Epidural anesthesia is usually better tolerated than general anesthesia. Cesarian section performed for obstetric indications only.

Penicillin prophylaxis is continued in young patients who had previous history of rheumatic carditis as they did in the nonpregnant women.

2. **Mitral regurgitation (MR):** The most common cause of MR during pregnancy is either rheumatic heart disease or mitral valve prolapse.

Regurgitant lesions are usually well tolerated in pregnancy because the fall in systemic vascular resistance leads to a decreased left ventricular after-load. Atrial fibrillation and hypertension may sometimes cause acute symptomatic decompensation.

Asymptomatic patients are managed conservatively without any medication but in patient with LV dysfunction and decompensated heart failure require digoxin and diuretics.

In the peripartum period increased venous return and systemic vascular resistance sometimes lead to decompensation requiring diuretics and afterload reduction.

Direct vasodilators like hydralazine may be used in patients with MR and hypertension for afterload reduction. ACEI are contraindicated during pregnancy because of their teratogenic effect.

Acute MR due to ruptured chordae tendineae is rare in pregnancy and usually cannot be well tolerated. This requires intra-aortic ballon pump placement and emergency surgery.

3. **Aortic stenosis (AS):** The most common cause in childbearing age is a congenitally bicuspid valve. Insolated rheumatic AS is less common and may occur in association with MS.

Mild-to-moderate AS with persevered LV function is usually well tolerated during pregnancy.

Severe aortic stenosis with <1 cm^2 valve area, mean gradient <50 mm Hg significantly increases the risk of pregnancy and may lead to significant hemodynamic deterioration, heart failure, and premature delivery. So, patients with severe AS should undergo prompt intervention before surgery. Symptoms of dyspnea, angina, or syncope attacks usually seen in late 2nd trimester. Percutaneous aortic ballon valvuloplasty (PABV) may reduce the risk of pregnancy as a temporary measure until valve replacement.

Patients with bicuspid aortic valve, root dilation especially those with associated coarctation of aorta are at increased risk for spontaneous aortic dissection, usually in the 3rd trimester and during labor.

Aortic insufficiency that occur after PABV is usually well tolerated during labor and delivery.

Close invasive monitoring is required during labor and delivery as in MS.

Spinal and epidural anesthesia is discouraged during labor and delivery as they cause vasodilatory effects.

4. **Aortic regurgitation (AR):** In young women it can be caused by congenital bicuspid valve or dilated aortic annulus, infective endocarditis, connective tissue disease (SLE, RA).

Atrial fibrillation without LV dysfunction is usually well tolerated owing to decrease in vascular resistance and increased heart rate causing a shorter diastole thereby reducing regurgitation.

In symptomatic patients with decompensated heart failure, diuretics, digoxin, and hydralazine for afterload reduction may be used.

5. **Hypertrophic obstructive cardiomyopathy (HOCM):**
(See K-2, 19 and 28)
Overall morbidity and mortality with HOCM is still higher in pregnancy.
Women should receive genetic counseling before conception whenever possible. The risk of inheriting disease may up to 50% in certain familial forms of HOCM.
Most asymptomatic patient with HOCM have a favorable outcome during pregnancy.
Management depends on severity of symptoms and severity of LV outflow obstruction. Blood loss and vasodilators should be avoided.
β-blockers are usually the drugs of choice for symptomatic patients with supraventricular arrhythmias, AF, with hemodynamic deterioration and fetus distress requires cardioversion.
Patients with ventricular fibrillation needing defibrillation also reported.
Patients with history of syncope, life-threatening arrhythmias or a family history of sudden cardiac death should be considered for prophylactic implantable defibrillator prior to pregnancy due to potential arrhythmogenic effect of pregnancy. Vaginal delivery is considered safe.
Tocolytic with β-adrenogenic properties and prostaglandins should be avoided.
Epidural anesthesia should be used with caution because of peripheral vasodilator effect and excessive blood loss should be avoided. Prompt IV fluids and blood transfusion is needed.
The rapid diuresis in immediate postpartum period may lead to a rapid decrease in circulating volume and therefore asymptomatic increase in outflow tract gradient. This can be avoided by IV hydration decreasing over 24–48 hours postpartum to achieve euvolemic state.

6. **Marfan's syndrome:**
(see L-215)
The CVS abnormalities included aortic root dilation with or without AR, aortic dissection and MVP.
Aortic dissection is the most feared complication of pregnancy in Marfan's syndrome and most likely to occur during 3rd trimester, including labor and delivery. Women without any symptoms have low risk and can tolerate vaginal delivery.
Medical management consists of use of β-blockers throughout pregnancy to reduce the risk of aortic rupture.
Cesarean section is preferred in patients with aortic dilation or evidence of dissection.

7. **Prosthetic heart valve:**
(See I-250 to 257)
Selection of suitable prosthetic valve during childbearing age is controversial. The patient's own valve should be conserved or repaired where possible. When valve replacement is necessary bioprosthetic and homograft valves are preferable as they are safer to mother and child, although their use is associated with increased risk of degeneration in younger people that can be aggravated by pregnancy.
Mechanical valves need anticoagulation which are at increased risk of maternal mortality and morbidity and fetal loss.
Risk of complications during pregnancy depends on:
   i. Type of valve
   ii. Position of valve
   iii. Prepregnancy cardiac function
   iv. Functional capacity.
The management is similar to that of native valve in pregnant women with well functioning bioprosthetic valves.
Pregnancy should be discouraged in patients with mechanical valves since the management of anticoagulation is challenging.
Pregnancy is a thrombogenic state and thromboembolism has been reported in up to 10–15% in pregnant women with mechanical prosthetic valve with high incidence of valve thrombosis and death. The incidence is high particularly with older generation valves (Bjork-Shirley, Start-Edwards), in mitral position but complications have been reported with newer generation valves in the aortic position.
Patients with prosthetic valves and poor LV function are also at high-risk for heart failure from volume overload during pregnancy and arrhythmias.

8. **Patients with NYHA class III or IV symptoms should be strongly advised against pregnancy as there is a chance of high mortality and fetal loss.**

22. Peripartum cardiomyopathy (PPCM): (See K 5-1)

The PPCM is more common in women older than 30 years age Incidence is almost 1 in 3000–4000 live births.

Following risk factors are proposed:
1. Multi gravida
2. Multiple fetuses
3. History of pre-eclampsia
4. History of eclampsia
5. Postpartum hypertension
6. African descent
7. History of maternal cocaine abuse
8. Selenium deficiency.

23. PPCM—this type of dilated cardiomyopathy is diagnosed when there is:

1. History of HF in the last month of pregnancy or within 5 months after delivery.
2. Absence of any cause of heart failure (Vs hypertension).
3. Absence of any recognizable heart disease prior to the last month of pregnancy (e.g. Valvular disease).
4. Echocardiographic evidence of LV dysfunction with low ejection fraction.

50% of women recover completely within 6 months of delivery.

The remaining women have stable LV dysfunction are continue to experience clinical deterioration. Estimated maternal mortality ranges from 10–15%.

These women should be strongly discouraged for subsequent pregnancy which has to face high-risk of complications.

24. Patients with heart failure should be treated vigorously with:

1. Oxygen
2. Diuretics
3. Digitalis
4. Vasodilators.

ACEI are definitely contraindicated. Vasopressors like dopamine, dobutamine, and milrinone have been used in pregnancy but data over there use is limited.

Volume overload should be avoided by careful monitoring during labor and delivery.

Patients with severe cardiac dysfunction and decompensation are evaluated for cardiac transplantation after pregnancy.

Primary Pulmonary Hypertension

25. This is associated with:

1. Very high maternal mortality (30–40%) and poor fetal outcome.
2. Worsening of symptoms occur more in 2nd and 3rd trimester.
3. Right ventricular failure (RVF).
4. Arrhythmias.

26. Management:

1. Early therapeutic medical termination of pregnancy is considered for those who become pregnant.
2. Anticoagulation throughout pregnancy or at least 3rd trimester, during labor and delivery.
3. Oxygen + inhaled nitrous oxide.
4. Prostaglandins (inhaled or IV) may be used.

27. Pregnancy after cardiac transplantation—

1. It is considered very high-risk for mother and fetus.
2. Increased maternal mortality from hypertension, pre-eclampsia, renal failure, premature rupture of membranse and infection.
3. Preterm labor is also a concern.
4. Fetal effects due to immunosuppressive medication.

In one study of 47 pregnancies in 35 transplant recipients noticed no increase in maternal mortality but there were increased infant mortality.

RECOGNITION AND MANAGEMENT OF CARDIAC EMERGENCIES IN PREGNANCY

28. Common cardiac emergencies encountered in pregnancy are:

1. Congestive cardiac failure
2. Acute pulmonary edema
3. Arrhythmias
4. Thromboembolism
5. Infective endocarditis
6. Aortic dissection and rupture
7. Coronary artery disease
8. Sudden death.

Common causes of death are congestive cardiac failure (36%) and pulmonary edema (23.5).

CONGESTIVE CARDIAC FAILURE

29. There are 4 factors contributing to CCF and death during and after delivery:

1. Oxygen consumption is increased by 15–20%.
2. Cardiac output is increased by 50% but tends to fall after 36th week.
3. Retention of sodium and water results in hemodilution, which is maximum by 32nd week.
4. Venous pressure rises due to increased blood volume. Compression of inferior vena cava in supine position is an important hemodynamic factor in reducing cardiac output during pregnancy and sudden increase of cardiac inflow in the immediate postpartum period.

30. The following 4 precipitating causes of heart failure in pregnancy should be identified:

1. *Anemia:* Marked anemia (Hb 2–3 g%) can result in decompensation of a normal heart in nonpregnant state. In all critically ill patients, the hemoglobin level is best maintained at least 10 g% for adequate tissue oxygenation.
2. *Endocarditis:* Sepsis or infective endocarditis should be sought for and managed with appropriate antibiotics.

3. *Arrhythmias:* Should be identified and managed accordingly.
4. *Venue thrombus with embolism:* Should be identified and managed accordingly.

31. Correct the underlying cardiac illness if possible, in the following 4 conditions:

1. *Mitral stenosis:* Patients with critical mitral stenosis may be subjected to balloon mitral valvuloplasty.
2. *Aortic stenosis:* Balloon valvuloplasty can also be performed if symptoms of failure do not progress with medical management.
3. *Atrial septal defect (ASD):* Transfemoral catheter closure by using a prosthesis Rashkind—umbrella device (RUD).
4. *Patent ductus arteriosus (PDA):* Transfemoral catheter closure by using a prosthesis.

All procedures are deferred as far as possible in view of the risk to fetus due to irradiation or transient hypotension.

32. Management of the congestive state:

4 general measures:

1. Absolute bed rest with head end elevation of 30–40 is a must. Excessive physical activity should be avoided. Patient is advised to lie in left lateral position at frequent intervals.
2. Restriction of salt.
3. Avoid fluid overload: Over enthusiastic IV fluids for mild to moderate diarrhea failing to recognize minimal underlying cardiac illness can result in decompensation.
4. Fever: Every 1°C rise in temperature increases metabolic demand by about 15% and poses a strain on the heart. Antipyretics and tepid sponging should be resorted to.

33. 4 specific measures:

1. Digoxin can be used safely.
2. Diuretic therapy should be monitored with daily weight checks, serial measurement of hematocrit, electrolytes and serum creatinine.
3. Vasodilators like nitroglycerin, hydralazine can be used.
4. Prophylactic heparin 5000 IU/SC/BD is administered. Low molecular weight heparin (LMWH) can also be used. In very severe failure, interventional procedures like intra-aortic balloon counter pulsation can be resorted to.

34. Know about the following 4 drugs before administering in pregnancy:

1. Sodium nitroprusside is best avoided because it causes fetal cyanide poisoning with harmful side effects.
2. Dopamine-dobutamine combination can be safely and effectively used.
3. ACE inhibitors are contraindicated. They may cause intrauterine growth retardation (IUGR).
4. ACE receptor blockers like losartan: Their safety is yet to be established.

ACUTE PULMONARY EDEMA

35. Acute pulmonary edema is precipitated by:

1. Increased venous return
2. Increased blood volume
3. Increased heart rate
4. Decreased pulmonary vascular resistance.

36. Pulmonary edema is commonly seen in:

1. Mitral stenosis
2. Systemic hypertension
3. Pulmonary thromboembolism
4. Atrial fibrillation.

37. Management of acute pulmonary edema:

Conventional management is effective. It includes:

1. Back rest
2. Oxygen
3. Anticongestive therapy—digoxin and diuretics
4. IV nitroglycerin is beneficial
5. Pressor amines like dopamine, dobutamine may be needed
6. Electrolyte abnormalities have to be corrected. Measurement of pulmonary artery wedge pressure will give a good guideline.
7. Treatment of precipitating causes like:
   i. Infection
   ii. Arrhythmias
   iii. Thromboembolism
   iv. Acute myocardial infarction—has to be done.
8. Lastly, medical and surgical venesection has to be considered in resistant cases.

   If facilities are available and symptoms are unremitting despite medical therapy, balloon mitral valvuloplasty or surgical mitral commissurotomy may be required. When decided for surgery, closed mitral commissurotomy is the procedure of choice.

   In mitral stenosis, patients are at great risk of pulmonary edema during 32 week of pregnancy or soon after delivery.

ARRHYTHMIAS

38. Cardiac arrhythmias during pregnancy are not unknown.

Clinical experience suggests a 'gestational arrhythmogenic effect'

Incidence: In 24-hours Holter monitoring—

1. Ventricular premature beats (VPB's) and atrial premature beats (APB's) are detected in 18% of pregnant women.
2. SVT 1.5–3% of women with heart disease. AV nodal reentrant tachycardia (AVNRT) is the common supraventricular tachycardia.
3. Atrial flutter and fibrillation are usually associated with mitral valve disease.
4. Ventricular tachycardia and fibrillation are rare in pregnancy and usually associated with structural heart disease. Ventricular tachycardia may be presenting manifestation of peripartum cardiomyopathy (PPCM), VT is also associated with thyrotoxicosis and hyperemesis gravidarum. Antiarrhythmic medicines used to treat VT are safe during pregnancy except amiodarone.

39. Complete heart block has been described in pregnancy, though rare.

It may be congenital/acquired. It may present as a result of:

1. Myocarditis
2. Myocardial infarction
3. Infective endocarditis
4. Congenital heart disease.

40. Management of arrhythmia's in pregnancy is similar to that of nonpregnant women except to avoid toxic drugs. Some of the following drugs are used depending on the type of arrhythmia:

1. Calcium blockers are ideal.
2. Quinidine is one of the safest antiarrhythmic drugs during pregnancy.
3. Lidocaine and mexiletine are equally safe for ventricular arrhythmias.
4. Digoxin can be used but higher than usual doses may be needed to achieve therapeutic goals. Rate control may be safely achieved with digoxin and β-blocker.
5. Sotalol (antithyroid like effect) and β-blockers are considered safe, but asphyxia neonatorum may be precipitated.
6. Disopyramide may trigger uterine contractions. Adenosine may be administered safely in AVNRT for the diagnosis and therapeutic purpose.
7. Amiodarone and phenytoin have definite teratogenic effects on fetus. Amiodarone should be used with caution and only for arrhythmias and responding to other medications. It may lead to neonatal hypothyroidism.
8. Cardioversion in atrial fibrillation and ventricular tachycardia is safe and does not increase fetal morbidity or mortality.

41. Protocol:

Step I

Cardiac Arrhythmia

Normal cardiovascular status

Organic heart disease

Step II

Treat underlying disease

Rule out other causes including:

1. Pulmonary disease
2. Electrolyte disturbance
3. Thyroid disorders
4. Arrhythmogenic drugs
5. Alcohol
6. Caffeine
7. Cigarette smoking
8. Drug abuse

Drug therapy only if arrhythmias are symptomatic or threatening to mother and/or fetus

Step III

Drug therapy only if arrhythmias persist

Treat underlying cause

Step IV

Antiarrhythmic therapy only if arrhythmias persist

Use smallest dosage required
Use drugs known to be safe to the fetus
Reevaluate periodically the indication for continuation of therapy

THROMBOEMBOLISM

42. Hypercoagulable state of pregnancy significantly increases the risk of thromboembolism. Uterine pressure on inferior vena cava is an added factor. Clinical presentation may be that of an acute massive pulmonary embolism with classical picture of the following 4 symptoms and signs:

1. Acute retrosternal discomfort
2. Shock
3. Cardiac failure or precipitation of cardiac failure
4. Arrhythmias in an existing cardiovascular disease.

Pulmonary thromboembolism has to be considered in any pregnant lady with or without underlying cardiac disease. It is most common during delivery and in immediate post-partum period. Usually, it is diagnosed clinically. X-ray chest, ECG, Echo will be of help to show an acute right ventricular outflow obstruction. Confirmation of diagnosis is by angiography and radionuclide scan.

43. Management of thromboembolism:

1. Hemodynamic monitoring
2. Volume replacement
3. Pressor amines for shock
4. Diuretics if pulmonary edema is present
5. Vasodilators
6. Correction of arrhythmias
7. Anticoagulants.
   a. Oral anticoagulants are effective but may cross placenta and cause high fetal loss and developmental abnormalities.
   b. Heparin—because of its large molecular size it does not cross the placenta. Intravenous heparin for emergency will be the sheet anchor.
8. Thrombolytic therapy is not safe.

Management of patients on anticoagulant therapy during pregnancy is a special exercise. These patients are ideally managed with regular subcutaneous heparin twice daily adjusted to APTT. In certain countries, anticoagulant therapy is given only to those subset of patients on a high-risk of thromboembolism, e.g. patients with atrial fibrillation, past history of thromboembolism and those with prosthetic valves.

There is another regimen where heparin is used for initial 3 months, oral anticoagulants for the later 6 months. Near term switch over to subcutaneous heparin. Heparin should be stopped with the onset of labor and again started after 2 hours after delivery. Oral anticoagulants should be restarted 24 hours after delivery and overlapped with heparin for 4 days.

INFECTIVE ENDOCARDITIS

The committee on bacterial endocarditis formed by the AHA has recommended routine prophylaxis for anticipated normal delivery only for patients with prosthetic heart valves. Antibiotic prophylaxis against infective endocarditis to all susceptible individuals should be a routine in our country because the bacteremia is unpredictable even in a normal vaginal delivery and the sterilization aspect is also unpredictable. Not only for patients with prosthetic valves but for all patients of congenital heart disease. RVHD, HOCM, MVP with thickened MV and MR should also be given the prophylactic antibiotic therapy. Antibiotic prophylaxis may not be necessary in patents with isolated secundum ASD and corrected PDA.

44. Infective endocarditis presents with:

1. Fever
2. Appearance of newer murmurs mostly diastolic
3. Congestive heart failure
4. Embolic manifestations.

Clinical suspicion, blood culture and echocardiography both transthoracic and transesophageal approach form the cornerstone of diagnosis. Treatment is initiated with crystalline penicillin or ampicillin or vancomycin with streptomycin or gentamicin. Change of antibiotic is done after getting the culture and sensitivity. Surgical intervention is needed in very rare situations. Infective endocarditis in pregnancy carries a high mortality.

Hypertensive emergencies are dealt separately at the end.

(A brief mention is made here for the sake of completion. Read the portion of hypertension in pregnancy in this chapter from V-63).

45. Hypertension in pregnancy can be described in 4 types.

1. Chronic hypertension
2. Pregnancy induced hypertension
3. Preeclmpsia
4. Eclampsia.

46. All the hypertensive urgencies and emergencies can occur during pregnancy but more common ones are eclampsia and pulmonary edema due to altered physiology. Management consists of:

1. General measures
2. Sedative management
3. Hypotensive management
4. Obstetrical management.

47. Management mainly depends on the urgent control of blood pressure toward safe levels, diastolic levels between 90–100 mm Hg and control and prevention of convulsions.

1. Sedation
2. Diuretics with frusemide IV
3. Hydralazine IV if available or oral l5–10 mg every 20–30 minutes to avoid a precipitous fall
4. Magnesium sulfate IM or IV. It is the drug of choice and should be continued for 12–24 hours postpartum.

SUDDEN DEATH

48. It may be one of the cardiac emergencies during pregnancy. It is commonly seen in:

1. Tight mitral stenosis
2. Primary pulmonary hypertension

3. Congenital cyanotic heart diseases
4. Massive pulmonary embolism
5. Severe aortic stenosis
6. Marfan's syndrome
7. Cardiomyopathy
8. Acute myocardial infarction.

49. Pathophysiology:

1. Thrombus occluding diseased mitral valve resulting in sudden low cardiac output
2. Dissection or rupture of aorta or rupture of heart
3. Tamponade
4. Malignant arrhythmias.

50. Recognition and management of sudden cardiac death.

1. CPR and advanced cardiac life support
2. Pharmacotherapy
3. Electrical therapy
4. Treat primary cause, if possible.

AORTIC DISSECTION

51. Aortic dissection is reported in patients with:

1. Marfan's syndrome
2. Long standing systemic hypertension
3. Coarctation of aorta
4. Aortoarteritis.

It is also noted in patients with crack cocaine use.

52. Patients with aortic root more than 40 mm are vulnerable.

During pregnancy the blood pressure rises, cardiac output increases and tissue softening occurs which make the aorta suffer this entity. Isometric strain performed during delivery increases the chances of rupture and hence cesarian section is preferred.

53. Diagnosis: 4 features—

1. Aortic dissection has to be considered in any pregnant lady with central tearing chest pain with radiation across the chest to the arm, back and along the thigh
2. Absent or diminished peripheral pulses
3. Mediastinal widening in chest X-ray
4. Echocardiography both TTE and TEE confirms the diagnosis.

54. Management:

1. Vigorous antihypertensive treatment. Adequate control of blood pressure with β-blockers or calcium blockers reduce the chances of aortic dissection or rupture
2. Stabilizing hemodynamic status
3. Total cardiopulmonary bypass
4. Surgical correction.

During pregnancy in coarctation of aorta, not only aortic dissection but rupture of cerebral Berry aneurysm can occur and present as subarachnoid intracerebral hemorrhage.

CORONARY ARTERY DISEASE (SEE CAD/IHD)

CAD is rare among women with child bearing age. Heavy smoking and concurrent use of oral contraceptives have been proved to be strong predictors of AMI.

55. Management:

1. Low dose aspirin, vasodilators, methyldopa, α-β blocker, and calcium channel blockers can be used safely.
2. Heparin can be used safely. Short-term heparin administration has not been associated with increased maternal or fetal adverse effects.
3. Antiplatelet agent cannot be used.
4. Thrombolytic therapy, PTCA and CABG have their limitations and should be decided upon individual case explaining the risk of radiation and CP bypass upon the fetus.

Acute myocardial infarction is associated with high maternal mortality during the third trimester and labor. Management of AMI needs adequate hemodynamic monitoring, adequate analgesics, reducing the second stage of labor with low forceps or elective cesarean section. Epidural anesthesia is safe and halothane is avoided if GA is desired. Atropine and ketamine are used with caution to prevent tachycardia.

Pregnancy with cardiac disease puts the additional hemodynamic stress on the diseased heart. Isometric strain performed during labor, possibility of bacteremia, and drugs used during labor increase the risk of cardiac complication. Regular medical supervision and safe pharmacotherapy make the pregnancy safe. Greater care is needed during the labor to choose the type of delivery. Care is extended to the first 4 days of delivery too.

56. Drugs in pregnancy: The common drugs and their potential side effects are shown in the following table:

Table V-2

Drug	Indication	FDA Category	Potential maternal and fetal adverse effect
1. Adenosine	Arrhythmia (PAT)	C	Limited data available
2. Amiodarone	Arrhythmia	C	↓ or ↑ thyroidism, IUGR, congenital goiter
3. Aspirin	CAD	C/D	IUGR, bleeding in mother and neonate

Contd...

Contd...

Drug	*Indication*	*FDA Category*	*Potential maternal and fetal adverse effect*
4. β-blockers	Arrhythmia, HTN, MI, HOCM, hyperthyroidism, MS, Marfan's	C/D	Fetal bradycardia, IUGR, hypoglycemia
5. Calcium channel blocker	Hypertension	C	Maternal hypotension causing fetal distress reported
6. ACEI/ARBI	Hypertension	D/X	C/I, IUGR, oligohydramnios, renal failure, fetal death
7. Digoxin	Arrhythmias, heart failure	C	Safe, no evidence of adverse effects
8. Diuretics	Hypertension	C	Hypovolemia and decreased uteroplacental circulation
9. Nitrates	Hypertension	C	Maternal Hypertension causing fetal distress reported
10. Xylocaine	Arrhythmias	C	Neonatal CNS depressant
11. Quinidine	Arrhythmias	C	Neonatal thrombocytopenia, oxytocic effect
12. Procainamide	Arrhythmias	C	No adverse effects reported
13. Flecainide	Arrhythmias	C	Limited data
14. Propafenone	Arrhythmia	C	Limited data
15. Sotalol	Arrhythmias	B	Fetal bradycardia, IUGR, limited data
16. Sodium nitroprusside	HTN, aortic dissection	C	Fetal thiocyanate toxicity

FDA category: (A) Controlled studies show no risk; (B) No evidence of risk in humans; (C) Risk cannot be ruled out; (D) positive evidence of risk, X-means contraindication pregnancy; IUGR-intrauterine growth retardation

Anticoagulation During Pregnancy

57. 4 common conditions that require anticoagulation during pregnancy are:

1. Mechanical prosthetic valve
2. Chronic atrial fibrillation
3. Acute thromboembolism
4. Eisenmenger's syndrome.

Rare causes included antiphospholipid antibody syndrome, and inherited deficiencies predisposing to thromboembolism (prothrombin gene mutation, factor V, Leiden deficiency).

58. 4 commonly used anticoagulants during pregnancy are:

1. Unfractionated heparin (UFH)
2. Low molecular weight heparin (LMWH)

Oral

3. Warfarin (Indanedione derivative)
4. Nicoumalone (Acitron-coumarin derivative).

The choice of anticoagulants depends on the preference of the patient and physician after considering the maternal and fetal risks associated with each drug.

59. Anticoagulants option during pregnancy:

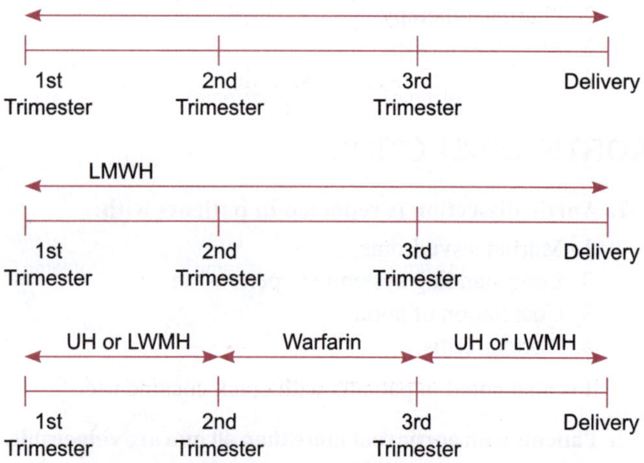

60. Unfractionated heparin (UFH): It does not cross the placental barrier and considered safe.

However, it is associated with:

1. Maternal osteoporosis.
2. Thrombocytopenia or thrombosis (HITT syndrome).
3. High incidence of thromboembolic events with older generation of mechanical valves.
4. Spontaneous hemorrhages are having bleeding preterm labor, in case of preterm labor, spontaneous hemorrhages are heavy bleeding/during delivery may be reversed by protamine sulfate. It can be given parenterally or subcutaneously throughout pregnancy.

Dose depends on PTT of 2.0–3.0 times the control level. High doses of UFH may be needed to achieve the goal of PTT because of the hypercoagulable state associated with pregnancy. IV infusion should be stopped 4 hours before cesarian operation.

61. Low molecular weight heparin (LMWH): Its use is still controversial as it has not been studied adequately. It does not cross the placenta so safer to the fetus.

The advantage over the UFH are:

1. More predictable anticoagulation response
2. Less incidence of HITT
3. Low-risk of heparin associated maternal osteoporosis
4. Low-risk of bleeding complications.

62. Warfarin: Freely passes across the placenta so it can badly affect the fetus. It is associated with:

1. High incidence of spontaneous abortion
2. Prematurity/stillbirth
3. Fetal bleeding
4. When given 6 to 12 weeks of pregnancy it is associated with warfarin embryopathy (i.e. abnormalities of fetal bone and cartilage formation) is about 4% to 10%. When given during 2nd or 3rd trimester, it causes CNS abnormalities such as optic atrophy, microencephalopathy, mental retardation, spasticity, and hypotonia. It is safe during lactation.

When women taking warfarin prior to pregnancy, should be counseled about the harmful effects of warfarin, if pregnancy is contemplated; once she becomes pregnant changing over to UFH or LMWH should be considered. Acitron oral anticoagulant is similar to warfarin in pregnancy.

THE HYPERTENSIVE DISORDERS OF PREGNANCY

The hypertensive disorders of pregnancy remain an enigma. Confidential esquires into maternal deaths in the United Kingdom have identified hypertension in pregnancy as the most frequent cause of maternal death. Pre-eclampsia remains the single most common cause of maternal death in UK and other developed countries. Maternal mortality is at high rate in developing countries like India and other underdeveloped countries. Hypertensive disorders are among the leading causes of maternal and perinatal mortality in developed countries. Hypertension occurs in well over 5% of all pregnancies and in 5% women who take oral contraceptives for 5 years.

There is an increasing evidence that low birth weight babies are more likely to develop hypertension in adult life gives greater search and emphasis to the need for prevention of pre-eclampsia, a leading cause for intrauterine growth retardation.

Pregnant women with hypertension is commonly seen by the family physician particularly at the periphery in PHCs, where he/she has to attend to all the complications unlike they are seen mostly by the obstetricians in metropolitan cities. This subject is dealt here to help the family physicians who take antenatal care and conduct deliveries.

Its cause is still unknown so it cannot be prevented or treated rationally.

63. Research problems in the etiology of hypertensive disorders of pregnancy: No definitive cause is found. So, the probable causes are discussed here under:

1. *Genetic:* There is a genetic predisposition to develop pregnancy induced hypertension (PIH) and pre-eclampsia but the mode of inheritance is uncertain. "pre-eclampsia gene" is most likely to lie on chromosome 1,3,9, or 18 and described a mutation in the angiotensin gene (chromosome 1). A positive history of hypertension or pre-eclamptic toxemia (PET) for their mothers and a further enquiries may reveal a positive history of grandmother(s) or sister(s) need an extra-care during pregnancy.
2. *Interaction between embryo and decidua:* Pre-eclampsia can occur in women with hydatidiform mole, which contains placental tissue without fetus. Development of placenta is impaired from the start. The trophoblast fails fully to invade and thus the spiral arteries dilate to only about 40% of that in normal pregnancy, which impairs the massive increase in the uteroplacental perfusion in the second half of pregnancy. This failure of dilatation in later pregnancy cause placental hypoxia, which may itself result in the systemic manifestations of the disease. This feature of dilatation is also seen in intrauterine growth retardation cases, so something else is also going wrong with pregnancy induced hypertension.
3. *Lipid peroxidation:* General lipid peroxidation is increased in pregnancies with established PET. Free oxygen radicals in the body cause various types of damage, including lipid peroxidation and subsequent endothelial cell injury, and damage to proteins and nucleic acids. Cells and tissues are usually protected from the effects of lipid peroxidation by several naturally occurring antioxidants. Combined serum measurements of antioxidant activity suggest that the normal rise during pregnancy is diminished with pre-eclampsia. Some antioxidant activities are significantly reduced in pre-eclampsia but not in pregnancy induced hypertension. A balance between peroxide generating and peroxide removing mechanisms exists. This may control cyclooxygenase activity and thus the rate of production of prostaglandins. Prostacyclin is an extremely potent vasodilator and antiaggregatory agent synthesized in the vascular endothelium. Its actions are delicately balanced by thromboxane, a potent locally acting vasoconstrictor and pro-aggregatory agent. Peroxide inhibits prostacyclin synthase but do not influence thromboxane synthase. The overall effect is a clear diminution in the vasodilator effect. Inhibition of prostacyclin synthesis cause the formation

of foam cells, accumulation of cholesterol esters and atherogenesis.

The fall in prostacyclin produced in pre-eclampsia, and the observation that low dose of aspirin (50 to 150 mg od) inhibits thromboxane synthase but not prostacyclin synthase led to the suggestion that aspirin might be a suitable prophylaxis. Prophylactic low dose aspirin of 60 mg od is advised, starting between 13 and 26 weeks of gestation and continued through the term. Aspirin does not reduce the incidence of preeclampsia, preterm birth or fetal growth retardation in high-risk cases.

Acetaminophen, an analgesic, widely used during pregnancy reduced the production of prostacyclin but not thromboxane when given to pregnant women.

4. *Endothelial dysfunction:* Another endothelial derived free radical is nitric oxide also called endothelially derived relaxation factor (EDRF). Superoxide easily breaks down nitric oxide. A delicate balance is maintained between superoxide and nitric oxide in the control of vascular tone. Disruption of endothelial integrity account for the loss of vasodilator capacity, which result in enhanced pressor response to angiotensin II and noradrenaline, which was first described more than 30 years ago, in pre-eclamptic women and repeatedly confirmed since.
5. *Membrane fluidity:* Membrane fluidity is altered in established pregnancy induced hypertension and pre-eclampsia. Plasma concentrations of polyunsaturated fatty acids are lower in established disease than in normal pregnancy which might contribute to the change.
6. *Calcium*: Lipid peroxidation in cell membrane increases their permeability to calcium. Prospective studies have shown a slow rise in platelet intracellular free calcium concentration with gestation in normotensive primigravidas, the concentration being significantly raised by the third trimester in women with pre-eclampsia.

   This may be the reason that contribute to the efficacy of calcium channel blockers in the treatment of hypertension in pregnancy.

   The rise in intracellular free calcium concentration in hypertensive pregnant women is interesting in another context. In established pregnancy induced hypertension (PIH) and pre-eclampsia, urinary calcium excretion (usually expressed in relation to urinary creatinine concentration) falls in direct proportion to the severity of the condition. Some groups have identified a fall in the ratio of urinary calcium to creatinine concentration in the second trimester as being a predictor of PIH and pre-eclampsia., while others have failed to do so. The mechanism for the presumed calcium retention has not been found.

   Intracellular calcium is raised, plasma ionized calcium is lower and urinary calcium excretion is decreased with pre-eclampsia. Decreased plasma ionized calcium would stimulate parathyroid hormone (PTH) and thereby increase distal tubular reabsorption of calcium resulting in hypocalciuria. This suggests that supplemental calcium prevents the development of pre-eclampsia but only in women on a low calcium diet. Increase intake of calcium would presumably raise the plasma calcium level, reduce parathyroid hormone secretion and thereby lowers blood pressure.
7. *Changes in CVS:* They occur mostly during second half of pregnancy and are hormonally driven rather than mediated by the sympathetic nervous system. In established pre-eclampsia before treatment, the cardiac index (Cardiac output in relation to body surface area) is reduced by some 22% while the systemic vascular resistance is noticeably raised. The raised vascular resistance of established pre-eclampsia is not sympathetically mediated. It was found more than 40 years ago that ganglion blockade with tetraethylammonium chloride was shown to be less effective in women with pre-eclampsia than in normotensive pregnant women.

   Therefore, it could be deduced that the treatment should be with direct vasodilators and not with agents that reduce the sympathetic neuron system activity.
8. *Renin-angiotensin system*: Pressor agents such as angiotensin II, stimulates the synthesis of vasodilators such as nitric oxide and prostacyclin, especially in the uterus. The pregnant uterus contains an autonomous renin-angiotensin-system. In PIH, impaired utero-placental circulation stimulates the uteroplacental renin-angiotensin system, which both increases peripheral vascular resistance, and hence perfusion pressure directly and stimulates vasodilator synthesis within the pregnant uterus, allowing increased perfusion.

   The fact that the administration of angiotensin converting enzyme inhibitors (ACE-I) to pregnant women lowers maternal pressure but at the cost of fetus. ACE-I are contraindicated in pregnancy because of their adverse effects on the fetus. It can cause oligohydramnios, stillbirth, and neonatal anuria.

64. Hypertension in pregnancy can be described in 4 types:

1. Chronic hypertension: It is suspected when there is: H/o HT in the family.

H/o HT in the preceding pregnancy
HT appearing before 20th week of gestation or
HT persisting after delivery in multipara and
In obese women (20% of women over 200 lbs weight, age above 30 years or more) systolic BP >200 mm Hg have HT
Cardiac enlargement
Absence of proteinuria.
Fundus examination shows retinal hemorrhages and exudates, tortuosity, narrowing of retinal arteries.
Serum urate levels are normal when there is superimposed pregnancy induced hypertension.
Placental abruption occurs in 5–10% of cases.
It is difficult to differentiate essential HT from pregnancy induced hypertension when the patient is seen in second trimester.

2. Pregnancy induced hypertension (PIH)
It is defined as the occurrence of a blood pressure of 140/90 mm Hg or above on at least two occasions four hours or more apart after the 20th week of pregnancy in a woman known to be normotensive before this time and in whom blood pressure has returned to normal by the sixth postpartum week. However, this definition does not distinguish borderline essential hypertension from true pregnancy induced hypertension.
Complicates 5–7% of pregnancies in otherwise normal primigravida women. More prevalent in Negroes, 30% black primiparous women are affected.
The BP more than 140/90 mm Hg after 20 weeks of gestation or SBP >30 mm Hg and/or DBP > 15 mm Hg over the baseline. This rise should be maintained for 6-hour period.
Serum urate level > 5.5 mg% is a strong biochemical indication of PIH or superimposed PIH on chronic HT
Placental abruption occurs in 2–10% of cases.

65. Pre-eclampsia: Hypertension appearing after 20 weeks of gestation usually accompanied by proteinuria and edema.

Chronic HT or PIH + Proteinuria + edema

Many writers use the term "Toxemia of Pregnancy" as a synonym for pre-eclampsia. Some describe all hypertensive disorders of pregnancy as toxemia of pregnancy, a term that is not logical and ambiguous as there is no toxin in the blood. Pre-eclampsia occurs during gestation or 7 days of delivery. Usually begins after 32 weeks of pregnancy, but can occur earlier, in women with pre-existing renal disease or HT. More in underdeveloped countries, more than 30% in Puerto Rico.
Peak incidence is in young primipara or in multiparous women over 35 years. Occurs in first trimester in hydatidiform mole.

Predisposing factors of pre-eclampsia are:
1. Primipara
2. Multipara over 35 years
3. Family H/o of pre-eclampsia or eclampsia
4. Chronic HT
5. Hydatidiform mole
6. Diabetes mellitus
7. Fetal hydrops
8. Multiple fetuses.

Pre-eclampsia is to be suspected when the HT is associated with symptoms of:
1. *Headache:* It is a frequent forerunner of first convulsion and is resistant to ordinary treatment.
2. *Visual disturbance:* From slight blurring to blindness due to retinal arteriolar spasm, ischemia, edema, etc. Scanty urine as a result of renal impairment. Epigastric distress or pain is a late symptom, may be the result of stretching of hepatic capsule by hemorrhage or of CNS origin. Apprehension, etc. Usually indicates imminent convulsions.
3. *Proteinuria:* Albumin traces to 2+ for 6 hours period of more than 300 mg in 24 hour urine collection, granular or hyaline casts are present. RBC and cellular casts are infrequent.
4. *Edema:* It is difficult to assess as 8.3 % of normal healthy pregnant women have some degree of edema. If the weight gain is more than 4 to 5 lbs in one week, edema is to be suspected (normal weight gain is 1 lb per week). Fundus shows retinal arterial spasm. Segmental arterial narrowing and a glistening retinal sheen are indicative of edema. Hemorrhage and exudates occur late and only in severe cases.
High blood uric acid level is common, reflecting a reduction in urate clearance.
Pre-eclampsia is further divided into mild and severe.
The ominous signs and symptoms of severe pre-eclampsia are:
   - SBP >160 mm Hg or more, DBP > 110 mm Hg or more for at least 6 hour after bed rest
   - Proteinuria of 5 g or more in 24 hour (3 or 4 + on qualitative test)
   - Oliguria (400 mL or less in 24 hour)
   - Platelet count <10 × 10^9 L or evidence of microangiopathic hemolytic anemia
   - Cerebral or visual disturbances due to retinal hemorrhages, exudates and papilledema
   - Pulmonary edema or cyanosis.
   - Severe epigastric pain
   - Fetal growth retardation
5. Eclampsia:
Pre-eclampsia (severe HT + proteinuria + edema)+ convulsions and coma in whom there is no coincidental neurological disorder like epilepsy, etc.

Maternal mortality ranges from 0–17% with majority of fatalities secondary to cerebral hemorrhage.

Fetal mortality rate is 10–37%.

66. Chronic hypertension in pregnancy threatens bad prognosis when the following 4 signs are present:

1. When cardiac enlargement or ECG changes are present, it indicates a grave outlook in pregnancy, as the cardiac failure is the most common cause of death in hypertensive vascular disease.
2. When renal function is markedly impaired—life expectancy of the mother is poor regardless of pregnancy.
3. When fundus examination shows old retinal hemorrhage or fresh hemorrhages usually indicates renal impairment or superimposed preeclampsia. It suggests grave prognosis and needs special care.
4. When initial SBP > 200 or DBP > 120 mm Hg, indicates higher risk of perinatal mortality in excess of 50% and higher incidence of maternal complications than milder chronic hypertensives. Chances of superimposed pre-eclampsia are greater if there is history of pre-eclampsia in previous pregnancy or pregnancies.

67. Pregnancy induced hypertension (PIH) is 20–40% more common in women with the following 4 underlying diseases:

1. Chronic renal disease
2. Essential hypertension
3. Diabetes mellitus
4. Systemic lupus erythematosus (SLE).

68. Following features favor the diagnosis of primary hypertension over pregnancy induced hypertension (PIH):

1. Onset of hypertension before 20 weeks of gestation.
2. Age over 30 years
3. Hypertension not caused by pre-eclampsia in a previous pregnancy
4. No hypertension during first pregnancy, but its appearance in subsequent ones
5. Absence of proteinuria and edema
6. Evidence of sustained and severe hypertension (SBP = 200 mm Hg)
7. Evidence of left ventricular hypertrophy
8. Evidence of retinal hemorrhages or exudates.

69. The following 4 predisposing factors contribute to the reduction of uteroplacental blood flow in pre-eclampsia:

1. Chiefly primigravida (70%) has more tense abdominal walls leading to increased intra-abdominal pressure which could be enhanced by obesity or short stature.
2. More space occupying conditions which increase the intra-abdominal pressure, such as multiple pregnancy, hydromnios, vesicular mole.
3. Maternal diseases that cause vasoconstriction such as diabetes mellitus, hypertension, renal diseases.
4. Production of vasospasm—either general or locally on the uterus as in emotional stress. More number of cases are seen in working women who are prone to more stress at home and outside.

70. Some other risk factors of pre-eclampsia include:

1. Limited exposure using condoms: Immunologic mechanisms—there may be an association with the duration and degree of exposure to antigen in the father's sperm. Women who develop pre-eclampsia tend to have shorter durations of cohabitation than women who do not have hypertension during pregnancy, suggesting that repeated exposure to male ejaculate may prevent pre-eclampsia. Similarly, the risk is great in women who use contraceptions that block exposure to sperm.
   There may be risk in women with oral sex and in women who have more interval between two pregnancies.
   Women with previous miscarriages or prior blood transfusion have reduced risk of pre-eclampsia due to altered maternal immune reactions.
2. Smoking
3. Stress
4. Family h/o pre-eclampsia
5. Obesity
6. Urinary tract infections
7. Diabetes type I
8. Hyperhomocysteinemia.

71. It is observed that larger the trophoblastic or placental mass the greater the incidence of pre-eclampsia as seen in the following 4 categories of patients:

1. Multiple pregnancy
2. Diabetes mellitus
3. Hydrops fetalis
4. Hydatidiform mole.

Accelerated dissemination of trophoblastic tissue fragments into maternal circulation also occurs.

72. Placenta plays the following adverse roles in toxemia of pregnancy:

1. Thromboplastin is liberated from placenta by ischemia.
2. Causes diminished uteroplacental flow leading to anoxia.
3. Ischemia or injury again liberates thromboplastin.
4. It indicates intravascular coagulation (some lesions in placenta are more extensive in pre-eclampsia)—like syncitial knots, increased number of true infarcts, loss

of syncytium, proliferation of cytotrophoblast, villous necrosis, acute fibrinoid degeneration of maternal dicidual arteries.

73. Pathogenesis of pre-eclampsia/eclampsia shows the following differences from the normal pregnancy:

Table V-3

	Normal pregnancy	*Pre-eclampsia/ eclampsia*
Hemodynamics		
1. Plasma volume	increased	decreased
2. Extracellular fluid volume	increased	decreased
3. Cardiac output	increased	decreased
4. Peripheral vascular resistance	decreased	increased
Vascular reactivity		
5. To vasopressin	unchanged	increased
6. To epinephrine	unchanged	increased
7. To norepinephrine	unchanged	increased
8. To angiotensin	decreased	increased
Renal function		
9. Blood flow	increased	decreased
10. Glomerular filtration rate	increased	decreased
11. Plasma uric acid	decreased	increased
12. Excretion of sodium load	normal	unchanged
Hormonal changes		
13. Plasma renin substrate	increased	unchanged
14. Plasma renin activity	increased	decreased
15. Plasma angiotensin II	increased	decreased
16. Angiotensin II receptor	decreased	increased
17. Plasma aldosterone	increased	decreased
18. Mineralocorticoid receptors	increased	decreased
19. Plasma insulin	increased	increased
20. Prostacyclin synthesis	increased	decreased
21. Thromboxane synthesis	increased	increased
22. Gonadotrophin	normal	increased
23. Estrogen	increased	decreased
24. Progesterone	increased	decreased

From the above features, it is deduced that the normal pregnancy is associated with increase in plasma volume, extracellular fluid volume with rise in cardiac output which are likely adaptations to progressive vasodilatation induced by hormonal milieu. Various factors help in vasodilatation—placenta imposes an arteriovenous shunt on the maternal circulation, the endothelial cells make more vasodilatory prostaglandins and nitric oxide, and increased levels of progesterone and estrogen may contribute.

As a result of these vasodilatory forces, the pressor response to exogenous angiotensin II becomes progressively lessened. Plasma levels of atrial natriuretic factor are increased, providing further evidence that despite an increased fluid volume the central circulation is not over expanded.

Peripheral edema is common along with the increased blood volume, but this often arises from interference of venous return by the enlarged uterus.

It is inferred now that normal pregnancy is a low blood pressure state associated with marked vasodilatation that reduces peripheral resistance, along with an expanded volume that increases cardiac output. Renal blood flow is markedly increased and the renin-aldosterone system is activated.

In pre-eclampsia/eclampsia, the basic abnormality seems to be profound vasoconstriction that reduces the intravascular capacity even more than blood volume. Intense vasospasm often can be seen in the nail beds, retina and coronary arteries. The hypoxia resulting from vasospasm leads to various changes in tissue structure and function. Structural alterations include, increased thickness of media, deposition of fibrin products resulting in diminution of blood flow. In severe cases of preeclampsia, plasma volume is reduced by 10–40%. Cardiac output is low, peripheral resistance is increased.

There is an increased response to pressor substances like vasopressin, epinephrine, norepinephrine, angiotensin in pre-eclampsia. Increased response to angiotensin precedes the development of hypertension. However, there is a controversy over the role of angiotensin in hypertension of pre-eclampsia.

74. Maternal consequences of pre-eclampsia/eclampsia:

1. HELLP syndrome

   A few women may develop serious complications of pre-eclampsia in the HELLP syndrome which involves ***h***emolysis, ***e***levated ***l***iver enzymes, and ***l***ow ***p***latelet counts. This syndrome has many similarities with the hemolytic syndrome and thrombotic thrombocytopenic purpura. Maternal and prenatal mortality increases with severity of thrombocytopenia below 150000/mL.
2. Disseminated intravascular coagulation (DIC)
3. Renal failure
4. Acute left ventricular failure
5. Cerebrovascular accidents

6. Acute yellow atrophy
7. Retinal detachment
8. Adult respiratory distress syndrome (ARDS).

75. Fetal consequences of pre-eclampsia/eclampsia

1. Decrease in fetal ballotment
2. Intrauterine growth retardation (IUGR)
3. Chronic fetal distress
4. Fetal death.

Chronic fetal distress in pre-eclampsia can give rise to cerebral palsy.

76. Renal lesions in preeclampsia/eclampsia show the following changes:

1. Reversible generalized swelling of glomerular tufts.
2. Thickening of basement membrane.
3. Increase in cytoplasm of endothelial cells resulting in narrowing of the capillary lumen.
4. Sub or interendothelial fibrinoid deposition.

1,2,3 are combinedly known as glomerular endotheliosis. As a result of these lesions, leakage of plasma proteins occur in the urine and they coagulate to form hyaline casts.

Narrowing of the capillary lumen causes reduction in glomerular filtration rate and renal blood flow. If the lesions are severe oliguria results. Reduced glomerular filtration rate and other hormonal changes of pregnancy causes retention of sodium and water.

The fibrinoid deposition is the result of slow relatively chronic disseminated intravascular coagulation.

77. The following biochemical tests are to be done in toxemia of pregnancy to know the severity BUN and urea clearance are within normal limits:

1. Rise in uric acid levels indicates the severity of toxemia
2. Delay of sodium excretion as a result of sodium retention. Blood chlorides increase
3. Hemoconcentration
4. Serum proteins decrease and the albumin factor is being most affected.

78. Following 4 pathological changes occur in eclampsia:

1. Rate of dissemination of intravascular coagulation is more rapid and more severe than in pre-eclampsia.
2. Fatal cases show multiple platelet emboli and fibrin emboli with perivascular hemorrhages in the brain.
3. Small petechial hemorrhages in the nuclei and white matter surrounding the ventricles are seen.
4. Such lesions together with severe vasoconstriction and tissue hypoxia cause convulsions and coma.

Repeated platelet count should be done in pre-eclampsia patients. In severe cases of very low platelet counts, (less than 50,000 to 100,000) platelet transfusion is advised.

79. Eclampsia is more frequent during the last trimester of pregnancy. It may occur in the following situations:

1. Antepartum—occurring before the onset of labor.
2. Intrapartum—occurring when the women is in labor.
3. Postpartum—occurring for the first time after delivery.
4. Antenatal—(intercurrent eclampsia) where the patient recovers from an attack and pregnancy continues.

80. When a woman suffering from hypertension becomes pregnant, the prognosis depends on:

1. A drop of 10–20 mm Hg SBP in the middle of second trimester, begins to rise again in the third trimester and may not reach higher than the pressure present at the start of pregnancy, there will be good prognosis.
2. When pressure continues to rise throughout pregnancy, there will be bad prognosis.
3. When toxemia supervenes—when SBP is over 160 mm Hg, proteinuria appears—edema develops, there will be bad prognosis.
4. When SBP is 180–200 or more even without proteinuria, there will be bad prognosis.

Prognosis is also bad when patient starts her pregnancy with SBP of 160 mm Hg or more and where the pressure steadily rises during pregnancy.

81. The objectives of treatment in pregnancy with hypertension are:

1. Prevention of convulsions, i.e. to prevent eclampsia
2. Delivery of a surviving child—Higher incidence of fetal morality, 10–40%.
   Fetal mortality rate starts increasing from diastolic pressure of > 85–90 mm Hg.
3. Safe delivery with minimum trauma (higher incidence of maternal mortality in eclampsia, majority are secondary to cerebral hemorrhage).
4. Prevention of residual hypertension.

82. The management of toxemia of pregnancy is discussed under the following 4 heads:

1. General management
2. Sedative management
3. Hypertensive management
4. Obstetrical management.

83. General management consists of:

1. Modified bed rest
2. Diet
3. Record maintenance
4. Elimination.

Encourage absolute bed rest with good nursing. Encourage to lie on one side or other rather than rest in supine position to improve urinary output. It helps in the control of hypertension and edema.

Diet should consists of more carbohydrates, less of protein and little of fats with total calories of about 2500. Encouraged to take more fluids such as barley water, fruit juice or diluted milk. As the patient starts improving, fluid diet is gradually replaced by ordinary diet.

Restriction of salt is debated (average daily salt in ordinary diet is 15–20 g which may be reduced to 5 to 6 g). Dietary supplements with calcium and magnesium is of some help.

84. Rest in left lateral position in toxemia of pregnancy helps in the following 4 ways:

1. Reduces aortocaval compression by gravid uterus thereby improving circulation to the lower limbs and return of blood to the heart.
2. Prevents supine hypertension syndrome.
3. Improves uteroplacental circulation.
4. Prevents aspiration of secretions in case the patient is under sedation.

85. Following records should be maintained:

1. Record of blood pressure 4th hourly
2. Daily intake and output chart
3. Daily weight
4. Daily urinary test for proteins.

Transient Hypertension

Blood pressure is elevated during pregnancy or in the first 24 hour of postpartum with no other signs of pre-eclampsia or pre-existing hypertension. This may be a manifestation of latent chronic hypertension, usually recurs in subsequent pregnancies and is responsible for most misdiagnosis of pre-eclampsia in multiparous women. However, this is not especially helpful as a predictor because of the "white coat hypertension", effects of hospitals, the normal fluctuations in blood pressure over short time, especially when there is apprehension. The blood pressure is high when it is taken by the superior-head of the unit—because of more fear and may be normal when a nurse is taken.

Inadequacies in blood pressure measurements may be found though it is within the normal range.

Reliable readings of maternal blood pressure are needed from early in pregnancy, certainly before 20 weeks of gestation. This will provide baseline record from which to assess the rise in pressure as the pregnancy progresses. This will also identifies the women with borderline and previously undiagnosed chronic hypertension. Women who develop pre-eclampsia have significant high systolic and diastolic blood pressures in second trimester.

Recording blood pressure in pregnancy should be measured with the woman seated or lying on her left side. Profound hypotension can occur in late pregnancy if a woman lies supine because of the mechanical obstruction of the inferior vena cava by the gravid uterus.

Roll-over-test in pregnant women: Record the blood pressure in left lateral position. After 5 to10 minutes, record the blood pressure in supine position. If the diastolic blood pressure goes up by 20 mm Hg, she may go into toxemia. It starts after 24 weeks of pregnancy. If positive, 90% may go into toxemia of pregnancy.

General practitioner and clinician should provide two sizes of cuff with an inflation bladders of 35 cm and 42 cm length. The cuff should depend on the arm circumference, with the bladder length being at least 80% of that circumference. Cuff width is not important above a minimum width of 11 cm. The center of the bladder must be placed directly over the artery to be compressed.

The question of whether to use Korotkoff sound IV or V remains highly controversial. The disappearance of sound phase V is more accurate, reliable, and less variable than the muffling phase 4. The use of the 4th sound avoids the problem of the occasionally encountered failure of disappearance of sound in pregnancy, but the frequency of occurrence of this problem is disputed. Better to follow anyone accurately in a hospital setting. Consistency in measurement throughout pregnancy should be the aim.

The rounding of blood pressure measurements (200/100, 180/80, 140/90/150/70) should be avoided as it can lead to wide variability. It is preferable to attempt record the blood pressure as accurately as possible, even though such accuracy will vary between observers.

The systolic blood pressure level is a better guide to the fetal outcome than the diastolic blood pressure. Every increment in maternal blood pressure at 28 or 36 weeks gestation was associated with a significant decrease in fetal birthweight.

The woman's weight and height should be measured at least at the first visit. The initial body mass index (weight (kg) /(height)(m^2)) is quite a useful predictor of hypertension having higher body mass indices.

Normal and abnormal may overlap. Hypertension identified from body mass index is likely to indicate the development of chronic hypertension (Normal weight gain is 1 lb per week).

Urine test for proteins is not accurate with dipsticks, though values designated +++ and ++++ do indicate severe disease. Proteinurea is best monitored in 24 hour urine collection, a value in excess of 500 mg/L being clinically important and helps in identifying in the progression of proteinuria.

86. Elimination: As the plasma volume is reduced and poor placental perfusion exists in severe pre-eclampsia, it seems illogical on scientific grounds to use diuretics unless the disease has progressed to renal failure, in which case, extra care should be taken.

Thiazide diuretics in women are used with chronic hypertension if prescribed before gestation or if the patient appeared salt sensitive. Thiazide diuretics can cause thrombocytopenia, so they are avoided. Loop diuretics such as furosemide may be given if necessary. Of late, the use of diuretics in the management of toxemia of pregnancy is also debated.

Diuretics are used only when there is definite need with great caution.

1. Hydrochlorothiazide 50–100 mg od
2. Chlorthalidone 50–100 mg od
3. Furosemide—40 mg od
4. Hypertonic glucose—20% glucose of 100–500 mL IV or more daily to promote diuresis.

87. The improvement is noticed by the following 4 changes:

1. Control of hypertension
2. Loss of weight
3. Disappearance of edema
4. Disappearance of urinary proteins.

Most of the mild cases are followed in these lines.

88. Sedative management of pregnancy with HT consists of any of the following 4 drugs usually depends on physician's preference:

1. Diazepam—10–20 mg IV in severe cases.
   Continuous sedation is to be given by 40 mg in 500 cc of 5% dextrose IV drip and not more than 300 mg in 24 hours. It is a good sedative and anticonvulsant. So, useful in eclampsia also.
2. Pethidine 100 mg IM—may be repeated 50 mg every 4 to 6 hours.
3. Magnesium sulfate 10–20 mL of 15–20% solution IM/IV may be repeated every 4 hours with usual precautions and not more than 20 gm given in 24 hours. It is a sedative as well as anticonvulsant. So useful in eclampsia.
4. Chlorpromazine—25 to 50 mg po or IM may be repeated. It is a sedative as well as hypotensive. So useful in eclampsia. Chlorpromazine 50 mg IM + phenergan 25 mg IM combination also may be given.

Pritchard's regime, Zuspan's regime, Sibai regime, Menomi's regime, etc. are mentioned with various combinations of magnesium sulfate, pethidine, phenergan, diazepam, chlorpromazine, etc. in the control of convulsions in eclampsia.

Diazepam infusion can cause respiratory distress syndrome. Magnesium sulfate is found to be good. Corticosteroids 2 mg × 6th hourly is given to control the cerebral edema.

89. Drugs in hypertension management: When considering the use of any drugs in pregnancy, doctors must always remember that they are treating two patients, one of whom has immature hepatic and renal function while the other may develop impaired hepatic and renal function. The following 4 hypotensive drugs are used in pregnancy in order of preference:

1. Methyldopa
2. Hydralazine
3. Labetalol
4. Nifedipine.

Control of Hypertension

When the BP is high during labor—it is to be immediately controlled by hydralazine 20 mg in 20 mL of 5% dextrose IV slowly.

A reasonable drop in BP occurs in 15 to 30 minutes in majority of cases and to be maintained for varying periods.

Chlorpromazine—Hypotensive and sedative affect 25 mg po every 4 to 6 hours.

Their main use is to get immediate action especially in labor when it is likely to rise to higher levels. So, it should have immediate action, prolonged effect without any side effects on either mother or child.

None of the routinely used antihypertensive drugs are teratogenic.

The hypotensive drugs should not be routinely used.

There is abnormal fall of BP in second trimester and decreases the need of hypotensive agents.

90. Choice of antihypertensive drugs in pregnancy:

Table V-4

Drug	*Mechanism of action*	*Dose*	*Comments*
1. Alpha methyldopa	Central α 2 agonists	250 mg tid up to 4 g per day	Safe, most commonly used drug of choice
2. Hydralazine	Direct vasodilator	5–10 mg IV every 15–30 minutes	Efficacious and safe, during pregnancy and lactation. Treatment of choice in eclampsia
3. Labetalol	α-β adrenergic blocker	20–80 mg IV every 10–20 minutes up to 300 mg	Second line of treatment appears efficacious widely used; scant safety data

Contd...

Contd...

Drug	Mechanism of action	Dose	Comments
4. Nifedipine/ Ramipril	Calcium channel blocker	10 mg qid up to 120 mg per day Ramipril 5–10 mg od or bid	Second line of treatment fetal distress from maternal hypertension is a concern

Sympatholytic agents especially methyldopa and labetalol are widely used in pregnancy induced hypertension and pre-eclampsia. They have a limited effect on the hypertension, which is not mediated by the sympathetic nervous system but it may be sufficient to allow useful prolongation of gestation. Their comparatively short-term use is not associated with intrauterine growth retardation, although growth retardation has been reported after longer use of β-blockers (atenolol) in pregnant women with chronic hypertension.

α 2-methyldopa, a drug that has been largely abandoned in the treatment of hypertension in every setting save pregnancy, reduces mid trimester abortions, perinatal deaths without causing any physical or mental abnormalities in the offspring followed for more than seven years. Rarely, hepatotoxicity may occur.

Vasodilators seem to be a more logical treatment. Direct vasodilator hydralazine is mostly used in cases of emergency in eclampsia. Hydralazine is also used as an adjunctive therapy with methyldopa.

α-and β-blockers, labetalol appears to be as effective as methyldopa, but there is little or no follow-up information on children born to mothers treated with labetalol. There is growing experience with parenteral preparations in pre-eclampsia/eclampsia.

Calcium channel blockers are increasingly used, especially nifedipine, nitrendipine or nimodipine.

The ACEI are contraindicated in pregnancy because of the adverse effects on the fetus. Their use in pregnant women has been associated with oligohydramnios, stillbirth, and neonatal anuria.

The fall in prostacyclin produced in pre-eclampsia and the observation that low doses of aspirin (60–150 mg od) inhibit thromboxane synthase but not prostacyclin synthase led to the suggestion that aspirin might be a suitable prophylactic agent against pre-eclampsia. However, aspirin may have a place in treating women with a history of pre-eclampsia before 30 to 32 weeks of gestation. Such women should probably start prophylactic treatment early in the second trimester. It has no role in high-risk women.

91. Antihypertensive drugs to be used with caution/avoid/ contraindicated in pregnancy:

Table V-5

Drug	Safety	Recommendations
1. Diuretics	Possible risk of compromising utero-placental circulation	To be used with caution
2. β-blockers	Should not be given in first trimester May be efficacious in late pregsnancy Use in late pregnancy can cause neonatal asphyxia, hypoglycemia, bradycardia. Atenolol has been associated with intrauterine growth retardation. It is the drug of choice in pregnancy with stenotic lesions (MS, AS) and in HOCM, Marfans' syndrome	Avoid (should not be given in first trimester)
3. ACE-I	Dangerous as they may cause oligohydramnios, intrauterine growth retardation, and renal dysfunction specially after using in second or third trimester. Can induce neonatal renal failure and hypotension	Contraindicated
4. Angiotensin receptor antagonists	Same as ACEI	Contraindicated

92. Clinical management of patients with pregnancy induced hypertension (PIH) is described in 4 types depending on the severity of HT and maturity of the fetus.

Table V-6

Clinical condition	Treatment
1. Mild PIH and immature fetus. Compliant patient and improvement	Expectant Ambulatory management a. General management consists of rest, diet, records, diuretics b. The patient is to be observed twice a week c. Fetal surveillance d. Educate about the increasing severity of the disease.

Contd...

Contd...

Clinical condition	*Treatment*
2. Noncompliant patient or lack of improvement	Hospitalization a. General management b. Fetal surveillance c. Patient is to be evaluated for headache, visual disturbances, epigastric pain or rapid weight gain d. No salt restriction (debated)
3. Severe PIH and immature fetus in the presence of fetal growth retardation or fetal jeopardy	Definitive a. Prevent convulsions ($MgSO_4$) b. Control hypertension (Hydralazine) c. Delivery by vaginal or Cesarean operation depending upon fetal and maternal condition
4. Severe PIH and mature fetus	Definitive a. Prevention of convulsions ($MgSO_4$) b. Control BP (Hydralazine) c. Delivery by vaginal or Cesarean operation, depending upon fetal and maternal conditions

93. Malignant hypertension is a grave condition. It is risky for both mother and fetus. Better terminated as soon as possible. The following 4 steps may be followed:

1. General treatment with complete bed rest—and careful watching.
2. Reserpine 0.25 mg bd.
   If possible, may be stopped 7 to 10 days before delivery.
3. Methyldopa 250 mg tds.
4. Sympathectomy in hypertension in selected cases, if diastolic pressure is high or pulse pressure is low.

Consider if the outlook for a successful pregnancy is poor.
Bilateral lumbodorsal sympathectomy—T8 to L3—sympathetic trunk.
A time interval of at least one year after operation is desirable before next pregnancy. Pregnancy is safe in a patient, who had a successful sympathectomy for hypertension.

94. Fetal surveillance is defined as tests of fetal well-being. It includes (but not limited) the following 4 records that are to be maintained:

1. Fetal movement charts
2. Contraction stress tests
3. Nonstress tests
4. Biophysical profiles.

A. Urinary estriol below 4 mg in 24 hours after 34 weeks of pregnancy is suggestive of fetal distress. Unwise to depend on a single test. Falling estriol levels as pregnancy advances would seem to be more significant.

B. Human placental lactogen (HPL) useful in assessment of placental function. HPL levels in PET are always low when intrauterine death occurs. Serum HPL levels are found to be related to severity of hypertension. Repeated estimation is necessary to have correct assessment than a single one.

95. The following 4 indications of fetus status are to be considered for induction of labor in pregnancy with hypertension.

1. Fetal maturity
2. Fetal distress
3. Fetal growth retardation
4. Progression to severe PIH.

When early onset severe pre-eclampsia is accompanied by ominous signals such as blurred vision, laboratory evidence of coagulation and fetal distress, termination of pregnancy may be considered best for mother and fetus.
Fetal Doppler studies are now available to know the cerebral blood flow, fetal distress, etc.
Middle cerebral artery flow, transcerebral flow, umbilical artery flow are now studied. Decrease in blood flow indicates fetal distress symptoms.

96. The management of a patient with PIH or chronic HT who presents in labor with a matured fetus consists of prevention of convulsions and the treatment of hypertension.

1. Magnesium sulfate IM or IV 5 g IM every 4 hours.
   Since eclampsia is most likely to come during labor, all women in labor with PIH should receive prophylaxis for convulsions. It should be maintained for 24 hours after delivery or 24 hours after the last convulsion, if eclampsia develops after postpartum. Magnesium sulfate causes dilatation of small intracranial vessels and relieves cerebral ischemia and has been found superior to other anticonvulsants. Its use has been associated with decreased cardiovascular damage in preterm infants.

University of Tennessee guidelines for intravenous magnesium sulfate administration:

Loading dose

Give 30 mL of 20% magnesium sulfate solution (6 g) in 100 mL of 5% dextrose over 10–15 minutes period.

Maintenance dose

Add 20 g of magnesium sulfate (four 10 mL ampoules of 50% solution) to 1000 mL of 5% dextrose and give intravenously at the rate of 100 mL/hr (2 g/hr). Obtain serum magnesium level 4–6 hours later and adjust the rate of infusion to keep the serum magnesium level between 4.8 and 9.6 mg/dL.

If the serum magnesium levels are not available the dose is adjusted according to the patellar reflex and the urine output during the last 4 hours period.

Pritchard's guidelines for intramuscular magnesium sulfate administration to patients with pre-eclampsia.

Intramuscular loading dose

Administer 10 mL of 50% magnesium sulfate solution (5 g) deeply in the outer quadrant of each buttock using 3 inch 20 gauge needle. The IM dose should immediately follow the intravenous dose in the patients with convulsions. Patients without convulsions receive only the intramuscular loading dose.

Maintenance dose

Give 5 g (10 mL of 50% solution) deep by IM injection in alternate buttock every 4 hours if the following criteria are met:

The patellar reflex is present. The urine output has been at least 100 mL during the preceding 3 hours. The respiration rate is normal (at least 14/min).

2. Injection hydralazine 5 to 10 mg IV slowly with additional 5 to 10 mg boluses every 20 min as necessary to control HT

   Acts directly on vascular resistance.

   Hypertension is treated when the DBP is over 110 mm Hg. Caution is taken to avoid over treatment. Placental circulation is impaired if diastolic goes below 90 mm Hg.

   Side effects include tachycardia and headache if there is no response.
3. Diazoxide in cases resistant or unresponsive to hydralazine. 30 mg of mini boluses are given since precipitation of hypotension may result with higher doses. Side effects include arrest of labor and neonatal hypoglycemia.
4. Injection nitroglycerin is tried in resistant cases. Refrain from using sodium nitroprusside because fetal cyanosis poisoning has been reported in experimental animals. However, maternal safety should dictate the choice of therapy.

   Parentral hydralazine is not available in India. Instead calcium channel blockers like nifedipine 10 mg doses or nimodipine 60 mg are giving promising results. Nimodipine improves the fetal cerebral blood flow also. There may be synergism between the calcium blockers and magnesium sulfate which may lead to precipitous declines in blood pressure levels, especially when used to control severe hypertension during labor.

97. Magnesium sulfate score more advantages in pre-eclampsia/eclampsia by the following 4 reasons:

1. Increases prostaglandins
2. Increases vasodilatation
3. Increases uterine blood flow
4. Increases bronchi dilatation.

   It decreases platelet aggregation also.

98. The following 4 precautions are to be taken while giving repeated doses of magnesium sulfate:

1. Check the knee-jerks before each injection. The drug is to be given only if they are active.
2. Check the respiration. It should be given only if they are 14 or more/min.
3. Check the urinary output for successive injections after initial dose. It should be at least 100 mL during preceding 3 hours, because it is excreted through kidneys only.
4. Always keep the injection calcium gluconate (1 g in 10 mL) by the side as an immediate antidose. If the patient is on digitalis, calcium is injected very slowly and cautiously.

The development of hyper-reflex or clones, or both, a fall in platelet count to below 10×100^9/L; and any rise in plasma transaminase are important warning features of deterioration in maternal or fetal condition.

99. Hydralazine acts in the following 4 ways:

1. Prevents vascular damage by relieving vascular spasm.
2. Prevents rupture of damaged vessels in the brain or elsewhere by marked reduction of hypertension.
3. Prevents strain on heart by reducing the after load.
4. Increases renal blood flow.

100. Hydralazine is to be preferred for the following 4 reasons:

1. It does not affect the cardiac output.
2. It increases renal blood flow.
3. It increases cerebral blood flow.
4. Side effects are less and no harmful effect either on the mother or the child.

It is useful for immediate control of BP especially during labor when it is likely to raise to very high levels.

101. Management of eclampsia: Delivery is delayed until convulsions are stopped, blood pressure is controlled, fluid and electrolyte balance is maintained.

1. Magnesium sulfate to control convulsions.
2. Control of severe hypertension (DBP 110 mm Hg) with intermittent intravenous hydralazine.
3. Limitation of fluid intake, unless fluid loss was excessive. Avoidance of diuretics and hyperosmotic agents.
4. Delivery once convulsions are arrested and consciousness is regained.

W Miscellaneous Subjects Related to Cardiology

CARDIOVASCULAR MANIFESTATIONS OF SYSTEMIC DISEASES

DIABETES AND HEART

Diabetes is a potent and independent cardiovascular risk factor. About 80% of all deaths and 75% of all hospitalization in diabetic patients are due to cardiovascular disease (CVD).

1. **Diabetes and heart could be discussed under 4 headings.**
   1. *Diabetes and coronary heart disease:*
      Ischemic heart disease account about 20% of deaths in diabetes in countries like India (about 40% in the West). Ischemic heart disease is two and five times more common in diabetic men and women, respectively compared to the general population. Sudden deaths due to cardiac arrest are more common in diabetes. Comorbidities including renal insufficiency peripheral and cerebrovascular diseases that are more prevalent in patients with diabetes are often worsen outcomes.
   2. *Diabetic cardiomyopathy:*
      Cardiomyopathy and left ventricular dysfunction in diabetes can be independent of coronary heart disease. Left ventricular dysfunction and cardiac decompensation are common in diabetics and may manifest in the form of exertional dyspnea, paroxysmal nocturnal dyspnea and congestive cardiac failure.
      Recurrent congestive heart failure may be an indicator of diabetic cardiomyopathy.
      Infants born to diabetic mothers may have temporary cardiomyopathy (thickening of interventricular septum diagnosed by echocardiogram).
   3. *Diabetic autonomic neuropathy and heart:*
      Both sympathetic and parasympathetic may be involved.
      Resting tachycardia is the commonest symptom.
      It is associated with silent heart attacks and with high mortality.
   4. *Effect of heart disease on carbohydrate metabolism:*
      Stress hyperglycemia particularly during acute myocardial infarction is an important abnormality.
      Stress ketosis also may occur in myocardial infarction.

Diabetes, Hypertension and Coronary Artery Disease

Hypertension and diabetes appear to increase coronary heart disease risk in part by causing an abnormality in lipid metabolism. Most affected are patients with familial dyslipidemic hypertension (FDH) and noninsulin dependent diabetes mellitus (NIDDM). The lipid disorders most often encountered in these patients are increased levels of triglycerides, very low-density lipoprotein (VLDL) cholesterol, and small, dense low-density lipoprotein (LDL) cholesterol, and low-levels of high-density lipoprotein (HDL) cholesterol. These abnormalities appear to result from increased hepatic secretion of VLDL particles due to increased concentrations of free fatty acids and glucose, reduced VLDL clearance due to reduced activity of lipoprotein lipase, and reduced LDL clearance due to glycosylation of proteins. Treatment of the dyslipidemia associated with FDH should follow the guidelines from the National Cholesterol Education Program of USA. Treatment in men and women with NIDDM should be considered when LDL cholesterol levels are 130 mg/dL or above, triglyceride levels are 200 mg/dL or above, or non-HDL cholesterol levels are 160 mg/dL or greater. Aggressive lifestyle changes should be initiated: first, including weight loss in obese patients, control of glucose levels in those with NIDDM, avoidance of antihypertensive drugs that may worsen lipid levels in patients with FDH, and eating a diet restricting saturated fat and cholesterol. Addition of lipid altering drugs should be considered if such changes do not achieve effective lipid control. The agent should be tailored to the patient's lipid profile, in general by using bile acid resins, niacin, or reductase inhibitors to lower LDL cholesterol and gemfibrozil or niacin to lower triglycerides. Niacin should be avoided in patients with NIDDM.

Vascular complications of diabetes mellitus manifests mainly as microvascular and macrovascular complications.

Duration of diabetes mellitus is an important factor in the pathogenesis of complications. Other risk factors like hypertension, cigarette smoking, obesity, hypercholesterolemia interact with diabetes to affect the clinical course of microangiopathy and macroangiopathy.

Microangiopathy include retinopathy, nephropathy and neuropathy.

Macroangiopathy include coronary artery disease, stroke, peripheral vascular disease.

Macrovascular complications: Atherosclerosis in diabetes accounts for most of the excess mortality. In the UK prospective diabetes mellitus study, fatal cardiovascular events were 70 times more common than deaths from microvascular complications. Hypertension affects at least half of the patients with diabetes.

2. There are 4 features of atherosclerosis in coronary artery disease in diabetic patients:

1. Prevalence of fatal and nonfatal coronary artery disease events are 2–20 times higher than for non-diabetics of similar age.
2. Protective effect of female sex is lost.
3. Higher incidence of diffuse, multivessel disease.
4. Plaque rupture and superimposed thrombosis leading to unstable angina and myocardial infarction is more common.

3. 4 features of acute myocardial infarction in diabetic patients:

1. In hospital and six-month follow-up mortality is double that in non-diabetic
2. Complications like arrhythmias, heart failure, death are more common.
3. Reperfusion rates after thrombolysis are similar to those of non-diabetic but reocclusion and reinfarction rates are higher.
4. Mortality is reduced by insulin-glucose-infusion immediately after myocardial infarction.

5-year survival better after coronary artery bypass graft than percutaneous coronary angioplasty because of higher rates of restenosis with angioplasty (81% vs 60%).

5-year survival rates after bypass graft or angioplasty are lower than non-diabetes.

4. Severity of the CAD in DM is due to:

1. Higher incidence of multivessel involvement.
2. More severe in the single vessel disease.
3. More diffuse.
4. More incidence of acute myocardial infarction.

5. Accelarated atherosclerosis is the cause of increase in incidence of IHD.

1. Painless infarctions are more common.
2. Larger infarcts are more common.
3. Greater frequency of shock and congestive cardiac failure.
4. High morbidity and mortality.

6. There are 4 contributing factors in the pathogenesis of atherosclerosis of coronary artery disease in diabetes:

1. Obesity:
   Visceral obesity is associated with macrophages infiltration that secretes TNF-α, IL-6, IL-8. Cytokines play a crucial role in initiation and progression of atherosclerotic lesions, may induce platelet aggregation, activation of platelets.
2. Hyperglycemia.
3. Hyperinsulinism.
   Elevation of inflammatory makers like CRP, IL-6, are observed in insulin resistance and type II diabetes.
4. Coagulopathy:
   Hyperglycemia, insulin resistance and oxidative stress. Hyperglycemia effects endothelial function and nitric oxide (NO) bioavailability. The nitric oxide causes vasodilation and platelet inhibition and thereby prevents vasoconstriction and thrombus. In the presence of cardiovascular risk factors and excessive production of super oxide occurs, inactivating nitric oxide and leading to the formation of peroxynitrite, a powerful antioxidant, mitochondrial production of superoxide increases the intracellular advanced glycation products impair endothelial function by increasing ROS and inflammatory cytokines and enhancing expression of adhesion molecule implicated in atherosclerosis. Hyperglycemia alters endothelial matrix production, which leads to basement membrane thickening. There is increased concentration of glycated end products and increased expression endothelium.

Diabetics have an increased levels of plasminogen activator inhibitor (PAI) which inhibits fibrinolysis and has associated with hyperinsulinemia and hypertriglyceridemia. The increase in PAI levels predisposes patients to recurrent MI. There are decreased levels of antithrombin III, protein C, protein S, all of which increase thrombotic events. The procoagulant state is associated with increased levels of Von Willi brand factor especially with endothelial injury, micro- and macrovascular damage and hyperglycemia. Levels of fibrogen, factor VII, and thrombin, antithrombin complexes are increased leading to increased clot generation and decreased resolution of clots on injured endothelium. Platelet adhesions and aggregability is increased in diabetics. Nitric oxide is produced by platelets which inhibits platelet aggregation and adhesion to endothelial cells which is defective in diabetics. The platelets in diabetes also secrete more vasoconstrictor prostanoids and vasodilator prostanoids.

7. Histologically, the myocardial interstitium shows increased amounts of:

1. Collagen
2. Glycoprotein
3. Triglycerides
4. Cholesterol.

and in some patients intimal thickening, hyaline deposition and inflammatory changes in small intramural arteries. These changes contribute to the excessive cardiovascular morbidity and mortality of diabetics.

8. Diabetic patients may have myocardial dysfunction characteristic of:

1. Restrictive cardiomyopathy in the absence of large vessel coronary artery disease.
2. Elevated left ventricular filling pressures.
3. Abnormally large fall in stroke volume.
4. Increase in after load.

9. The autopsy findings of diabetics revealed 4 times (4 to 5 times) increase in coronary arterial disease (CAD) in comparison to non-diabetics.

10. Following 4 recommendations are made for prevention of coronary heart disease in clinical practice for diabetic patients:

1. Change in lifestyle, regular exercise, dietary control.
2. Glycemic control:
   - Target—Glycosylated hemoglobin ≥7.0%; Fasting blood glucose 4–7 mmol/L
   - Metformin (first-line if body mass index >25)
   - Sulfonyurea
   - Acarbose
   - Glitazones
   - Insulin
   - Combination therapy.
3. Blood pressure control:
   - Target—≤140/80 mm Hg without macroangiopathy
   - ≤130/80 mm Hg with macroangiopathy
   - Angiotensin-converting enzyme inhibitors (ACEI) and angiotensin receptor blockers (ARBs) are renoprotective but caution in renal artery stenosis
   - (17% of hypertension diabetics)
   - Diuretics
   - β-blockers
   - α-blockers
   - Long-acting calcium antagonists
   - 50% of patients will require ≥ 3 drugs for optimum control.
4. Lipid control:
   - Serum cholesterol <5.0 mmol/L in patients with established coronary artery disease
   - Primary prevention in those with > 30% risk of coronary artery disease over 10 years, statins (regular monitoring of liver function).

Niacin would be an ideal agent because of its ability to increase HDL and decrease triglycerides levels. However, the effect on cardiovascular outcomes is still unproven in diabetics. Troublesome side-effects especially cutaneous flushing make niacin a second-line agent.

11. Affects of diabetic autonomic neuropathy on CVS:

1. Fixed rate tachycardia—Resting tachycardia.
2. More likely to have abnormal or absent pain response to myocardial ischemia probably as a result of generalized autonomic nervous system dysfunction.
3. Non-responsive to physiological stimuli or drugs. May develop orthostatic hypotension due to absence of circulatory reflexes.
4. Increased frequency of ventricular arrhythmias secondary to QT prolongation that may cause sudden death.

The associated diseases are related to the severity, duration, degree, and control of blood supply.

12. Management of coronary artery disease in patients with diabetes mellitus.

1. Lifestyle modification includes smoking cessation which is strongly recommended for all diabetics. Weight loss and increased physical activity are also strongly recommended because of their beneficial effects in improving lipid profile, insulin resistant, glycemic control, hypertension, obesity, and platelet and coagulation abnormalities.
2. Control of hyperglycemia: It is highly effective in preventing and retarding microvascular and to lesser degree macrovascular complications in both type I and type II diabetes mellitus.
3. Lipid lowering therapy: Statins showed marked reduction of major coronary artery disease and related atherosclerotic events.

4. Control of hypertension: Showed marked reduction in cardiovascular events related to macrovascular complications to some extent microvascular events.

13. Adverse prognostic features in diabetics with coronary artery disease:

1. Endothelial dysfunction with reduced coronary flow reserve.
2. Endothelial cell multiplication and migration abnormalities.
3. Increased platelet activity/increased platelet activated fraction.
4. Increased thromboxin A2 secretion.
5. Higher fibrinogen and factor VIII levels.
6. Lower antithrombin III and plasma fibrinolytic activity.
7. Role of insulin and insulin-like growth factor.
8. High plasmogen activator inhibitor.

Clinical

1. Older patients.
2. Female gender.
3. Obese.
4. High prevalence of high blood pressure.
5. Severe angina.
6. Congestive heart failure antecedents.
7. Previous MI/worse post-MI prognosis.
8. Previous CABG.

Angiographic

1. Extensive disease with angiographically small reference vessels diffuse distal CAD.
2. Multivessel disease.
3. Frequent left main vessel disease.
4. Poor collateral vessel development.

COR PULMONALE

Cor pulmonale or chronic pulmonary heart disease may be defined as right ventricular hypertrophy resulting from diseases affecting the function and structure of the lungs, except when they are the result of left-sided heart diseases of congenital cardiac defects. This also includes the diseases of the pulmonary arteries which are not accompanied by parenchymal disease of the lungs.

Primary disease of left side of the heart and congenital heart disease must be excluded before making the diagnosis of cor pulmonale.

Cor pulmonale does not automatically mean heart failure. Right ventricular failure is a complication rather than an essential feature of cor pulmonale.

Pulmonary arterial hypertension invariably precedes cor pulmonale. If the pulmonary hypertension that caused right ventricular hypertrophy is not relieved by treatment, cor pulmonale will become associated with right heart failure. The treatment and prognosis depend more on the relieving respiratory disease than on improving the performance of the right ventricle.

14. There are 4 groups of respiratory disorders which predispose to chronic cor pulmonale:

1. Intrinsic disease of the lungs and intrapulmonary airways
   a. Chronic obstructive lung disease (COLD).
   b. Diffuse pulmonary interstitial disease, e.g. pulmonary fibrosis, granulomatous and infiltrative lung disorders, fibrosing alveolitis, cystic lung disease.
   c. Pulmonary vascular disease, e.g. primary or secondary pulmonary hypertension.
   d. Parasitic—Schistosomiasis seen in middle-east countries also can lead to multiple pulmonary embolism, pulmonary endarteritis and pulmonary hypertension.
2. Upper respiratory obstruction:
   a. Tracheal stenosis
   b. Obstructive sleep apnea syndrome
   c. Congenital anatomic abnormalities of oropharynx.
3. Malfunctioning of chest bellows when they cause hypoventilation:
   a. Kyphoscoliosis
   b. Neuromuscular incompetence
   c. Marked obesity (Pickwickian syndrome).
4. Inadequate ventilatory drive from respiratory centers:
   a. Primary or idiopathic alveolar increase in total blood volume hypoventilation ('Ondine's curse').
   b. Chronic mountain sickness:
      Pulmonary hypertension of high altitude if sustained for a long time may result in right-sided heart failure.
   c. Central sleep apnea syndrome:
      Commonest cause of pulmonary heart disease is chronic obstructive lung disease (COLD).
      Severe chronic bronchitis is an invariable cause of congestive cardiac failure in the middle-aged men. This is strongly associated with cigarette smoking and air pollution. Less frequently bronchial asthma and emphysema also lead to cor pulmonale.
      Alveolar hypoventilation results in hypoxia in chronic bronchitis and is reversible if hypoxia can be reversed. Rarely pulmonary polyarteritis and cystic fibrosis of pancreas and very occasionally certain drugs like aminorex may cause pulmonary hypertension.

THIAMINE DEFICIENCY (BERIBERI)

(Ref. Chapter K-30, 31)

OBESITY

(Ref. Chapter B-38, E-186)

15. Although it is not defined as a disease per se, severe obesity is associated with hypertension, coronary artery diseases with an increase in cardiovascular morbidity and mortality.

There are 4 characteristic features of cardiovascular system in obesity:

1. Increase in total blood volume.
2. Increase in central blood volume.
3. Increase in cardiac output.
4. Increase in left ventricular filling pressure.

Cardiac output is elevated in order to supply the metabolic needs of the excessive adipose tissue.

Left ventricular filling pressure is often at the upper limit and rise excessively with exercise. Ventricular dysfunction develops as a result of chromic volume and pressure overload. This gives rise to left and in some right ventricular hypertrophy; and generalized cardiac enlargement, which is not due simply to fatty infiltration of myocardium.

16. Clinical features consists of:

1. Hypertension
2. Pulmonary congestion
3. Peripheral edema
4. Exercise intolerance.

Weight reduction is the effective therapy and results in reduction in blood volume and normal cardiac output. Sodium restriction, digitalis and diuretics may also be helpful.

17. This should be distinguished from the Pickwian syndrome, which may have similar cardiovascular features, but in addition have the following 4 features:

1. Central apnea
2. Hypoxemia
3. Pulmonary hypertension
4. Cor pulmonale.

THYROID DISEASE

Thyroid hormone exerts a major influence on the cardiovascular system in direct or indirect way. They are prominent in both hyper- and hypothyroidism.

18. Thyroid hormone causes:

1. Increase in body metabolism and oxygen consumption which indirectly increases cardiac workload.
2. Exerts direct inotropic and chromotropic effects which are similar to adrenergic stimulation, e.g. tachycardia, increased cardiac output.
3. Increases the synthesis of myosin and of sodium/potassium ATPase.
4. Increase the density of myocardial β-adrenergic receptors.

HYPERTHYROIDISM

19. It increases:

1. Heart rate.
2. Cardiac output.
3. Pulse pressure.
4. High output cardiac failure.

20. Patients may present with any of the following 4 symptoms:

1. Palpitation.
2. Fatigue.

In patients with underlying heart disease:

3. Angina.
4. Heart failure.

Both angina pectoris and congestive heart failure are unusual, unless there is coexisting underlying heart disease which may resolve with treatment of hyperthyroidism.

Sinus tachycardia is present in about 40% of patients and atrial fibrillation in about 15%. (Ref. Chapter D-79).

Thyrotoxicosis is an important curable cause of atrial fibrillation.

21. Following 4 signs are present in hyperthyroidism:

1. Hyperactive pericardium as evidenced by forceful apex beat.
2. Increase in intensity of first heart sound and pulmonary second sound.
3. Third heart sound.
4. Mid-systolic murmur heard best at the left sternal border with or without systolic ejection click.

A systolic scratchy sound, Means-Lerman and scratch may; occasionally present at the second intercostal space during expiration and is thought to be due to rubbing of pericardium against the pleura.

Elderly patients with hyperthyroidism may present with only the cardiovascular manifestations of thyrotoxicosis which may be resistant to therapy until the hyperthyroidism is controlled. On the causes of resistant or refractory heart failure is marked thyrotoxicosis (Ref. Chapter C-217 –refractory heart failure).

HYPOTHYROIDISM

22. There is reduction in:

1. Cardiac output
2. Stroke volume
3. Heart rate
4. Blood pressure.

In some cases, there may be pericardial effusion which only rarely results in tamponade.

23. Clinical features include:

1. Cardiomegaly
2. Bradycardia
3. Weak arterial pulse
4. Distant heart sounds.

24. The following 4 biochemical abnormalities can occur:

1. ↓T3 T4 , ↑TSH
2. ↑CK
3. ↑SGOT
4. ↑LDH

2,3,4 may lead to a mistaken diagnosis of myocardial infarction.

25. ECG generally shows:

1. Low voltage.
2. Sinus bradycardia.
3. Prolongation of AV conduction as evidenced by increase in PR interval.
4. Intraventricular conduction disturbances.
5. Prolongation of QT interval.
6. Decreased P voltage.
7. Flat or inverted T wave.
8. Non-specific ST-T changes.

26. Chest X-ray may show:

1. Cardiomegaly.
2. Sometimes a “water bottle” configuration.
3. Pleural effusion/pericardial effusion.
4. Evidence of congestive heart failure.

27. Pathologically heart may be:

1. Pale, dilated and flabby.
2. Myofibrillar swelling.
3. Loss of striations.
4. Interstitial fibrosis.

Patients with hypothyroidism frequently show increased cholesterol and triglycerides and severe atherosclerotic coronary artery disease.

Patients of hypothyroidism, especially in elderly should be cautiously treated with thyroid hormone replacement therapy, starting with very small doses which are increased gradually. These patients are prone to angina after treatment which is not present prior to administration of thyroid hormone. Extreme care is needed to prevent angina and myocardial infarction during hormone replacement therapy.

MAGNESIUM AND CORONARY ARTERY DISEASE

28. Introduction: Magnesium is:

1. the most abundant intracellular ion in plants
2. the second most common cation in the ocean
3. the third most common on land
4. the fourth most abundant metal in the living human body.

29. Normal: In the adult:

1. 1000 mmol (24 g) of which about
2. 39% is the intracellular of which
3. 20% in the skeletal muscle
4. Normal serum level is 0.7 to 1.0 mmol (1.5 to 2.3 mEq/L) and it lacks correlation to total body magnesium.

Intracellular magnesium has good correlation to intracellular potassium. It is important for more that 300 different enzyme systems.

30. Magnesium deficiency may lead to:

1. Atherosclerosis—Coronary artery disease
2. may increase intra-arterial coagulation
3. Hypertension
4. Arrhythmias leading sudden cardiac death.

Recently magnesium administration has been proven to be of definite value in acute myocardial infarction.

Aging, stress, type-A personality also predispose to magnesium deficiency. Subjects with type-A personality, who have increased urinary catecholamines and circulating free fatty acid levels have been shown to have lower erythrocyte magnesium levels.

31. Cardiac arrhythmias with and without magnesium.

Deficiency responsive to magnesium administration:

1. Sinus tachycardia.
2. Atrial fibrillation in rheumatic heart disease.
3. Intractable ventricular tachycardia and ventricular fibrillation with or without hypomagnesemia.
4. Torsades de pointes ventricular tachycardia.
5. Ventricular tachyarrhythmia due to digitalis toxicity/ intoxication.
6. Paroxysmal atrial tachycardia, flutter and fibrillation with hypomagnesemia.
7. Multifocal atrial tachycardia with or without hypomagnesemia.
8. Ventricular premature beats with or without hypomagnesemia.

The protective effect of parenteral magnesium in control of arrhythmias has been reported in intervals during the past decades.

The decrease in potassium and magnesium due to diuretics and aldosterone increases arrhythmias which are intensified by aldosterone secretion and potentiation of the sympathetic nervous system. When both cations are deficient, repletion of magnesium is necessary for the repair of magnesium and potassium tissue levels and the cardiac arrhythmias. It has been suggested that the only antiarrhythmic intervention needed to prevent recurrence of cardiac arrest, sudden death may be repletion of potassium and magnesium in patients with cardiac disease having a history of deficit of these cations.

MAGNESIUM AND ACUTE MYOCARDIAL INFARCTION (AMI)

There is growing evidence that magnesium deficiency may be a predisposing factor for myocardial infarction and subsequent complications.

Addition of magnesium to the postmyocardial infarction regimen parenterally in the early phase and orally subsequently may be useful.

Recent controlled studies have verified the improvement in management and survival after acute myocardial infarction achieved by intravenous therapy with magnesium. Renal failure is the only contraindication to magnesium administration and treatment regimes are safe.

Increase in serum magnesium levels has been found to limit the infarct size, decrease cardiac arrhythmias and improved left ventricular failure.

8 mmol of magnesium sulfate was administered intravenously over 5 minutes followed by 65 mmol over 24 hours.

The beneficial effect was independent of thrombolysis or aspirin or of previous treatment with β-blockers.

Oral magnesium 15 mmol/day of magnesium hydroxide in acute myocardial infarction showed no benefit.

400–600 g/day of fruits, vegetables and legumes and a few nuts may provide adequate dietary magnesium for primary and secondary prevention of coronary artery disease, magnesium therapy may also potentiate the action of antioxidants which may decrease free radical production.

HIV/AIDS

Cardiac disease may occur at any stage of human immnuno-deficiency virus (HIV) infection/acquired immuno deficiency syndrome (AIDS). HIV infection has resulted in a low but significant morbidity (6–7%) and mortality (1–6%) based on reports from US and Europe. Important manifestations are more frequent with advanced AIDS.

32. Some historical perspectives of AIDS:

1. In 1981—First reported case of AIDS from USA.
2. In 1983—AIDS virus was identified. First documentary reports of cardiac involvement in AIDS were published with pathological findings in 10 patients. Reichert and associates reported one case of Kaposi's sarcoma (KS) adjacent to the right coronary artery.
3. In 1984—Welch and colleagues reported cardiac involvement at autopsy in 11 of 36 AIDS patients; findings included myocardial infiltrates and necrosis, KS of the epicardium and myocardium, and cytomegalovirus (CMV) infection of the myocardium.
4. In 1989—Lewis reported cardiac involvement in 59 of 115 autopsies that include pericardial effusion, secondary right ventricular hypertrophy, KS of the pericardium and myocardium, non-bacterial thrombotic endocarditis, myocardial infiltration, congestive cardiomyopathy and focal abscess.

Human immunodeficiency virus (HIV) can affect all parts of the heart including the pericardium, myocardium and endocardium.

33. Pericardial disease in AIDS patients:

1. *Viral infections:* Cytomegalovirus, herpes simplex virus.
2. *Bacterial infections:* Tuberculosis, *Mycobacterium avium* complex, *Nocardia asteroides*, *Staphylococcus aureus*.
3. *Disseminated fungal infection:* Aspergillus.
4. *Neoplasis:* Kaposi's sarcoma, lymphoma.

34. Myocardial disease in AIDS patients:

1. HIV myocarditis/cardiomyopathy.
2. Disseminated opportunistic infections: Tuberculosis, *Cryptococcus myocarditis, Histoplasma capsulatum, Pneumocystitis carinii, Candida albicans, Aspergillus fumigatus*.
3. Neoplasia: Kaposi's sarcoma, lymphoma.
4. Medications: Pentamidine, α-interferon, antiretroviral therapy.

Not all myocarditis associated with AIDS is the result of opportunistic infections. The AIDS virus may cause myocytic degeneration without inflammation.

35. Endocardial disease in AIDS patients:

1. Viral endocarditis.
2. Bacterial endocarditis: *Staphylococcus aureus, Streptococcus pneumoniae* and *Haemophilus influenza*.
3. Non-bacterial thrombotic endocarditis.
4. Disseminated fungal infections: *Candida* species, *Aspergillus*.

It is surprising that endocarditis is relatively infrequent, despite the fact that intravenous drug users (IDUs) account for the second largest population with HIV infection. It is possible that HIV infected IDUs with endocarditis die from bacterial infections before they become significantly immunocompromised or they succumb prematurely to other diseases related substance abuse.

Multiple opportunistic infections bode a poor prognosis. It appears that tuberculous pericarditis in HIV patients is less likely to respond to therapy than extracardiac tuberculosis.

36. Investigations:

1. Routine blood and urine tests: CBC, Hb, ESR, urine for albumin, sugar, microscopic examination blood culture.
2. HIV diagnostic tests: Elisa-Tridot, Western blot.
3. CD4, CD8 counts.
4. X-ray chest: Cardiomegaly with left atrial and ventricular dilatation and pulmonary vascular redistribution, pulmonary infiltrates.
5. ECG: Arrhythmias, pseudoinfarct pattern may occur if focal patches infiltrates or neoplasm are present, LVH, non-specific ST-T changes.
6. Echocardiogram/Doppler echocardiogram/Trans-esophageal Echo: For pericardial effusion, cardiac tamponade, Kaposi's sarcoma, vegetations, myocarditis/cardiomyopathy.
7. CT scan/MRI: Gallium scanning is non-specific, but may be useful in selected cases.
8. Biopsy.

37. Management: Non-HIV related causes must be excluded before proceeding to treatment.

Consider the hypersensitivity and drug interactions:

1. In intravenous drug users (IDUs), cocaine has been shown to produce myocarditis as well as a myopathy due to coronary spasm and ischemia.
2. Amphotericin may cause dysrhythmias, hypertension and cardiac arrest.
3. HIV related therapies, pentamidine, both intravenous or intramuscular has been associated with *torsades de pointes* with or without potassium, calcium, magnesium deficiency. This is treated by withdrawal of the drug followed by repletion of electrolytes with a possible role of type IB antiarrhythmics, overdrive atrial or ventricular pacing or isoproterenol administration. Zidovudine, didanosine may cause exacerbation of pre-existing cardiac disease.
4. α-interferon, used in the treatment of Kaposi's sarcoma may produce reversible cardiomyopathy.

38. Currently available antiretroviral agents are 1. Nucleoside reverse transcriptase inhibitors (NRTIs)—zidovudine, lamivudine, stavudine, didanosine, zaicitabine, abacavir; 2. Non-nucleoside reverse transcriptase inhibitors (NNRTIs)—nevirapine, delavirdine, efavirenz; 3. Protease inhibitors (PIs)–ritonavir, squinavir, indinavir, nelfinavir, amprenavir.

Several factors need to be considered when choosing a specific initial regimen. This is not appropriate place to discuss details. It advised to refer on HIV/AIDS literature. However, it is mentioned formally about treatment.

Specific treatment for HIV/AIDS—antiretroviral regime.

Clinical setting of CD4 count:

1. 500–200/mm³	Zidovudine 100 mg x 5/day or 200 mg tid
2. < 200/mm³	ZDV as above and pneumocystis pneumonia prophylaxis (PCP)
3. Complicated cases	Combination therapy with ZDV + ddI or ZDV + ddC
4. Disease progression	Change to didanosine (ddI) or dideoxycytidine (ddC) on ZDV.

39. Any one of the following 4 combinations may be used in complicated cases with two NRTIs and one NNRTI:

2 NRTIs	1 NNRTI	No. of pills/day
1. Lemivudine 150 mg + Zidovudine 300 mg	Nevirapine 200 mg	4
2. Stavudine 30 mg + Lamivudine 150 mg	Nevirapine 200 mg	6
3. Didanosine 100 mg + Stavudine 30 mg	Nevirapine 200 mg	8
4. Didanosine 100 mg + Zidovudine 300 mg	Nevirapine 200 mg	8

Conventional treatment of congestive heart failure with bed rest, inotropic agents, vasodilators, diuretics and where indicated antiarrhythmic drugs and anticoagulants should be given. Most HIV patients can undergo successful valve replacement, but those with continued bacteremia at the time of surgery do badly.

PRIMARY TUMORS OF THE HEART

40. Historical perspective:

Before the introduction of 2D echocardiography, the primary tumors of the heart are rarely reported.

1. In 1952, Goldberger et al reported the first angiographic diagnosis of a left atrial myxoma.
2. In 1954, Crafoord did the first successful excision of left atrial myxoma, using the cariopulmonary bypass under direct vision.

3. In 1959, a cardiac tumor was first demonstrated by M-mode echo.
4. With the introduction of 2D echocardiography, radionuclide blood pool scanning, digital substraction angio, CT, MRI, it is now possible to diagnose the cardiac tumors even in asymptomatic stage and successfully treat cardiac tumors by surgery.

Clinical Features

Systemic findings: Fever, cachexia, arthralgia, Raynaud's rash, clubbing, episodic bizarre behavior.

41. Cardiac manifestations are more related to anatomical location:

1. Epicardial—hemorrhagic pericardial effusion.
2. Myocardial tumors—disturbances of conduction or rhythm in AV node—angiomas, mesotheliomas, → AV conduction disturbances.
3. Intramural—simulate congestive/restrictive CM by impairing ventricular function.
4. Left atrial—most common is benign myxoma, usually solitary mimic mitral valve disease, but sudden in onset, intermittent, related to patient's body position.
   - Mobile pedunculated, prolapsed variable degree into the mitral orifice → MS
   - Valve traumatized → MR
   - Tumor plop may be heard.
5. Right atrial—sarcomas more commonly found → right heart failure.
6. Right ventricular → Right heart failure as result of obstruction to right ventricular filling or outflow, usually rapidly progressive systolic ejection murmur at left sternal border, delayed P2.
7. Left ventricular—often asymptomatic, conduction disturbances, arrhythmias, interference of ventricular function, left ventricular outflow obstruction—syncope, atypical chest pain—murmur and the BP may vary with position.
8. Embolic phenomena—because of friable consistency and intracavitary location depends on location of the tumor and any intracardiac shunt.

Systemic emboli: Left → Systemic circulation—infarct and hemorrhage of viscera, peripheral limb ischemia, vascular aneurysms.
Diagnosis by skin biopsy (petechiae) or muscle/histological examination of systemic emboli material.
Pulmonary emboli: Right-sided/left-sided with proximal to LR intracardiac shunts.

Benign Cardiac Tumors

About 75% are benign histologically. Majority of benign cardiac tumors are myxomas.

Almost all malignant cardiac tumors are angio and rhabdomyosarcomas. They cause local mediastinal invasion, distant metastases, pericardial pain, hemorrhagic pericardial effusion.

42. Some features of myxoma:

1. 93% sporadically.
2. Around 51 years of age.
3. 70% in females .
4. 86% left atrium—usual site of attachment in area fossa ovalis.
5. Over 90% solitary.
6. Other – RA, RV, LV, MV – more likely to have multiple myxomas involving chambers other than LA.
7. 7% familial—autosomal dominant, relatively young age.
8. With lentigines, pigmented nevi or both, primary nodular cortical disease with or without Cushing's syndrome. Myxomatous mammary fibroadenomas, testicular tumors, pituitary adenomas with gigantism or acromegaly.

NAME (nevi, atrial myxoma, myxoid neurofibroma, ephelides).
LAMB (lentigines, atrial myxoma, bleu nevi).

43. Pathology:

1. Generally pedunculated.
2. Average 4–8 cm in diameter.
3. Gelatinous and polypoid.
4. Histology—cells uniform small polygonal with round or oval nuclei, moderate amount of cytoplasm, surrounded by myxomatous stroma composed of mainly an eosinophilic matrix—which appears to be of acid mucopolysaccharide similar to chondroitin C.

44. There are 4 investigations:

1. Echo: M-mode—a mass behind the anterior leaflet of the MV during diastole when the tumor extends into the AV canal, post-descent of the AMV. 2D Echo is more sensitive.
2. CT—high degree of tissue discrimination, degree of intramural tumor extension, extracardiac structure.
3. MRI.
4. Cardiac catheterization.

45. 2D Echo is more sensitive and the tumors are classified into 4:

Class 1—Small, prolapse through MV
Class 2—Small, non-prolapse
Class 3—Large, prolapse
Class 4—Large, non-prolapse.

46. Invasive procedure is needed because:

1. Non-invasive evaluation has not been fully adequate in defining tumor location or attachment.
2. All four chambers have not been adequately visualized non-invasively.
3. A malignant cardiac tumor is likely.
4. Other cardiac lesions may coexist and dictate a different surgical approach.

47. Following features may be found in 2D Echo:

1. Compression or displacement of cardiac chambers.
2. Compression or displacement of large vessels.
3. Deformity of cardiac chambers.
4. Intracavitary filling defects.
5. Marked variation in myocardial thickness.
6. Pericardial effusion.
7. Local alterations in wall motion.
8. Visualization of vascular supply of tumor.

Treatment: Operative excision which gives complete cure

- Operative mortality is 5%.
- 5% may recur due to incomplete excision of the original tumor, growth from a second pretumorous focus, or intracardiac implantation from the original tumor.
- In high-risk patients, careful search for multiple tumors preoperatively and more extensive resection of underlying endocardium, atrial septum recommended.
- Careful and long-term follow-up by 2D Echo is advised.

Family screening is advised for 1st degree of relative.

COMPUTER IMAGING/TOMOGRAPHY

48. The following techniques are included in this section:

1. Cardiac computed tomography (cardiac CT).
2. Computerized axial tomographic scan (CAT scan).
3. Electron-beam computed tomography (EBCT or Ultrafast CT).
4. Digital cardiac angiography (DCA).
5. Digital subtraction angiography (DSA).
6. Magnetic resonance imaging (MRI).
7. Radionuclide imaging or radionuclide angiography.
8. Single photon emission computed tomography (SPECT).

49. Cardiac computed tomography (cardia CT), computerized axial tomographic scan (CAT scan).

It is an imaging technique that provides cross-sectional images of the chest, including the heart and great vessels. It has high spatial resolution, three-dimensional registration and minimal blurring caused by motion. In general, it is useful in:

1. Coronary artery scanning.
2. Aortic disease such as aortic dissection.
3. Cardiac masses.
4. Pericardial disease.

It provides clinically relevant anatomic and functional information relatively non-invasively, and with extremely low associated short- and long-term risks. (If the well-known potential hazards are avoided).

This is mostly used to examine the brain. This test helps to define the problem created by stroke.

50. Electron-beam computed tomography (EBCT or Ultrafast CT)

EBCT is the 'ultrafast' form of imaging technology. It is particularly useful in evaluating:

1. Bypass graft patency.
2. Intra and congenital cardiac lesions.
3. Quantify right and left ventricular muscle mass, chamber volume.
4. Systolic and diastolic dysfunction such as cardiac output and ejection fraction.

EBCT can also be used to measure calcium deposits in the coronary arteries. The amount of calcium detected by the EBCT is relative to the amount of underlying coronary atherosclerosis. This is useful in predicting the occurrence of fatal and non-fatal heart attacks or the need for coronary bypass surgery or coronary (balloon) angioplasty over the next one or two years. A negative calcium score implies a very low risk for obstructing coronary lesions and has a high negative predictive value for coronary events.

The increased predictive value of EBCT of the coronary arteries relative to traditional risk factor assessment is not yet completely defined. EBCT is not a substitute for cardiac catheterization. EBCT measurement of calcium is of no known value in patients who have already sustained a heart attack or undergone coronary bypass graft or coronary angioplasty.

51. Cardiac positron emission tomography (PET)

(See Nuclear Cardiology 55–57)

PET of the heart allows the study and quantification of various aspects of heart tissue function. It combines tomographic imaging with radionuclide isotopes of blood flow, metabolism, and receptors. The tracer kinetic principles are used in this technique. It is useful in:

1. Quantifying regional myocardial blood flow.
2. Substrate fluxes.
3. Biochemical reaction.
4. Neuronal control.

Its use in research has provided novel observations in cardiac physiology and pathophysiology.

Clinically, it is highly accurate for non-invasively detecting, localizing and describing coronary artery disease that impairs blood flow to myocardium. It accurately identifies injured but viable myocardium such as reversible ventricular dysfunction.

Many improvements have occurred in PET scanners including cyclotron production of tracer labels and radiotracer synthesis which have enhanced the function of cardiac PET studies. Cardiac studies can also be performed without an onsite cyclotron, using generator-produced isotopes such as rubidium-82 and/or off-site produced tracers of metabolism.

Digital Cardiac Angiography, Digital Subtraction Angiography (DCA or DSA)

This modified form of imaging records pictures by computer of the major blood vessels to the heart or brain. It helps in identifying any blockages and their severity. In this test, a dye is injected into a vein in the arm, and an X-ray machine quickly takes a series of pictures of the chest or head and neck.

52. Magnetic resonance imaging (MRI).

It is also called nuclear magnetic resonance (NMR) imaging. The advantages are:

1. It is non-ionizing and has no known biological hazards.
2. It can provide high-resolution images of the cardiac chambers and large vessels without the need for contrasts agents.
3. It is intrinsically three-dimensional and has high tissue contrast.
4. It produces images of cardiovascular structures without interference from adjacent bone or air.

53. MRI is an acceptable technique for evaluating:

1. Congenital heart diseases before or after surgical repair.
2. Cardiac muscle diseases, including those affecting the right ventricle such as dysplasia.
3. Cardiac masses such as intracardiac tumor or invasive lung malignancy.
4. Diseases of the pericardium such a constrictive pericarditis, pericardial effusion, or hematoma.
5. Disease of the aorta such as coarctation, aortic aneurysm, dissection.

   Less common applications of MRI include evaluation of:

6. Cardiac chamber morphology such as ventricular mass.
7. Global or regional ventricular function.
8. Valve regurgitation.

54. Other potential applications are currently under active investigation. They include:

1. Evaluation of coronary artery anatomy and flow.
2. Evaluation of myocardial blood flow.
3. Assessment of myocardial viability with pharmacologic stress.
4. Assessment of myocardial metabolism by spectroscopic techniques.

In summary, MRI is useful in evaluating clinically relevant anatomic and functional information non-invasively and with minimal risk, if the well-known contraindications (such as pacemakers) and potential hazards (such as attraction of metallic objects) are avoided.

Radionuclide Imaging or Radionuclide Angiography (Includes such test as Thallium test, MUGA scan or acute Infarct Scintigraphy)

These tests involve injecting substances called radionuclides into the bloodstream. Computer-generated pictures can then find them in the heart. These tests show how well the heart muscle is supplied with blood, how well the heart's chambers are functioning, or identify a part of the heart damaged by heart attack.

This is used a nuclear brain scan. Radioactive compounds isotopes are injected into a vein in the arm, and a machine similar to a Geiger counter creates a map as showing their uptake into different parts of the heart. The pictures show how the brain functions rather than the structure. This test can detect blocked blood vessels and areas where the brain is damaged.

Single Photon Emission Computed Tomography (SPECT)

(See Nuclear Cardiology 55 to 57)

Several large, published studies have demonstrated the quantitative methods of interpretation. When SPECT is used to image the technetium-based myocardial perfusion tracers, global and regional function of the ventricle can be obtained in addition to regional perfusion. SPECT imaging of the heart can also be used in conjunction with newer agents that evaluate metabolism, but these applications are at present investigational. SPECT myocardial perfusion imaging is a well-established, clinically useful technique for diagnosing coronary artery disease and for managing patients with known CAD.

NUCLEAR CARDIOLOGY

There are latest non-invasive technique using radioactive isotopes. These include radionuclide imaging or radionuclide angiography (includes such tests as thallium test, MUGA scan or acute infarct scintigraphy), single photon emission computed tomography (SPECT).

55. There are 4 clinical nuclear medicine procedures in current use:

1. Assessment of myocardial perfusion by means of ionic tracers, principally thallium 201.
(Ref. Chapter E-107)
2. Assessment of damage in acute myocardial infarction by means of infarct-avid radionuclides.
3. Assessment of ventricular function by means of radionuclide ventriculography.
4. Identification and quantification of intracardiac shunts.

Acute infarct scintigraphy: It is based on the principle that tachnetium-99m stannous pyrophosphate (^{99m}Tc PYP), a bone imaging agent has property to bind to calcium deposits as well as to organic macromolecules in necrotic myocardium. It is concentrated by acutely necrotic tissue but not by normal myocardium. It gives a scintigraphic image of a 'hot spot' of radioactivity.

56. Acute infarct scintigraphy is particularly useful in the following 4 situations:

1. Diagnosis of myocardial infarction after cardiac surgery.
2. In acute myocardial infarction with left bundle branch block where the ECG diagnosis is difficult.
3. In patients with atypical chest pain and equivocal enzymatic or electrocardiographic changes.
4. In suspected myocardial contusion.

57. Radionuclide ventriculography (RVG): Radioactive isotope, usually technetium-99m attached to RBC is used in radionuclide ventriculography (RVG). This is useful in the diagnosis of following 4 conditions:

1. RVG diagnosis of ischemic (coronary) heart disease.
The scans are taken before and after exercise. Ventricular performance noted. Development of regional wall motion abnormality is characteristic of ischemic heart disease. Impaired global function of the left ventricle occurs in other conditions like dilated cardiomyopathy, aortic regurgitation, etc.
Severity of the disease is assessed from magnitude of the fall in global ejection fraction before and after exercise.
2. RV congestive cardiac failure: Symptoms of heart failure may be due to cardiac and noncardiac conditions. Assessment of biventricular function provides important information for distinguishing the different causes. It is a useful guide for the differential diagnosis of dyspnea. In dyspnea, due to pulmonary congestion by left ventricular dysfunction shows decrease in left ventricular ejection fraction and normal right ventricular ejection fraction. Dyspnea due to pulmonary disease shows normal left ventricular ejection fraction. Dyspnea due to increased stiffness of left ventricle caused by myocardial hypertrophy shows normal ejection fraction of both ventricles.
3. Myocardial infarction: Left ventricular ejection fraction is more depressed in anterior infarction than in inferior infarction. Right ventricular dysfunction is predominant in inferior infarction.
In cardiogenic shock of acute myocardial infarction, RVG distinguishes between extensive left ventricular damage from right ventricular infarction. It is helpful in the treatment and to know the prognosis.
4. RVG can distinguish between left ventricular aneurysm and diffuse myocardial damage.
RVG is useful in determining the changes in ventricular function produced by various drugs like vasodilators, positive inotropic agents and cardiac depressants such as doxorubicin and disopyramide.

Shunt scintigraphy is done by modified method of RVG in which a bolus of radioactive traces are injected intravenously and its passage through the heart chambers and great vessels are recorded.

TELEMEDICINE

Telemedicine is medicine carried out at a distance—images are transmitted so that the patient and doctor no longer have to be present in the same place at the same time.

The defining aspect of telemedicine is the use of electronic signals to transfer information from one site to another. Telemedicine systems can be characterized by the type of information sent (such as ECG, radiographs, CT scans, MRIs or clinical findings) and by the means used to transmit it.

Today, telemedicine is a diverse collection of technologies and clinical applications.

Presently however, "store-and-forward" technologies are the most promising. In these systems, static images or audio-video lips are transmitted to a remote data storage devise, from which they can be retrieved by a medical practitioner for review and consultation.

The Future

What impact will telemedicine have on medical practice in the year 2000? The crystal ball reveals that remote consultation will be commonplace in the image-based specialities, both for non-specialist centers to get specialist opinions and for specialists to get second opinions. In radiology, pathology and ultrasound the two centers will interact electronically in real time to obtain image or specimen positioning and will highlight relevant areas. In other specialities such as dermatology, accident and emergency, and fetal medicine, concomitant video conferencing will then allow the doctor in the specialist center to counsel the patient directly.

Sometimes, it will be more appropriate to discuss management confidentially with the referring practitioner (via headphones) who in turn may be better placed to counsel his or her patient.

Yet, a technology of this magnitude is likely to have drawbacks. Early reports suggested that diagnosis based on transmitted images may be less accurate than the originals. Patients may increasingly demand specialist consultation and thereby overburden provision. There will be pressure on specialist centers to provide services with rapidity. Confidentiality may be an issue.

The medical community should treat telemedicine as both a means of communication and a new diagnostic or therapeutic modality. Research into safety, efficacy, cost-effectiveness, and satisfaction must be a high priority, and providers should be kept up-to-date with telemedicine developments. Using the lowest cost and most conventional technology that will meet clearly identified needs also seems prudent. Finally, decisions about large-scale implementation should be based on the services to be provided rather than the technology used. Telemedicine systems are simply one more method of providing needed medical services to patients and other medical care consumers.

SCIENCE, MEDICINE AND THE FUTURE

Recent advances in molecular genetics and genome sequencing has lead to the emergence of various technologies that permit rapid screening for specific polymorphisms, genetic sequence of target genes, such as those coding for enzymes, ion channels, and other types of receptors.

This has made advances in identifying specific genes and gene products associated with various diseases which may act as targets for new drugs and identifying genes and allelic variants of genes that affect our response to current drugs.

Number of research programs are developing from the human genome project, including genome-wide screens to identify single nucleotide polymorphisms—that is, differences between individuals of a single base pair in their DNA. These can be used to map and identify specific genes associated with various diseases such as diabetes, hypertension, dyslipidemias, cancer, arthritis and many familial or congenital diseases. Many of these proteins encoded by these genes are expected to become targets for new drugs. Identification of these genes by polymorphism analysis indicates that these drugs are directed to act on specific gene variants to have the maximum benefit. This leads in future to the concept of drug stratification, or individualized drug treatment in which the choice of drug is influenced by a patient's genetic status.

58. Possible future developments are:

1. Establishment and recording of individual patient genotypes—that is "personal pharmacogenetic profiles".
2. Development of new drugs for patients with specific genotypes—that is, 'drug stratification'.
3. Establishment of prescribing guidelines, based on clinical studies, for drugs that are subjected to substantial polymorphic metabolism. The drug dose will relate to genotype and will highlight the possibility of drug interactions when multiple drugs are prescribed concomitantly.
4. Pharmacogenetic testing will substantially reduce the need for hospitalization, and its associated costs, because of adverse drug reactions.

Clinically, many cases are noticed where the drug response varies from failure to respond to a drug to adverse drug reactions and drug-drug interactions when several drugs are used concomitantly. The clinical consequences ranges from patient discomfort through serious illness to occasional mortality. One UK study has suggested that 1 in 15 hospital admissions are due to adverse drug reactions and recent US study estimated that 106,000 patients die and 2.2 millions injured each year by adverse drug reaction to prescribed drugs.

It is now clear that much individuality in drug response is inherited which is genetically determined. Pharmacogenetics deals with the study of variability of genetic response to drugs.

Genomic analysis will generate an enormous information in human polymorphism and several hundred thousands single nucleotide polymorphism will probably be identified in the next few years. However, function of each polymorphic gene or to be more exact, of the gene product and its variants forms have to be determined. In particular, it will be necessary to determine whether a gene product is of pharmacological or toxicological importance and whether individual allelic variants are of therapeutic importance. It will take many years to overcome these hurdles. However, the future diagnosis and treatment may follow 'genomic' approach.

Modern DNA based tests which require only a sample of tissue—blood from a finger prick, cells from a mouth wash or hair follicle cells—enable the rapid and unequivocal determination of the 'pharmacogenetic profile' or genotype of a patient.

DNA based testing can be applied to populations, but we are still a long way from having a pharmacogentic DNA chip that general practitioners/family physicians can use to identify all the drugs to which any particular patient is sensitive. However, there is increasing evidence that 'pharmacogenetics' or 'genotype' of a patient will be extremely important in the future for health care services. Pharmacogentic or genotype of a patient is currently used in only a few limited number of teaching hospitals and specialist academic centers. It is currently most advanced in Scandinavian countries.

HEART DISEASES—WHAT *AYURVEDA* SAYS!

Though the modern concepts of anatomy and physiology of the heart are exhaustive the metaphysical concept of heart is not conceived, whereas the *Ayurvedic* concept of heart is very exhaustive and the ancient wisdom stresses on the importance of the metaphysical concept. The metaphysical concept deals with Mind and Heart, Heart and Mind link. The emotions and some thought waves which generate from 'Mind' *(Manasu)* have great impact on the heart. The negative thought waves and negative emotions worsen the ailing heart, whereas positive thought waves and positive emotions restores the ailing heart to its normalcy. This concept is well-explained in Ayurveda and Yoga treatises.

Susrutacharya is the first who discovered the circulation of blood in the body thousands of years back than Harvey.

Nonetheless Ayurveda has described "Anginal pain' as *Hruschoola* (Bhava Prakasa) and infective endocarditis as *Krimija-Hrudroga*, etc.

Primary Prevention

"Heavy and fatty meals, sedentary habits and over indulgence in sleep are the causes of heart diseases."

Charaka 600 BC

Coronary Artery Disease

'Those who wish to protect this great organ—the heart and its roots (coronary arteries) must scrupulously avoid all that causes mental affliction."

Charaka 600 BC

These are only few Examples

The nomenclature given to the organ that is pumping blood by the ancient saints as "Hridaya" (heart) is a generic name and not coined name. Each letter in the word contributes its meaning explaining its physiology. *"Hru" (Hruth)* means 'Receive', "Da" (Dath-Danam) means 'Give', *"Ya" (yath)* 'Move' in a circle. Thus it sets blood for circulation.

In those days of *samhita* period when the philosophy and science of life (Ayurveda) was written, the people were self-disciplined with regard to the norms of Food *(Aahara)*, Sleep *(Nidra)* and Celebracy *(Brahmacharya)*. Therefore, they were free from the 4 risk factors that now responsible for the most of the heart diseases. If one traces back to find out the real causative factor or factors responsible for the vulnerability of these people who are afflicted with the four risk factors, it is nothing but the one's own behavior, in other words it is a mental phenomenon. When the mind is surrendered to the one's vagaries of the five senses, the self-discipline is affected. So much so the normal physiological activities turn into pathological activities.

Indian Ayurveda emphasizes on the importance of self-discipline. It gives the code of rules to be followed in day-to-day activities. The central core of Ayurveda is its philosophy on which the foundation of its science is laid. Philosophy is the science of mind and the subtle form of life science is philosophy. Mind influences the sciences of the physical body. This fact was realized by the propounders of Ayurveda. Therefore, Ayurveda is defined as philosophy and science of life.

Philosophy is the subtle form of life science. Lack of self-discipline is responsible for one's ill-health and ill-health of the society!

'HEART-TO-HEART'

The phrase 'Heart-to-Heart' generally means closeness, love, compassion and faith. This has relavance in medicine specially in the management and prevention of heart disease. This is a concept to remove communication gap, difference of opinions.

Between spouses
Between the members of the family
Between the personnel at places of work
Between the patient and physician.

A physician's job does not end by treating the sick alone but he should keep the healthy ones away from the disease of body as well as mind.

With recent enormous growth of specialities and super-specialities, we have cardiologists, neurologists, nephrologists, endocrinologists, gastroenterologists, hapatologists, rheumatologists and many other specialists but very few doctors who can have comprehensive care of the person as a whole and not just his heart or liver alone.

This lacuna is realized specially in America and in some developed countries and started a new speciality of 'Family Practice'. National Board of Examinations in India has started 'Family Medicine' speciality similar to that of old family physician, with whom the patients have a dialog of 'Heart-to-Heart' without any fear in order to make his problems well understood by the person who does the comprehensive medical care of his health problem. This doctor who has holistic approach has knowledge of the person as a whole and some knowledge about the surroundings in which the patient lives.

Hurry, Worry, Curry are risk contributing factors.

Man today is a victim of worry. What is the cause of this worry? Lack of contentment is the cause for worry. The rich man is not contented in spite of the accumulation of wealth. A discontented man looses, whereas, a contended man gains. Living on ill-gotten money also causes ill-health to some extent. The living made by unjust means causes many unknown diseases to take root in us. Worry causes hurry and both of them together bring about ill-health. So Hurry, Worry and Curry (Fatty foods) are the root causes of cardiac ailments.

It is not only the unbridled passion which damages the health of man, but the consumption of meat, liquor, fatty foods, etc. also causes equal damage.

As is the food, so is the mind.
As is the mind, so are the thoughts.
As are the thoughts, so is the conduct.
As is the conduct, so is the health.

Faults in food habits (taking 'Rajasa' and 'Tamasa' foods), 'Acharas' (conduct, character) causes bad thoughts (Vicharas —thought process) in the mind—increases the desire, lust, anger, passion, selfishness, proud. By taking 'Satwika' Ahara (food that does not cause bad thoughts), improves the good thoughts resulting in peaceful living. Today, many people say "I want peace". Where is the answer. The answer is in his words itself. If one removes "I", i.e. selfishness, "want", i.e. excessive desire, he is left with peace. The peaceful living in harmony with others lessen the number of heart attacks in the population.

Doctors usually ridicule certain risk factors like smoking, obesity, hypertension, diabetes factors. The treating physician generally advises the patient to keep on:

Do regular exercise
Do not smoke
Do not drink
Do not worry.

But about 1/4th to 1/3rd of heart attack patients may not show any of these risk factors. So, the doctors duty lies in unmasking the hidden risk factors responsible for the heart attack.

The physician and family members should realize that habits like sedentary lifestyle, smoking and drinking are not the maladies from which an individual suffers but rather enjoys them and hence it is difficult for him to leave these.

The treating physician and family members instead of ordering to stop smoking or drinking should gently deal with the situation giving moral and psychic support. At this juncture, the concept of 'Heart-to-Heart' care comes in while involving the family members especially, the spouse. This is where one should understand why he is smoking or drinking and gently dealing psychological problems with it gives better results. At an individual level, our ancient Ayurveda stresses.

Achaara (Conduct, character)
Vichaara (Thought process)
Vyavahara (Interpersonal dealings)
Aahaara and Nidra (Eating habits and sleep)
for the well-being of human body.

Role of spouse in the heart care: Coronary risk factors such as smoking, hypertension, mental tension and high cholesterol are now known in many houses and there is no controversy that they should be adequately controlled.

The heart attacks occur more in men paradoxically called the strong sex. Being repeatedly told not to smoke and not to drink, may itself at times cause over protection and may create more tension and more problems. Since the spouse is the well-wisher, convincing with deep concern, affection, compassion brings very good results. Here is a situation where 'Heart-to-Heart' dialogue helps to sort out the problem.

Alcohol: Excessive drinking over 3 to 4 ounces daily could increase the incidence of heart attacks by increasing blood pressure and blood lipids. The additional harmful effects like social, economic and cognitive aspects are burdensome to the individual and as well as the family and society. Alcohol permit is sometimes canceled by the wife without discussing with the treating physician. This is another situation where the spouse can play a greater role in keeping him away from alcohol by love and affection.

We often see the writings like 'I ♥ you'. Figure of heart '♥' is written instead of love. Inner meaning of it is that the heart is filled with love.

Heart '♥' is symbolic of	love
Heart '♥' is symbolic of	compassion
Heart '♥' is symbolic of	kindness
Heart '♥' is symbolic of	forgiveness

One should love each other. Today, we see narrowness in love (contraction of love) instead of expansion of love. See with love '♥', spread the love '♥', you live in peace. Loving each other, living in harmony and peace will bring down the number of heart attacks in population.

Positive emotions like loving and being loved, affection and forgiveness are beneficial to the body and mind in general and heart in particular. Negative emotions like anger, anxiety, tension and jealousy increase the heart rate and blood pressure which are harmful to the heart. A very important protective factor for the human heart could be perfect interpersonal relationship. An in-depth understanding of each other feelings, needs and aspirations and cooperating with each other with a little sacrifice and at times forgiveness on either side go a longway to prevent many a heart attack. Strained family environment specially interspouse relationship, strained conditions at working places can lead to heart disease.

The initial prevention of heart attacks thus could start at this level.

The lady as a:
mother or mother-in-law
daughter or daughter-in-law
sister or sister-in-law
as a wife, friend or secretary.
And the gentleman as a
father or father-in-law
son or son-in-law
brother or brother-in-law
as a husband, friend or secretary.

Modifying interpersonal relationship, dealing and reacting in a positive direction may prevent heart attacks. So, the concept of 'Heart-to-Heart', loving each other should be well-practical to prevent heart attacks.

Index

L

M

N

O

P

Q

R

S